Head and Neck Imaging
Excluding the Brain

Head and Neck Imaging

Excluding the Brain

Edited by

R. THOMAS BERGERON, M.D.

Professor of Radiology,
New York University School of Medicine,
New York, New York

ANNE G. OSBORN, M.D.

Professor of Radiology,
University of Utah College of Medicine,
Salt Lake City, Utah

PETER M. SOM, M.D.

Professor of Radiology,
Mount Sinai School of Medicine,
New York, New York

With 1467 illustrations

The C. V. Mosby Company

ST. LOUIS   TORONTO   1984

MOSBY

A TRADITION OF PUBLISHING EXCELLENCE

Editor: **Samuel E. Harshberger**
Assistant editor: **Anne Gunter**
Manuscript editor: **Mark Spann**
Design: **Jeanne Bush**
Production: **Linda R. Stalnaker, Barbara Merritt**

The C.V. Mosby Company
11830 Westline Industrial Drive, St. Louis, Missouri 63146

Library of Congress Cataloging in Publication Data
Main entry under title:

Head and neck imaging excluding the brain.

    Includes index.
    1. Head—Radiography.   2. Neck—Radiography.
3. Tomography.   4. Imaging systems in medicine.
I. Bergeron, R. Thomas. II. Osborn, Anne G. III. Som,
Peter M. [DNLM: 1. Head—Radiography. 2. Neck—Radiography. 3. Tomography, X-Ray Computed. WE 705 H4305]
RC936.H43   1984   617'.5107572   83-11447
ISBN 0-8016-0622-5

C/CB/MV 9 8 7 6 5 4 3   02/C/253

Contributors

ALEX BERENSTEIN, M.D.

Associate Professor of Radiology,
New York University School of Medicine,
New York, New York

R. THOMAS BERGERON, M.D.

Professor of Radiology,
New York University School of Medicine,
New York, New York

DONALD P. BLASCHKE, D.D.S.

Department of Oral and Maxillofacial Surgery,
University of Tennessee Memorial Hospital,
Knoxville, Tennessee

R. NICK BRYAN, M.D., Ph.D.

Associate Professor of Radiology,
Baylor College of Medicine;
The Methodist Hospital,
Houston, Texas

JOHN A. CRAIG, M.D.

Assistant Professor of Ophthalmology,
Baylor College of Medicine,
Houston, Texas

HENK DAMSMA, M.D.

University Hospital Utrecht,
Utrecht, The Netherlands

JON H. EDWARDS, M.D.

Assistant Professor of Radiology,
Cornell University Medical College,
Manhasset, New York

AJAX E. GEORGE, M.D.

Professor of Radiology,
New York University School of Medicine,
New York, New York

C. KEITH HAYDEN, JR., M.D.

Assistant Professor of Radiology and Pediatrics,
University of Texas Medical Branch,
Galveston, Texas

IRVIN I. KRICHEFF, M.D.

Professor of Radiology,
New York University School of Medicine,
New York, New York

PIERRE L. LASJAUNIAS, M.D.

Associate Professor of Radiology,
Hospital du Kremlin-Bicetre,
Paris, France

JOSEPH P. LIN, M.D.

Professor of Radiology
New York University,
Bellevue Medical Center,
New York, New York

ANTHONY A. MANCUSO, M.D.

Associate Professor,
Department of Radiology,
University of Utah Medical Center,
Salt Lake City, Utah

JACQUES MORET, M.D.

Service de Radiologie,
Fondation Ophthalmologique A. de Rothschild,
D'Utilite Publique,
Paris, France

ARNOLD M. NOYEK, M.D., F.R.C.S.(C), F.A.C.S.

Professor of Otolaryngology,
Associate Professor of Radiology,
University of Toronto,
Toronto, Ontario, Canada

ANNE G. OSBORN, M.D.

Professor of Radiology,
University of Utah College of Medicine,
Salt Lake City, Utah

RICHARD S. PINTO, M.D.

Associate Professor of Radiology,
New York University School of Medicine,
New York, New York

PIERRE RABISCHONG, M.D., PH. D.

Professor of Anatomy,
I.N.S.E.R.M. Unité de Recherches Bio-Mecaniques,
Montpellier, France.

DEBORAH L. REEDE, M.D.

Assistant Professor of Radiology,
New York University School of Medicine,
New York, New York

DOUGLAS E. SANDERS, M.D.

Professor of Radiology,
University of Toronto,
Toronto, Ontario, Canada

CHARLES J. SCHATZ, M.D.

Associate Clinical Professor of Radiology and Otolaryngology,
University of Southern California,
Los Angeles, California

HARRY S. SHULMAN, M.D., F.R.C.P.(C)

Associate Professor of Radiology,
University of Toronto,
Toronto, Ontario, Canada

PETER M. SOM, M.D.

Professor of Radiology,
The Mount Sinai School of Medicine,
New York, New York

MARVIN I. STEINHARDT, M.A., M.D., F.R.C.P.(C)

Associate Professor of Radiology,
University of Toronto,
Toronto, Ontario, Canada

LEONARD E. SWISCHUCK, M.D.

Professor of Radiology and Pediatrics,
University of Texas Medical Branch,
Galveston, Texas

JACQUELINE VIGNAUD, M.D.

Chef du Service de Radiologie,
Fondation Ophthalmologique A. de Rothschild,
D'Utilite Publique,
Paris, France

PAUL F.G.M. van WAES, M.D., PH. D.

Professor of Radiology,
University Hospital Utrecht,
Utrecht, The Netherlands

MARGARET A. WHELAN, M.D.

Assistant Professor of Radiology,
New York University School of Medicine,
New York, New York

JUDAH ZIZMOR, M.D., F.A.C.R.

Clinical Professor of Radiology,
New York University School of Medicine,
New York, New York

FRANS W. ZONNEVELD, M.Sc.

Phillips Medical Systems Division,
Eindhoven, The Netherlands

TO
OUR FAMILIES

Preface

The introduction of computed tomography (CT) and the subsequent spectacular refinement of x-ray imaging technology over the past decade have revolutionized the workup of patients with head and neck disease. Although these afflictions have always existed in abundance, radiologists have been able to attend only a few of them, reflecting tacit acknowledgement of the limited benefits this specialty had to offer. Technologic advancement has changed that. As a consequence, an enormous reservoir of once elusive pathology has suddenly become susceptible to the probing inquiry of modern invention. But even the most dedicated radiologist has discovered himself ill-equipped to address the challenge of contemporary head and neck radiology. For the most part he finds himself insecure in his understanding of basic anatomy, unaware of pathology, uncertain of clinical course, and unprepared to advise on the preferred imaging technique to best demonstrate suspected disease.

The imaging modalities that are now available—and CT is pre-eminent among them—provide more visual information than many radiologists know how to use. All of the intellectual resources of even the best of interpreters are challenged regularly by this extraordinary technology. In many ways the goal of this book is to make the interpreter as good as his images.

The editors and contributors in this work have approached their task with certain goals in mind: to familiarize the newcomer in the field with developmental anatomy when it is important in understanding anomalies and developmental variants; to stress surgical anatomy when those landmarks are the best way to communicate the location and extent of disease; to relate pathologic anatomy with recognizable clinical disease states; to refine approaches to differential diagnoses based not only on radiologic criteria but also on clinical nuances; and ultimately to give direction on the method of diagnostic approach, leading to the most efficient method of arriving at the most likely diagnosis with the greatest degree of certainty.

This book is meant to serve as a teaching resource for the newly interested as well as a source of in-depth information for the more sophisticated reader. There is a strong emphasis on anatomy; however, it has been placed in the context of relevance to the interpretation of images and to the understanding of progression of disease.

The more traditional imaging modalities have not been neglected or ignored because they have not always been replaced by newer ones. These conventional techniques are presented and their place in the evaluation of patients with head and neck disease is emphasized.

The editors give public thanks to their distinguished contributors, many of whom are unchallenged experts in their particular field of endeavor. Their excellent work has helped this book become a reality. Each of the editors also carries a debt to many associates and fellow workers who have helped bring this work to fruition, and we express our thanks to them.

R. Thomas Bergeron, M.D.
Anne G. Osborn, M.D.
Peter M. Som, M.D.

Contents

Head and Neck Imaging
Excluding the Brain

1 □ The paranasal sinuses

PETER M. SOM

Understanding paranasal sinus pathology is based in part on a thorough familiarity with the local anatomy. This anatomy, in turn, can be appreciated best if the pertinent embryology is reviewed. To this end, a brief summary of the anatomic development of the paranasal sinuses will precede a discussion of the gross anatomy as it pertains to the radiology of the paranasal sinuses.

□ Embryology
■ The stomodeum

The facial region develops from mesodermal tissues ventral to the developing forebrain. Externally, the facial area is covered by ectoderm that extends into a slit-like mouth cavity called the *stomodeum*. As the stomo-deum deepens, it approaches the developing foregut region. The junction between the ectoderm, which covers the stomodeum, and the endoderm, which covers the foregut, is called the *buccopharyngeal membrane* (Fig. 1-1). This membrane disappears in the early somite stages; its position roughly parallels the level of the lymphoid tissue composing the future Waldeyer's ring.[30]

The pharyngeal arches develop concurrently. The first branchial arches bifurcate into maxillary and mandibular processes. The mandibular processes occupy a position caudal to the stomodeum; the maxillary processes flank the stomodeum laterally and cranially. The ectoderm and mesoderm covering the overhanging forebrain form the cephalic abutment (Fig. 1-2).

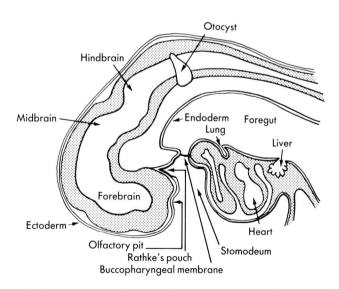

Fig. 1-1. Longitudinal section line drawing of anterior portion of human embryo in early somite stage. Note relationship of stomodeum to buccopharyngeal membrane and foregut. (After Davies, J.: Embryology and anatomy of the face, palate, nose and paranasal sinuses. In Paparella, M.M., and Shumrick, D.A., editors: Otolaryngology, vol. 1, Philadelphia, 1973, W.B. Saunders Co.)

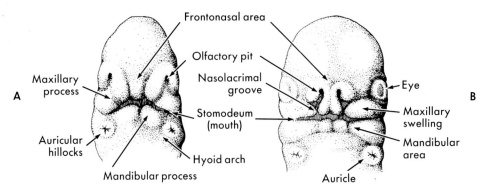

Fig. 1-2. Ventral view of human embryo face at, **A,** 10 mm, 33 day, and, **B,** 15 mm, 37 day stages. (After Davies, J.: Embryology and anatomy of the face, palate, nose and paranasal sinuses. In Paparella, M.M., and Shumrick, D.A., editors: Otolaryngology, vol. 1, Philadelphia, 1973, W.B. Saunders Co.)

■ Olfactory pits

Coincident with the progressive development of the stomodeum, thickenings of ectoderm (nasal placodes) appear on either side of the midline overlying the forebrain. These olfactory placodes sink into the underlying mesoderm and form the olfactory (nasal) pits (Fig. 1-2). As the olfactory pits progressively deepen, they also migrate toward the midline. The intervening mesoderm is compressed into what will constitute the future nasal septum.

The ectoderm covering the olfactory pits migrates progressively closer to the ectoderm covering the stomodeum. In the region of the eventual posterior nares, these two ectodermal coverings fuse and form the oronasal (bucconasal) membrane. With progressive fetal maturation, this membrane disappears and the posterior choanae result. The embryology of the nose is considered in greater detail in Chapter 2.

Ventral to the olfactory pits is a mass of mesoderm that will eventually constitute the upper lip. The upper portion of this mesoderm is continuous with the nasal septum and is called the primordial palate. It forms the premaxillary portion of the palate in which the incisor teeth will develop.[129]

■ Further development of the face

As the facial area develops (10 mm or 33 days), grooves between the mandibular and maxillary arches and the frotonasal area become modified. One of these grooves extends from the lateral edge of the olfactory pit to the inner aspect of each developing eye. These grooves deepen and the overlying ectoderm merges to form the future *nasolacrimal ducts* (Fig. 1-2).

The eyes are progressively displaced from their early lateral positions to anterior positions on the face. This displacement is the result of pressures exerted by me-sodermal masses behind the eyes that develop at a disproportionately faster rate than the eyes.[30]

The maxillary shelves or processes appear on the lateral walls of the oronasal cavity and grow toward the midline, where they fuse with each other and with the developing nasal septum. This fusion occurs along the ventral three quarters of the nasal septum (ninth week). Dorsally, these shelves fail to fuse with the nasal septum and form the soft palate. The nasal cavities thus become surrounded by the condensation of the differentiating mesenchyme. Processes along the lateral nasal walls emerge, giving rise to the turbinates.[2]

■ The paranasal sinuses

All the paranasal sinuses originate as evaginations from the nasal fossae.[107] The *maxillary sinus* is the first to form. After each nasal fossa and its turbinates are established, a small ridge develops above the inferior turbinate that marks the future uncinate process. An evagination starts just above this ridge and enlarges laterally from the nasal cavity. By birth a rudimentary sinus approximately 7 × 4 × 4 mm is present with its longest dimension in the anteroposterior axis.[103] The developing maxillary sinus initially lies medial to the orbit. The growth rate of maxillary sinuses has been estimated to be 2 mm vertically and 3 mm anteroposteriorly each year.[100] By the end of the first year the lateral margin of the sinus extends laterally under the medial portion of the orbit. The sinus reaches the infraorbital canal by the second year and passes inferolaterally to it during the third and fourth years. By the ninth year the lateral margin extends to the malar bone. Lateral growth ceases at the fifteenth year.

In infancy, the maxillary sinus floor lies at the level of the middle meatus. By the eighth to ninth year the floor is at the same level as the nasal fossa floor.[1] There is considerable variability at this level, and the sinus floor may not reach the plane of the nasal cavity floor until age 12 years if, in fact, it ever reaches this level.[100,107] The final descent of the sinus, signaling the cessation of sinus growth, does not end until the third molar has erupted. In 20% of adults the most dependent portion of the maxillary sinus is above the nasal cavity floor; it lies at the same level in 15% of adults and below this level in 65% of adults.[1] The mean dimensions of the adult maxillary sinuses are 34 mm deep, 33 mm high, and 23 mm wide. The average volume of the adult maxillary sinus is 14.75 ml.[107]

The *ethmoid sinuses* begin formation in the fifth fetal month, when numerous separate evaginations arise from the nasal cavity. They subsequently dissect into the primitive ethmoid bone. Expansion of these cells continues until late puberty or until the walls of the sinuses reach a layer of compact bone. The adult ethmoid block contains 3 to 15 paired cells[103] and averages 3.3 × 2.7 × 1.4 cm in size.

Developmentally, *frontal sinuses* represent displaced anterior ethmoid cells.[107,133] The frontal recess is an evagination of the anterosuperior portion of the middle meatus. If a frontal sinus develops from this frontal recess, it drains directly into the middle meatus. If a frontal sinus develops directly from an anterior ethmoid cell, a nasofrontal duct drains it via the ethmoid cells into the superior portion of the hiatus semilunaris.

Development of the frontal sinuses is quite variable. They fail to develop in 4% of the population. On the average, by the age of 4 years the upward growth of the frontal sinuses reaches half the height of the orbit; it reaches the level of the orbital roof by age 8 years. By age 10 years the sinuses extend above the orbital roof and into the vertical portion of the frontal bone.[15]

The *sphenoid sinuses* emerge in the fourth fetal month. They enlarge progressively and at birth measures 2 × 2 × 1.5 mm. This growth continues within the sphenoid bone until adulthood.

Because the paranasal sinuses develop as diverticula of the nasal cavity, they are covered by similar mucosa. This mucosa consists of pseudostratified ciliated columnar epithelium and mucous-secreting goblet cells. It contains both mucous and seromucinous glands, which together with the goblet cells secrete almost 2 liters of fluid daily, half of which is used to humidify the inspired air. The sinus mucosa has slightly fewer mucous glands than the nasal mucosa. The epithelial cilia beat towards the various sinus ostia. The mucosa is firmly attached to the periosteum of the surrounding sinus. This mucoperiosteum regenerates readily after infection, injury, or surgery. The regenerated mucosa, however, contains fewer cilia and glands and contains scar tissue as well. These factors lessen resistance to infection.

□ **Normal gross anatomy**
■ Frontal sinuses

The *frontal sinuses* are two usually asymmetric cavities that lie between the inner and outer tables of the frontal bone above the supraorbital margins and the nasion.[35] Each frontal sinus is one main cavity, often incompletely subdivided by numerous intrasinus septae. The main cavity can have both vertical and horizontal extensions. Whereas the vertical extension lies between the anterior and posterior cortical plates of the frontal bone the horizontal extension lies between the roof of the orbit and the floor of the anterior cranial fossae. The frontal sinuses can open either directly into the nasal cavity just above and anterior to the hiatus semilunaris (about one half the cases) or into the anterior ethmoid cells, which in turn open into the hiatus semilunaris.

■ Ethmoid sinuses

The *ethmoid sinuses* consist of multiple thin-walled cavities in the ethmoidal labyrinth. They vary in number and size from 3 large to 18 small cells on each side and their openings into the nasal cavity are highly variable.[52] The size and number of the ethmoid cells are inversely related. In general, the posterior cells are both larger and fewer than the anterior cells.

Most anatomists divide the ethmoid cells into anterior, middle, and posterior groups. The three groups are not sharply delineated from one another, however, and the anterior and middle groups are occasionally combined into a single "anterior" group. The anterior ethmoid sinuses are separated from the medial orbital wall by the lacrimal bone. The posterior ethmoid sinuses are separated from the orbits by the lamina papyracea.[52]

The anterior group, which can have up to 11 cells, opens into the ethmoidal infundibulum or into the hiatus semilunaris.[52] The middle group opens into the middle meatus above the hiatus semilunaris, and the posterior group opens by one or more ostia into the superior meatus.[92]

The fovea ethmoidalis, or ethmoid roof, separates the ethmoid sinuses from the anterior cranial fossa. It is elevated in various areas by the underlying ethmoid air cell expansion. The fovea lie immediately on either side of, and slightly higher than, the midline cribriform plates. Inferiorly, the ethmoid bone articulates with the maxilla.

The lacrimal bone is frequently pneumatized by some of the adjacent anterior ethmoid cells. The turbinates may be pneumatized by an anterior extension of the posterior ethmoidal cells.

Further considerations of the ethmoid bone and its relationships to the nasal fossae are discussed in Chapter 2.

■ Maxillary sinuses

The paired *maxillary sinuses* lie within the body of the maxillary bone. Behind the orbital rims, each sinus roof slants obliquely upward, separating the antrum below from the orbit above. The highest point of the antrum is in the posteromedial apex, which lies under the orbital apex. The medial wall of each maxillary sinus is also the inferolateral wall of each nasal cavity. The posterolateral antral wall is formed by the curved infratemporal bony wall of the maxilla. The anterior wall of the antrum is the anterior wall of the maxilla. The posterior wall on its medial aspect forms the anterior border of the pterygopalatine fossa.

Each central sinus cavity has zygomatic, alveolar, and palatine extensions. The floor of the maxillary sinus is lowest near the second premolar and first molar tooth[35] and usually lies 3 to 5 mm below the nasal floor. The roots of the three molars therefore often form conical elevations that project into the sinus floor.[103] Sometimes the overlying bone is absent and only mucosa covers the roots.

The maxillary sinus ostium opens into the hiatus semilunaris below the bulla ethmoidalis and above the uncinate process (Fig. 1-3). It is therefore far above the sinus floor and opens relatively high on the lateral nasal wall. An accessory ostium is present just above the posterior aspect of the inferior turbinates in 30% to 40% of specimens. Although the main ostium has a relatively large bony opening, it is partially filled by mucosa and

several adjacent overlapping bones. The functional diameter of the maxillary sinus ostium is therefore reduced and can be as small as 2.4 mm.[1]

Each antrum is usually a single cavity. The maxillary sinus rarely has true septae; these are often vertically oriented and functionally divide the antrum into separate, smaller cavities, each with its own ostium.

■ Sphenoid sinuses

The *sphenoid sinuses* are paired structures lying posterior to the upper part of the nasal cavity within the sphenoid bone. These cavities are frequently asymmetric. Although the intersinus septum that separates the sphenoidal sinuses anteriorly is usually located near the midline and aligned with the nasal septum, its posterior course is often oblique. This can result in one sinus being significantly larger than the other. As with the other paranasal sinuses, extensions from the main sinus cavity are commonplace. Lateral extension along the skull base into the greater and lesser sphenoidal wings and into the roots of the pterygoids may be seen.

Anterosuperiorly, the sinus is separated from the anterior cranial fossa by the roof of the sinus or the planum sphenoidale; more posteriorly the sinus is related to the floor of the sella turcica. Anteroinferiorly, the sinus forms the roof of the posterior nasal cavity and, more posteriorly, the roof of the nasopharynx. The lateral margins of the sphenoidal sinuses are related in their anterior aspects to the optic canals and the supe-

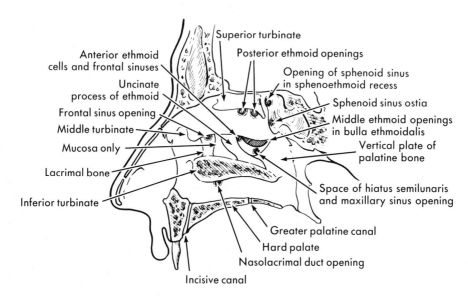

Fig. 1-3. Schematic drawing of lateral nasal cavity wall with turbinates partially removed. Note the bones composing this wall and the one segment composed only of mucosa. Also note sinus ostia. (After Davies, J.: Embryology and anatomy of the face, palate, nose and paranasal sinuses. In Paparella, M.M., and Shumrick, D.A., editors: Otolaryngology, vol. 1, Philadelphia, 1973, W.B. Saunders Co.)

rior orbital fissures. On their more posterior aspects the sinuses are related laterally to the cavernous sinuses and middle cranial fossa.

The two sphenoidal sinuses rarely communicate with one another. Their drainage normally is into the two sphenoethmoidal recesses, through openings in the anterosuperior part of the sinus base. As with the maxillary antra, the ostia of the sphenoidal sinuses are placed nearer the roof of each sinus than the floor. Thus when the head is in the upright position, fluid may accumulate within the sphenoidal sinuses.

□ Radiographic technique

Although numerous views are available for radiographic evaluation of the paranasal sinuses, four projections are included consistently in the routine examination. These consist of two frontal projections, the Caldwell view and the Waters view; a base (submento vertex) view; and a lateral view. Supplemental studies may also occasionally be employed. These include the oblique projection (Rhese view), other craniocaudal angulations of the frontal projection (transorbital, posteroanterior projections), the Towne view, the Granger view, and the modified Waters view.[35,80]

Radiographic examination of the paranasal sinuses should always include a horizontal beam view in order to identify the possible presence of fluid levels within a sinus cavity. This requisite may be met if the patient is erect during examination. If the patient is lying down, then it is mandatory to obtain at least one cross-table (horizontal beam) lateral view.

Use of a head holder is imperative. Some radiologists prefer the patient to suspend respiration during exposure; others hold the opinion that the air–soft tissue interfaces are displayed to better advantage if the patient is engaged in quiet nasal inspiration during exposure.

Beam restriction (use of a cylinder cone *and* shutter diaphram), a focal spot size of 0.6 mm or less, and the use of a grid (movable or fixed) will all contribute to improved imaging.

■ Horizontal beam 5° off-lateral view

The head is placed in a lateral position relative to the cassette. The nose is then rotated 5° toward the cassette from the true lateral position. If the patient is seated, the cassette is usually placed in the vertical position. If the patient is lying down, he is placed in either the semiprone or the prone position and the cassette is positioned horizontally. The central ray enters perpendicular to the cassette and is centered at the outer canthus of the eye in the middle of the film. The orbitomeatal line is parallel to the base of the film (Fig. 1-4). The purpose of using the 5° off-lateral view rather than the

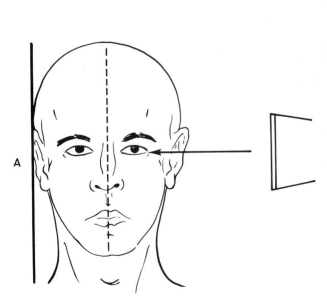
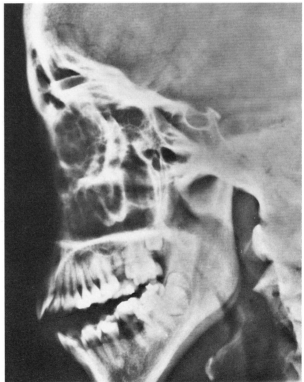

Fig. 1-4. Lateral view. **A,** Positioning diagram. **B,** Sample radiograph.

true lateral view is to rotate the posterior walls of the maxillary antra slightly so that they do not superimpose on one another in this projection. This permits evaluation of the integrity of the bony margins of the posterior aspect of the maxillary antra individually.

■ Modified Caldwell view

The patient is positioned directly facing the cassette in either the sitting or the prone position. The midsagittal plane is perpendicular to the film. The orbitomeatal line is perpendicular to the cassette and the central ray is angled 15° caudally as it enters the posterior skull. The nasion is used as the centering point of the central ray and also serves as the centering point of the skull on the cassette. The purpose of this view is to project the petrous pyramids at, or slightly below, the level of the orbital floors (Fig. 1-5).

■ Modified Waters view

The patient is positioned facing the cassette in either the erect or the prone position. The orbitomeatal line is angled 37° to the plane of the cassette. The central ray is centered on the film perpendicular to the cassette, emerging at the anterior nasal spine of the patient (Fig. 1-6, A).

Variations in the positioning angle may be required to give the "perfect" Waters view. On one hand, if the head is not extended sufficiently, the petrous structures will be projected over the maxillary sinuses, thereby obscuring sinus detail. On the other hand, if the head is hyperextended, the maxillary sinuses become distorted and foreshortened, thus obscuring sinus disease. The "perfect" Waters view has the petrous pyramids projected just below the floor of the sinus cavities. Another variation is to use the Mahoney modification with the mouth open.[80] The open-mouth Waters view normally allows good visualization of the lower posterior sphenoid sinus margins (Fig. 1-6, B).

■ Modified base (submentovertical or submentovertex) view

The modified base view was described by Schuller and Pfeiffer.[80] The reference line used is the infraorbital line, which runs from the infraorbital margin to the center of the external auditory meatus. The goal of the positioning is to have the infraorbitomeatal line parallel to the film plane. This projection is considerably easier to obtain in either the sitting (erect) or the prone position. Patients with cervical or thoracic degenerative disease, or with a short neck or obesity will have difficulty

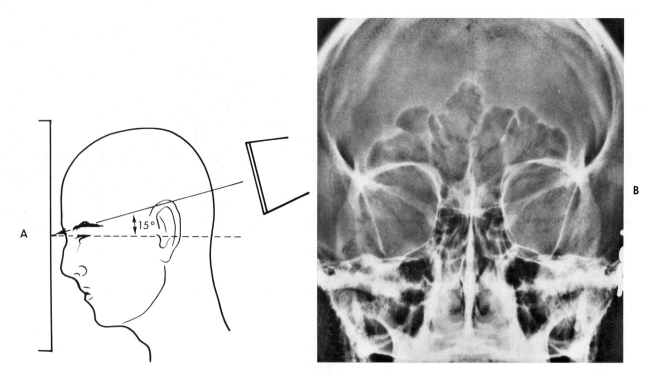

Fig. 1-5. Caldwell view. **A,** Positioning diagram. **B,** Sample radiograph.

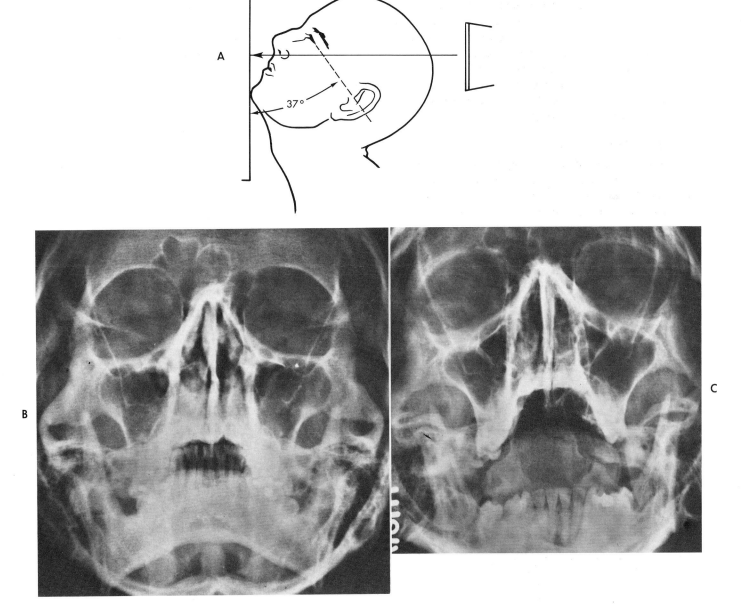

Fig. 1-6. Waters view. **A,** Positioning diagram. **B,** Sample standard (closed mouth) radiograph. **C,** Open-mouth radiograph.

extending their head sufficiently if the examination is attempted with the patient supine. The central ray is directed perpendicular to the infraorbitomeatal line and centered ¾ inch anteriorly to the plane of the external auditory meatus (Fig. 1-7). A modification, with the centering 1½ inches in front of the external auditory meatus, has also been suggested.[35]

A variation of the traditional submentovertex view is the Welin or overangulated base view.[35] The view results in an average angle of 120° open posteriorly between the infraorbitomeatal line and the cassette. This overangulation is accomplished by tilting the cassette top toward the patient with the patient's head fully extended in the modified base projection. The central ray is directed to the level of the frontal sinus. This position is a useful adjunct view for evaluation of the anterior and posterior walls of the frontal sinuses (Fig. 1-8).

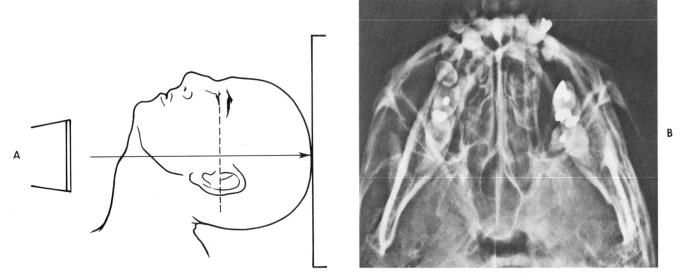

Fig. 1-7. Modified base view. **A,** Positioning diagram. **B,** Sample radiograph.

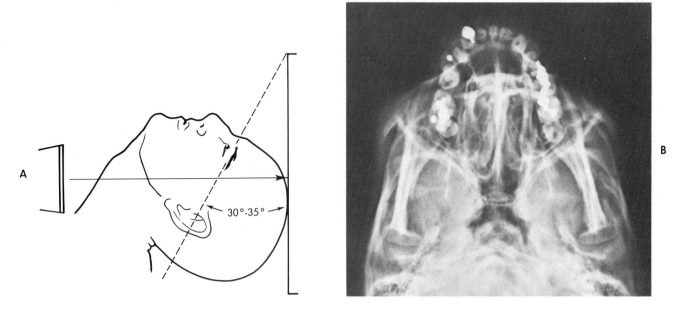

Fig. 1-8. Overangulated base view. **A,** Positioning diagram. **B,** Sample radiograph.

■ Rhese or oblique view

The Rhese view is excellent for study of the posterior ethmoid air cells, which are otherwise obscured by superimposition of the anterior cells in frontal views. Superimposition of the anterior right and left ethmoid cells in the Rhese view, however, tends to limit its usefulness in paranasal sinus examination. Correct positioning will have the optic canal placed just off the midorbit in the lower outer quadrant. Each side is taken separately and then compared (Fig. 1-9).

■ General considerations in regard
to projections used to define
the paranasal sinuses

The lateral view offers great utility in demonstrating the degree of development of the sphenoid and frontal sinuses, and to a lesser extent the maxillary and ethmoid sinuses. It is the best view for demonstrating fluid levels in the sphenoid sinuses, provided of course that it is obtained with a horizontal beam. The lateral view is an excellent view for assessing the integrity of the roof of the sphenoid sinuses, the roof of the ethmoid sinuses, and the roof, floor, and posterior wall of the maxillary sinuses.

The modified Caldwell view gives the best view of the frontal sinuses and is the optimum projection for assessing the status of the "mucoperiosteal white line." Many of the ethmoid cells are demonstrated in this view, but the anterior, middle, and posterior groups are superimposed on one another.

The modified Waters view is the premier projection for assessing the maxillary sinuses. Asymmetry in development, with a small antrum mimicking a "clouded" antrum in the Waters projection, however, may be easily identified as such in the base view. The base view also allows the best evaluation of the anteroposterior dimensions of the maxillary antra and gives an uninterrupted view of their posterolateral walls. The ethmoid sinuses are again partially obscured in the base view by the turbinates and associated soft tissues within the nasal cavity. Providing that the mandibular shadow is projected away from the frontal bone and that the central ray is directed far enough anteriorly, the anterior and posterior walls of the frontal sinuses may also be well defined on the base view.

Despite the most careful positioning and meticulous attention to all of the details that go into careful plain filming of the paranasal sinuses, it must be stressed that plain films occasionally fall short of accurately defining bony and soft tissue anatomy of the paranasal sinuses. In that circumstance, either complex motion tomography or computed tomography (CT) or both must be pursued. This situation is particularly true when there is ethmoid or sphenoid sinus disease that may be almost completely obscured despite every reasonable attempt to define this anatomy using conventional plain film radiography.

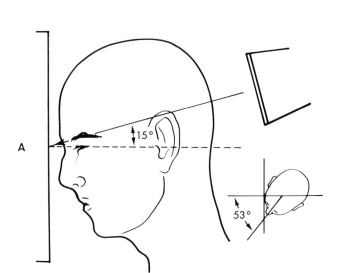
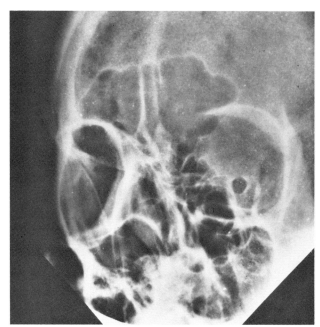

Fig. 1-9. Rhese (oblique) view. **A,** Positioning diagram. **B,** Sample radiograph.

□ Normal radiographic anatomy

Radiography provides the most thorough noninvasive evaluation of the nasal cavity and the paranasal sinuses. Direct observation of the nasal cavity is essentially limited to the lower nasal septum, inferior turbinates, and portions of the middle turbinates. The remainder of the nasal cavity and of course the sinuses are not visualized.

The knowledgeable interpreter of radiographs moves through the realm of normal anatomy and anatomic variants with ease. Facility in this regard must be achieved first before mastery in the analysis of the pathologic case is possible. This section addresses the normal anatomy of the paranasal sinuses as seen on plain films, complex motion tomography, and CT scans. It is important to emphasize that the complex, curved surfaces of the paranasal sinuses and nasal cavity, along with the overlying adjacent osseous and soft tissue structures, make it imperative to examine all radiographic projections before offering a diagnosis. Unfortunate errors in diagnosis may be avoided by first confirming an observation in other views.

■ Plain films
The frontal sinuses

The superior and lateral extents of the frontal sinuses are best evaluated in the Caldwell and Waters views. Occasionally the Rhese views can be useful. The anterior and posterior sinus walls are best appreciated on the lateral and submentovertex (base) views.

Because the frontal sinuses develop from anterior ethmoid air cells, hypoplasia may result in frontal sinuses that project only slightly above the upper ethmoid level (Fig. 1-10). Unilateral hypoplasia is not uncommon (Figs. 1-11 and 1-12). Bilateral aplasia occurs in only about 4% of the cases. In the small or poorly developed frontal sinus, the contours are smooth and rounded, while in the well-developed frontal sinus the margins are scalloped and septae project from the periphery toward the sinus cavity proper (Figs. 1-13 and 1-14). These septae are thin and may extend in length up to one third of the vertical dimension of the sinus cavity.

Marginal contour and the presence of septae are important considerations when entertaining the possibility of a frontal sinus mucocele, for as a mucocele enlarges it will erode these septae, consequently the sinus contour becomes smoothly ovoid or circular in configuration. The normal frontal sinus can abut on the superomedial orbital margin. It does not encroach, however, on this orbital contour or flatten the normal orbital rim concavity. If these findings are seen, an expanding mucocele must be considered.

The superomedial walls of the orbits frequently appear indistinct in the Waters view. This should not be interpreted as pathologic unless this area of suspected destruction is confirmed in the Caldwell view.

Asymmetry of the frontal sinuses is the rule. At its superior peripheral margin, the intersinus septum usually is far to either side of the midline. However, at its "central" or inferior margin it is always in or very near the midline (Fig. 1-14). Any intersinus septum deviated from the midline *at the frontoethmoidal level* may therefore indicate displacement by a mass lesion. The intersinus septum is almost always intact; however, an

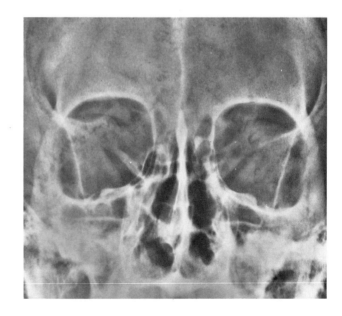

Fig. 1-10. Caldwell view of patient with bilateral hypoplastic frontal sinuses.

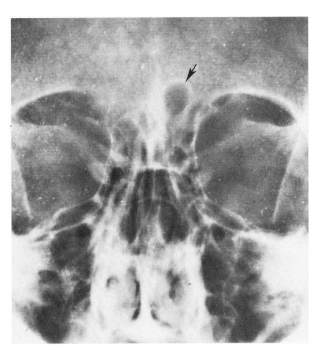

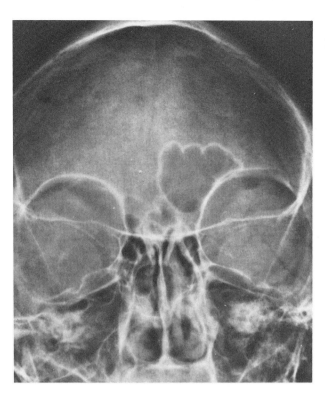

Fig. 1-11. Caldwell view of patient with aplastic right frontal sinus and hypoplastic left frontal sinus. Note smooth round contour of hypoplastic sinus *(arrow)*.

Fig. 1-12. Caldwell view of patient with hypoplastic right frontal sinus and moderately developed left frontal sinus. Note scalloping of left frontal sinus contours.

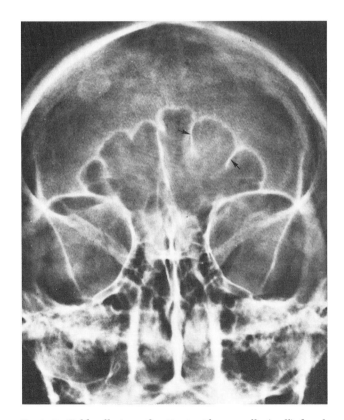

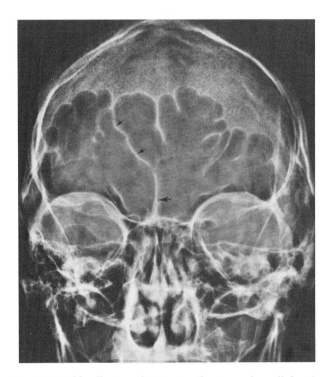

Fig. 1-13. Caldwell view of patient with normally (well) developed frontal sinuses. Note scalloped contour resulting in sinus septa *(arrows)*.

Fig. 1-14. Caldwell view of patient with extremely well-developed frontal sinus. Intersinus septum is near midline at frontoethmoid level and over to right side peripherally *(arrows)*.

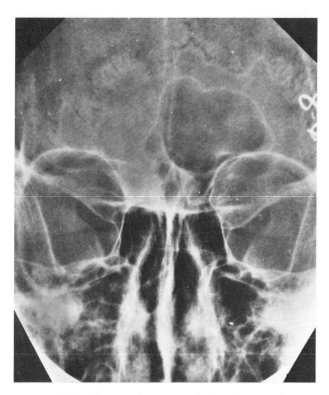

Fig. 1-15. Caldwell view of patient with hypoplastic right frontal sinus and moderately well-developed left frontal sinus. Perisutural sclerosis of lambdoid suture may mimic a clouded right frontal sinus margin.

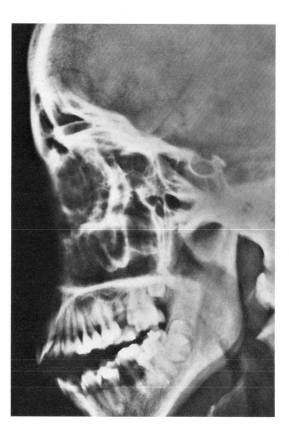

Fig. 1-16. Lateral view demonstrating anterior and posterior frontal sinus walls near midline. In large sinuses, lateral margins are not seen because of normal frontal bone curvature and resulting obliquity to incident beam.

acquired or congenital septal defect allowing herniation of mucosa from the contralateral side through this defect has been described.[35]

The margins of each frontal sinus should have a thin (1 mm) dense rim, the mucoperiosteal margin (the mucoperiosteal white line), separating it from the adjacent frontal bone. There should be no zone of reactive sclerosis in the adjacent frontal bone. This would suggest chronic infection. In the Caldwell view, lambdoidal perisutural sclerosis (a normal finding) can be projected over the frontal sinus margin, which could suggest an erroneous diagnosis of mucoperiosteal thickening or reactive sclerosis of the frontal bone margin (Fig. 1-15). A comparison of the Caldwell and Waters views is helpful.

Differentiation between a completely clouded frontal sinus and a hypoplastic frontal sinus can be difficult. With good quality films, some frontal sinus margin can almost always be seen, albeit poorly, in extensive inflammatory disease.

The lateral and the base views both allow evaluation of the anterior and posterior sinus walls[145,146] (Figs. 1-16 and 1-17). Only those portions of the sinus walls tangential to the x-ray beam will be seen. Oblique margins

will not be visualized. Thus a fracture or a displaced fragment of the sinus wall can easily be overlooked unless appropriate oblique views or tomograms are obtained. Occasionally, bony ridges can be seen projecting from the anterior or posterior sinus walls on the lateral view. These are the sinus septae seen from the side.

On the lateral view there is a bone density area often seen at the base of the frontal sinuses anteriorly near the level of the nasion (Fig. 1-18). This represents the overlapping lower sinus walls and the superomedial orbital margins. The nasofrontal suture is seen anteriorly at this level. This dense-appearing, overlapping bone should not be confused with an osteoma. In the Caldwell view, an osteoma would still appear dense, whereas this normal bone region seen en face will not appear any denser than the other surrounding normal bony structures.

Anterior ethmoidal air cells can extend superiorly and posterolaterally, pneumatizing the orbital plates of the frontal bone, and radiographically resembling frontal sinuses. They are seen as slightly curvilinear radiolucencies paralleling the superior orbital margins on the Caldwell view (Fig. 1-19). Their posterior extent is best

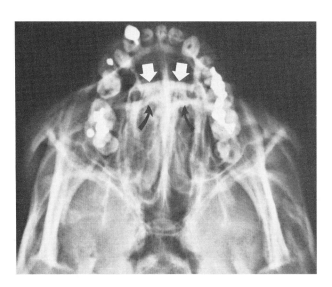

Fig. 1-17. Base view showing anterior frontal sinus wall *(white arrows)* and posterior sinus wall *(black arrows).*

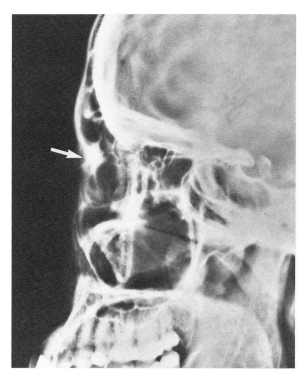

Fig. 1-18. Lateral view with white arrow pointing to "pseudo-osteoma" that is a result of overlapping of normal bone and will not be seen on Caldwell or PA view.

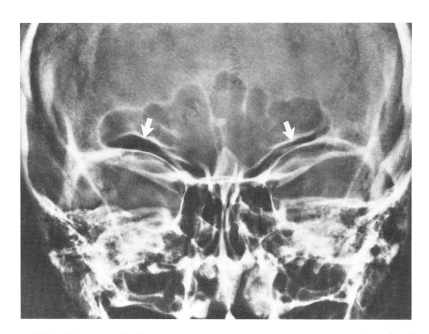

Fig. 1-19. Caldwell view with white arrows pointing to symmetric anterior ethmoid cell pneumatization of orbital plates of frontal bone. They are superimposed on normal frontal sinuses.

appreciated on the lateral and the Waters views. These supraorbital extensions, unlike the frontal sinuses, tend to be bilaterally symmetrical.

The ethmoid sinuses

The *ethmoid sinuses* are best evaluated in the Caldwell view. The lateral ethmoidal cortex forms the medial wall of the orbit. This thin plate of bone, the lamina papyracea, is oriented obliquely to the incident beam, with the posterior margin being lateral to the anterior margin. Thus the slightly concave line usually thought of as representing the entire medial wall of the orbit is in reality only the lamina papyracea overlying the posterior ethmoid cells (Fig. 1-20). The absence of clearly delineated septa may represent mucoperiosteal thickening, which results in blurring of the thin bony interfaces. Without additional roentgenographic findings (such as clouding of the sinus cavities) the clinical significance of these minimally blurred ethmoid septa is questionable. Focal osteoporosis from previous inflammatory disease may also result in poorly defined ethmoidal septa with or without associated active inflammatory disease.

If the anterior ethmoid sinuses are of specific interest, the Waters view, which projects the posterior ethmoid sinuses inferiorly, can give more selective visual isolation of the anterior cells (Fig. 1-21). In the Waters view, the medial wall of the orbit overlying the anterior ethmoid sinuses is formed by the lacrimal bone and not by the lamina papyracea. Little detailed evaluation is possible in the lateral and base views because the ethmoid cells overlap. However, gross localization of pathologic processes can be obtained to good advantage in both these projections. The posterior ethmoid cells can be isolated in the oblique view, but the anterior cells overlap and detail is poor. Overlapping of adjacent bony structures can also obscure ethmoid sinus detail. On the submentovertex view the palatal structures, nasal septum, turbinates, and anterior calvarium are projected over the ethmoid sinuses.

On the lateral view, the lateral orbital margins can project as a diffuse area of clouding over the middle ethmoid sinuses. The frontal processes of the maxillary bone may give a dense appearance just in front of the true anterior ethmoid margin (Fig. 1-22). These should not be misinterpreted as pathologic processes.

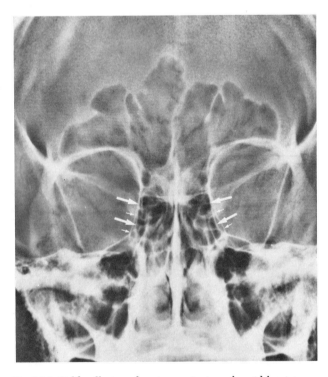

Fig. 1-20. Caldwell view showing posterior ethmoid lamina papyracea *(small white arrows)* and middle or more anterior ethmoid lamina papyracea *(larger white arrows)*. Medial orbital wall runs obliquely between them. Note horizontal normal ethmoid septa.

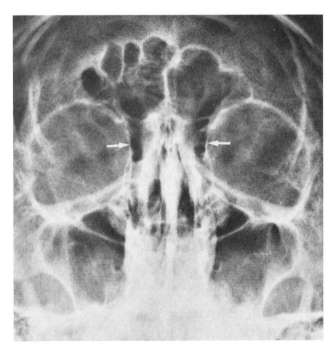

Fig. 1-21. Waters view isolating anterior ethmoid cells and overlying lacrimal bones *(white arrows)*.

On the Caldwell view, a narrow, groovelike indentation is occasionally seen at the superior margin of the ethmoidal cells on both the left and right sides (Fig. 1-23). These indentations are the anterior ethmoid canals and are surgical landmarks. They delimit the ethmoid roof and serve to identify the sinus cavities from the overlying anterior cranial fossa. Embryologically, the canals' upper surfaces are formed from the frontal bones and their lower surfaces develop from the ethmoid bones. They can sometimes be useful reference points when localizing tumor processes because they are constant surgical landmarks. The anterior canal transmits the nasociliary nerve and anterior ethmoidal vessels. More posteriorly, similar-appearing posterior ethmoid canals can rarely be seen. These latter canals are less constant landmarks and are usually better identified on tomograms. The posterior canals transmit the posterior ethmoidal nerve and vessels.

The ethmoidomaxillary plate is the posterior boundary between the ethmoid and maxillary bones. It is best seen in the Caldwell view and again is a useful landmark in tumor localization (Fig. 1-24). Occasionally the nasal ridge ethmoid cells (agger nasi) are identified lying anterior to the middle turbinates along the superolateral nasal wall.

The maxillary sinuses

The *maxillary sinuses* are best evaluated in the Waters view.[143,152] Unlike the frontal and sphenoid sinuses, the maxillary sinuses tend to be quite symmetric in size and configuration, although minor degrees of asymmetry are commonplace. Unilateral hypoplasia is present in 1.7% of patients and bilateral hypoplasia in 7.2% of patients.[63] Hypoplasia can occur with thalassemia in cases in which the demand for increased marrow space

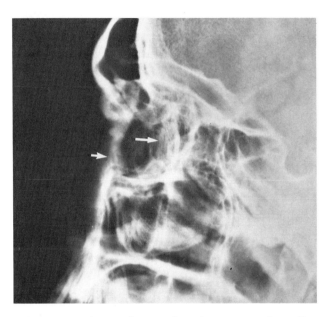

Fig. 1-22. Lateral view showing frontal processes of maxillary bones (*small white arrow*) and lateral orbital rims (*large white arrow*) projected over ethmoid cells.

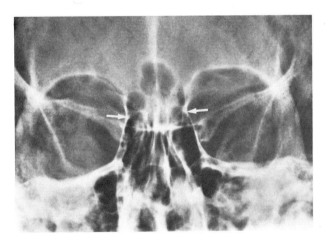

Fig. 1-23. Caldwell view with white arrows indicating anterior ethmoid canals. Slight midline deviation of medial orbital walls is best way of locating these surgical landmarks, which mark floor of the anterior cranial fossa.

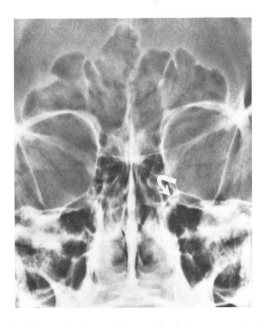

Fig. 1-24. Caldwell view with curved white arrow pointing to ethmoidomaxillary plate. This is posterior junction between ethmoid and maxillary bones.

Fig. 1-25. A, Waters view of patient with hypoplastic left maxillary sinus. Note oblique angle of orbital floor, which is depressed laterally, and small sinus dimensions in all directions. **B,** Frontal tomogram of another patient with hypoplastic left maxillary sinus. Note oblique orbital floor and thick maxillary sinus walls.

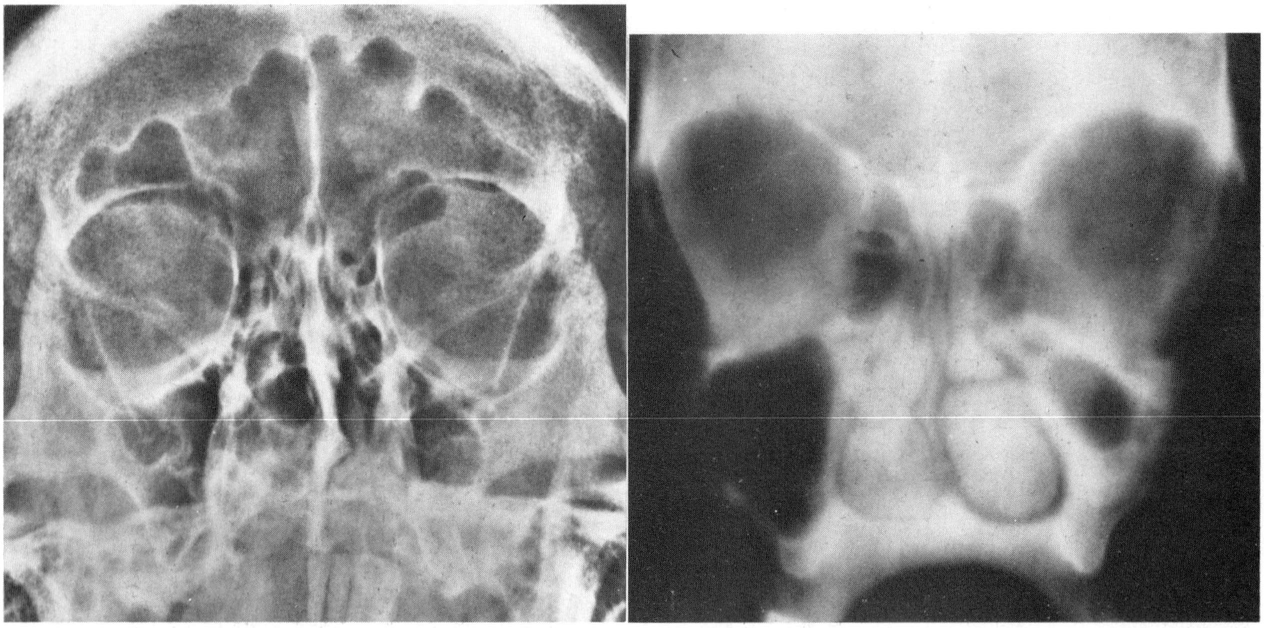

does not allow much, if any, postnatal sinus development. Unilateral maxillary hypoplasia may have several causes. Trauma, infection, surgical intervention, or radiation therapy (occurring during development of the sinus) all can result in a unilateral small maxilla and thus a hypoplastic sinus. The exact cause cannot be ascertained radiographically. First and second branchial arch anomalies such as Treacher Collins' syndrome and mandibulofacial dysostosis can also result in sinus hypoplasia. The normal slanting of the orbital floor is accentuated in these hypoplastic sinuses (Fig. 1-25). This results in an apparent depressed lateral margin of the sinus roof, which can be misinterpreted as a depressed fracture. Clinical history assists in the differential diagnosis.

Differentiation between a hypoplastic maxillary sinus and a sinus whose walls have become thickened with resulting encroachment on the sinus cavity (ossifying fibroma, fibrous dysplasia, "brown" tumors, etc.) may at times be difficult. Hypoplastic sinuses are smaller than normal not only in their vertical dimension but also in their horizontal development under the orbital floors. In contradistinction, a previously normal sinus whose walls have thickened secondary to acquired disease that subsequently encroached on the sinus cavity will usually have normal lateral development under the orbit (Fig. 1-26).

The lateral wall as projected on the Waters view rep-

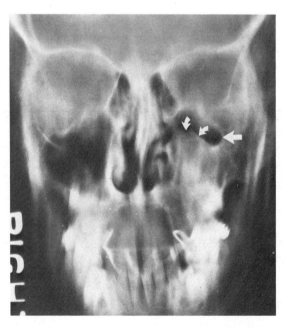

Fig. 1-26. Frontal tomogram of patient with ossifying fibroma of lateral maxillary wall. Curved small white arrows point to mass indenting into sinus cavity, simulating hypoplastic sinus. Large white arrow points to lateral sinus margin with normal obliquity to orbital floor.

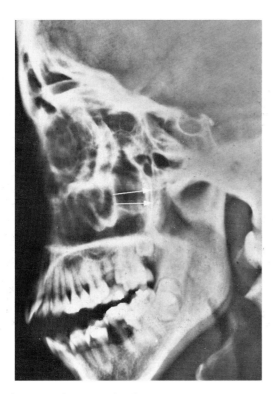

Fig. 1-27. Lateral view with white arrows indicating posterior maxillary sinus wall and anterior margin of pterygomaxillary fissure.

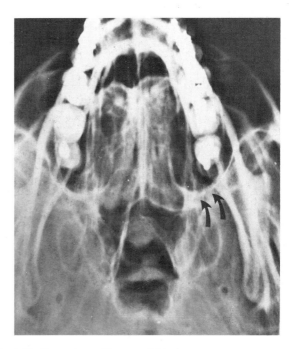

Fig. 1-28. Base view with curved black arrows on pterygomaxillary fissure. Maxillary sinus lies anteriorly and sphenoid bone posteriorly.

resents only the anterior segment of the maxillary sinus. The main portion of the posterolateral wall is oblique to the frontal incident beam and is best seen in the base view. This oblique portion of the sinus wall often casts a slight haze over the lateral portion of the sinus on frontal views. This finding is frequently misinterpreted as "clouding" of the maxillary sinus. In this circumstance, however, actual mucoperiosteal thickening is not present, and the base view will demonstrate the absence of disease.

The most medial portion of the posterior maxillary sinus wall (and its related structures) can be seen on both the lateral and the base projections. Thus the (off) lateral view also allows one of the best evaluations of the sphenomaxillary (pterygomaxillary) fissure. However, minimal rotation projects one fissure anterior to the other and final localization of a pathologic process, if present, will require comparison of both the lateral and the submentovertex views (Figs. 1-27 and 1-28) (see Chapter 3).

The medial wall of the maxillary sinus is best seen in the Caldwell view. The medial wall is slightly concave in its midportion. The overlying nasal structures anteriorly and the sphenoidal sinus and base of the skull posteriorly obscure considerable detail, although the inferior turbinates are consistently identified (Fig. 1-

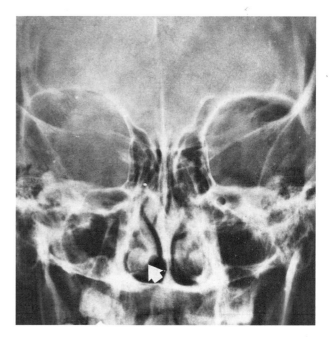

Fig. 1-29. Caldwell view with white arrow on right inferior turbinate.

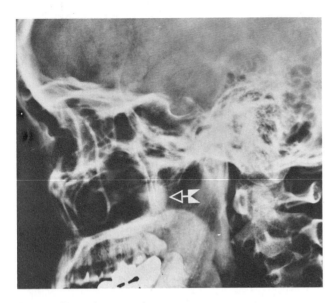

Fig. 1-30. Lateral view with arrow pointing to posterior margin of inferior turbinate. Note that it extends just posterior to hard palate and that it does not reach into main space of nasopharynx.

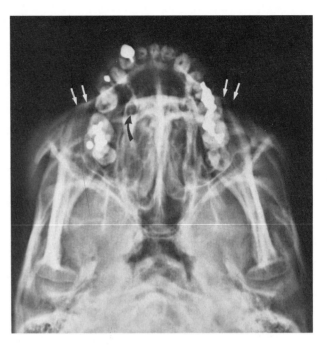

Fig. 1-31. Base view with white arrows indicating anterior wall of maxillary sinuses. Only those portions of walls tangent to incident beam are seen. Curved black arrow points to nasolacrimal duct and fossa.

29). Slight asymmetry or minimal rotation can make one nasal turbinate appear larger than the other and thereby suggest an erroneous diagnosis of an inflammatory process. The posterior portions of the inferior turbinates are usually best seen on the lateral projection (Fig. 1-30). The middle turbinates are smaller and, although they can be seen, little detail is consistently evident.

The anterior sinus wall is not visualized well on any view. Both the lateral and overangulated base views (Fig. 1-31) show portions of this wall, although the bony concavity allows only small segments to be seen in tangent at any one time.

The lateral view best delineates extension of the maxillary sinus below the hard palate. In addition, partially unerupted teeth are seen to best advantage in this projection. In the Waters view, unerupted teeth can simulate air-fluid levels or localized mass lesions in the base of the antra.

In the Caldwell view the roof of the maxillary sinus is almost in tangent. Although most of the roof is superimposed, the posterior medial apex of the maxillary sinus can usually be identified (Fig. 1-32). Because of the superimposition of bony shadows, the Waters view is helpful. Unfortunately, however, with the Waters view the sinus roof is seen obliquely and posterior

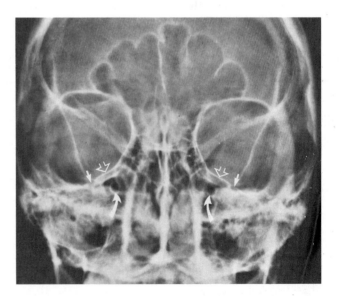

Fig. 1-32. Caldwell view. Open arrowheads point to posterior medial wall of maxillary sinus (orbital floor). White arrowhead points to posterior portion of infraorbital canal, seen as notch in orbital floor. Curved white arrows point to foramen rotundum.

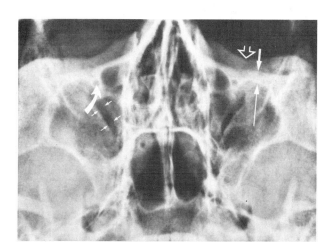

Fig. 1-33. Waters view. Open arrowhead points to soft tissue line over inferior orbital rim. Medium white arrow points to bony inferior orbital rim, and thin long white arrow points to lowest point of orbital floor. Four small white arrows outline superior orbital fissure seen through right maxillary sinus. Curved white arrow indicates infraorbital foramen.

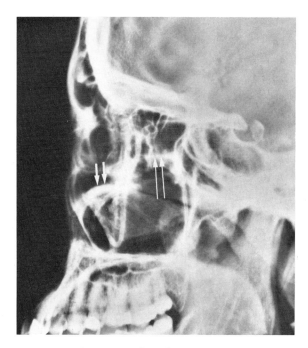

Fig. 1-34. Lateral view. Smaller white arrows point to anterior inferior orbital floor on one side. Longer thin white arrows point to posterior superior orbital floor on opposite side.

masses or a focally depressed fracture may occasionally be overlooked. The infraorbital canal appears as a notch in the orbital floor in the Caldwell view (Fig. 1-32). The infraorbital foramen, the anterior opening of the canal, is best seen in the Waters view and lies just below the orbital rim (Fig. 1-33).

Three parallel lines can be seen near the inferior orbital margin in the Waters view (Fig. 1-33). The most superior of these lines is the soft tissue margin overlying the anterior inferior orbital rim. The middle line is the actual bony rim of the orbit and the inferior line is the antral roof (at a plane about 1 cm behind the rim). Because the orbital floor is oriented obliquely so that its highest point lies in the posteromedial portion of the orbit, two lines can be seen in the lateral view: a posterosuperior line that represents the orbital floor near the orbital apex and an anteroinferior line that represents the flatter portion of the orbital floor (Fig. 1-34). The actual infraorbital canal is not usually seen on the routine lateral film.

Occasionally a canal-like lucency is seen in the lateral maxillary sinus wall in the Waters view. This is the posterior superior alveolar canal and should not be confused with a fracture line (Fig. 1-35).

The lateral (zygomatic) recess is a variable extension of the maxillary sinus into the body of the zygoma. This

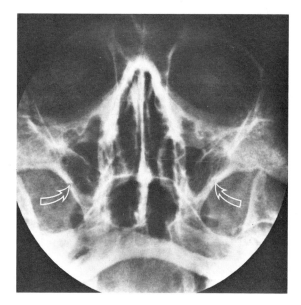

Fig. 1-35. Waters view. Open curved arrows point to posterior superior alveolar neurovascular canals.

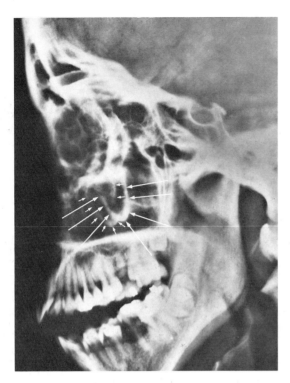

Fig. 1-36. Lateral view. Large white arrows outline zygomatic recess of one maxillary sinus cavity and small white arrows outline this recess on opposite side.

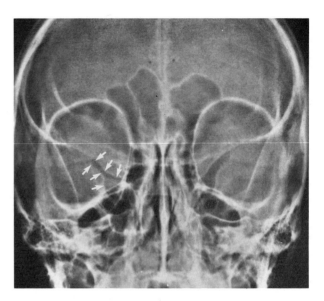

Fig. 1-37. Caldwell view. White arrows outline right superior orbital fissure. Slight asymmetry with left side is normal. Cranial nerves and vascular structures all pass through medial wider portions of these fissures.

portion of the sinus is smaller than the main body of the sinus cavity. Because of this, it may appear less dense and suggest mucoperiosteal thickening. The entire sinus should be evaluated before a diagnosis of inflammatory disease is suggested. On the lateral view these zygomatic recesses are seen as overlapping V's projected over the main body of the maxillary sinus (Fig. 1-36). Their margins should always be carefully evaluated in order to detect early destruction.

Structures that are projected through or are in relationship to the maxillary sinuses

The foramen rotundum is best seen on the Caldwell view and is projected over the superomedial portion of each maxillary sinus (Fig. 1-32). The superior orbital fissure has a slightly concave lateral configuration, or **C** shape, which points at its inferior extent to the foramen rotundum. The foramen is usually separated from the fissure by a small bony ridge. This ridge can occasionally be absent. The maxillary nerve (V2) runs through this foramen, crosses the sphenomaxillary fissure and enters the infraorbital canal.

The superior orbital fissures are usually somewhat asymmetric. They are best seen in the Caldwell and Waters views. The fissures have a narrow lateral portion and a wider medial portion (Fig. 1-37). The cranial

nerves and vascular structures course through the medial portion. In the Waters view, the fissures appear as obliquely oriented lines running superolaterally to inferomedially (Fig. 1-33). Occasionally the lesser sphenoid wing cortex margin is also seen; this should not be confused with a maxillary sinus septum, which is a rare finding. When the fissure is projected over the inferior orbital rim, it should not be confused with a fracture line. In the Waters view the infraorbital canal ridge appears either as a cortical line or as a pair of parallel lines, projected over the upper sinus. These are not true septa and can easily be distinguished from the superior orbital fissure lines because of their different orientation and their parallel rather than divergent configuration.

The oblique orbital (innominate) lines are seen consistently in the Waters and Caldwell views.[142,144-146] They represent the most anterior portion of the temporal fossa. At its lower margin each oblique orbital line curves sharply medially, indicating the beginning of the infratemporal fossa. Occasionally this line is seen to bend inferiorly again, where it represents the lateral pterygoid plate (Fig. 1-38).

The superior rim of the middle cranial fossa is constituted by the lesser wing of the sphenoid bone and the anterior clinoid process medially and the orbital plate

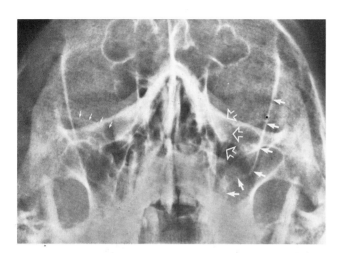

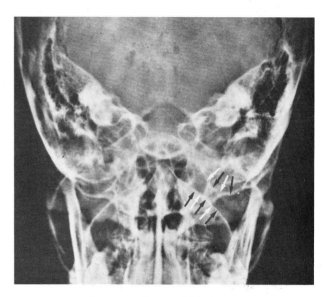

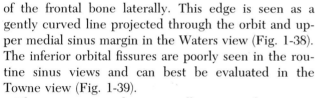

Fig. 1-38. Waters view. White arrows point to left oblique orbital line. Note its lower medial curve horizontally to delimit the beginning of the infratemporal fossa and vertical bend downward to outline lateral pterygoid plate. Small white arrows point to superior rim of right middle cranial fossa. Open arrowheads outline left nasal cartilages that can mimic cyst or polyp in antrum.

Fig. 1-39. Towne's view. White and black arrows outline inferior orbital fissure. Superior line is sphenoid bone border and inferior line is maxillary bone border.

of the frontal bone laterally. This edge is seen as a gently curved line projected through the orbit and upper medial sinus margin in the Waters view (Fig. 1-38). The inferior orbital fissures are poorly seen in the routine sinus views and can best be evaluated in the Towne view (Fig. 1-39).

The zygomatic arches are well seen on the Waters view. The underpenetrated base view and the "jug handle" view also project the arches well. The posterior portions of the arches are well seen in the Towne view. The zygomaticotemporal suture is easily identified and should not be confused with a fracture line. Occasionally a small canal, the zygomaticofacial canal, can be seen in the body of the zygoma near the level of the lateral orbital wall. This canal transmits the zygomaticofacial nerve.

The soft tissue shadow of the upper lip is often seen projected across the lower antral margins of the Waters view (Fig. 1-40). Mustaches also can produce soft tissue artifacts. The lateral margins of these shadows extend beyond the sinus walls. They should not be confused with retention cysts of the sinuses. Soft tissue swelling of the cheek can mimic clouding of the underlying antrum; this is usually accompanied by swelling of the soft tissue infraorbital line. The nasal alae can mimic a medial wall polyp or retention cyst in the Waters view

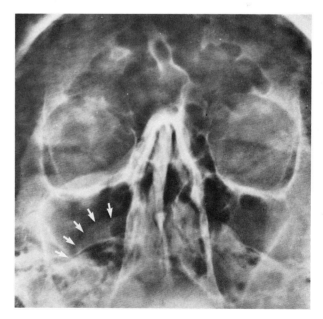

Fig. 1-40. Waters view. White arrows outline lip shadow projected over maxillary sinus.

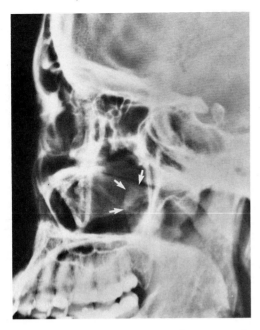

Fig. 1-41. Lateral view. White arrows outline coronoid process of mandible projected over posterior maxillary sinus cavity.

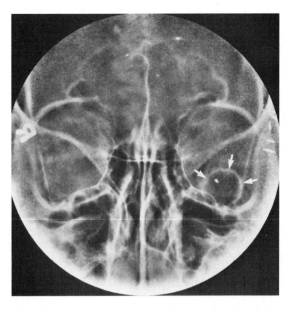

Fig. 1-42. Caldwell view. White arrows outline lateral sphenoid sinus recess, which has extended up into greater wing of sphenoid bone. Note that inferior medial margin is not seen because this margin connects with sinus proper.

(Fig. 1-38). In the lateral view, the coronoid processes of the mandible project over the inferoposterior sinus margin (Fig. 1-41), especially if the mouth is closed. If the coronoid processes are blunt and rounded, they may simulate retention cysts or polyps in the maxillary sinus. When the coronoid processes are sharply pointed, they may simulate a fractured bone segment or an unerupted tooth.[144]

The sphenoid sinuses

The *sphenoid sinuses* are probably the most difficult sinuses to evaluate by routine films because they are surrounded by the facial bones and nasal cavity on the frontal views and by the base of the skull on the lateral views. Along with the frontal sinuses, the sphenoid sinuses are the most variable in configuration. Approximately one half of the population (48%) have lateral recesses, and these show great variability between the left and right sides.[38] The base, lateral, and open-mouth Waters views are the best views with which to evaluate the posterior sinus wall and the lateral extent of the sinus recesses. The lateral recesses frequently extend into the greater wing of the sphenoid bone and appear as a lucent orbital defect in the Caldwell view (Fig. 1-42). This extension has a thin mucoperiosteal line. Although the inferior margin of the recess will not be definable in the Caldwell view, the Waters or base view will confirm the presence of a lateral recess.

The lateral recesses can also extend into the ptery-

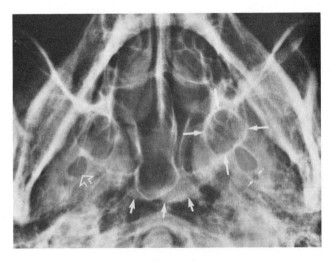

Fig. 1-43. Base view. Large white arrows outline pneumatized pterygoid fossa. Medium white arrows outline posterior margin of tongue. Small white arrows point to foramen spinosum and open arrow points to foramen ovale.

goid plates, resulting in a triangular lucency in the lateral and Caldwell views. This appears as an oval lucency on the base view in the pterygoid fossa (Fig. 1-43). The pterygoid processes are pneumatized in 25% of cases and are extensively pneumatized in 8%.[38]

The posterior limit of sphenoidal sinus development is variable. In 60% of cases, the sinuses extend posteriorly to the anterior sella wall and lie under the sella

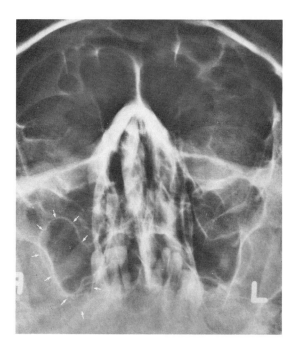

Fig. 1-44. Waters view. Small white arrows outline lateral recess of sphenoid sinus projected through maxillary sinus.

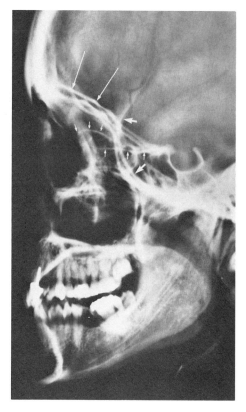

Fig. 1-45. Lateral view. Small white arrows pointing upward indicate planum sphenoidale in midline. Small white arrows pointing downward outline roof of ethmoid sinuses and long white arrows point to orbital roofs. White arrowhead delimits curved anterior margin of middle cranial fossa.

floor. In 40% of cases, the sinuses extend only to the anterior wall of the sella turcica. In less than 1% of cases, the sphenoid sinuses do not develop posteriorly enough to reach the anterior sella wall.[143] Although the posterior margin is variable and can be asymmetric, unilateral aplasia is a rare occurence. Significant asymmetry is therefore an indication of possible sphenoid sinus pathology.

The open-mouth Waters view projects the posterior sphenoidal sinus wall and the lateral extensions through the maxillary sinuses. The margins of the lateral extensions can simulate antral trabeculations, and pathologic changes in these recesses can be mistaken for antral pathology (Fig. 1-44).

The lateral view delineates the sphenoidal sinus roof and the posterosuperior wall. The inferior portions of the sinus are obscured by the overlapping skull base and zygomatic arches. The anterior walls of the middle cranial fossa are seen as paired curvilinear lines that are projected over the posterior sinus cavity (Fig. 1-45).

Lack of sphenoidal sinus pneumatization beyond the age of 10 years should strongly suggest the presence of "occult" sphenoid sinus pathology.[49] Between 67% and 75% of patients with maxillary sinus inflammatory disease have associated sphenoid sinus disease.[49] Involvement of the sphenoid sinus alone is uncommon.

■ **Associated structures surrounding the paranasal sinuses**

Soft tissues. The nasopharyngeal soft tissue should be carefully examined on the lateral view because sinus disease can extend into the nasopharynx as well as vice versa. The soft palate is well seen in the lateral view. If the patient is not phonating or breathing nasally, the soft palate may abut on the roof of the nasopharynx and create the impression of a nasopharyngeal mass. The uvula and posterior soft palate also can cast a transverse soft tissue shadow in the base view. This too can mimic a nasopharyngeal or sphenoid sinus mass.

The posterior margin of the tongue and soft palate can be easily confused in the base view (Fig. 1-43) but are easily separated in the lateral view. In the base view a density can be seen overlying the sphenoid sinus running from left to right. This usually represents the posterior tongue margin rather than the soft palate. These shadows should not be confused with those caused by sinus disease. The lateral walls of the nasopharynx and oropharynx can also produce shadows over the sphenoid sinus and lateral sphenoid recesses.

Occasionally the pinna of the ear can be projected over the sphenoidal sinus and nasopharynx in the lateral view, simulating a mass lesion. This can usually be differentiated by tracing out the entire lower ear pinna.

Bony structures. In the lateral view the planum sphenoidale is clearly seen as a dense straight line. The cribriform plate is rarely visualized. A line drawn from the anterior planum to the nasion closely approximates the actual cribriform plate level. The fovea ethmoidalis, which are just lateral to the cribriform plate, and the orbital roofs (which lie even more superolaterally) are all above the cribriform plate and planum and are usually well seen in the lateral view (Fig. 1-45). The crista

galli is best seen in the Caldwell view (Fig. 1-46). The bony portion of the nasal septum is not optimally visualized on any projection. The cartilaginous portion of the septum, which makes up the majority of the anterior septum, is not well demonstrated radiographically and is only seen on CT scans.

In the lateral projection, the anterior nasal spine has a sharp triangular appearance. A bright light is usually necessary to properly visualize this structure. Destruction of the anterior nasal spine is almost always a result of previous trauma or surgery. Hansen's disease (leprosy) also destroys the anterior nasal spine. Midline lethal granuloma does not.

The hard palate is best seen in the lateral view. Its nasal surface is flat and normally has a well-delineated cortical margin. The oral surface is slightly concave downward.

In the base view three pairs of lines are consistently seen. The most posterior lines are concave posteriorly and represent the greater sphenoid wing, i.e., the anterior margin of the middle cranial fossa (Fig. 1-47). Slight rotation of the head or asymmetry between the sphenoid bones can result in poor visualization of these curved lines. The second line is relatively straight and is obliquely oriented to the midsagittal plane. It represents the posterior orbital wall and is formed by the greater sphenoid wing and orbital surface of the zygoma (Fig. 1-47). It ends medially at the pterygoid fossa apex. The thinnest portion of this line will lie in its lateral

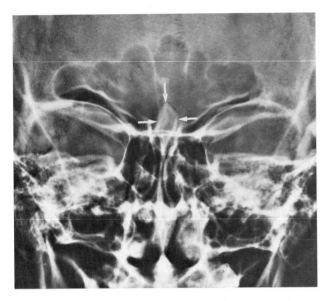

Fig. 1-46. Caldwell view. White arrows outline crista galli.

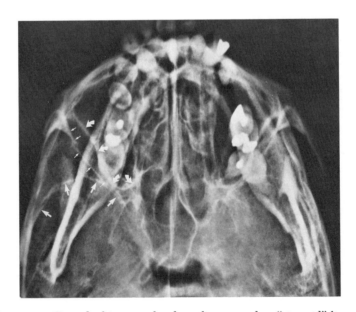

Fig. 1-47. Base view. Curved white arrowheads outline curved or "sigmoid" line of posterior maxillary sinus wall. Small white arrows outline posterior orbital wall. Those arrows pointing upward delimit sphenoid bone portion and those arrows pointing downward outline zygomatic bone portion. Their junction represents suture line. Larger white arrows point to curved anterior margin of middle cranial fossa.

half and represents the suture line between these two bones. The third line is the sigmoid or S-shaped line of the posterior maxillary sinus wall. Depending on film angulation, the sigmoid line can be anterior to, overlapping and crossing, or posterior to the orbital line (Figs. 1-43 and 1-47). More of this posterior sinus wall is seen in the base view than in any other view.

In the base view, the pterygoid fossa is a V-shaped space with its apex directed anteriorly. The medial and lateral pterygoid plates cast three shadows (Fig. 1-48). A medial line represents the medial pterygoid plate; two lateral lines represent the lateral pterygoid plate. The caudal margin of the lateral pterygoid plate forms the most lateral line and the cephalad margin of the lateral plate, near the base of the skull, forms the middle pterygoid line. Occasionally, the hamulus of the medial plate can be seen on plain films. The pterygoid fossa is thus the space between the middle and medial lines near the base of the skull, and more caudally near the mouth, the boundaries are the lateral and medial lines. (See Chapter 3.)

In the base view, the frontal bone casts two transverse lines across the anterior portion of the ethmoid and maxillary sinuses. These lines correspond to the anterior and posterior cortical tables of the frontal bone (Fig. 1-17). In addition, the zygoma and the anterior wall of the maxillary sinus cast a transverse line across the same region (Fig. 1-48). The relationship of the frontal table lines to the zygomaticomaxillary line depends on the angulation of the base view. In the more markedly angled base view, the lacrimal canals can be seen projected through the hard palate.

■ Complex motion tomography

The extent of both soft tissue disease and bony destruction are consistently underestimated on even the best quality plain films, and therein lies the justification for complex motion tomography. Tomograms are usually obtained in straight anteroposterior (AP) or lateral views, for these provide "anatomy book" depiction of the structures and permit ready comparison of symmetry between the left and right sides. The special angulations and rotations of plain films required to project an area of interest free of superimposed structures or to show the sinuses in tangent are made superfluous by the tomographic technique. Tomograms in the horizontal plane are useful but difficult to obtain consistently because of the problems inherent with patient positioning. CT, on the other hand, demonstrates anatomy in this projection with ease.

In routine cases, zero degree AP tomographic sections are obtained at 5 mm intervals. Because the section thickness is usually under 1.5 mm using this technique, intercalated cuts at 1 to 3 mm intervals may be necessary in selected instances.

Far anteriorly, the *frontal processes of the maxillary bones* form the slightly curved lateral margins of the nasal cavity. The *perpendicular plate of the ethmoid*

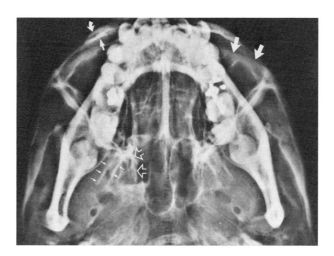

Fig. 1-48. Base view. Open arrows point to line of medial pterygoid plate. Two small white arrows (directed laterally) outline cephalad line of lateral pterygoid plate. Three small white arrows (directed medially) outline caudad line of lateral pterygoid plate. Large white arrows delimit anterior wall of left maxillary sinus. Frontal bone outer table (*medium curved arrow*) and inner table (*medium straight arrow*) are seen on right side.

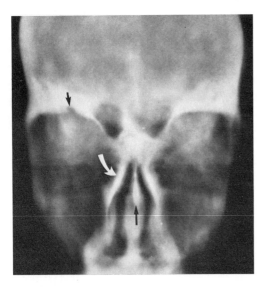

Fig. 1-49. Short black arrow points to supraorbital notch. Most anterior and basal portions of the frontal sinus are seen. Curved white arrow indicates frontal process of maxilla, and straight longer black arrow points to perpendicular plate of ethmoid bone.

bone forms the anterosuperior nasal septum, while cartilage and soft tissues form the lower nasal septum. Minimal asymmetry or midline deviation of the septum is normal (Figs. 1-49 and 1-50). The *premaxilla* and the *incisive crest* are seen on the anterior floor of the nasal cavity (Figs. 1-50 and 1-51). The incisive canals, which lie on either side of the nasal septum base, form the incisive foramen (Fig. 1-52). This foramen contains branches of the sphenopalatine artery and the nasopalatine nerve, a branch of the maxillary nerve.[52,99] (See Chapter 2.)

The soft tissues and bony concha of the *inferior turbinates* are also visualized (Fig. 1-51). The space between the lateral aspect of the inferior turbinate and the nasal wall, and that space immediately under it, constitute the *inferior meatus*. The *nasolacrimal duct* opens into the inferior meatus (Figs. 1-52 to 1-54). If these structures are patent, therefore, the act of crying is accompanied by tears welling from the nose as well as down the cheeks. The space above the inferior turbinate and anterior to the *middle turbinate* is called the *nasal atrium* (Fig. 1-52). Small bony thickenings

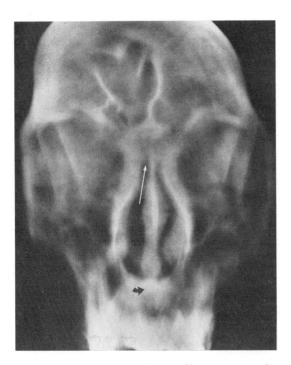

Fig. 1-50. Long white arrow indicates olfactory recess. Curved black arrow rests on premaxilla and points to base of incisive crest.

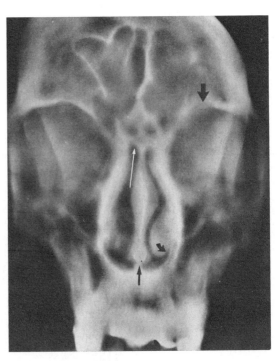

Fig. 1-51. Long white arrow indicates olfactory recess. Curved black arrow rests on left inferior turbinate and points to inferior meatus just lateral to turbinate. Thin black arrow rests on premaxilla and points to incisive crest. Large black arrow points to region of supraorbital notch.

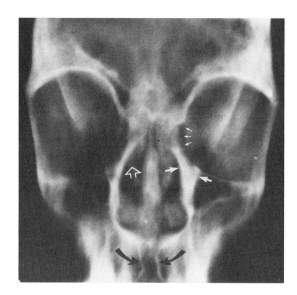

Fig. 1-52. Curved black arrows indicate incisive foramen. Open arrow rests on space anterior to middle turbinate called nasal atrium. Small white arrows indicate lacrimal fossa area and larger white arrows delimit upper margins of nasolacrimal duct.

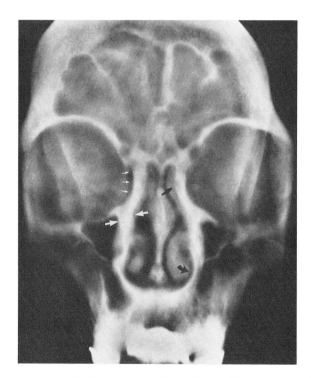

Fig. 1-53. Small white arrows indicate lacrimal fossa area, and larger white arrows point to margins of upper nasolacrimal duct. Straight black arrow points to agger nasi region of upper lateral nasal cavity. Curved black arrow rests on inferior turbinate and points to air in inferior meatus.

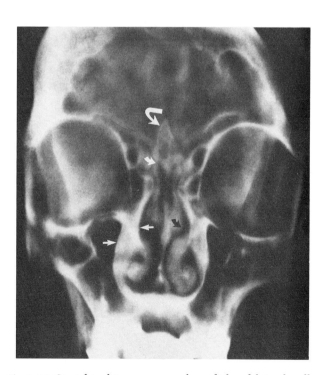

Fig. 1-54. Straight white arrows mark medial and lateral walls of lower nasolacrimal duct. Curved black arrow rests on middle turbinate and points to middle meatus. Curved white arrow points to superior attachment of middle turbinate and marks lateral extent of cribriform plate. Angled white arrow indicates anterior crista galli.

along the upper lateral nasal wall constitute the *agger nasi,* or nasal ridge. Occasionally, these bony thickenings may have small lucencies within them that represent pneumatization by the anterior ethmoid cells (Fig. 1-53).

Anteriorly, the nasal roof contains two shallow, slightly divergent grooves that are called the *olfactory sulci* (Figs. 1-50 and 1-51). The frontomaxillary suture lies anterosuperiorly, and the frontal bone and beginning of the frontal sinus are seen more posteriorly (Fig. 1-49).

The degree of frontal sinus development determines its tomographic appearance. Additionally, because the frontal surface is curved, the superior midline portions of the main body of the frontal sinus are encountered anterior to the lateral extensions. The base (floor) of the sinus is demonstrated slightly posteriorly. The intersinus septum and septa should be clearly defined and measure 1 to 2 mm in thickness. The base of the sinus septum should be midline. The posterior sinus wall is not well visualized in the AP view because its cortical margin is parallel to the film plane.

At about the same sections as the agger nasi, the superior nasolacrimal canal and the *lacrimal fossa* above are in focus (Figs. 1-52 and 1-53). Because the canal courses posteroinferiorly at an average tilt of 20°, the inferior portions are seen more posteriorly. The canal walls can be parallel although they usually diverge slightly at their inferior extent. The lacrimal bone forms the medial wall of the nasolacrimal canal and lacrimal fossa as well as the anteromedial orbital wall. The inferior portion of the medial canal wall ends near the inferior turbinate base. The lateral canal wall is continuous with the lower lateral nasal cavity wall (Fig. 1-54).

The lacrimal fossa is slightly concave laterally and averages 1 mm in thickness. The lamina papyracea is slightly thinner and straighter than the concave lacrimal bone (Figs. 1-53, 1-55 and 1-56).

On anterior cuts, the medial orbital wall and superomedial orbital margin are in the plane of focus. The middle and lateral margins are clearly seen 1.5 to 2.0 cm more posteriorly (Fig. 1-51 to 1-56).

The frontal notch and then the more lateral *supraorbital notch* can be seen in the superior orbital margin (Fig. 1-51). They transmit the frontal artery and nerve and the supraorbital artery and nerves respectively. They are not to be confused with focal destructive lesions. Occasionally, the supraorbital notch is a complete foramen (Fig. 1-49).

The *olfactory sulci* lie under the cribriform plates as they course posteriorly. They terminate in the sphenoethmoidal recesses into which the sphenoid sinus ostia

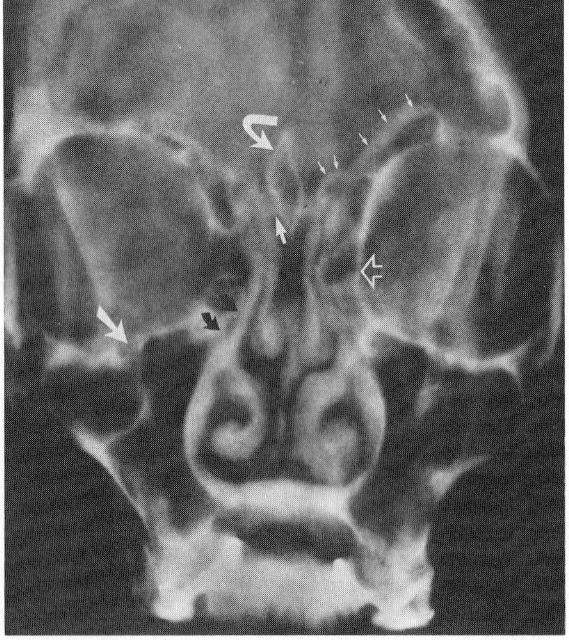

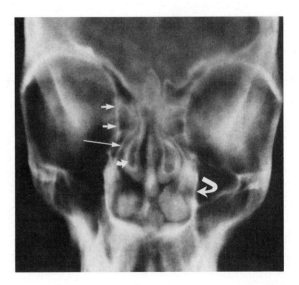

Fig. 1-55. Larger white arrow points to infraorbital canal. Angled white arrow points to crista galli. Small white arrows indicate ethmoid roof (fovea ethmoidales) medially and roof of supraorbital ethmoid cell laterally. Medium white arrow points to level of cribriform plate, and open arrow indicates lamina papyracea.

Fig. 1-56. Curved white arrow points to pneumatization of middle turbinate, and straight white arrows indicate lamina papyracea. Angled white arrow points to membranous portion of medial antral wall. This is seen as thinning or "absence" of medial bony wall. Long white arrow indicates uncinate process of ethmoid bone.

also open. The *cribriform plates* are identified as very thin horizontal densities located to either side of the nasal septum. They are outlined by air in the olfactory sulci.

The cribriform plates are lower than and medial to the fovea ethmoidalis, or ethmoid roof (Figs. 1-55 to 1-58). The orbital roofs lie lateral to and above the fovea ethmoidalis. Grooves or areas of thinning in the orbital roofs may mimic dehiscent bone on tomographic sections.

The *crista galli* is seen as a biconvex crest anteriorly that narrows posteriorly to a vertical plate (Figs. 1-54 to 1-58). It is often pneumatized. Asymmetry in the base of the crista galli (concavity on one side and the normal convexity on the other side) or in the medial portions of the fovea ethmoidalis is highly suggestive of a mass lesion in the cribriform area. Exact identification of the cribriform plate may be impossible, even on optimal films. This thin bone is perforated by numerous olfactory nerve foramina and may not be sufficiently dense to be identified between the soft tissue density of the anterior cranial fossa above and the soft tissues of the nasal cavity below. The film interpreter should be circumspect in making the diagnosis of cribriform plate destruction solely on the basis of poor visualization of the actual plate or because of the presence of a soft tissue mass underlying the cribriform plate in the nasal cavity.

The middle turbinate attaches to the lateral cribriform plate margin (Figs. 1-54 and 1-55). The middle turbinates are often pneumatized by posterior ethmoid cells (Fig. 1-56). The lateral nasal wall is an exquisitely sculptured structure. Its contour bulges inward at the level of the middle turbinates, sweeping over a group of anterior ethmoid cells that constitute the lateral margin of the nasal wall at that level. The bulge is the *ethmoid bulla* (Figs. 1-57 and 1-58). The undersurface of the ethmoidal bulla in turn forms the superolateral wall of an inverted, funnel-like canal, the *ethmoid infundibulum*. The inferomedial wall of this canal is formed by the uncinate process of the ethmoid, a slightly curved thin bone that forms most of the middle meatus (Figs. 1-56 to 1-58).

The superior opening of the funnel-shaped ethmoid infundibulum is the *hiatus semilunaris*. This region of the medial maxillary wall is covered only by mucosa (see anatomy section) and the bony hiatus thus formed just above the inferior turbinate attachment should not be confused with a focal destructive process.

The superior turbinate forms a vertically oriented, platelike structure on the sections through the mid-and posterior portions of the middle turbinates (Fig. 1-59).

On progressively more posterior cuts, the membranous nasal septum recedes and the perpendicular plates of the ethmoid bones come into focus, along with their articulation with the vomer. The articulation can some-

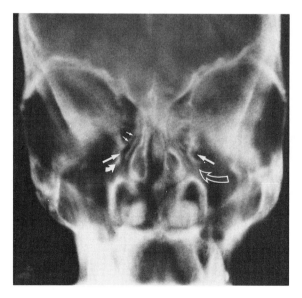

Fig. 1-57. Large straight white arrows indicate ethmoid infundibulum. Open arrow points to membranous portion of medial maxillary sinus wall. Curved white arrow points to tip of uncinate process of ethmoid bone, and small white arrows indicate border of ethmoid bulla.

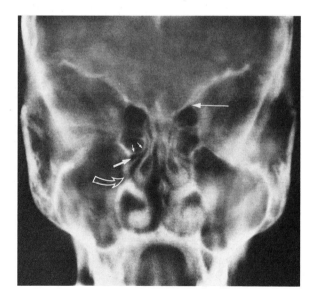

Fig. 1-58. Medium white arrow lies on ethmoid infundibulum, which opens into hiatus semilunaris. Small white arrows delimit ethmoid bulla. Open arrow points to membranous portion of medial wall of antrum. Long white arrow points to anterior ethmoid canal.

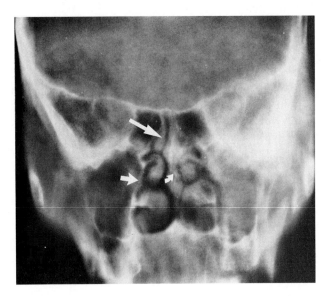

Fig. 1-59. Large white arrow points to superior turbinate. White arrowhead indicates thin mucosal portion of medial antral wall. Curved white arrow points to septal angulation, which indicates junction of ethmoid and vomer bones.

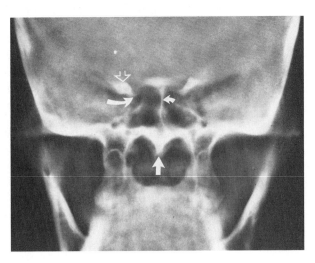

Fig. 1-60. Open arrowhead points to anterior clinoid process. Long curved white arrow indicates region of optic canal and anterior margin of carotid sulcus. Small curved white arrow rests on left sphenoid sinus proper and points to sphenoid septum. White arrow points to rostrum of sphenoid to which vomer attaches.

times be identified by a small crestlike projection[99] (Fig. 1-59). The vomer composes most of the posterior septum. The posterosuperior septum also thickens to form the rostum of the sphenoid bone (Fig. 1-60).

The ethmoid cells are clearly visualized with sharply delineated intercellular septa. The *anterior ethmoidal canal* is seen bilaterally near the posterior segment of the crista galli (Figs. 1-58 and 1-61). The posterior ethmoidal canal is identified on more posterior cuts. If supraorbital ethmoid extensions are present, they are seen paralleling the orbital roofs (Figs. 1-55 and 1-56).

Like the orbit, the contours of the maxillary sinus are not seen in their entirety on any single tomographic section. Anteriorly, the medial wall and roof are in the plane of focus. More posteriorly, the middle roof, part of the lateral wall, and zygomatic recess are seen (Figs. 1-54 and 1-55). Farther posteriorly, the superomedial recess or *ethmoidomaxillary plate (maxilloethmoidal bar)* region is in focus (Figs. 1-58 and 1-61). The *inferior orbital fissure* separates the roof of the maxillary sinus from the lateral wall of the orbit and is usually seen as two laterally divergent bony lines. The upper line is the lower margin of the greater sphenoid wing; the lower line is the maxillary sinus roof (Fig. 1-62). The fissure is narrowest in its midportion and diverges both medially and laterally. The lateral margins are continuous with the infratemporal fossa. The "oblique orbital line" and its medial extension to delimit the infratemporal fossa are also seen on these posterior sections.

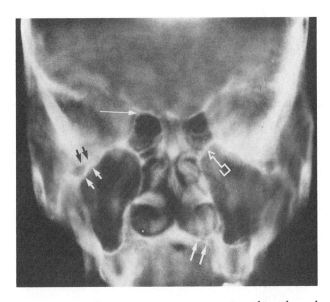

Fig. 1-61. Long white arrow points to posterior ethmoid canal. Fancy white arrow indicates ethmoid maxillary plate. Medium white arrows point to palatine grooves. Short white arrows point to maxillary side of inferior orbital fissure, and short black arrows point to sphenoid side of inferior orbital fissure.

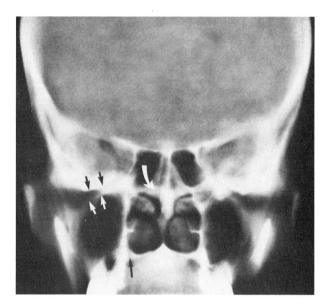

Fig. 1-62. Long black arrow points to greater palatine foramen, which is lower opening of pterygopalatine canal. Small white arrows point to maxillary side and small black arrows point to sphenoid side of inferior orbital fissure. Curved white arrow indicates region just behind superior turbinate and in front of anterior sphenoid sinus wall. This is region of sphenoethmoid recess.

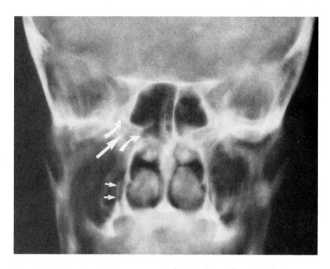

Fig. 1-63. Small white arrows indicate lateral wall of pterygopalatine canal. Large white arrow lies in region of pterygopalatine fossa. Lower curved white arrow indicates connection with nasal cavity by way of sphenopalatine canal and upper curved white arrow indicates communication with superior orbital fissure.

The maxillary sinus roof is horizontal anteriorly but slopes upward and medially toward the orbital apex (Fig. 1-61). The orbit has a circular configuration anteriorly but becomes more triangular near its apex (Figs. 1-54 and 1-59). The lamina papyracea, almost vertically oriented in its anterior segments, also slants superomedially. The maxillary sinus cavity diminishes in size posteriorly. Its configuration changes from triangular anteriorly to a vertically oriented rectangle posteriorly (Figs. 1-55 and 1-61).

The infraorbital canal runs in the orbital floor and emerges from the anterior maxillary wall as the infraorbital foramen (Fig. 1-55). The bone over the lower margin can be very thin or dehiscent.

The sphenopalatine canal orifice is seen as a horizontal discontinuity of the upper nasal cavity wall (Fig. 1-63). It lies just behind the superior turbinate and connects the nose with the pterygopalatine fossa (Fig. 1-63). About 5 mm anteriorly the pterygopalatine canal is seen as a vertically oriented canal just lateral to the nasal cavity wall (Figs. 1-62 and 1-63).

The pterygoid plates are clearly seen farther posteriorly. The medial plate and hamulus are vertically oriented, and the lateral plate is slightly divergent at its lower margin (Fig. 1-64). The *pterygoid fossa* is the space between the two pterygoid plates. Its anterior

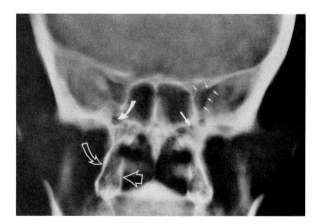

Fig. 1-64. Small white arrows indicate lesser sphenoid wing side *(two arrows)* and the greater sphenoid wing side *(three arrows)* of superior orbital fissure. Curved white arrow points to foramen rotundum at lower medial margin of superior orbital fissure. Straight medium white arrow points to vidian canal. Open curved arrow indicates lateral pterygoid plate, and open arrowhead indicates medial pterygoid plate.

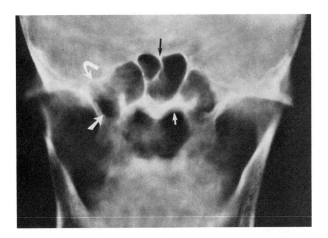

Fig. 1-65. Angled white arrow illustrates extension of lateral recess of sphenoid sinus into greater sphenoid wing. Large white arrow indicates extension of recess into pterygoid fossa. Small white arrow points to thin soft tissue line of nasopharyngeal roof mucosa under sphenoid bone. Black arrow points to planum sphenoidale at level of sphenoid sinus septum.

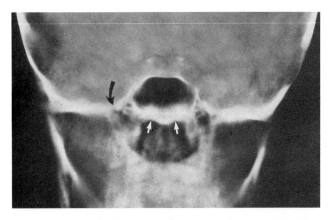

Fig. 1-66. Curved black arrow points to foramen lacerum. Sphenoid sinus cavity is behind lateral attachment of sinus septum and thus appears to have no septum. Sinus roof is now floor of sella turcica or lamina dura. White arrows indicate soft tissues of nasopharyngeal roof under sphenoid bone.

wall and the horizontally oriented fossa floor (the pyramidal process) are both formed by the palatine bone.

The sphenoid sinus cortical margins should be sharply defined. The intersinus septum is normally in the midline anteriorly (Figs. 1-60, 1-63, and 1-64). When the intersinus septum deviates far from the midline, sections behind its posterior septal attachment demonstrate only one sinus cavity (Fig. 1-65). The lateral recesses into the greater sphenoid wing or pterygoid processes are also clearly seen (Fig. 1-66). They are frequently asymmetric.

The nasopharyngeal soft tissues should be carefully assessed (Figs. 1-65 and 1-66). A suspect focal irregular-

ity should be confirmed on lateral films. The posterolateral sphenoid sinus walls abut against the cavernous sinuses. The sinus roof is the floor of the sella turcica (Fig. 1-66). The relative thickness of the roof and lateral walls depends on the degree of pneumatization and development of the main sphenoid sinus cavity. The cortical bone of the floor of the sella turcica or lamina dura should be white, bright, and sharply marginated. The foramen lacerum is seen just lateral to the sinus base as a defect in the floor of the middle cranial fossa (Fig. 1-66). Just posterior and slightly lateral to the foramen lacerum is the much smaller foramen spinosum.

The optic canals are seen bilaterally between the superolateral sphenoid sinus margins and the anterior clinoid processes (Fig. 1-60). The superior orbital fissures can be somewhat asymmetric although usually this is not the case. Their lateral portions are narrow or slitlike spaces; the medial portions appear wider and more oval (Fig. 1-64). The foramen rotundum lies near the inferomedial margin of the superior orbital fissure, and the small bony septum separating them is occasionally absent. The vidian (pterygoid) canal lies inferomedial to the foramen rotundum (Figs. 1-60 and 1-64). The vidian canal is a conduit between the middle cranial fossa near the foramen lacerum and the pterygopalatine fossa. It transmits the vidian nerve, which carries secretomotor functions for the lacrimal glands and nasal mucosa. The pterygopalatine fossa is a roughly rectangular space just above the pterygoid plates and inferolateral to the floor of the sphenoid sinus (Fig. 1-63) (see Chapter 3).

■ Computed tomography

The air-containing cavities of the face are particularly well suited for exploiting the peculiar capability of computed tomography (CT) to delineate bone and soft tissue concurrently. In the presence of soft tissue disease, the potential of bony involvement is omnipresent. Moreover, soft tissue disease is defined with remarkable clarity and fidelity by CT to a degree never before approachable.

In the axial projection the scans should run from above the frontal sinuses to below the hard palate. The scans should be reviewed at both bone window (1000 or more) and soft tissue (200 to 400) settings. Ideally this should be done at the console by the radiologist.

Axial projection

In all the paranasal sinuses, normal mucosa is not seen. The sinus cavity air appears to abut directly on the bony sinus walls.

The most superior portions of the paranasal sinuses are the frontal sinuses. Although the sinuses are highly variable in shape and extent, they appear as air-containing cavities with well-delineated anterior and posterior cortical plates (Figs. 1-67 to 1-71). Adjacent intracranial

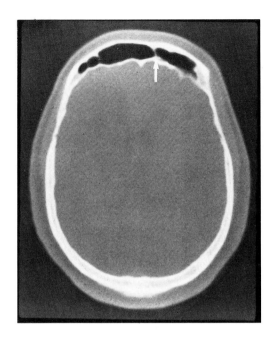

Fig. 1-67. Axial CT scan. White arrow points to normal frontal sinus septum. Notice how well anterior and posterior sinus walls are seen.

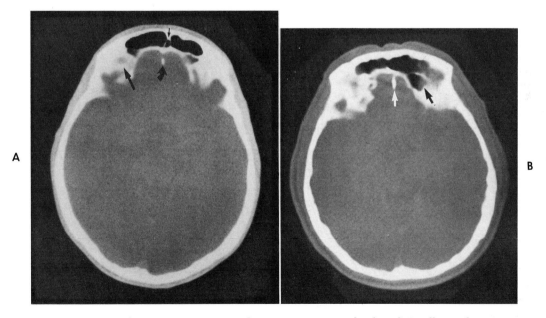

A   B

Fig. 1-68. A, Axial CT scan. Large straight arrow points to orbital roof. Small straight arrow points to intersinus septum. Curved arrow points to tip of crista galli. **B,** Axial CT scan. White arrow points to crista galli. Notice extension of frontal sinus into orbital roof on left side (*black arrow*).

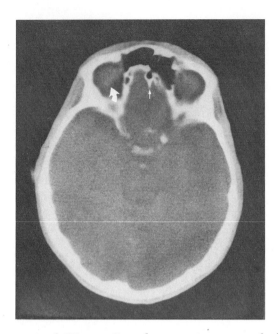

Fig. 1-69. Axial CT scan. Curved arrow points to top of orbit. Straight arrow points to posterior tip of partially pneumatized crista galli. Top of sella turcica is seen more posteriorly, just starting to come into scan plane.

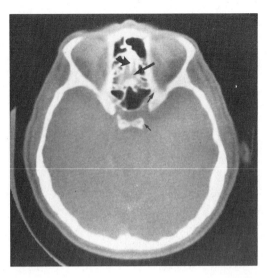

Fig. 1-70. Axial CT scan. Small black arrow points to posterior clinoid process. Medium black arrow rests on region of optic canal and superior orbital fissure. Large black arrow points to soft tissues of midline intracranial structures and this area should not be confused with ethmoid sinus clouding. Curved black arrow points to crista galli.

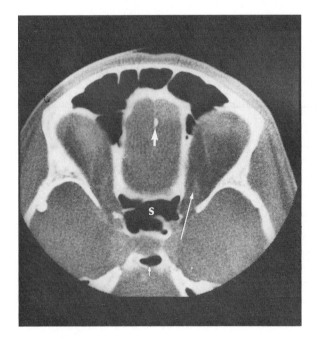

Fig. 1-71. Axial CT scan. Long thin arrow lies on optic canal and superior orbital fissure region. Medium arrow points to crista galli and lies on normal midline anterior cranial fossa structures. Small arrow points to sphenoid sinus pneumatization of dorsum sellae. *S,* Sphenoid sinus.

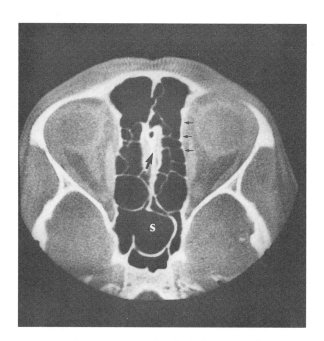

Fig. 1-72. Axial CT scan reveals ethmoid septa and lamina papyracea *(small arrows)*. Sphenoid sinus *(S)* and curved intersinus septum are well seen. Larger arrow points to top of nasal septum.

structures should also be examined for extension of frontal sinus disease. Soft tissue CT settings demonstrate any asymmetry of the overlying scalp and forehead. The frontal sinus septa and the intersinus septum usually can be identified. A nonaerated, diseased frontal sinus may at times be difficult to see in the surrounding normal bone. Whenever only one frontal sinus or no frontal sinuses are seen, the examination should be reviewed at the console of the scanner, with manipulation of window widths and levels. A careful review at wide windows will usually reveal whether the sinus is diseased or merely hypoplastic.

The ethmoid sinuses are clearly delineated in the axial projection.[22] The thin lamina papyracea is well seen although it can normally appear discontinuous (Figs. 1-72 to 1-74). The intercellular ethmoid septa are well seen, as is the upper nasal septum. More posteriorly, the sphenoid sinus can be clearly identified although several serial scans may be required for complete delineation (Figs. 1-71 to 1-74). Pneumatization of the greater sphenoid wing or the pterygoid region should not be misinterpreted as a destructive lesion. The sphenoid sinus and its recesses may also show considerable asymmetry.

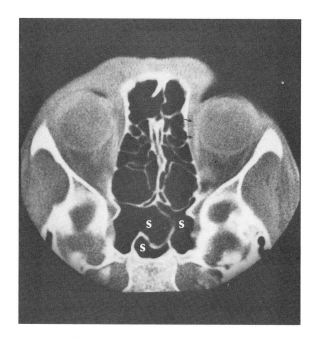

Fig. 1-73. Axial CT scan. Arrows indicate medial rectus muscle, which normally is clearly separated from lamina papyracea in its anterior and middle thirds by extra conal fat. Sphenoid sinus compartments *(S)* and ethmoid cells are well seen.

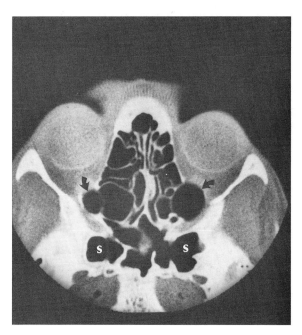

Fig. 1-74. Axial CT scan. Curved arrows point to most superior tips of maxillary sinuses. Ethmoid cells and sphenoid sinus are well seen. Sphenoid sinus lateral recesses *(S)* are easily identified.

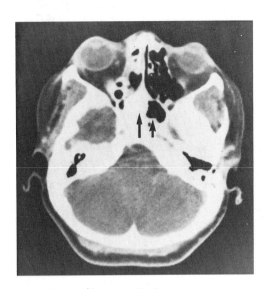

Fig. 1-75. Axial CT scan. Short black arrow points to an apparently solitary left sphenoid sinus cavity. Large black arrow rests on an apparently nonpneumatized portion of right sphenoid bone.

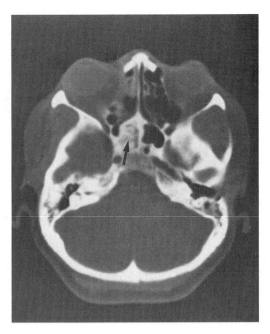

Fig. 1-76. Axial CT scan. Same patient and scan as in Fig. 1-75 but reviewed at different settings. Black arrow points to clouding of normally developed right sphenoid sinus cavity.

The sphenoid intersinus septum can appear very thin but usually is well seen. While the right and left sphenoid sinus cavities can vary in size, particularly in their posterior extension, a unilaterally well-developed sinus does not occur with an aplastic or markedly hypoplastic contralateral sinus. If only one main sinus cavity is seen, the settings should be checked to evaluate clouding of the opposite side (Figs. 1-75 and 1-76).

A depressed and enlarged sella floor may protrude into the sphenoid sinus, mimicking a sinus polyp (Fig. 1-77). Because the axial scans are performed with the patient supine, a true polyp usually falls to the posterior sinus wall and appears simply as a clouded sinus cavity. The main sphenoid sinus cavity and its recesses are well seen (Figs. 1-78 and 1-79).

The maxillary sinus roofs (orbital floors) usually appear quite asymmetric. The sinus apex appears as a round or ovoid lucency in the posteromedial portion of the orbital floor (Figs. 1-74 and 1-79). The slightly flatter anterolateral floor is more easily seen in the AP view (Fig. 1-80). Occasionally portions of the infraorbital canal can also be identified. The anteroinferior orbital wall is often poorly seen because it is sectioned obliquely. More caudal scans show a clear, well-defined anterior maxillary sinus wall. The overlying facial soft tissues, posterolateral wall, and medial (nasal) wall all appear sharply defined. Some thinning of the posterior wall near the pterygoid plates is often observed and

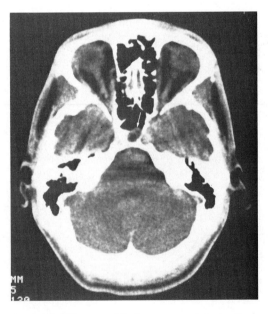

Fig. 1-77. Axial CT scan. Black arrow points to "polypoid" depression of sella floor into sphenoid sinus cavity secondary to pituitary tumor.

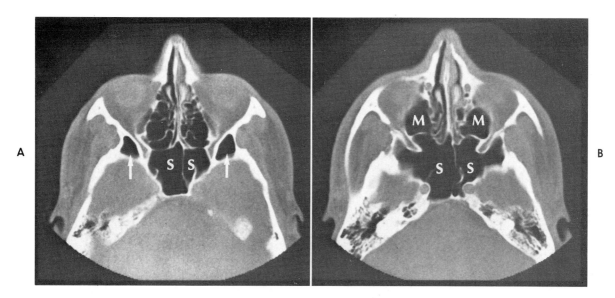

Fig. 1-78. A, Axial CT scan. Main sphenoid sinus cavity (S) is well seen. Arrows point to sphenoid sinus pneumatization of greater wings of sphenoid bone as it forms posterior orbital wall. **B,** Axial CT scan slightly more caudal than **A.** Lateral extensions of sphenoid sinus are clearly seen as they go into greater sphenoid wings. Main sphenoid sinus cavities (S) and apices of maxillary sinuses (M) are clearly seen.

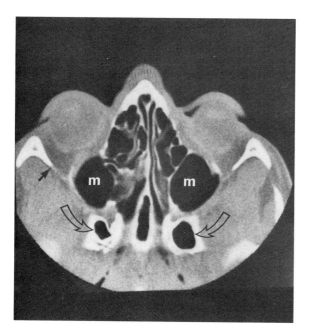

Fig. 1-79. Axial CT scan. Curved arrows point to sphenoid sinus pneumatization of pterygoid plates. Black arrow indicates zygomaticosphenoid suture in posterior orbital wall. *M* denotes maxillary sinus.

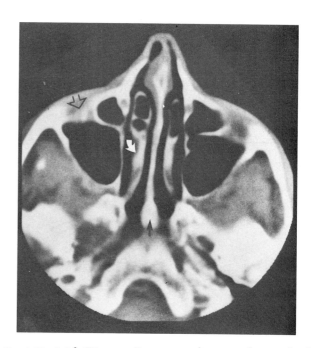

Fig. 1-80. Axial CT scan. Open arrow lies on inferior orbital rim. Apparent bone destruction or soft tissue mass results from curved orbital rim and periorbital soft tissues. Curved white arrow rests on midline meatus and points to middle turbinate. Black arrow points to rostrum of sphenoid and posterior nasal septum.

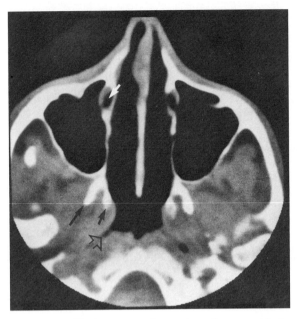

Fig. 1-81. Long black arrow indicates lateral pterygoid plate, and short black arrow indicates medial pterygoid plate. Open arrow points to fossa of Rosenmüller. White arrow indicates nasolacrimal duct. All antral walls are clearly seen.

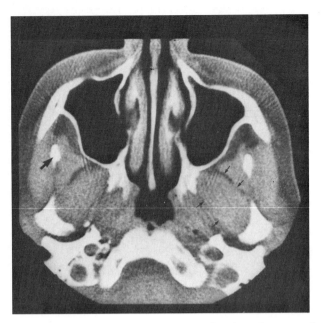

Fig. 1-82. Axial CT scan. Small arrows outline lateral pterygoid muscle. Large arrow points to coronoid process of mandible. Inferior turbinates, nasal septum, and antral walls are all clearly seen.

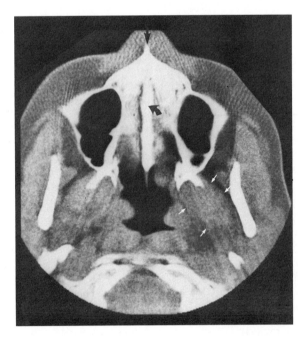

Fig. 1-83. Axial CT scan through lowermost nasal cavity. Curved arrow indicates lower nasal septum resting on hard palate. Lowest portions of maxillary sinuses are easily seen. Small arrows outline medial pterygoid muscle. Arrow at top points to anterior nasal spine.

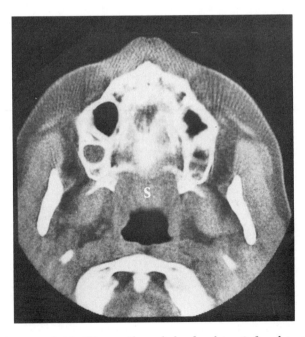

Fig. 1-84. Axial CT scan through hard palate. Soft palate is seen (S) and alveolar recesses are identified.

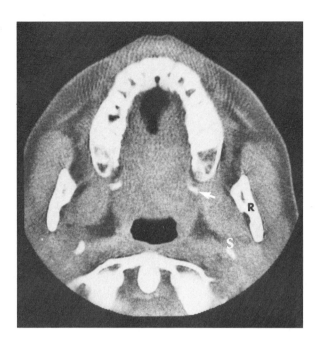

Fig. 1-85. Axial CT scan just below hard palate. Hamulus of pterygoid is seen *(arrow)*. Styloid process *(S)* and mandibular ramus *(R)* are identified.

should not be mistaken for bone destruction (Figs. 1-81 and 1-82). The alveolar recess can be seen if both the proper bone settings are used and tooth filling–caused artifacts do not degrade the image (Figs. 1-83 and 1-84). The hard palate often is clearly visualized and the "rule of symmetry" allows detection of bone destruction (Figs. 1-83 to 1-85).

Coronal scans should be taken whenever the integrity of a bony plate that lies in a plane parallel to the axial scans is questioned. If disease has spread from the mouth to the nose (across the hard palate), from the antrum to the orbit (across the orbital floor), or from the orbit, ethmoid, nasal cavity or sphenoid into the anterior cranial fossa (across the bony roofs), a coronal CT scan should be obtained to better delineate the extent of the disease.

Coronal computed tomography

It is essential to have a machine with a tilting gantry in order to reliably obtain coronal scans. The coronal scans will vary somewhat in appearance because the scan angles will vary from 50° to 90°. Because the teeth lie under the maxillary sinus, nasal cavity, and frontal and ethmoid sinuses, fillings or metal caps can degrade the coronal images. This problem can often be solved by reducing the coronal CT scan angle. The anatomic orientation is similar to that discussed in the section on complex motion tomography.

Coronal CT scans far anteriorly reveal the frontal sinuses, the frontal processes of the maxillary bones, and the anterior nasal cavity (Figs. 1-86 to 1-89). The orbital

roofs and occasionally the supraorbital notch are seen at these levels.

Slightly more posterior scans demonstrate the crista galli and cribriform plates (Figs. 1-88 to 1-91). Intracranial tumor extension through the cribriform plates or the fovea ethmoidalis can usually be well delineated in this projection.

The maxillary sinuses are also well demonstrated (Figs. 1-90 to 1-93). They often appear somewhat foreshortened if the scan angle is less than 90°. The roof and the medial and lateral sinus walls are all clearly delineated. Although the superior meatus and turbinate and the sphenoethmoidal recess are often obscured, the inferior and middle turbinates and meati are seen consistently. The nasal septum, the olfactory grooves, and the hard palate can also be readily identified. Occasionally, the palatine grooves and pterygopalatine canals are visualized. The soft tissues over the oral surface of the hard palate can only be seen if the tongue is depressed away from the palate (Figs. 1-93 and 1-94).

The ethmoid sinuses are exquisitely delineated in the coronal plane (Figs. 1-88 to 1-92). Proper window settings are necessary to visualize the intercellular septa and lamina papyracea.

The sphenoid sinus and its margins and recesses are also consistently well seen (Figs. 1-93 to 1-97). The pterygoid plates and fossa, the osseous roof of the nasopharynx, and the floor of the middle cranial fossa are all clearly demonstrated. The pterygoid canals, the anterior clinoid processes, and the sella turcica should be identified on each complete scan series.

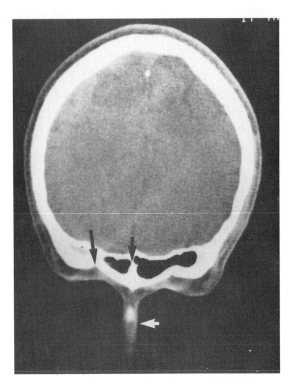

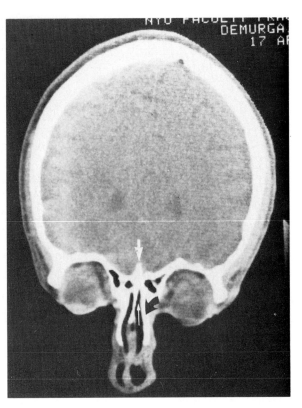

Fig. 1-86. Coronal CT scan. Frontal sinuses and intersinus septum *(short arrow)* are seen far anteriorly. Supraorbital notch *(long arrow)* in anterior superior orbital rim is seen. White arrow points to most anterior portion of nose.

Fig. 1-87. Coronal CT scan. Curved black arrow indicates frontal process of maxilla. Long white arrow indicates crista galli. Thin white arrow lies in olfactory recess of nasal cavity.

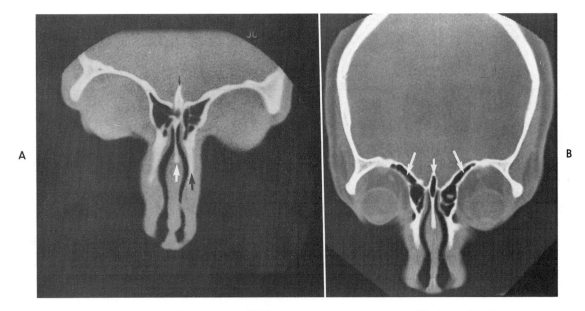

Fig. 1-88. A, Coronal CT scan. Small black arrow points to crista galli. Long black arrow indicates frontal process of maxilla. Anterior ethmoid cells are clearly seen, as is cartilaginous nasal septum and perpendicular plate of ethmoid bone *(white arrow)*. **B,** Coronal CT scan. Long white arrows indicate supraorbital ethmoid cells as they extend up into orbital roofs. Short white arrow points to pneumatization of crista galli.

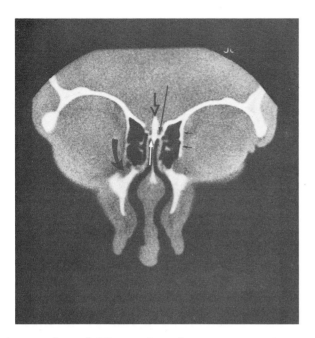

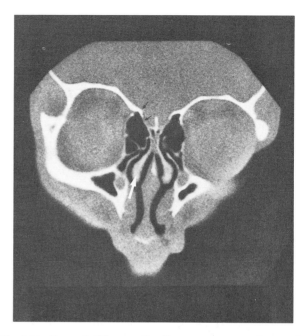

Fig. 1-89. Coronal CT scan. Curved arrow points to lacrimal fossa and small arrows indicate lamina papyracea. Long black arrow points to cribriform plate, on which rests crista galli *(open arrow)*. White arrow lies on olfactory recess and points to cribriform plate.

Fig. 1-90. Coronal CT scan. Small arrows point to fovea ethmoidalis, lateral to and above cribriform plate. White arrow points to middle turbinate. Most anterior portions of maxillary sinus are just coming into view.

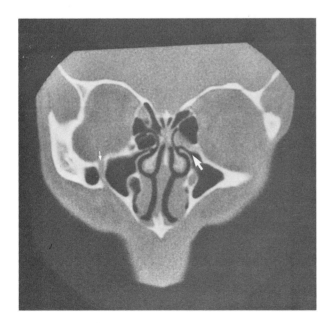

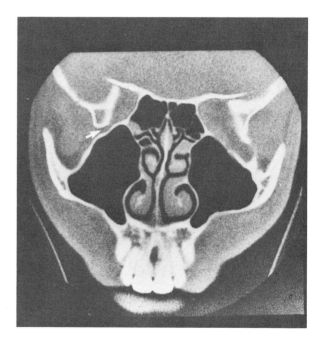

Fig. 1-91. Coronal CT scan. Infundibulum, or drainage canal of antrum, is seen *(large arrow)*. Small arrow indicates portion of infraorbital canal. Middle and inferior turbinates and nasal septum are clearly seen.

Fig. 1-92. Coronal CT scan. More posterior scan clearly shows antral walls and nasal cavity structures. Inferior orbital fissure is also seen *(arrow)*.

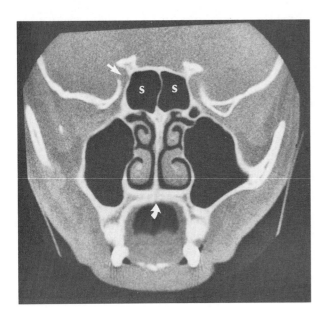

Fig. 1-93. Coronal CT scan. Anterior sphenoid sinus is seen (S). Planum sphenoidale forms its roof. Optic canal (*arrow*) and portions of superior orbital fissure are visualized. Tongue is depressed and normal mucosa over hard palate (*curved arrow*) is seen.

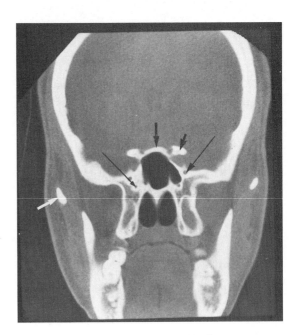

Fig. 1-94. Coronal CT scan. Large black arrow points to planum sphenoidale with underlying sphenoid sinus cavity. Short black arrow points to left anterior clinoid process. Large long arrow points to left foramen rotundum. Small long arrow points to right vidian canal. White arrow points to coronoid process of mandible.

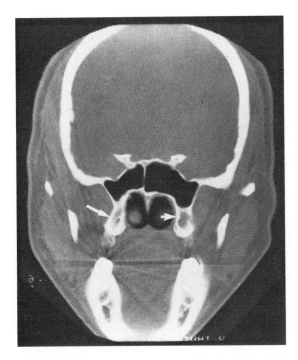

Fig. 1-95. Coronal CT scan. Lateral recesses of sphenoid sinus are clearly seen to extend into floor of middle cranial fossa and down into pterygoid plates. Large white arrow points to lateral pterygoid plate. Small white arrow points to medial pterygoid plate.

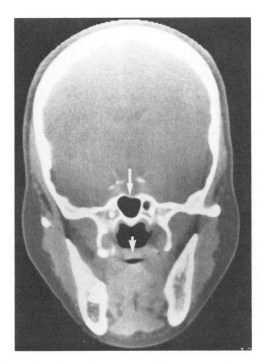

Fig. 1-96. Coronal CT scan. Large white arrow points to sella floor that forms posterior roof of sphenoid sinus. Small white arrow points to soft palate.

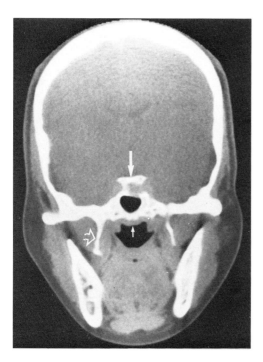

Fig. 1-97. Coronal CT scan. Large white arrow points to top of dorsum sellae. Small white arrow points to soft tissues of nasopharyngeal roof. Open arrow points to posterior edge of lateral pterygoid plate.

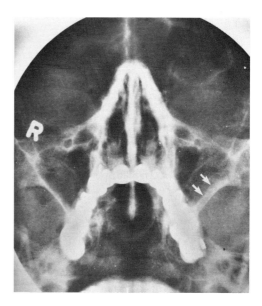

Fig. 1-98. Waters view. Minimal mucoperiosteal thickening is seen in left maxillary sinus *(arrows)*. This uniform soft tissue thickening parallels sinus wall contours.

□ Pathology

■ Inflammatory disease

Acute sinusitis

Mild mucosal inflammatory changes of *viral upper respiratory tract infections* are completely reversible. If secondary bacterial infection occurs, the inflammatory changes will subside with complete return of the mucosa to its normal histologic pattern and physiologic function as long as adequate sinus drainage is maintained. Once interference with the normal sinus drainage occurs, a mucopurulent exudate can accumulate within the sinus cavity. The sinus obstruction is usually secondary to inflammatory edema at the ostia, although congenital or acquired ostial narrowing may have similar results. Sinus involvement is usually secondary to extension from the nasal passages. Between 10% and 20% of cases of recurrent sinusitis are secondary to chronic dental infections or occur as complications of tooth extractions.[133]

Accurately determining the involved pathogens in bacterial infections requires either direct sinus puncture or open surgical biopsy.[21] Nasal and ostial cultures do not correlate well with these more accurate surgical techniques. The pathogens most commonly encountered in *acute sinusitis* are *Streptococcus pneumoniae* (pneumococcus) and *Haemophilus influenzae*. Patho-

genic anaerobes are rare. In contradistinction, anaerobes predominate in chronic sinusitis. Low oxygen tension in the obstructed sinus cavity probably favors growth of these anaerobes. The predominant isolates are peptostreptococci, *Bacteroides* sp., and fusobacteria.[39,45]

The maxillary sinuses are most frequently involved in inflammatory disease, followed by the ethmoid and frontal sinuses. Clinically, the sphenoid sinuses are least often affected.

Clinical manifestations

The primary symptom of infection in the paranasal sinuses is local pain. Extensive polyposis with expansion of the nasal cavity and paranasal sinus walls is not associated with pain unless an infection supervenes. This is also true of bone expansion and destruction secondary to mucoceles and tumors. However, infection may be superimposed on an underlying malignancy. Only 3% of patients with sinusitis complain of headaches.[136]

Radiographic findings

Plain films of uncomplicated *viral sinusitis* usually reveal minimal changes, if any. There may be some swelling of the turbinates. The mucosa of the maxillary sinuses may be slightly edematous. This is seen as a uniformly thickened soft tissue layer just inside the thin dense bony line of the mucoperiosteum (Fig. 1-98). This layer varies from 1 to 10 mm in thickness (Fig. 1-99). Less often, a diffuse haze will be seen in one or both maxillary sinuses. This represents both mucosal edema and antral fluid. A true air-fluid level may or may not be present.

In *acute bacterial sinusitis*, air-fluid levels are commonly seen (Figs. 1-100 and 1-101). Involvement of the paranasal sinuses is usually asymmetric. The maxillary sinus is most frequently involved; mucosal thickening and fluid retention are the typical roentgenographic findings. If both maxillary sinuses are involved, one usually has more marked changes than the other (Figs. 1-102 and 1-103). Although pansinusitis can occur in acute bacterial sinusitis, it is much more commonly seen in allergic sinusitis. Unilateral involvement of the sinuses is also more common in bacterial sinusitis than in allergic sinusitis, and if only one sinus is involved it is almost never allergic in origin. *Inflammatory polyps* are rarely seen and when present are associated with chronic bacterial sinusitis.

Allergic sinusitis

Approximately 10% of the population has allergic rhinitis and sinusitis. The most common form is seasonal pollinosis and (in North America) the prevalent form is ragweed allergy. Spores from molds are also important antigens.[126]

Allergic reactions are manifestations of type I immunologic disorders represented by an IgE reagin-antibody reaction with a resulting release of mediators that produce symptoms of sneezing, nasal obstruction, and watery rhinorrhea. Profuse secretions associated with nasal obstruction can result in retained secretions and eventual infection.[126]

Mucoperiosteal (mucosal) hypersecretion and hyperplasia result in a mild to markedly thickened mucosa that can obscure the sinus cavity. These changes are bilateral and primarily involve the maxillary sinuses (Fig. 1-104), although symmetric involvement of the ethmoid, frontal, and sphenoid sinuses is common. The secretions are normally clear and mucoid in character. Purulent secretions from the sinus cavity indicate the presence of secondary infection. The hypertrophic mucosa is less capable of resisting subsequent infections.[126]

The thickened mucosa can become heaped in irregular folds. True polypoid hypertrophy may be present. Radiographically, these changes appear as hypertrophic polypoid mucosal thickening and when present are far more suggestive of allergic sinusitis than bacterial infection. Although there is a diffuse hypersecretion, air-fluid levels are rarely seen in allergic sinusitis. Bilateral edema of the nasal turbinates, pansinusitis, polyp for-

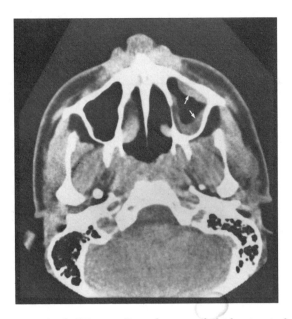

Fig. 1-99. Axial CT scan. Smooth mucosal thickening in left maxillary sinus *(arrows)* is typical of inflammation.

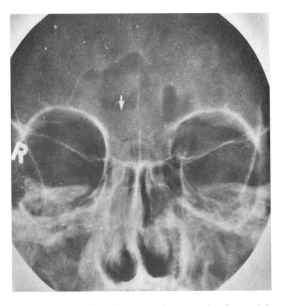

Fig. 1-100. Erect Caldwell view. There is clouding of frontal and right ethmoid sinuses. Arrow points to air-fluid level in right frontal sinus. *Acute bacterial sinusitis.*

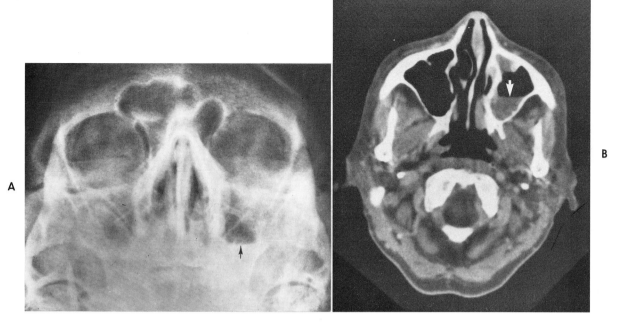

Fig. 1-101. A, Erect Waters view. There is marked mucoperiosteal thickening in both maxillary sinuses with air-fluid level on left *(arrow)*. *Acute bacterial sinusitis.* **B,** Axial CT scan. Air-fluid level is seen *(arrow)* in left antrum. Notice normal right antrum. *Acute bacterial sinusitis.*

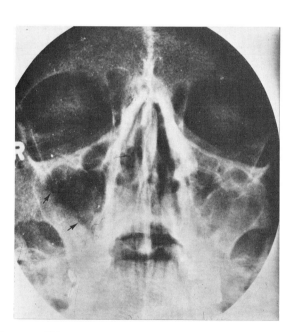

Fig. 1-102. Waters view. Asymmetric mucoperiosteal thickening of maxillary sinuses. Diffuse haziness is present on left side, and polypoid mucosal thickening is seen on right side *(arrows)*. *Bacterial sinusitis.*

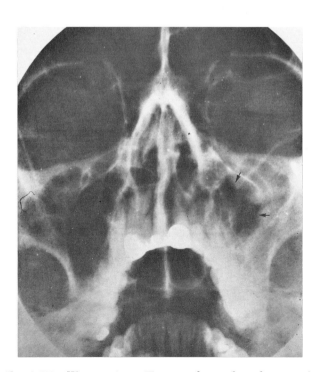

Fig. 1-103. Waters view. Hypertrophic polypoid mucosal changes in left maxillary sinus *(arrows)*. Asymmetry suggested bacterial etiology.

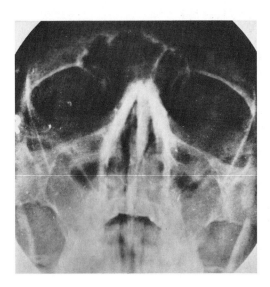

Fig. 1-104. Waters view. Bilateral, symmetric, marked muco-periosteal thickening in allergic sinusitis.

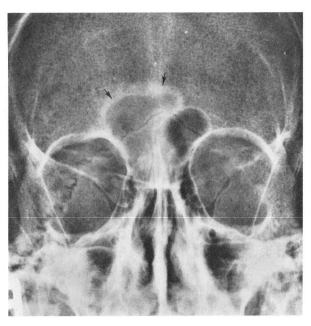

Fig. 1-105. Caldwell view. Chronic right frontal sinusitis is indicated by zone of reactive sclerosis seen in frontal bone adjacent to right frontal sinus *(arrows)*. Clouding of this sinus cavity may represent chronic or acute disease or both. Minimal clouding is also present in right posterior ethmoid cells.

mation, or diffuse polyposis is far more common in allergic disease then in bacterial sinusitis.

Chronic sinusitis

Chronic sinusitis results from either persistent acute inflammation or repeated bouts of acute sinusitis. Chronic disease can result in atrophic, sclerosing, or hypertrophic polypoid mucosal change. The sclerosing changes result in areas of squamous metaplasia and dense connective tissue reaction, coupled with sclerosis of the mucosal vessels. The atrophic type may coexist with the hypertrophic type and as such cannot be differentiated radiographically. Differentiating between chronic (inflammatory) hypertrophic polypoid sinusitis and chronic allergic polypoid sinusitis may be a moot task because both allergic and infectious sinusitis can and usually do coexist in the chronic stages.

The roentgenographic findings of either focal decalcification or a reactive sclerosing osteitis (Fig. 1-105) are uncommonly seen in the antibiotic era. When identified, such findings suggest chronic infection, sometimes granulomatous or fungal, rather than allergic sinusitis.

Pansinusitis and nasal polyps can have a different significance in the newborn and pediatric ages. At birth, only rudimentary maxillary sinuses and the ethmoid sinuses are present. Failure to aerate these sinuses may

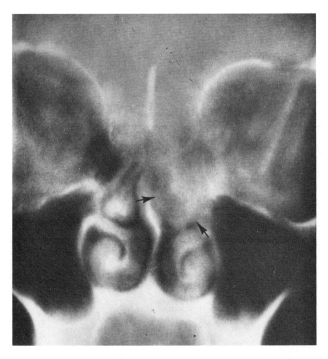

Fig. 1-106. Coronal tomogram. Polypoid soft tissue mass is extending into left ethmoid sinus and upper nasal cavity *(arrows)*. Although thinned, left lamina papyracea is intact. *Encephalocele.*

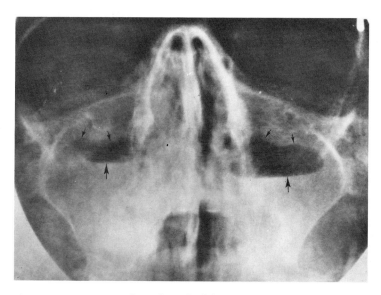

Fig. 1-107. Erect Waters view. Bilateral air-fluid levels are present in maxillary sinuses 24 hours after bilateral antral lavage *(large arrows)*. Mucoperiosteal thickening in both antra is also seen along antral roofs *(small arrows)*.

cause them to appear opacified for several weeks. This is probably caused by retained secretions. Persistent opacification or recurrent episodes of sinusitis by the age of 1 year may indicate the presence of cystic fibrosis (mucoviscidosis). Because of persistent nasal obstruction, probably a result of polyposis, the frontal sinuses are often hypoplastic. In addition, any condition that alters the host immune responses, such as immunoglobulin abnormalities and blood dyscrasias, can also appear as recurring sinusitis.

The presentation of a "nasal polyp" in the first few years of life should suggest the possibility of an *encephalocoele* (Fig. 1-106).[7] (This subject is considered in detail in Chapter 2.)

Air-fluid levels

The most common cause of an air-fluid level is acute bacterial sinusitis. The next most common cause is recent antral lavage (Fig. 1-107). For at least 2 to 3 days following lavage, enough fluid remains in the sinus cavities to produce an air-fluid level.

Trauma can result in an air-fluid level or air-blood level with or without an accompanying fracture. A history of direct trauma will suggest this cause. The trauma, however, need not be physical. Barotrauma can also cause both mucoperiosteal edema and an air-fluid level; this almost always occurs in the antra. Inexplicably, most of the symptoms are referable to the frontal sinuses, which show little roentgenographic abnormality.[41]

Hemorrhage as a result of bleeding disorders such as von Willebrand's disease and other coagulation or platelet disorders may be associated with sinus bleeding. Occasionally, sinusitis with air-fluid levels has ben reported in chemically induced sinusitis. Chromates and other industrial pollutants have been implicated in such cases.

Complications of sinus infections

Complications of inflammatory sinusitis can be divided into two main groups: (1) those that affect the sinus mucosa directly and (2) those that affect neighboring structures outside the sinus cavity.

The most common complication occurring in the sinus itself is the *mucous retention cyst*, seen in approximately 10% of routine examinations.[42] Mucous retention cysts result from obstruction of a seromucinous gland, with resulting cystic expansion.[148] The wall of the retention cyst is therefore lined by the epithelium of the specific gland involved. Mucous retention cysts appear as homogenous soft tissue masses that usually are on the floor or lateral wall of the maxillary sinus

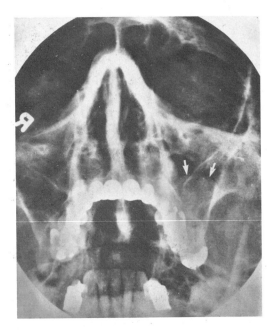

Fig. 1-108. Waters view. Arrows outline upper curved contour of homogeneous soft tissue mass in left antrum. This is a retention cyst, but radiographically it could also be a polyp.

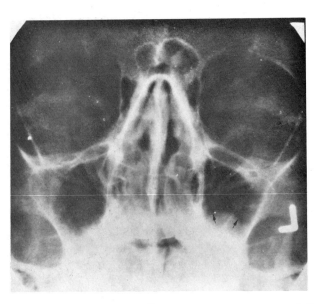

Fig. 1-109. Waters view. Small retention cyst is present in left maxillay sinus *(arrows)*. There is mucoperiosteal thickening in both antra.

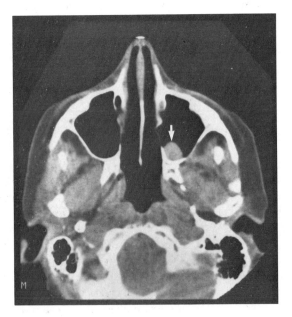

Fig. 1-110. Axial CT scan reverals incidental finding of retention cyst *(arrow)* in posterior left maxillary sinus.

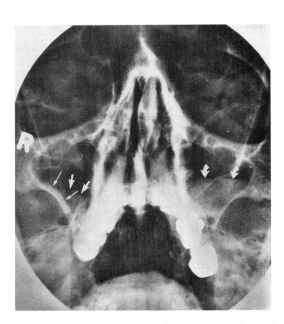

Fig. 1-111. Waters view. Curved white arrows indicate large "flat" retention cyst in left maxillary sinus that may simulate an air-fluid level if careful attention is not paid to its contour. Thin arrows point to uniform mucoperiosteal thickening in right antrum, and straight medium arrows outline small retention cyst in right antrum.

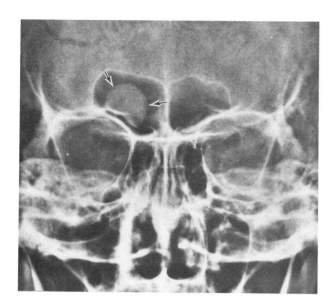

Fig. 1-112. Caldwell view. Solitary retention cyst in right frontal sinus *(arrows)*.

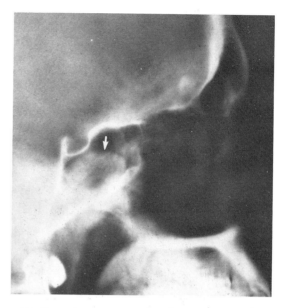

Fig. 1-113. Lateral tomogram. Arrow points to large asymptomatic retention cyst in sphenoid sinus.

(Figs. 1-108 to 1-110). The medial wall and roof are less frequently involved. The dome-shaped or spherical configuration is usually diagnostic although some cysts are quite broad-based and can simulate an air-fluid level (Fig. 1-111). An erect frontal view with the head tilted is helpful in those circumstances. Because of the effects of gravity, the air-fluid level will remain parallel to the ground irrespective of position of the head. On the other hand, the air–soft tissue contour of a cyst is virtually independent of gravity and tilting of the head may cause the cyst to shift position slightly while maintaining its overall configuration.

Retention cysts sometimes occur in the frontal and ethmoid sinuses (Fig. 1-112). The true incidence of retention cysts in the sphenoid sinus is difficult to estimate because small cysts are easily obscured on routine sinus films. They are usually incidental findings when tomography is performed on neighboring structures such as the sella turcica or the base of the skull (Fig. 1-113). Retention cysts are clinically silent unless they completely fill the sinus cavity. In this case, they are one of the causes of a completely opaque sinus cavity on plain films. On tomograms, a thin rim of air often can be seen surrounding the homogeneous cysts, suggesting the diagnosis (Figs. 1-114 and 1-115). Associated inflammatory disease may obscure even this air. Because retention cysts usually mold themselves to the sinus, actual expansion of the cavity is rare. When expansion does occur, it is usually in the sphenoid sinus. Pain clinically referable to this sinus (suboccipital, be-

tween the eyes, or deep central in location) is invariably present.

When a retention cyst occurs in the roof of the maxillary sinus, it may be difficult to distinguish from a small blow-out fracture of the orbit with local herniation of periorbital tissues (Fig. 1-116). This is a trying circumstance, for the asymptomatic cyst may be first demonstrated only at the time of radiologic pursuit of the diagnosis of the blow-out fracture. Lateral tomography usually is definitive.

In the Waters view, a smooth, homogeneous soft tissue mass is sometimes also seen in relationship to the infraorbital canal. This is a normal variant, caused by mucosa overlying an unusually low-lying infraorbital canal.

A *serous cyst* results from fluid accumulation and loculation in the *submucosal* layers of the mucoperiosteum. The serous cyst therefore does not have a single epithelial lining, as does the mucous retention cyst. As the serous cyst enlarges, it pushes the overlying mucosal layers in front of it and these layers then form the cyst wall. Serous cysts usually occur in the maxillary sinus floor. Differentiation between the mucous and serous cysts is impossible radiographically although statistically the vast majority are mucous retention cysts. It is therefore reasonable to refer to all such roentgenographic densities as mucous retention cysts. Unerupted molar teeth, the nasal alae, the lips, and the mandibular coronoid processes can also mimic the appearance of an antral cyst, particularly in the Waters view.

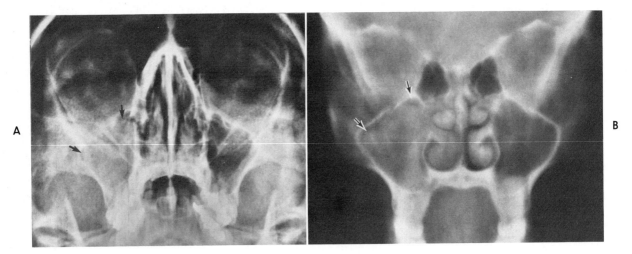

Fig. 1-114. A, Waters view. Complete opacification of right maxillary sinus. Thin rim of air can be seen in sinus cavity at top of mass *(arrows)*. Some mucoperiosteal thickening is present in left antrum. **B,** Coronal tomogram on same case as **A.** Large retention cyst is well seen molding to shape of sinus cavity *(arrows)*. Air is seen over medial and superior margins of cyst.

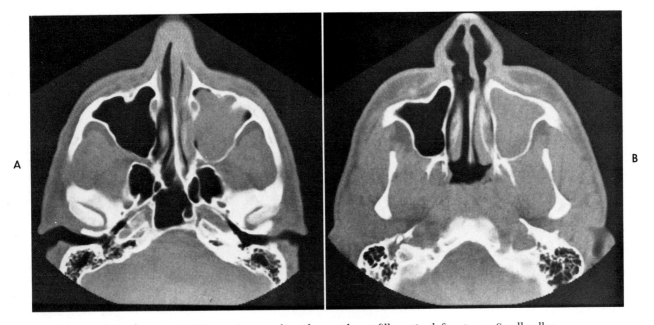

Fig. 1-115. A, Axial CT scan. Large polypoid mass almost fills entire left antrum. Small collections of air at periphery outline mass. **B,** Axial CT scan more caudal than **A** reveals total opacification of left antrum. Visualization of air on **A** was necessary to make diagnosis of large polyp or retention cyst.

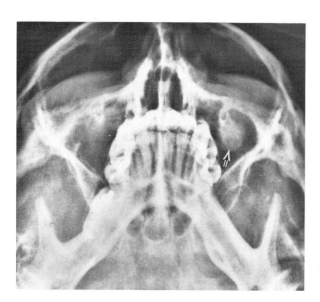

Fig. 1-116. Waters view. Retention cyst in roof of left maxillary sinus *(arrow)*.

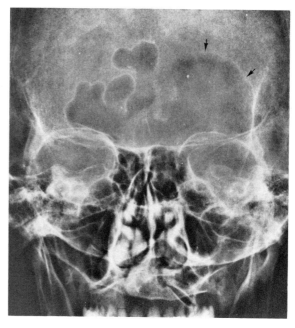

Fig. 1-117. Caldwell view. Right frontal sinus has normal scalloped margin with sharp mucoperiosteal line. Left frontal sinus is slightly clouded when compared to normal right side; however, overall appearance on left is that of "lucent" defect. Contour is smooth and mucoperiosteal line is hazy or absent *(arrows). Mucocele of left frontal sinus.*

Mucoceles and other benign expansile masses

The most clinically important cystic complication of inflammatory disease is the *mucocele* because it can expand and destroy adjacent structures. A mucocele is the most common expansile lesion affecting the paranasal sinuses. If infection occurs, it is called a *pyocele.*

The origin of mucoceles is controversial, but the fundamental direct cause is obstruction of the ostium of the sinus.[118] The initial ostial obstruction is usually secondary to inflammation, although trauma, allergy, or tumor can also be the cause of obstruction.[11]

Mucous secretions accumulate and eventually fill the entire sinus. The mucous mass abuts on the mucoperiosteum of the sinus cavity, which now functions as the cyst wall. As the mucocele slowly increases in size, thinning and remodeling of the sinus walls occur, resulting in expansion of the sinus cavity. No air margin remains between the mucous mass and the sinus wall (a theoretical differentiating point between the mucocele and the large retention cyst). Pressure atrophy, erosion, and destruction of the sinus walls are late findings. The association of mucoceles with tumors is probably more common than the paucity of reports in the literature suggests. Proptosis secondary to an antral mucocele can be the presenting symptom of an antral carcinoma.[120] Frontal sinus mucoceles may be the presenting symptom of ostial obstruction caused by an underlying frontal carcinoma.[37,54,104] About 65% of all mucoceles involve the frontal sinuses, 25% involve the ethmoid sinuses, and 10% involve the maxillary sinuses; only rarely do lesions involve the sphenoid sinuses. Radiographically identifiable calcifications occur in 5% of the cases.

Radiographic findings

In the frontal sinus, the earliest radiographic signs are clouding of the sinus and effacement of the normal mucoperiosteal line. Erosion of the sinus septa as a result of pressure then follows and eventually results in a smooth-walled sinus cavity (Fig. 1-117). As the mucocele starts to expand, a zone of reactive sclerosis in the adjacent frontal bone becomes apparent.

In a hypoplastic frontal sinus (which normally does not develop septation) the only findings may be clouding with loss of the mucoperiosteal margin (white line) and reactive sclerosis in the adjacent frontal bone (Fig. 1-118). It should be recalled that, regardless of size, a normal frontal sinus does not encroach on the orbital margin. Any erosion or downward displacement of the orbital rim must be considered secondary to a mucocele until proven otherwise. This rule also applies to displacement of the frontal intersinus septum at its base.

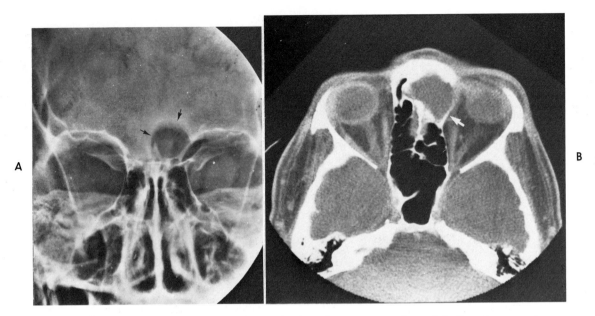

Fig. 1-118. A, Caldwell view of aplastic right frontal sinus. Hypoplastic left frontal sinus is rounded with smooth contours and there is zone of reactive sclerosis in adjacent frontal bone (*arrow*). Left inferior contour abuts on left orbital rim. *Mucocele.* **B,** Axial CT scan. Nonenhanced expansile mass is seen in lower left frontal sinus. Notice displacement of sinus wall (*arrow*). *Mucocele.*

The net effect of the bone destruction (with resulting decreased radiodensity) and the increased soft tissue density of the mucocele itself makes most frontal mucoceles actually appear radiolucent when compared to the adjacent frontal bone. The increased density of the sinus cavity that occurs early in the process and is associated with the initial infection usually disappears as bone erosion progresses.

Frontal mucoceles can expand in several directions. If they expand into the vertical portion of the frontal bone, the anterior table can be displaced and a mass lesion is present on the forehead (Fig. 1-119). If the posterior table is displaced, the mass extends into the anterior cranial fossa and displaces the frontal lobe posteriorly. In either instance, the periosteal lining of the frontal bone covers the mass lesion. Occasionally, separated but intact pieces of the frontal tables are identified lying over the surface of the mass. Frontal mucoceles can also extend into the horizontal extensions of the frontal sinus. The orbital roof is displaced inferolaterally and proptosis usually is present (Figs. 1-120 and 1-121).

Ethmoid mucoceles involve the anterior cells more often than the posterior group[73,103] and account for about 25% of all mucoceles.[119] Because ethmoid sinuses have the smallest ostia of all the paranasal sinuses, the

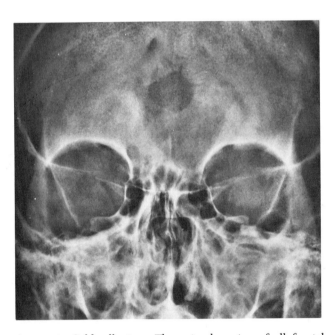

Fig. 1-119. Caldwell view. There is obscuring of all frontal sinus margins with areas of sclerosis marking sinus limits. There is vague oval lucency in left frontal sinus and smaller, more sharply defined circular lucency at superior sinus margin. *Frontal sinus mucocele with focal perforation of anterior table presenting as soft tissue mass under forehead.*

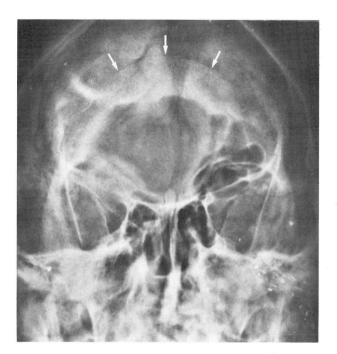

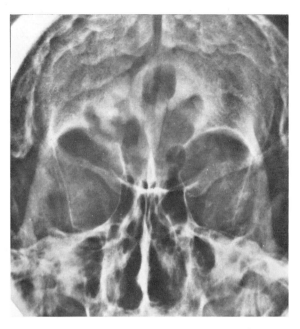

Fig. 1-120. Caldwell view. There is smoothly contoured, enlarged frontal sinus with zone of reactive sclerosis in adjacent frontal bone. Only a small portion of left frontal sinus appears normal overlying left orbit. Superomedial right orbital margin is flattened and destroyed. Mound of soft tissue elevation on forehead can be appreciated by soft tissue rim that surrounds entire mass *(arrows)*. *Right frontal sinus mucocele that is elevating the forehead and causing proptosis.*

Fig. 1-121. Caldwell view. Reactive sclerosis surrounds clouded frontal sinuses (compared to normal ethmoid air cell density). Superomedial right orbital margin is flattened and destroyed. *Chronic frontal sinusitis with right frontal mucocele.*

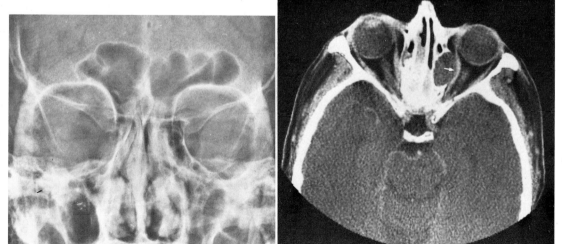

Fig. 1-122. A, Caldwell view. Clouding of right ethmoid sinuses. Posterior right ethmoid lamina papyracea is destroyed. Eye was clinically proptotic and laterally displaced. *Right ethmoid mucocele.* **B,** Axial CT scan of different patient. There is expansile, nonenhanced left ethmoid sinus mass that has bowed medial rectus muscle laterally *(arrow). Mucocele.*

viscosity of mucus has been suggested as playing an additional role in their development. This may explain why ethmoid mucoceles predominate in patients with cystic fibrosis.[19]

Ethmoid mucoceles primarily expand the lamina papyracea, resulting in proptosis and lateral displacement of the globe. Although clinically obvious, they may be very difficult to diagnose by plain film examinations (Fig. 1-122). Ethmoid mucoceles can either be relatively radiolucent or appear slightly clouded on plain films. The most consistent findings are those of local ethmoid septa demineralization and destruction. The examination of choice is the CT scan, which localizes the process as well as defines the integrity of the lamina papyracea.[119]

If the entire ethmoid complex is expanded by a non-enhancing process and many of the ethmoid septa are preserved, polypoid mucoceles are present. These essentially are individual ethmoid mucoceles with polypoid mucosa and usually occur in patients who have a history of allergy (Fig. 1-123).[118]

Maxillary sinus mucoceles represent about 10% of all mucoceles.[120] They invariably cause a totally opaque sinus (Figs. 1-124 and 1-125), and early in their devel-

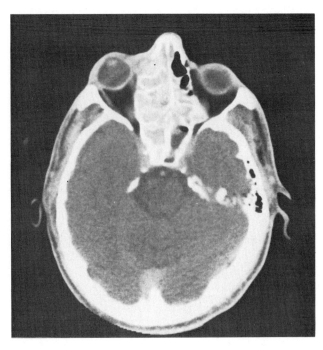

Fig. 1-123. Axial CT scan reveals enlargement of ethmoid complex with preservation of the lamina papyracea and most ethmoid septa. *Polypoid mucocele.*

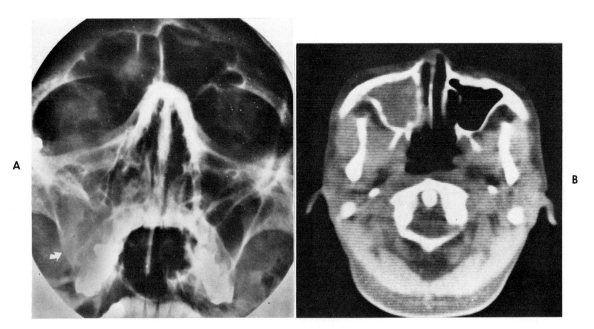

Fig. 1-124. A, Waters view. Completely clouded right maxillary sinus with minimal thinning and expansion of lateral wall *(arrow). Mucocele.* **B,** Axial CT scan of same case as Fig. 1-129. Completely filled right maxillary sinus with slightly expanded walls (compare to normal left side). *Mucocele.*

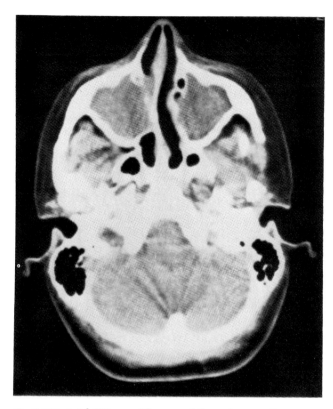

Fig. 1-125. Axial CT scan. There are bilateral expansile, nonenhanced maxillary sinus masses. *Bilateral mucoceles.*

opment they cannot be differentiated from routine inflammatory disease. Eventually the sinus cavity walls are expanded, and later bone erosion secondary to pressure atrophy occurs (Fig. 1-126). In these later stages, differentiation from a tumor may be extremely difficult. If any areas of sinus wall displacement can be identified, the diagnosis of a maxillary sinus mucocele should be considered.

The orbital floor can be elevated with resulting upward displacement of the globe and concomitant diplopia (Fig. 1-127, *A* to *C*). In rare cases, extensive destruction of the orbital floor allows the globe to sink downward, with resulting enophthalmos and diplopia. Expansion of the anterior wall results in clinically evident deformity of the cheek and face. Antral mucoceles occurring after surgery are discussed on page 96.

Sphenoid sinus mucoceles are uncommon and result in an opaque sinus. Superior expansion can mimic a pituitary tumor. Although the lamina dura is destroyed, the major bone erosion and soft tissue mass are in the sphenoid sinus itself (Fig. 1-128). In rare cases, the mucocele can expand inferiorly, eroding the roof of the nasopharynx and appearing as a nasopharyngeal tumor.

Most sphenoid mucoceles expand anteriorly into the posterior ethmoid sinuses and recesses of the sphenoid sinuses (Fig. 1-129). Because of their location, they may

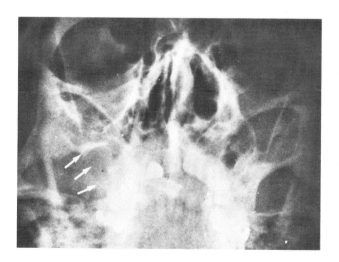

Fig. 1-126. Waters view. There is opacification of right antrum with destruction of lateral wall *(arrows)*. This could be antral carcinoma; however, it proved to be *mucocele.*

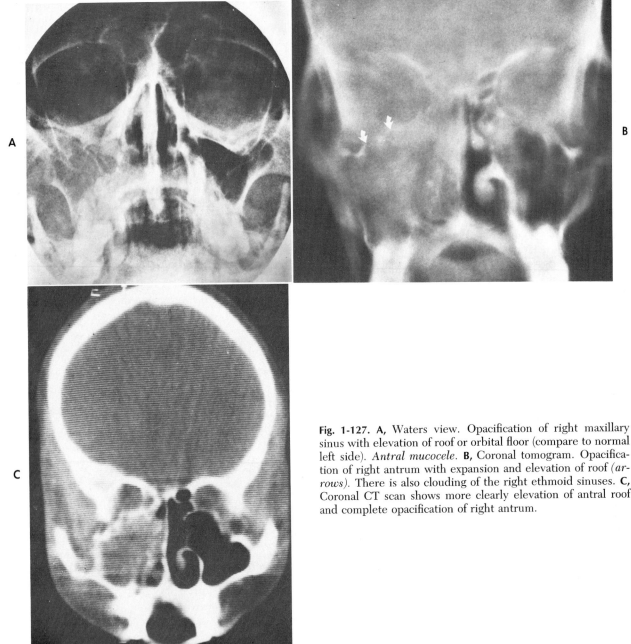

Fig. 1-127. A, Waters view. Opacification of right maxillary sinus with elevation of roof or orbital floor (compare to normal left side). *Antral mucocele.* **B,** Coronal tomogram. Opacification of right antrum with expansion and elevation of roof (*arrows*). There is also clouding of the right ethmoid sinuses. **C,** Coronal CT scan shows more clearly elevation of antral roof and complete opacification of right antrum.

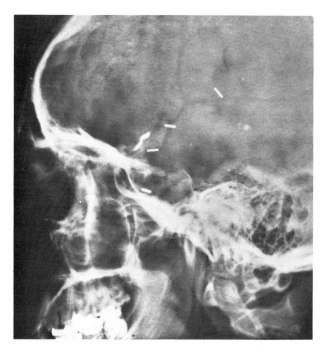

Fig. 1-128. Lateral view. There is destruction of anterior wall and sella floor. Anterior clinoid processes and upper dorsum are intact. Sphenoid sinus is clouded. Surgical clips are laterally placed, unrelated, and secondary to previous surgery. Findings suggest either pituitary mass or sphenoid lesion. *Sphenoid mucocele.*

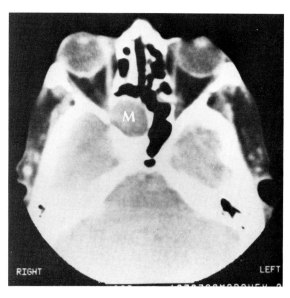

Fig. 1-129. Axial CT scan. There is expansile nonenhanced right sphenoid sinus mass *(m)* that encroaches on right orbital apex. *Sphenoid sinus mucocele.*

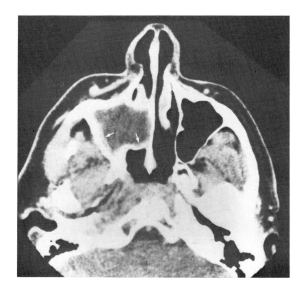

Fig. 1-130. Axial CT scan. There is expansile right antral mass. Mass itself is nonenhanced; however, there is rim of enhancement around margin of mass *(arrows)*. *Pyocele.*

present clinically with an orbital apex syndrome. Because of the diminished lucency of the sinus cavity and bone destruction, radiographic differentiation from a malignancy may be impossible. Bone remodeling and expansion should suggest the correct diagnosis.

When a mucocele of any sinus becomes infected, a *pyocele* occurs. Pyoceles can occur in any sinus but are most common in the frontal area. In the early stages, systemic manifestations of the infectious process dominate the clinical picture. Radiographically, unless a mucocele was initially nonopaque (frontal and *some* ethmoid mucoceles) and then became opaque, a pyocele cannot be differentiated from a mucocele on plain films or multidirectional tomograms. The development of an air-fluid level or the recent demineralization or destruction of a margin of the mucocele also can suggest the presence of a pyocele (Figs. 1-130 and 1-131).[152]

Because extension of the mucoceles can be intracranial, intraorbital, nasopharyngeal, and parasellar, CT scans allow a more complete evaluation of the mucocele margins than tomography or plain film examination. In CT scanning, mucoceles are nonenhancing expansile masses. If a rim of enhancement is seen, a pyocele is more likely present.[118]

There are several entities that should be included in the differential diagnosis of a mucocele. These entities will vary according to the specific sinus involved. *Primary cholesteatoma* is an uncommon cystic lesion of epithelial origin that is filled with keratin-containing material (Fig. 1-132). It probably arises from a congenital rest. Epidermoid cysts originate either in the diploë or, less frequently, in the outer table of the skull. The net effect of frontal bone loss and the increased density of the keratin material results in a lucent, expansile lesion. An epidermoid cyst usually has a thin, dense border that appears similar to the normal mucoperiosteal sinus margin. In a mucocele, this line is obscured early and a zone of reactive sclerosis surrounds the lesion. Primary cholesteatomas do not induce reactive sclerosis. Mucoceles also have smooth margins, but cholesteatomas usually have a slightly scalloped appearance.[150] These are primary bone lesions and only secondarily encroach on the sinuses.

A cholesteatoma may destroy part of the adjacent frontal sinus margin, but these lesions are usually eccentric and the remaining sinus itself appears normal. Depression or destruction of the orbital rim can also be present.

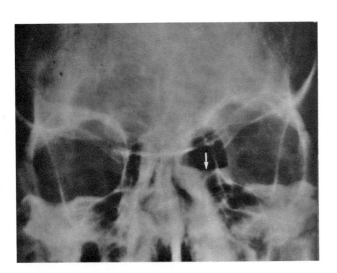

Fig. 1-131. Caldwell view. Expanded mid- and anterior left ethmoid sinuses bulging lamina papyracea into left orbit. Air-fluid level *(arrow)* indicates an *ethmoid pyocele*. There is also *chronic and acute bifrontal sinusitis.*

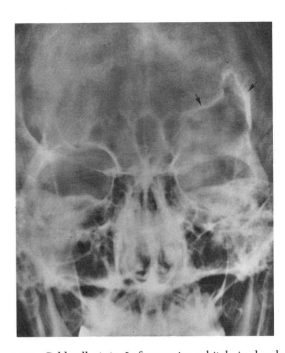

Fig. 1-132. Caldwell view. Left superior orbital rim has been depressed and partially eroded by lytic lesion in left frontal bone *(arrows)*. Lesion abuts on frontal sinuses, which are essentially normal. There is well-defined sclerotic rim around mass, and lesion has partially lobulated contour. *Primary cholesteatoma.*

Secondary cholesteatomas are rare. They are usually located in the maxillary sinus and develop after a fracture or oroantral fistula.[150] The affected sinus is opaque and the surrounding walls are either expanded or destroyed. Secondary cholesteatomas can mimic an antral mucocele or carcinoma.

Pneumosinus dilatans is also a rare entity that has been reported to occur in all sinuses. It affects only a few cells of a particular sinus cavity. These cells are expanded but have normal septal walls and cell architecture with a normal sinus mucosa. There is an unusual male/female ratio of 16:1, and the peak age incidence is 20 to 40 years. When it occurs in the ethmoid sinuses, pneumosinus dilatans can be distinguished from an ethmoid mucocele by normal intact septa and no central point of origin for the air-cell expansion.[74]

Alteration in the contour of the planum sphenoidale from a straight, nearly horizontal line to a curved surface that suggests upward bowing of the roof of that sinus should not be confused with pneumosinus dilatans.[70] Rather, this finding most commonly represents the so-called "blister" reaction of the planum to an overlying meningioma.[74]

A pneumocele of the maxillary sinus is a very rare entity. Abnormal expansion of the sinus walls presumably results from a one-way check valve mechanism at the ostia. Repeated air trapping, secondary to events such as sneezing, results in expansion that can lead to focal areas of bone dehiscence. The sinus is normally aerated or hyperlucent and has an intact mucoperiosteal margin.[84,87] The bony sinus walls may be thinned or destroyed. Pneumoceles are cured by a Caldwell-Luc and antrostomy procedure.

Also included in the differential diagnosis of benign expansile masses are inflammatory and allergic polyps. Most inflammatory polyps are nasal. Given sufficient time to grow, polyps will expand, thin, and eventually destroy the nasal vault walls (Fig. 1-133).[148] The main radiographic findings are a homogeneous soft tissue mass (or masses) with expansion of the nasal walls. If dehiscence occurs, it is usually along the medial wall of the maxillary sinus. When multiple polyps are present, air can sometimes be seen outlining the lesions (Fig. 1-134, *A* and *B*).

Polyps commonly occur in the maxillary sinus as well. These lesions only rarely fill the sinus cavity completely (Fig. 1-135), and differentiation from a retention cyst is usually impossible.

Occasionally, an antral polyp expands sufficiently to reach the sinus ostia. A portion of the polyp can herniate through the ostia and appear as a nasal polyp. This combined antral and nasal polyp is called an *antrochoanal polyp*. This type of polyp represents between 3.7% and 6.2% of all nasal polyps. Although the polyps

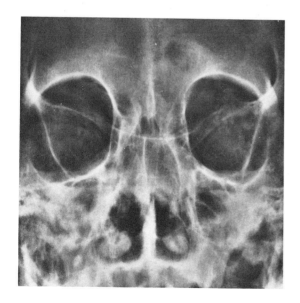

Fig. 1-133. Caldwell view. Clouding of frontal, ethmoid, and maxillary sinuses as well as upper nasal cavity. There is some widening of ethmoid space (hypertelorism). *Chronic sinusitis with inflammatory nasal and ethmoid polyps.*

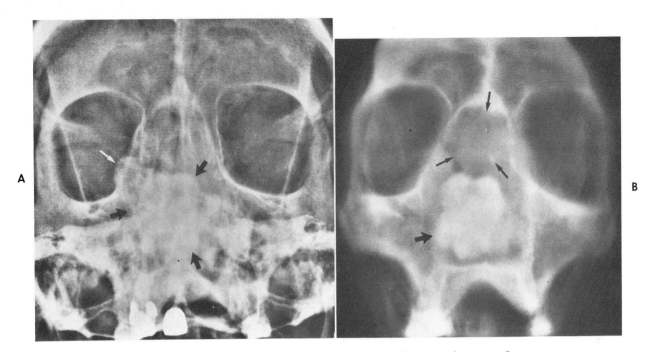

A

B

Fig. 1-134. A, Caldwell view. Clouding of ethmoid sinuses and antra with some inflammatory changes in frontal sinuses. There is hypertelorism with localized bulge into inferomedial right orbit *(white arrow)*. Nasal cavity is filled with bone density mass *(black arrows)* and soft tissue masses. *Nasal osteoma with inflammatory polyps.* **B,** Coronal tomogram of same patient as in Fig. 1-138. Nasal osteoma is clearly seen *(large arrow)* and soft tissue masses are identified in nasal, ethmoid, and maxillary spaces. Air surrounding these masses *(black arrows)* was identified on serial tomograms.

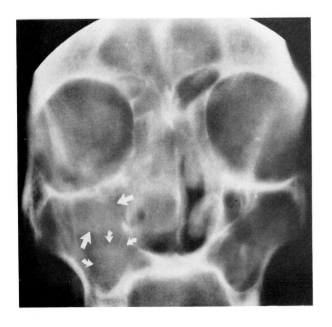

Fig. 1-135. Coronal tomogram. Soft tissue density is seen in roof of right antrum *(large arrows)* and in floor of this antrum *(small arrows)*. Similar densities are seen in ethmoid sinuses and right nasal cavity. *Multiple polyps.*

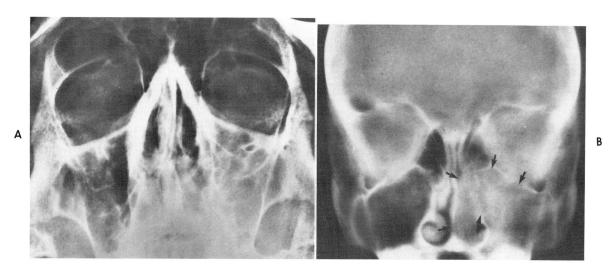

Fig. 1-136. A, Waters view. Complete opacification of left maxillary sinus with no bone destruction. Differential diagnosis should consider large retention cyst or polyp with or without associated infection. Tumor must also be excluded. *Antrochoanal polyp.* **B,** Coronal tomogram. Same patient as in Fig. 1-136, *A.* Homogeneous mass extends from left antrum through widened infundibulum into left nasal cavity *(arrows). Antrochoanal polyp.*

are usually unilateral, solitary lesions, bilateral maxillary sinus disease is seen radiographically in 30% to 40% of the cases. The majority of cases of antrochoanal polyps occur in teenagers and young adults. Of the patients with antrochoanal polyps, 7½% also have other nasal polyps. No association with allergic disease has been proven.[113]

Radiographically, a homogeneous soft tissue polypoid nasal mass is seen with an ipsilateral opaque maxillary sinus (Fig. 1-136 *A* and *B*). Sometimes the infundibulum is seen to be widened. Rarely is there actual expansion of the sinus cavity. Differentiation of the nasal portion from an inferior turbinate can be difficult on plain films but usually can be accomplished with CT scans (Fig. 1-137). The polyp usually extends well into the nasopharynx and can reach the nasopharyngeal roof. A normal turbinate usually extends only just posterior to the hard palate.

Allergic polyps have the same origin as serous cysts (Fig. 1-138). Submucosal fluid gradually accumulates and causes expansion of these polyps, which therefore collapse dramatically at surgery when the fluid escapes. Allergic polyps are usually multiple and cannot be differentiated radiographically from multiple inflammatory polyps.

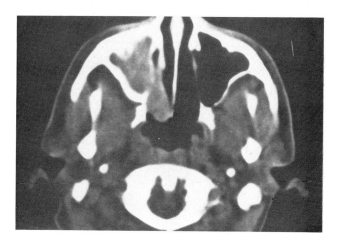

Fig. 1-137. Axial CT scan. Polypoid mass is seen to fill right antrum and extend into nasal cavity. *Antrochoanal polyp.*

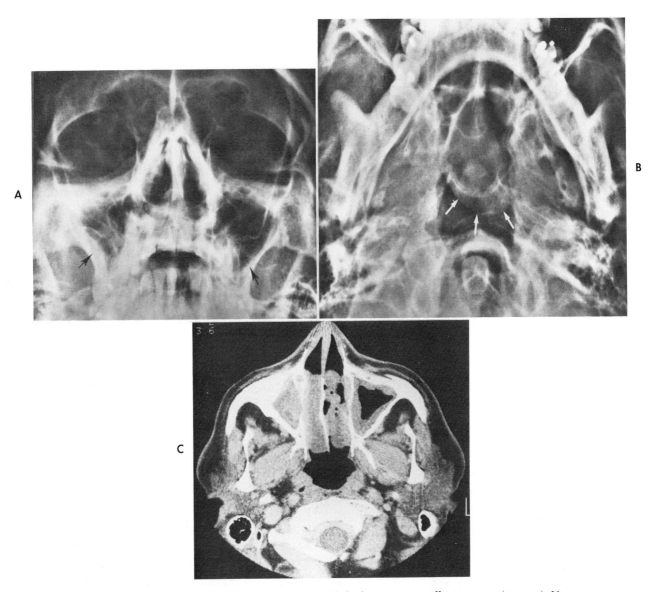

Fig. 1-138. A, Waters view. Mild mucoperiosteal thickening in maxillary sinuses *(arrows).* No mass seen in sinuses or nasal cavity. **B,** Base view. Same patient as in Fig. 1-142, A. Polypoid mass is seen in posterior nares and nasopharynx *(arrows).* It could be allergic polyp or inflammatory polyp. Clear antra rule out antrochoanal polyp. *Allergic nasal polyp.* **C,** Axial CT scan of different patient. Multiple polypoid nasal cavity masses are seen. There is no bone destruction. Inflammatory changes are seen in both maxillary sinuses. *Allergic polyposis.*

Complications of sinus inflammatory disease affecting adjacent structures

In the antibiotic era, most acute paranasal sinus infections are successfully treated. However, delay in treatment or resistant organisms can lead to a variety of complications stemming from an initially localized infective process.

Because the frontal, ethmoid, and maxillary sinuses form portions of the orbital roof, medial wall, and floor respectively, they can be viewed as "paraorbital" sinuses. The most frequent complications from inflammatory paranasal sinus disease (outside of the sinus proper) occur in the orbit and periorbital tissues. Because the ophthalmic veins do not contain valves but communicate directly with the veins of the face, nasal and paranasal cavities, and cavernous sinus, there is a ready tract for spread of infection.

Inflammatory processes in the paraorbital sinuses can result in painless reactionary edema of the eyelids and orbital contents. Actual orbital infection is absent. Compression with impeded venous drainage is postulated as the cause and minimal proptosis can be present. Radiographs and CT scans may reveal some soft tissue and periorbital edema associated with underlying sinusitis. No bone erosion is present.[66,147]

The next stage of complication is a true orbital cellulitis. Edema, proptosis, pain, and chemosis can be present and there is no focal collection of pus. This complication requires aggressive intravenous antibiotic therapy. Again, the radiographs and CT scans reveal sinusitis with periorbital and orbital edema without bone destruction (Fig. 1-139, *A* and *B*).

A subperiosteal or orbital abscess is a more serious complication. Such abscesses most commonly are secondary to ethmoid sinusitis. Both types produce pain and varying degrees of proptosis, ophthalmoplegia, and visual impairment. Surgical intervention and drainage by means of a subtotal ethmoidectomy is indicated for a subperiosteal abscess, while the orbital abscess requires orbital decompression and possible exploration. In addition to proptosis, edema, and sinusitis, radiographs and CT scans demonstrate a mass. Posterior extension of the abscess into the skull can result in septic thrombophlebitis and cavernous sinus thrombosis. The mortality of this complication is estimated to be 80% with a morbidity of 75% among survivors.[66] Radiographically, only the inflammatory changes in the paranasal sinuses may be evident.

The superior orbital fissure syndrome is related specifically to sphenoid sinus disease and clinically involves all the structures running through this fissure. Progressive involvement of cranial nerves VI, III, and IV occurs. The ophthalmic nerve, (V_1), the ophthalmic vein, and the cavernous sinus sympathetics are involved later. Radiographically, mucosal thickening and diminished aeration of the sphenoid sinus can be associated with either reactive sclerosis or erosion and destruction of the adjacent lesser and greater sphenoid wings.

Local involvement of the optic nerve can also result from inflammation in the sphenoid, ethmoid, or poste-

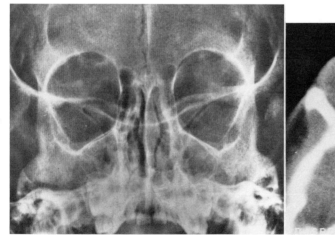
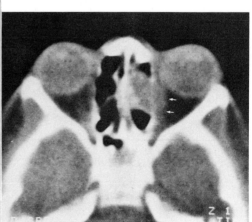

Fig. 1-139. A, Waters view. There is clouding of left ethmoid and both maxillary sinuses. Inflammatory process is most likely diagnosis. Lateral proptosis of left eye and associated inflammation cannot be appreciated. **B,** Axial CT scan of same patient as in **A.** Localized soft tissue mass is seen in left middle and anterior ethmoid sinuses. There is also widening and infiltration of medial periorbital tissues with lateral displacement of medial rectus muscle *(arrows)*. *Orbital cellulitis and subperiosteal abscess.*

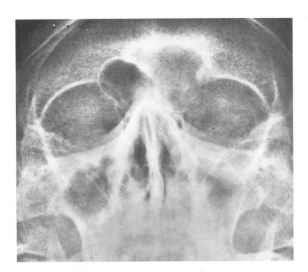

Fig. 1-140. Waters view. There is clouding of left frontal sinus with thickened zone of reactive bone around cavity. There are also mild inflammatory changes in maxillary, ethmoid, and sphenoid sinuses. *Acute and chronic sinusitis and osteomyelitis in frontal bone.*

rior maxillary sinuses. Sinusitis in these areas is said to be the cause in 15% to 20% of cases of retrobulbar neuritis.[35] Radiographs may reveal little if any pathology, and only focal sinus disease may be evident on tomography or CT.

A brain abscess represents the most serious complication of paranasal sinus inflammatory disease. Intracranial abscesses originate from nasal cavity and paranasal sinus disease in 3% of cases. They tend to occur in the frontal lobes; relatively few are reported in the temporal and parietal lobes. Clinically, signs and symptoms of generalized systemic infection may be absent. An associated meningitis can dominate the clinical picture.[66]

Another complication of paranasal sinus inflammatory disease is osteomyelitis. This is usually related to frontal sinus disease (Fig. 1-140). Rarely, osteomyelitis of the maxillary sinus can occur after dental infections (Fig. 1-141). The clinical evidence of osteomyelitis precedes the radiographic manifestations by 7 to 14 days. Radiographically, spotty areas of rarefaction in the sinus wall are seen. These can proceed to areas of sclerosis and sequestrum formation. A superficial subgaleal abscess can form on the forehead in rare cases. There may be no roentgenographic evidence of intervening bone destruction. This is the so-called Pott's puffy tumor.[93]

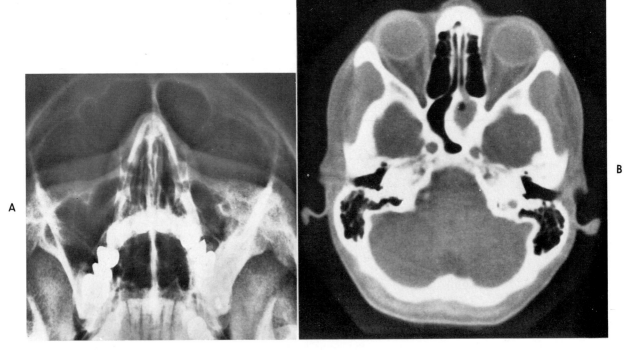

Fig. 1-141. A, Waters view. Markedly thickened reactive bone around left antrum and extending into left zygoma. *Chronic osteomyelitis.* **B,** Axial CT scan. There is opacification of left sphenoid sinus. Notice thickened, sclerotic bone surrounding this sinus. *Chronic sinusitis and reactive osteitis.*

All of these intracranial and intraorbital complications are more likely to occur in acute sinusitis rather than in chronic inflammatory disease.

■ Higher bacterial forms

Actinomycosis is a noncontagious suppurative or granulomatous disease produced most commonly by the anaerobic organism *Actinomyces israelii.* Less often *A. bovis* or *A. eriksonii* is the causitive agent. *A. israelii* is a normal constituent of the human mouth flora. It is a pleomorphic, slow-growing bacterium with a tendency toward branching that produces a characteristic mycelium. The cell walls of *A. israelii* contain muramic acid and lysine, both of which are not found in the cell walls of fungi. The cell walls also lack chitin and glucons, which are characteristic in the cell walls of fungi.[44] Sulfur granules form when actinomyces become cemented together by a protein-polysaccharide substance that is produced in response to tissue inflammation.[98] Actinomycosis is a chronic infection that primarily involves the head and neck region. Soft tissue inflammation with a granulomatous reaction is common, as are multiple draining sinuses.

Radiographically, the changes are nonspecific except that, unlike most bacterial diseases, actinomycosis is al-most always a unilateral disease. Adjacent osteomyelitis can develop subsequently. The combination of bone destruction with diminished aeration makes differentiation from a malignancy impossible (Fig. 1-142). If untreated, the infection can spread to the thoracic or abdominal viscera. Only rarely is the central nervous system involved. The method of spread is either by direct extension or by hematogenous dissemination from a secondary focus in the chest or abdomen. The treatment of choice is penicillin.

Nocardiosis is caused by *Nocardia asteroides*, a grampositive bacterium that can also exhibit branching. It may even produce sulfur granules. *Nocardia* is weakly acid-fast and can grow aerobically. In addition, it has distinctive biochemical reactions. All of these distinguish nocardiosis from actinomycosis in the laboratory. Clinically and radiographically the two infections are indistinguishable from one another.

■ Fungal disease

Rhinocerebral mucormycosis is caused by fungi of the class Phycomycetes that have nonseptated mycelia. The genera involved are *Rhizopus*, *Mucor*, and *Absidia;* the vast majority of infections are caused by *Rhizopus arrhizus* or *R. oryzae*. In 50% to 75% of cases the pa-

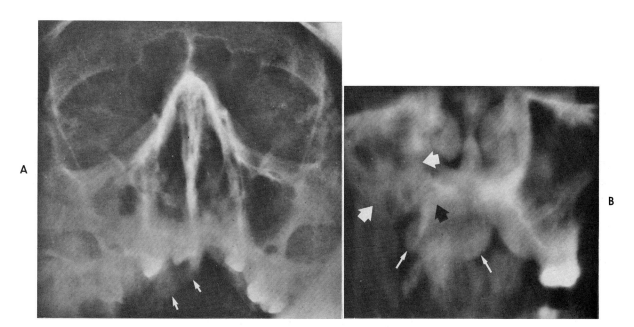

Fig. 1-142. A, Waters view. Mucoperiosteal thickening is seen in right maxillary sinus with possible destruction of lateral wall and roof. Soft tissue mass is also seen projected into mouth *(arrows)*. This could be squamous cell carcinoma. *Actinomycosis.* **B,** Coronal tomogram. There is destruction of medial and lateral right maxillary sinus walls *(large white arrows)* and alveolar process and right hard palate *(large black arrow)*. There is reactive sclerosis of right antral roof. A nodular soft tissue mass extends into mouth *(smaller white arrows)*. This could be carcinoma, but mass in mouth would be uncharacteristic. *Actinomycosis.*

tients also have poorly controlled diabetes mellitus.[66,97] Mucormycosis is also seen, although much less frequently, in patients with chronic renal failure and acidosis, as well as in patients with malnutrition, cancer, and cirrhosis, and patients on prolonged antibiotic, steroid, or cytotoxic drug therapy.

The fungus is part of the normal respiratory flora. It spreads by first invading the nasal cavity and maxillary sinuses and then extends into the ethmoid sinuses and orbits. The fungi invade the arterioles and arteries, causing endothelial damage that initiates thrombosis. This leads in turn to areas of ischemic infarction. The pathway for intracranial spread is by way of the ophthalmic artery.[66]

Radiographically, there is nodular mucoperiosteal thickening of the maxillary sinuses. The ethmoid sinuses can be clouded. The frontal sinuses are spared and no air-fluid levels are seen (Fig. 1-143). Multiple focal areas of bone destruction can be seen, involving multiple sinuses.[53]

Clinically, black-crusting, necrotic tissue is seen over the turbinates, septum, or palate. Although the literature reports cases of survivors, the mortality is extremely high. Among these survivors there is a high incidence of blindness, cranial nerve palsies, and hemiparesis. The limited therapy available consists of surgery to debride the destroyed tissue and the administration of heparin and amphotericin B.

Mucormycosis can manifest itself somewhat differently in the nondiabetic immunosuppressed patient. Minimal ischemic changes are seen in the nasal cavity instead of the black crusting, and pulmonary and disseminated infection are more common.

Aspergillosis is caused by the fungus *Aspergillus*, a member of the Ascomycetes class. It is a ubiquitous organism frequently found in soil, decaying food, fruits, and plants. The spores are common contaminates of the respiratory tract, and *Aspergillus* can be frequently found in the external auditory canal. *A. fumigatus* and *A. flavis* are pathogens in humans, with 90% of the infections caused by *A. fumigatus*. Infection of the paranasal sinuses is rare, except in the Sudan, where it may be endemic.[83,135]

Involvement of the paranasal sinuses usually occurs in otherwise healthy patients, and there is no relationship between the paranasal sinus infection and pulmonary aspergillosis, which occurs most often in debilitated patients. Local infection and stagnation are also favorable conditions for this fungal disease to develop.

The paranasal infection usually is confined to one sinus, and most of the time that is the maxillary antrum. Ethmoid infection is the next most common; sphenoid sinus and frontal sinus disease are rare (Fig. 1-144).[127] Sinus irrigation reveals a greenish white, foul-smelling membrane that may be related to the anaerobic conditions in the sinus. An immune response to the fun-

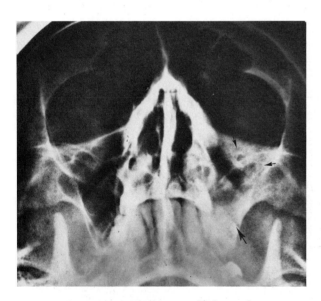

Fig. 1-143. Waters view. Thickening of left antral mucoperiosteum. There are multiple lucencies seen in bone of left antral roof and lateral wall suggesting focal areas of destruction. Remaining paranasal sinuses are normal. These are nonspecific inflammatory changes with possible osteomyelitis. *Mucormycosis.*

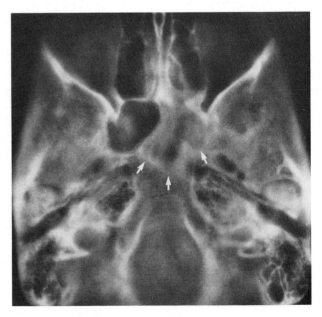

Fig. 1-144. Base tomogram. Right sphenoid sinus is clear. There is clouding of left sphenoid sinus with blurring of mucoperiosteal line *(arrows)*. Ethmoid sinuses are normal. This is a nonspecific inflammatory type picture. *Aspergillosis.*

gus may also play a causative role.[82] Less commonly the orbit is involved, resulting in proptosis and decreased vision.[138] Skin involvement has also been reported.

The *Aspergillus* fungus causes a vasculitis similar to that in mucormycosis, with resulting thrombosis. Hematogenous intracranial spread can lead to areas of hemorrhagic infarction. Early in the disease, the signs and symptoms are nonspecific and the infection resembles any chronic bacterial infection except that it is resistant to normal conservative therapy. In the late stages, bone destruction occurs and the infection is indistinguishable from malignancy. Wide surgical excision is the treatment of choice.

Candidiasis is caused by the yeastlike organism *Candida albicans.* It is an opportunistic infection that is usually seen in diabetic patients and otherwise healthy people after the use of broad-spectrum antibiotics. Candidosis occasionally occurs after maxillary trauma. The maxillary sinus is almost exclusively involved. Radiographically, candidosis cannot be differentiated from other types of chronic bacterial or fungal sinusitis. Orbital and intracranial complications are rare.[23] Antral lavage with topical nystatin is the treatment of choice.

■ Granulomatous disease

Granulomatous diseases of the paranasal sinuses and nasal cavity are uncommon. All of these diseases tend to involve the sinuses after first involving the nasal cavity and nasal septum. The primary CT findings are nasal soft tissue nodules and thickening. As the disease progresses, spread into the sinuses is seen (Fig. 1-145). Late in the disease, bone destruction and soft tissue masses can simulate malignancy and again are nonspecific findings. The diagnosis is established by pertinent history and clinical testing.

A convenient classification of granulomatous disease involving the nasal and paranasal cavities is as follows:

Group 1. Lesions that occur in response to chronic irritation and result in a foreign body–type reaction such as that seen in berylliosis or with chromate salts

Group 2. Granulomas secondary to an infectious process such as tuberculosis, leprosy, actinomycosis, rhinosporidiosis, rhinoscleroma, syphilis, yaws, glanders, leishmaniasis, and blastomycosis

Group 3. Autoimmune diseases such as Wegener's granulomatosis

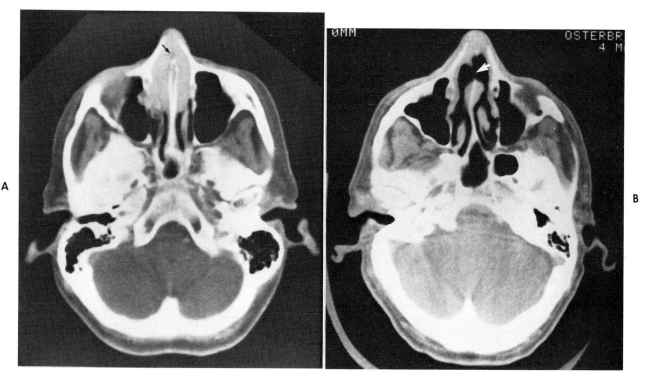

Fig. 1-145. A, Axial CT scan. There is enhanced bilateral nasal cavity mass. Some bone erosion of anterior nasal septum is present *(arrow)*. *Wegener's granulomatosis.* **B,** Axial CT scan. Nodular soft tissue thickening is present on nasal septum. Focal erosion of cartilaginous portion of septum *(arrow)* has occurred. *Granuloma in cocaine addict.*

Group 4. Idiopathic midline granulomas (probably lymphoma related)

Group 5. Unclassified, as in sarcoid[75]

Chronic beryllium granulomas are related to inhalation and primarily involve the nasal cavity. The granulomas can be indistinguishable from those seen in sarcoidosis.[54a]

Chromate salts have been implicated in nonspecific granuloma formation; however, they also appear related to inhalation and primarily involve the nasal cavity. Involvement of the sinuses is a late and unusual event in these group 1 lesions.

Tuberculosis is caused by *Myobacterium tuberculosis*, which stains acid-fast and is a strict aerobe. The disease is worldwide in distribution. Tuberculosis rarely involves the sinuses; when it does the maxillary and ethmoid sinuses are most frequently involved. In the late stages, with bone involvement, pain can be the dominant symptom. Paranasal sinus disease is always secondary to a primary tuberculous infection elsewhere in the body (usually pulmonary). Most frequently, hematogenous spread rather than direct extension accounts for the sinus disease (Fig. 1-146, *A*).

Leprosy is a chronic granulomatous disease caused by the pleomorphic acid-fast bacterium *Mycobacterium leprae*. It is found in Asia, Africa, and Central and South America. Early in the disease, the roentgenographic findings are those of nonspecific sinusitis with the primary changes confined to the nasal cavity. Later, changes in the nasal mucosa and paranasal sinuses resemble any of the chronic granulomatous diseases *with the exception that the anterior nasal spine is destroyed*. If trauma, previous surgery, and congenital maxillonasal dysplasia can be ruled out, this latter finding is pathognomonic of leprosy (Fig. 1-146, *B*). The treatment of choice is the administration of sulfone derivatives.

Actinomyosis and Nocardia have already been discussed in detail on p. 65.

Rhinosporidiosis is caused by the fungus *Rhinosporidium seebri*.[68] It is found most frequently in India and Sri Lanka as well as in Brazil. The presenting symptom is usually nasal obstruction secondary to soft pinkish,

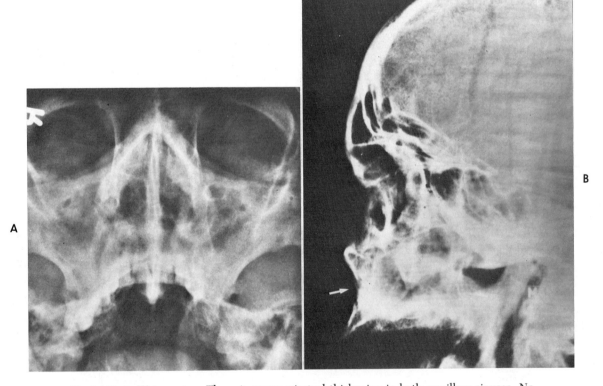

Fig. 1-146. A, Waters view. There is mucoperiosteal thickening in both maxillary sinuses. No bone destruction is present. These are nonspecific findings. *Tuberculosis*. **B,** Lateral view. Anterior nasal spine is destroyed. Ethmoid and maxillary sinuses are clouded. On frontal films there was soft tissue thickening of nasal structures. Sinus and nasal structure findings are nonspecific. Anterior nasal spine destruction indicates leprosy.

sessile, or pedunculated nasal polyps that are primarily unilateral. The sinuses show diminished aeration. The treatment is simple surgical excision or electrocautery.

Rhinoscleroma is a chronic inflammatory disease producing nasal obstruction and indurated nonulcerative inflammatory nodules. The disease is common in the Mediterranean countries and in Asia, Indonesia, and Latin America and is caused by the bacillus *Klebsiella rhinoscleromatis*. The paranasal sinuses are rarely involved. Disease extension from the nasal cavity results in nonspecific sinusitis. The treatment of choice is surgical excision.

Syphilis has worldwide distribution and is caused by *Treponema pallidum*. The early stages produce no consistent roentgenographic findings. In the late stages, gummas in the mucous membrane of the nose can produce painful destruction of the palate, the nasal septum, and rarely the sinus walls.[54a]

Yaws is a tropical infection caused by *T. pertenue*. This spirochete gives positive Wasserman and flocculation tests, as does *T. pallidum*. Later in the disease, destructive granulomas produce severe ulcerations of the nasal region (gangosa) and proliferative exostoses along the medial wall of the maxillary sinus (goundou). The treatment of choice is penicillin.

Glanders is found in Asia, Africa, and South America but not in the United States. It is caused by the bacterium *Pseudomonas mallei*. Human infection commonly is secondary to contact with horses. The disease can be a fulminant process leading to death or it can be a chronic granulomatous disease. Involvement is primarily confined to the nasal cavity and septum, with the sinuses involved only rarely. The bacteria are sensitive to sulfadiazine.

American mucocutaneous *leishmaniasis* is caused by *Leishmania brasiliensis*. It occurs primarily in Central and South America, with the exception of Chile. In the espundia type, the mucosal surface of the mouth and nose become involved with painful, mutilating erosions that can secondarily involve the sinuses.[54a]

South American *blastomycosis* is caused by the fungus *Blastomyces (Paracoccidioides) brasiliensis*. It can produce destructive, painful granulomas of the nasal cavity that rarely involve the sinuses.[54a] Amphotericin B is the treatment of choice.

Wegener's granulomatosis is a disease characterized by a triad of necrotizing granulomatous vasculitis of the upper and lower respiratory tracts, necrotizing glomerulonephritis, and varying degrees of disseminated small vasculitis.[43] The mean age at onset is 40 years, and there is a male/female ratio of 2:1. The maxillary sinus is most frequently involved although pansinusitis is also common. The roentgenographic findings are nonspecific. Mucoperiosteal thickening and sometimes destruction of the sinus walls and nasal septum occur (Fig. 1-147). Secondary bacterial infection further complicates the roentgenographic picture. Cyclophosphamide is the drug of choice and some long-term remissions have been achieved.

Idiopathic midline granuloma is characterized by chronic necrotizing inflammations of the nose, sinuses, midline facial tissues, and upper airways. The lungs, kidneys, and other organs are uninvolved. The histopathology is nonspecific and reveals acute and chronic inflammation with or without granulomas. Radiographic findings are nonspecific and resemble those of other granulomatous diseases. Because local irradiation (5000 rads) has been shown to produce long-term remissions, the word "lethal" has been dropped from the old name "lethal midline granuloma."[43] This disease is probably lymphoma related.

Sarcoidosis is a systemic disease characterized by noncaseating epithelioid granulomas. The granulomas are not limited to sarcoid and can be seen in tuberculosis, leprosy and berylliosis.[51] Sarcoid has a predilection for the Scandinavian countries and for rural southeastern United States. It is more common in black females and the median age is 25 years.

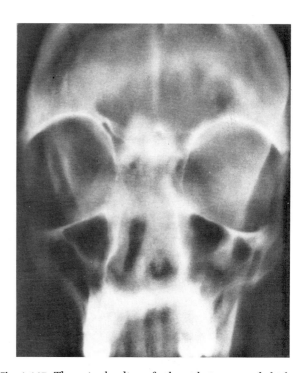

Fig. 1-147. There is clouding of ethmoid sinuses and thickening of soft tissues of nasal cavity, especially on left side. Mucoperiosteal thickening is also present in left maxillary sinus. Some destruction is present in lamina papyracea of right ethmoid sinus. These are nonspecific findings of either tumor or fungal type of chronic inflammation. *Wegener's granulomatosis.*

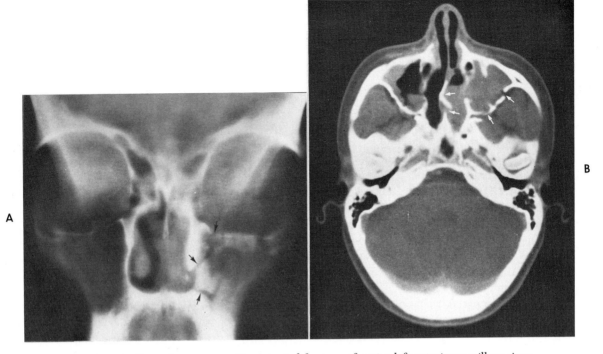

Fig. 1-148. A, Coronal tomogram. Comminuted fracture of entire left anterior maxillary sinus wall. There is hemorrhage in left nasal cavity. **B,** Axial CT scan. There are fractures of left maxillary sinus wall and nasal septum *(arrows)*. There is opacification of left antrum and left nasal cavity. There is some mucosal thickening in right antrum.

Nasal sarcoid occurs in 3% to 20% of cases of systemic sarcoidosis. When it occurs, there are multiple small granulomas of the septum and turbinates. Polypoid degeneration of the mucosa can occur. Rarely, one or more sinuses can be affected and the nonspecific roentgenographic changes are those of chronic inflammation. Bone destruction may occur. The association with chest roentgenogram findings usually suggests the diagnosis. Steroid therapy may suppress the inflammatory reaction and provide symptomatic improvement.

□ Trauma

Because the maxilla is the largest bone in the midfacial skeleton, it is involved most frequently in facial trauma.[108] Fractures involving the maxilla can be divided into those that involve the maxilla alone and those that involve the maxilla as well as several adjacent facial bones.

■ Isolated maxillary fractures

The most common maxillary fracture involves the alveolar process of the maxilla and is the result of a force applied upwards against the mandible. These force vectors thrust the mandible against the maxilla and push the maxillary teeth both upward and outward. Fracture of the alveolar process ensues. Because of the strong supporting soft tissue attachment over the alveolus, there is rarely displacement of the alveolar process.

Direct impact on the maxilla from a narrow object such as an automobile steering wheel or hammer can force the anterior wall of the alveolar ridge inward (lingually). The same force applied to the maxillary teeth can also displace the alveolar process inward. These partial fractures of the maxilla almost always involve the anterior or anterolateral portions of the bone and leave the main body of the maxilla still attached to the cranium (Figs. 1-148 to 1-150).

Vertical or sagittal fractures of the maxilla are also occasionally encountered. They result from an impact directed from the side against either the anterior portion of the maxilla or the palate. The fracture results in separation of the maxilla by a sagittally oriented fracture line that usually passes through the weakest portion of the palatine process of the maxilla. This region is just lateral to the midline. The midline itself is reinforced by the attachment of the vomer, and the lateral portions are strengthened by the alveolar process. They are therefore resistant to direct lateral trauma. Vertical fractures are often associated with fractures of the horizontal plate of the palatine bone, the posterior wall of

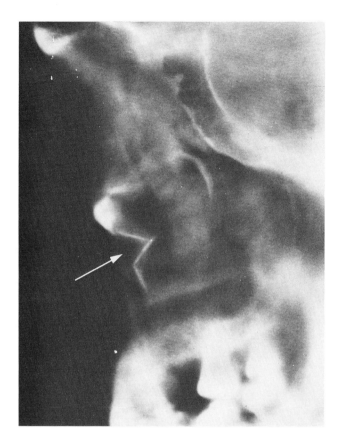

Fig. 1-149. Lateral tomogram. Anterior maxillary sinus wall is buckled inward *(arrow)*. This isolated type of fracture is secondary to blow from narrow object.

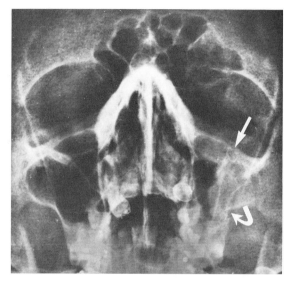

Fig. 1-150. Waters view. Vertical type of fracture of left maxilla without an associated zygoma fracture. Fracture line runs from infraorbital canal *(straight arrow)* to lower lateral wall *(curved arrow)*. Hemorrhage partially fills sinus cavity.

the maxillary sinus, and the ethmoid bone. The frontal process of the maxilla and the nasal bones occasionally are involved. An isolated fracture in this area is rare.

■ Fractures involving the maxilla and adjacent facial bones

Areas of relative structural weakness in the midportion of the facial skeleton were extensively studied by LeFort to determine the common sites of facial fracture.[69] Although his experiments were carried out with modest impact forces compared to those encountered in a high-speed car crash today, the essential classifications still apply. These greater forces have resulted in only mild variations in the level and direction of the fracture lines initially determined by LeFort.

Lefort I fracture (transverse or Guerin's fracture)

The fracture line is oriented transversely through the maxilla above the line of dentition. The nasal septum and lower portions of the pterygoid plates are also involved. The fracture segment thus is composed of the lower portions of the maxillary sinus, the alveolar process, the entire palate, and lower portions of the pter-

oyoid plates. This "floating palate" usually is displaced posteriorly and results in malocclusion (Fig. 1-151). Hemorrhage into the antra may also result in an opaque sinus with air-fluid levels (Figs. 1-152 to 1-155). These fractures are the result of a local impact delivered over the upper lip region.

LeFort II (pyramidal) fracture

The fractureline begins as a transverse line through the upper nasal bones and through the frontal processes of the maxillary bones. The fracture line continues backward across the lacrimal bones and then angles forward through the roofs of the maxillary sinuses to the anterior inferior orbital rims. It then descends through the anterior maxillary walls very near the zygomaticomaxillary sutures, extends through the posterior maxillary sinus walls and across the pterygomaxillary fissures, and ends in the lower pterygoid plates. The zygomatic bones remain attached to the cranium, and the fracture line gives rise to a "floating" maxilla (Figs. 1-156 to 1-158). There are various degrees of malocclusion. Epistaxis is almost always present and paresthesia or anesthesia over one or both of the infraorbital nerve distri-

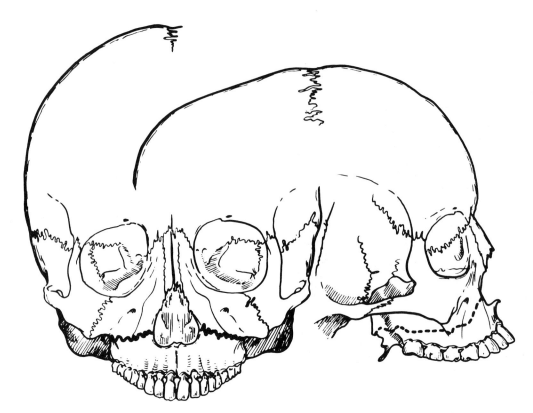

Fig. 1-151. Diagram of LeFort I fracture. (Modified from Converse, 1968.)

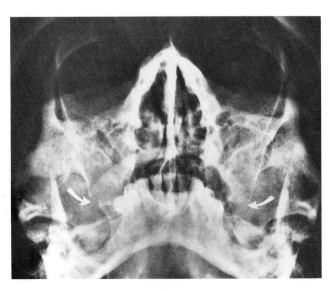

Fig. 1-152. Waters view of LeFort I fracture. Arrows indicate lateral margins of transverse fracture. Hemorrhage is present in both antra.

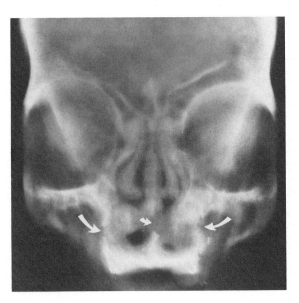

Fig. 1-153. Coronal tomograms. LeFort I fracture line is seen through medial antral walls and nasal structures (*arrows*).

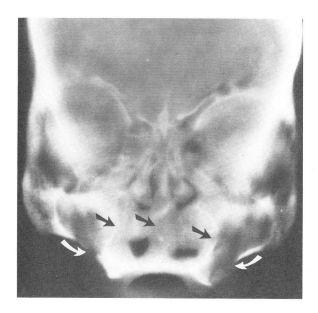

Fig. 1-154. Coronal tomograms. LeFort I fracture line is seen extending completely across nasal cavity and both antra *(arrows)*.

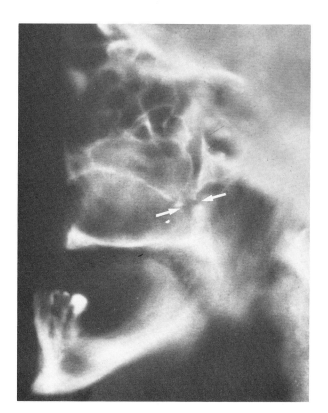

Fig. 1-155. Lateral tomogram. LeFort I fracture line is seen to extend posteriorly through pterygoid plates *(arrows)*.

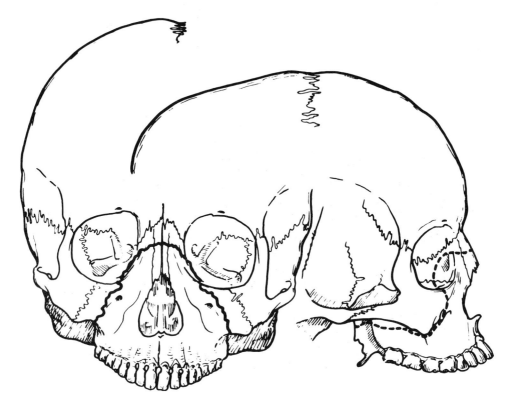

Fig. 1-156. Diagram of LeFort II fracture. (Modified from Converse, 1968.)

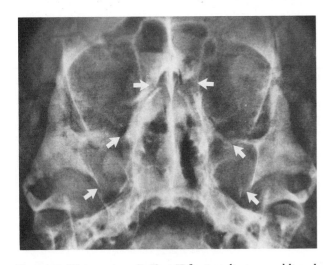

Fig. 1-157. Waters view. LeFort II fracture line runs obliquely across both maxilla and up across ethmoid sinuses and nasal bones *(arrows)*. In addition this patient has separation of left zygomaticofrontal suture.

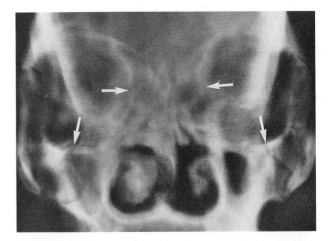

Fig. 1-158. Coronal tomogram of LeFort II fracture. Arrows indicate upper maxillary fracture lines and ethmoid fracture level.

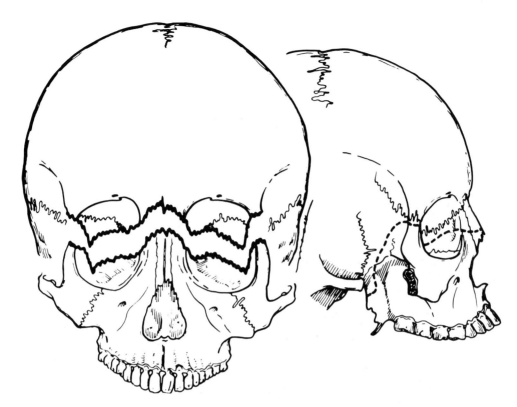

Fig. 1-159. Diagram of LeFort III fracture. (Modified from Converse, 1968.)

butions may be present. Backward displacement of the nasoorbital area and splaying of the fracture segments may result in a "dishface" deformity. This fracture is caused by a strong, broad impact over the central facial area.

LeFort III fracture (craniofacial disjunction)

The fracture line runs across the nasofrontal region, then backwards across the frontal process of the maxilla, the lacrimal bones, and the ethmoid bones (upper medial orbital walls). It extends posteriorly across the orbital fissure. From this point, the fracture line extends in two different directions. One line runs upward across the lateral orbital wall and ends near the zygomaticofrontal suture. The second line extends backward into the sphenomaxillary fissures and ends in the lower pterygoid plates.

If there is excessive posterior displacement, the cribriform plate and ethmoid cells are fractured. This can result in cerebrospinal fluid leakage. A marked dishface deformity is present and usually there is some damage to the lacrimal apparatus. Bleeding into the orbits is from injury to the ethmoidal arteries. Open-bite malocclusion is frequent.

These fractures result from a strong, broad impact

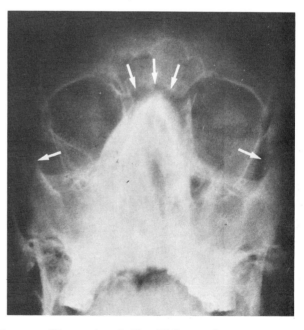

Fig. 1-160. Waters view. LeFort III fracture line is seen across nasofrontal region and lateral orbital rims *(arrows).*

over the nasal area, across the orbital rims and zygomas. LeFort III fractures also include the zygomas, a differentiating point from the LeFort II fracture. The facial skeleton is therefore detached from the cranium (Figs. 1-159 and 1-160).

• • •

Fractures of the maxilla are less common in children, probably because of the greater flexibility and resilience of the bones. These fractures can be very difficult to identify. The inability to evaluate damage done to the maxillary growth centers is a major radiographic and clinical problem. Damage to these centers will result in facial asymmetry and deformity in adulthood. Dental development can also be impaired.

■ Orbital floor fractures

The term "blow-out fracture" does not refer to a specific fracture but instead defines a specific mechanism that results in a fracture. A blow-out fracture is caused by a rapid increase in intraorbital pressure resulting from a traumatic force applied to the orbital contents.[142] The object inflicting this force must be larger than the orbital rim (fist, ball, etc.) and thus does not actually enter the orbit. It pushes the orbital contents backward into the smaller cone-shaped orbital apex. This increased intraorbital pressure is exerted on the orbital walls and the fracture occurs at the weakest region, the middle orbital floor. The orbital rim itself is not fractured. This classical type of blow-out fracture is called a pure blow-out fracture (Fig. 1-161).[26] The globe is usually undamaged.

In the typical car injury, the face is thrown violently against the dashboard. This impact fractures the thick inferior orbital rim, which is displaced backwards, resulting in a comminuted orbital floor fracture. However, the continuing forward momentum of the face against the dashboard raises the intraorbital pressure and results in a superimposed blow-out fracture. This type of combined blow-out fracture and inferior orbital rim fracture is termed an impure blow-out fracture.[26] This type of fracture can also be associated with LeFort II and LeFort III fractures. Either the medial or the lateral third of the orbital floor is involved in these impure blow-out fractures. Medial fractures are associated with medial orbital wall fractures and nasoorbital fractures. Lateral fractures are associated with zygomatic fractures. The fractured segment can be comminuted, with a sagging, hammocklike appearance (Fig. 1-162) or of the trapdoor variety (Fig. 1-163), with a displaced segment hanging into the antrum by a periosteal hinge.

Herniation of orbital fat, the inferior rectus, and sometimes the inferior oblique muscles into the fractured orbital floor occurs (Figs. 1-164 and 1-165). This is accompanied by hematoma and edema. Displacement of these orbital tissues is one cause of enophthalmos. Retention of the globe in the orbital apex, enlargement of the orbital cavity, and orbital fat necrosis secondary to pressure, hematoma, or a low-grade inflammatory process also can contribute to enophthalmos.

Diplopia on upward gaze not only is a result of muscle entrapment in the fracture line but also is secondary to rotation of the globe by the orbital antagonist muscles. Diplopia may also be secondary to edema of the intraorbital tissues as well as to edema of the eyelids and adjacent facial soft tissues in the absence of tissue herniation. Rarely, a depressed fracture of the orbital roof can impinge on the globe, resulting in diplopia on

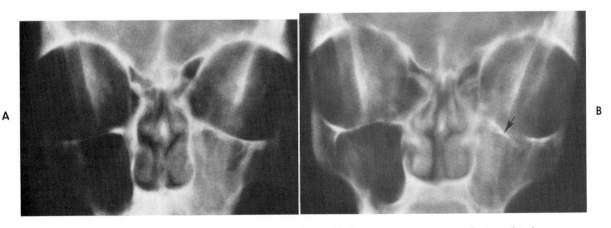

Fig. 1-161. A, Coronal tomogram reveals clouding of left antrum with intact inferior orbital rim. **B,** Coronal tomogram 1 cm posterior to Fig. 1-161, **A,** reveals depressed medial orbital floor fracture. This is pure blow-out fracture *(arrow).*

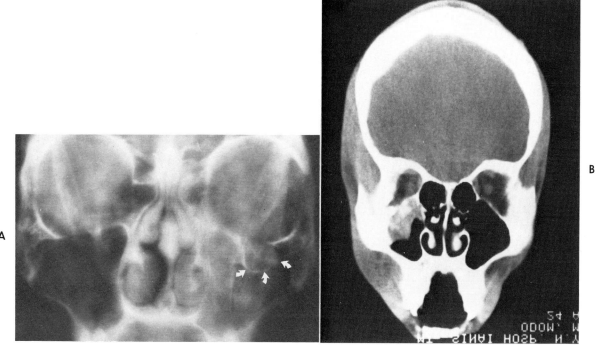

Fig. 1-162. A, Coronal tomogram reveals hemorrhage in left antrum with left blow-out fracture. Fracture segments and orbital tissues sag into underlying sinus cavity *(arrows).* **B,** Coronal CT scan. There is right comminuted orbital floor fracture with hemorrhage in underlying antrum. No abnormality is present in orbit itself.

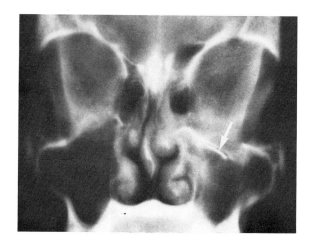

Fig. 1-163. Coronal tomogram. Trapdoor type of blow-out fracture with fracture segment *(arrow)* "hinged" medially by periosteum.

upward gaze and simulating a blow-out fracture (Fig. 1-166).[76] The resulting communication with the anterior cranial fossa may lead to cerebrospinal fluid leakage. Rarely, herniation of tissue can occur through a medial orbital wall fracture.[31] If the inferior orbital rim or the zygoma or both are fractured, these usually can be identified on plain films. The actual blow-out fracture fragments are visualized less often.

Indirect signs of orbital floor fracture include opacification of the antrum caused by hemorrhage and mucosal edema. An air-fluid (air-blood level) will occasionally be seen. Orbital emphysema only extremely rarely occurs with a pure blow-out fracture because the orbital contents are wedged within the bony dehiscence and effectively plug the hole. Further bleeding and edema seal the hole tightly.

Air within the orbit (orbital emphysema) indicates there is a communication with a paranasal sinus, most probably with the ethmoid sinus. Because the lamina papyracea is so thin, fractures of the medial orbital wall may be radiographically undetectable. Associated soft tissue density indicating either submucosal or mucosal edema or hemorrhage within the affected ethmoid cells may be the only clue. When nose blowing increases the orbital emphysema and causes orbital crepitus, the fractures are usually ethmoidal.

Air within the orbit may also arise from complex frac-

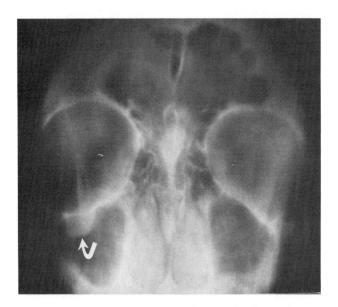

Fig. 1-164. Coronal tomogram. Inferior orbital muscles are herniated into right maxillary antrum through blow-out fracture *(arrow)*.

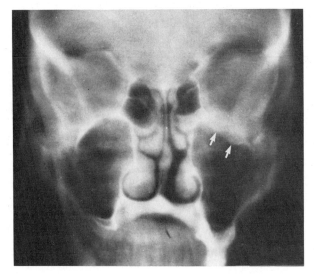

Fig. 1-165. Coronal tomogram. There is mildly depressed orbital floor fracture *(arrows)* and clouding of lower posterior ethmoid sinuses. At surgery there was entrapment of medial orbital tissues in associated ethmoid fracture.

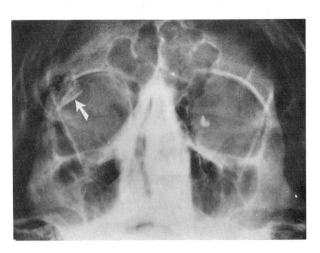

Fig. 1-166. Waters view. Clinically this patient had blow-out fracture and was unable to elevate right globe. Depressed orbital roof fracture is seen *(arrow)*, which was impinging on globe and thus preventing its elevation. Foreign body is seen in left eye.

tures involving the frontal sinus, orbital roof, and maxilla; however, these are usually obvious radiographically.

Tomography plays a quintessential role in the radiographic assessment of facial trauma, and blow-out fractures are no exception. The plain film Waters view is a laudable beginning of the radiologic assessment, but hardly the end. Fracture fragments are frequently en face in the frontal view alone and sometimes cannot be detected even with the finest tomography. Lateral tomography is the best single approach for assessing the contour and integrity of the orbital floor (Figs. 1-162 to 1-164). CT scanning also allows good visualization of the fracture segments.

Zygomatic fractures are closely related to maxillary fractures. The zygoma forms the anterolateral orbital rim as well as the lateral portion of the orbital floor. It has sutural attachments to the frontal, maxillary, and temporal bones. A classification of isolated zygomatic fractures based on rotation and displacement of the body of the zygoma has been clinically helpful and is as follows:[34,65]

Group 1 (69%). Fractures with no significance displacement

Group 2 (10%). Isolated zygomatic arch fractures; there is inward buckling of the arch, and the orbit and maxillary sinus are uninvolved

Group 3 (33%). Fractures with downward and medial or inward displacement of the zygoma but no rotation

Group 4 (11%). Fractures with downward, inward, and backward displacement of the zygoma with medial rotation

Group 5 (22%). Fractures with downward, inward, and backward displacement with lateral rotation of the zygoma

Group 6 (18%). Additional fracture lines cross the main fragment

The Waters view is the single best projection for evaluating zygomatic fracture lines and separation of the zygomaticofrontal suture. The zygomatic arch is also well seen on this view. Tomograms will give better details, especially if the orbital floor is involved. Opacification of the maxillary antrum indicates hemorrhage and edema. Bleeding from the nose may indicate blood escaping through the maxillary sinus ostrium into the middle meatus. These zygomatic fractures are caused by direct impact forces applied directly to the zygoma or to one of its processes. Fractures that involve the orbital floor (zygomaticomaxillary suture), the zygomaticofrontal suture, and the posterior zygomatic arch are also called tripod or trimalar fractures (Figs. 1-167 to 1-173).

Nasoorbital fractures involve the bones that form the

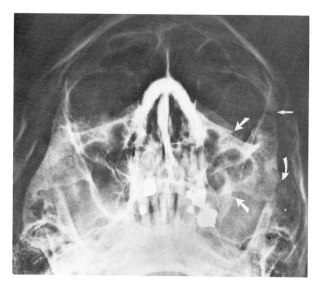

Fig. 1-167. Waters view of typical "tripod fracture". Angled arrows indicate zygomaticomaxillary fracture. Curved arrow points to zygomatic arch fracture and small arrow indicates zygomaticofrontal suture separation. There is depression of zygoma with little if any rotation.

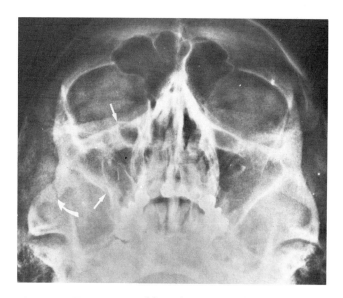

Fig. 1-168. Waters view of less obvious tripod fracture. Zygomaticomaxillary (*straight arrows*) and zygomatic arch (*curved arrow*) fractures are clearly seen. Zygomaticofrontal separation is quite often not seen if there is no rotation or permanent diastasis.

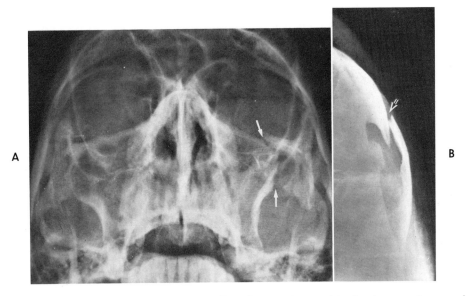

Fig. 1-169. A, Waters view. Zygomaticomaxillary fracture *(arrows)* is clearly seen. Increased density over anterior zygomatic arch only suggests fracture and zygomaticofrontal suture looks normal. **B,** Underpenetrated base view reveals zygomatic arch fracture.

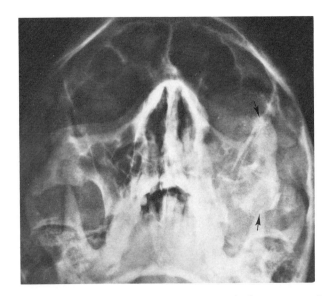

Fig. 1-170. Waters view. Tripod fracture with depression and marked lateral rotation of zygoma *(arrows)*.

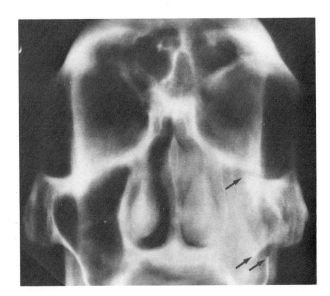

Fig. 1-171. Coronal tomogram of zygomatic fracture *(arrows)*. There is depressed left zygoma with inward displacement (overlapping of inferior orbital rim). Zygomaticofrontal and zygomatic arch fractures are not in plane of focus.

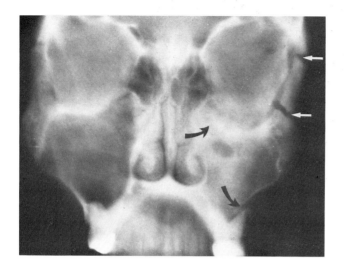

Fig. 1-172. Coronal tomogram. There is unusual fracture of frontal process of zygoma *(white arrows)* and additional maxillary fracture *(black arrows)* with depression of orbital floor. Hemorrhage fills left antrum.

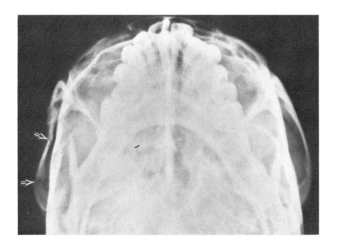

Fig. 1-173. Underpenetrated base view. There is depressed right zygomatic arch fracture *(arrows)*. No other fractures were present.

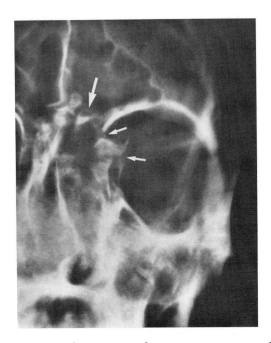

Fig. 1-174. Coronal tomogram. There is extensive naso-orbital fracture with disruption of ethmoid sinuses, medial orbital wall *(small arrows)*, and frontal bone *(large arrow)*.

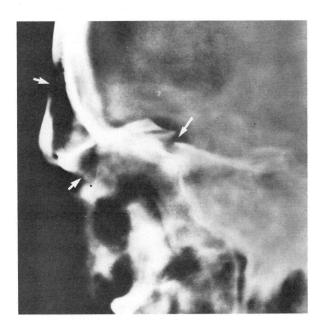

Fig. 1-175. Lateral tomogram. There is crushing-type comminuted naso-orbital fracture *(small arrows)* with rotation of cribriform plate and disruption of posterior ethmoid sinuses *(large arrow)*. There is localized pneumocephalus at this latter point.

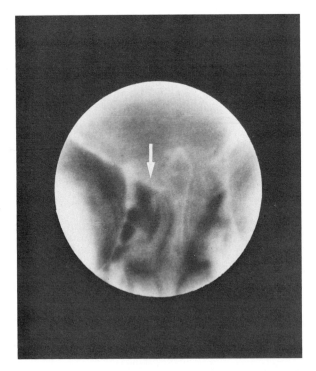

Fig. 1-176. Coronal tomogram. There is fracture of left cribriform plate. Disrupted segment can be best appreciated when compared to normal intact right side *(arrow)*.

skeletal framework of the nose. The upper nasal bones, lacrimal bones, and lower frontal bone are projected backward between the orbits when a strong impact force is directed over the bridge of the nose. This results in a crushing type of comminuted fracture of the cribriform plate and anterior ethmoid air cells (Figs. 1-174 to 1-176). Cerebrospinal fluid rhinorrhea may result. As the nasoorbital structures are displaced backward, they can produce traumatic hypertelorism. The nasal septum and anterior ethmoid cells can be extensively shattered. The nasolacrimal apparatus can also be damaged by disrupted fracture segments.

■ Frontal sinus fractures

Fractures of the frontal sinuses are the result of either direct trauma to the sinus region or extension of a calvarial fracture into the frontal sinuses (Figs. 1-177 and 1-178). These fractures have been grouped into two types.[132] The first, more common type is a linear fracture of the anterior wall (Fig. 1-179). This type of fracture produces opacification of the sinus secondary to hemorrhage and edema. The fracture line frequently involves the superomedial orbital rim. The second type is a comminuted fracture with a depressed anterior wall

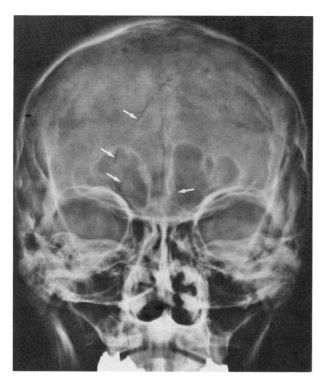

Fig. 1-177. Caldwell view. There is comminuted frontal bone fracture *(arrows)* with involvement of frontal sinus. Only minimal clouding of right frontal sinus is present.

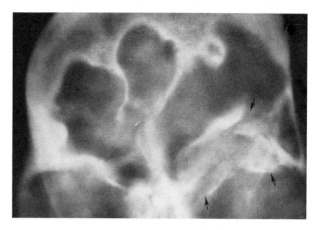

Fig. 1-178. Coronal tomogram. There is comminuted fracture of left frontal sinus and superior orbital rim *(arrows)*.

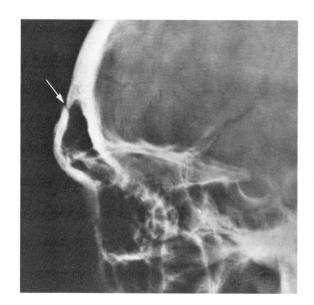

Fig. 1-179. Lateral view. There is linear fracture of anterior frontal sinus wall *(arrow)*. This film was taken 1 month after trauma and sinus has almost completely cleared.

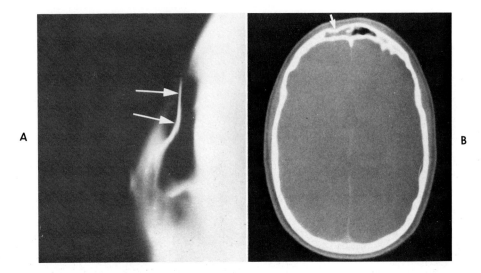

Fig. 1-180. A, Coned-down lateral tomogram of depressed anterior frontal sinus wall fracture. Depressed segment (*arrows*) reflects shape of object causing fracture. **B,** Axial CT scan. There is fracture of right anterior frontal sinus wall (*arrow*). Hemorrhage fills sinus. Posterior wall is intact.

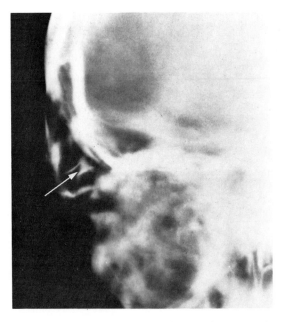

Fig. 1-181. Lateral view. There is depressed anterior frontal sinus wall fracture. Part of fracture segment is seen lying within sinus cavity (*arrow*).

that may reflect the overall shape of the object that caused the fracture (Figs. 1-180 and 1-181).

Complex fractures may involve both the anterior and posterior frontal sinus walls. Isolated fractures of the posterior wall without involvement of the anterior wall are very rare. Bergeron and Rumbaugh[9] have shown a number of "internal compound fractures" of the skull wherein a fracture of the skull enters one of the paranasal sinuses and communication is established with the subarachnoid space. In frontal sinus fractures of this type, the posterior wall alone may be affected. Tearing of dura may cause cerebrospinal fluid rhinorrhea, meningitis, and brain damage to the frontal lobes. Pneumocephalus may be evident on plain films. Involvement of the sinus floor can lead to orbital emphysema.

Isolated ethmoid fractures are rare. They usually are associated with multiple facial bone fractures. Blow-out fractures of the orbit have associated medial orbital wall fractures (through the lamina papyracea of the ethmoid bone) in at least 20% of cases.[26] These ethmoid fractures are difficult to demonstrate on plain films. Opacification of the ethmoid sinuses indicates hemorrhage, edema, or rarely, entrapped orbital tissues (Figs. 1-182 and 1-183).

Sphenoid sinus fractures are rare. They are usually associated with basilar skull fractures. These fractures may be difficult to visualize. Secondary findings are opacification of the sphenoid sinus resulting from edema and hemorrhage. An air-fluid level may also indicate leakage of cerebrospinal fluid into the sinus cav-

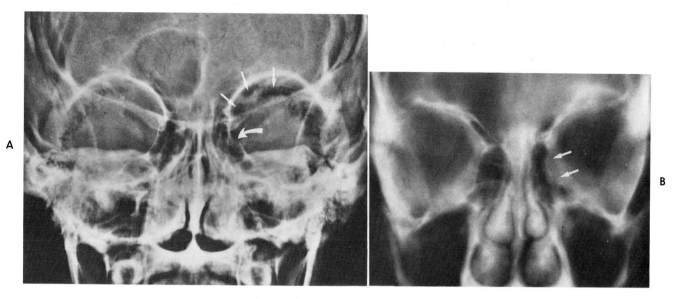

Fig. 1-182. A, Caldwell view. There is left orbital emphysema *(straight arrows).* There is no clouding of ethmoid sinuses; however, there is disruption of medial orbital wall *(curved arrow).* **B,** Coronal tomogram. Orbital soft tissues *(arrows)* are seen herniated into left ethmoid fracture.

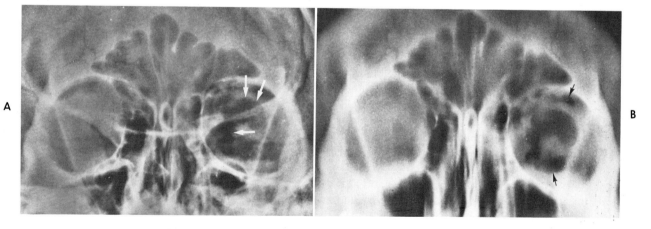

Fig. 1-183. A, Caldwell view. There is left orbital emphysema *(straight arrows)* and clouding of left ethmoid sinuses. **B,** Coronal tomogram. Orbital emphysema and ethmoid clouding are seen better than on plain film *(arrows),* however, fracture line is not evident. This is not an uncommon finding.

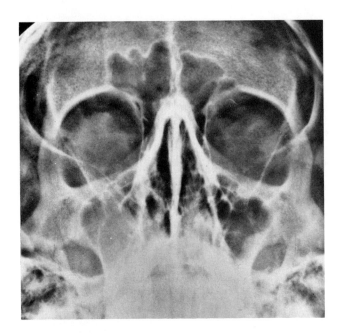

Fig. 1-184. Waters view. Nodular thickening of the mucosa on the lateral wall of the left antrum and marked thickening of the entire mucosa in the right antrum all secondary to hemorrhage. Remaining sinuses are normal. These changes were secondary to barotrauma, however, they are nonspecific findings and could represent inflammatory disease.

ity. As has been noted by others,[9,90a] the presence of an air-fluid level alone in one of the supramaxillary paranasal sinuses is not equivalent to the diagnosis of a cerebrospinal fluid fistula. Trauma to the sinus mucosa may be responsible for collections of blood (submucosal or intraluminal hematomas) and subsequent air-fluid levels within the sinus may occur in the absence of any fracture or fistula. It should be remembered that the sinus mucosa normally produces secretions, and if the patient remains in one position for any long period of time (more than 12 to 24 hours), the normal secretions may pool in the dependent portions of the sinus. If drainage is interfered with, as with nasal intubation in the comatose patient, an air-fluid level appears within the sphenoid sinus within a day or so. We have been able to demonstrate this phenomenon frequently in patients who have no history of head injury and no possibility of cerebrospinal fluid fistula or sinus trauma.

Mastoid fractures may be the source of cerebrospinal fluid rhinorrhea. The fluid courses through the mastoid antrum into the middle ear, down the eustachian tube, and into the pharynx. This may best be manifested when the patient's head is placed in a dependent position. This type of rhinorrhea can occur only if the tympanic membrane is intact. If this membrane is ruptured, the patient will have cerebrospinal fluid otorrhea. Pneumocephalus is usually not seen and loss of mastoid cell aeration may be the only radiographic finding.

■ Barotrauma

Barotrauma is the result of sudden markedly negative intrasinus pressure. This condition is encountered in both airplane pilots and deep-sea divers. The low pressure causes rupture of mucosal vessels and results in subepithelial hematomas as well as free intrasinus bleeding. Radiographically, these changes may take 3 to 10 weeks to completely resorb. Clinically, the frontal sinuses are involved most often, with 92% of patients experiencing pain referable to the frontal region. Epistaxis is the second most commonly exhibited symptom. Radiographically, and somewhat inexplicably, the maxillary sinuses and not the frontal sinuses are affected in almost all patients. The frontal sinus shows changes in only 25% and the ethmoid sinuses in less than 20% of cases. The changes are primarily those of mucosal thickening, which can be nodular in appearance (Fig. 1-184). Only 12% of patients have air-fluid levels.[41]

□ **Analysis of postoperative films**

Before embarking on the analysis of postoperative films of the paranasal sinuses, the interpreter should be knowledgeable of the following:

1. The operative procedures, i.e., what bone, or part thereof, is normally removed as part of the procedure? Is a boneflap made for entrance into the sinus and is it replaced over the surgical approach site? Is any foreign material inserted into the sinus cavity during the operation? Is the sinus packed with a foreign substance at the conclusion?

2. The period that has elapsed from time of surgery to the time of the radiographic examination. Edema, secretions, and hematomas obscure almost all detail in the early postoperative period.

3. The normal postoperative appearance of the paranasal sinuses. Only rarely does a sinus return to a com-

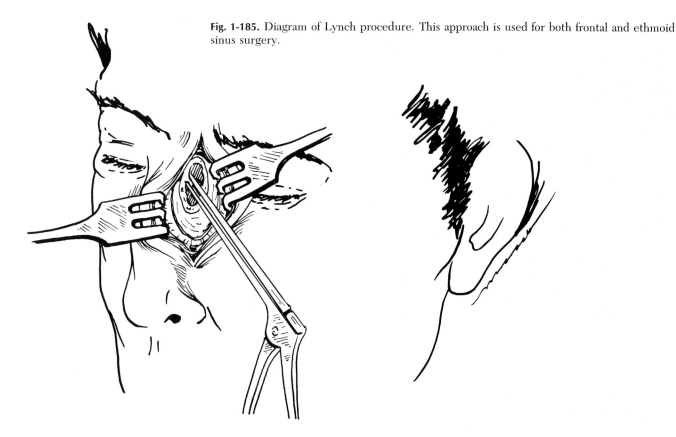

Fig. 1-185. Diagram of Lynch procedure. This approach is used for both frontal and ethmoid sinus surgery.

pletely normal preoperative roentgenographic appearance. What are the changes of the normal healing process that are to be anticipated on the postoperative examination?

4. The radiographic evaluation of recurrent disease. Ideally all patients, and specifically patients with tumors of the paranasal sinuses, must have postoperative examinations that serve as a baseline for the future evaluation of recurrent disease. This baseline study must be obtained in the stable postoperative period. To a lesser extent, the same admonition holds for patients operated on for inflammatory disease.

■ The frontal sinuses

With the advent of the antibiotic era, surgical intervention for frontal sinus inflammatory disease markedly diminished. In passing, it must be stressed that acute frontal sinusitis is a serious disease and that the identification of an air-fluid level in the frontal sinus secondary to acute infection demands urgent treatment because of the imminent possibility of intracerebral complications. In this respect the implication of an air-fluid level within the frontal sinuses is vastly different from that within the maxillary antra.

There are a variety of available surgical procedures; the one used is based on both clinical assessment and the developmental size of the sinus cavity.

These surgical procedures can be divided into two main groups: (1) those that do not obliterate the sinus and therefore require reconstruction of frontonasal drainage and (2) those that do obliterate the sinus cavity so that frontonasal drainage need not be maintained. The *Lynch* and *Killian* procedures belong to the former group, and the *Reidel* and the more recent, cosmetically acceptable osteoplastic flap procedure belong to the latter group.[4] (In all of these procedures, a strong effort is made to remove the sinus mucosa. If mucosa remains, the mucosal cells can give rise to a postoperative mucocele.)

In acute sinusitis a trephine procedure can be used to accomplish immediate sinus drainage. No attempt to remove or destroy the sinus mucosa is made. The procedure is performed with an incision in the superomedial margin of the orbit behind the orbital rim. The trephine makes a hole in the sinus floor and drainage is accomplished. This procedure usually has no roentgenographic manifestations because the small drainage hole rarely can be identified, even by tomography. This is primarily because of the marked curvature of the frontal bone in this region and the resulting consistent lack of a tangential surface to the incident x-ray beam.

The Lynch procedure removes an actual segment of the frontal sinus floor by means of an approach similar to that used in trephination (Fig. 1-185). The radiographic picture is that of a normal sinus or a sinus without a well-defined mucoperiosteal line. Tomography may fail to visualize the defect in the floor. This procedure is used for small, shallow, chronically infected sinuses. In the larger sinuses, all the sinus mucosa may not be removable through the floor incision. An external ethmoidectomy is almost always performed and a polyethylene tube (only some of which are radiopaque) is used to create a drainage pathway between the frontal sinus and the middle meatus. The tube is left in place approximately 6 to 8 weeks and then removed. With all frontal sinus operations, at least 6 to 8 weeks should elapse before a baseline study is obtained, provided the postoperative course is uneventful. This period allows the edema and other operative changes to resolve completely. The polyethylene tube will therefore not be visualized because it has been removed before the first baseline study.

If the frontal sinus is large or has some minimal reactive osteitis in the adjacent frontal bone, greater access into the sinus cavity is desirable. The Killian procedure provides an additional opening in the anterior sinus wall (Fig. 1-186). An intact superior orbital rim separates the two incisions. Following surgery, the soft tissues of the forehead form the anterior sinus wall. Because the orbital rim is intact, this forehead depression is small and does not obliterate the sinus cavity. Plain films or tomograms and CT scans will demonstrate this anterior wall bony defect. This sinus cavity will show diminished lucency secondary to the partially depressed soft tissues of the forehead displacing the sinus air. An external ethmoidectomy for drainage is performed as in the Lynch procedure.

Reidel's procedure is reserved for cases of more extensive osteitis, osteomyelitis, and chronic sinusitis. It is an extension of the Killian procedure to include the intervening bone of the superior orbital rim (Fig. 1-187). The anterior wall defect (and when necessity dictates, a posterior wall defect up to the dura) is seen on plain films, tomograms, and CT scans. The orbital rim defect is also well seen on the Caldwell and Waters views. A sizeable depression in the forehead is evident clinically as it sinks into the bony defect and obliterates the sinus cavity air. Without history, the bone destruc-

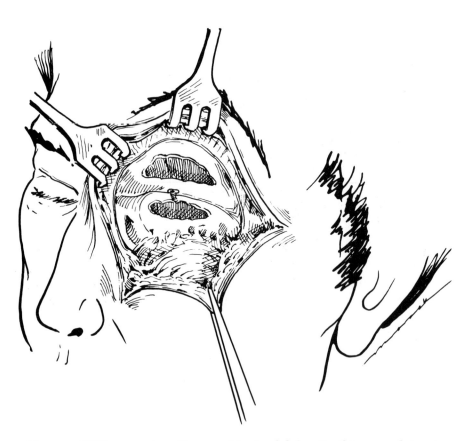

Fig. 1-186. Diagram of Killian procedure. Because of forehead deformity, this approach is not commonly employed today.

tion and soft tissue sinus mass can mimic a malignant process.

Presently, if a trephine for simple acute drainage or a Lynch approach will not suffice, the osteoplastic flap has become the procedure of choice. As a result, the more disfiguring Killian and Reidel procedures are rarely seen.

The osteoplastic flap is a more recent and cosmetically satisfactory operation that obliterates the sinus cavity and does not leave the deformity of the Reidel procedure. The osteoplastic flap is patterned from a template of the frontal sinus traced from a Caldwell view. Using the template as a guide, the anterior sinus wall margin is traced out with a saw, leaving the inferior periosteum intact over the orbital rims and nasion, the anterior wall is then fractured at this basal attachment and bent downward to expose the entire sinus cavity (Fig. 1-188). After all the mucosa is removed, a piece of abdominal muscle or fat or both is placed in the sinus cavity and the anterior bony wall is lifted back into its original place. No depression of the forehead tissues is present.

This procedure gives several consistent roentgenographic findings (Figs. 1-189 to 1-192). The surgical bone flap is best seen on the lateral films and appears as an anterior sinus wall fracture. A soft tissue polypoid mass in the sinus cavity or partial opacification of the sinus and areas of minimal diminished lucency in adjacent portions of the cavity are seen. This is the result of the muscle and fatty tissue placed into the sinus superimposed on the bony flap. If several years have elapsed after surgery, calcifications can appear in these soft tissues (Fig. 1-193).

In nonobliterative frontal sinus surgery, delayed roentgenographic examinations may demonstrate the persistence of the mucoperiosteal white line; however, more frequently this line is ill-defined. Most postoperative frontal sinuses have a vague, hazy quality secondary to fibrosis that can mimic mucosal thickening. Usually the sinus is not opaque or even clouded sufficiently to suggest an active sinusitis or mass lesion. Less commonly, the sinus can appear radiographically normal. Air-fluid levels are not to be expected and will usually indicate postoperative infection.

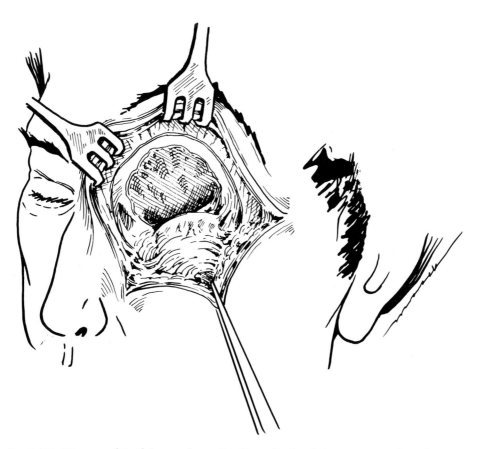

Fig. 1-187. Diagram of Reidel procedure. Significant forehead depression resulting from removed anterior sinus wall has made this procedure unpopular today.

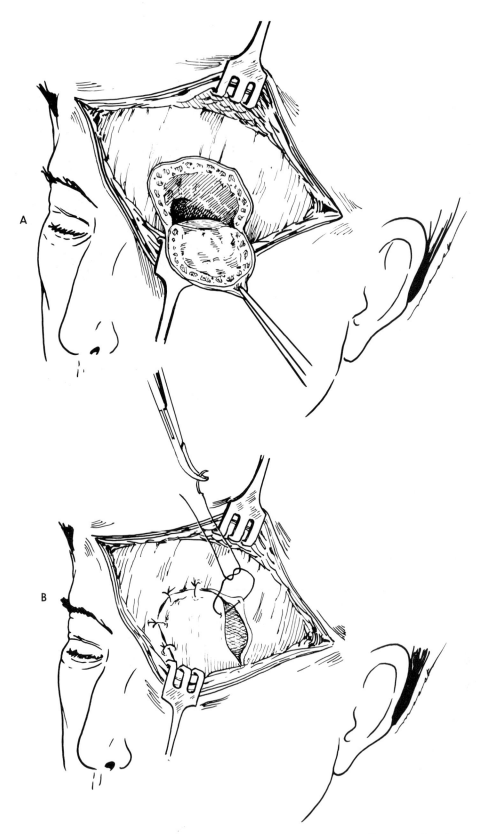

Fig. 1-188. A, Diagram of osteoplastic flap procedure. Anterior sinus wall is opened with lower periosteum intact. **B,** Diagram of osteoplastic flap closure showing intact periosteum and no bony defect to cause cosmetic depression.

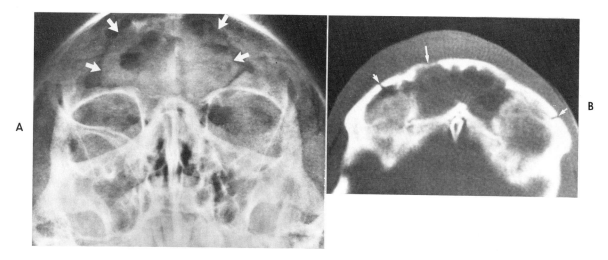

Fig. 1-189. A, Caldwell view of bilateral osteoplastic flap *(arrows)*. This should not be confused with "clouded sinus" or sinus mass. **B,** Axial CT scan. Osteoplastic flap procedure has been performed. Surgical fracture lines are seen *(small arrows)*. Area of osteomyelitis has developed *(large arrow)* with overlying inflammation in forehead.

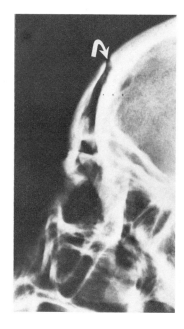

Fig. 1-190. Lateral view. Arrow points to surgical incision for osteoplastic flap. Note that sinus cavity is not obliterated. This surgical defect should not be confused with fracture.

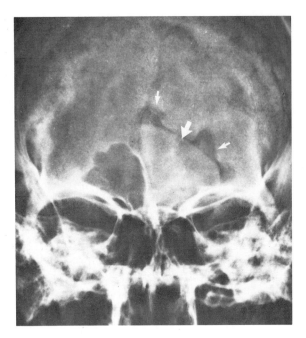

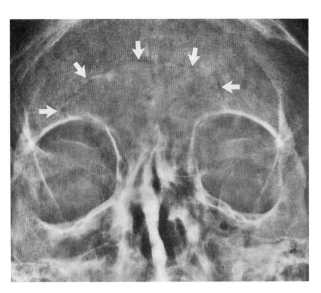

Fig. 1-191. Caldwell view of unilateral (left) osteoplastic flap *(large arrow)*. Smaller arrows point to outer sinus margin, which is slightly larger than flap.

Fig. 1-192. Caldwell view of bilateral osteoplastic flap that fits the surgical defect almost exactly *(arrows)*. This should not be mistaken for hypoplastic frontal sinuses or complete sinus clouding.

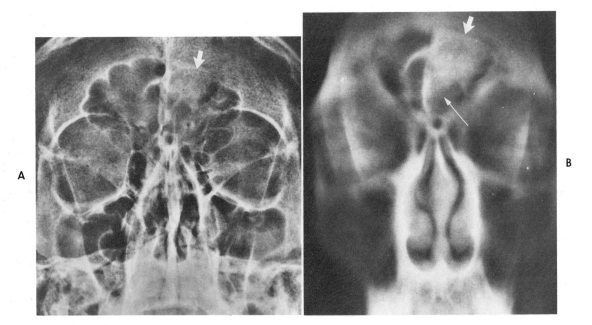

Fig. 1-193. A, Caldwell view of vague localized soft tissue density in the left frontal sinus *(arrow)*. **B,** Frontal tomogram reveals a partially calcified fatty-muscle block inserted in frontal sinus as part of previous osteoplastic flap procedure *(short arrow)*. Circular lucent defect *(long arrow)* represents small recurrent mucocele.

■ The ethmoid sinuses

Ethmoidectomy is performed by means of three basic approaches: external, internal, and transantral. Irrespective of the operative approach, the goal is to remove the septae and mucous membrane of the intervening ethmoid cells, leaving one single, large "sinus" cavity behind. The mucosa must be completely removed in order to assure that no postoperative mucoceles develop. The procedure can be limited to an anterior ethmoidectomy or it can be a complete anterior and posterior ethmoidectomy. One may approach the posterior cells only by exenteration of the anterior cells. If an external approach is used, the lamina papyracea is removed. This will be manifested on the Caldwell and Waters views as absence of the medial orbital wall. Because the lamina papyracea is normally thin, careful examination is necessary to avoid overlooking its absence (Fig. 1-194). The ethmoid sinus cavity itself, now having the intercellular septa removed, usually appears as clear and radiolucent as a normal sinus. Careful inspection, however, will reveal the absence of these septa, which suggests either minimal infection with blurring of these septa or previous surgery. The combination of this finding and an absent lamina papyracea strongly indicates previous surgery.

The internal ethmoidectomy, approached through the nose, can leave the lamina papyracea intact. The middle turbinate, however, may be surgically removed. This approach is often used when surgery also involves the nasal cavity and the sphenoid sinus. Destruction of these medial ethmoid structures can simulate disease because of the mucosal scarring that can persist in the naturally occurring crevices of this region. If only the middle turbinate is missing and the other turbinates are intact, previous surgery should be suspected.

It should be remembered that the surgical landmarks in an external ethmoidectomy are the anterior and posterior ethmoidal artery canals, which delimit the floor of the anterior cranial fossa. Postoperative bleeding can occur and a large hematoma can fill the exenterated ethmoid cavity. En bloc fibrosis and scarring of this hematoma can occur without apparent postoperative resolution of the hematoma. Complete opacification of an ethmoid sinus with poor visualization of the lamina papyracea or adjacent nasal structures may suggest the presence of a tumor (Fig. 1-195). Axial CT scans usually demonstrate a sharp demarcation between present and absent laminae that suggests previous surgery (Fig. 1-196). This can be a very difficult diagnosis without a history.

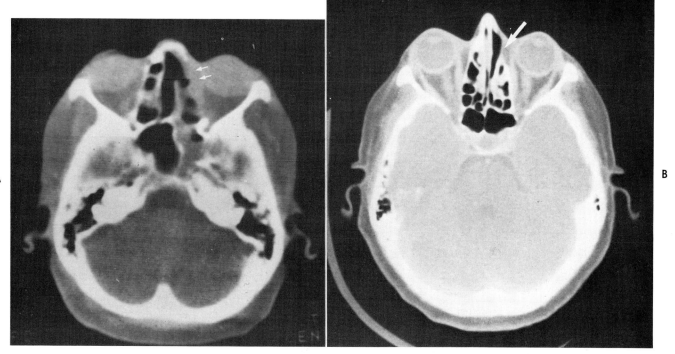

Fig. 1-194. A, Axial CT scan. Arrows indicate absent lamina papyracea of left ethmoid sinuses. Intercellular septa are missing, and some postoperative fibrosis is present. There is no intraorbital mass. Changes in the ethmoid (and sphenoid) sinuses are normal postoperative findings. **B,** Axial CT scan after external ethmoidectomy. Lamina papyracea is absent anteriorly *(arrow)* and ethmoid septa have been removed.

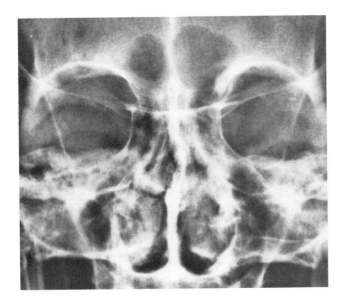

Fig. 1-195. Caldwell view. Clouding of left ethmoid sinus suggests infection or mass. This was postoperative en bloc fibrosis and could not be radiographically differentiated.

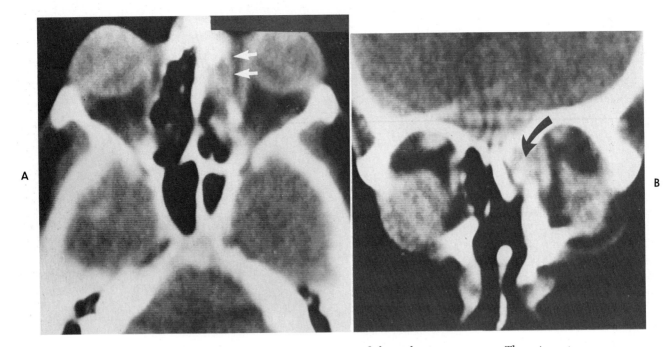

Fig. 1-196. A, Axial CT scan. Arrows point to area of absent lamina papyracea. There is postoperative scarring but no recurrent disease. **B,** Coronal CT scan. Arrow points to postoperative ethmoid scarring that could not be differentiated from recurrent disease.

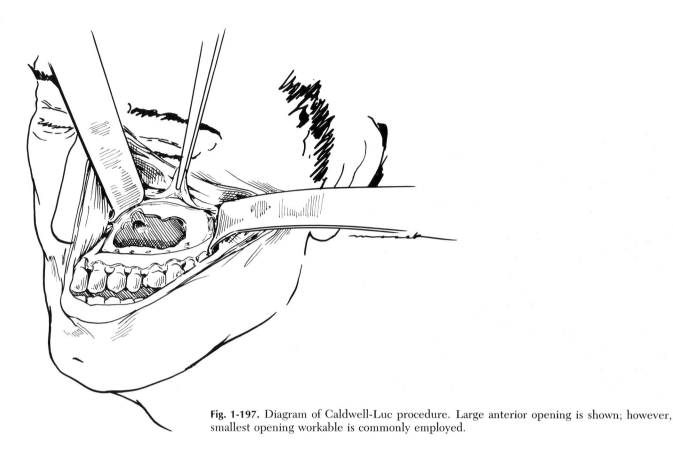

Fig. 1-197. Diagram of Caldwell-Luc procedure. Large anterior opening is shown; however, smallest opening workable is commonly employed.

Occasionally a transantral ethmoidectomy is performed with combined surgery of the maxillary and ethmoid sinuses. The ethmoidomaxillary plate is removed to allow entrance into the ethmoid cavity. Absence of this plate in a patient with en bloc ethmoid scarring and postoperative maxillary changes could erroneously suggest tumor or recurrent inflammatory disease throughout the area. Prior postoperative baseline studies may help in evaluating recurrent disease.

■ The maxillary sinuses

The most common surgical procedure of the maxillary sinuses is the Caldwell-Luc procedure. It is used for both diagnostic and therapeutic purposes. The Caldwell-Luc procedure creates an anterior opening into the maxillary sinus between the roots of the upper canine and first molar teeth (canine fossa) (Fig. 1-197). Postoperatively, the hematoma in the surgical window usually becomes fibrous and closes the bone defect. New bone formation is common. Axial CT scans clearly demonstrate the anterior wall defect (Fig. 1-198). In rare instances, the hematoma breaks down or becomes infected and an oroantral fistula is created. This occurs between the first and second postoperative weeks and usually closes without surgery.

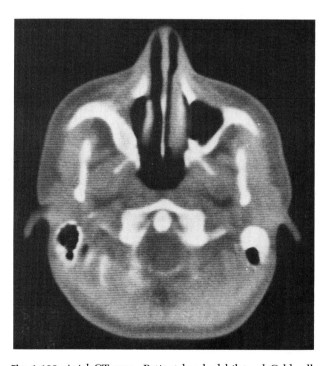

Fig. 1-198. Axial CT scan. Patient has had bilateral Caldwell-Luc procedures. Posterolateral antral walls are slightly thickened on left and markedly thickened on right secondary to recurrent infection. Scarring has almost obliterated right antrum.

Following removal of the diseased sinus mucosa, the last part of the Caldwell-Luc procedure calls for a nasoantral window or antrotomy. The window is made in the inferior meatus just above the nasal floor. It must be large enough so that it will not close postoperatively. The antrotomy is at a lower level than the normal sinus infundibulum and as such is a more efficient drainage outlet. When closure of the antrotomy occurs secondary to mucosal overgrowth and fibrous scarring, it is not well demonstrated radiographically and is better evaluated clinically.

On baseline postoperative studies 10% to 20% of the antra appear radiographically normal with no evidence of surgery. The sinuses appear opaque in 30% to 40% of cases.[151] The sinuses have some degree of fibrosis that simulates mucosal disease in 40% to 60% of cases. This fibrosis results from two factors: (1) the extent of resorption of the secretions and bleeding that occurs in the immediate postoperative period and (2) the degree of reepithelialization and the histology thereof. In the severely diseased sinus almost all the mucosa will have been removed surgically. In less severe cases, the mucosal stripping is limited to mucosa that is irreversibly damaged. If this is a small mucosal island at the base of a cyst, then the broad surrounding mucoperiosteum will reepithelialize as normal mucosa. However, particularly in the more extensively involved cases, the new epithelium may be either atrophic or even hypertrophic. The apparently thickened mucoperiosteum on the sinus film represents both mucosa and fibrosis (Figs. 1-199 and 1-200). The normal mucoperiosteal line may be poorly seen or absent altogether in the more extensively stripped sinuses.

During the first 2 postoperative weeks, air-fluid levels and opacification from edema and blood can dominate the roentgenogram. After this period an air-fluid level may indicate the presence of an infectious process. The baseline examination can usually be obtained within 6 to 8 weeks. In rare cases, calcifications, osteoma, or even complete ossification of the sinus cavity occur (Fig. 1-201, A and B).[87,151] Unusual fibrotic compartmentalization of the sinus has also been reported.

Wide variation in the postoperative appearance of the antrum necessitates comparison with a baseline study if recurrent disease is to be evaluated accurately. Empyema, osteomyelitis, and extension of disease beyond the confines of the antrum may require the correlation of close clinical and radiographic observation to effect an early diagnosis.

A postoperative mucocele may occur in the lateral portion of the sinus, in the presence of a small, medially aerated sinus cavity. The mucocele abuts on the lateral wall, which is locally thinned or destroyed. The secondary mucocele arises from retained antral mucosa and fibrosis that block off the lateral portion of the sinus. Primary mucoceles develop from sinus osteal obstruction and thus involve the entire sinus cavity (Figs. 1-202 and 1-203).

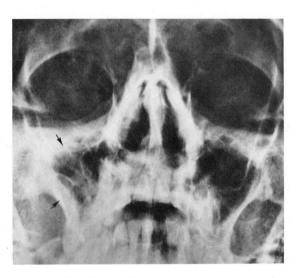

Fig. 1-199. Caldwell view. Postoperative scarring in right antrum mimics inflammatory disease (*arrows*).

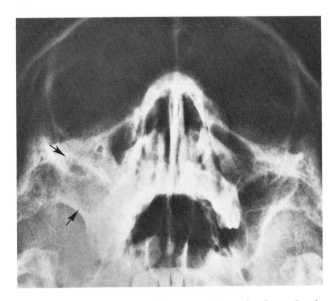

Fig. 1-200. Caldwell view. Almost complete clouding of right antrum represents normal postoperative appearance (*arrows*).

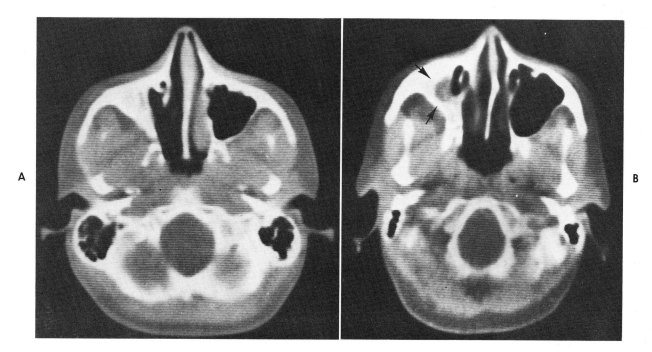

Fig. 1-201. A, Axial CT scan reveals postoperative ossification of most of right antrum. **B,** Axial CT scan reveals partial postoperative ossification *(arrows)* of right antrum.

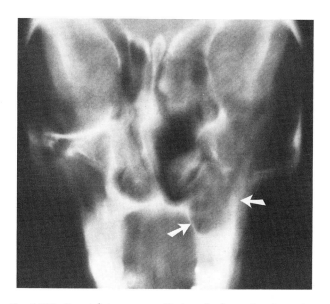

Fig. 1-202. Frontal tomogram. Patient had previously undergone both partial left maxillectomy and transnasal ethmoidectomy. Note absence of left middle turbinate. Arrows outline a localized postoperative mucocele extending into and expanding alveolus.

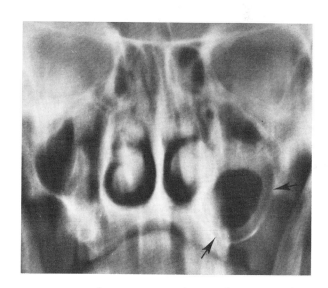

Fig. 1-203. Frontal tomogram reveals expanding cavitary lesion of lower left antrum *(arrows)*. Central portion had been evacuated in an office transnasal biopsy. *Postoperative mucocele.*

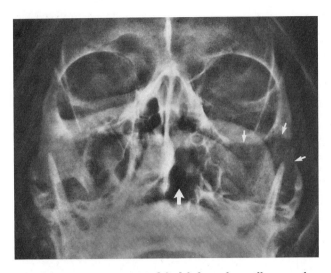

Fig. 1-204. Waters view. Modified left total maxillectomy has been performed. Portions of orbital floor, zygoma, zygomatic arch *(small arrows)*, and lateral and medial antral walls have been resected. In addition, left hard palate has been removed *(large arrow)*.

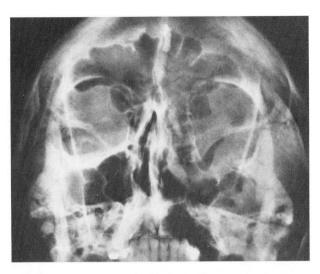

Fig. 1-205. Waters view. Total left maxillectomy has been performed. Left orbital floor, medial and lateral antral walls, and portion of hard palate have been resected. Only bony margins (or absence of bone) can be clearly identified.

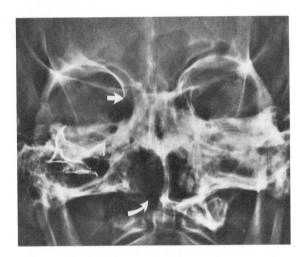

Fig. 1-206. Caldwell view. Right ethmoidomaxillary resection was performed. Right ethmoid margin is clearly seen *(arrow)*. Mesh stent was placed for orbital support. Right half of palate was also resected *(curved arrow)*. Clouding of ethmoid sinuses was stable in appearance for many years and represents postoperative scarring, not recurrence.

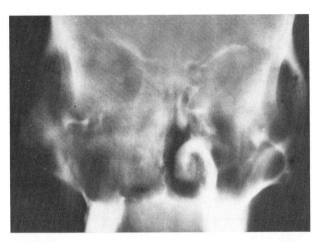

Fig. 1-207. Coronal tomogram after right ethmoidopartial maxillary resection. Recurrent disease is best evaluated by examination of bony margins and any new soft tissue masses. Patient had inflammatory changes with no tumor recurrence.

■ Partial and total maxillectomies

In complete maxillectomy for neoplasm, the involved antrum is removed intact to avoid the risk of contamination of the surgical field. The floor of the orbit, the medial portion of the body of the zygoma, the ethmoidomaxillary plate, the lateral nasal wall, and a variable portion of the hard palate are extirpated (Fig. 1-204). The pterygoid plates are usually left intact. Considerable variation exists, depending on the extent of the tumor mass. The soft tissues of the cheek may be held in position by a prosthesis, and skin grafting of the surgical cavity is always done. The baseline radiographic studies are thus very confusing (Figs. 1-205 to 1-207). Only the bone margins can be properly evaluated, and extension of osseous destruction will necessitate future comparison with this examination. The soft tissue component may be partially or totally obscured on the plain film examination. CT scans allow evaluation of both the

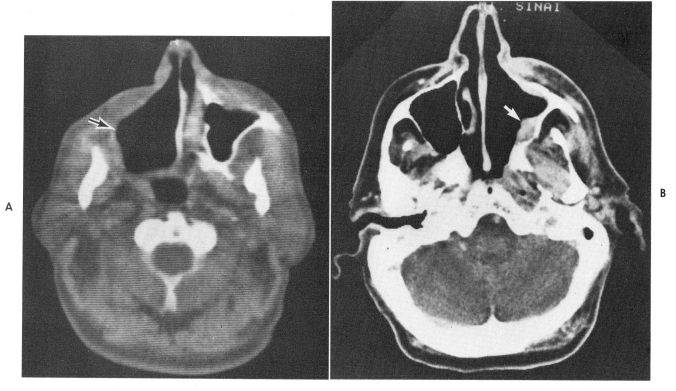

Fig. 1-208. A, Axial CT scan after right maxillectomy. Soft tissues around postoperative antral defect are smooth, with no evidence of recurrence. Contour of these structures cannot be clearly appreciated on radiographs. **B,** Axial CT scan after left partial maxillectomy. Nodular recurrence *(arrow)* is seen in posterior antral wall.

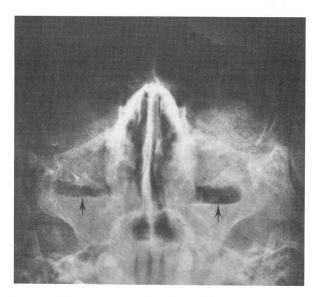

Fig. 1-209. Waters view. Bilateral antral air-fluid levels with apparent bilateral blow-out fractures. Patient had bilateral orbital decompressions for malignant exophthalmus.

surgical cavity and soft tissues (Fig. 1-208). The cavity should normally be smooth. Focal nodular masses or a localized region of soft tissue thickening normally indicate recurrent disease. Again a baseline study is suggested to assist evaluation.

Orbital exenteration as well as en block ethmoid resection can also be performed. An orbital decompression operation may mimic a blow-out fracture. This postoperative appearance requires the history for diagnosis (Fig. 1-209).

■ The sphenoid sinus

The "hidden sinus" requires surgical intervention less frequently than any of the other paranasal sinuses. Because of its relationship to the skull base, radical surgery for tumors is unrealistic. More commonly, diagnostic or therapeutic procedures (for cysts, polyps, benign tumors, mucoceles, etc.) are the reasons for surgical entry. The sphenoid sinus may be reached by means of several approaches: transethmoid, transseptal, transantral, and transpalatal.

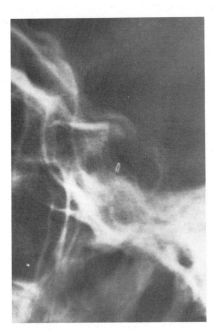

Fig. 1-210. Lateral film. Surgical clip and abnormally shaped sella indicate that previous transsphenoidal hypophysectomy accounts for absence of the anterior lamina dura.

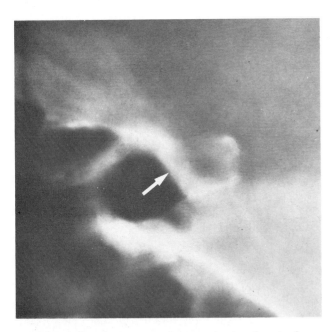

Fig. 1-211. Lateral tomogram. Anterior lamina dura is absent (*arrow*) secondary to transsphenoidal hypophysectomy for microadenoma. Sphenoid sinus is clear.

The sphenoid sinus usually does not appear clouded on baseline studies postoperatively, irrespective of surgical approach, provided that the radiologic examination is performed after the acute postoperative period. This probably is a reflection of the difficulty in evaluating this sinus rather than the uniqueness of the sphenoid sinus. The mucoperiosteal margins can be poorly defined. On lateral tomograms the site of surgical bone removal may be apparent. CT scans and frontal tomograms allow evaluation of the sinus roof and lateral walls. Thinning or local areas of dehiscence must be noted for future comparison.

Postoperative studies of patients who have had transsphenoidal hypophysectomy reveal a focal area of destruction in the anterior lamina dura. Some diminished aeration of the adjacent sinus cavity may persist. If surgical clips are placed in the pituitary bed, one may make the diagnosis of previous sinotomy with ease, even in the absence of clinical history (Fig. 1-210). Without clips, a destructive lesion in the sinus roof may be misdiagnosed (Fig. 1-211).

□ Radiation therapy

Many tumors that involve the paranasal sinuses are surgically incurable. In such cases radiation therapy is often used as either a curative or a palliative treatment. Changes related to radiation therapy can be superimposed on any previously performed diagnostic or surgical procedures. Initially a nonspecific radiation-induced edematous reaction occurs in the involved mucoperiosteum—a sterile mucositis. Infectious disease during treatment can further complicate the roentgenographic picture. Thus a thickened mucosa may represent tumor, infection, nonspecific radiation-induced edema, or all three. Of these, tumor is clinically the most important to diagnose, and several examinations compared to a baseline study may be the only effective means of roentgenographic evaluation. Any nodular mucosal mass seen on CT scanning must be held highly suspect as being a tumor.

Radiation osteitis can occur in the facial bones and is most often seen in the mandible, where it has a specific radiographic appearance.[125] Changes of radiation osteitis in the paranasal sinuses are rare. Occasionally a thickened, sclerotic bone segment can be seen, suggesting osteitis. This is a nonspecific finding and may be related to infectious osteitis. The diagnosis of radiation osteitis is primarily based on severe localized pain in the presence of these radiologic changes.

The entity of irradiation-induced sarcoma is now well established. It is estimated that the incidence is 0.1% of the 5-year survivors with a latent period between 3 and 40 years.[35] The radiographic characteristics of the sarcomas (osteosarcoma, fibrosarcoma, and chondrosarcoma) will be discussed in the tumor section. Such sarcomas can develop in either normal bone or bone involved with either benign or malignant disease.

□ Tumors

Destructive lesions of the nose and paranasal sinuses comprise a diverse group of diseases that classically have been grouped together with little hope of arriving at a specific radiographic diagnosis. With the advent of complex motion tomography and high resolution multiplanar CT, a systematic approach to differential diagnosis and treatment planning has been attempted. It is only with a combined clinicoradiographic approach that a meaningful prebiopsy differential diagnosis is truly possible.

Accurate anatomic mapping of a lesion also has important therapeutic implications. The size of the lesion and extent of bone destruction are consistently underestimated on plain films. Complex motion tomography is performed in the Caldwell view because of reproducibility and because this single view reveals the most overall information compared to the lateral, base, Waters, and straight AP frontal views. The CT scans are performed if possible without and with contrast enhancement and in both the axial and coronal projections (see p. 39).

Tumors of the paranasal sinuses are classified on the basis of bone destruction. Although a specific diagnosis can be offered in only a few individual cases, certain disease groups can be ruled out or placed low on the list of differential diagnosis—particularly when the radiologic information is coupled with clinical history. In selected cases the radiographic findings can actually dictate the treatment planning.

■ Important clinical correlates

It is worthwhile to make some general statements regarding monosinus disease because this condition offers the greatest challenge in tumor diagnosis. Allergic sinusitis rarely if ever affects only one sinus cavity, and unilateral multisinus disease is also uncommon. Inflammatory sinusitis often affects only one sinus and is frequently asymmetric or unilateral. Ostia obstruction may be a result of edema and inflammatory mucosal changes. Occasionally, a tumor that can be obscured by an inflammatory response may be the true cause of osteal obstruction.[119] Careful clinical and radiographic evaluation of unilateral or solitary sinusitis is therefore necessary. If the clinical course is either prolonged or unusual, further clinical and specific radiographic evaluation is indicated.

The presence of pain denotes infection. Although an adequate explanation is lacking, extensive bone remodeling or destruction, whether caused by benign or ma-

lignant disease, is unaccompanied by either local or diffuse pain *unless* infection is also present. The absence of pain must not be interpreted as a sign of tumor absence but merely as the lack of an active infection, either bacterial or fungal.

■ Bone destruction

The concept that radiographic patterns of bone destruction are related to tumor growth rate is not new.[37,120] Aggressive, growing neoplasms comprise group 1 lesions. These lesions destroy the surrounding bone rapidly and do not allow remodeling or expansion. The bone is focally destroyed, demineralized, or both. Its original presence is often demonstrable only microscopically. A soft-tissue nodular mass, usually the tumor process itself, is associated (Fig. 1-212). This can be helpful in differentiating between bone loss secondary to previous surgery and tumor destruction. Postoperative fibrosis can mimic the soft-tissue tumor mass. Usually, however, postoperative fibrosis is smooth in contour, unlike the nodular tumor (Fig. 1-224).

Group 2 destructive lesions have two main radiographic findings: *focal destruction* coupled with *hyperostotic* or reactive bone (Fig. 1-213). Superimposed chronic infection with osteomyelitis makes up the vast majority of this group. The combination of these roentgenographic findings reflects the alternating character of the disease process. There are periods of aggressive

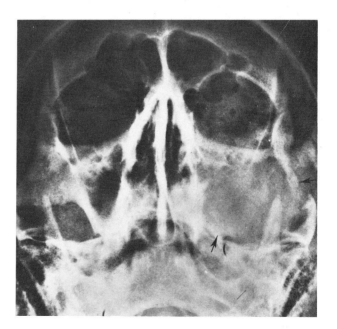

Fig. 1-212. Waters view of group 1 aggressive bone destruction. There is soft tissue mass in left antrum with complete destruction of lateral antral wall and portions of zygoma (*arrows*). *Squamous cell carcinoma of antrum.*

tumor growth interspersed with periods of relative quiescence, allowing the reactive bone to form. Rarely, anaplastic carcinomas and lymphoepitheliomas can cause an unexplained osteoblastic bone reaction. Sclerotic bone may also be seen in recurrent tumors after previous radiation therapy. On the whole, the association of tumor and dense bone is far less frequent than that seen in infectious diseases.

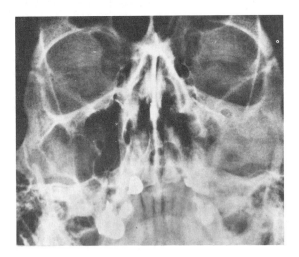

Fig. 1-213. Waters view of group 2 bone destruction. There is soft tissue mass in left antrum with destruction of lateral wall and thickening of antral roof. *Chronic osteomyelitis.*

A group 3 lesion has as its primary finding an expansion of the involved cavity that may or may not be associated with areas of bone destruction. The expansion is at the margins of the tumor, and any destruction within the confines of the mass is not considered critically because the soft tissue mass often obscures the bone and simulates destruction (Figs. 1-214 and 1-215). Occasionally, segmental bone destruction can be seen at the periphery; even in these instances, however, the lesion should be classified as a group 3 lesion if there are other areas of intact bone around an expanded cavity. The cavity expansion is the result of bone remodeling; i.e., new bone is laid down on the outer bony margin while the inner margin is destroyed by pressure or tumor invasion.

It should be noted that there is little relationship between the radiographic appearance of lack of aggressiveness implied by the rate of tumor growth, allowing bone remodeling, and the biologic aggressiveness of the tumor process. With the exception of mucoceles and benign polyps, all the other lesions causing group 3 changes are malignant, and most are *highly* malignant, having 5-year survival rates lower than those of squamous cell carcinoma of the sinuses.

Because a number of these diseases can vary in their clinical presentation and course, their roentgenographic appearance, and even the histologic evaluation of their aggressiveness, the designation of "benign" or "malignant" is inappropriate for this presentation. Certain tumors that look alike on roentgenographic examination and are histologically similar behave biologically quite

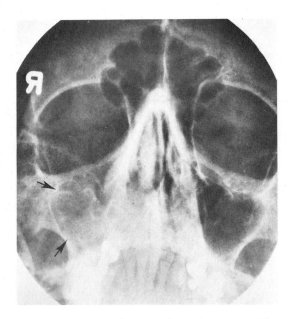

Fig. 1-214. Waters view of group 3 bone destruction. There is complete clouding of the right antrum *(arrows)*, which may be minimally enlarged compared to left side. No bone destruction is seen. *Antral mucocele.*

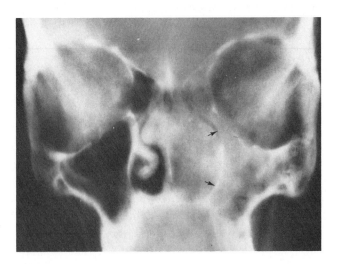

Fig. 1-215. Coronal tomogram of group 3 bone destruction. There is an expansile left nasal cavity mass that has bowed lateral nasal wall outward *(arrows)*. Clouding of left ethmoid sinuses and antrum is secondary to obstruction. *Chronic nasal polyp.*

differently. The true malignant nature of some tumors rests finally with the particular patient.

A classification based on the cell of origin and the particular organ system has been chosen. When applicable, if a specific roentgenographic appearance is not identified with a tumor, the grouping of its destructive patterns will be given according to the earlier discussion.

■ Ectodermal neoplasm

There are a few benign ectodermal neoplasms. The adenoma is a rare, localized polyplike tumor of glandular origin that occurs in the nasal cavity, paranasal sinuses, and nasopharynx. It should not be confused with the adenomatous polyp (already discussed in the section on inflammatory diseases).

The keratotic or fungiform papilloma occurs at the mucocutaneous junction of the cartilagenous septum and is a small, wartlike growth with no roentgenographic manifestations.[13]

The inverting papilloma is the most common of these lesions although it comprises only about 4% of the tumors of the nasal cavity and paranasal sinuses. There is a male predominance and a lack of an allergic history. Inverting papillomas arise from the transitional or Schneiderian epithelium of the lateral nasal wall near the junction of the ethmoid and maxillary sinuses,[134] and they commonly extend into these sinuses. As with all papillomas, there is a high tendency to recur, with between 25% to 50% recurring at least once; 70% of patients have a history of prior nasal surgery.[136] Alarmingly 10% to 13% percent of patients have either cellular atypia or associated invasive squamous cell carcinoma.[6,60]

Radiographically, inverting papillomas are almost always expansile, unilateral nasal masses. If the tumor is unusually large, it may displace the nasal septum, but it usually will not extend across the midline. Extension into the ipsilateral ethmoid sinus and maxillary antrum is common (Figs. 1-216 to 1-218).

The cylindrical cell papilloma is quite rare and has the same distribution, malignant potential, and roentgenographic appearance as the inverting papilloma.

Of the premalignant lesions, leukoplakia has no roentgenographic manifestations and is a purely clinical diagnosis, as is the malignant carcinoma in situ.

Squamous cell carcinomas are the most common malignant tumors of the paranasal sinuses and nasal cavity. They comprise between 80% to 90% of all neoplasms affecting these areas. Tumors of the nasal cavity repre-

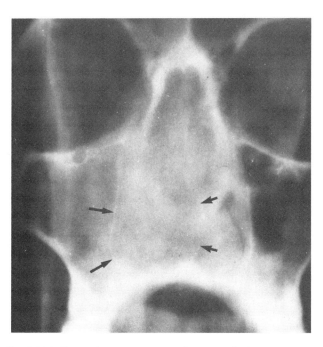

Fig. 1-216. Coronal tomogram reveals expansile homogeneous right nasal mass with secondary obstruction and clouding of antrum. Nasal septum *(small arrows)* and lateral nasal wall *(large arrows)* are bowed outwards by mass. *Inverting papilloma.*

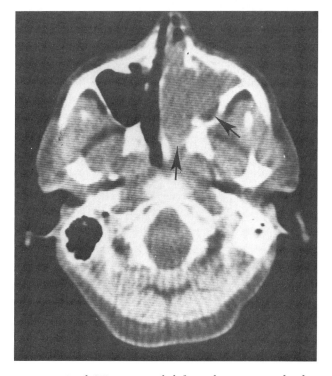

Fig. 1-217. Axial CT scan reveals left nasal cavity mass that has broken into left antrum and extends posteriorly into nasopharynx *(arrows)*. Mass stops at midline and has preserved nasal septum. *Inverting papilloma.*

sent about 10% of these squamous cell tumors. The disease primarily affects males (a 2:1 ratio), and 95% of patients are over the age of 40 years. Chronic sinusitis or nasal polyps precede or are associated in about 15% of cases. Squamous cell carcinomas arise on the lateral wall (turbinates) in 50% of cases.[3] About 80% of all cancers in the paranasal sinuses arise in the maxillary antra.[124] Eighty percent of the antral neoplasms are squamous cell carcinomas. All the tumors have a soft tissue mass in the sinus cavity on initial roentgenographic examination. There is roentgenographic evidence of bone destruction in 70% to 90% of cases.[25,67] This bone destruction represents the classic group 1 lesions, i.e., aggressive destruction with no cavity expansion (Figs. 1-212 and 1-219 to 1-226).[121]

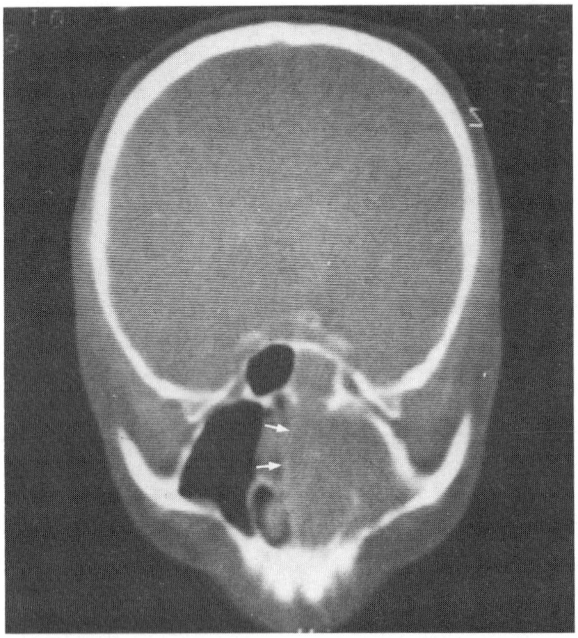

Fig. 1-218. Coronal CT scan of left-sided mass extending into posterior ethmoid and sphenoid sinuses as well as left antrum. Bony margins are all preserved, as is nasal septum *(arrows)*, which is slightly bowed to right. *Inverting papilloma.*

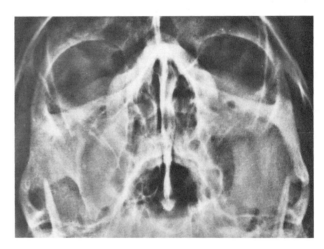

Fig. 1-219. Waters view reveals extensive group 1 destruction of the left lateral antral wall. *Squamous cell carcinoma of antrum.*

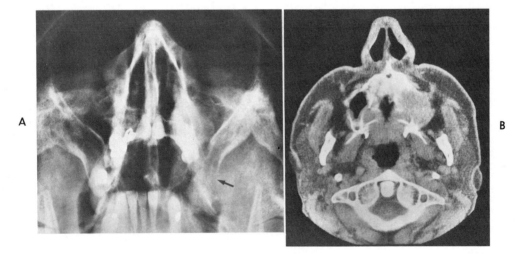

Fig. 1-220. A, Waters view reveals destruction of lower left lateral antral wall *(arrow)* and alveolus with clouding of antrum. *Squamous cell carcinoma.* **B,** Axial CT scan. There is aggressively destructive lesion of lower left antrum and hard palate. Bone is not displaced around mass and lesion infiltrates soft tissues of cheek.

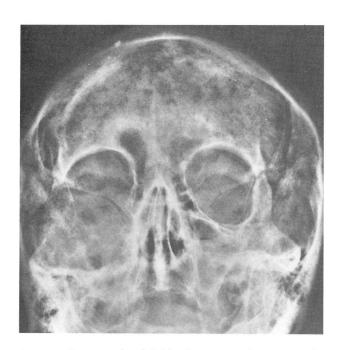

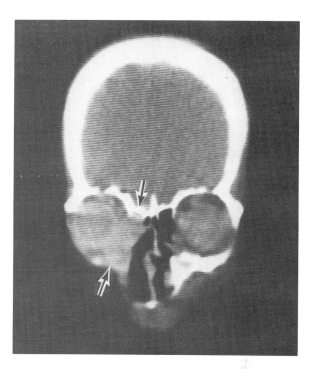

Fig. 1-221. Over-angulated Caldwell view reveals extensive destruction of right orbital floor and lateral wall. Body of right zygoma and right antrum are also destroyed. Chronic reactive sclerosis is seen around frontal sinuses, indicating chronic infection. *Squamous cell carcinoma of right antrum with extension.*

Fig. 1-222. Coronal CT scan reveals destructive lesion of right orbital floor, maxilla, and ethmoid. Mass has invaded orbital structures, pushing globe laterally and effacing periorbital fat planes. *Squamous cell carcinoma.*

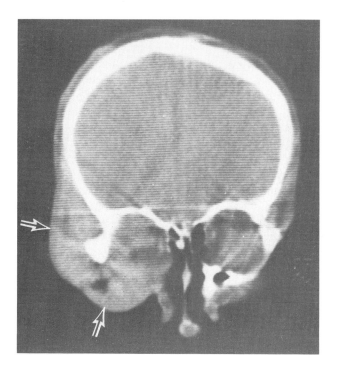

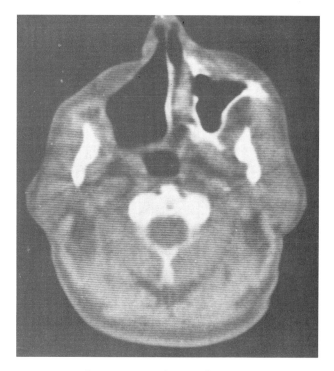

Fig. 1-223. Coronal CT scan after right maxillectomy with tumor present over maxillary region and lateral orbital wall on right. Tumor extends into right temporal fossa *(arrows)*. *Squamous cell carcinoma.*

Fig. 1-224. Axial CT scan reveals normal postoperative appearance after right maxillectomy. Note smooth soft tissue contour.

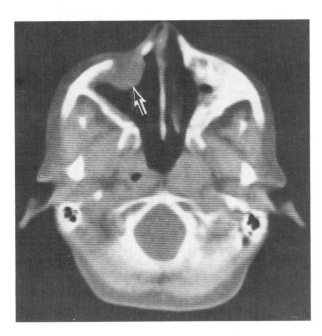

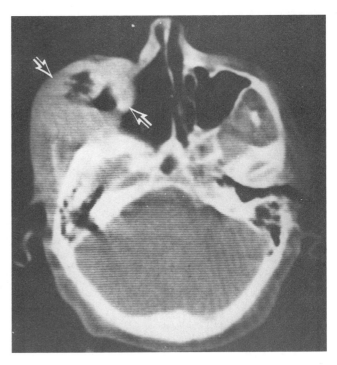

Fig. 1-225. Axial CT scan after partial maxillectomy. Soft tissue nodular mass is seen anteriorly *(arrow)* (compare to smooth contour of Fig. 1-227). *Recurrent squamous cell carcinoma.* Note reactive bone in left antrum after infection and radiation.

Fig. 1-226. Axial CT scan after radical right maxillectomy. Soft tissue mass has nodular contour on antral side and extends into temporal fossa *(arrows)*. *Recurrent squamous cell carcinoma.*

Thus a clouded antrum with group 1 type of bone destruction has about an 80% chance of being a squamous cell carcinoma.

Between 10% and 20% of squamous cell carcinomas occur in the ethmoid sinuses; only isolated cases occur in the frontal and sphenoid sinuses. Frontal ostial obstruction by carcinoma can result in a frontal mucocele that may disguise the underlying tumor.[37,54,104] Statistically, patients with frontal and sphenoid carcinomas have the poorest prognosis, with few patients surviving 2 years. The overall 5-year survival rate for all patients with squamous cell carcinomas is between 25% and 30%. This indicates the inability to establish an early diagnosis. The best results appear to be from combined radiotherapy and surgery.[6,134]

The anaplastic squamous cell carcinoma can be confused histologically with melanoma, plasmacytoma, embryonal rhabdomyosarcoma, histiocytic lymphoma, and esthesioneuroblastoma. Under electron microscopy, desmosomes identify the cells as carcinoma cells.

Between 4% and 8% of tumors in the nasal cavity and paranasal sinuses arise from glandular elements of the mucosa.[81] The majority of these tumors are either adenoid cystic carcinomas (cylindromas) or adenocarcinomas. Benign and malignant mixed tumors and other glandular tumors are extremely rare. Approximately

one half (4%) of glandular tumors are tumors of minor salivary gland origin. The minor salivary glands are distributed throughout the oral cavity, nasal cavity, sinuses, larynx, trachea, bronchi, and lacrimal glands.[102]

The cylindroma (or adenoid cystic carcinoma) is the most common malignant tumor of the minor salivary glands. There is no sex predominance and the peak age incidence is 40 to 50 years. Most cylindromas occur in the palate (50%). The maxillary sinus is next most frequently affected. Between 20% and 30% of cylindromas have distant metastases, primarily to bone and lung. The 5-year survival rate for patients with cylindromas is only 5% to 10%, and 10-year survivors are extremely rare. Cylindromas have been found to contain two distinct cell types, i.e., the myoepithelial (type A) and the secretory (type B). The type A cells have been shown to survive irradiation.[101] Early invasion of the perineural tissues is also common, and this may occur at some distance from the tumor bed.[5] Thus a normal tumor margin on a surgical specimen may be deceiving and may explain the low cure rate. Surgery is still the treatment of choice. Radiographically, this is a group 3 destructive lesion (Figs. 1-227 and 1-228). In rare cases this tumor exhibits group 1 aggressive destruction, but far more often some cavity expansion is evident.

The true incidence of *primary adenocarcinoma* is dif-

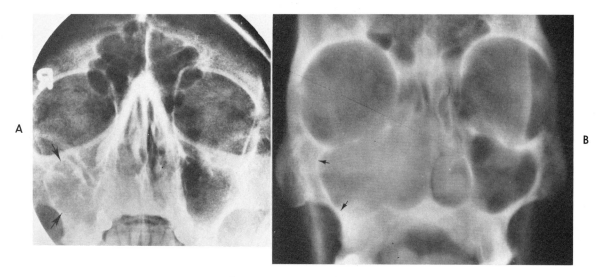

Fig. 1-227. A, Waters view reveals opacification of right antrum and no obvious bone destruction. **B,** Coronal tomogram reveals clouding of right antrum and nasal cavity with destruction of intervening medial antral wall. Right antrum is slightly enlarged compared to left antrum (*arrows*), and most of bony tumor margins are intact (with exception of focal areas of orbital floor and medial wall). *Cylindroma.*

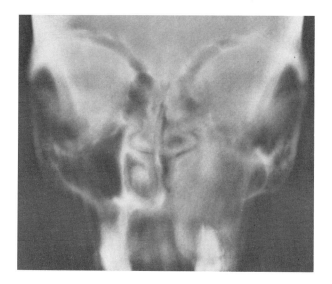

Fig. 1-228. Coronal tomogram reveals an expansile tumor of left antrum that has also destroyed portions of left alveolus and hard palate. Extension into left ethmoid sinuses is also present. *Cylindroma.*

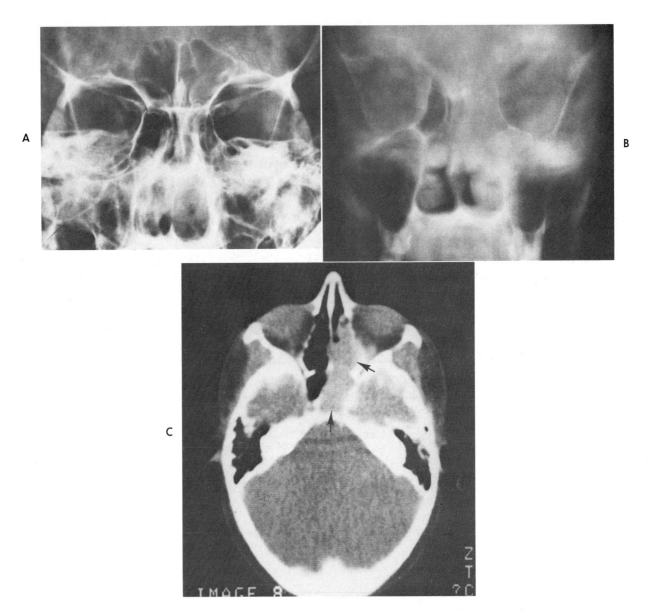

Fig. 1-229. A, Caldwell view reveals haziness of left ethmoid sinuses and upper nasal cavity. There is no obvious bone destruction. **B,** Coronal tomogram reveals tumor mass in left ethmoid sinuses, upper nasal cavity, and upper antrum. Lamina papyracea is intact. **C,** Axial CT scan reveals tumor mass in left ethmoid and sphenoid sinuses with preservation of nasal septum and lamina. *Adenocarcinoma of ethmoid sinus.*

ficult to assess because of confusion with adenoid cystic carcinoma. Probably close to 4% of the tumors in the nasal cavity and paranasal sinuses are true adenocarcinomas.

There is a distinct predilection of adenocarcinomas for involvement of the ethmoid sinuses. The frontal and sphenoid sinuses appear to be relatively immune to the development of these glandular neoplasms. The Bantu have a high incidence of antroethmoidal adenocarcinoma, presumably related to their use of carcinogenic snuff. Woodworkers in the hardwood furniture industry also have an inexplicably high incidence of adenocarcinoma.[134]

Adenocarcinomas are seen far less often with cervical nodes than are adenoid cystic carcinomas, and the 5-year survival rate is intermediate between squamous cell carcinoma and cylindroma (20%). There is a tendency toward intracranial metastasis. The ethmoid

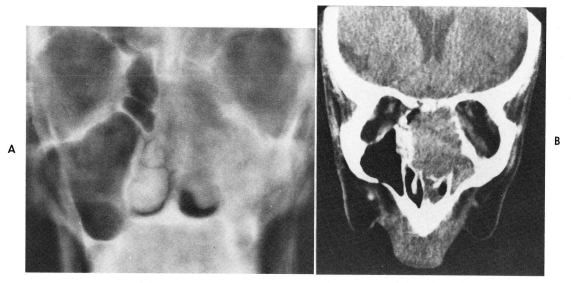

Fig. 1-230. A, Coronal tomogram reveals tumor mass in left nasal cavity and ethmoid and maxillary sinus. Lamina papyracea, orbital floor, and most remaining antral margins are intact. *Malignant mixed tumor of minor salivary gland origin.* **B,** Coronal CT scan. There is expansile nonenhanced tumor of left nasal cavity and ethmoid and maxillary sinuses. *Cylindroma.*

opacification is usually associated with ipsilateral antral disease, with a group 3 destructive pattern (Fig. 1-229).

Rarely, a mixed tumor of minor salivary gland origin is reported. Its roentgenographic characteristics, whether benign or malignant, are those of a group 3 lesion. This same mixed tumor is the most common neoplasm of the major salivary glands (Fig. 1-230).

■ Neurogenic neoplasms

One difficulty in discussing tumors of the peripheral nervous system is the confusing and overlapping terminology in the older literature. As more sophisticated technology and the use of electron microscopy have emerged, some of the ambiguity has cleared. It appears that the terminology of Schwannoma, neurinoma, neurilemmoma, and perineural fibroblastoma all refer to the same tumor process.[6]

The schwannoma is a solitary, encapsulated tumor that arises in the nerve sheath and thus can often be dissected free of the nerve proper.[5] The schwannoma is often painful, and malignant change is extremely unusual. It is almost never associated with von Recklinghausen's disease. The *neurofibroma*, on the other hand, is a distinct tumor that is nonencapsulated, is intimately associated with the nerve proper, and cannot be dissected free of the involved nerve. Neurofibromas usually are multiple and have approximately an 8% chance of malignant degeneration.[89] Neurofibromas usually are

nontender and can occur as either solitary or multiple tumors with or without the association of von Recklinghausen's disease.

Neurofibromatosis is a hamartomatous disorder that is transmitted as an autosomal dominant trait with variable penetrance. The syndrome includes cafe au lait spots, acoustic "neuromas" (neurofibromas) and bone lesions, many of which are characteristic of von Recklinghausen's disease.[58]

The neurogenic sarcoma is usually firm, lobulated, and circumscribed. Pain and paresthesias can be associated if a large nerve is involved. The prognosis is poor in these malignancies and hematogenous metastases can occur.

Radiographically, all these tumors are slow growing and remodel adjacent bone structures (group 3 destructive lesions). These tumors can occur along major nerve trunks or along peripheral nerve branches. As such, the nerve or origin is often not identified. Because 44.8% of solitary neurofibromas and schwannomas occur in the head and neck region,[29] they must be considered in any differential diagnosis thereof. Most of these tumors occur outside of the sinus cavities. If they occur in the infratemporal fossa, bowing of the posterior antral wall can superficially mimic a juvenile angiofibroma (Fig. 1-231).[122] If they occur within the sinus cavity, differentiation from other group 3 lesions may be impossible (Fig. 1-232).[17] The radiographic differentiation of the

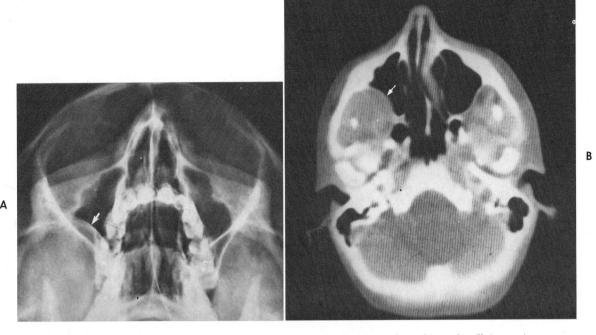

Fig. 1-231. A, Waters view reveals anterior bowing of right posterolateral antral wall *(arrow)*. **B,** Axial CT scan reveals right retromaxillary mass that has bowed posterior antral wall forward *(arrow)*. Absence of nasopharyngeal mass makes angiofibroma very unlikely. *Schwannoma of pterygomaxillary fossa.*

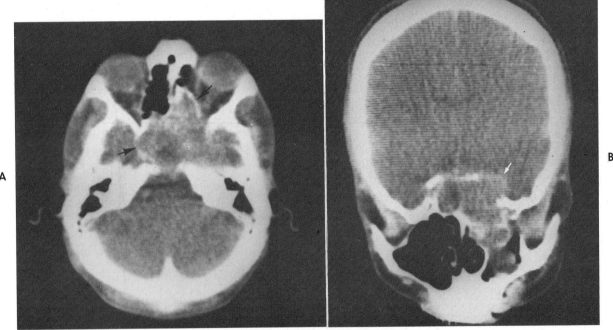

Fig. 1-232. A, Axial CT scan reveals mass in sphenoid sinus and left posterior ethmoid sinuses. Sinus margins are bowed outward and are intact with exception of left sphenoid sinus wall *(arrows)*. **B,** Coronal CT scan reveals sphenoid sinus mass that has pushed out sinus walls to extend intracranially *(arrow)*. It also has broken through sinus floor and extends into left antrum. *Schwannoma of sphenoid sinus.*

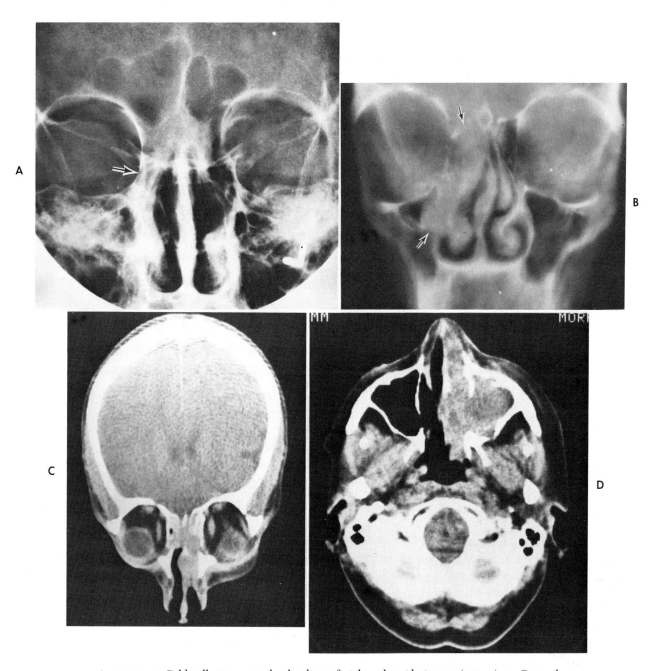

Fig. 1-233. A, Caldwell view reveals clouding of right ethmoid sinuses *(arrow).* **B,** Coronal tomogram reveals mass in right ethmoid sinus extending into right maxilla. Lamina papyracea is intact. Cribriform plate is obscured but was surgically proven intact. **C,** Coronal CT scan on different patient. There is soft tissue enhanced mass in left nasal cavity. Some ethmoid septal destruction is present on left, bone is intact on right side. *Esthesioneuroblastoma.* **D,** Axial CT scan. There is minimally enhanced expansile mass in left nasal cavity that extends into left antrum. *Esthesioneuroblastoma.*

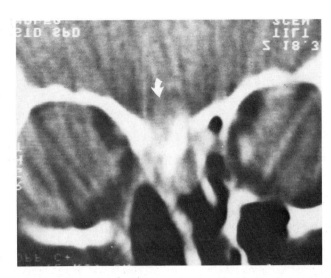

Fig. 1-234. Coronal CT scan with contrast enhancement reveals upper nasal cavity and ethmoid mass that extends intracranially *(arrow)*. Both lamina papyracea are intact. *Esthesioneuroblastoma.*

histologic type and the benignity or malignancy of the lesion is impossible. In CT scanning, most of these tumors enhance nonhomogeneously because of areas of hemorrhage and cystic degeneration within the tumor.

Other peripheral nerve tumors, such as granular cell myoblastomas (benign and malignant) and neuroepitheliomas, very rarely occur in the paranasal sinuses.

The *esthesioneuroblastoma* (olfactory neuroblastoma) is a neoplasm of neuroectodermal origin. It is a polypoid tumor that resembles an inflammatory nasal polyp. Most occur between 10 and 34 years of age. The tumors occur in the upper third of the nasal septum, the superior and supreme nasal turbinates, and the cribriform plate.[91] The ethmoid sinuses and then the maxillary sinuses are the most often involved secondarily (Figs. 1-233, *A* to *C* and 1-234). Rarely, extension into the other sinus cavities occurs.[8,90] Distant metastases (primarily to the cervical nodes and lungs) are reported in about 20% of cases. About 11% of cases have intracranial extension necessitating a combined otolaryngologic-neurosurgical approach.[91] No prediction as to the biologic behavior of the tumor can be made either radiographically or histologically. Some will be slow-growing and others will be markedly aggressive. There is a high incidence of late recurrences. Although some of these tumors may be radiosensitive, few if any are radiocurable, and combined radiation and surgery is the treatment of choice. This tumor can often be confused microscopically with anaplastic carcinoma, malignant melanoma, plasmacytoma, embryonal rhabdomyosarcoma, and histiocystic lymphoma. Electron microscopy demonstrates

secretory granules (catecholamine granules) characteristic of this tumor. The 5-year survival rate is about 50%; however, nearly 50% of these survivors die in the next 5-year period.

■ **Meningiomas**

In the vast majority of cases, extracranial meningiomas are actually extensions from intracranial tumors. However, primary extracranial meningiomas have been reported in the paranasal sinus, facial bones, skin, and nasal cavity.* The present theory of meningioma origin is that arachnoid cell rests are left behind during embryonic development.

Nasal or sinus meningiomas are seen radiographically as soft tissue masses that expand the involved space and remodel the adjacent bony walls as a group 3 lesion (Figs. 1-235 and 1-236). The hyperostotic reaction that often accompanies meningioma can simulate a group 2 lesion, although the primary finding is one of cavity expansion rather than aggressive bone destruction. Calcification may be present and suggest the diagnosis. CT scans not only aid in detecting calcification but also delineate any intracranial component of the tumor. A rare osteoblastoma of the ethmoid sinuses (Fig. 1-252) can closely mimic the roentgenographic appearance.[116]

Malignant melanomas comprise about 3.6% of nasal cavity and paranasal sinus neoplasms.[91] These represent less than 1% of all malignant melanomas and 10% of the mucous membrane melanomas. The peak age inci-

_____
*References 55, 71, 91, 95, 130.

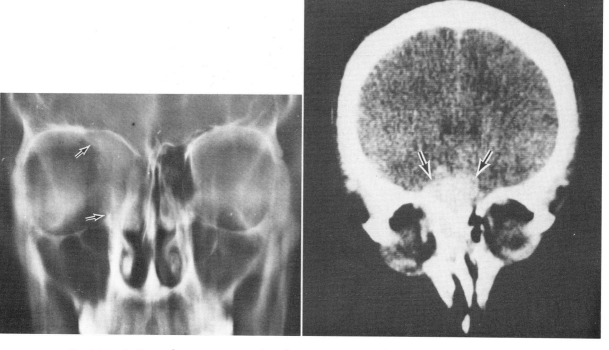

Fig. 1-235. A, Coronal tomogram reveals soft tissue mass in right frontal and ethmoid region that has broken through into orbit. **B,** Coronal CT scan with contrast enhancement reveals densely staining mass in right frontoethmoid area that extends intracranially. *Meningioma extending into paranasal sinuses.*

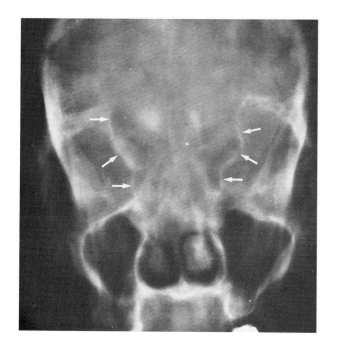

Fig. 1-236. Coronal tomogram reveals widening of orbital roofs and ethmoid complex *(arrows)* by soft tissue mass with calcification. *Meningioma extending into nasal cavity.*

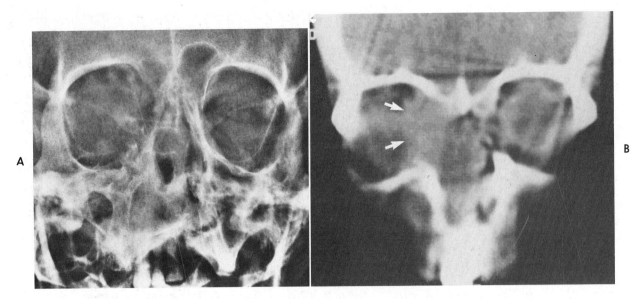

Fig. 1-237. A, Caldwell view reveals clouding of right ethmoid and maxilla with destruction of medial orbital wall and portion of floor. **B,** Coronal CT scan reveals mass in nasal cavity and right ethmoid sinuses with destruction of right lamina *(arrow). Malignant melanoma.*

dence is the fourth to sixth decades. Unilateral nasal obstruction or epistaxis is the usual presenting symptom. Malignant melanomas have a lower incidence of regional lymph node metastases than tumors arising in the skin. The 5-year survival rate is 11% or less. The average survival is only 2 to 3 years and the 10-year survival rate is 0.5%.[50]

The majority of paranasal sinus melanomas arise in the nasal cavity, primarily over the anterior nasal septum and the middle and inferior turbinates. No precursor lesion has been found. They derive de novo from ectodermal crest elements, namely, ectopic melanocytes. The mucous membranes of the nose and paranasal sinuses are rarely involved by metastatic melanomas.

Approximately one third of melanomas are amelanotic, and differentiation from anaplastic carcinoma, esthesioneuroblastoma, plasmacytoma, embryonal rhabdomyosarcoma, and histiocystic lymphoma may be difficult histologically. Final pathologic diagnosis may require electron microscopy, with which intracytoplasmic melanosomes can be demonstrated. This tumor is radioresistant and combined surgery and chemotherapy are the treatments of choice.

Radiographically, these lesions tend to be group 3 lesions with some elements of expansion, although pure group 1 aggressive destruction can also be seen (Figs. 1-237 and 1-238).

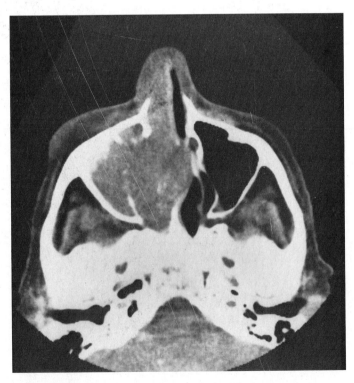

Fig. 1-238. Axial CT scan reveals expansile right nasal cavity mass obstructing right antrum. *Malignant melanoma.*

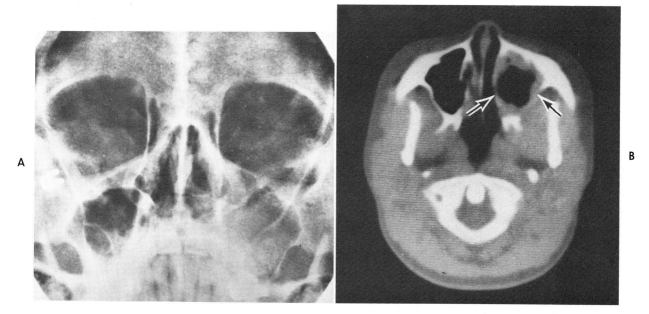

Fig. 1-239. A, Waters view reveals clouding of left antrum with thinning of lateral wall. **B,** Axial CT scan performed after surgical drainage of presumed mucocele reveals thinning or destruction of medial and posterolateral left antral walls, with fairly uniform soft tissue thickening around entire antrum. *Chordoma of antrum.*

Chordomas are dysontogenetic tumors that arise in remnants of the embryonic notochord. There are three major anatomic groups: cranial (clivus), spheno-occipital, and sacrococcygeal. Rarely, chordomas have been reported in the maxilla and mandible.[110] Small derivatives of the distintegrating notochord can become separated and form ectopic rests in the paranasal sinus region.[6,141] Most of the chordomas involving the paranasal sinus are extensions from clivus or high cervical-nasopharyngeal tumors, although isolated chordomas can occur (Fig. 1-239). The combination of bone destruction, soft tissue mass, occasional calcification, and classical location should suggest the diagnosis.

■ **Mesodermal neoplasms**

True mesodermal neoplasms of the nasal cavity and paranasal sinuses are rare. The benign tumors are slightly more common (60% of the cases) than their malignant, sarcomatous counterparts. As a group these sarcomas represent almost 10% of the nasal and paranasal sinus tumors.[13] Approximately 80% of this group are *lymphosarcomas.* They have an equal sex distribution and only 15% have preceding or associated nasal polyposis and sinusitis. They are radiosensitive and as such are the only sarcomas to be radiocurable.[13] The soft tissue sarcomas as a group are not radiosensitive, are more common in females, and have a high association with sinusitis and nasal polyposis. Surgery and chemotherapy are at present the best modes of therapy. Of

the nonepithelial tumors involving this region, 25% are osseous and fibro-osseous lesions.[48] Nonepithelial tumors constitute a heterogenous group of conditions including osteomas, fibrous dysplasia, ossifying fibroma, osteoblastoma, giant cell tumor, and osteogenic sarcoma.

Osteomas have several histologic patterns. The "ivory" type is composed of hard, dense, mature bone, containing only small amounts of fibrous tissue. The "mature" osteomas have mature cancellous bone without dense ivory bone. These tumors are radiographically very dense and well demarcated.

The *fibrous osteoma* contains abundant mature lamellar bone but also a greater amount of intertrabecular fibrous tissue. As a result they are less radiodense and more likely to be confused with a cyst although most fibrous osteomas are not as exquisitely smooth as a cyst or polyp. These osteomas almost always arise at the junction of the membranous and enchondral bone at the frontoethmoidal suture (Figs. 1-240 to 1-243). They remain within the confines of the frontal or ethmoid sinus cavities, abutting on but rarely expanding the sinus walls. They are usually asymptomatic unless they cause obstruction of the sinus ostia with resulting secondary infection (17% of cases).[48] Osteomas in the maxillary and sphenoidal sinuses are rare (Fig. 1-244). If multiple osteomas of the facial bones and calvarium are seen, Gardner's syndrome should be considered (Fig. 1-245). Of all the benign paranasal sinus tumors, only

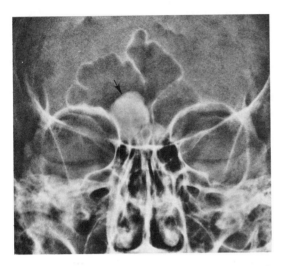

Fig. 1-240. Caldwell view. Dense bony lesion in right frontal sinus extends upward from the frontoethmoid plate *(arrow)*. *Osteoma.*

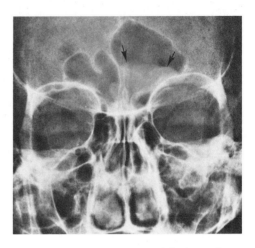

Fig. 1-241. Caldwell view reveals ground glass soft tissue mass in left frontal sinus growing upward from frontoethmoid plate *(arrow)*. This is too dense to be polyp or cyst. *Soft osteoma.*

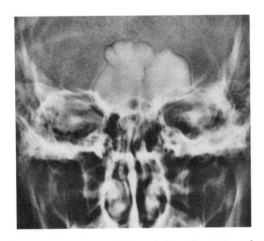

Fig. 1-242. PA view reveals large bilateral osteoma that has conformed to sinus contour.

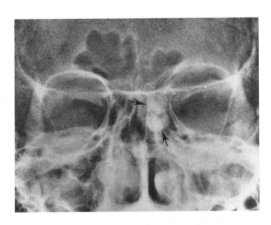

Fig. 1-243. Caldwell view reveals dense mass in left ethmoid extending downward from frontoethmoid plate. *Osteoma.*

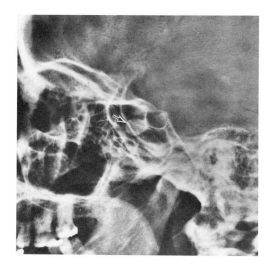

Fig. 1-244. Lateral view reveals dense spherical lesion in sphenoid sinus growing off posterior wall. *Osteoma.*

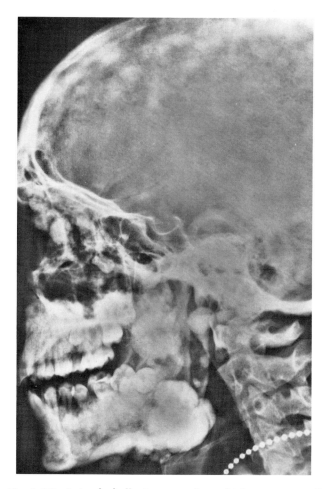

Fig. 1-245. Lateral skull view reveals multiple osteomas of mandible and facial bone as well as calvarium. *Gardner's syndrome.*

the osteoma is associated with spontaneous cerebrospinal fluid rhinorrhea.[110]

Fibrous dysplasia histologically has fibrous bone and no osteoblasts. It may represent a hamartomatous malformation.[48] Fibrous dysplasia can be monostotic or polyostotic. This latter form may be associated with the systemic manifestations of Albright's syndrome. The monostotic lesions are 20 to 30 times more common. They are first noticed early in life, grow rapidly in childhood, and tend to stabilize in adult life.[134] The patients usually exhibit facial asymmetry that can become quite severe (leontiasis ossea).

Radiographically, the tissue density of the lesions depends on the degree of fibrous tissue present. Either a "ground glass" appearance or a dense bony appearance is seen. Facial bone involvement is almost always asymmetric (Figs. 1-246 to 1-248). Secondary encroachment by this expansile process into the sinus cavities, nasal cavity, and orbit can simulate dense soft tissue masses or the reactive changes associated with a meningioma.

The *ossifying fibroma* has highly cellular fibrous tissue with less mature and less organized osseous tissue than the fibrous osteoma. There is also more osteoblastic activity present. These lesions occur mainly in the maxilla but have been reported in all the facial bones.[48] Painless soft tissue swelling and redness have been reported in the overlying facial tissues. Radiographically, these lesions tend to encroach into the sinus cavity rather than expand the outer table and deform the facial structures. Gross calcifications can be seen and the sinus mucoperiosteum, pushed inward into the sinus cavity by the expanding sinus wall lesion, can appear as

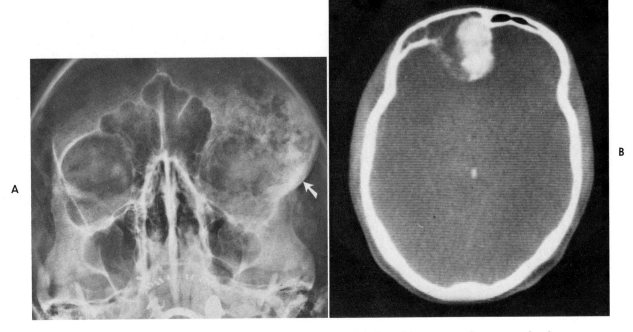

Fig. 1-246. A, Waters view reveals mottled lesion of left frontal bone extending into orbital roof. Thickening of lateral calvarium can be well seen *(arrow)*. *Fibrous dysplasia.* **B,** Axial CT scan. There is widening of right frontal bone. Diplöe is thickened by both bone density and soft tissue density (fibrous) material. *Fibrous dysplasia.*

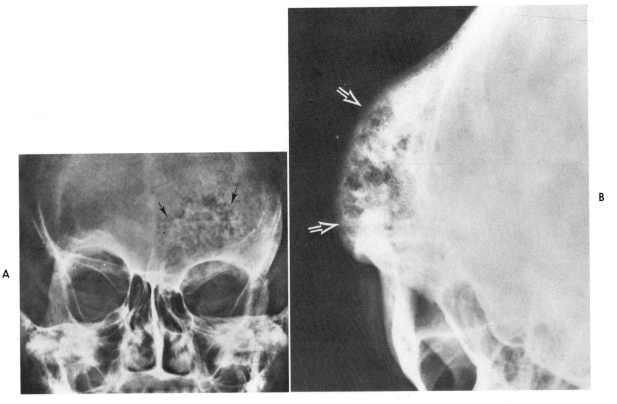

Fig. 1-247. A, Caldwell view reveals mottled lesion of left frontal bone (arrows), which has depressed left orbital roof. **B,** Coned-down lateral skull view reveals mottled expansile process in frontal bone *(arrows)*.

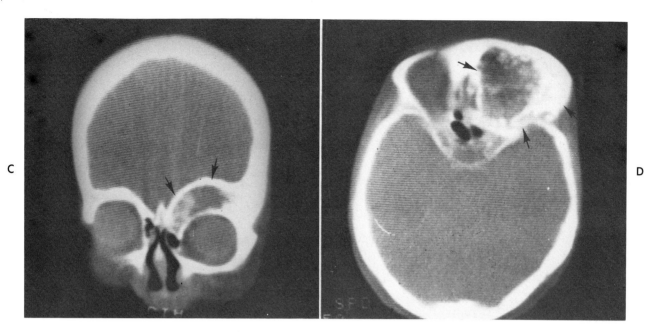

C

D

Fig. 1-247, cont'd. C, Coronal CT scan reveals expansion of left orbital roof with areas of decreased and increased density in diplöe *(arrows)*. **D,** Axial CT scan reveals expansion of left frontal bone with mottled appearance *(arrows)*. *Fibrous dysplasia.*

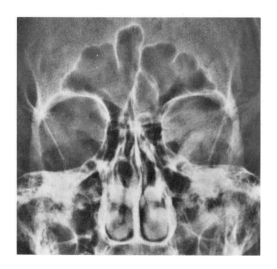

Fig. 1-248. Caldwell view reveals areas of increased density over left posterior orbital wall with narrowing of superior orbital fissure. This could represent hyperostotic reaction to a meningioma; however, this was *fibrous dysplasia.*

a calcified rim. A rim of air remaining in the sinus can almost always be identified, which is a differential point from a mucocele (Figs. 1-249 and 1-250).

Occasionally the bone expansion can be subtle, particularly in a thick bone such as the zygoma, and only a vague alteration in the appearance of the bone will suggest an abnormality (Fig. 1-251, *A* and *B*).

Both the pathologist and radiologist may have great difficulty in differentiating between certain cases of fibrous dysplasia and ossifying fibroma.

Osteoblastoma is a rare tumor in the paranasal sinuses.[12] Most frequently it affects the vertebral neural arches, long bones, and small bones of the hands and feet, although several cases have been found in the ethmoid sinuses.[40,46,48,116] Clinically, pain is present that is often quite severe and may be insidious in onset. It is often worse at night and unlike the pain of an osteoid osteoma, it is not relieved by aspirin. Frequently, soft tissue swelling and erythema may overlie the lesion.

Osteoblastomas have been classified as either benign or aggressive. The benign type rarely recurs; the aggressive type tends to recur locally but does not have distant metastases as does osteogenic sarcoma. Radiographically, these are soft tissue expansile masses with scattered areas of calcification or bone formation. Gross areas of organized bone formation can also be seen (Fig. 1-252). The differential diagnosis must include meningioma and osteogenic sarcoma.

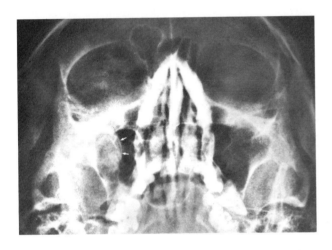

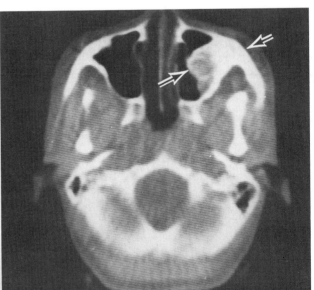

Fig. 1-249. Waters view reveals thickening of entire right lateral antral wall, which has pushed sinus mucoperiosteal line medially *(arrows)*. There was no facial deformity. *Ossifying fibroma.*

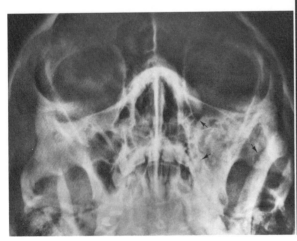

Fig. 1-250. A, Waters view reveals mottled expansile lesion of left maxilla and zygoma *(arrows)*, which has pushed lateral sinus wall medially. **B,** Axial CT scan reveals bony, mixed-density expansile lesion of left maxilla and zygoma with no significant external facial deformity *(arrows)*. *Ossifying fibroma.*

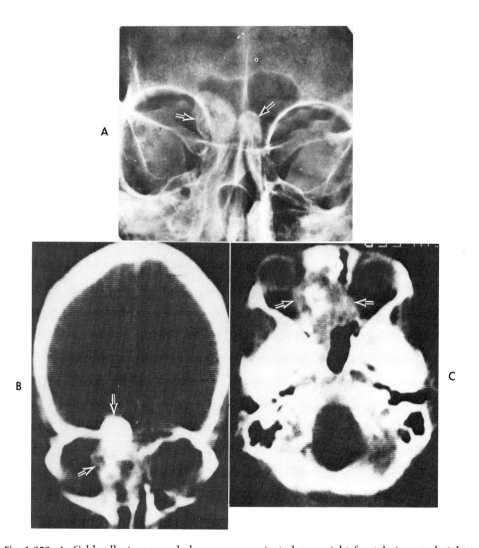

Fig. 1-251. A, Waters view reveals soft tissue swelling over right zygoma and inferior orbital rim *(arrows).* **B,** Coronal tomogram reveals expansile lytic lesion of right zygoma *(arrows).* This could be fibrous dysplasia but was read as *ossifying fibroma.*

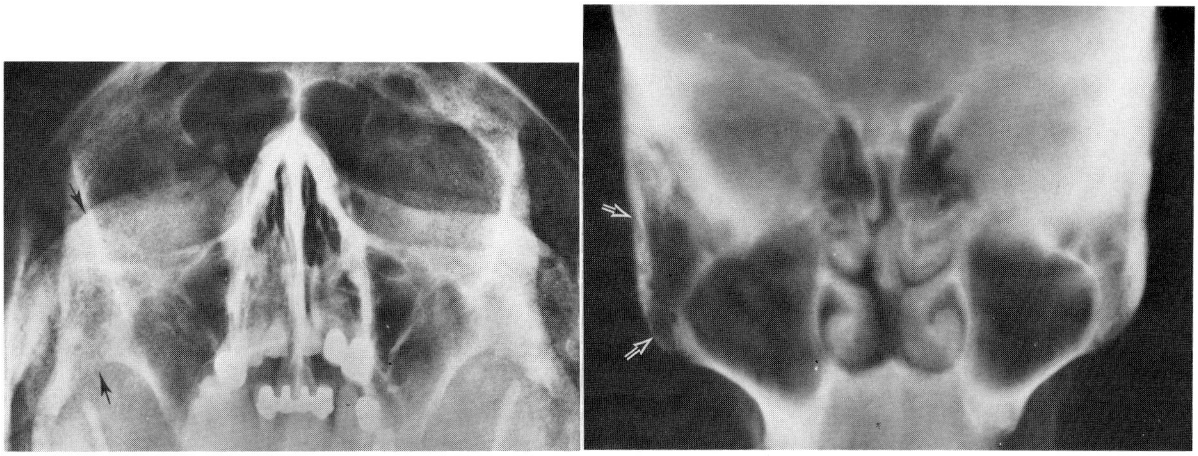

Fig. 1-252. A, Caldwell view reveals bony mass projected over right frontal sinus and right orbit *(arrows).* Clouding of right ethmoid sinus is also present. **B,** Coronal CT scan without contrast enhancement reveals dense bone density lesion extending intracranially but extradurally and mixed dense and lytic lesion of ethmoid sinuses and nasal cavity that has broken into right orbit *(arrows).* **C,** Axial CT scan reveals ethmoid mass of mixed density extending into orbit *(arrows). Osteoblastoma.*

Osteogenic sarcoma involving the nasal cavity and paranasal sinuses is rare. It is a nonhomogeneous soft tissue destructive (group 1 type) mass. The maxillary sinuses (most commonly) and ethmoid sinuses are involved most often.[48,72] CT scans delineate both the ossified and nonossified components. Although these findings are highly suggestive of osteogenic sarcoma, the plain film finding of a "sun burst" periosteal reaction is diagnostic (Fig. 1-253, *A* and *B*). These tumors are highly aggressive, and combined radiation therapy, chemotherapy, and radical surgery have had little success in preventing metastases.[6,48] The 5-year survival rate is reported to vary between 11% and 30%.

Giant cell tumors involving the paranasal sinuses primarily affect the maxilla and are usually in relationship to the alveolar ridges. They occur in two clinical forms that are histologically indistinguishable. The peripheral (soft tissue) type is four times more common than the central type and involves the alveolar mucosa. It is usually related to previous tooth extraction and the underlying bone is uninvolved. In the less common central (bone) type, extensive bone destruction may be present and there is often a history of antecendent trauma.

The radiographic findings in cases of giant cell tumors are those of a purely lytic expansile lesion that cannot be differentiated radiographically or histologically from the "brown tumor" of hyperparathyroidism (Fig. 1-254).

Only laboratory testing can resolve the differential diagnosis. The brown tumors are more common in primary than in secondary hyperparathyroidism.[47] The "true" giant cell tumor that affects the peripheral skeleton is extremely rare in the maxilla. It generally occurs after the age of 20 years whereas the giant cell reparative granulomas tend to occur before age 20 years. These two tumors can be differentiated histologically although they are radiographically similar.[114] Curettage is the treatment of choice for all these lesions. The odontogenic reparative granuloma is an inflammatory lesion that is a separate entity related to the roots of the teeth and that is only confused because of its name.

Cherubism is a genetic condition affecting bilaterally first the mandible and then, in two thirds of the cases, the maxilla. The lesions appear between 2 and 4 years of age, increase in size until about 7 years of age, and then tend to slowly regress.[134] Histologically and radiographically they resemble the reparative granulomas. The symmetric appearance of the lesions suggests the diagnosis.

Ewing's sarcoma is an uncommon malignancy that arises from the primitive mesenchyme of the medullary cavity of bone. In about 2% of cases the mandible is involved; the maxilla is involved only one eighth as often.[117] Characteristically, there is an "onion skin" type of periosteal reaction that reflects aggressive tumor el-

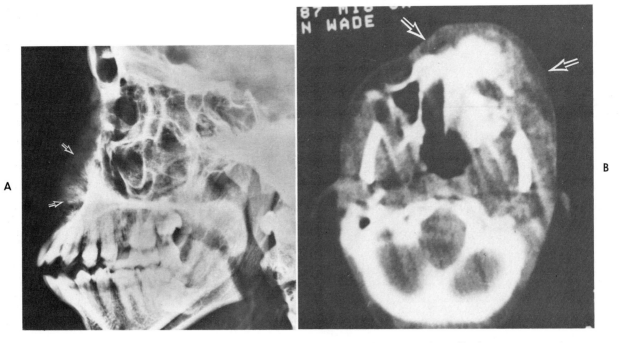

Fig. 1-253. A, Lateral skull view reveals "sunburst" periosteal reaction of maxilla characteristic of osteogenic sarcoma (*arrows*). **B,** Axial CT scan reveals not only dense osseous portion of tumor but also extensive noncalcified extension over face and cheek (*arrows*). *Osteogenic sarcoma.*

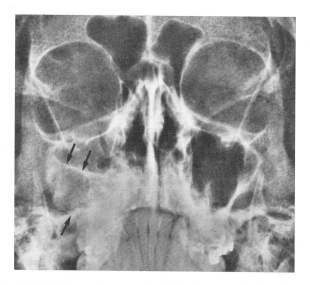

Fig. 1-254. Waters view reveals thickening of right lateral antral wall *(arrows)*. This could be ossifying fibroma or fibrous dysplasia; however, this was *healed "brown tumor" of maxilla.*

evation and penetration of the periosteum. These are destructive lesions that can be cystic or lobulated. The 5-year survival rate is 8% and the 10-year survival rate is 4%.[117] Because this tumor occurs primarily in children and young adults, it may be considered in the differential diagnosis of osteogenic sarcomas of the maxilla. Recent chemotherapeutic regimens have given promise of much improved survival statistics.[59,96,106]

Paget's disease (osteitis deformans) tends to appear after the fourth decade and increases in frequency with increasing age. Whenever the maxilla and mandible are involved, the skull is affected.[6] Clinically, there is an ache over the affected area with gradual enlargement of the jaws and spreading of the teeth that results in malocclusion.

Although the disease exhibits lytic, mixed, and blastic stages in the calvarium, it is the blastic stage that primarily is seen in the facial bones (Fig. 1-255). The involvement tends to be more symmetric than with fibrous dysplasia. The sinus cavities, nasal cavity, and orbits can eventually be obliterated. If early sinus ostial

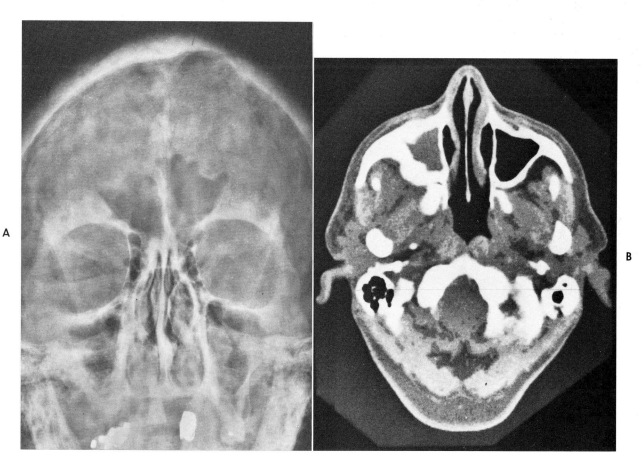

Fig. 1-255. A, Caldwell view reveals increased density of orbital rims and maxilla and nodular densities throughout calvarium. *Paget's disease.* **B,** Axial CT scan. There is dense thickening of right antral walls and lateral pterygoid plate. Bone appears somewhat unsharp. Obstruction of right antral ostium has occurred. *Paget's disease.*

obliteration occurs, secondary infection can further complicate the clinical picture. Dense, expanded facial bones are seen over the classic "cotton wool" changes in the calvarium. There is a reported 2% incidence of sarcomatous degeneration into osteogenic sarcoma.[6,86]

Chondroma of the facial bones is extremely rare.[28] Some physicians contend that a pathologic diagnosis of benign chondroma in the facial area should never be accepted[16] because the chondrogenic tumors are more often malignant (a ratio of 2:1).[24] The benign chondromas are locally invasive with a strong tendency to recur. They have been reported in the ethmoid bones, maxilla, and nasal cartilages. Wide surgical excision is suggested.

Chondrosarcomas are very rare in the maxilla and occur primarily in the anterior alveolar area. In the mandible they tend to occur in the ramus and in the premolar and molar regions. The peak incidence occurs in the third to fifth decades. Chondrosarcomas are less common than osteogenic sarcomas.[7] Their margins may be difficult to evaluate radiologically.[77] The treatment of choice is radical surgery, however, the survival figures are worse than those of osteogenic sarcoma.

The fibrous lesions affecting the paranasal sinuses and nasal cavity are a diverse group that have often proved confusing to both pathologist and surgeon. The true malignant potential of a tumor may be difficult to evaluate histologically, and encapsulation of the tumor has all too often been mistakenly interpreted as a sign of benignity.

The dermoid tumor occurs primarily in the abdominal wall. Only about 2% occur in the head, primarily in the masseteric aponeurosis, where they can simulate parotid masses.[6] Because they can have an aggressive character and a tendency to recur locally, they have been classified by some as grade I fibrosarcomas.[14]

Nodular (pseudosarcomatous) fasciitis is probably a reactive nonneoplastic response to an injury. Although it has a rapid clinical onset, it is a benign process.[128]

The benign fibroma is a rare lesion in the head and neck that usually occurs at the posterior portion of the inferior or middle turbinate. It is a polypoid mass that can protrude into the nasopharynx and in diagnosis it must be differentiated from a nasal polyp and an antrochoanal polyp. Usually the fibroma does not have any associated ipsilateral antral disease (Fig. 1-256).

Fibrosarcoma is an uncommon tumor in the paranasal region constituting only 0.5% of all malignancies and 5.5% of the malignant soft tissue sarcomas.[131] Most occur in the fourth and sixth decades and between 30% and 60% recur locally. Distant metastases are unusual. The overall 5-year survival rate for all grades is only 33%. Radiographically, fibrosarcomas tend to be both slow growing and expansile. Almost all the low-grade tumors arise as a late manifestation of long-standing chronic inflammation.

Rhabdomyosarcoma is primarily a disease of the young. Approximately 75% of these tumors occur in the first decade and 7% in the second decade. Thereafter, 2% to 4% occur in each subsequent decade. The orbit and eyelid account for 32% of the cases and only 9% to 10% occur in the maxillary sinuses. Most rhabdomyosarcomas appear to arise from unsegmented and undifferentiated mesoderm and only a relatively small number arise from myotome-derived skeletal muscle.[6] The most common type is the embryonal variety. The pleomorphic type occurs most frequently in adults. With chemotherapy, the 5-year survival rate has increased from 5% to 40% and even better results are anticipated. Electron microscopy shows actinomycin filaments in the cytoplasm. Histologically, embryonal rhabdomyosarcoma can be confused with melanoma, plasmacytoma, esthesioneuroblastoma, histiocytic lymphoma, and anaplastic carcinoma.

Radiographically, most of these lesions are aggressive group 1 lesions although occasionally a group 3 lesion is seen. Usually the clinical picture, age, and roentgenographic findings suggest the diagnosis (Figs. 1-257 to 1-259).

The *myxoma* is a benign mesenchymal tumor that

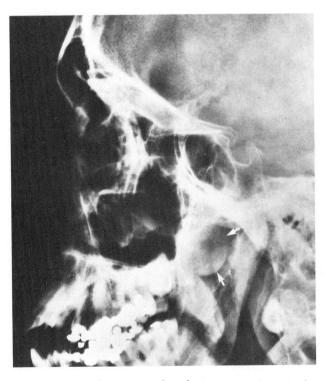

Fig. 1-256. Lateral view reveals soft tissue mass in posterior nares *(arrows)*. This is larger than normal posterior margin of inferior tubinate. *Benign fibroma of turbinate.*

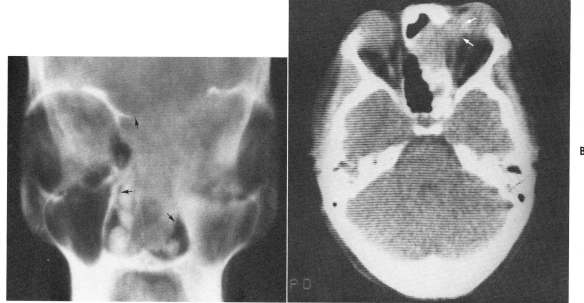

Fig. 1-257. A, Coronal tomogram reveals destruction of left superomedial and inferior orbital rim with tumor in ethmoid sinuses and nasal cavity *(arrows).* **B,** Axial CT scan reveals breakthrough into left medial orbit by ethmoid tumor mass *(arrows). Embryonal rhabdomyosarcoma.*

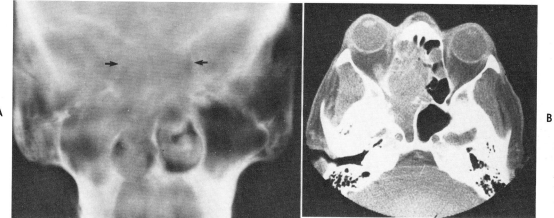

Fig. 1-258. A, Coronal tomogram reveals an ethmoid, nasal cavity, and right antral mass that has widened ethmoid complex with intact lamina papyracea *(arrows)* and intact orbital floor. *Embryonal rhabdomyosarcoma.* **B,** Axial CT scan. There is expansile right sphenoethmoid mass. Right lamina papyracea is laterally displaced but intact. *Embryonal rhabdomyosarcoma.*

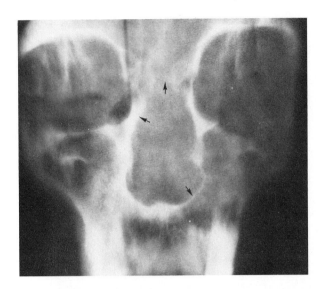

Fig. 1-259. Coronal tomogram reveals nasal cavity mass that has widened nasal vault and invaded ethmoid complex. *Embryonal rhabdomyosarcoma.*

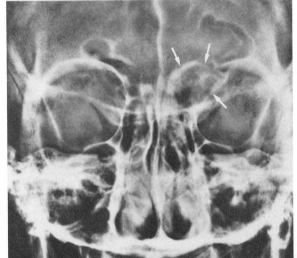

Fig. 1-260. A, Caldwell view reveals expansile and destructive lesion of left superomedial orbit *(arrows)*. **B,** Coronal CT scan reveals that expansile ethmoid mass has broken through into orbit *(arrow)*. **C,** Axial CT scan confirms expansile nature of mass that bulges into orbit *(arrows). Leiomyosarcoma.*

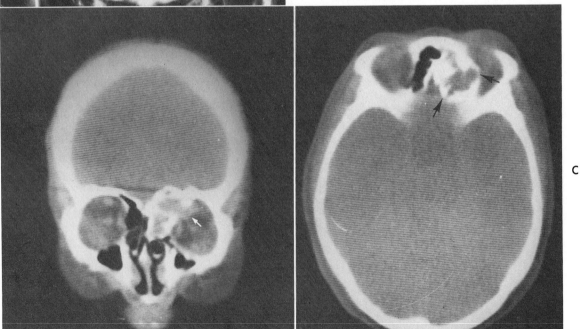

rarely occurs in the head and neck region. Most have been reported in the jaws, and isolated cases have occurred in the paranasal sinuses. They are slow-growing group 3 lesions that tend to recur even after wide surgical excision. Usually only an incomplete capsule is present.[19]

Leiomyosarcomas can occur in the head and neck region. Approximately 25% of the superficial soft-tissue tumors have been reported in the cheek, tongue, and mandible. Although many can be easily shelled out surgically, 60% to 70% recur locally. Direct involvement of the paranasal sinuses is extremely rare. Leiomyosarcomas most probably originate from blood vessels; 50% of patients do not survive 5 years. Leiomyosarcomas are group 3 destructive lesions and the treatment of choice is radical surgery (Fig. 1-260).[36]

The *mesenchymoma* is a rare and unusual tumor that is composed of two or more mesenchymal elements not ordinarily found together in a tumor. The benign variety is rarely found in the head and neck; however, the malignant variety does occur in this region. Most commonly, rhabdomyosarcomatous and vasoformative malignant elements are found. Our case showed a group 1 destructive pattern (Fig. 1-261).

Malignant fibrous histiocytomas of the paranasal sinuses are rare, representing 1% of the nonepithelial malignancies. Those that occur in the maxilla are not as aggressive and tend not to metastasize as much as the more common lesions that occur in the extremities. Radical surgical resection is the treatment of choice.

These lesions have a high local recurrence rate and they occur primarily in the fourth and fifth decades.* These malignancies tend to be group 1 destructive lesions that are enhanced on CT scans.

Primary malignant vascular tumors are rare. The diagnosis may be made too frequently, whenever a poorly differentiated sarcoma of bone manifests a prominent vascular pattern. A variety of terms have been used synonymously: hemangiosarcoma, angiosarcoma, angioblastic sarcoma, and hemangioendothelioma. These lesions have a more indolent clinical behavior than the soft tissue angiosarcomas, and radiographically they tend to be aggressive group 1 lesions. Rarely, a metastatic tumor in a sinus cavity may appear as a "vascular tumor." This is especially true of metastatic hypernephromas (Fig. 1-281).[6]

Hemangiopericytomas are vascular tumors that typically occur in the soft tissues of the extremities and trunk. They only rarely involve the paranasal sinuses. Hemangiopericytomas may be clinically benign or malignant and can metastasize to the lungs, liver, bone, and regional lymphatics. They are polypoid lesions of the group 1 or group 3 type that usually cause antral destruction. Radical surgery may produce a cure rate of 53% (Fig. 1-262).

Hemangiomas of bone represent 50.7% of osseous neoplasms and 10% of the primary benign neoplasms of the skull.[6] Most hemangiomas occur in the parietal and

---

*References 27, 33, 78, 123, 128.

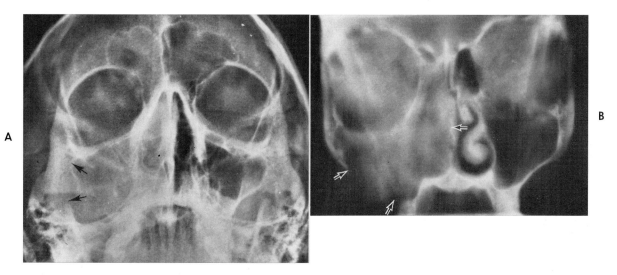

Fig. 1-261. A, Waters view reveals clouding of right antrum with destruction of lateral wall *(arrows)*. **B,** Coronal tomogram reveals right antral, nasal cavity, and ethmoid mass that has destroyed inferior orbital margin and medial and lateral antral walls. *Mesenchymoma.*

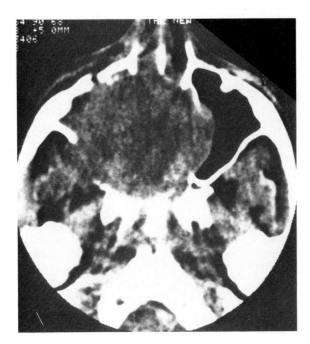

Fig. 1-262. Axial CT scan reveals nonuniformly enhanced expansile nasal cavity and right antral mass. *Hemangiopericytoma.*

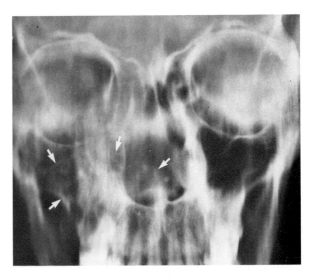

Fig. 1-263. Coronal tomogram reveals faintly defined expansile mass of right maxilla extending into right nasal cavity *(arrows)*. Focal calcifications are seen throughout mass and lucent spaces appear to be scattered in portions of alveolus. *Hemangioma.*

frontal bones. The involvement of the jaws is rare and the zygoma has been involved in two cases.[137] The most common roentgenographic appearance is that of a "honeycomb" or "soap bubble" sharply defined, expansile destructive lesion (Fig. 1-263).

Juvenile angiofibromas account for approximately 0.5% of all neoplasms of the head and neck. The incidence has been estimated to be between 1:5000 and 1:6000 otolaryngologic admissions.[6,57] Juvenile angiofibromas are highly vascular, locally invasive, nonencapsulated tumors that occur almost exclusively in adolescent males.[94] The symptoms include severe recurrent epistaxis, nasal obstruction, facial deformity, and nasal speech. All lesions start in the nasopharynx and extend outward from this point. The most consistent and suggestive roentgenographic findings are a nasopharynx mass and anterior bowing of the posterior wall of the ipsilateral maxillary sinus.[56] These findings, however, are not pathognomonic and can be seen in other slow-growing lesions in this region, such as lymphoepitheliomas, schwannomas, and fibrous dysplasia.[109] There is rarely actual tumor breakthrough into the antrum. Expansion of the nasal cavity by a homogeneous soft tissue mass is also common, but upward bowing of the floor of the sphenoid sinus is uncommon. Instead, the tumor mass frequently is seen as already having broken

through into the sphenoid sinus cavity. The CT scans may suggest the diagnosis, showing an enhanced nasopharyngeal mass that extends into the pterygopalatine fossa and sphenoid sinus in an adolescent male[139]; however, angiography remains the most accurate means of establishing a definitive radiologic diagnosis (Figs. 1-264 to 1-269). Delayed CT scanning will miss the marked enhancement of the tumor, so scanning should be performed immediately after a bolus injection. Although hormonal therapy and radiation therapy have played various roles in treatment, surgery remains the treatment of choice. Recent embolization techniques may hold the promise of markedly reducing the surgical dangers by almost eliminating blood loss.

Tumors of the hemopoietic system are rare in the nasal cavity and paranasal sinuses. Most are secondary to leukemic invasion. *Extramedullary plasmacytomas* are rare and usually occur in males (a 4:1 male/female ratio) over the age of 40 years. It has been estimated that between 10% and 30% of patients will develop multiple myeloma.[91] Approximately 80% of all these lesions occur in the head and neck region and about 15% exhibit amyloid microscopically. The behavior of these tumors is correlated with their pathologic appearance. Extramedullary plasmacytomas may be confused histologically with melanoma, histiocytic lymphoma, esthesio-

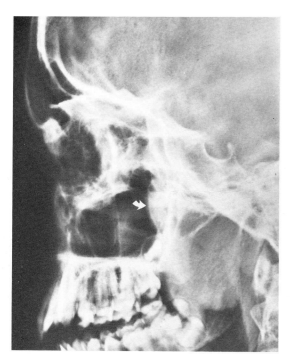

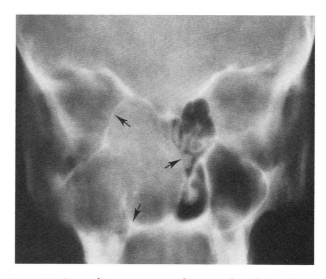

Fig. 1-264. Lateral view reveals large nasopharyngeal mass that fills sphenoid sinus and bulges posterior antral wall anteriorly (*arrow*). *Juvenile angiofibroma.*

Fig. 1-265. Coronal tomogram reveals expansile right nasal cavity mass that extends into ethmoid and antrum (*arrows*). *Juvenile angiofibroma.*

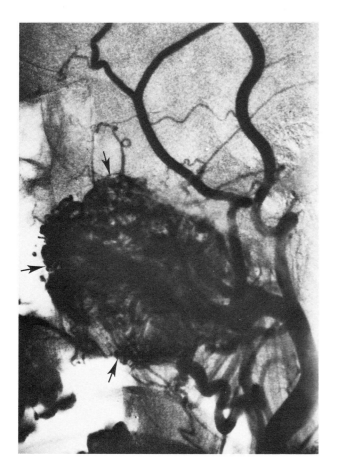

Fig. 1-266. Lateral angiogram reveals characteristic angiographic appearance of juvenile angiofibroma (*arrows*).

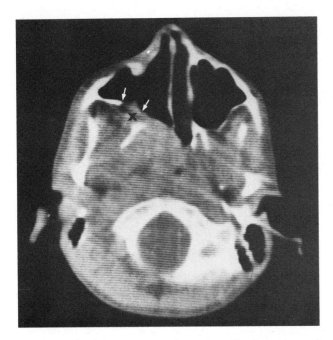

Fig. 1-267. Axial CT scan reveals anterior displacement and thinning of right posterior antral wall *(arrow)* with widening of pterygopalatine space *(x)* and destruction of medial pterygoid process. There is a large nasopharyngeal mass. *Juvenile angiofibroma.*

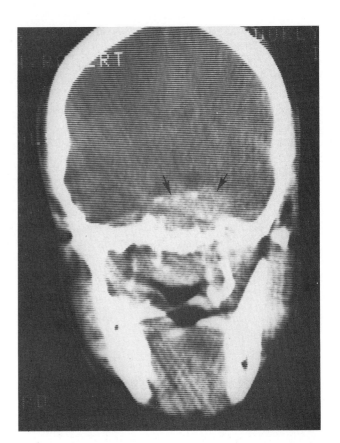

Fig. 1-268. Coronal CT scan reveals contrast-enhanced nasopharyngeal mass that extends intracranially *(arrows)*. There is erosion of right pterygoid plates. *Juvenile angiofibroma.*

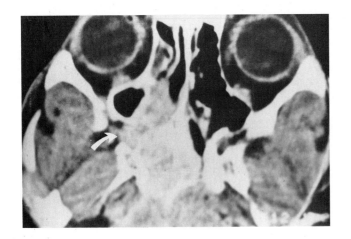

Fig. 1-269. Axial CT scan reveals enhanced nasopharyngeal mass that widens right pterygopalatine space *(arrow)* and extends into nasal vault. *Juvenile angiofibroma.*

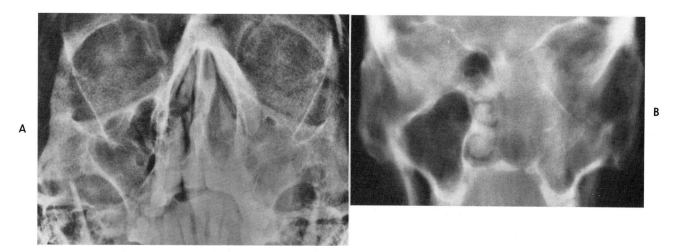

Fig. 1-270. **A,** Waters view reveals clouding of left antrum with no obvious bone destruction. **B,** Coronal tomogram reveals expansile soft tissue density tumor of left nasal cavity, ethmoid, and maxillary sinuses. Lamina papyracea and orbital floor are intact. *Extramedullary plasmacytoma.*

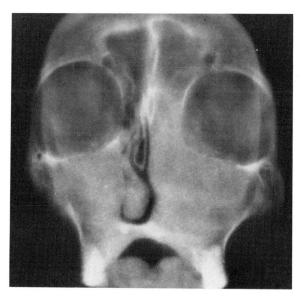

Fig. 1-271. Coronal tomogram of partly expansile, uniformly homogeneous tumor mass in left nasal cavity, ethmoid, and maxillary sinuses. Lamina papyracea, orbital floors, and lateral antral walls are intact. *Histiocytic lymphoma.*

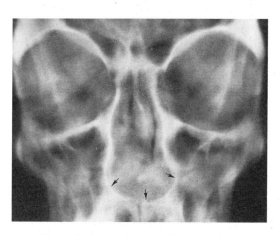

Fig. 1-272. Coronal tomogram reveals expansile lower nasal cavity mass. *Histiocytic lymphoma.*

neuroblastoma, embryonal rhabdomyosarcoma, and anaplastic carcinoma. Histochemically they stain with methyl green pyronine. Radiation therapy followed by surgery, if necessary, is the present treatment of choice. Radiographically, extramedullary plasmacytomas tend to be expansile group 3 lesions (Fig. 1-270).

Histiocytic lymphomas (reticulum cell sarcomas) are rare in the paranasal sinuses. The 5-year survival rate in this extranodal region is between 53% and 57%.[115] Chemotherapy and radiation therapy are the treatments

of choice, and the nasal cavity and antrum are the most common sites of involvement. Disease in the ethmoid sinuses is the next most common, and frontal and sphenoid sinus involvement is rare. Local spread beyond the confines of the sinus does not seem to portend a poorer prognosis, and concurrent generalized lymphoma is unusual. Histologically, it can be confused with melanoma, plasmacytoma, embryonal rhabdomyosarcoma, esthesioneuroblastoma, and anaplastic carcinoma. Radiographically, there is classic group 3 bone destruction (Figs. 1-271 and 1-272).

■ Odontogenic lesions

Dental cysts as a group are uncommon. The vast majority remain periapical in location and confined to the maxillary alveolus. A small group, however, can enlarge sufficiently to extend into the maxillary sinus. These are all extrinsic cysts and do not directly involve the maxillary sinus mucosa.[32] (This subject is considered in greater detail in Chapter 7.)

Primordial (follicular) cysts develop from the tooth sac while it is still in the embryonal stages and before any calcified structures have been laid down. Primor-

dial cysts are quite rare and occur most often in the maxillary sinus, elevating an intact mucoperiostium (see Chapter 7).

Dentigerous cysts are epithelium-lined sacs that develop from the enamel organ in association with crowns of unerupted teeth. The teeth most often involved are the third molars, canines, and second premolars. Most dentigerous cysts occur in the early decades of life and grow in size if the eruption of the involved tooth is retarded or prevented. When the capsule around an unerupted tooth is larger than 2 cm in diameter, there is a

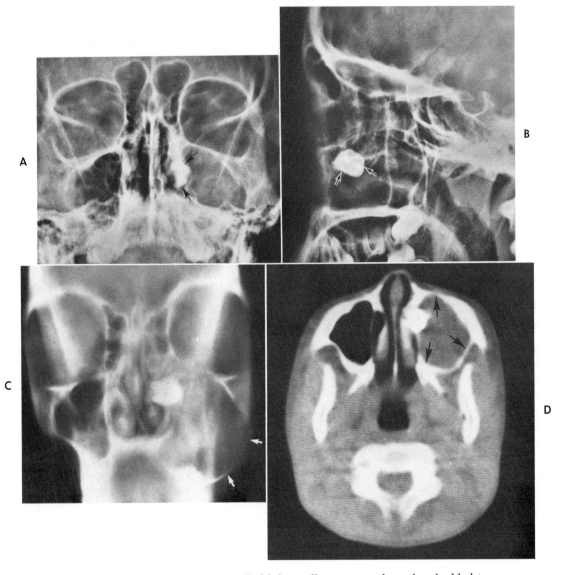

Fig. 1-273. A, Waters view reveals opacified left maxillary sinus with tooth enbedded in medial antral wall *(arrows).* **B,** Lateral view clearly shows tooth displaced into upper anterior medial wall *(arrows).* **C,** Coronal tomogram reveals expansile nature of lesion *(arrows)* and clearly defines tooth roots in medial antral wall. **D,** Axial CT scan confirms expansile left antral mass *(arrows)* with tooth in medial antral wall. *Dentigerous cyst.*

high probability that a dentigerous cyst will develop in that tooth. Their growth rate is quite variable. Radiographically they are cystic, expansile, but well-circumscribed lesions usually with the tooth crown projecting into the cyst cavity. Later in development, portions of the tooth enamel will remain attached to the cyst wall while the major portion of the crown becomes situated outside the cyst wall. Although benign in appearance, a small percentage of these cases can have ameloblastic degeneration of the cyst wall (Fig. 1-273).[125]

Radicular or periodontal cysts are the most common of the dental cysts and occur after the eruption of the involved tooth. They are epithelium-lined sacs, usually at the apex of the tooth root, and are derived from the epithelial remnants of the periodontal membrane. The stimulus to growth is probably inflammation and these cysts occur in association with carious teeth. They occur more often in the maxilla than in the mandible (a ratio of 3:2) and radiographically are round to ovoid, radiolucent lesions that can also be destructive. Their growth rate is variable, and because of the associated infection and destruction there is a predisposition to develop oroantral fistulas after dental extraction (Fig. 1-274).

Odontogenic tumors arise from abnormal proliferation of the cells and tissues involved in odontogenesis. They have been classified as either epithelial or mesodermal tumors. The epithelial tumors have been further subdivided according to whether or not inductive changes are present in connective tissues.[125]

The radiographic appearance of these tumors is variable, depending on their location, stage of develop-

ment, and histology. Ameloblastomas, odontogenic myxomas, and ameloblastic fibromas may resemble the dentigerous cysts, whereas cementifying fibromas (cementomas), especially in their early stages, may resemble radicular cysts.

When calcifications are present (mixed odontogenic tumors and cementomas) they characteristically do not merge with the normal adjacent bone but are encapsulated by connective tissue, exhibiting a thin radiolucent border on radiographs.[125]

Ameloblastomas (adamantinomas) are epithelial tumors without inductive connective tissue changes. The ameloblasts they contain can arise from the enamel organ, follicle, periodontal membrane, epithelium that lines a dentigerous cyst, or the marrow spaces of the jaws. Ameloblastomas occur four times more frequently in the mandible than in the maxilla, where the canine region is the most common location. They appear primarily in the third to fifth decade and have no sex predilection.

These lesions are locally aggressive and tend to recur. Surgery is the treatment of choice. The true metastatic nature of this tumor appears debatable.[32] Radiographically, they are typically loculated or honeycombed multicystic tumors. Portions of the involved tooth may be seen embedded in the lesion. Bone destruction can be aggressive (group 1 type) and simulate antral carcinoma; however, most exhibit group 3 type of bone destruction (Fig. 1-275). Whenever a dentigerous cyst is seen, the possibility that a portion of its wall may have degenerated into an ameloblastoma must be

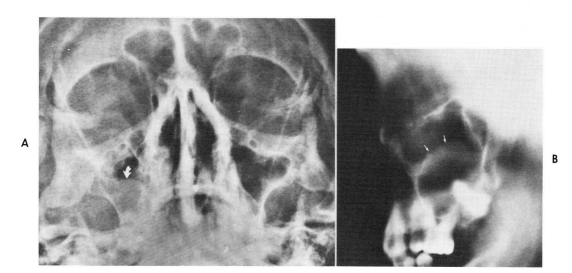

Fig. 1-274. A, Waters view reveals smooth soft tissue mass in right antrum. Mucoperiosteal margin has been elevated *(arrow)* by expansile mass in maxillary alveolus. **B,** Lateral tomogram reveals cystic expansile mass bulging into antrum *(arrows)* with tooth root in its lower margin. *Radicular cyst.*

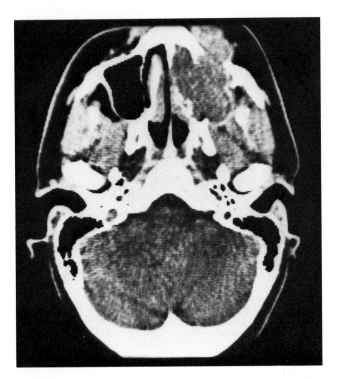

Fig. 1-275. Axial CT scan reveals expansile left antral mass that has eroded anterior antral wall and bulges into left cheek. *Ameloblastoma.*

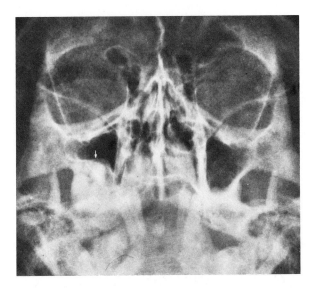

Fig. 1-276. Waters view reveals mottled, dense expansile mass in right maxillary alveolus that has elevated the sinus muco-periosteum *(arrow). Complex odontoma.*

seriously noted. This change may only be in a microscopic focus and radiographically a benign dentigerous cyst should remain the diagnosis.

The odontomas are epithelial tumors with inductive connective tissue changes. They can occur in two distinctive forms. The less common tumor is the *complex odontoma,* which has less dental differentiation and is seen radiographically as an amorphous, calcified, expansile mass than can fill the maxillary sinus (Fig. 1-276).

The more common *compound odontoma* represents almost full dental differentiation, resulting in a mass of formed dental structures. Commonly, innumerable tiny mature teeth (denticles) are seen within the mass.[32] The tumor can also invade the maxillary sinus (Fig. 1-277).

Mesodermal tumors that involve the maxillary sinus are rare. Most commonly, odontogenic myxomas (fibromyxomas) should be considered primarily because these expansile lesions can achieve sufficient size to involve the maxillary antrum. The roentgenographic findings are nonspecific and may resemble ameloblastomas, giant-cell reparative granulomas, fibrous dysplasia, or dentigerous cysts. The treatment of choice is surgical eradication (see Chapter 7).

Cementifying fibromas (cementomas) are mesodermal tumors that may reflect a localized form of fibrous dysplasia. They occur more frequently in the mandible

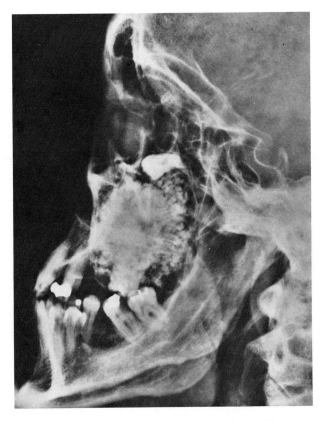

Fig. 1-277. Lateral view reveals large expansile maxillary mass with multiple discrete tooth densities *(denticles). Compound odontoma.*

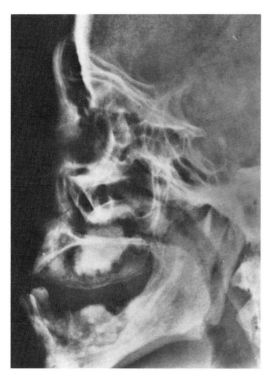

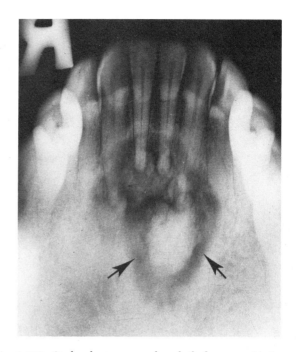

Fig. 1-279. Occlusal view reveals calcified mass with lucent zone separating it from surrounding palate *(arrows).* Note small radiopaque densities surrounding tooth roots (hypercementosis). *Cementoma.*

Fig. 1-278. Lateral view reveals densely calcified mass with lucent zone separating it from adjacent maxillary alveolus. Lesion has expanded alveolus and elevated sinus floor. *Cementoma.*

than in the maxilla (a 15:1 ratio) and there is a strong tendency for multiple occurrences. Cementifying fibromas have their origin from the proliferation of connective tissue of the periodontal membrane and their roentgenographic appearance depends on the stage of development. In the early stage they are radiolucent periapical lesions resembling radicular cysts; however, the involved tooth is usually healthy. The next stage occurs when there has been sufficient calcification to produce a radiopaque image within the original lucent area. There may be associated hypercementosis of the roots (deposition of cementum on the surface of the root); however, no resorption of the root occurs. The last stage of development occurs with almost complete calcification of the lesion, resulting in an ovoid or round radiopaque mass that is surrounded by a radiolucent space separating it from the surrounding normal bone (Figs. 1-278 and 1-279).[125]

Fissural cysts are extrinsic cysts that have their origin in the embryonic fusion of the frontonasal process and the two maxillary processes. It is believed that residual islands of ectoderm at the lines of fusion may later form these cysts. The cysts that occur along the midline fusion of the maxillary processes (incisive canal, nasopalatine cysts) do not involve the paranasal sinuses (Fig. 1-280). The lateral cysts are divided into those lying in

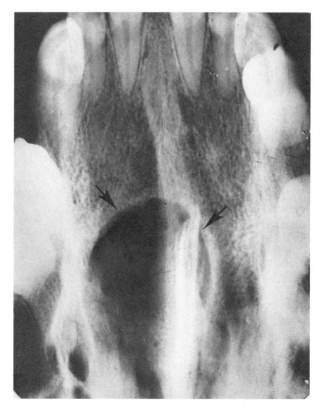

Fig. 1-280. Occlusal view reveals midline lucent cystic lesion of the palate *(arrows). Fissural cyst.*

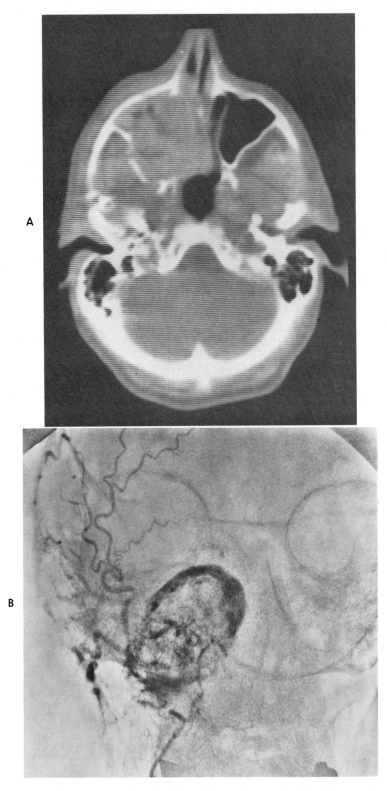

Fig. 1-281. A, Axial CT scan reveals expansile right antral mass that has destroyed portions of medial antral wall. Lucency within mass is an artifact secondary to surgery. **B,** Frontal angiogram reveals vascular stain in right antrum. *Metastatic hypernephroma.*

the superficial soft tissues and those lying in the underlying bone. The nasoalveolar cysts are soft tissue cysts that appear as small swellings in the upper lip or lateral nasal floor. They rarely produce bone destruction or involvement of the maxillary sinuses. Globulomaxillary cysts, or lateral bony fissural cysts, lie in the incisive suture near the lateral incisor tooth and canine tooth. As they enlarge, they push the roots of the canine and incisor teeth apart and encroachment into the maxillary sinus lumen occurs.[105]

■ Metastatic disease

Metastatic disease in the head and neck region can occur either from primary lesions of this region or from distant malignancies below the clavicles. Metastatic cervical lymph nodes clearly occur most often in association with head and neck primary tumors; of these the nasopharynx is the most common seeding source. The occult primary tumors that exhibit only cervical nodal disease may remain unknown until the patient's death. However, within a 5-year period after initial presentation between 28% and 45% percent of these occult primary tumors will finally reveal themselves.[6] In this group the vast majority occur in the upper respiratory tract (nasal cavity, mouth, naso-oro-hypopharynx, and larynx).

Metastases to the paranasal sinuses and nasal cavity rarely occur with primary lesions below the clavicles. However, when metastases are present the vast majority of them are from renal cell carcinomas. Local symptoms referable to the metastases precede the discovery of primary renal lesions in 50% to 60% of cases.[10,85] The renal cell lesions commonly exhibit epistaxis and nonspecific swelling, pain, or nasal obstruction. The combination of an expansile sinus lesion that is vascular should suggest metastatic hypernephroma (Fig. 1-281).

The next most common primary sites to metastasize to the sinonasal cavities are the lungs and breasts, and rarely the gastrointestinal and distal urogenital tracts. Radiographically, these are destructive, nonspecific lesions that most often cannot be differentiated from primary malignancies (Figs. 1-282 and 1-283). If skip areas of bone destruction are seen, metastases should be suspected because primary lesions destroy bone contiguously without skip areas (Fig. 1-284).

True metastases to the mandible (not from contiguous spread from oral malignancies) occur most often from malignant breast tumors with the kidneys and lungs being the next most common sites. Primary head and neck malignancies were initially thought to rarely metastasize below the clavicles. More recent studies, however, suggest that approximately 50% of the cases at necropsy showed distant metastases.[62] The majority of these were metastatic to the lungs and mediastinal lymph nodes. The lumbosacral spine and ribs were involved less often. In the vast majority of these cases (80%) there was failure to control the local disease.

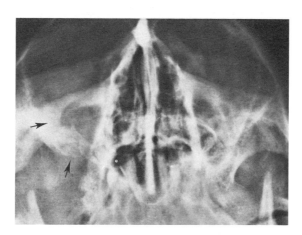

Fig. 1-282. Waters view reveals destruction of right lateral antral wall with clouding of sinus (*arrows*). This could be squamous cell carcinoma; however, it was *metastatic ovarian carcinoma*.

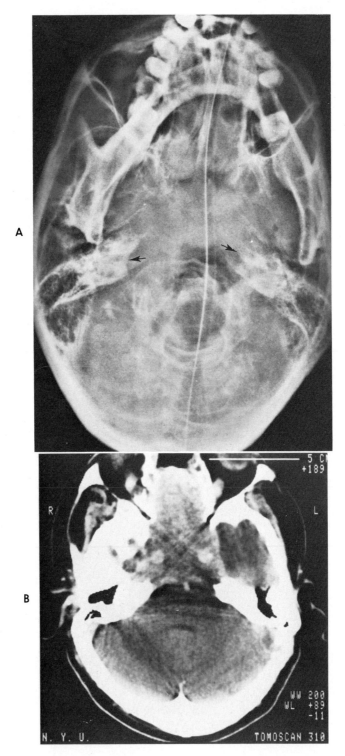

Fig. 1-283. A, Base view with nasogastric tube in place. There is large destructive lesion of clivus and both petrous apices *(arrows).* **B,** Axial CT scan reveals enhanced lesion that has destroyed central skull base and both petrous apices. *Metastatic hypernephroma.*

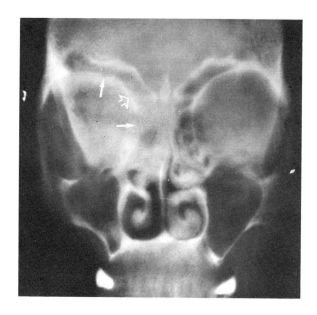

Fig. 1-284. Coronal tomogram. Two separate areas of bone destruction *(solid arrows)* are separated by segment of normal bone *(open arrow)*. Soft tissue mass fills right ethmoid sinus and supraorbital cell. *Metastatic lung adenocarcinoma.*

□ References

1. Alberti, P.W.: Applied surgical anatomy of the maxillary sinus, Otolaryngol. Clin. North Am. **9**(1):3-20, 1976.
2. Arey, L.B.: Developmental anatomy, Philadelphia, 1962, W.B. Saunders Co.
3. Badib, A.O., Kurohara, S.S., Webster, J.H., and Shedd, D.P.: Treatment of cancer of the nasal cavity, Am. J. Roentgenol. **106**:824-830, 1969.
4. Ballenger, J.J.: Diseases of the nose, throat and ear, ed. 12, Philadelphia, 1977, Lea & Febiger.
5. Batsakis, J.G.: Mucous gland tumors of the nose and paranasal sinuses, Ann. Otol. **79**:557, 1970.
6. Batsakis J.G.: Tumors of the head and neck: clinical and patological considerations, ed. 2, Baltimore, 1979, The Williams & Wilkins Co
7. Batsakis, J.G., and Dito, W.R.: Chondrosarcoma of the maxilla, Arch. Otolaryngol. **75**:55-61, 1962.
8. Becker, M.H. and Jacox, H.W.: Olfactory esthesioneuroepithelioma: experience in the management of rare intranasal malignant neoplasm, Radiology **82**:77-83, 1964.
9. Bergeron, R.T., and Rumbaugh, C.L.: Skull trauma. In Newton, T.H., and Potts, D.G.: Radiology of the skull and brain, St. Louis, 1971, The C.V. Mosby Co.
10. Bernstein, J.M., Montgomery, W.W., and Balogh, K.: Metastatic tumors to the maxilla, nose and paranasal sinus, Laryngoscope **76**:621, 1966.
11. Bordley J.E., and Bosley, W.R.: Mucoceles of the frontal sinus: causes and treatment, Ann. Otol. Rhinol. Laryngol. **82**:696-702, 1973.
12. Borello, E.D., Argentina, R., and Sedano, H.O.: Giant osteoid osteoma of the maxilla, Oral Surg. **23**:563-566, 1967.
13. Bortnick, E.: Neoplasms of the nasal cavity, Otolaryngol. Clin. North Am. **6**(3):801-812, 1973.
14. Butler, J.J.: Fibrous tissue tumors: nodular fascities, dermatofibrosarcoma protuberans and fibrosarcoma, grade I, desmoid type. In Tumors of bone and soft tissues, Chicago, 1965, Year Book Medical Publishers, Inc., p. 397.
15. Caffey, J.: Pediatric x-ray diagnosis, ed. 5, Chicago, 1967, Year Book Medical Publishers, Inc.
16. Cahn, L.R.: Cartilage tumors of the jaws: report of three cases, Oral Surg. **7**:1320, 1954.
17. Calcaterra, T.C., Rich, J.R., and Ward, P.W.: Neurilemoma of the sphenoid sinus, Arch. Otolaryngol. **100**:383-385, 1974.
18. Caldarelli, D.D., and Sperling, R.L.: Hemangiopericytoma of maxilla, Arch. Otolaryngol. **102**:49-50, 1976.
19. Canalis, R.F., Smith, G.A., and Konrad, H.R.: Myxomas of the head and neck, Arch. Otolaryngol. **102**:300-305, 1976.
20. Canalis, R.F., Zajtchuk, J.T., and Jenkins, H.A.: Ethmoid mucoceles, Arch. Otolaryngol. **104**:286-291, 1978.
21. Carpenter, J.L., and Artenstein, M.S.: Use of diagnostic microbiologic facilities in the diagnosis of head and neck infections, Otolaryngol. Clin. North Am. **9**(3):611-629, 1976.
22. Carter, B.L., Morehead, J., Wolpert, S.M., Hammerschlag, S.B., Griffiths, H.J., and Kahn, P.S.: Cross-sectional anatomy: computed tomography and ultrasound correlation, New York, 1977, Appleton-Century-Crofts.
23. Chapnick, J.S., and Bach, M.C.: Bacterial and fungal infections of the maxillary sinus, Otolaryngol. Clin. North Am. **9**(1):43-54, 1976.
24. Chaudhry, A.P., Robinovitch, M.R., Mitchell, D.F., and Vickers, R.A.: Chondrogenic tumors of the jaws, Am. J. Surg. **102**:403, 1961.
25. Conley, J.: Concepts in head and neck surgery, Stuttgart, 1970, Georg Thieme Verlag, KG.
26. Converse, J.M.: Reconstructive plastic surgery: principles and procedures in correction, reconstruction and transplantation, Philadelphia, 1964, W.B. Saunders.
27. Crissman, J.D., and Henson, S.L.: Malignant fibrous histiocytoma of the maxillary sinus, Arch. Otolaryngol. **104**:228-230, 1978.

28. Dahlin, D.C.: Bone tumors: general aspects and an analyses of cases, Springfield, Ill., 1957, Charles C Thomas Publisher.

29. Das Gupta, T.K., Brasfield, R.D., Strong, E.W., and Hajdu, S.L.: Benign solitary schwannomas (neurilemomas), Cancer **24**:355, 1969.

30. Davies, J.: Embryology and anatomy of the face, palate, nose and paranasal sinuses. In Paparella, M.M., and Shumrick, D.A.: Otolaryngology, vol. 1, Philadelphia, 1973, W.B. Saunders Co.

31. Davidson, T.M., Olesen, R.M., and Nahum, A.M.: Medial orbital wall fracture with rectus entrapment, Arch. Otolaryngol. **101**:33-35, 1975.

32. Dayal, V.S., Jones, J., and Noyek, A.M.: Management of odontogenic maxillary sinus disease, Otolaryngol. Clin. North Am. **9**(1):212-222, 1976.

33. Del-Rey, E., and De la Torre, F.: Fibrous histiocytoma of the nasal cavity, Laryngoscope **90**:1686-1692, 1980.

34. Dingman, R.O., and Natvig, P.: Surgery of facial fractures, Philadelphia, 1964, W.B. Saunders Co.

35. Dodd, G.D., and Jing, B.S.: Radiology of the nose, paranasal sinuses and Nasopharynx, Baltimore, 1977, The Williams & Wilkins Co.

36. Dropkin, L.R., Tang, C.K., and Williams, J.R.: Leiomyosarcoma of the nasal cavity and paranasal sinuses, Ann. Otol. Rhinol. Laryngol. **85**:399-403, 1976.

37. Dubois, P.J., Schultz, J.C., Perrin, R.L., and Dastur, K.J.: Tomography in expansile lesions of the nasal and paranasal sinuses, Radiology **125**:149-158, 1977.

38. Etter, L.E.: Atlas of roentgen anatomy of the skull, Springfield, Ill., 1955, Charles C Thomas, Publisher.

39. Evans, F.O., and others: Sinusitis of the maxillary antrum, N. Engl. J. Med. **293**:735-739, 1976.

40. Reference deleted in proofs.

41. Fagan, P., McKenzie, B., and Edmonds, C.: Sinus barotrauma in divers, Ann. Otol. Rhinol. Laryngol. **85**:61-64, 1976.

42. Fascenelli, F.W.: Maxillary sinus abnormalities: radiographic evidence in an asymptomatic population, Arch. Otol. Laryngol. **90**:190-193, 1969.

43. Fauci, A.S., and Wolff, S.M.: Wegener's granulomatosis and related diseases, DM **23**(7):1-36, 1977.

44. Fradis, M., Zisman, D., Podoshin, L., Wellisch, G.: Actinomycosis of the face and neck, Arch. Otolaryngol. **102**:87-89, 1976.

45. Frederick, J., and Braude, A.I.: Anaerobic infection of the paranasal sinuses, N. Engl. J. Med. **290**:135-137, 1974.

46. Freedman, S.R.: Benign osteoblastoma of the ethmoid bone: report of a case, Am. J. Clin. Pathol. **63**:391-396, 1975.

47. Friedman, W.H., Pervez, N., and Schwartz, A.E.: Brown tumor of the maxilla in secondary hyperthyroidism, Arch. Otolaryngol. **100**:157-159, 1974.

48. Fu, Y-S., and Perzin, K.H.: Nonepithelial tumors of the nasal cavity, paranasal sinuses, and nasopharynx: a clinicopathologic study, Cancer **33**:1289-1305, 1974.

49. Fujioka, M., and Young, L.W.: The sphenoidal sinuses: radiographic patterns of normal development and abnormal findings in infants and children, Radiology **129**:133-136, 1978.

50. Gallagher, J.C.: Upper respiratory melanoma pathology and growth rate, Ann. Otol. **70**:551-556, 1970.

51. Gordon, W.W., Cohn A.M., Greenberg, S.D., Komorn, R.M.: Nasal sarcoidosis, Arch. Otolaryngol. **102**:11-14, Jan 1976.

52. Goss, C.M., editor: Gray's anatomy, ed. 27, Philadelphia, 1963, Lea & Febiger.

53. Green, W.H., et al.: Mucormycosis infection of the craniofacial structure, AJR **101**:802-806, 1967.

54. Guerry, R.K., and Smith, J.L.: Paranasal sinus carcinoma causing orbital mucocele, Am. J. Ophthalmol. **80**:943-945, 1975.

54a. Harrison, T.R.: Harrison's principles of internal medicine, ed. 9, New York, 1980, McGraw-Hill Book Co.

55. Hill, C.L.: Meningioma of the maxillary sinus, Arch. Otolaryngol. **76**:547-549, 1962.

56. Holman, C.B., and Miller, W.E.: Juvenile nasopharyngeal fibroma roentgenologic characteristics, AJR **94**:292-298, 1965.

57. Hora, J.F., and Brown, A.K.: Paranasal juvenile angiofibroma, Arch. Otolaryngol. **76**:457, 1962.

58. Hunt, J.C., and Pugh, D.G.: Skeletal lesions in neurofibromatoses, Radiology **76**:1961.

59. Hustu, H.O., Pinkel, D., and Pratt, C.B.: Treatment of clinically localized Ewing's sarcoma with radiotherapy and combination chemotherapy, Cancer **30**:1522-2527, 1972.

60. Hyams, V.J.: Papillomas of the nasal cavity and paranasal sinuses, Ann. Otol. Rhinol. Laryngol. **80**:192, 1971.

61. Isselbacher, K.J., et al.: Harrison's principles of internal medicine, ed. 9, New York, 1980, McGraw-Hill Book Co.

62. Ju, D.M.C.: A study of the behavior of cancer of the head and neck during its late and terminal phases, Am. J. Surg. **108**:552, 1964.

63. Karmody, C.S., Carter, B., and Vincent, M.E.: Developmental anomalies of the maxillary sinus, Trans. Am. Acad. Ophthalmol. Otolaryngol. **84**(4, part I):723-728, 1977.

64. Kent, J.N., Castro, H.F., and Girotti, W.R.: Benign osteoblastoma as nasal polyps, Cancer **29**:153-156, 1972.

65. Knight, J.S., and North, J.F.: The classification of malar fractures: an analysis of displacement as a guide to treatment, Br. J. Plast. Surg. **13**:325, 1961.

66. Kutnick, S.L., and Kerth, J.D.: Acute sinusitis and otitis: their complications and surgical treatment, Otol. Clin. North Am. **9**(3):689-701, 1976.

67. Larsson, L.G., and Martensson, G.: Maxillary antral cancers, J.A.M.A. **219**:342, 1972.

68. Lasser, A., Smith, H.W.: Rhinosporidiosis, Arch. Otolaryngol. **102**:308-310, May 1974.

69. Lefort, R.: Etude experimentale sur les fractures de la machoire superieure, Rev. Chir. **23**:208-227, 1901.

70. Leonardi, M., and Fabris, G.: Pneumosinus dilatans: sign closely related to meningioma of the planum sphenoidale, Ann. Radiol. **19**:803-806, 1976 (French).

71. Lindstrom, C.G., and Lindstrom, D.W.: On extracranial meningioma: case of primary meningioma of nasal cavity, Acta Otolaryngol. **68**:451, 1969.

72. LiVolsi, V.A.: Osteogenic sarcoma of the maxilla, Arch. Otolaryngol. **103**:485-488, 1977.

73. Lloyd, D.M., Bartram, C.I., and Stanley, P.: Ethmoid mucoceles, Br. J. Radiol. **47**:646-651, 1974.

74. Lombardi, G.: Radiology in neuro-opthamology, Baltimore, 1967, The Williams & Wilkins Co.

75. Maillard, A.A.J., and Geopfert, H.: Nasal and paranasal sarcoidosis, Arch. Otolaryngol. **104**:197-201, 1978.

76. McClury, F.L., and Swanson, P.J.: An orbital roof fracture causing diplopia, Arch. Otolaryngol. **102**:497-498, 1976.

77. McCoy, J.M., and McConnel, F.M.S.: Chondrosarcoma of the nasal septum, Arch. Otolaryngol. **107**:125-127, 1981.

78. Merrick, R.E., Rhone, D.P., and Chilist, J.: Malignant fibrous histiocytoma of the maxillary sinus: case report and literature review, Arch. Otolaryngol. **106**:365-367, 1980.

79. Merrell, R.A., Jr., and Yanagisawa, E.: Radiographic anatomy of the paranasal sinuses. I. Water's view, Arch. Otolaryngol. **87**:184-195, 1968.

80. Merrill, V.: Atlas of roentgenographic positions, ed. 3, St. Louis, 1967, The C.V. Mosby Co.

81. Mesara, B.W., and Batsakis, J.G.: Glandular tumors of the upper respiratory tract, Arch. Surg. **92**:872, 1966.
82. Miglets, A.W., Saunders, W.H., and Ayers, L.: Aspergillosis of the sphenoid sinus, Arch. Otolaryngol. **1-4**:47-50, 1978.
83. Milosev, B., et al.: Primary aspergilloma of paranasal sinuses in the Sudan, Br. J. Surg. **56**:132-137, 1969.
84. Morrison, M.D., Tchang, S.P., and Maber, B.R.: Pneumocele of the maxillary sinus, Arch. Otolaryngol. **102**;306-307, 1976.
85. Nahum, A.M., and Bailey, B.J.: Malignant tumors metastatic to the nose and paranasal sinuses: case report and review of the literature, Laryngoscope **73**:942, 1963.
86. Newman, F.W.: Paget's disease: statistical study of 82 cases, J. Bone Joint Surg. **28**:798, 1946.
87. Noyek, A.M., and Zizmor, J.: Pneumocele of the maxillary sinus, Arch. Otolaryngol. **100**:155-156, 1974.
88. Noyek, A.M., and Zizmor, J.: Radiology of the maxillary sinus after Caldwell-Luc surgery, Otolaryngol. Clin. North Am. **9**(1):135-151, 1976.
89. Oberman, H.A., and Sullenger, G.: Neurogenous tumors of the head and neck. Cancer **20**:1992, 1967.
90. Oberman, H.A., and Rice, D.H.: Olfactory neuroblastomas: a clinicopathologic study, Cancer **38**:2494-2502, 1976.
90a. Ogawa, T.K., Bergeron, R.T., Whitaker, C.W., et al.: Air-fluid levels in the sphenoid sinus in epistaxis and nasal packing, Radiology **118**:351-354, 1976.
91. Ogura, J.H., and Schenck, N.L.: Unusual nasal tumors problems in diagnosis and treatment, Otol. Clin. North Am. **6**(3):813-837, 1973.
92. Paff, G.H.: Anatomy of the head and neck, Philadelphia, 1973, W.B. Saunders Co.
93. Paparella, M.M., and Shumrick, D.A.: Otolaryngology, vol. 3, Head and neck, Philadelphia, 1973, W.B. Saunders Co.
94. Patterson, C.N.: Juvenile nasopharyngeal angiofibroma, Can. J. Surg. **13**:228, 1970.
95. Pendergrass, E.P., and Hope, J.W.: Extracranial meningioma with no apparent intracranial source: report of a case, Am. J. Roentgenol. **70**:967-970, 1953.
96. Phillips, R.R., and Higinbotham, N.L.: The curability of Ewing's endothelioma of bone in children, J. Pediatr. **70**:392-397, 1967.
97. Pillsbury, H.C., and Fischer, N.D.: Rhinocerebral mucormycosis, Arch. Otolaryngol. **103**:600-604, 1977.
98. Pollock, P.G., and others: Cervico-facial actinomycosis, Arch. Otolaryngol. **104**:491-494, 1978.
99. Potter, G.D.: Sectional anatomy and tomography of the head, New York, 1971, Grune & Stratton, Inc.
100. Proetz, A.W.: Essays on the applied physiology of the nose, ed. 2, St. Louis, 1953, Annals Publishing Co.
101. Ramsden, D., Sheridan, B.F., Newton, N.C., and DeWilde, F.W.: Adenoid cystic carcinoma of the head and neck: a report of 30 cases, Aust. N.Z. J. Surg. **43**:102-108, 1973.
102. Ranger, D., Thackray, A.C., and Lucas, R.B.: Mucous gland tumours, Br. J. Cancer **10**:1-16, 1976.
103. Ritter, F.N.: The paranasal sinuses: anatomy and surgical technique, St. Louis, 1973, The C.V. Mosby Co.
104. Robinson, J.M.: Frontal sinus cancer manifested as a frontal mucocele, Arch. Otolaryngol. **101**:718-721, 1975.
105. Rogers, J.H., Fredrickson, J.M., and Noyek, A.M.: Management of cysts, benign tumors, and bony dysplasia of the maxillary sinus, Otolaryngol. Clin. North Am. **9**(1):233-247, 1976.
106. Rosen, G., et al.: Proceedings: disease-free survival in children with Ewing's sarcoma treated with radiation therapy and adjuvant four-drug sequential chemotherapy, Cancer **33**:384-393, 1974.
107. Schaeffer, J.P.: The embryology, development and anatomy of the nose, paranasal sinuses, naso-lacrimal passageways and olfactory organ in man, Philadelphia, 1920, P. Blakiston's Son & Co.
108. Schultz, R.C.: Facial Injuries, Chicago, 1970, Year Book Medical Publishers, Inc.
109. Shaffer, K., Huaghton, V., Farley, G., and Friedman, J.: Pitfalls in the radiographic diagnosis of angiofibroma, Radiology **127**:425-428, 1978.
110. Shugar, J.M.A., Som, P.M., Krespi, Y.P., Arnold, L.M., and Som, M.L.: Primary chordoma of the maxillary sinus, Laryngoscope **90**(11):1825-1830, 1980.
111. Shugar, J.M.A., Som, P.M., Eisman, W., Biller, H.F.: Non-traumatic cerebrospinal fluid rhinorrhea, Laryngoscope **41**(1)114-120, 1981.
112. Smith, B., and Regan, W.F., Jr.: Blowout fractures of the orbit: mechanism and correction of inferior orbital floor fracture, Am. J. Ophthalmol. **44**:733, 1957.
113. Smith, C.J., Echevarria, R., and McLelland, C.A.: Pseudosarcomatous changes in antrochoanal polyps, Arch. Otolaryngol. **99**:228-230, 1974.
114. Smith, G.A., and Ward, P.H.: Giant cell lesions of the facial skeleton, Arch. Otolaryngol. **104**:186-190, 1978.
115. Sofferman, R.A., and Cummings, C.W.: Malignant lymphoma of the paranasal sinuses, Arch Otolaryngol. **101**:287-292, 1975.
116. Som, P.M., Bellot, P., Blitzer, A., Som, M.L., and Geller, S.A.: Osteoblastoma of the ethmoid sinus: the fourth reported case, Arch. Otolaryngol. **105**:623-625, 1979.
117. Som, P.M., Krespi, Y.P., Hermann, G., and Shugar, J.M.A.: Ewing's sarcoma of the mandible, Ann. Otol. **89**(1,Part 1):20-23, 1979.
118. Som, P.M., and Shugar, J.M.A.: The CT classification of ethmoid mucoceles. J. Comput. Assist. Tomogr. **4**(2):199-203, 1980.
119. Som, P.M., and Shugar, J.M.A.: The significance of bone expansion associated with the diagnosis of malignant tumors of the paranasal sinuses, Radiology **136**:97-100, 1980.
120. Som, P.M., and Shugar, J.M.A.: Antral mucoceles: a new look, J. Comput. Assist. Tomogr. **4**(4):484-488, 1980.
121. Som, P.M., and Shugar, J.M.A.: When to question the diagnosis of anaplastic carcinoma, Sinai J. Med. **48**(3):230-235, 1981.
122. Som, P.M., Shugar, J.M.A., Cohen, B.A., and Biller, H.F.: The non-specificity of the antral bowing sign in maxillary sinus pathology, J. Comput. Assist. Tomogr. **5**(3):350-352, 1981.
123. Spector, G.J., and Ogura, J.H.: Malignant fibrous histiocytoma of the maxilla, Arch. Otolaryngol. **99**:385-387, 1974.
124. Spratt, J.S., Jr., and Mercado, R. Jr.: Therapy and staging in advanced cancer of the maxillary antrum, Am. J. Surg. **110**:502, 1965.
125. Stafne, E.C., and Gibilisco, J.A.: Oral roentgenographic diagnosis, ed. 4, Philadelphia, 1975, W.B. Saunders Co.
126. Stahl, R.H.: Allergic disorders of the nose and paranasal sinuses, Otolaryngol. Clin. North Am. **7**(3):703-718, 1974.
127. Stevens, M.H.: Aspergillosis of the frontal sinus, Arch. Otolaryngol. **104**:153-156, 1978.
128. Stout, A.P.: Tumors of the soft tissues: an atlas of tumor pathology, sect. II, fascimile 5, Washington, D.C., 1953, Armed Forces Institutes of Pathology.
129. Streeter, G.L.: Developmental horizons in human embryos 1948. In Paparella, M.M., and Shumrick, D.A.: Otolaryngology, vol. 1, Philadelphia, 1973, W.B. Saunders Co.
130. Suzuki, H., Gilbert, E.F., and Zimmerman, G.: Primary extracranial meningioma, Arch. Pathol. **84**:202-206, 1967.
131. Thompson, D.E., Frost, H.M., Hendrick, J.W., and Horn, R.C., Jr.: Soft tissue sarcomas involving the extremities and the limb girdles, South Med. J. **64**:33, 1971.

132. Valvassori, G.E., and Hord, G.E.: Traumatic sinus disease, Semin. Roentgenol. 3:160-171, 1968.

133. Van Alyea, O.E.: Nasal sinuses: anatomic and clinical consideration, Baltimore, 1942, The Williams & Wilkins Co.

134. Van Nostrand, A.W.P.: Pathologic aspects of osseous and fibroosseous lesions of the maxillary sinus, Otolaryngol Clin. North Am. 9(1):35-42, 1976.

135. Veress, B., et al.: Further observations on the primary paranasal aspergillus granuloma in the Sudan: a morphological study of 46 cases, Am. J. Trop. Med. Hyg. 2216:765-772, 1973.

136. Vrabec, D.P.: The inverted Schneiderian papilloma: a clinical and pathological study, Laryngoscope 85(1):186-220, 1975.

137. Walker, E.A., Jr., and McHenry, L.C.: Primary hemangioma of the zygoma, Arch. Otolaryngol. 81:199, 1965.

138. Warder, F.R., Chikes, P.G., and Hudson, W.R.: Aspergillosis of the paranasal sinuses, Arch. Otolaryngol. 683-685, 1975.

139. Weinstein, M.A., Levine, H., Duchesneau, P.M., and Tucker, H.M.: Diagnosis of juvenile angiofibroma by computed tomography, Radiology 127:703-795, 1978.

140. William, H.L.: Vasotonic headache associated with chronic maxillary sinusitis, Arch Otolaryngol. 88:95-97, 1968.

141. Wright, D.: Nasopharyngeal and cervical chordoma:–some aspects of their development and treatment, J. Laryngol. 81:1337-55, 1967.

142. Yanagisawa, E., and Smith, H.W.: Radiographic anatomy of the paranasal sinuses. IV. Caldwell view, Arch. Otolaryngol. 87:311-322, 1968.

143. Yanagisawa, E., and Smith, H.W.: Normal radiographic anatomy of the paranasal sinuses, Otolaryngol. Clin. North Am. 6(2):429-457, 1973.

144. Yanagisawa, E., and Smith, H.W.: Radiology of the normal maxillary sinus and related structures, Otolaryngol Clin North Am. 9(1):55-81, 1976.

145. Yanagisawa, E., Smith, H.W., and Merrell, R.A.: Radiographic anatomy of the paranasal sinuses. 3. Submentovertical view, Arch. Otolaryngol. 87:299-310, 1968.

146. Yanagisawa, E., Smith, H.W., and Thaler, S.: Radiographic anatomy of the paranasal sinuses. II. Lateral view, Arch. Otolaryngol. 87:196-209, 1968.

147. Zimmerman, R.A., and Bilaniuk, L.T.: CT of orbital infection and its cerebral complications, Am. J. Roentgenol. 134:45-50, 1980.

148. Zizmor, J., and Noyek, A.M.: Inflammatory diseases of the paranasal sinuses, Otolaryngol. Clin. North Am. 6(2):459-472, 1973.

149. Zizmor, J., and Noyek, A.M.: Fractures of the paranasal sinuses, Otolaryngol. Clin. North Am. 6(2):473-485, 1973.

150. Zizmor, J., and Noyek, A.: Radiology of the nose and paranasal sinuses. In Paparella, M.M., and Shumrick, D.A., Otolaryngology, vol. 1, Philadelphia, 1973, W.B. Saunders Co.

151. Zizmor, J., and Noyek, A.M.: The radiologic diagnosis of post surgical disease of the sinuses and mastoids, Otolaryngol. Clin. North Am. 7(1):25-279, 1974.

152. Zizmor, J., Noyek, A.M., and Chapnik, J.S.: Mucocele of the paranasal sinuses, Can. J. Otolaryngol. 3(suppl. 1):1, 1974.

2 □ The nose

ANNE G. OSBORN

No facial feature has received so much attention in folk sayings and literature (and so little notice in diagnostic radiology) as the nose. "Just follow your nose," "sticking your nose into somebody else's business," and "paying through the nose" are phrases in our ordinary daily vocabulary. Cyrano de Bergerac and Pinocchio not only are literary figures but have become part of our language and culture as well.[7] The nose, that "bone and gristle penthouse" (Steward Robertson), is a surprisingly interesting radiographic subject.

□ Normal and abnormal embryologic development

■ Normal development

The development of the human face occurs chiefly between the fourth and eighth weeks of fetal development. By the age of 12 weeks the face has approximated typical human proportions, although it continues to undergo gradual modifications throughout gestation and the postnatal period into adulthood.[25,57]

The nose itself has a complex origin. At 4 weeks' gestation a slight midline bulge appears just above the stomodeum (Fig. 2-1, A). This bulge, called the frontonasal prominence, slowly elevates into the dorsum and apex of the nose. The nasal (olfactory) placodes are thickened ovoid discs of epidermal ectoderm that develop on the inferolateral aspects of the frontonasal prominence (Fig. 2-1, A). During the fifth week of gestation these placodes invaginate, forming central depressions called the nasal pits (Fig. 2-1, B). Rapid mesenchymal proliferation at the margins of the nasal pits produces horseshoe-shaped elevations called the medial and lateral nasal processes (Fig. 2-1, C).[32,57]

During the fifth and sixth weeks of development the upper jaw also emerges. As the embryonic maxillary processes become increasingly more prominent, they grow toward the midline, crowding the nasal elevations together (Fig. 2-1, C and D). The paired medial nasal processes subsequently fuse with each other in the midline. Their caudal ends also merge inferolaterally with the developing maxillary processes. Externally, this tissue fusion gives rise to the bridge of the nose and the medial aspect of the upper lip (Fig. 2-1, E and F). Under the bridge of the nose it forms the nasal septum.[11] The alae of the nose are derived from the lateral nasal prominences.

The nasal pits gradually deepen and grow dorsocaudally, ventral to the developing brain. By the seventh fetal week the primitive nasal cavities are separated from the oral cavity by a double layer of epithelium called the oronasal membrane. The oronasal membrane then ruptures and the nasal pits open freely into the oral cavity. These regions of continuity are the primitive choanae that lie posterior to the primary palate.

The lateral palatine processes, two horizontal mesodermal projections arising from the inner surfaces of the maxillary prominences, soon fuse with each other and with the medial palatine processes and the nasal septum. Thus the oral and nasal cavities again become separated. This fusion also results in separation of the two nasal cavities.

Elevations on the lateral walls of the nasal chambers develop into the superior, middle, and inferior conchae. The epithelial lining of the nasal cavity is composed predominantly of typical respiratory epithelium. However, ectodermal epithelium in the medial roof of each nasal cavity and nasal septum becomes specialized as the olfactory region. Cells of this epithelium form axonic processes that synapse with cells in the olfactory bulb.

The paranasal sinuses develop during late fetal life and infancy as diverticula of nasal mucosa that evaginate into the surrounding bone. The resulting excavations become the expanding paranasal sinuses. The sphenoid sinuses are formed postnatally, and the frontal, ethmoid, and maxillary sinuses first appear during the fourth or fifth month of fetal life.[11]

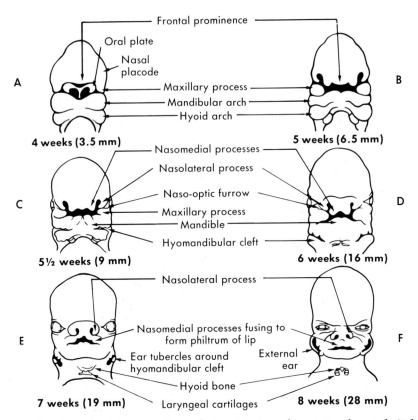

Fig. 2-1. Embryologic development of nose during 4 to 8 week gestational period. (Adapted from Morris' Human Anatomy ed. 12, by Barry J. Anson, editor. Copyright © 1966, McGraw-Hill Book Co. Used with the permission of McGraw-Hill Book Co.)

□ Gross anatomy
■ Bony framework

The skeleton of the external nose contains both osseous and cartilaginous elements. Its bony components are the two nasal bones and part of the frontal processes of the maxillae. The major cartilaginous structures include the septal, lateral, and greater alar cartilages.

The nasal cavity itself is divided by the nasal septum into two approximately equal chambers (Fig. 2-2, *A*). The septum consists of the perpendicular lamina of the ethmoid bone, the vomer, and the septal cartilage as well as the medial crura of the two greater alar cartilages (Fig. 2-2, *B*). The roof of the nasal fossa is formed, from front to back, by the nasal cartilage, the nasal bone, the nasal process of the frontal bone, the cribriform plate of the ethmoid bone, and the body of the sphenoid bone. The floor of the nasal cavity is formed by the palatal process of the maxilla and the horizontal segment of the palatine bone.[14]

The lateral walls of the nasal cavities are complex. The middle and superior conchae are parts of the ethmoid bone and project into the lumen of the nasal cavity. The inferior concha, usually the largest and longest of the three conchae, is a separate bone. The maxilla, lacrimal bone, ethmoid bone, and perpendicular plate of the palatine bone all form part of the lateral nasal wall (Fig. 2-2, *C*).

A number of important foramina open into the nasal fossa: (1) the cribriform plate foramina; (2) the incisive canal, (3) the nasolacrimal duct, (4) the orifices of the paranasal sinuses, (5) the sphenopalatine foramen, and (6) the hiatus maxillaris. The nasolacrimal duct opens into the inferior meatus. The sphenopalatine foramen lies just behind the middle turbinate and connects the nasal cavity with the pterygopalatine fossa. The hiatus maxillaris is a large, irregular opening extending from the nose into the maxillary sinus. It is normally covered by a thin membrane plus parts of the inferior concha and the palatine, ethmoid, and lacrimal bones. The maxillary sinus ostium opens into the posterior corner of the middle meatus. The frontal sinus drains by way of the frontonasal duct into the frontal recess of the middle meatus. The sphenoid sinus opens into a portion of the nasal cavity called the sphenoethmoid recess, which lies posterior to and above the superior concha (Figs. 2-2 to 2-4).[40]

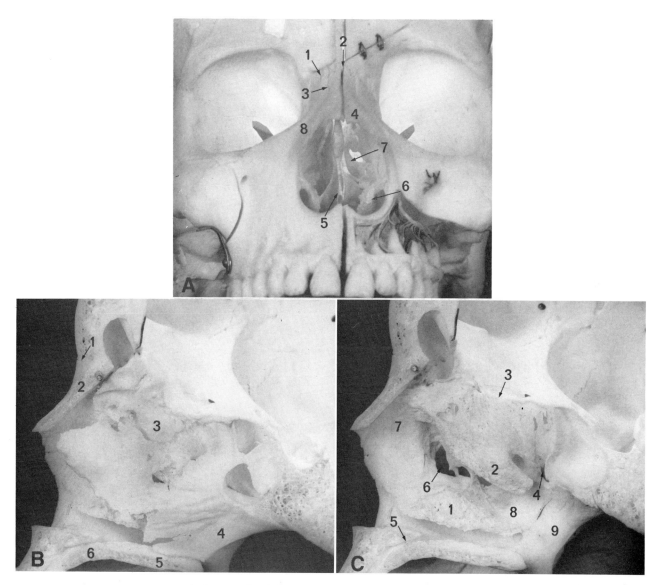

Fig. 2-2. A, Frontal photograph of dried skull. *1,* Nasofrontal suture; *2,* internal suture between two nasal bones (cut across); *3,* nasomaxillary suture; *4,* nasal bone; *5,* osseous nasal septum; *6,* inferior nasal concha; *7,* middle nasal concha; *8,* frontal process of maxilla. **B,** Photograph of bisected dried skull, medial view, showing bony nasal septum. *1,* Nasofrontal suture; *2,* nasal bone; *3,* perpendicular lamina of ethmoid bone; *4,* vomer; *5,* horizontal lamina of palatine bone; *6,* horizontal lamina of maxilla. **C,** Same case as **B.** Nasal septum has been removed to show lateral walls of nasal fossa. *1,* Inferior nasal concha; *2,* middle nasal concha; *3,* cribriform plate; *4,* sphenopalatine foramen; *5,* incisive canal; *6,* hiatus maxillaris; *7,* frontal process of the maxilla; *8,* perpendicular plate of the palatine bone; *9,* medial pterygoid plate.

■ Vascular anatomy

The vascular anatomy of the nasal fossa is complex, involving both external and internal carotid arterial supply. Five arteries supply the mucoperiosteum of the nasal cavity; the sphenopalatine artery is the most important of these vessels.[37]

The sphenopalatine artery originates from the third, or pterygopalatine, segment of the maxillary artery. Prior to its exit from the pterygopalatine (pterygomaxillary) fossa, the sphenopalatine artery occasionally gives origin to a posterior nasal branch. More commonly, it first exits from the superomedial aspect of the pterygopalatine fossa by way of the sphenopalatine foramen (Fig. 2-2, C). The sphenopalatine artery then enters the nasal fossa behind and slightly above the middle concha (Fig. 2-3).

The sphenopalatine artery has two major groups of branches: the posterior lateral nasal branches and the posterior septal branches. The posterior lateral nasal arteries ramify over the nasal conchae, first giving off branches that supply the inferior turbinate and then giving rise to superior branches that supply the middle and superior turbinates (Fig. 2-3, A). These lateral nasal branches also assist in supplying the maxillary, ethmoid, and sphenoid sinuses.

After giving origin to the posterior lateral nasal branches, the main trunk of the sphenopalatine artery continues medially along the roof of the nasal cavity.

When it reaches the nasal septum, the sphenopalatine artery gives origin to its medial branches, the posterior septal arteries. These branches course anteriorly along the nasal septum (Fig. 2-3, B). The most inferior of these branches becomes the nasopalatine artery. This vessel runs through the incisive canal to become continuous with the greater palatine artery.

The anterior and posterior ethmoid arteries originate from the ophthalmic artery and send numerous small branches through the cribriform plate to anastomose with nasal branches of the sphenopalatine artery (Fig. 2-3, B, arrow 2). This rich anastomotic network provides an important potential collateral pathway between the internal and external carotid circulations.

Two other arteries also provide some blood supply to the nasal fossa. The terminal branch of the greater palatine artery enters the incisive foramen, where it anastomoses with the nasopalatine artery (a septal branch of the sphenopalatine artery). The final artery supplying the nasal fossa is the septal branch of the superior labial artery. It originates from the facial artery and supplies the medial wall of the nasal vestibule.

"Little's area" is a portion of mucosa on the anteroinferior wall of the nasal septum just above the intermaxillary bone (Fig. 2-3, B). This area is supplied by Kisselbach's plexus, which in turn is composed of branches from the facial, sphenopalatine, and greater arteries. Little's area is a common site of nosebleed.

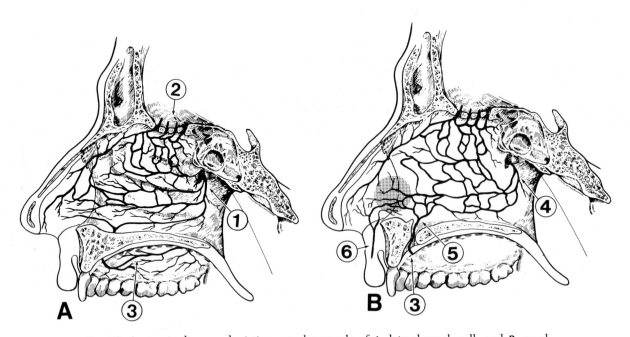

Fig. 2-3. Anatomic diagram depicting vascular supply of **A,** lateral nasal wall, and **B,** nasal septum. *1,* Posterior lateral nasal branches of sphenopalatine artery; *2,* anterior and posterior ethmoid arteries; *3,* greater palatine artery; *4,* posterior septal branches of sphenopalatine artery; *5,* nasopalatine artery; *6,* septal branch of superior labial artery. (From Osborn, A.G.: AJR **130:**89-97, 1978. Copyright © 1978, American Roentgen Ray Society.)

■ Nerve supply

Specialized receptor cells in the olfactory mucosa send bundles of nerve fibers through the cribriform plate of the ethmoid bone to enter the olfactory bulb. Pain, temperature, and touch are transmitted by the anterior ethmoid nerve (a branch of the ophthalmic division of cranial nerve V). Nasal branches of the sphenopalatine ganglion also contain parasympathetic fibers from the facial nerve that carry secretory impulses to the nasal mucosa and sympathetic fibers from the T_1 to T_3 segmental nerves to blood vessels of the nasal fossa.[40]

□ Normal radiographic anatomy
■ Nasal bones

The nasal bones themselves are best seen in either the lateral or occlusal view. Occasionally, a Waters view may also demonstrate the nasal bones and nasal septum. In the lateral view the nasofrontal and nasomaxillary sutures are often seen (Fig. 2-4, A). Londitudinal radiolucent lines paralleling the axis of the nose represent bony grooves for the nasociliary nerve and should not be mistaken for a fracture. The nasal septum and nasal spine of the maxilla are often best seen in the occlusal view (Fig. 2-4, B).

■ Nasal fossa

The nasal cavity, septum, and turbinates are clearly demonstrated in the routine PA Caldwell view. The posterior aspects of the inferior and middle turbinates are often quite prominent in lateral films of the facial bones and should not be mistaken for an oropharyngeal mass (Fig. 2-5). AP hypocycloidal tomograms demonstrate the bony margins of the nasal cavity and the turbinates in exquisite detail (Fig. 2-6) (see also Chapter 1).

Axial CT scans through the midorbital level include the perpendicular lamina of the ethmoid bone plus portions of the frontal sinuses and frontonasal duct (Fig. 2-7, A). Sections 5 mm more inferiorly include the superior meatus (Fig. 2-7, B). The adjacent ethmoid air cells, nasal bone, and lamina papyracea are also well seen in the axial plane (Fig. 2-7, C). Cuts through the pterygopalatine fossa and vomer sometimes demonstrate the sphenopalatine foramen (Fig. 2-7, D). The nasolacrimal duct, middle meatus, and middle turbinate are seen at the level of the inferior orbital fissure (Fig. 2-7, E). The hiatus semilunaris is a window between the maxillary sinus and the nose that should not be mistaken for an area of bone destruction (Fig. 2-7, F).

Coronal sections through the anterior aspect of the nasal fossa include the perpendicular plate of the eth-

Text continued on p. 152.

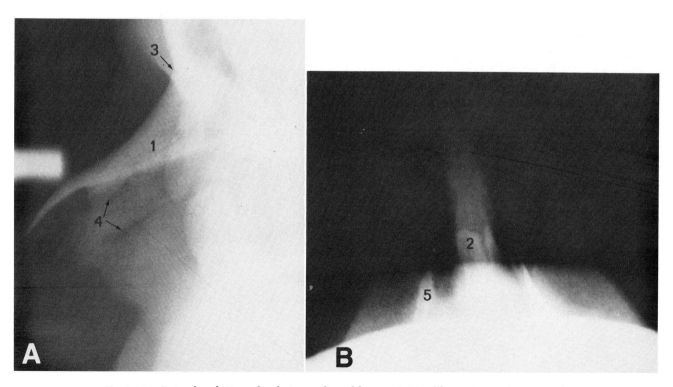

Fig. 2-4. A, Lateral and, **B,** occlusal views of nasal bones. *1,* Nasal bone; *2,* nasal septum; *3,* nasofrontal suture; *4,* grooves for nasociliary nerve; *5,* frontal process of maxilla.

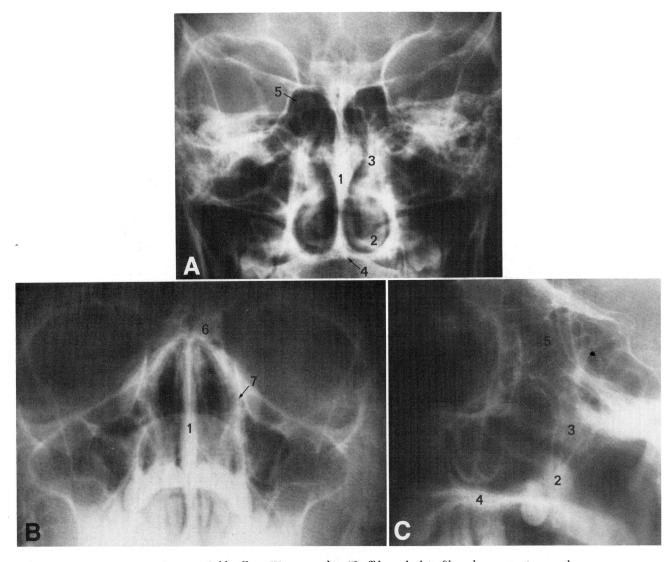

Fig. 2-5. A, Routine Caldwell, **B,** Waters, and **C,** 5° off-lateral plain films demonstrating nasal fossa and its contents. *1,* Nasal septum; *2,* inferior turbinate; *3,* middle turbinate; *4,* hard palate; *5,* ethmoid sinus; *6,* nasal bone; *7,* lateral wall of nasal cavity (medial wall of maxillary sinus).

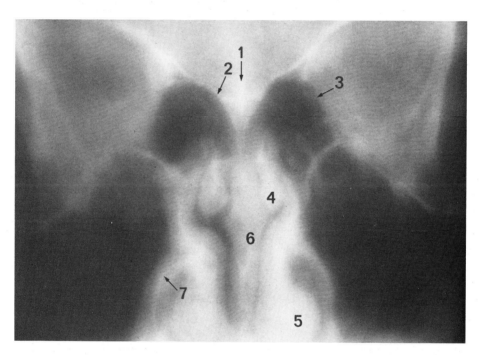

Fig. 2-6. AP hypocycloidal tomogram through nasal fossa at level of crista galli. *1,* Crista galli; *2,* lateral wall of the olfactory fossa; *3,* lamina papyracea of ethmoid bone; *4,* middle turbinate; *5,* inferior turbinate; *6,* nasal septum; *7,* medial wall of maxillary sinus.

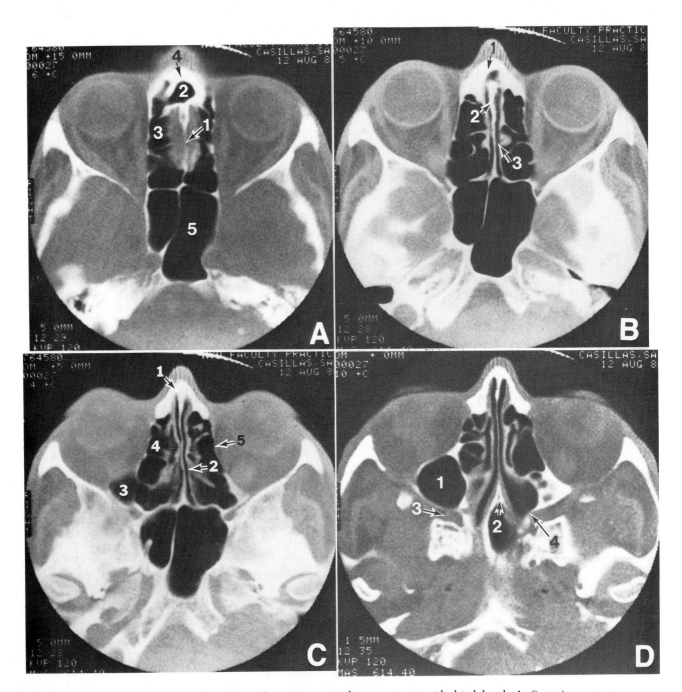

Fig. 2-7. A, Axial CT scan without contrast enhancement at midorbital level. *1,* Superior attachment of perpendicular plate of ethmoid; *2,* inferior portion of frontal sinus; *3,* ethmoid labyrinth; *4,* nasal process of frontal bone (glabella); *5,* sphenoid sinus. **B,** Axial CT scan 5 mm below **A.** *1,* Nasal bone; *2,* osseous nasal septum (perpendicular plate of ethmoid); *3,* sphenoethmoid recess. **C,** Axial CT scan 5 mm below **B.** *1,* Nasal bone; *2,* osseous nasal septum; *3,* apex of right maxillary sinus; *4,* ethmoid labyrinth; *5,* lamina papyracea. **D,** Axial CT scan 5 mm below **C.** *1,* Maxillary sinus; *2,* base of sphenoid with attachment of vomer; *3,* pterygopalatine fossa; *4,* sphenopalatine foramen. (From Osborn, A.G., and McIff, E.B.: Head Neck Surg. **4:**182-192, 1982.)

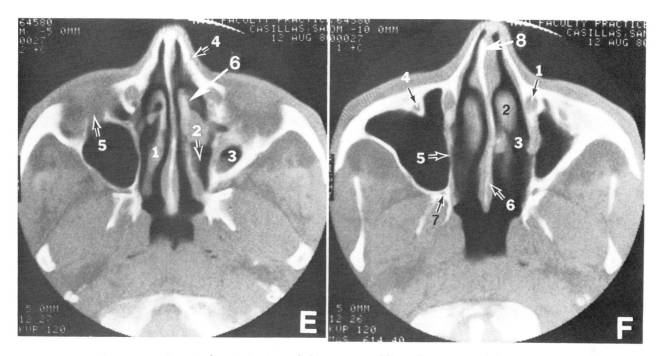

Fig. 2-7, cont'd. E, Axial CT scan 5 mm below **D.** *1,* Middle turbinate; *2,* middle meatus; *3,* apex of hypoplastic left maxillary sinus; *4,* suture between nasal bone and frontal process of maxillary bone; *5,* inferior orbital fissure (obliquely sectioned); *6,* inferior meatus (anterior aspect). **F,** Axial CT scan 5 mm below **E.** *1,* Nasolacrimal duct; *2,* middle turbinate; *3,* middle meatus; *4,* infraorbital canal; *5,* hiatus semilunaris; *6,* suture between vomer and perpendicular plate of ethmoid; *7,* pterygopalatine canal; *8,* cartilaginous nasal septum.

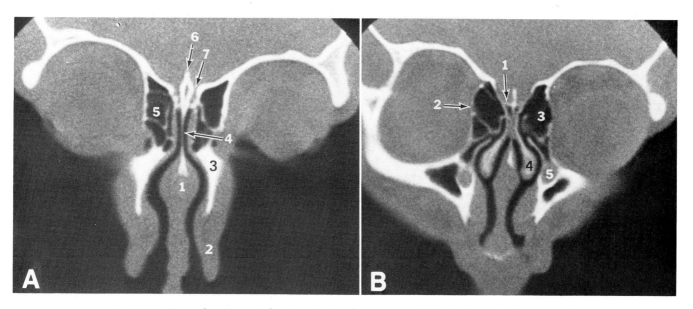

Fig. 2-8. A, Coronal CT scan without contrast enhancement. *1,* Cartilaginous nasal septum; *2,* lateral crus, greater alar cartilage; *3,* frontal process of maxilla; *4,* perpendicular lamina of ethmoid; *5,* ethmoid sinus; *6,* crista galli; *7,* olfactory fossa. **B,** Coronal CT scan 8 mm posterior to **A.** *1,* Cribriform plate; *2,* lamina papyracea; *3,* ethmoid sinus; *4,* middle concha; *5,* nasolacrimal duct (obliquely sectioned). (From Osborn, A.G., and McIff, E.B.: Head Neck Surg. **4:**182-192, 1982.)

Continued.

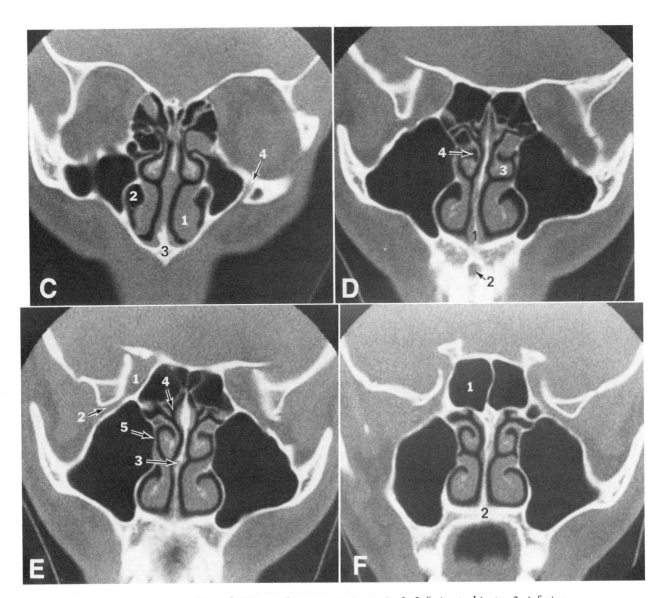

Fig. 2-8, cont'd. C, Coronal CT scan 8 mm posterior to **B.** *1,* Inferior turbinate; *2,* inferior meatus; *3,* nasal spine of maxilla; *4,* inferior orbital fissure (obliquely sectioned). **D,** Coronal CT scan 10 mm posterior to **C.** *1,* Vomer; *2,* incisive canal; *3,* middle turbinate; *4,* middle meatus. **E,** Coronal CT scan 6 mm posterior to **D.** *1,* Superior orbital fissure; *2,* inferior orbital fissure; *3,* suture between ethmoid and vomer; *4,* sphenoethmoidal recess; *5,* hiatus semilunaris. **F,** Coronal CT scan 6 mm posterior to **E.** *1,* Sphenoid sinus; *2,* hard palate.

moid, the cartilaginous septum, the nasal alae, and the frontal processes of the maxillae (Fig. 2-8, *A*). The nasolacrimal ducts and the olfactory fossae lie just behind this level (Fig. 2-8, *B*). The olfactory fossa is an important landmark in detecting subtle intracranial extension of nasal tumors. The middle and inferior turbinates are well seen at the level of the nasal spine (Fig. 2-8, *C*). The incisive canal lies at the anterior aspect of the hard palate (Fig. 2-8, *D*). The junction between the vomer

and the perpendicular plate of the ethmoid is often seen in the coronal plane as an apparent discontinuity. It should not be mistaken for a fracture (Fig. 2-8, *E*). The hiatus semilunaris is also included in these midmaxillary sections. The sphenoid sinus and sphenoethmoid recesses are seen in more posterior sections (Fig. 2-8, *F*).[39]

CT scans clearly demonstrate soft tissue as well as osseocartilaginous anatomy (Figs. 2-7 and 2-8).[36]

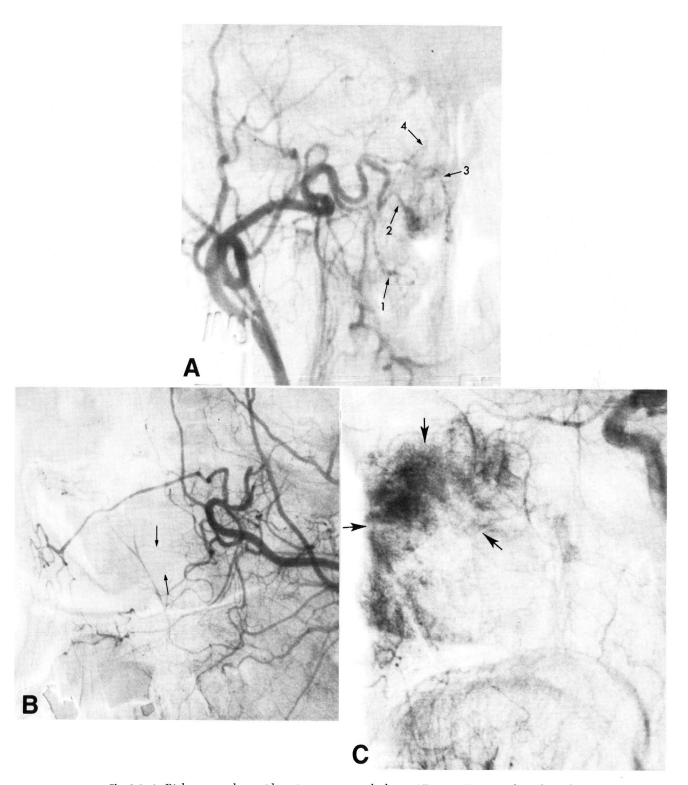

Fig. 2-9. A, Right external carotid angiogram, arterial phase, AP view. Posterior lateral nasal branch of sphenopalatine artery supplies inferior *(1)* and middle *(2)* turbinates. After giving off its lateral branches, main trunk of sphenopalatine artery continues medially, where it terminates in its septal branch *(3)*. Arrow *4* indicates sphenopalatine anastomosis with nasal branch of ethmoid artery. **B,** Normal left external carotid angiogram, arterial phase, lateral view. Branches of sphenopalatine artery are indicated by small arrows. **C,** Left common carotid angiogram, late arterial phase, lateral view. Prominent nasal mucosal vascular blush is present *(arrows)*. Patient had acute rhinitis. (From Osborn, A.G., and McIff, E.B.: Head Neck Surg. **4:**182-192, 1982.)

■ Nasal arteries

Angiography in the human usually reveals relatively sparse nasal vascularity. The posterior lateral nasal and posterior septal branches of the sphenopalatine artery are clearly seen on routine AP external carotid angiograms (Fig. 2-9, *A* and *B*). The septal branches course anteromedially along the nasal septum. Occasionally, small ethmoid branches of the sphenopalatine artery can be visualized as they course superiorly toward the cribriform plate. The anterior and posterior ethmoid arteries, which are branches of the internal carotid artery, are inconsistently visible on normal cerebral angiograms.

Because the mucosal blood flow varies widely, the nasal vascularity on late arterial or early capillary phase films may range from sparse to striking. On occasion, a distinct vascular blush may be present. Sometimes the mucosal vascularity can be marked, erroneously giving the impression of a vascular lesion (Fig. 2-9, *C*). Administration of a topical vasoconstrictor to the normal nasal mucosa reduces this vascular blush significantly.[37]

□ **Pathologic anatomy**
■ Congenital malformations

Developmental defects affecting the nasal cavity and adjacent structures usually are located along lines where fusion normally occurs. *Cleft palate*, the most common malformation affecting the nose, results from failure of the lateral palatine processes to fuse with each other, with the nasal septum, or with the primary palate.[32] Cleft palate is seen in a continuum of severity ranging from bifid uvula (an incidental finding seen in 1% of the population) to complete cleft palate, which may include the alveolar ridge. A complete cleft palate may also (although not necessarily) be associated with cleft lip and cleft anterior maxilla (Fig. 2-10).

The various nasal fusion anomalies may also be associated with disturbances in the development of other midline facial structures (Fig. 2-11). These median cleft syndromes are more uncommon than isolated midface defects.[7]

Facial anomalies other than fusion failure syndromes are unusual. *Hypoplasia* of the nose may be seen in achondroplasia, congenital syphilis, ectodermal dysplasia, some of the mucopolysaccharidoses, snub-nose dwarfism, and other syndromes.[7] If the embryonic nasal elevations continue to develop, cylindrical soft tissue masses that project from the face may be formed. These *proboscoid noses* usually occur with complete absence of the nasal cavities and underdevelopment of the maxillary process.[46]

If the oronasal membrane fails to perforate during the

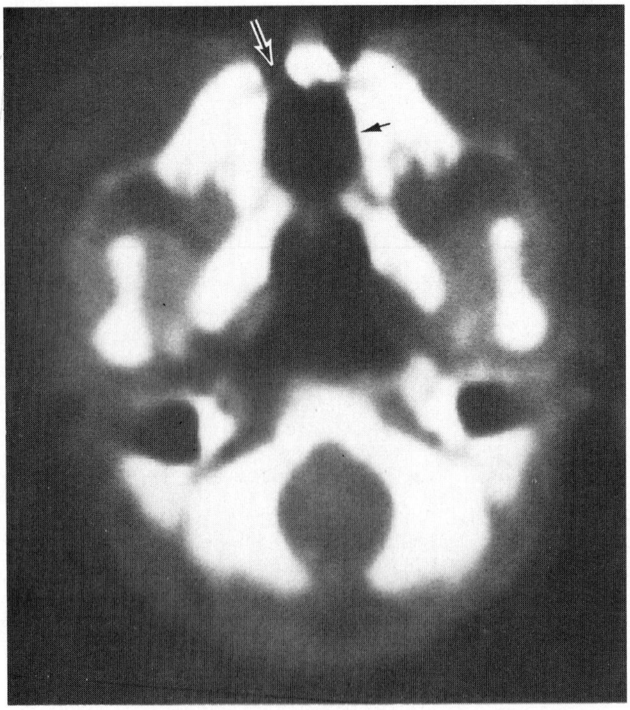

Fig. 2-10. Axial CT scan of newborn with complete cleft palate (*black arrow*). Cleft extends into premaxilla (*outlined arrow*). (From Osborn, A.G., and McIff, E.B.: Head Neck Surg. **4:**182-192, 1982.)

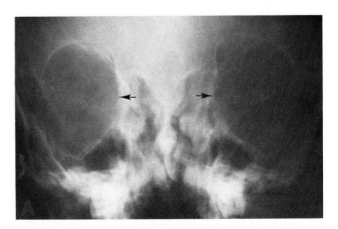

Fig. 2-11. AP plain film radiographs of paranasal sinuses (**A**) and mandible (**B**) in patient with midline cleft face. Note extreme hypertelorism (*arrows*) and partial duplication of alveolar ridges.

seventh fetal week, no choanal aperture into the oropharynx develops. The resulting *choanal atresia* may be unilateral or bilateral, partial or complete, purely membranous, membranosseous, or osseous.[11,14] Contrast nasopharyngogram is the preferred method of demonstrating this lesion. With complete atresia, pooling of the contrast medium in the posterior segment of the nasal cavity occurs (Fig. 2-12).

Other congenital abnormalities of unknown cause,

such as histiocytosis X, may have dramatic manifestations in the skull and facial bones, including the nasal fossa (Fig. 2-13).

■ Foreign bodies

A wide variety of foreign bodies have been found in the nasal fossae. Those that are radiopaque can be identified on plain films (Fig. 2-14). Longstanding foreign bodies may become encrusted with mineral salts, form-

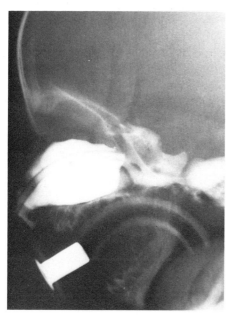

Fig. 2-12. Contrast nasopharyngogram, lateral view, in patient with choanal atresia. Note pooling of contrast material within nasal cavity. No communication with oropharynx is present.

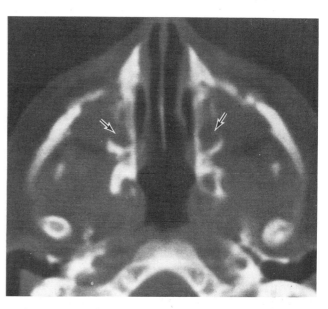

Fig. 2-13. Axial CT scan in patient with diffuse histiocytosis X. Note multiple lytic, expansile lesions involving nasal fossa (*arrows*).

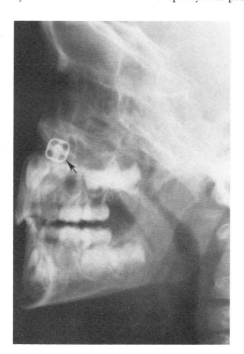

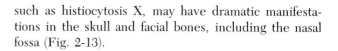

Fig. 2-14. Plain film radiograph, lateral view, in child with radiopaque foreign body in nose (*arrow*).

ing a rhinolith that appears as a calcified mass in the nasal cavity.[42,47a]

■ Trauma

Fractures of the nasal bones vary with the site of impact as well as with the direction and intensity of the applied force.[14] Isolated nasal fractures vary from the simple, nondisplaced linear type to comminuted lesions with depression of the septum and lateral splaying of the fracture fragments (Fig. 2-15). Fractures of the adjacent maxilla and orbit as well as of the lacrimal, ethmoid, and frontal bones may accompany severe facial trauma. AP and lateral tomograms are helpful in delineating the full extent of complex multisinus facial fractures (Fig. 2-16), although CT is usually superior to tomography in the evaluation of facial trauma.[59a]

With severe nasofrontal-ethmoid or naso-orbital injuries the nasal bones are often shattered and the entire midface is displaced posteriorly. Traumatic hypertelorism may be present. The ethmoid labyrinth, turbinates, and septum are often fragmented, and the cribriform plate is disrupted. Axial and coronal CT scans are also useful in evaluating these complicated cases (Fig. 2-16, E). Complications of nasofrontal-ethmoid injuries include frontal sinus injuries, cerebrospinal fluid rhinorrhea, impaired vision or olfaction, pseudohypertelorism, and facial deformity.[27]

■ Inflammatory lesions

Allergic rhinitis is a perennial or recurrent seasonal disease. The nasal mucosa becomes edematous and pale. Plain films may disclose swollen, boggy turbinates that often completely fill the nasal cavity. Patients with longstanding allergic sinusitis can occasionally develop polypoid changes in the nose and paranasal sinuses. *Chronic purulent sinusitis* may occasionally cause decalcification and osteolysis of the paranasal sinus walls.

Granulomatous diseases that can involve the nose include syphilis, leprosy, tuberculosis, sarcoid, yaws, and rhinoscleroma.[60] Destruction of the nasal bones, septum, turbinates, and adjacent sinuses may be present and in advanced cases can mimic mucormycosis or other aggressive fungal infections. Occasionally, extensive sclerosis of the skull base can occur.[34] Absence of the anterior nasal spine of the maxilla is considered pathognomonic of leprosy in the absence of maxillonasal dysplasia, trauma, or surgery.[60]

A number of fungal diseases can involve the nasal fossa. In humans, *Aspergillus fumigatus* can exist as a saprophyte, parasite, or frank pathogen. Aspergillosis occurs either as a focal process unassociated with any underlying disease (common in agricultural communities with a hot, humid climate) or in patients with altered host resistance. Noninvasive aspergillosis starts as a unilateral sinusitis that does not respond to routine therapy and is roentgenographically indistinguishable from chronic bacterial sinusitis.[29] The aggressive form of aspergillosis occurs as a nasal or sinus soft tissue mass with bone destruction that may be quite extensive and can therefore mimic neoplasia, mucormycosis, granulomatous disease, or chronic sinusitis with osteomyelitis

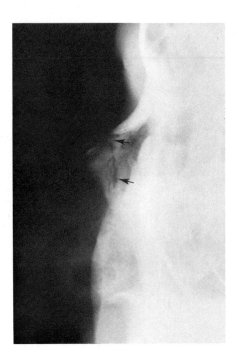

Fig. 2-15. Comminuted fracture of nasal bone *(arrows)*, lateral view.

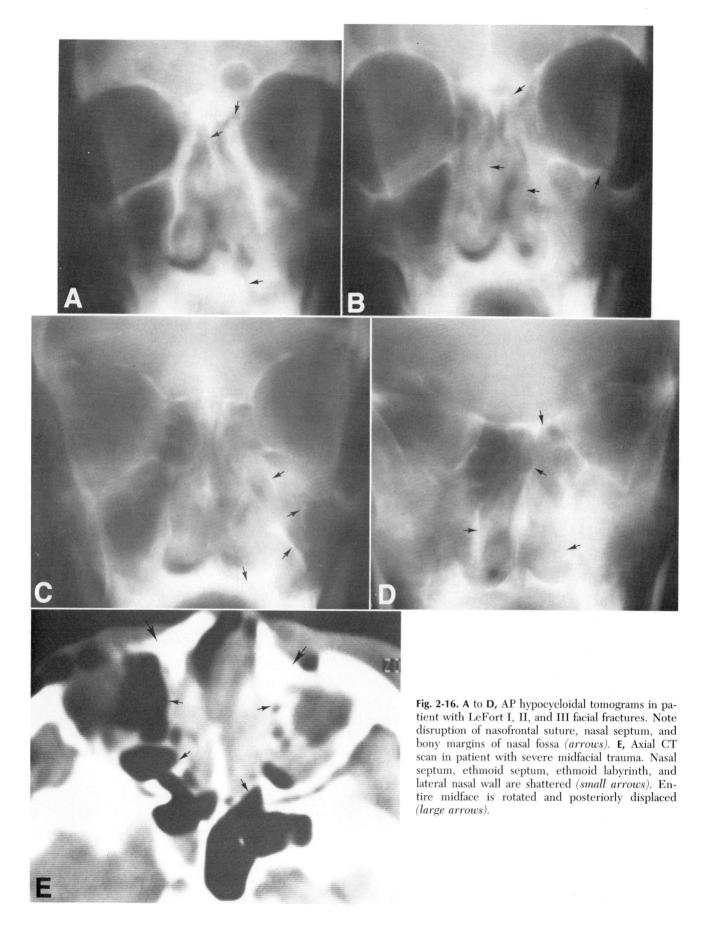

Fig. 2-16. A to **D,** AP hypocycloidal tomograms in patient with LeFort I, II, and III facial fractures. Note disruption of nasofrontal suture, nasal septum, and bony margins of nasal fossa *(arrows).* **E,** Axial CT scan in patient with severe midfacial trauma. Nasal septum, ethmoid septum, ethmoid labyrinth, and lateral nasal wall are shattered *(small arrows).* Entire midface is rotated and posteriorly displaced *(large arrows).*

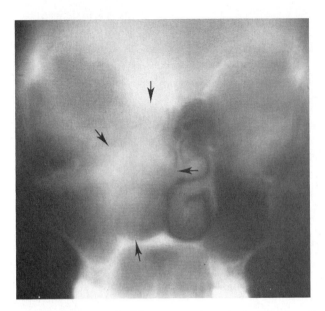

Fig. 2-17. AP hypocycloidal tomogram in patient with aspergillosis. Unilateral nasal and paranasal sinus soft tissue mass with bone destruction is present *(arrows)*. (From Osborn, A.G., and McIff, E.B.: Head Neck Surg. **4:**182-192, 1982.)

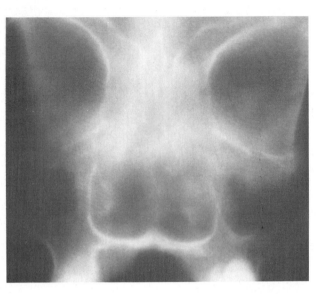

Fig. 2-18. AP hypocycloidal tomogram in patient with mucormycosis. Note destruction of turbinates, nasal septum, ethmoid septa, and superomedial walls of maxillary sinuses. (From Osborn, A.G., and McIff, E.B.: Head Neck Surg. **4:**182-192, 1982.)

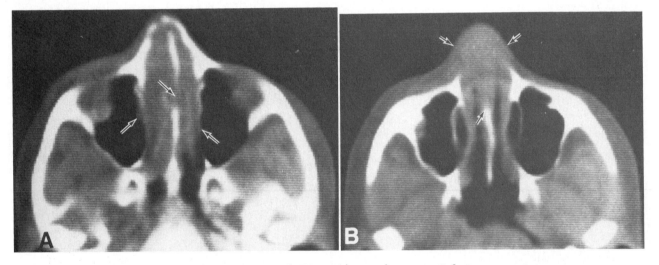

Fig. 2-19. Axial CT scans in patient with Wegener's granulomatosis. Soft tissue mass is associated with destruction of nasal bone, septum, and cartilage *(arrows)*. (Courtesy P. Som, M.D.; from Osborn, A.G., and McIff, E.B.: Head Neck Surg. **4:**182-192, 1982.)

(Fig. 2-17).[28] If present, bone thickening and sclerosis are helpful differential diagnostic features.

Rhinocerebral mucormycosis is caused by ubiquitous fungi that are normally saprophytic. Under some conditions they may become opportunistic, producing mucosal thickening and focal bone destruction in the nasal fossa that initially follows natural foramina and fissures.[1] These lesions tend to be relatively symmetric (Fig. 2-18). The differential diagnosis includes carcinoma, gran-

ulomatous and fungal diseases, osteomyelitis, necrotizing granuloma, and the midline reticuloses.[56]

Wegener's granulomatosis is actually a spectrum of diseases characterized by the presence of necrotizing granulomas with vasculitis. Roentgenographic findings include pansinusitis with destruction of the nasal septum and turbinates (Fig. 2-19). The differential diagnosis is similar to that for mucormycosis. Idiopathic midline granuloma and the closely related lymphoreticular

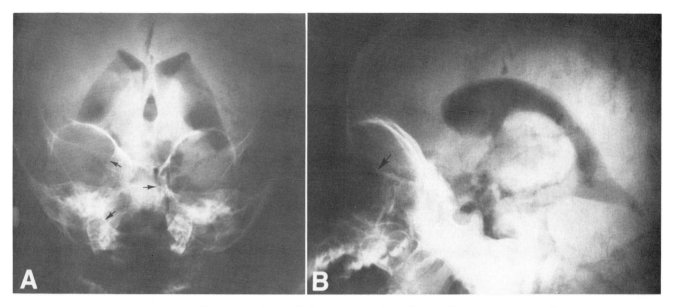

Fig. 2-20. Patient with intranasal encephalocele. **A,** AP view shows soft tissue mass expanding right ethmoid sinuses and nasal fossa *(arrows).* **B,** Lateral view demonstrates anterior dehiscence of cribriform plate *(arrow).*

disorders can have a similar roentgenographic appearance.[2]

■ Nonneoplastic mass lesions involving the nasal cavity

Meningoceles and *encephaloceles* may involve the nasal cavity. Both result from congenital herniation of either intracranial meningeal and neural tissue or meninges alone into the nasal fossa. The herniation occurs through open suture lines or defects in the cribriform plate. Encephaloceles contain primitive neural and supporting tissue; meningoceles contain arachnoid, dura, and cerebrospinal fluid. The radiographic findings with encephaloceles include bony dehiscence and soft tissue mass in the nose or paranasal sinuses (Fig. 2-20). The so-called *nasal glioma* is not a neoplastic lesion but rather a sequestered gliomatous mass with or without an intracranial connection.[61]

Dermoid cysts are developmental lesions that may be found at any point from the nasofrontal suture to the base of the columella along the midline of the nose or nasal septum. A dimple or fistula containing a hair may be present over the dorsum of the nose. Radiographic findings include broadening or disruption of the bridge of the nose, a sharply demarcated bony defect in the region of the nasofrontal suture or nasal bone, and a fusiform soft tissue mass within the nasal septum.[14]

Benign polyps are the most common nasal masses in children. Contrary to common belief, allergy is an unusual cause. Unilateral polyps (Fig. 2-21) and antro-

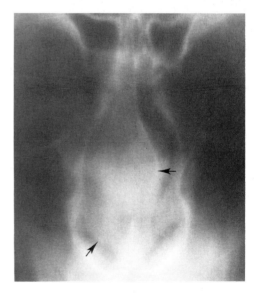

Fig. 2-21. AP hypocycloidal tomogram. Large inflammatory nasal polyp is present *(arrows).*

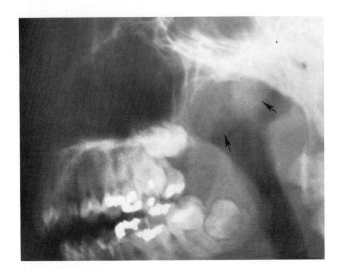

Fig. 2-22. Lateral plain film of 10-year-old child with nasopharyngeal soft tissue mass *(arrows). Large antrochoanal polyp.*

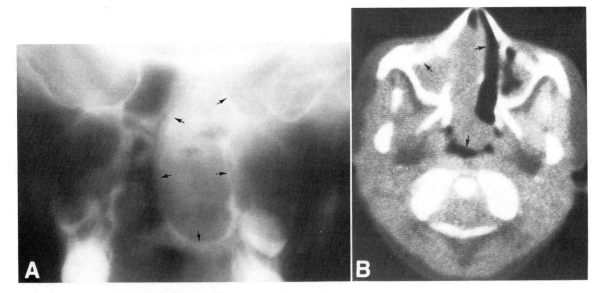

Fig. 2-23. A, AP hypocycloidal tomogram, and **B,** axial CT scan in 7-year-old child with huge left antrochoanal polyp *(arrows).* Note pressure erosion of medial wall of maxillary sinus plus expansion of left bony nasal fossa.

choanal polyps (Fig. 2-22) are more often inflammatory. Patients with cystic fibrosis commonly have bilateral nasal polyps.[54]

Antrochoanal polyps are a benign solitary polypoid lesions that usually arise in the maxillary sinus and pass through its ostium into the choana (Fig. 2-23). From there they may extend into the posterior nasopharynx. These polyps characteristically opacify and enlarge the sinus cavity without bone destruction.[54] Occasionally, a large nasopharyngeal soft tissue mass may be present (Fig. 2-22).

Chronic hypertrophic polypoid rhinosinusitis is characterized by polypoid mucosal hypertrophy and chronic

superimposed infection. When extensive (Fig. 2-24), benign nasal polyposis can cause expansion of the nasal cavity and bone erosion that may suggest a more ominous diagnosis, such as tumor, osteomyelitis, or necrotizing granuloma.[58,59] The presence of associated bone expansion plus a clinical history of vasomotor instability and rhinitis, chronic sinusitis, and nasal polyps should be helpful in the radiographic differential diagnosis.[59]

Large frontal or ethmoid *mucoceles* may occasionally extend into the nasal fossa. Opacification of the nasal and paranasal sinuses, with thinning and expansion or pressure deformity of their bony walls, is characteristic.[13,44] Nasopharyngeal encroachment is unusual but

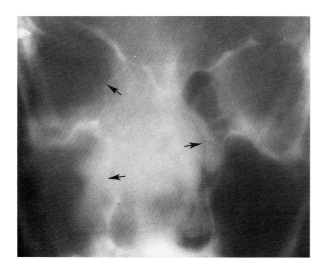

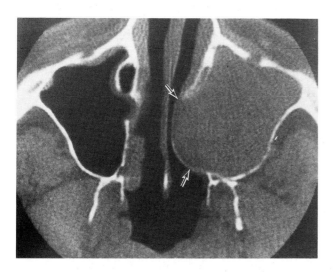

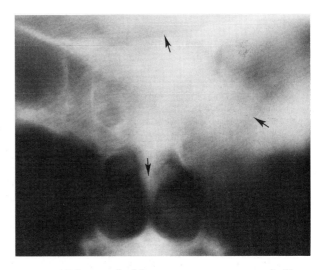

Fig. 2-24. AP hypocycloidal tomogram in patient with hypertrophic polypoid rhinosinusitis. Bony margins of opacified nasal fossa and right paranasal sinuses are thinned and expanded *(arrows)*. (From Osborn, A.G., and McIff, E.B.: Head Neck Surg. **4:**182-192, 1982.)

Fig. 2-25. Axial CT scan in patient with large right maxillary mucocele. Lesion has expanded into nasal fossa *(arrows)*. (Courtesy R.T. Bergeron, M.D.)

Fig. 2-26. AP hypocycloidal tomogram in patient with fibrous dysplasia. Note involvement of sphenoid bone as well as septum and roof of nasal fossa *(arrows)*.

does occur.[52] Multiplanar computed tomography is often helpful in delineating the precise intracranial and extracranial extent of these lesions.[18,39] Antral mucoceles, once thought to be extremely rare, may represent up to 10% of all paranasal sinus mucoceles.[54] If sufficiently large, they can erode the medial maxillary wall and extend directly medially into the nasal fossa (Fig. 2-25). A unique subgroup termed ethmoidal *polypoid mucocele* has recently been described. These lesions differ from the more common variety of mucoceles in that they involve and expand the entire ethmoid complex; no single central mass is present. Most of the laminae papyracea and ethmoid septae are preserved.[20a]

Fibrous dysplasia of the facial bones or skull base may affect the nasal cavity. The thickened, sclerotic bone can produce varying degrees of nasal mass and obstruction (Fig. 2-26).

■ Benign tumors of the nasal cavity

Hemangiomas, neurofibromas, lipomas, and meningiomas may involve the nose. *Hemangiomas* initially arise in the ethmoid region. Growth is slow and therefore signs of both bone expansion and destruction are usually present along with a soft tissue mass. Hemangiomas and tumors of neural derivation are relatively common in children (Fig. 2-27).[49] Primary nasal and

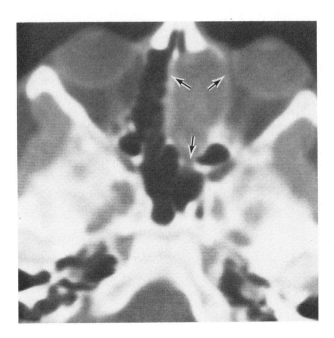

Fig. 2-27. Axial CT scan in 14-year-old boy with cribriform plate neurofibroma *(arrows)* that extends inferiorly into nasal apex. Note presence of bone expansion as well as destruction. (From Osborn, A.G., and McIff, E.B.: Head Neck Surg. **4:**182-192, 1982.)

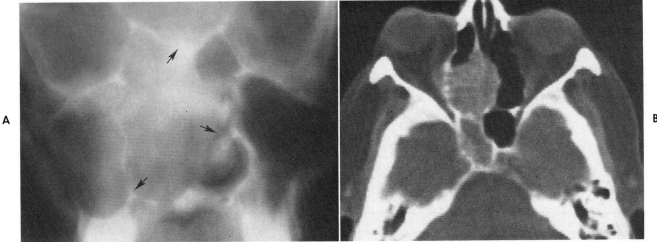

A   B

Fig. 2-28. A, AP hypocycloidal tomogram of large nasal fossa meningioma *(arrows).* **B,** Axial CT scan with contrast in different patient. Large cribriform plate meningioma extends inferiorly into nasal apex. (**B** from Osborn, A.G. and McIff, E.B.: Head Neck Surg., **4:**182-192, 1982.)

paranasal sinus *meningiomas* (Fig. 2-28, *A*) probably arise from embryonal arachnoid nests, although they more commonly occur as extensions of intracranial lesions that have a predominantely extracranial growth pattern (Fig. 2-28, *B*). Benign osteocartilaginous tumors do occur in the nasal fossa but are uncommon in this location (Fig. 2-29).

Juvenile nasopharyngeal angiofibroma is a highly vascular tumor of adolescent males that arises in the nasopharynx and pterygopalatine fossa. It initially bows

the posterior wall of the maxillary sinus anteriorly and the pterygoid plates posteriorly (Fig. 2-30, *A*). Angiofibromas tend to spread along natural fissures and foramina, extending anteromedially through the nasopharynx or sphenopalatine foramen into the nose, posterosuperiorly through the foramen rotundum into the sphenoid sinus and middle cranial fossa, laterally through the pterygomaxillary fissue into the infratemporal fossa, and anteriorly into the maxillary sinus.[17,21] Vascular supply can be from branches of the internal or

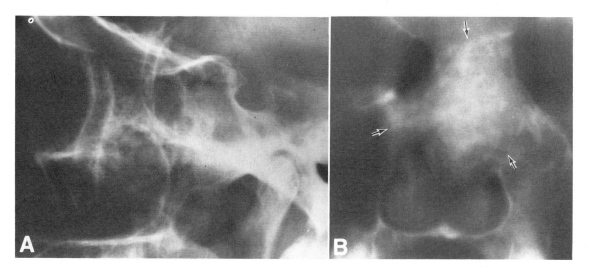

Fig. 2-29. A, Lateral plain film and, **B,** AP hypocycloidal tomogram of patient with sphenoid osteochondroma extending into nasal apex *(arrows)*.

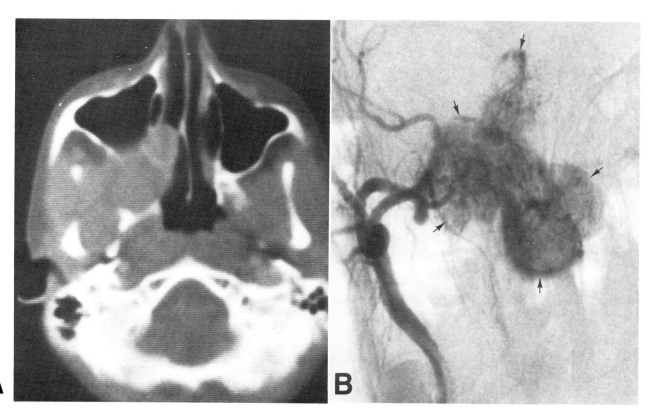

Fig. 2-30. A, Axial CT scan with contrast enhancement in patient with angiofibroma involving nasal and pterygopalatine fossae sinuses. **B,** Right external carotid angiogram, arterial phase, AP view, demonstrating lobulated vascular mass *(arrows)* in another patient with angiofibroma *(arrows)*. (From Osborn, A.G., and McIff, E.B.: Head Neck Surg. **4:**182-192, 1982.)

external carotid artery or the vertebral artery and may be unilateral or bilateral (Figure 2-30, *B*). Preoperative embolization significantly reduces intraoperative blood loss.[23,45] Recent authors have stressed the usefulness of CT in the radiographic staging of juvenile angiofibroma.[50]

The so-called angiomatous polyp may superficially resemble an angiofibroma. The lesions are avascular or hypovascular at angiography. On CT they may show enhancement. In contrast to angiofibroma, angiomatous polyps occur either as isolated nasal masses without a nasopharyngeal mass or appear as a bulky nasopharyngeal mass that does not invade the pterygopalatine fossa or sphenoid sinus. Unlike angiofibromas, angiomatous polyps are easily removed surgically. Radiation therapy and embolization are inappropriate.[52a]

Inverted papilloma is an uncommon benign epithelial tumor that involves the nasal fossa and paranasal sinus mucosa.[9] Irregular verrucous polyps are present. Inverted papillomas are primarily lesions of the lateral nasal wall but have also been observed on the nasal septum.[22] The radiographic findings are nonspecific, although a common finding is a unilateral nasal mass with opacification of the contiguous maxillary sinus. Pressure deformity or erosion of the bony sinus walls and nasal cavity may be present (Fig. 2-31). The nasal cavity is often filled with a tumor that may extend into the nasopharynx. Advanced cases can closely resemble carcinoma of the paranasal sinuses.[3,31] Recurrence after incomplete surgical removal is common.

■ Malignant tumors

Most primary malignant tumors involving the nasal fossa are epithelial or fibro-osseous in origin. *Squamous cell carcinoma* is the most common, accounting for 80% to 90% of tumors.[4] It often begins in the maxillary sinus and involves the nose by contiguous spread. Distant metastases are not uncommon.[12] High-resolution axial and coronal CT scans have essentially replaced plain film tomography in the evaluation of malignant facial lesions because they accurately delineate posterior, superior, orbital, intracranial, and infratemporal tumor extension (Fig. 2-32).[23,31]

Adenocarcinoma of the nose is less common than the squamous cell variety; cylindroma is the most frequent variant. Radiographic findings are usually an asymmetric or unilateral soft tissue mass exhibiting a purely destructive, aggressive growth pattern. Adenocarcinoma usually originates in minor salivary glands located in the nasal fossa (Fig. 2-33), along the palate (Fig. 2-34), or in other mucosal surfaces.[30]

Bone expansion is uncommon in malignant facial tumors and is rarely if ever caused solely by squamous cell carcinoma. Its presence should suggest either a coexisting mucocele or a slowly progressive malignant lesion such as lymphoma or esthesioneuroblastoma.[54]

Sarcomas are the predominant nasal malignancy in children. Most are embryonal or alveolar rhabdomyosarcomas.[2,49] Nearly 80% of these tumors are found in children under 12 years of age. Sarcomas usually exhibit a purely destructive growth pattern, extending

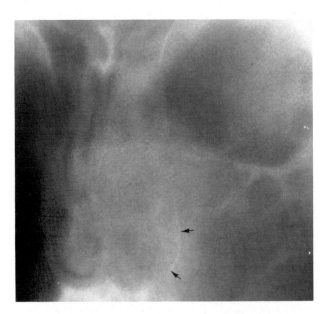

Fig. 2-31. AP hypocycloidal tomogram in patient with large inverting papilloma in left nasal fossa. Lesion extends into ethmoid and maxillary sinuses. Note combined bone expansion (*arrows*) and pressure erosion. (From Osborn, A.G., and McIff, E.B.: Head Neck Surg. **4:**182-192, 1982.)

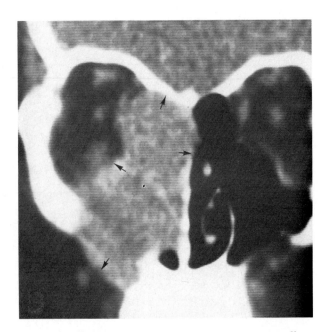

Fig. 2-32. Coronal CT scan in patient with squamous cell carcinoma of right maxillary sinus (*arrows*). Note destruction of adjacent sinus walls with direct extension into nasal fossa, ethmoid, and orbit.

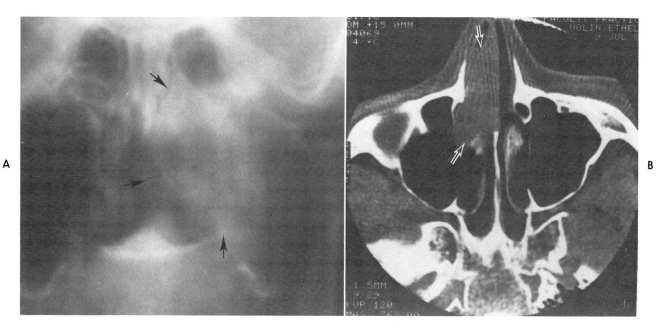

Fig. 2-33. A, AP hypocycloidal tomogram showing adenoid cystic carcinoma that originated in lateral nasal wall *(arrows)*. **B,** Axial CT scan of minor salivary gland adenocarcinoma originating in nasal septum *(arrow)*.

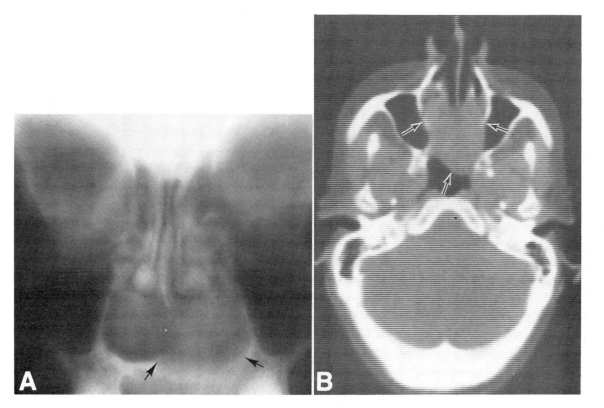

Fig. 2-34. A, AP hypocycloidal tomogram in patient with adenoid cystic carcinoma originating in hard palate *(arrows)*. **B,** Axial CT scan demonstrating involvement of nasal cavity, left maxillary sinus, and nasopharynx *(arrows)*. (From Osborn, A.G., and McIff, E.B.: Head Neck Surg. **4:**182-192, 1982.)

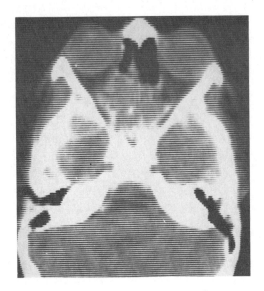

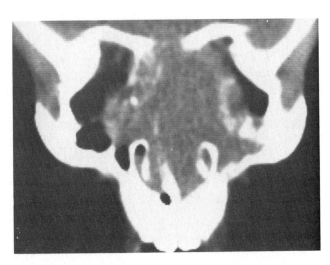

Fig. 2-35. Axial CT scan without contrast enhancement in 6-year-old boy with rhabdomyosarcoma of nasal fossa *(arrows)*. (From Osborn, A.G., and McIff, E.B.: Computed tomography of the nose, Head Neck Surg. **4:**182-192, 1982.)

Fig. 2-36. Coronal CT scan in 8-year-old boy with primary nasal and paranasal sinus lymphoma. Note extensive bone destruction.

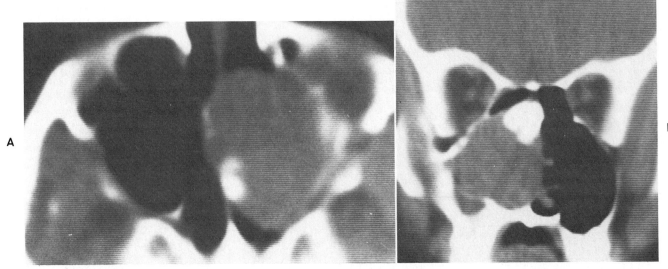

Fig. 2-37. Axial **(A)** and coronal **(B)** CT scans in 33-year-old woman with 15-year history of nasal "stuffiness". Slow-growing nature of lesion is indicated by associated calcification and bone expansion. Grade I fibrosarcoma. (From Osborn, A.G., and McIff, E.B.: Head Neck Surg. **4:**182-192, 1982.)

from the nose into adjacent structures such as the orbits and ethmoid sinuses (Fig. 2-35). Metastases can be widespread and multiple. Primary lymphoma of the upper aerodigestive tract is not uncommon in children[20] and can be radiographically indistinguishable from rhabdomyosarcoma (Fig. 2-36). Fibrosarcomas do occur in adults but are uncommon (Fig. 2-37).

Olfactory neuroblastomas or esthesioneuroblastomas are rare neurogenous tumors of the nasal cavity and paranasal sinuses. They arise high in the nasal fossa and

probably originate from sensory receptor cells of the olfactory mucosa. When they are small, their location may provide a clue to the diagnosis (Fig. 2-38). However, neither the clinical nor the radiographic findings are specific. Unilateral opacification of the ethmoid sinuses (with or without accompanying bone destruction) is often present, along with a soft tissue mass in the nose. Extension into the sphenoid and maxillary sinuses, orbit, and cranial vault is frequent. When the tumor becomes so extensive, it is indistinguishable from

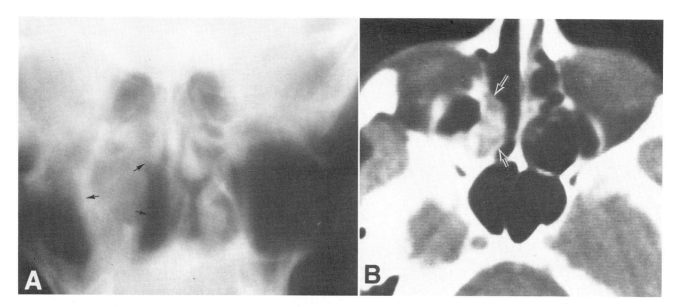

Fig. 2-38. A, AP hypocycloidal tomogram in patient with relatively focal esthesioneuroblastoma *(arrows)*. B, Contrast-enhanced axial CT scan in another patient with small biopsy-proven esthesioneuroblastoma *(arrows)*.

A

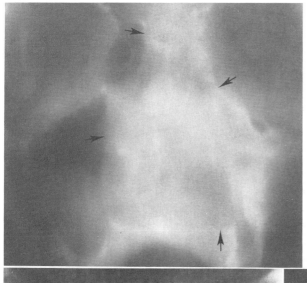

Fig. 2-39. A, AP hypocycloidal tomogram in patient with large esthesioneuroblastoma *(arrows)*. Soft tissue mass and bone destruction are extensive, but slight expansion of nasal fossa indicates relatively slow-growing process. B, Coronal CT scan in another patient with extensive esthesioneuroblastoma. C, Axial CT scan of partially calcified esthesioneuroblastoma that expands nasal fossa and maxillary sinus. This appearance is somewhat atypical. (C from Osborn, A.G., and McIff, E.B.: Head Neck Surg. 4:182-192, 1982.)

B

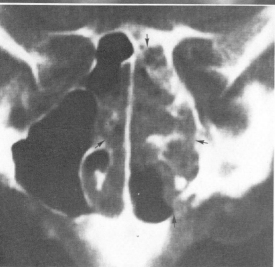

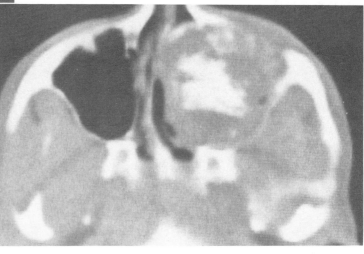

C

A

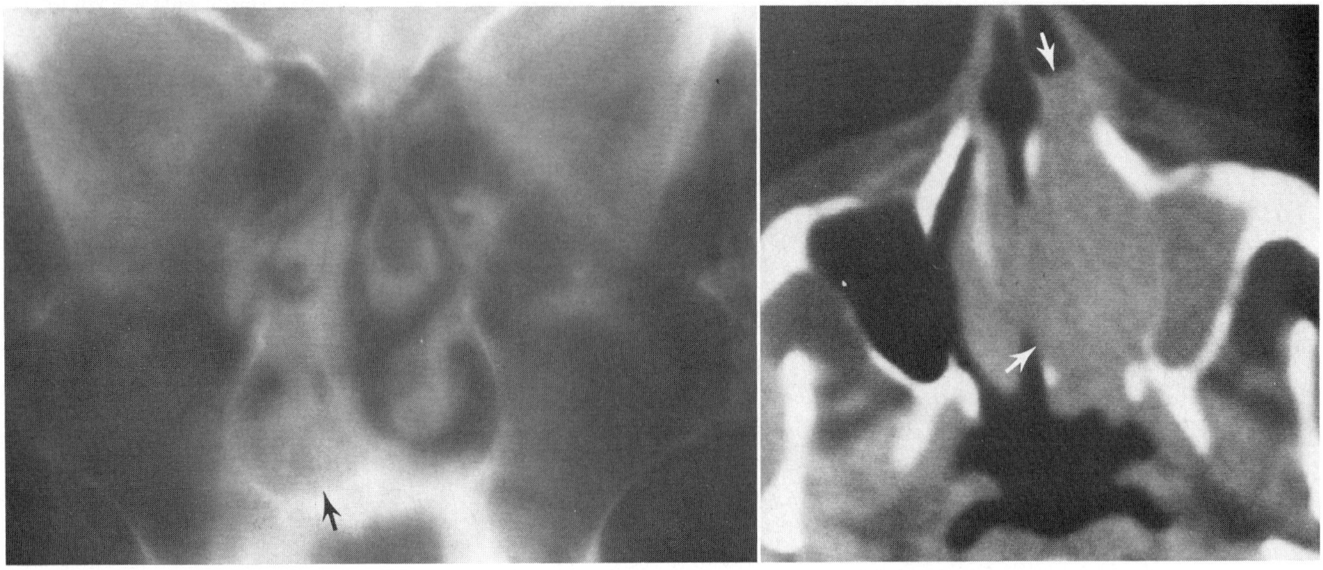

B

Fig. 2-40. A, AP hypocycloidal tomogram in 47-year-old man with lymphomatous masses in both maxillary antra and nasal fossa *(arrows).* **B,** Contrast-enhanced axial CT scan in patient with primary lymphoma of nasal fossa *(large arrows).* Lateral nasal wall is expanded, indicating either benign or slow-growing malignant lesion. Adjacent maxillary sinus is obstructed but not involved by tumor. Difference in attenuation coefficient permits this important distinction.

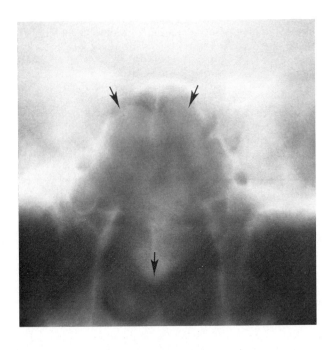

Fig. 2-41. AP hypocycloidal tomogram in patient with chordoma extending into sphenoid sinus and superior aspect of nasal fossa *(arrows).*

other nasal malignancies (Fig. 2-39). Distant metastases are not uncommon. Angiographic findings vary from definite hypervascularity with early draining veins to a faint but discrete tumor blush. CT shows a contrast-enhancing mass and delineates the extent of the soft tissue component. It may also help distinguish tumor mass from secondary or reactive sinusitis (Fig. 2-25).[8,26,41,47]

Extramedullary plasmacytoma, a rare form of plasma cell dyscrasia in which malignant plasma cell tumors originate outside the bone marrow, may arise in the nasal fossa, paranasal sinuses, or upper airway. Tomography usually demonstrates the presence of a soft tissue mass with associated bone destruction.[48] Primary *lymphoma* usually appears as soft tissue masses in the nasal fossa and paranasal sinuses (Fig. 2-40).

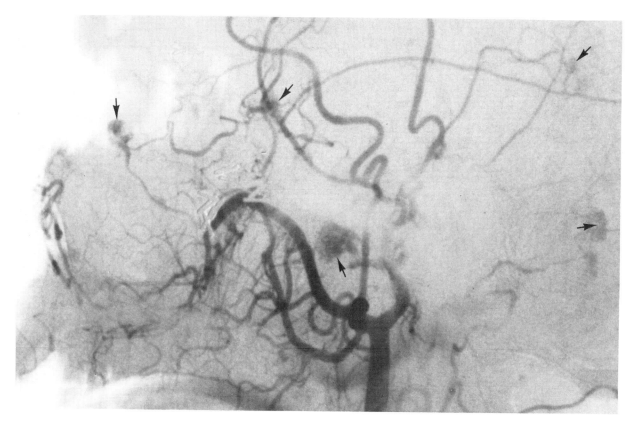

Fig. 2-42. Selective left external carotid angiogram, arterial phase, lateral view in patient with recurrent epistaxis secondary to Rendu-Osler-Weber disease. Numerous telangiectasias involving scalp and nasopharyngeal mucosa are indicated by arrows.

Metastatic disease of the nasal cavity is uncommon. Occasionally, metastases from vascular lesions, such as renal cell carcinoma, may cause intractable epistaxis. Malignant tumors from other sites may secondarily involve the nasal fossa (Fig. 2-41). Uncommonly, chordoma may appear initially with sinonasal symptoms caused by nasal and paranasal extension of the tumor.[10,15]

■ Epistaxis and vascular malformations

Hereditary hemorrhagic telangiectasis (Rendu-Osler-Weber disease) is a congenital disorder characterized by small arteriovenous fistulae or capillary telangiectasias that involve the skin, mucous membranes, and viscera.[35] Selective internal and external carotid angiography in these cases may disclose multiple small vascular nests in the nasal and oropharyngeal mucosa (Fig. 2-42).

Of all cases of *epistaxis,* 90% occur in Little's area and result primarily from atrophic rhinitis, hypertension and aging, or atherosclerotic disease involving the sphenopalatine artery.[51] Many investigators have advo-cated careful angiographic evaluation of the maxillary and internal carotid arteries, particularly in recurrent or posterior epistaxis.[16,37] More recently, a variety of therapeutic embolization procedures have been used in the treatment of recurrent or intractable epistaxis (see Chapter 9).*

□ **An algorithmic approach to the evaluation of nasal and paranasal lesions**

As is evident from the preceding discussion, the roentgenographic findings in a variety of nasal masses are quite similar and in many instances can be virtually indistinguishable. Therefore the radiologist's role should be to delineate the presence and precise extent of the mass and provide a reasonable differential diagnosis, rather than attempt to establish a specific histologic diagnosis on the basis of radiographs alone.

Initial evaluation of the patient with a probable mass in the nose or paranasal sinuses should begin with high-quality plain films. If these demonstrate definite bone

*References 5, 6, 19, 24, 33, 43.

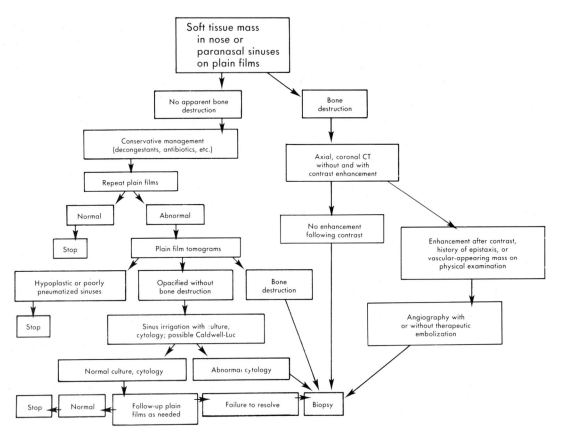

Fig. 2-43. Suggested algorithmic approach to evaluation of soft tissue masses in nose or paranasal sinuses. (From Osborn, A.G., and McIff, E.B.: Head Neck Surg. **4:**182-192, 1982.)

destruction, the workup can proceed directly to axial and coronal CT, performed both without and with contrast enhancement. If there is a history of epistaxis, or if the scans show marked increase in attenuation of the lesion following intravenous contrast, cerebral angiography should precede biopsy (Fig. 2-43).

If no apparent bone destruction is identified on initial plain films, conservative medical management can be instigated and followed up at an appropriate interval by repeat plain films. If these are persistently abnormal, plain film tomography is often helpful. The presence of bone destruction indicates the need to perform a CT scan. If abnormal cells are found with sinus washing, a CT scan can also be performed, or the referring clinician may proceed directly to biopsy.[39]

□ **References**

1. Addlestone, R.B., and Baylin, G.J.: Rinocerebral mucomycosis, Radiology **115:**113-117, 1975.
2. Batsakis, J.G.: The pathology of head and neck tumors. Part 5. Nasal cavity and paranasal sinuses, Head Neck Surg. **2:**410-419, 1980.
3. Batsakis, J.G., Regezi, J.A., and Rice, D.H.: The pathology of head and neck tumors. Part 8. Fibroadipose tissue and skeletal muscle, Head Neck Surg. **3:**145-168, 1980.
4. Batsakis, J.G., Solomon, A.R., and Rice, D.H.: The pathology of head and neck tumors. Part 11. Carcinoma of the nasopharynx, Head Neck Surg. **3:**511-524, 1981.
5. Bernstein, A., and Kricheff, I.I.: Catheter and material selection for transarterial embolization: technical considerations. I. Catheters, Radiology **132:**619-630, 1979.
6. Berenstein, A., and Kricheff, I.I.: Catheter and material selection for transarterial embolization: technical considerations. II. Materials, Radiology **132:**631-639, 1979.
7. Bergstrom, L.B.: Anomalies of the nose and paranasal sinuses. In English, G.M., editor: Otolaryngology, New York, 1976, Harper & Row, Publishers, Inc.
8. Burke, D.P., Gabrielsen, T.O., Knake, J.E., et al.: Radiology of olfactory neuroblastoma, Radiology **137:**367-372, 1980.
9. Calcaterra, T.C., Thompson, J.W., and Paglia, D.E.: Inverting papillomas of the nose and paranasal sinuses, Laryngoscope **90:**53-60, 1980.
10. Campbell, W.M., McDonald, T.J., Unni, K.K., and Laws, E.R., Jr.: Nasal and paranasal presentations of chordomas, Laryngoscope **90:**612-618, 1980.
11. Corliss, C.E.: Patten's human embryology, New York, 1976, McGraw-Hill Book Co.
12. Dennington, M., Carter, D.R., and Meyers, A.D.: Distant metastases in head and neck epidermoid carcinoma, Laryngoscope **90:**196-201, 1980.

13. Diaz, F., Latchow, R., Duvall, A.J., III, et al.: Mucoceles with intracranial and extracranial extensions, J. Neurosurg. **48**:284-288, 1978.

14. Dodd, G.D., and Jing, B.S.: Radiology of the nose, paranasal sinuses and nasopharynx Baltimore, 1977, The Williams & Wilkins Co.

15. Eisemann, M.L.: Sphenooccipital chordoma presenting as a nasopharyngeal mass, Ann. Otol. Rhinol. Laryngol. **89**:271-275, 1980.

16. Ericsson, J.S., and Lindell, D.: Selective carotid angiography in patients with intractable epistaxis, Rhinology **13**:47-50, 1975.

17. Fitzpatrick, P.J., Briant, T.D.R., and Berman, J.M.: The nasopharyngeal angiofibroma, Arch. Otolaryngol. **106**:234-236, 1980.

18. Hesselink, J.R., Weber, A.L., New, P.F.J., et al.: Evaluation of mucoceles of the paranasal sinuses with computed tomography, Radiology **133**:397-400, 1979.

19. Hilal, S.K., and Michelsen, J.W.: Therapeutic percutaneous embolization for extra-axial vascular lesions of the head, neck, and spine, J. Neurosurg. **43**:275-287, 1975.

20. Hunter, D.W., L'Heureux, P.R., and Latchaw, R.E.: Malignant facial tumors in children: radiologic examination, Pediatr. Radiol. **10**:2-8, 1980.

20a. Jacobs, M., and Som, P.M.: The ethmoidal "polypoid mucocele," J. Comput. Assist. Tomogr. **6**:721-724, 1982.

21. Jafek, B.W., Krekorian, E.A., Kirsch, W.M., and Wood, R.P.: Juvenile nasopharyngeal angiofibroma: management of intracranial extension, Head Neck Surg. **2**:119-128, 1979.

22. Kelly, J.H., Joseph, M., and Carroll, E., et al.: Inverted papilloma of the nasal septum, Arch. Otolaryngol. **106**:767-771, 1980.

23. Lasjaunias, P.: Nasopharyngeal angiofibromas: hazards of embolization, Radiology **136**:119-123, 1980.

24. Latchaw, R.E., and Gold, L.H.A.: Polyvinyl foam embolization of vascular and neoplastic lesions of the head, neck, and spine, Radiology **131**:669-679, 1979.

25. Lavell, C.L.B.: An analysis of fetal craniofacial growth, Ann. Hum. Biol. **1**:269-287, 1974.

26. Manelfe, C., Bonafe, A., Fabre, P., and Pessey, J.J.: Computed tomography in olfactory neuroblastoma: one case of esthesioneuroepithelioma and four cases of esthesioneuroblastoma, J. Comput. Asst. Tomogr. **2**:412-420, 1978.

27. May, M.: Nasofrontal-ethmoidal injuries, Laryngoscope **87**:948-953, 1977.

28. McGill, T.J., Simpson, G., and Healy, G.B.: Fulminant aspergillosis of the nose and paranasal sinuses: a new clinical entity, Laryngoscope **90**:748-754, 1980.

29. McGuirt, W.F., and Harrill, J.A.: Paranasal sinus aspergillosis, Laryngoscope **89**:1563-1568, 1979.

30. Miller, R.H., and Calcaterra, T.H.: Adenoid cystic carcinoma of the nose, paranasal sinuses, and palate, Arch. Otolaryngol. **106**:424-426, 1980.

31. Momose, K.J., Weber, A.L., Goodman, M., et al.: Radiological aspects of inverted papilloma, Radiology **134**:73-79, 1980.

32. Moore, K.L.: The developing human, Philadelphia, 1977, W.B. Saunders Co.

33. Moseley I: Therapeutic embolization of the carotid arteries: a review, Head Neck Surg. **1**:519-532, 1979.

34. Nemir, R.L., Branom-Genieser, N., and Balasubramanyam, P.: Extensive sclerosis of the base of the skull due to primary nasal tuberculosis, Pediatr. Radiol. **8**:42-44, 1979.

35. Newton, T.H., and Troost, B.T.: Arteriovenous malformations and fistulae. In Newton, T.H., and Potts, D.G., editors: Radiology of the skull and brain, vol. 2, St. Louis, 1974, The C.V. Mosby Co.

36. Nicholson, R.L., and Dreel, L.: CT anatomy of the nasopharynx, nasal cavity, paranasal sinuses, and infratemporal fossa, CT **3**:13-22, 1979.

37. Osborn, A.G.: The nasal arteries, AJR **130**:89-97, 1978.

38. Osborn, A.G.: The vidian artery: normal and pathologic anatomy, Radiology **136**:373-378, 1980.

39. Osborn, A.G., and McIff, E.B.: Computed tomography of the nose, Head Neck Surg. **4**:182-192, 1982.

40. Paff, G.H.: Anatomy of the head and neck, Philadelphia, 1973, W.B. Saunders Co.

41. Parsons, C., and Hodson, N.: Computed tomography of paranasal sinus tumors, Radiology **132**:641-645, 1979.

42. Price, H.I., Batnitzky, S., Karlin, C.A., and Norris, C.W.: Giant nasal rhinolith, AJNR **2**:371-373, 1981.

43. Quisling, R.G.: Intrapetrous carotid artery branches: pathological application, Radiology **134**:109-113, 1980.

44. Roberson, G.H., Patterson, A.K., Deeb, M.E., et al. Sphenoethmoidal mucocele: radiographic diagnosis, AJR **127**:595-599, 1976.

45. Roberson, G.H., Price, A.C., Davis, J.M., and Bulati, A.: Therapeutic embolization of juvenile angiofibroma, AJR **133**:657-663, 1979.

46. Rontal, M., and Duritz, G.: Proboscis lateralis: case report and embryologic analysis, Laryngoscope **87**:996-1006, 1977.

47. Rosengren, J.E., Jing, B.S., Wallace, S., and Danziger, J.: Radiographic features of olfactory neuroblastoma, AJR **132**:945-948, 1979.

47a. RSNA Case of the day. Case IV: rhinolith, Radiology **146**:251-252, 1983.

48. Schabel, S.I., Rogers, C.I., Rittenberg, G.M., and Bubany, R.: Extramedullary plasmacytoma, Radiology **128**:625-628, 1978.

49. Schramm, V.L., Jr.: Inflammatory and neoplastic masses of the nose and paranasal sinus in children, Laryngoscope **89**:1887-1897, 1979.

50. Sessions, R.B., Bryan, R.N., Naclerio, R.M., and Alford, B.R.: Radiographic staging of angiofibroma, Head Neck Surg. **3**:279-283, 1981.

51. Shaheen, O.: Studies of the nasal vasculature and the problems of arterial ligation for epistaxis, Ann. R. Coll. Surg. Engl. **47**:30-44, 1970.

52. Siegel, M.J., Shackelford, G.D., and McAlister, W.H.: Paranasal sinus mucoceles in children, Radiology **133**:623-626, 1979.

52a. Som, P.M., Cohen, B.A., Sacher, M., et al.: The angiofibroma: two different lesions, Radiology **144**:329-334, 1982.

53. Som, P.M., and Shugar, J.M.A.: Antral mucoceles: a new look, J. Comput. Asst. Tomogr. **4**:484-488, 1980.

54. Som, P.M., and Shugar, J.M.A.: The significance of bone expansion associated with the diagnosis of malignant tumors of the paranasal sinuses, Radiology **136**:97-100, 1980.

55. Towbin, R., Dunbar, J.S., and Bove, K.: Antrochoanal polyps, A.J.R. **132**:27-31, 1979.

56. Wetmore, S.J., and Patz, C.E.: Idiopathic midface lesions, Ann. Otol. Rhinol. Laryngol. **87**:60-69, 1978.

57. Wilson, D.B.: Embryonic development of the head and neck. Part 3. The face, Head Neck Surg. **2**:145-153, 1979.

58. Wilson, McC.: Chronic hypertrophic polypoid rhinosinusitis, Radiology **120**:609-613, 1976.

59. Winestock, D.P., Bartlett, P.C., and Sondheimer, F.K.: Benign nasal polyps causing bone destruction in the nasal cavity and paranasal sinuses, Laryngoscope **88**:674-679, 1978.

59a. Zilkha, A.: Computed tomography in facial trauma, Radiology **144**:545-548, 1982.

60. Zizmor, J.: An atlas of otolaryngologic radiology, Philadelphia, 1978, W.B. Saunders Co.

61. Zizmor, J., and Noyek, A.M.: Cysts, benign tumors, and malignant tumors of the paranasal sinuses, Otolaryngol. Clin. North Am. **6**:487-508, 1973.

3 □ The pterygopalatine (sphenomaxillary) fossa

ANNE G. OSBORN

The pterygopalatine (sphenomaxillary) fossa is the primary distribution center for both the parasympathetic innervation and the vascular supply of deep facial structures. It is also a major anatomic "crossroad" between the nasal and oral cavities, infratemporal fossa, orbit, pharynx, and middle cranial fossa. As such, it provides a natural pathway for dissemination or spread of a wide variety of disease processes to contiguous structures within the face and calvaria.[27]

□ Normal gross anatomy
■ Bony margins

The pterygopalatine fossa is a small, slightly elongated triangular compartment that lies just behind the posterior wall of the maxillary sinus and in front of the pterygoid plates. It is bounded anteriorly by the corpus maxillae and superiorly by the body of the sphenoid bone. The medial margin of the pterygopalatine fossa is formed by the orbital process of the palatine bone. Its posterior border consists of the fused anterior mass of the medial and lateral pterygoid plates (Fig. 3-1).

■ Communications

Through a variety of fissures and foramina the pterygopalatine fossa communicates with the nasal and oral cavities, infratemporal fossa, orbit, pharynx, and middle cranial fossa. Eight passageways lead directly to or from the pterygopalatine fossa itself.[2,3,29] It is through these bony canals that branches of the pterygopalatine ganglion and terminal maxillary artery are distributed (Fig. 3-2). In most instances both the vessels and accompanying nerves are named for the canal through which they pass (see below).

Laterally, the pterygopalatine fossa is continuous with the intratemporal fossa by way of the pterygomaxillary fissure. The pterygopalatine and nasal fossae communicate with each other by way of the sphenopalatine foramen, an opening in the orbital process of the palatine bone. Anterosuperiorly, the pterygopalatine fossa is connected to the orbital apex through the posteromedial aspect of the intraorbital fissure. Inferiorly, the lesser and greater palatine canals communicate with the oral cavity, transmitting their respective nerves and arteries.

Three posteriorly directed foramina exit from the pterygopalatine fossa in an obliquely oriented line within the root of the sphenoid bone. From lateral to medial they are (1) the foramen rotundum, (2) the pterygoid (vidian) canal, and (3) the pharyngeal or palatovaginal canal.

The foramen rotundum lies above and lateral to the pterygoid canal, connecting the pterygopalatine and middle cranial fossae. It runs laterally as it courses anteriorly. The pterygoid or vidian canal lies within the body of the sphenoid between the roots of the medial and lateral pterygoid plates. The vidian canal connects the pterygopalatine fossa with the foramen lacerum. In contrast to the foramen rotundum, the vidian canal runs medially as it courses anteriorly. The palatovaginal (pharyngeal) canal is formed by the junction of the processus vaginalis of the sphenoid bone and sphenoid process of the palatine bone. The palatovaginal canal connects the vault of the nasopharynx with the pterygopalatine fossa[38] and transmits the pharyngeal nerve. Because the similarity in terminology may be confusing, by way of review the reader is encouraged to take note of the following distinctions:

1. Pterygopalatine *fossa:* this term is synonymous with sphenomaxillary fossa. It is a large triangular space situated between the posterior wall of the maxillary antrum and the anterior wall of the pterygoid fossa.
2. Pterygomaxillary *fissure:* the lateral extension of the pterygopalatine fossa, which serves as the

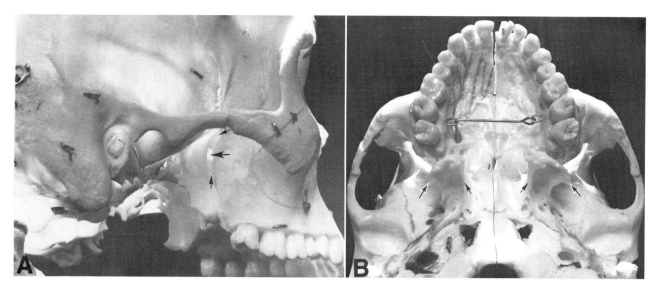

Fig. 3-1. Photographs of dried skull. **A,** Lateral view. Teardrop-shaped pterygopalatine fossa *(small arrows)* lies just in front of pterygoid plates. Sphenopalatine foramen, indicated by large arrow, lies within depths of fossa. **B,** Submentovertex view. Medial and lateral pterygoid plates are indicated by black and outlined arrows respectively. (Reproduced from Osborn, A.G.: AJR **132:**389–394, 1979. Copyright © 1979, American Roentgen Ray Society.)

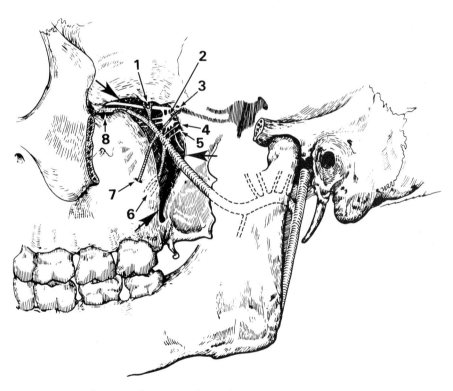

Fig. 3-2. Anatomic diagram of pterygopalatine fossa and its major contents. Segments of zygomatic arch and mandible have been removed to show fossa *(large black arrows)*. Fossa narrows inferiorly to become pterygopalatine canal. Maxillary artery is seen entering fossa by way of pterygomaxillary fissure. *1,* Sphenopalatine foramen, with branches of sphenopalatine artery exiting medially to supply nasal cavity; *2,* sphenopalatine (pterygopalatine) ganglion; *3,* foramen rotundum. Maxillary nerve passes anteriorly from semilunar ganglion, exits through foramen, and passes through superior part of pterygopalatine fossa. Artery of foramen rotundum courses posterosuperiorly through foramen rotundum. *4,* Vidian artery (artery of pterygoid canal); *5,* pharyngeal artery; *6,* greater and lesser palatine arteries; *7,* posterior superior alveolar artery; *8,* inferior orbital fissure. Infraorbital artery and nerve course anteriorly thorugh fissure to enter orbit. (From Osborn, A.G.: AJR **132:**389–394, 1979. Copyright © 1979, American Roentgen Ray Society.)

communication between the pterygopalatine fossa (medially) and the infratemporal fossa (laterally).

3. Pterygopalatine *canal:* the narrow inferior extension of the pterygopalatine fossa.
4. Pterygoid canal: synonymous with vidian canal. This is a conduit between the pterygoid fossa and the foramen lacerum.
5. Pharyngeal canal: synonymous with the palatovaginal canal. This is a conduit between the pterygopalatine fossa and the nasopharynx.
6. Pterygopalatine ganglion: synonymous with the sphenopalatine ganglion.

■ Nerves of the pterygopalatine fossa

The most important contents of the pterygopalatine fossa are the sphenopalatine ganglion and the maxillary artery and nerve. The maxillary nerve (the second division of cranial nerve V) exits from the middle cranial fossa and courses anteriorly through the foramen rotundum to enter the pterygopalatine fossa. As it crosses the fossa the maxillary nerve gives off zygomatic and posterior superior alveolar nerves and sends branches to the sphenopalatine ganglion (Fig. 3-2). It then continues anteriorly as the infraorbital nerve. After passing through the inferior orbital fissure and canal, it emerges from the infraorbital foramen and is distributed to the skin of the face, nose, lower eyelid, and upper lip.

The sphenopalatine ganglion, one of four parasympathetic ganglia of the head, lies in the superomedial portion of the pterygopalatine fossa. Parasympathetic fibers from the facial nerve synapse in the sphenopalatine ganglion. All other fibers pass through this structure and its branches without synapsing. The sphenopalatine ganglion relays secretomotor impulses to the lacrimal gland and nasopharyngeal mucosa.[16,29]

■ Arteries of the pterygopalatine fossa

The third or pterygopalatine portion of the maxillary artery courses through the pterygomaxillary fissure, loops within the pterygopalatine fossa, and gives rise to terminal branches that leave the fossa by passing into a bony canal or foramen (Figure 3-2). Each vessel bears the name of the canal that transmits it.[2]

The posteriorly directed branches of the distal maxillary artery are the artery of the foramen rotundum, the artery of the pterygoid canal, and the pharyngeal artery. The artery of the foramen rotundum is the most lateral of these three branches. It passes posterosuperiorly through its canal to anastomose with the artery of the inferior cavernous sinus (infero-lateral trunk of the internal carotid artery).[21] The vidian artery runs posterolaterally through the pterygoid canal, then exits through the foramen lacerum to supply rami to the oropharyngeal mucosa. Its main trunk may also continue

posteriorly to anastomose with the petrous segment of the internal carotid artery.[28] The most medial of the three posterior maxillary artery branches is the pharyngeal artery. It exits from the pterygopalatine fossa through the palatovaginal (pharyngeal) canal and is distributed to the oropharynx and eustachian tube orifice.

The anteriorly directed branches of the distal maxillary artery are distributed around the maxillary sinus. The posterior superior alveolar artery arises just as the maxillary artery passes into the pterygopalatine fossa. It courses inferiorly to supply the mucosa of the cheek and the buccinator muscle, maxillary antrum, alveolar ridge, and teeth.[11] The infraorbital artery, an anterosuperior branch of the maxillary artery, runs through the inferior orbital fissure and canal, emerging from the infraorbital foramen to supply branches around the nose, orbit, and cheek.

The greater (descending) palatine artery courses inferiorly within the pterygopalatine fossa, defining the posterior and inferior aspects of the maxillary sinus. It anastomoses with branches of the facial artery to supply the hard palate.[21] The sphenopalatine artery is the major terminal branch of the maxillary artery. It leaves the pterygopalatine fossa through the sphenopalatine foramen, coursing medially to supply the mucosa of the nasal fossa.[26]

■ Normal radiographic anatomy

The pterygopalatine fossa itself is surprisingly variable in size and shape (Fig. 3-3). The transverse diameter as well as overall length of the fossa vary considerably from side to side and from patient to patient.[27] The configurations range from an elongated, slitlike crevasse to a somewhat more triangular, teardrop-shaped opening (Fig. 3-3). In all normal cases the surrounding cortical margins of the fossa are well delineated.[30]

Plain film radiographs and lateral hypocycloidal tomograms through the pterygopalatine fossa and medial pterygoid plate demonstrate the broad superior portion of the fossa as it narrows inferiorly to become the pterygopalatine canal (Figs. 3-4 and 3-5, *A*). The base of the

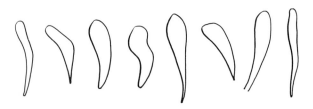

Fig. 3-3. Variations in configuration of pterygopalatine fossa. Drawn from actual radiographs. (From Osborn, A.G.: AJR **132:**389-394, 1979. Copyright © 1979, American Roentgen Ray Society.)

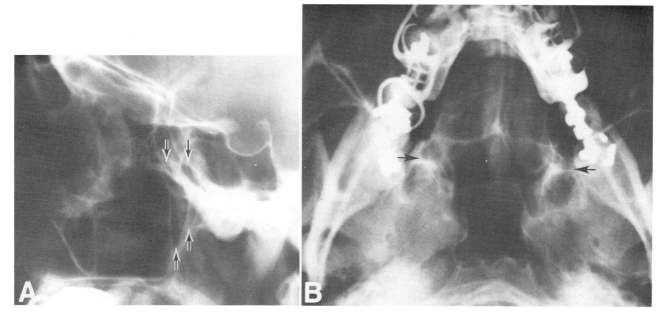

Fig. 3-4. A, Plain film radiograph of face, lateral view. Film is slightly rotated. Two pterygopalatine fossae *(arrows)* are clearly identified as elongated, teardrop-shaped openings lying behind maxillary sinuses. **B,** Plain film radiograph of skull, submentovertex view. Pterygoid fossae *(arrows)* lie just in front of pterygoid plates.

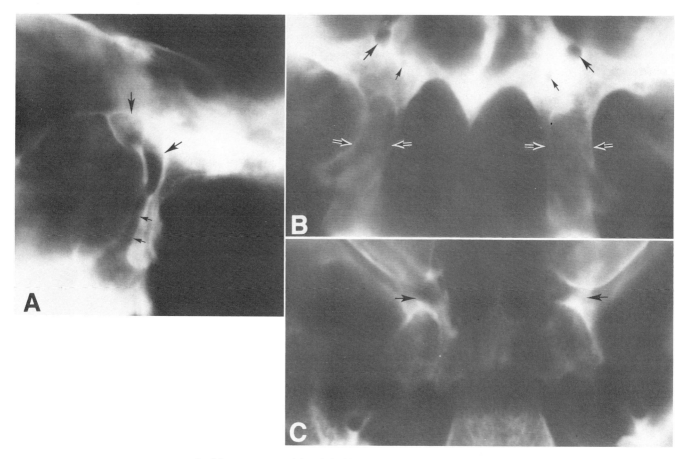

Fig. 3-5. Hypocycloidal tomograms of dried skull. **A,** Lateral view. Pterygopalatine fossa *(large arrows)* narrows inferiorly to become pterygopalatine canal *(small arrows).* **B,** AP view. Pterygoid plates are indicated by outlined arrows. Foramen rotundum *(large black arrow)* and pterygoid canal *(small black arrows)* are shown. **C,** Submentovertex view. Pterygopalatine fossa *(arrows)* is space formed by posterior wall of maxillary sinus and fused anterior mass of pterygoid plates. (From Osborn, A.G.: AJR **132:**389-394, 1979. Copyright © 1979, American Roentgen Ray Society.)

pterygoid plates and the pterygoid fossa, the V-shaped space contained between the two pterygoid plates, are both best appreciated on either AP (Fig. 3-5, *B*) or submentovertex (Fig. 3-5, *C*) tomograms. The foramen rotundum and pterygoid canal can also be identified on these views. The palatovaginal or pharyngeal canal is anatomically insignificant and is rarely visualized.

The pterygopalatine fossa and its adjacent structures are also clearly delineated on CT scans. Axial sections through the posterior lateral recess of the nasopharynx (fossa of Rosenmuller) demonstrate the characteristic inverted U appearance of the medial and lateral ptery-goid plates (Figs. 3-6, *A*, and 2-7, *E*). The pterygopalatine canal, the inferior continuation of the pterygopalatine fossa, is occasionally visualized as a small foramen in front of the fused anterior mass of the pterygoid plates. Horizontal scans 1 cm above this level pass through the pterygopalatine fossa itself. The fossa is seen as a curved, slitlike space contained between the posterior wall of the maxillary sinus and the base of the pterygoid plates (Figs. 3-6, *B*, and 2-7, *D*). Direct sagittal or reconstructed lateral scans through the pyterygoid plates clearly demonstrate the teardrop-shaped pterygopalatine fossa (Fig. 3-6, *C*).

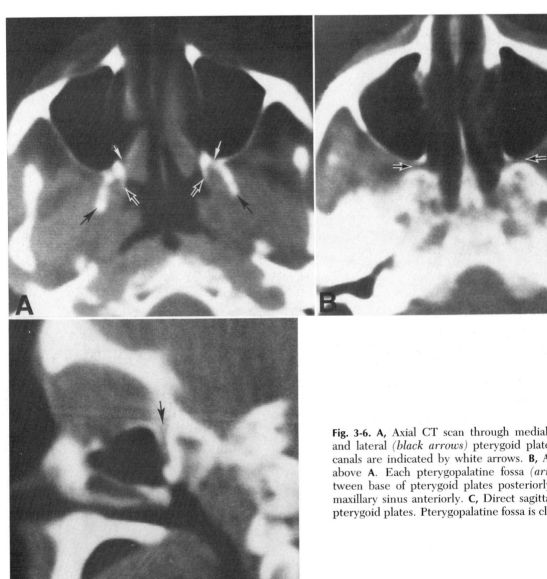

Fig. 3-6. A, Axial CT scan through medial *(outlined arrows)* and lateral *(black arrows)* pterygoid plates. Pterygopalatine canals are indicated by white arrows. **B,** Axial CT scan 1 cm above **A.** Each pterygopalatine fossa *(arrows)* is space between base of pterygoid plates posteriorly and back wall of maxillary sinus anteriorly. **C,** Direct sagittal CT scan through pterygoid plates. Pterygopalatine fossa is clearly seen *(arrow).*

□ Lesions involving the pterygopalatine fossa
■ Trauma

Severe facial trauma often involves the pterygoid plates. Complex zygomaticomaxillary[4,12,42] and LeFort or bilateral multisinus fractures may involve these structures. Because the middle and inferior portions of the pterygoid processes are fused to the posterior maxillary wall (Fig. 3-1, *A*), the application of lateral or frontal force to the maxilla may result in pterygoid plate interruption.[12,30] LeFort I and II (pyramidal) fractures usually extend through the pterygoid plates, often widening the pterygomaxillary fissure. LeFort III injuries (craniofacial dysjunction) interrupt the pterygoid plates near the apex of the pterygopalatine fossa at the junction of the plates and the body of the sphenoid. Multiple pterygoid plate fractures with widening, distortion, or compression of the pterygopalatine fossa are common in patients with severe facial injury. Plain film tomography has been used to delineate such fractures (Figure 3-7, *A*) although CT is now the diagnostic procedure of choice in complex facial trauma (Fig. 3-7, *B*).[41a] Traumatic pseudoaneurysm or occlusion of the distal maxillary artery within the pterygopalatine fossa is an occasional associated complication (Fig. 3-8).[8]

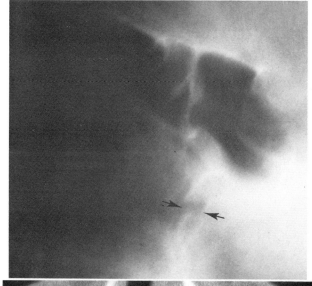

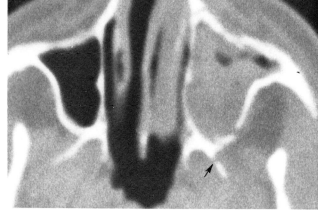

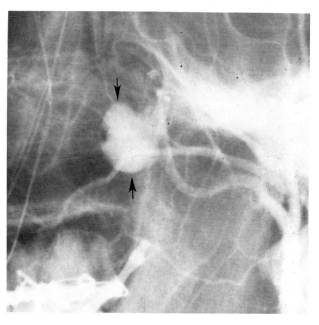

Fig. 3-7. A, Lateral hypocycloidal tomogram in patient with multiple facial fractures that involve pterygoid plates and maxillary sinus *(arrows)*. Note distortion of pterygopalatine fossa. **B,** Axial CT scan shows comminuted fracture through maxillary sinus. Note associated pterygoid fracture *(arrow)*. (**A** from Osborn, A.G.: AJR **132:**389-394, 1979. Copyright © 1979, American Roentgen Ray Society.)

Fig. 3-8. Left external carotid angiogram, arterial phase, lateral view in patient with LeFort II and III fractures and posttraumatic pseudoaneurysm *(arrows)* pterygopalatine segment of maxillary artery. (Courtesy Franklin J. Miller, Jr., M.D., University of Utah College of Medicine, Salt Lake City, Utah.)

■ Inflammatory lesions

Uncomplicated inflammatory lesions of the nose and paranasal sinuses do not usually involve the pterygopalatine fossa.[44] Chronic hypertrophic polypoid rhinosinusitis—a condition characterized by marked polypoid mucosal hypertrophy of the nasal fossa and paranasal sinuses—may be evidenced by extensive bony erosion or sclerosis.[13,41] In such instances the marked bone destruction may suggest a more ominous diagnosis, such as neoplasm, necrotizing granuloma, or fungal infection. The presence of associated bone expansion plus a clinical history of vasomotor rhinitis, chronic sinusitis, and nasal polyps should be helpful in the radiographic differential diagnosis.[13,41]

Necrotizing granulomas and fungal infections can and often do involve the pterygopalatine fossa. Focal bone destruction without expansion is present in the nasal cavity (Fig. 3-9). Multiple paranasal sinuses are usually involved[1,22,23] and the bone destruction initially tend to follow natural foramina and fissures.

■ Nonneoplastic mass lesions

The rare but unusually extensive sphenoethmoid mucocele may involve the pterygopalatine fossa (Fig. 3-10). Multiple curvilinear expansile deformities of the adjacent sinus walls (suggesting a benign, long-standing process), opacification, and focal areas of bone thinning or destruction are suggestive of the diagnosis.[10,32] CT

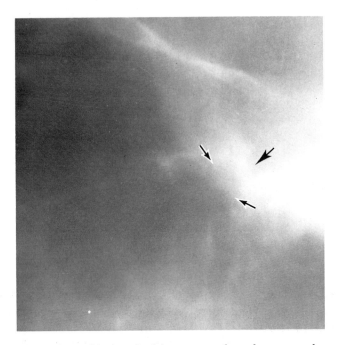

Fig. 3-9. Lateral hypocycloidal tomogram through pterygopalatine fossa in patient with extensive mucormycosis. Fungus has eroded fossa *(outlined arrows)* and foramen rotundum *(black arrow).*

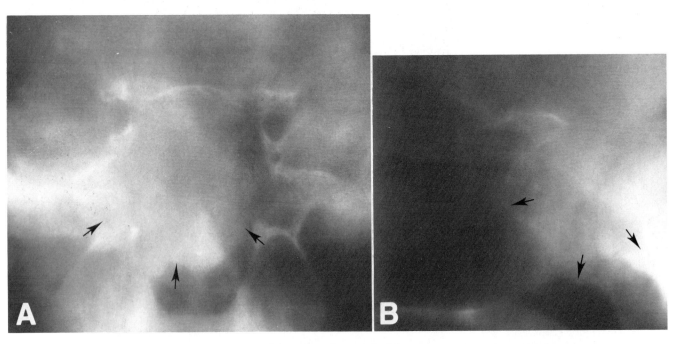

Fig. 3-10. Anteroposterior **(A)** and lateral **(B)** hypocycloidal tomograms in patient with huge sphenoethmoid mucocele that has destroyed sella turcica and extended into pterygopalatine fossa, eroding base of pterygoid plates.

scans are particularly helpful in delineating the extent of the soft tissue mass.[18]

Benign, nontumorous lesions such as giant carotid cavernous sinus or paraclinoid aneurysms may produce pressure erosion of the sphenoid sinus.[25] If the aneurysm is of sufficient size, the bone destruction may extend into the base of the pterygoid process and the apex of the pterygopalatine fossa.

Localized or regional fibrous dysplasia (leontiasis ossea) may involve several adjacent bones of the facial skeleton and anterior cranial fossa. Bone replacement by dense osteoid and fibrous tissue results in varying degrees of bone thickening and encroachment on the pterygopalatine fossa (Fig. 3-11). The differential diagnosis includes Paget's disease, meningioma, osteoblastic metastasis, epidermoid carcinoma, and chronic osteomyelitis.[43]

■ Benign tumors

A variety of benign tumors may involve the pterygopalatine fossa and its adjacent structures. The epithelial or inverting papilloma usually appears as a unilateral nasal soft tissue mass accompanied by simultaneous expansion and focal destruction of the affected paranasal sinuses.[5] Unusually large lesions can involve the pterygopalatine fossa and are radiographically indistinguishable from carcinoma.[9,24]

Juvenile nasopharyngeal angiofibromas are benign hamartomas that arise in the nasopharynx of adolescent males.[6,31] Plain films or tomography demonstrate a nasopharyngeal soft tissue mass and expansion of the pterygopalatine fossa (Fig. 3-12, A). Once considered pathognomic of angiofibroma, anterior bowing of the posterior antral wall and subsequent enlargement of the pterygopalatine fossa is nonspecific and reflects the presence of slow-growing retromaxillary space tumor.[37] Schwannoma, lymphoepithelioma, and fibrous histiocytoma should also be included in the differential diagnosis.

Angiofibromas are highly vascular lesions that have a reticulated appearance with a homogeneous blush persisting into the early venous phase of angiography (Fig. 3-12, B). Early draining veins are uncommon.[35] The angiographic appearance is quite characteristic although fibrous tumors, lymphoepitheliomas, and extracranial meningiomas may closely resemble angiofibromas.[34]

Angiofibromas spread locally by extension along natural foramina and fissures. Although they may extend widely, displacing bony septae and permeating natural foramina, they do not invade structures such as the carotid sheath.[7] The most common routes by which angiofibromas spread from the pterygopalatine fossa are posteriorly or superiorly into the cavernous sinus and middle cranial fossa; anteriorly into the maxillary sinus; and inferolaterally into the infratemporal fossa.[14,19,20]

Numerous authors have recently emphasized the role of CT in the radiographic staging of juvenile angiofibromas.[33,40] Characteristic findings on CT scans are those of a contrast-enhanced nasopharyngeal soft tissue mass with an expanded pterygopalatine fossa (Fig. 3-13), although other benign tumors, such as fibrous histiocytomas, can appear identical (Fig. 3-14). Enlargement or

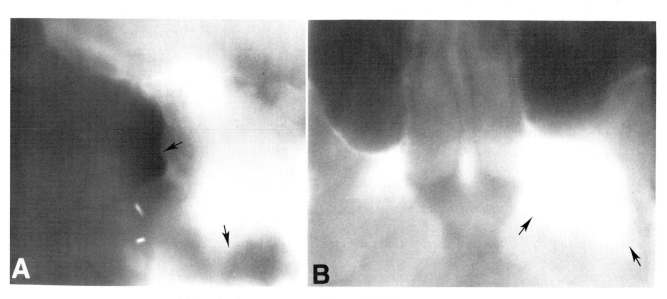

Fig. 3-11. Lateral (**A**) and submentovertex (**B**) hypocycloidal tomograms in patient with severe fibrous dysplasia *(arrows)* that involves pterygoid plates and sphenoid alae, obliterating pterygopalatine fossa.

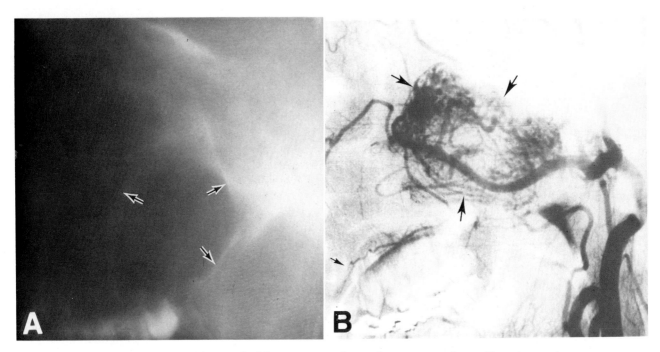

Fig. 3-12. A, Lateral hypocycloidal tomogram and, **B,** selective external carotid angiogram in patient with large angiofibroma *(black arrows)* that has expanded pterygopalatine fossa *(outlined arrows).*

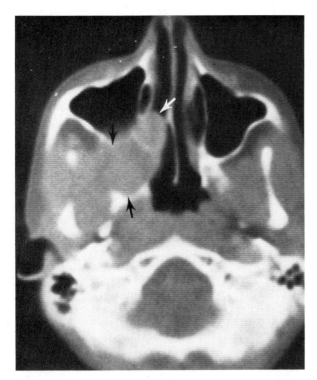

Fig. 3-13. Contrast-enhanced axial CT scan in 16-year-old boy with juvenile angiofibroma *(arrows).* Lesion extends medially through sphenopalatine foramen into nose and laterally into infratemporal fossa (note encroachment on retromaxillary fat pad). Pterygoid plates are deformed and displaced posteriorly.

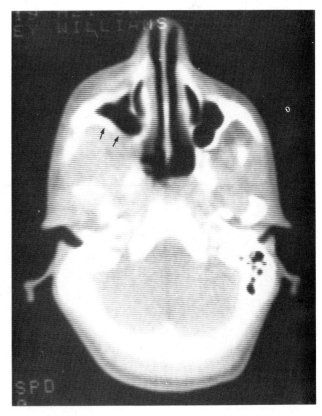

Fig. 3-14. Postcontrast CT scan shows an enhancing retromaxillary mass. Note enlargement of pterygopalatine fossa and anterior bowing of intact posterior sinus wall *(arrows). Fibrous histiocytoma.* (Courtesy of P.M. Som, M.D.)

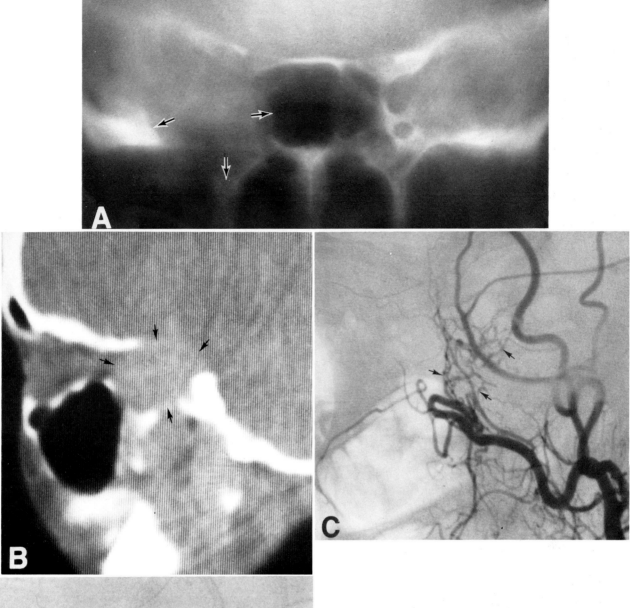

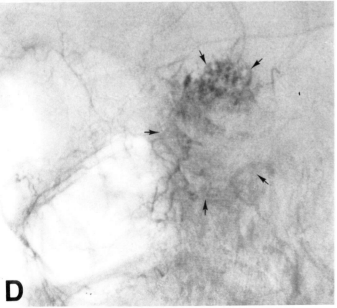

Fig. 3-15. Patient with large neurinoma of fifth cranial nerve. **A,** AP hypocycloidal tomogram. Tumor *(arrows)* has produced pressure erosion of sphenoid wing and extended into base of right pterygoid plates and sphenoid sinus. **B,** Contrast enhanced direct sagittal CT scan delineates both extra- and intra-cranial extension of lesion. **C,** External carotid angiogram, early arterial phase, lateral view. Note enlargement of multiple small branches of maxillary artery *(arrows)* that exit from pterygopalatine fossa to supply tumor. **D,** Late arterial phase film. Vascular tumor is outlined *(arrows)*. (**A** from Osborn, A.G.: AJR **132:**389-394, 1979. Copyright © 1979, American Roentgen Ray Society. **B** from Osborn, A.G., and Anderson, R.E.: Radiology **129:**81-87, 1978. Used by permission of The Radiological Society of North America.)

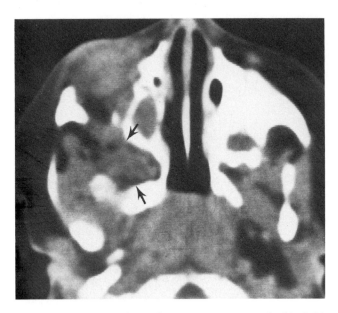

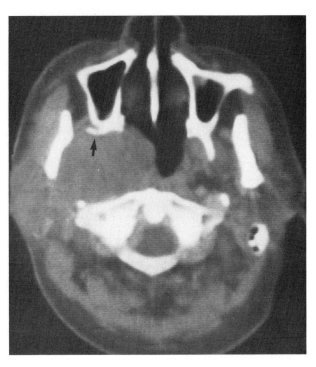

Fig. 3-16. Contrast-enhanced CT scan in 9-month-old child with huge plexiform neurofibroma originating in cavernous sinus. Direct extension into pterygopalatine fossa and infratemporal fossa is seen *(arrows)*.

Fig. 3-17. Axial CT scan of slow-growing tumor originating in deep lobe of parotid gland. Extension into nasopharynx, infratemporal fossa, and pterygopalatine fossa is seen *(black arrow)*. Note anterior displacement of lateral pterygoid plate *(outlined arrow)*.

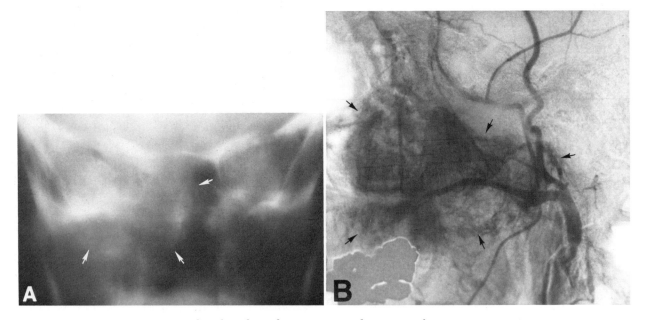

Fig. 3-18. Patient with right sphenoid wing intra- and extracranial meningioma. **A,** Anteroposterior hypocycloidal tomogram. Note striking sclerosis involving right pterygoid plates and pterygopalatine fossa *(arrows)*. Left pterygoid plates are normal. **B,** Selective external carotid angiogram, midarterial phase, lateral view. Large vascular tumor *(small black arrows)* displaces pterygopalatine segment of maxillary artery forward *(outlined arrows)*.

destruction of the numerous openings into the pterygopalatine fossa can be demonstrated by high resolution CT. Such studies are particularly helpful in delineating intracranial extension because it can occur in the absence of skull base abnormalities or without neurologic impairment.[40]

Other benign tumors, such as large pituitary adenomas or neurinomas of the trigeminal ganglion, may erode the sphenoid alae, extending into the base of the pterygoid plates and the apex of the fossa (Figs. 3-15 and 3-16). Benign extracranial soft tissue tumors arising from the parotid gland, deep cervical lymph nodes, and nasopharynx can also extend into the pterygopalatine fossa (Fig. 3-17).

The rare primary meningioma of the nasal fossa (as well as the more common sphenoid wing meningioma) may extend predominately extracranially, producing striking sclerosis involving the pterygopalatine fossa and pterygoid plates (Fig. 3-18, *A*). Angiography is helpful in delineating these lesions (Fig. 3-18, *B*). The differential diagnosis includes Paget's disease, fibrous dysplasia, and osteoblastic metastases.

■ Malignant tumors

Primary malignant tumors of the paranasal sinuses usually produce opacification and bone destruction without evidence of focal expansion of the sinus walls.[36,42] Squamous cell carcinoma, adenocarcinoma, melanoma, rhabdomyosarcoma, and the uncommon esthesioneuroblastoma may all involve the pterygopalatine fossa and its adjacent bony margins by direct extension (Figs. 3-19 and 3-20).

Metastatic lesions of the pterygoid plates and pterygopalatine fossa are uncommon. Osteoblastic metastases from prostate carcinoma may simulate meningioma, fibrous dysplasia, or Paget's disease (Fig. 3-21). Other common metastases are from hypernephroma, carcinoma of the breast, multiple myeloma, or melanoma.

Although multiplanar hypocycloidal tomography and superselective magnification angiography have been helpful in delineating malignant facial lesions involving the pterygopalatine fossa, CT permits imaging of both adjacent soft tissues and intracranial contents. Conventional radiography may fail to demonstrate the presence

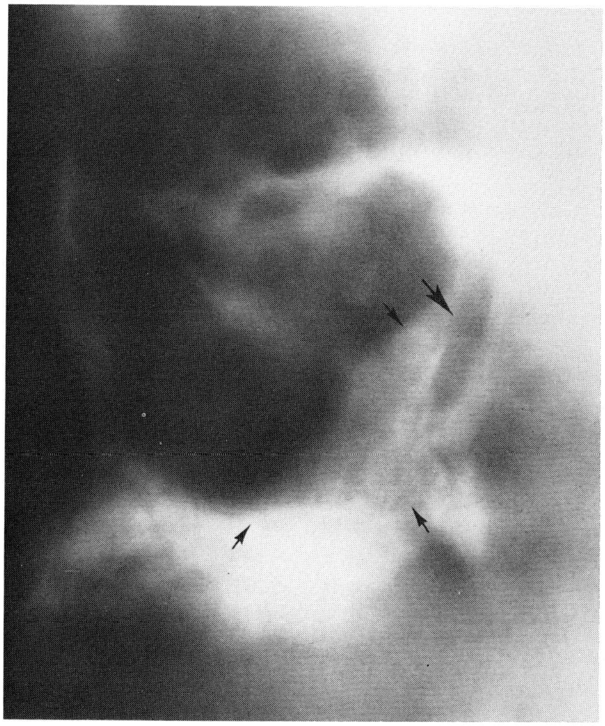

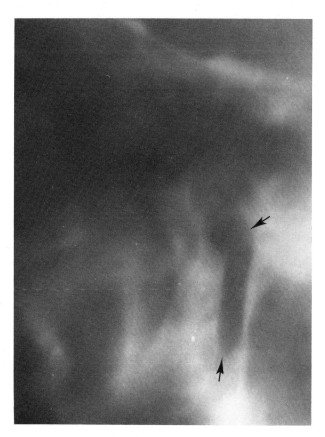

Fig. 3-19. Lateral hypocycloidal tomogram in patient with adenocystic carcinoma involving palate and maxillary sinus *(small arrows)*. Hard palate, pterygoid hamulus, and pterygopalatine fossa *(large arrow)* are all involved by permeative, destructive lesion.

Fig. 3-20. Lateral hypocycloidal tomogram in patient with esthesioneuroblastoma invading pterygopalatine fossa *(arrows)*. Note erosion and loss of cortical margin around fossa.

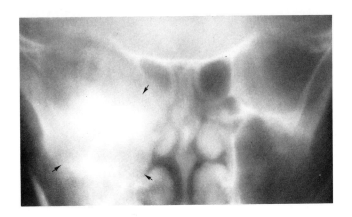

Fig. 3-21. AP hypocycloidal tomogram in patient with known prostatic carcinoma metastatic to right orbit, maxillary sinus, sphenoid wing, pterygoid plates, and pterygopalatine fossa (*arrows*).

or precise extent of disease processes in these areas, but multiplanar CT scans can often precisely delineate the abnormality, rendering both diagnosis and subsequent treatment planning more accurate.[15,17,39,40]

□ References

1. Addlestone, R.B., and Baylis, G.J.: Rhinocerebral mucormycosis, Radiology **115**:1137, 1975.
2. Allen, W.E., Kier, E.L., and Rothman, S.L.G.: The maxillary artery: normal arteriographic anatomy, AJR **118**:517, 1973.
3. Allen, W.E., Kier, E.L., and Rothman, S.L.G.: The maxillary artery in craniofacial pathology, AJR **121**:124, 1974.
4. Archer C.R., and Sunderain, M.: Uncommon sphenoidal fractures and their sequelae, Radiology **122**:157, 1977.
5. Batsakis, J.G.: The pathology of head and neck tumors. Part 5. Nasal cavity and paranasal sinuses, Head Neck Surg. **2**:410, 1980.
6. Batsakis, J.G., and Rice, D.H.: The pathology of head and neck tumors. Part 9a. Vasoformative tumors, Head Neck Surg. **3**:231-239, 1981.
7. Bohman, L., Mancuso, A., Thompson, J., and Hanafee, W.: CT approach to benign nasopharyngeal masses, AJNR **1**:513-520, 1980.
8. Braun, T.W., and Sotereanos, G.C.: Vascular changes in the pterygopalatine fossa after craniofacial dysjunction surgery, J. Oral Surg. **37**:88, 1979.
9. Calcaterra, T.C., Thompson, J.W., and Paglia, D.E.: Inverting papillomas of the nose and paranasal sinuses, Laryngoscope **90**:53, 1980.
10. Diaz, F., et al.: Mucoceles with intracranial and extracranial extensions, J. Neurosurg. **48**:284, 1978.
11. Djindjian, R., Merland, J-J.: Superselective arteriography of the external carotid artery, Berlin, 1978, Springer-Verlag.
12. Dolan, K.D., and Jacoby, C.G.: Facial fractures, Semin. Roentgenol. **13**:37, 1978.
13. Dubois, P.J., Schultz, J.C., Perrin, R.L., and Dastur, K.J.: Tomography in expansile lesions of the nasal and paranasal sinuses, Radiology **125**:149, 1977.
14. Fitzpatrick, P.J., Briant, T.D.R., and Berman, J.M.: The nasopharyngeal angiofibroma, Arch. Otolaryngol. **106**:234, 1980.
15. Forbes, W.S.C., et al.: Computed tomography in the diagnosis of diseases of the paranasal sinuses, Clin. Radiol. **29**:401, 1978.
16. Goss, C.M., editor: Gray's Anatomy of the human body, Philadelphia, 1973, Lea & Febiger.
17. Hesselink, J.R., et al.: Computed tomography of the paranasal sinuses and face. Part II. Pathological anatomy, J. Comput. Asst. Tomogr. **2**:568, 1978.
18. Hesselink, J.R., et al.: Evaluation of mucoceles of the paranasal sinuses with computed tomography, Radiology **133**:397, 1979.
19. Jafek, B.W., Krekorian, E.A., Kirsch, W.M., and Wood, R.P.: Juvenile nasopharyngeal angiofibroma: management of intracranial extension, Head Neck Surg. **2**:119, 1979.
20. Lasjaunias, P.: Nasopharyngeal angiofibromas: hazards of embolization, Radiology **136**:119, 1980.
21. Lasjaunias, P., Berenstein, A., and Doyon, D.: Normal functional anatomy of the facial artery, Radiology **133**:631, 1979.
22. McGill, T.H., Simpson, G., and Healy, G.B.: Fulminant aspergillosis of the nose and paranasal sinuses: a new clinical entity, Laryngoscope **90**:748, 1980.
23. McGuirt, W.F., and Harrill, J.A.: Paranasal sinus aspergillosis, Laryngoscope **89**:1563, 1979.
24. Momose, K.J., et al.: Radiological aspects of inverted papilloma, Radiology **134**:73, 1980.
25. Nutik, S.N.: Carotid paraclinoid aneurysms with intradural origin and intracavernous location, J. Neurosurg. **48**:526, 1978.
26. Osborn, A.G.: The nasal arteries, AJR **130**:89, 1978.
27. Osborn, A.G.: Radiology of the pterygoid plates and pterygopalatine fossa, AJR **132**:389, 1979.
28. Osborn, A.G.: The vidian artery: normal and pathologic anatomy, Radiology **136**:373, 1980.
29. Paff, G.H.: Anatomy of the head and neck, Philadelphia, 1973, W.B. Saunders Co.
30. Potter, G.D.: The pterygopalatine fossa and canal, AJR **107**:520, 1969.
31. Roberson, G.H., Price A.C., Davis, J.M., and Gulati, A.: Therapeutic embolization of juvenile angiofibroma, AJR **133**:657, 1979.
32. Roberson, G.H., et al.: Sphenoethmoidal mucocele: radiographic diagnosis, AJR **127**:595, 1976.
33. Sessions, R.B., Bryan, R.N., Naclerio, R.M., and Alford, B.R.: Radiographic staging of juvenile angiofibroma, Head Neck Surg. **3**:279-283, 1981.
34. Shaffer, K., Haughton, V., Farley, G., and Friedman, J.: Pitfalls in the radiographic diagnosis of angiofibroma, Radiology **127**:425, 1978.
35. Sinha, P., and Aziz, H.I.: Juvenile nasopharyngeal angiofibroma, Radiology **127**:501, 1978.
36. Som, P.J., and Shugar, F.J.A.: The significance of bone expansion associated with the diagnosis of malignant tumors of the paranasal sinuses, Radiology **136**:97, 1980.
37. Som, P.M., Shugar, J.M.A., Cohen, B.A., and Biller, H.A.: The nonspecificity of the antral bowing sign in maxillary sinus pathology, J. Comput. Assist. Tomogr. **5**:350-352, 1981.
38. Sondheimer, E.K.: Basal foramina and canals, In Newton, T.H.,

and Potts, D.G., editors: Radiology of the skull and brain, vol. 1, St. Louis, 1971, The C.V. Mosby Co.

39. Ter Brugge, K.G., Chiu. C.C., Leekham, R.N., and Lawson, V.G.: CT scanning of the pterygopalatine fossa, Presented at the seventeenth annual meeting, American Society of Neuroradiology, Toronto, May 20-24, 1979.

40. Vanel, D., Couanet, D., Grenier, P., et al.: Apport de la tomodensitometrie (TDM) dans le bilan des tumeurs du cavum et de la région ptérygo-maxillaire, Ann. Radiol. **22:**435-440, 1979.

41. Winestock, D.P., Bartlett, P.C., and Sondheimer, F.K.: Benign nasal polyps causing bone destruction in the nasal cavity and paranasal sinuses, Laryngoscope **88:**675, 1978.

41a. Zilkha, A.: Computed tomography in facial trauma, Radiology **144:**545-548, 1982.

42. Zizmor, J., and Noyek, A.M.: Cysts, benign tumors, and malignant tumors of the paranasal sinuses, Otolaryngol. Clin. North Am. **6:**487, 1973.

43. Zizmor, J., and Noyek, A.M.: Fractures of the paranasal sinuses, Otolaryngol. Clin. North Am. **6:**473, 1973.

44. Zizmor, J., and Noyek, A.M.: Inflammatory diseases of the paranasal sinuses, Otolaryngol. Clin. North Am. **6:**459, 1973.

4 □ The salivary glands

PETER M. SOM and DOUGLAS E. SANDERS

□ Embryology

All the salivary glands share a common basic embryologic development. They arise in glandular primordia that develop by proliferation of the oral epithelium (Fig. 4-1). As these buds enlarge they invade the adjacent mesenchyme. The salivary anlages become branching cords of cells that progressively enlarge and acquire lumens about the sixth month of fetal life. The distal, or terminal, ducts dilate to form the secretory acini. The proximal portion of the anlage becomes the main glandular salivary duct. The adjacent mesenchyme eventually divides the gland into multiple lobules and finally encases it in a glandular capsule.[14,18]

Although this overall embryogenesis is common to all the salivary glands, there are some important differences in the development of the individual glands. The parotid gland anlages are the first to develop at about the fourth to sixth week (10 mm stage) of fetal life. The submandibular glands arise late in the sixth week (18 mm stage) and the sublingual glands in the eighth week (22 mm stage) as paired rows of 10 to 20 primordia of small glands with individual ducts in the floor of the mouth. These multiple primordia are confluent and share a common mesenchymal capsule. The minor salivary glands develop late at about the twelfth week (62 mm stage).[33]

Although the parotid anlages are the first to appear, the submandibular and sublingual glands are the first to become arranged into encapsulated structures. The parotid gland develops in a loose condensation of mesenchymal tissue in which there is also the developing lymphatic system. The late encapsulation allows admixture of salivary and lymph tissue. Thus in the fully developed gland lymph nodes are entrapped within its capsule and salivary tissues are entrapped within the gland and the adjacent lymph nodes. This situation is

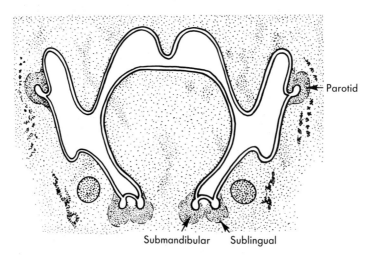

Fig. 4-1. Diagram of coronal section of human embryo at approximately 7 weeks. Epithelial buds of developing major salivary glands can be seen extending into adjacent mesenchyme. (Modified from Mason D.K., and Chisholm, D.M.: Salivary glands in health and disease, Philadelphia, 1975, W.B. Saunders Co.)

unique to the parotid gland and has not been reported to occur with either the submandibular or sublingual glands.

□ Anatomy

The major salivary glands consist of three bilaterally paired glands. Each set of glands has a unique size and shape.

■ Parotid gland

The parotid gland is the largest of the salivary glands, weighing between 14 and 28 gm.[18] The major portion of the gland (80%) lies on the outer surface of the masseter muscle and the angle and ramus of the mandible. It lies in front of the mastoid tip and below the zygomatic arch. A smaller portion (20%) extends medially between the posterior edge of the mandibular ramus anteriorly and the sternocleidomastoid muscle posteriorly (Fig. 4-2). The parotid gland presses against the posterior belly of the digastric muscle and rests lateral to the styloid muscles, internal carotid artery, internal jugular vein, and the last four cranial nerves. Finally, it abuts anteriorly on the medial pterygoid muscle. The facial nerve exits the skull base through the stylomastoid foramen, courses lateral to the styloid process, and descends on the lateral margin of the posterior belly of the digastric muscle. The main trunk of the facial nerve then pierces the posterior border of the gland. Within the substance of the parotid the facial nerve divides into its major branches (Fig. 4-3).[5,11]

Anatomically, there are no separate superficial and deep lobes in the parotid gland. Rather, this is an artificial division created by the plane of the facial nerve. However, because the portion of the gland under the facial nerve but lying over the masseter muscle is still referred to as the superficial lobe, a more practical definition is a division created by a plane extending between the site of the facial nerve's penetration into the posterior parotid gland and the posterolateral margin of the mandibular ramus. Any parotid tissue deeper than, or medial to, this plane is referred to as lying in the deep lobe of the parotid gland. The external carotid artery and the posterior facial vein (the major vessels traversing the parotid) both lie just inside the deep lobe.

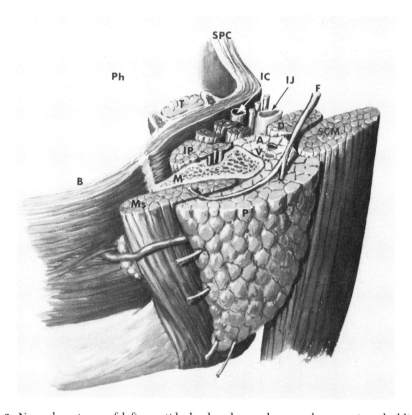

Fig. 4-2. Normal anatomy of left parotid gland and parapharyngeal space viewed obliquely and from above. *Ph*, pharynx; *SPC*, superior pharyngeal constrictor muscle; *T*, tonsil; *B*, buccinator muscle; *MS*, masseter muscle; *SCM*, sternocleidomastoid muscle; *D*, posterior belly of the digastric muscle; *IP*, internal pterygoid muscle; *M*, mandible; *IC*, internal carotid artery; *IJ*, internal jugular vein; *P*, parotid gland; *F*, facial nerve; *A*, external carotid artery; *v*, posterior facial vein. (From Som, P.M., and Biller, N.R.: Radiology **135:**387-390, 1980.)

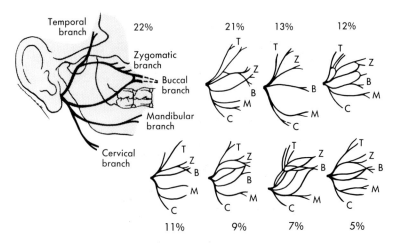

Fig. 4-3. Variations of facial nerve branching in parotid gland. (Modified from Davis, R.A., et al.: Surg. Gynec. Obstet. **102:**384, 1956.)

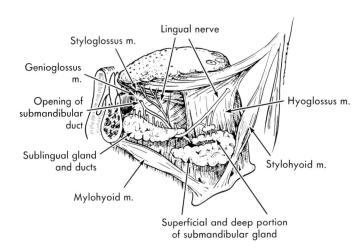

Fig. 4-4. Lateral view of sublingual and submandibular glands and their major anatomic relationships (Modified from Mason, D.K., and Chisholm, D.M.: Salivary glands in health and disease, Philadelphia, 1975, W.B. Saunders Co.)

The intraglandular parotid ducts converge anteriorly to form the main parotid duct (Stensen's duct), which exits the anterior gland and crosses the masseter muscle and buccal fat pad. It then turns medially to pierce the buccinator muscle and buccal mucosa to open intraorally opposite the second upper molar tooth. About 20% of people have small accessory glands that lie on or above (and drain into) Stensen's duct anterior to the main parotid gland.[1]

Lymph nodes are included within the parotid gland tissue. These nodes and those immediately adjacent to the gland all drain into the superior deep cervical nodal chain.

■ Submandibular gland

The submandibular gland is the second largest salivary gland, weighing between 10 and 15 gm, or about one half the size of the parotid gland. It is artificially divided into a superficial and deep lobe. The superficial lobe lies in the digastric triangle and is bounded anteriorly and inferiorly by the anterior belly of the digastric muscle, posteriorly by the posterior belly of the digastric and stylohyoid muscles, and laterally by the lower border of the mandible and medial pterygoid muscle (Fig. 4-4). Posteriorly, the stylomandibular ligament separates it from the parotid gland. The floor of the triangle is formed by the mylohyoid muscle in front

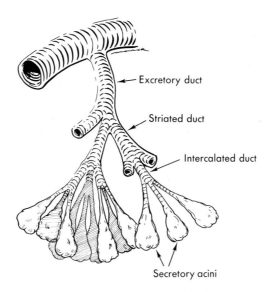

Fig. 4-5. Diagram of major salivary ductal system. (Modified from Batsakis, J.G.: Tumors of the head and neck: clinical and pathological considerations, ed. 2, Baltimore, copyright © 1979, The Williams and Wilkins Co.)

and the hyoglossus muscle behind. This portion of the submandibular gland is covered by the platysma muscle and is traversed by the anterior facial vein and marginal mandibular nerve. The facial artery runs upward on its posterior aspect, then turns downward and forward between the submandibular gland and the mandible.

The deep portion of the submandibular gland lies under the posterior edge of the mylohyoid muscle. The lingual nerve lies above it and the hypoglossal nerve below it. The main excretory duct is Wharton's duct, which exits the gland anteriorly and makes a sharp turn around the posterior edge of the mylohyoid muscle. The duct then runs forward and upward, lying medial to the sublingual gland and lateral to the genioglossus muscle. It opens into the anterior floor of the mouth on the sublingual papilla. As the duct courses upward, the lingual nerve winds around it, being first lateral, then inferior, and finally medial to it. The gland's lymph drains into the submandibular lymph nodes.

■ The sublingual glands

The sublingual glands are the smallest of the major salivary glands, weighing about 2 gm. They lie just under the sublingual mucosa in the floor of the mouth (Fig. 4-4). The sublingual glands rest on the mylohyoid muscle and the inner surface of the mandible in relationship to the genioglossus muscles and lie lateral to the styloglossus muscle. There are up to 20 individual minor ducts (ducts of Rivinus) that open independently into the floor of the mouth along the sublingual papilla and fold. Occasionally, some of these minor ducts fuse to form Bartholin's duct, which in turn opens into Wharton's duct.[14,18]

All of the major salivary glands have a similar treelike branching pattern of the ductal system. It progresses from the largest excretory ducts, through the striated ducts to the intercalated ducts, and finally to the acini, which are either serous or mucus producing (Fig. 4-5). The parotid gland has long, thin intercalated ducts and is essentially a serous gland. The submandibular gland has shorter and wider intercalated ducts and is predominantly a serous gland, although some mucous acini are present. The sublingual gland has very short intercalated ducts and is predominantly a mucous gland.

■ Minor salivary glands

The minor salivary glands lie beneath the mucosa of the oral cavity, palate, pharynx, larynx, trachea, and paranasal sinuses.[1] They are particularly concentrated in the buccal, labial, palatal, and lingual regions. The ratio of major to minor salivary gland tumors is about 5:1, with the majority of these minor gland lesions occurring in the palate and oral cavity.[1]

The total daily salivary flow is 1000 to 1500 ml. The parotid and submandibular glands contribute in equal amounts about 90% of this total. The sublingual glands contribute 5% and the minor salivary glands 5%.[33]

□ **Developmental anomalies**

Anomalies of the salivary glands are rare and when they occur they are generally associated with other facial abnormalities. Agenesis or hypoplasia of salivary tissue is causally related to xerostomia, sialadenitis, and dental caries.[18]

Familial parotid agenesis and agenesis associated

with hemifacial microstomia, mandibular facial dysostosis, cleft palate, and anophthalmia have all been reported.[18] Parotid hypoplasia has been observed in the Melkersson-Rosenthal syndrome.[34] Aberrant salivary tissue has been reported in the mandible, temporal bone, and neck. When aberrant submandibular gland tissue occurs in the inner surface of the angle of the mandible, it appears radiographically as a lucent cystic lesion with a thin sclerotic rim.[18,43] Congenital intraglandular cysts occur in a variety of forms (see p. 211).

□ Sialography

Sialography is the radiographic demonstration of the salivary glandular ductal system. This is accomplished by using a radiopaque contrast medium. Only the parotid and submandibular glands lend themselves to being studied by this technique. The sublingual glands and minor salivary glands are not routinely studied because they either do not have a single excretory duct or are too small to be cannulated. In 1913, Arcelin first demonstrated a submandibular stone by using bismuth as the contrast material.[33] In 1925, Barsony and Uslenghi independently introduced the sialogram as a diagnostic procedure.[18] Since their initial presentations many refinements have occurred that have improved the ease of the technique as well as its diagnostic accuracy.

■ Plain films

Before any contrast material is introduced into the salivary ducts, coned-down soft tissue technique films should be obtained to rule out the possibility of radiopaque sialolithiasis or dystrophic calcifications. For the parotid gland PA, extended chin open-mouth lateral, and oblique views should be obtained (Figs. 4-6 and 4-7). For views of the submandibular gland, two modifications are made. First, the lateral film should be taken with the chin extended, the mouth open, and the index finger pressing the tongue downward (Fig. 4-8). These maneuvers are designed to project a calculus away from the mandible. Secondly, an intraoral occlusal film can demonstrate a Wharton's duct stone in the floor of the mouth that may be radiographically silent

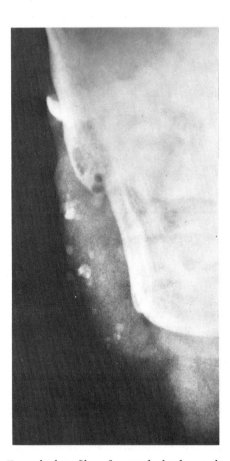

Fig. 4-6. Frontal plain film of parotid gland reveals multiple calcification in gland that will become obscured when contrast material is injected into gland. *Chronic recurrent sialadenitis.*

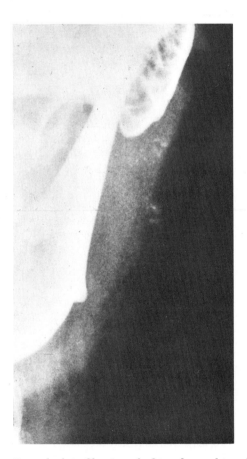

Fig. 4-7. Frontal plain film reveals faint dystrophic calcifications in parotid gland. *Mixed tumor.*

on the other conventional films (Figs. 4-9 and 4-10). If a small calculus is suspected in the region of Stensen's duct on a PA film, a film with the patient's cheeks blown out may confirm the finding or better demonstrate it. A variety of views can be tailored to individual cases.

A fluoroscopic unit with spot-filming capabilities adds the feature of allowing the physician to visibly monitor the injection process as well as the ability to spot-film rapidly in the most desirable positions.[15]

Xeroradiography films are not used very much today because of their relative lack of availability and their high radiation doses as compared to conventional radiography.

Regardless of whether conventional plain films or spot films are used, this initial examination should be used to correct exposure factors for the sialogram. In addition, these films should be carefully examined to obtain any information that may lead to a further refinement of the differential diagnosis. Specifically, the mandible may show evidence of local, systemic, or metastatic disease.

□ **Indications**

The sialogram may reveal information that clinical examination and plain film examinations cannot. The most common applications of sialography are as follows.

1. The detection or confirmation of small radiopaque or radiolucent sialolithiasis or foreign bodies
2. The evaluation of the extent of irreversible ductal damage that is secondary to recurrent inflammation; this information contributes to the decision-making process of whether surgery should or should not be performed
3. The further differentiation of diseases that are clinically similar (e.g., chronic sialadenitis, sialosis, granulomatous diseases, autoimmune diseases)

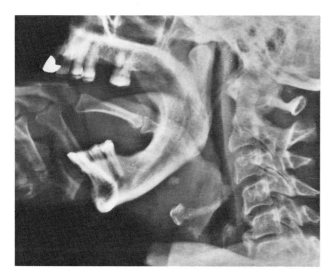

Fig. 4-8. Lateral film with index finger pressing tongue downward reveals submandibular calculus that was otherwise hidden by mandible.

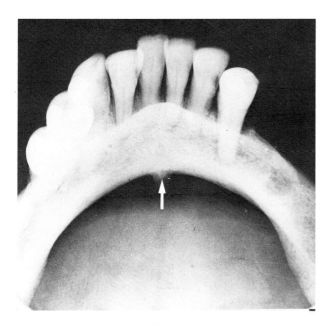

Fig. 4-9. Normal intraoral occlusal film. Arrow indicates mental spine(s), which is origin of genioglossus muscles.

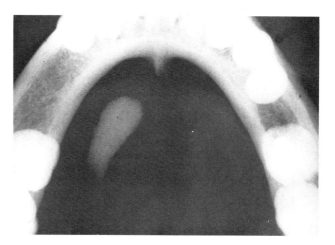

Fig. 4-10. Intraoral occlusal film reveals large calculus in Wharton's duct. Even calculi of this size can go unnoticed on other soft tissue views.

4. The further evaluation of suspected neoplasms as to size, location, extension into adjacent tissues, and if possible, malignancy
5. The evaluation of fistulae, strictures, or diverticuli, especially in posttraumatic cases
6. Although generally not accepted as a therapeutic modality, some physicians use the sialogram in this limited way. This distension sialography is especially used in cases of chronic sialadenitis and chronic stricture.[25]

■ Contraindications

There are two major contraindications to sialography: (1) known patient sensitivity to iodine compounds and (2) acute salivary inflammation.

Known patient sensitivity to iodine compounds is particularly contraindicative when the history reveals marked urticaria, dyspnea, asthmatic symptoms, or hypotension as the manifestations of the iodine allergy.

Acute salivary inflammation is a strong contraindication to performing a sialogram primarily because the examination will aggravate or spread the infection. In addition, the examination is severely painful and because of this the information obtained is often incomplete. Another potential problem is that leakage of contrast material into the gland's parenchyma can occur through the inflamed ductal epithelium and this may possibly elicit a parenchymal foreign body reaction.

■ Contrast material

There are two different classes of contrast materials to choose from: the water-soluble and the fat-soluble agents.

Fat-soluble agents have been used in sialography for many years. Of the three main agents used, Ethiodol is more desirable than either Lipiodol or Pantopaque. This is because the former agent has a much lower reported frequency of eliciting foreign body salivary parenchymal reactions.[33] This type of reaction can only take place if perforation of the ductal epithelium occurs. Although these reactions are reported pathologically, practically speaking they have clinically not been a major deterrent to the use of these agents and are almost always asymptomatic. The viscosity of Ethiodol is 50 to 100 centipoise at 15° C, which is less viscid than the other fat-soluble agents.[33] This allows an easier injection and better filling of the smallest caliber salivary ducts. The excellent roentgenographic visualization with Ethiodol makes it an attractive agent. In addition, because it is more viscid than the water-soluble agents, it is easier to keep in the ductal system. This is a desirable feature if a CT-sialogram is to be performed after the conventional sialogram. Because the opacification with Ethiodol is so good, small radiolucent stones may

be obscured if careful monitoring of the sialographic filling phase is not maintained.

The water-soluble agents in general give less opacification, are far less viscid (2.5 to 29.8 centipoise), and are more physiologic and miscible with saliva than the fat-soluble agents. In addition, no foreign body reactions have been reported with these substances. The low viscosity allows easier injections and greater filling of small caliber salivary ducts, and small radiolucent stones are less easily obscured. The drawbacks to use of water-soluble agents are the relatively low roentgenographic opacification and the rapid drainage and absorption from the ducts of this low viscosity material. The most commonly used agents are Hypaque and Renografin products. However, the most ideal of these agents may be Sinografin, which has the highest viscosity and best roentgenographic opacification of the water-soluble substances. These agents are cleared by the gland within minutes, whereas the fat-soluble agents are slowly eliminated and not absorbed.

Even though the iodine content of Sinografin and Ethiodol is approximately the same (38% and 37% respectively) Ethiodol usually produces a denser acinar opacification and a sharper ductal outline. This may reflect the admixture of Sinografin and saliva and the rapid absorption of the contrast agent.

■ Equipment

The following is a list of equipment necessary to perform a sialographic examination.

1. Sialographic cannulas. The most commonly used are the Rabinov cannulas with tips ranging from .012 to .033 inches (Fig. 4-11).[31] Variations, such as the Manashil modification of the Rabinov cannula and cannulas designed by Lowman and Belleza, are also available. The larger diameter needles are for the parotid gland, the smaller ones for the submandibular gland. No matter which cannula is used it is important that a flexible polyethylene tube connects the actual cannula with a syringe. This allows mobility during injection and a relative lack of artifacts on either the x-ray film or the CT scan.
2. Lacrimal dilators 0000 through 0 caliber.
3. A 5 or 10 ml syringe.
4. 4 × 4 inch gauze sponge pads.
5. Vials of Ethiodol and Sinografin.
6. Secretogogue such as fresh lemon, lemon extract, or lemon concentrate.
7. Head light.
8. High-power optic glasses.

Most physicians use a hand injection technique because of the finer injection control and the overall ease of use. A hydrostatic method of delivering the contrast

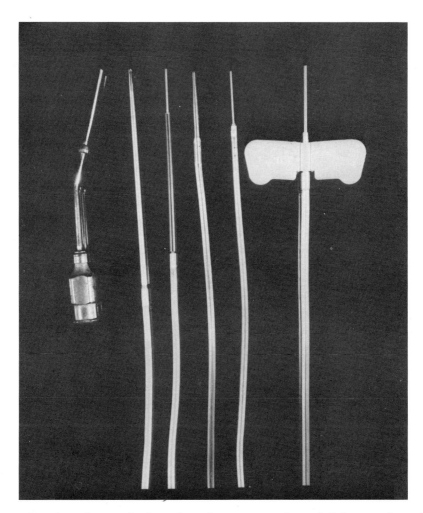

Fig. 4-11. Sampling of some of sialography catheters commonly used. Rabinov catheters have both end and side holes available.

material has been described, but is not commonly employed.[33] It consists of placing a filled syringe 70 cm above the level of the patient's mouth and allowing a continuous slow drip of contrast material into the gland.[16]

■ Technique

Parotid gland cannulization

The opening of Stensen's duct is opposite the second upper molar tooth. It may be difficult to see, especially if the patient has created a bite ridge on the buccal mucosa. Palpation of the gland along the course of Stensen's duct allows clinical evaluation of a parotid lesion (single or multiple, soft or rock-hard, etc.) and possible detection of a stone in the major duct. If the duct orifice cannot be seen, drying the buccal mucosa with a gauze pad and then milking the gland may produce a droplet of saliva that will locate the opening. The administration of a secretogogue may accomplish the same

thing. Slight abduction of the cheek with the thumb and index finger allows easier insertion of the lacrimal dilators. After they are removed, the cannula is inserted and between 0.5 and 1.5 ml of contrast material is slowly injected. The contrast-filled syringe is then taped to the patient's upper chest or shoulder so that it does not overlie the area of interest.

Submandibular gland cannulization

The orifice of Wharton's duct lies under the tip of the tongue on the sublingual papilla. The opening is smaller than that of Stensen's duct. The tongue should be pushed backward with a gauze sponge to put tension on the papillae as well as to dry the area. Either glandular milking or a secretogogue aids in identifying the orifice.[23] The duct is fairly straight, directed backward and downward at about a 45° angle.[16] Between 0.2 and 0.5 ml of contrast material is usually injected.

The main cause of failure to cannulate a salivary duct

is nonsecretion of saliva. This may reflect chronic infection, radiation, or even ductal occlusion from a stone, surgery, or trauma. Previous surgery in the floor of the mouth accounts for most failures of submandibular cannulization.

Once the cannula is in place, the injection of the contrast is performed. The patient should be warned that discomfort will be felt in the region of the injected gland, and a signal should be set up with the patient so that the physician will know when glandular filling begins. Most patients describe the sensation as being similar to the discomfort felt when trying to blow up a very hard balloon. Actual pain is not felt except in cases of persistant infection. The sensation lasts essentially during the injection phase and usually disappears within 2 to 5 minutes after the injection pressure stops.

■ The sialogram

The sialogram can be considered in three phases: ductal filling, acinar filling, and evacuation.

The parotid study

Stensen's duct is approximately 6 cm long. It has a small C-shaped curve anteriorly as it bends around the buccal fat pad and proceeds to lie on the outer surface of the masseter muscle (Fig. 4-12).

Its normal caliber is 1 to 3 mm and in a direct PA view the duct should be within 15 to 18 mm of the lateral cortex of the mandible. If it is more laterally dis-

placed, either the parotid gland is enlarged or there is a mass in or near the masseter muscle. There is no specific pattern of ductal distribution for the parotid gland, and the variance is not only from person to person but also from side to side in the same patient.[49] Usually there is a major excretory duct for the upper and lower poles of the superficial lobe. The overall pattern is that of a leafless tree. The farther away from Stensen's duct, the smaller the caliber of the side ducts, the more the branch points, and the more numerous the side ducts (Fig. 4-13).

As the ducts arch behind the mandible toward the deep lobe, they may appear stretched on a frontal film. However, on lateral and oblique films there is no spreading or crowding of the ducts to suggest a mass lesion. Virtually no area of the gland should be ductless.

Acinar filling can be accomplished in most patients and is a normal finding.[23] It is a good technique, particularly in the evaluation of small mass lesions (Fig. 4-14). Some indentations in the gland's periphery may be seen from the temporal bone or adjacent lymph nodes. There should normally be no areas with lack of paren-

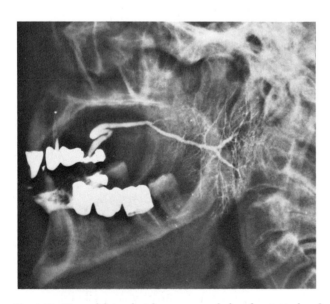

Fig. 4-12. Normal lateral sialogram reveals bend anteriorly of Stensen's duct around buccinator fat pad as it then procedes to lie on outer surface of masseter muscle. There is normal branching pattern to parotid ducts and no area of gland is "ductless".

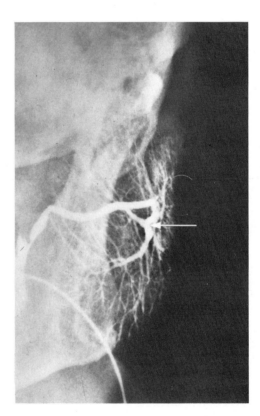

Fig. 4-13. Normal frontal sialogram. Hilum of gland *(arrow)* should not be more than 15 to 18 mm from lateral mandibular cortex. Posterior deep lobe ducts often appear stretched as they arch behind mandible.

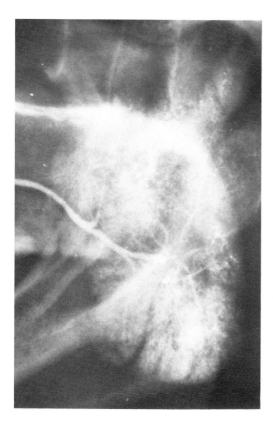

Fig. 4-14. Lateral sialogram of parotid gland with acinar filling. All of periphery is seen, however, ductal detail has become obscured.

chymal (acinar) filling. The evacuation films usually reveal complete ductal emptying within 5 to 15 minutes. Any delayed emptying or trapping of contrast material indicates a stricture or obstruction.[16] More complete evacuation can be obtained if a secretogoque is used.

Solitary or multiple accessory parotid glands can be seen and are situated above Stensen's duct and anterior to the main gland.

The submandibular study

Wharton's duct is about 5 cm long and has a caliber of 2 to 4 mm. Just before it enters the gland it makes a C-shaped curve around the posterior edge of the mylohyoid muscle. The duct has a relatively straight overall course directed from the sublingual papilla toward the angle of the mandible. The gland has shorter ducts than the parotid gland and they tend to taper more sharply in caliber (Figs. 4-15 and 4-16). The duct walls are thinner than those of the parotid gland and perforate easily with minimal overfilling. Occasionally, Bartholin's duct will fill on the submandibular study. In this case, the sublingual gland may be visualized and appears as an accessory gland with a normal branching ductal pattern.

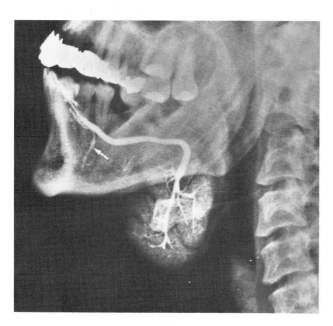

Fig. 4-15. Normal lateral submandibular sialogram with acinar filling. Bartholin's duct has been partially filled *(arrow)*. Notice that these are shorter, thicker, and more rapidly tapering ducts than seen in parotid gland. Wharton's duct is also wider than Stensen's duct and bend it makes around posterior edge of myohyoid muscle is clearly seen.

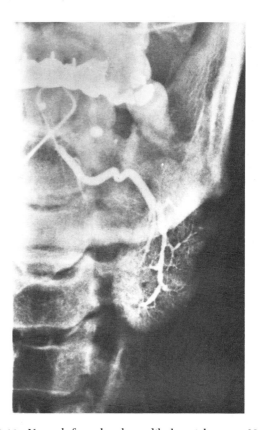

Fig. 4-16. Normal frontal submandibular sialogram. Notice how normally Wharton's duct runs from floor of mouth in midline outward and downward toward angle of mandible.

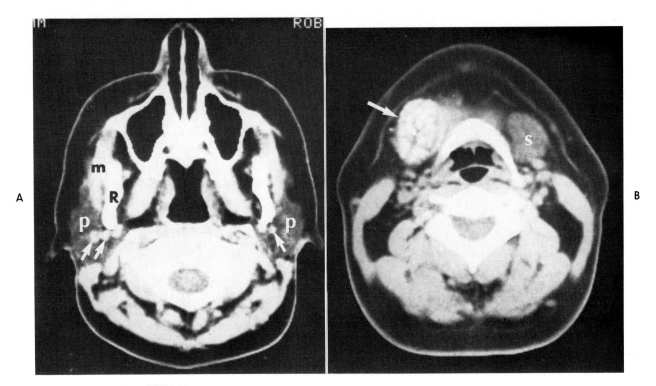

Fig. 4-17. A, Axial CT scan with intravenous contrast. Parotid glands *(P)* are seen to be lower density than adjacent muscles. External carotid arteries and posterior facial veins are seen *(arrows)*. *M,* Masseter muscle; *R,* ramus of mandible. **B,** Axial CT scan. Right submandibular sialogram has been performed. Contrast material is seen filling gland *(arrow)*. Left submandibular gland *(S)* is also well seen and is less dense than adjacent muscles.

■ CT scanning

The parotid glands usually are of lower attenuation than the adjacent muscles. The margins of the gland can be clearly delineated in most cases. The external carotid artery and posterior facial vein can easily be identified traversing the gland just posterior to the ramus of the mandible (Fig. 4-17, *A*).

The submandibular glands are easily identified in the submental triangles of the neck. These glands are of lower attenuation than muscle, although in many patients the glands are almost as dense as muscle. This may reflect the relatively lower fat content of the gland or subclinical infection (Fig. 4-17, *B*).

■ CT sialogram

If a CT sialogram is to be performed, the sialographic cannula is left in the duct and the patient is moved to the CT scanner. The cannula acts as a "stopper" and helps prevent the emptying of the contrast material from the ductal system. The patient can wait 30 to 60 minutes before the CT scan is performed. A more im-

mediate scheduling time is desirable primarily for the patient's comfort and convenience.

A small "touch-up" injection is given just before the scan is started if Ethiodol is used. This 0.2 to 0.3 ml injection ensures that the gland and duct are maximally filled. If Sinografin is used, a complete injection must be given in order to ensure maximal visualization of the salivary gland and duct[17] (Figs. 4-17 and 4-18).

The scan should be taken parallel to the inferior orbital meatal line (IOM) and run at 5 mm intervals from the lowest margin of the gland to its upper level. Artifacts from teeth fillings may require an alteration of the scan angle to the superior orbital meatal (SOM) or even coronally oriented planes. Intravenous contrast material is unnecessary for the further evaluation of intraglandular pathology because it will not affect the surgical or medical treatment.[39,40] At the conclusion of the scan the cannula is removed, a secretogogue is given, and the patient is sent home.

At the present time fine ductal changes, which can be seen on the conventional sialogram, are not appre-

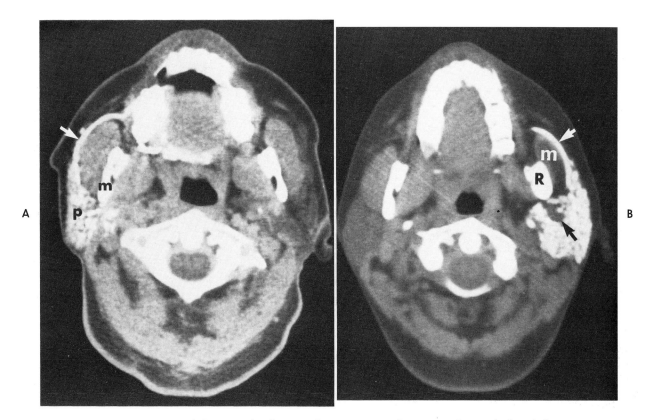

Fig. 4-18. A, Normal CT parotid sialogram. Contrast material is seen in Stensen's duct *(white arrow)* and parotid gland *(p)*. *M,* Mandible. **B,** Normal CT sialogram. Stensen's duct is seen *(white arrow)*. Location of vascular bundle is also seen *(black arrow)*. *M,* Masseter muscle; *R,* ramus of mandible.

ciated on the CT sialogram. Because of this, a sialogram is the examination of choice when ductal anatomy is important (inflammatory and autoimmune disorders). A contrast-enhanced CT scan is probably the examination of choice when evaluating glandular masses. A CT sialogram is necessary only if the gland is dense or the mass is small or if there is poor correlation between the CT scan and the clinical observations.

■ Complications

Complications from sialography are extremely rare. If allergy to the contrast material is excluded, only a rare possibility of postexamination infection need be considered. These infections usually occur as flare-ups in glands that have a subclinical infection or are predisposed to infection because of ductal obstruction. When they occur, the infections usually take 48 hours to manifest themselves clinically. The patient is alerted that in the normal circumstance any discomfort from the procedure, such as mild swelling or dull aching, should be resolved by 48 hours. If increasing discomfort is noted,

the patient should contact the referring physician in order to be placed on a short course of antibiotics. If rapid treatment is given, infections usually resolve themselves within an additional 48-hour period and are of little clinical inconvenience to the patient.

Ductal perforations are rare and virtually never lead to a significant clinical complication. This is especially true if Sinografin is used as the contrast material.

□ **Inflammatory disorders**

The salivary glands have a limited number and type of tissue responses to inflammation so that similar symptoms may be manifested by a variety of different lesions. This is not a particular clinical problem in those few diseases that are acute and usually a single event. However, in the chronic conditions the signs and symptoms of the obstructive and nonobstructive inflammatory diseases can merge with those of the granulomatous and autoimmune diseases, which in turn may be confused with certain neoplasms. It is important to remember that rarely does the clinically obvious case come to sialography. The cases that are examined have a diagnostic problem that the clinician needs help in resolving. Similarly, the radiologist should consider the clinical presentation when making a differential diagnosis.

■ Acute inflammatory disorders

The maintenance of a normal salivary flow plays a paramount role in preventing a retrograde glandular infection from the mouth. These ascending bacterial infections, both acute and chronic, are more common in the parotid gland than in the submandibular gland, for three reasons: (1) the orifice of Stensen's duct is larger than that of Wharton's duct, (2) the Stensen's duct orifice is more easily injured by dental prostheses, cheek biting, and other mechanical trauma, and (3) the caliber of the parotid ducts is smaller than the caliber of the corresponding ducts of the submandibular gland. This relates to a greater ease of salivary flow interruption, stasis of secretions, and an altered character of the secretions.[1] On the other hand, the submandibular gland is more susceptible to infection caused by obstruction of Wharton's duct secondary to stone formation, and abscesses can occur behind these obstructions.

Viral infections

Mumps. By far the most common cause of viral parotid swelling is mumps. Although this virus may involve the submandibular glands, the major clinical disease is in the parotids. The disease is most reliably diagnosed only during epidemics and can be confirmed by measuring serum antibody titers to mumps S and V antigens.[1] The disease can be subclinical, which may account for most misdiagnoses of the parotid enlargement. One attack of the disease provides immunity.

Other viruses can cause parotitis and may account for some of seriologically negative mumps findings.[1] Coxsackievirus, parainfluenzavirus, herpesvirus, echovirus, and influenzavirus type A have all been implicated.

Bacterial infections

Acute suppurative sialadenitis. This is an acute, painful, diffuse swelling primarily of the parotid gland. One or both glands are affected, and it is associated with local and systemic signs of sepsis.[48] About two thirds of the cases are associated with the postoperative period (surgical parotitis) and occur in debilitated dehydrated patients with poor oral hygiene.[47] Acute suppurative sialadenitis usually affects the elderly but also can occur de novo in infants. Good oral hygiene and hydration have markedly reduced its incidence. The cause is an ascending or retrograde bacterial infection originating in the mouth. *Staphylococcus aureus, Streptococcus viri-*

dans, and *Steptococcus pneumoniae* are implicated in most cases. If untreated, an abscess will form that can rupture into the external auditory canal, the parapharyngeal space, or the skin. The primary forms of treatment include antibiotics, local heat, hydration, and surgery.

Because of the acute nature of these illnesses, sialograms are rarely performed. If such a study is performed, areas of peripheral ductal narrowing and "pruning" as a result of cellular infiltration of the gland are seen. Focal areas of dilatation and narrowing of the major ducts can also be present. These probably reflect functional changes secondary to the inflammatory process.[33]

■ Chronic inflammatory disorders

The chronic inflammatory disorders of the salivary glands usually appear as recurrent acute or subacute attacks of painful glandular swelling. The periods in between these episodes are for the most part asymptomatic, and the involved gland may be virtually clinically normal.

A second form of chronic inflammatory disease is that of a slow progressive enlargement of the gland punctuated with periodic episodes of acute (usually painful) attacks.

Lastly, there may be a long history of a slow progressive, essentially painless glandular enlargement. It is this last group of inflammatory diseases that can cause clinical confusion with neoplasms. In general, an attempt to separate these chronic conditions into those caused or associated with obstruction and those that are nonobstructive should be made because the treatment and prognosis may vary considerably.

As with the acute inflammatory diseases, the chronic nonobstructive diseases involve the parotid gland with a greater frequency, whereas the obstructive disorders more often involve the submandibular gland. Chronic recurrent sialadenitis is characterized by recurrent diffuse or localized painful salivary gland swellings. Pus can be rapidly expressed from the duct orifice. Pathogens similar to those found in the acute diseases are implicated. Because of local ductal obstructions and stasis, the salivary secretions can precipitate within the duct lumens. This is associated with an increase in lysosomes that may account for the focal destruction of the duct walls that occurs with concommitant release of the duct's contents into the glandular parenchyma.[45] These nonobstructive, chronic sialadenitides can have one of the following sialographic appearances.

Chronic sialadenitis

The sialogram reveals focal areas of peripheral ductal dilatation and scattered globular or saccular accumula-

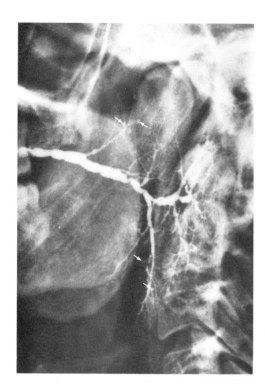

Fig. 4-19. Lateral sialogram of chronic inflammation (sialadenitis). Stensen's duct is abnormally widened, with narrowings occuring mainly at branch points. Some widening of major ducts is also present; however, peripheral ducts are almost normal. Scattered small globules of contrast material can be seen in gland *(arrows)* representing either small abcesses or focal sialectasis.

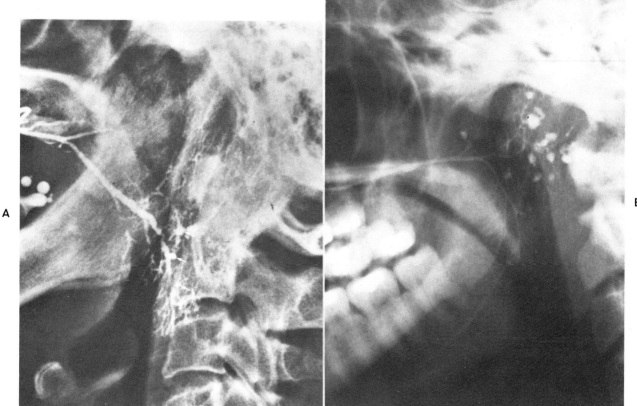

Fig. 4-20. A, Sialogram of chronic sialadenitis reveals widened Stensen's duct with several areas of narrowing within gland. Small abscess cavities can be identified *(arrows)*. **B,** Lateral sialogram showing multiple collections of contrast material of varying size primarily in posterior pole of gland. Most of remaining gland is normal. *Chronic sialadenitis.*

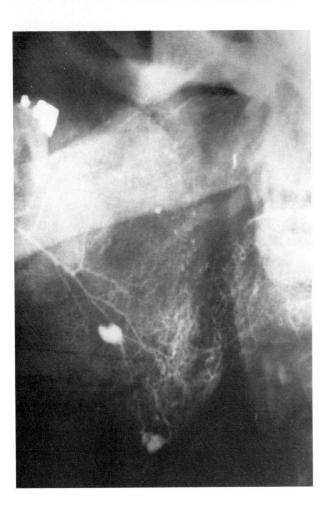

Fig. 4-21. Parotid sialogram of patient with vague mass (absence of ducts) in upper portion of superficial lobe and scattered abscess cavities in gland. *Tuberculosis.*

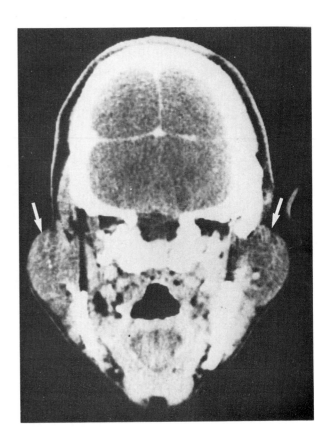

Fig. 4-22. Coronal CT scan. Both parotid glands *(arrows)* are more dense than normal and are slightly enlarged. *Chronic sialadenitis.*

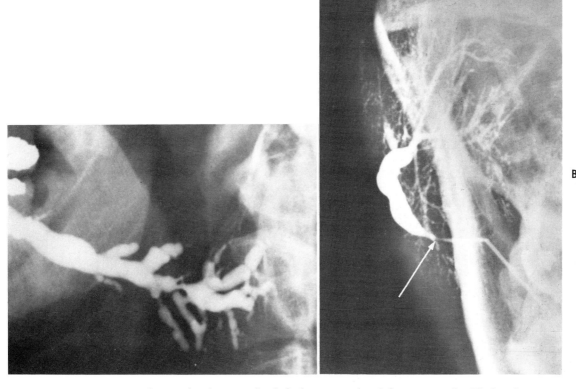

Fig. 4-23. A, Lateral parotid sialogram of sialodochitis. Peripheral ducts cannot be filled and only dilated main ductal system is seen. **B,** Frontal sialogram of parotid gland with main ductal dilatation secondary to stricture *(arrow)*. Films still looked the same 15 minutes after cannula was removed.

tions of contrast material. These occur at the level of the intercalated ducts and acini. They are not as uniform in size or distribution throughout the gland as the changes seen in the autoimmune diseases. Varying degrees of main ductal dilatation can occur, with narrowing at the branching points of the primary excretory ducts. There is a delayed emptying of the contrast material (Figs. 4-19 to 4-21).

On CT the glands usually have a nonhomogeneous higher attenuation than normal glands (Fig. 4-22). Although this appearance is suggestive of an inflammatory process of the parotid gland, it is nonspecific and can occasionally be seen in normal patients with no history of parotid gland disease.

Sialodochitis

In these cases there is a marked dilatation of the main duct. It has been described as fusiform or sausage shaped in appearance, and periodic areas of stricture or narrowing can give the main duct a "string of sausage"

look.[33] Branch point narrowings also occur. The peripheral ducts are either normal in size or narrow, in contradistinction to sialadenitis, in which the peripheral ducts are dilated or saccular. In advanced cases, the peripheral ducts become poorly filled and eventually nonvisualized. Thus in the end stage only a dilated deformed main duct with a few narrowed primary ducts is seen (Fig. 4-23, *A*).

These changes closely resemble those of ductal obstruction secondary to a calculus or stricture. One differentiating point is that although there is delayed emptying in the nonobstructive diseases, it is never as prolonged or complete as the delay seen in the obstructive diseases (Fig. 4-23, *B*).

□ Sialolithiasis

In contrast to most inflammatory conditions and salivary tumors that primarily involve the parotid glands, between 80% and 90% of all salivary gland calculi occur in the submandibular gland. Ten percent to 20% occur

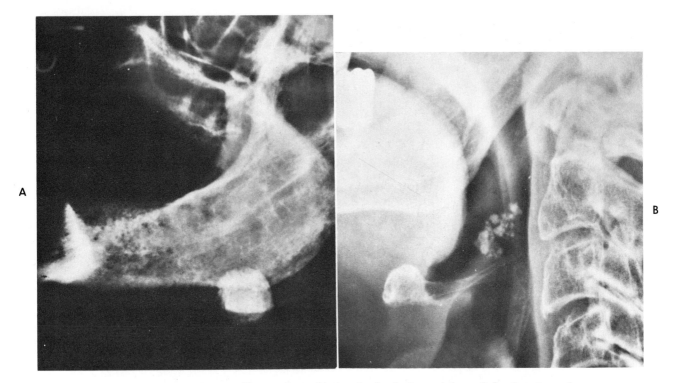

Fig. 4-24. A, Lateral view of large submandibular gland calculus in hilum of gland. **B,** Lateral view of multiple small parotid calcifications in peripheral ducts.

in the parotid gland, and 1% to 7% occur in the sublingual gland.[1,33] At least one calculus is present in about two thirds of the cases of chronic sialadenitis, and 25% of patients with at least one stone have multiple stones.[33] Eighty percent of the submandibular stones are radiopaque, whereas only 60% of parotid stones are radiopaque. Some of the reasons suggested for the higher incidence of stones in the submandibular gland are that (1) it has a mucous and serous secretion, whereas the parotid has only a watery serous secretion, (2) the submandibular gland contains more hydroxylapatite and phosphatase, which help precipitate salts in an alkaline pH, and (3) the orifice of Wharton's duct is smaller compared to the caliber of the duct than is the Stensen's duct orifice compared to Stensen's duct. This size difference allows easier obstruction at the orifice by a stone developing within the larger duct.

Submandibular stones tend to be located in Wharton's duct and the gland hilum, whereas parotid stones tend to occur in peripheral ducts and acini. Occasionally, these stones can erode through the ductal epithelium. This happens most often in Wharton's duct, in which the stones can be found in pseudodiverticuli lying in the floor of the mouth. As a general rule, stones do not obstruct unless they are larger than 3 mm (Fig. 4-24).

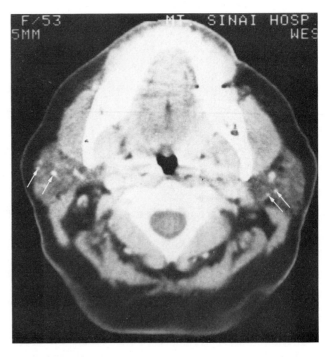

Fig. 4-25. Axial CT scan reveals several minute calcifications (*arrows*) in both parotid glands. These were not seen on plain film examination. *Chronic sialadenitis.*

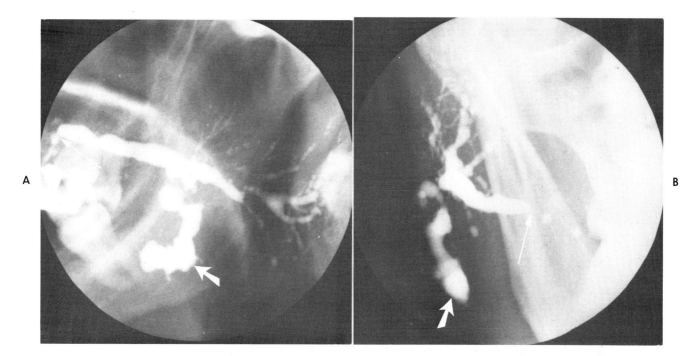

Fig. 4-26. A, Lateral sialogram of main duct dilation secondary to stricture near Stensen's duct orifice *(long arrow).* Abscess and fistulous tract have developed *(short arrow).* **B,** Frontal view of patient in **A.** Long arrow indicates stricture. Short arrow indicates abscess and fistulous tract.

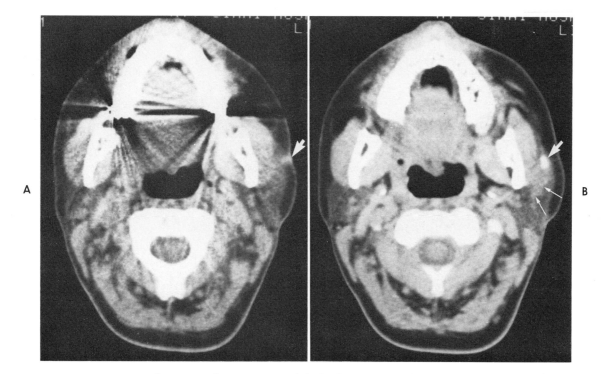

Fig. 4-27. A, Axial scan reveals sinus tract in left cheek *(arrow).* Patient was having clear fluid drain from this site. **B,** Axial CT scan just cephalad to **A** reveals small parotid calculus *(short arrow)* causing obstruction. This was not seen on plain film examination. Notice increased density of obstructed parotid ducts just posterior to stone *(long arrows).*

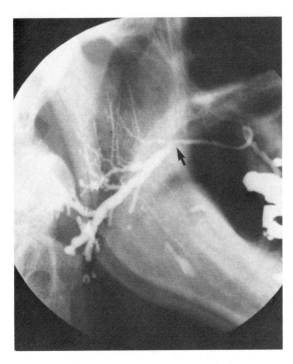

Fig. 4-28. Lateral view of ductal dilatation and obstruction secondary to radiolucent stone *(arrow)*. This type of stone can only be seen on sialographic study.

The opaque stones are better seen in plain film examination than in sialography because the contrast material may obscure the stones. In sialography the stones may either be fixed in position or mobile and may interfere with both ductal filling and ductal emptying. The stones are better seen with Sinografin than with Ethiodol. CT scanning, because of its increased contrast differentiation as compared to conventional filming, can often visualize small calculi not seen on plain films (Fig. 4-25). Behind the obstruction (whether complete or incomplete) changes of sialadenitis and sialodochitis can occur. If complete obstruction persists, abscess formation and fistulae can occur. Repeated passage of stones can cause areas of ductal fibrosis, which in turn may lead to focal strictures[33] (Figs. 4-26 to 4-28).

■ Sialodochitis fibrinosa (Kussmaul's disease)

This unusual disease is characterized by recurrent acute, but usually painless, attacks of parotid or submandibular gland swelling secondary to a mucous or fibrinous ductal plug. The appearance of such a plug in Stensen's or Wharton's duct orifice is diagnostic. It occurs primarily in dehydrated and debilitated patients and the treatment is massage and secretogogues to release the plug. Sialograms rarely are performed because of the clinical uniqueness of this entity.[48]

□ **Autoimmune diseases**

The autoimmune diseases form a clinically heterogeneous group of salivary gland disorders that all share a common histology. This specific histologic pattern is the single basic unifying factor for all these diseases.[1] The pathology initially involves a lymphocytic infiltration of the gland that is directed at the intercalated ducts, which become thinned and fragmented. The lymphocytes also progressively destroy the acini; eventually the only remaining ductal epithelium consists of isolated clusters of epithelial and myoepithelial cells surrounded by a dense lymphocytic infiltration. These have been described as epimyoepithelial islands in a sea of lymphocytes, and Godwin coined the term "benign lymphoepithelial lesion."[10] It represents the end stage of the disease process.

The sialographic findings of these autoimmune diseases reflect the underlying pathology and therefore are just as diagnostic as is the histologic picture. There is, however, controversy in the literature about the pathologic-radiographic findings that account for the characteristic roentgen sialographic appearance of these diseases. One group of investigators believe that the collections of contrast material seen on the sialogram are a result of paraductal extravasations through the weakened intercalated duct walls.[27,28,29] When a sialogram is performed the contrast material is injected under hand pressure in a retrograde manner into the ducts. This pressure allows the contrast material to perforate the damaged intercalated ducts and accumulate as droplets in the paraductal areas of the gland. Because the disease affects the entire gland uniformly, these paraductal extravasations occur uniformly throughout the gland. They do not occur under normal pressures in glands that are either normal or involved by any other pathologic entities.[32] Because these collections are extraductal, they remain in the gland after the ducts empty. If Ethiodol is used the collections can remain for months.

The other group of investigators believed that the collections of contrast material accumulate in localized dilatations of the intercalated ducts.[9] They postulate a trapdoor type of mechanism that allows the collections to form but not empty when the ducts empty. There are no significant sialectatic changes in the acini or more proximally in the ductal system.

Both groups agree that the accumulations occur at the intercalated duct level in a unique manner seen only in the autoimmune diseases. There may, in fact, be an element of both types of processes going on in each case. The important conclusions, however, are (1) the roentgen appearance is seen only with these diseases and (2) the changes are at the intercalated duct level and in either case do not reflect the classical concept of sialectasis, especially because the most terminal

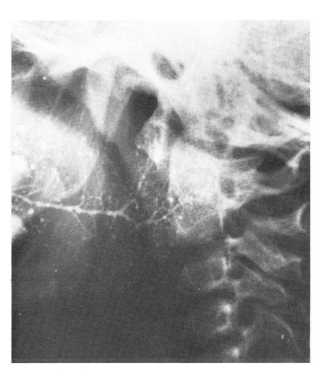

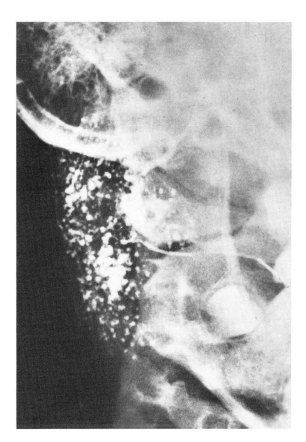

Fig. 4-29. Lateral sialogram of punctate pseudosialectasis. Notice that Stensen's duct is normal in caliber and all portions of gland are involved.

Fig. 4-30. Frontal view of patient with diffuse punctate pseudosialectasis. Stensen's duct is normal.

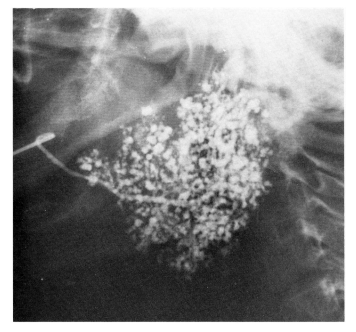

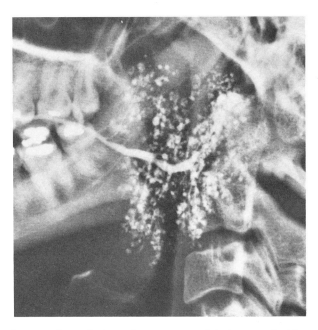

Fig. 4-31. Oblique sialogram view of patient with punctate to globular pseudosialectasis. Notice that entire gland is involved.

Fig. 4-32. Lateral view of punctate to globular pseudosialectasis with mild dilatation of Stensen's duct. This reflects early inflammatory changes of cavitary stage.

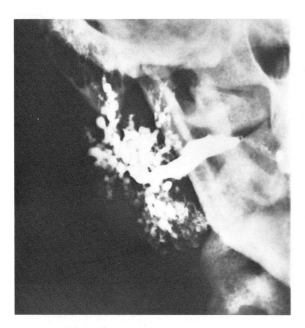

Fig. 4-33. Frontal oblique film of cavitary pseudosialectasis.

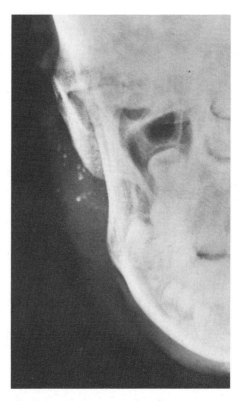

Fig. 4-34. Frontal postevacuation film of patient with punctate pseudosialectasis. Ducts have emptied, however, paraductal extravasations remain.

ductal regions (acini) are not ectatic. To emphasize these differences, the term *pseudosialectasis* seems more appropriate (Figs. 4-29 to 4-34).

The four progressive roentgenographic stages are as follows.

1. Punctate pseudosialectasis. This is the earliest roentgenographic pattern. There are spherical collections of contrast medium measuring 1 mm or less in diameter that are uniform in both size and distribution throughout the gland. The main ductal system is normal. After the administration of a secretogogue the ducts clear; however, the punctate collections remain.

2. Globular pseudosialectasis. This is the next stage of disease development. The spherical collections of contrast material now measure 1 to 2 mm in diameter. The main ducts are normal; however, most of the peripheral minor ducts are not seen. The appearance has been likened to a branchless, fruit-laden tree.[13] These collections remain after a secretogogue is given.

3. Cavitary pseudosialectasis. This is a still further progression of the disease process. There are irregular, larger globules of contrast material that are nonuniformly distributed throughout the gland. There is dilatation of the main ductal system.

4. Destructive pseudosialectasis. This represents the end stage of the disease. The contrast material dissects into the septa of the gland and into the subcapsular spaces. There is no recognizable peripheral ductal branching. The pattern can be so bizarre that differentiation from an aggressive malignancy may be impossible.[30]

It appears that only the punctate and globular changes truly reflect the characteristic underlying autoimmune pathology.[33] The cavitary and destructive changes reflect more the superimposition of secondary inflammatory disease on the underlying punctate and globular findings. This is most noticeable in the main duct system where inflammatory dilatation, functional change, and deformity are seen in progressive stages. In addition, patients with punctate or globular changes have nearly normal salivary flow rates, whereas patients with cavitary or destructive changes have secretory rates appreciably lower than normal.[13] Thus as the primary disease progresses salivary flow slowly decreases, ascending infection occurs, and further glandular damage ensues.

The clinical appearances of the autoimmune diseases vary considerably. There are two basic groups, those that are localized to the salivary and lacrimal glands and those that have an associated systemic component. The former group is referred to as Mikulicz' disease and has

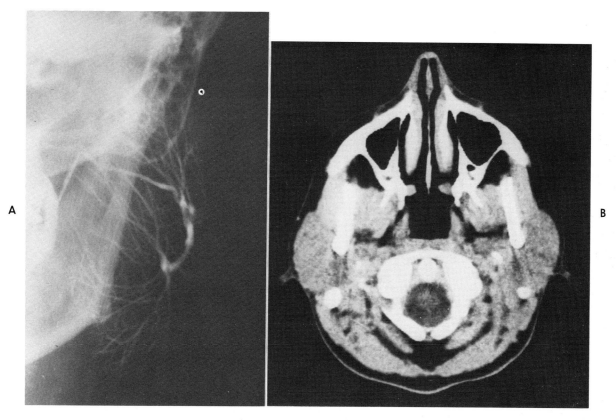

Fig. 4-35. A, Frontal sialogram of enlarged gland with normal but widely separated ducts. *Sialosis.* **B,** Axial CT scan reveals both parotid glands to be enlarged and uniformly increased in density. *Sialosis.*

two clinical forms: recurrent parotitis in children and recurrent parotitis in adults. Those diseases with a systemic component are referred to as Sjögren's syndrome and clinically there is xerostomia, keratoconjunctivitis sicca, and a collagen disease that is usually rheumatoid arthritis. About 15% to 30% of cases of Sjögren's syndrome have parotid involvement.[18] About 95% of cases are in women.

In recurrent parotitis in children, the majority of cases occur in males and most resolve spontaneously at puberty. Recurrent parotitis in adults occurs primarily in women and most cases progress to involve secondary infection.

The sicca syndrome refers to cases of xerostomia and keratoconjunctivitis sicca without a collagen disease. There is evidence that all of these clinical entities are manifestations of a single disease with a variable clinical penetrance.[2,4,19,20]

In all cases of Mikulicz' disease there are recurrent attacks of parotid swellings that usually affect one side at a time or, if both sides are involved, one side invariably is more affected than the other. Sjögren's syndrome tends to have less frequent, longer-lasting at-

tacks that are mainly bilateral. Sialographically, changes are invariably present bilaterally in all clinical forms of these autoimmune diseases.

There is a small group of patients that have persistently swollen glands or appear clinically with a localized mass. This is the so-called tumor simulating group.[6] The sialogram can differentiate between a tumor and an autoimmune disease.

There is an increased incidence of lymphoproliferative disorders in patients who have previously existing lymphoepithelial lesions,[1,33] and unlike primary parotid lymphomas, which have a good prognosis, these lymphoproliferative disorders have a very grave prognosis and are often rapidly fatal.

Mikulicz' syndrome refers to a group of disorders that clinically can mimic the autoimmune diseases. They are, however, caused by a specific, underlying disease such as one of the granulomatous diseases, the lymphoneoplasms, or the sialoses.

■ Sialosis or sialadenosis

This refers to a nonneoplastic, noninflammatory, nontender enlargement of the parotid glands that appears clinically as bilateral recurrent progressive swellings. Sialosis can be seen in metabolic disorders as well as with allergic and drug reactions. Conditions such as cirrhosis, diabetes, ovarian, thyroid, and pancreatic insufficiency, alcoholism, or malnutrition can cause sialosis. Drugs such as sulfisoxazole, phenylbutazone, catecholamines, and iodide-containing compounds have also caused sialosis.[18]

The sialogram reveals an enlarged gland with a sparse-appearing peripheral ductal system (Fig. 4-35, A). The sparse appearance is a result of the normal number of ducts being spread apart in the enlarged gland. The ducts themselves are otherwise normal. Histologically, there is serous acinar cell hypertrophy, interstitial edema, ductal atrophy, and fatty infiltration of the gland. On CT the salivary glands are enlarged and initially look denser than normal (Fig. 4-35, B). In the advanced stage of the process the glands look more fatty than normal as well as enlarged.

■ The granulomatous diseases

The evaluation of the multinodular or chronically enlarged gland is a challenging problem. In addition to chronic sialadenitis, sialosis, and autoimmune diseases, the physician must consider the granulomatous diseases, the lymphoneoplasms, and rare primary and metastatic tumors in the differential diagnosis.

The granulomatous diseases occur primarily in the intraparotid and paraparotid lymph nodes and in the glandular parenchyma. These granulomas can enlarge and may simulate neoplasms. Usually the gland is nontender and multinodular to palpation. A variety of diseases may thus secondarily involve the salivary glands. These diseases include sarcoid, tuberculosis, actinomycosis, cat-scratch fever, and atypical mycobacterial infection.[1]

Sarcoid is a systemic disease of undetermined cause that is characterized by noncaseating granulomatous invovement of multiple organ systems. Parotid gland involvement is reported to occur in 10% to 30% of patients with systemic sarcoidosis and in some of these cases the parotid enlargement may be the only clinical manifestation of the disease. Usually there is bilateral painless parotid gland enlargement (83%) and a decreased salivary flow. In addition, involvement of the minor salivary glands may result in xerostomia.[33] Parotid involvement may also occur as part of Heerfordt's syndrome, which consists of uveitis, parotid swelling, and facial nerve paralysis. Generally, sarcoid disease of the salivary glands tends to spontaneous regression, and only 30% of cases require treatment.

Primary tuberculous involvement of the salivary

glands is rare; when it does occur the parotid glands are affected more often than the submandibular glands. It is most likely that this form of the disease arises from a focus in the tonsils or teeth and then spreads by way of the regional lymph nodes to the gland.

Secondary salivary gland involvement in cases of generalized tuberculosis affects the submandibular glands more often than the parotid glands.[1]

Atypical mycobacterial infections can involve the neck and appear clinically as painless cervical adenopathy with subsequent secondary involvement of the salivary glands. Systemic symptoms are usually not present. Although this type of infection is unusual, it is being seen clinically today more often than tuberculosis.

Cat-scratch (animal) fever is a necrotizing granulomatous disease that is increasing in frequency as the number and variety of pets grows. It can involve the parotid lymph nodes and mimic primary parotid disease.[1]

Actinomycosis causes an indolent chronic inflammatory disease that usually results in the formation of sinus tracts. It often originates in the angle of the mandible and then spreads to the adjacent nodes and the parotid gland.[16]

The sialographic findings in all these diseases are similar. Early in the process the sialogram is usually normal. As the disease progresses there is "pruning" or a decrease in the number of minor duct radicles seen on the sialogram. Eventually, multiple (usually two to six) discrete benign-appearing masses are seen. Each one smoothly displaces the adjacent parotid ducts. The masses represent the enlarged lymph nodes or parenchymal granulomas. Rarely, a solitary intraparotid node will enlarge; in this instance it cannot be differentiated from a cyst or benign neoplasm. Less often, the conventional sialogram will appear normal or show a single benign lesion. The CT sialogram, however, will reveal multiple intraparotid and possibly paraparotid masses. This CT finding is a reliable indicator of disease that is too small to be visualized clearly on the conventional study. Masses as small as 5 mm have been identified in this manner (Figs. 4-36 to 4-42).[42]

The systemic lymphomas may involve the parotid gland nodes secondarily and as such they present a sialographic picture similar to the granulomatous diseases. Usually, other cervical adenopathy is present and is detected either clinically or on the CT scan (see section on tumors). Similarly, multiple Warthin's tumors or rare metastases to the parotid gland can give the same sialographic picture of multiple discrete masses (see section on tumors).

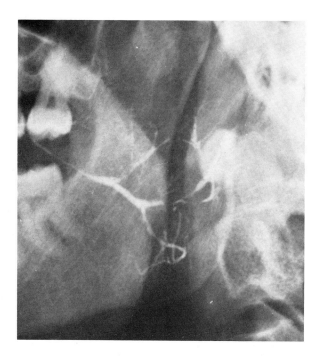

Fig. 4-36. Lateral sialogram of parotid gland. Ducts are "pruned" in appearance and displaced around several masses. *Sarcoid.*

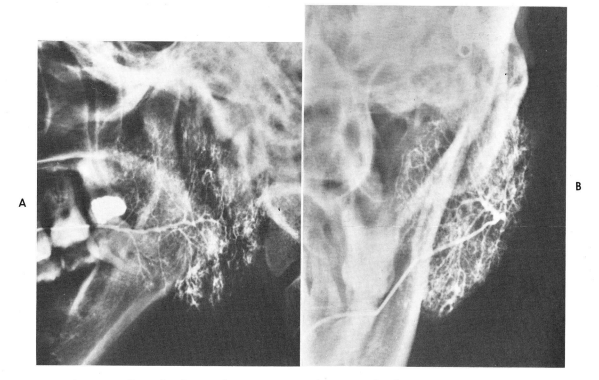

Fig. 4-37. A, Lateral sialogram that appears normal. B, Frontal sialogram film of same patient as in A. No mass lesions are seen.

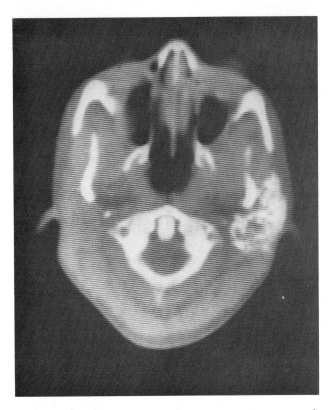

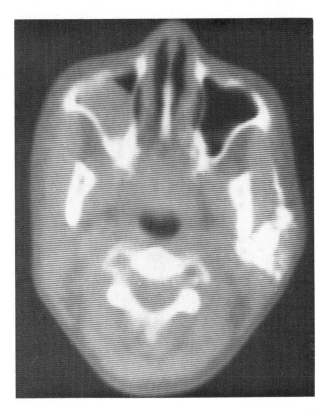

Fig. 4-38. CT sialogram of same patient as in Fig. 4-37 reveals two areas of nonfilling in posterior and deep portions of gland.

Fig. 4-39. CT sialogram of same patient as in Fig. 4-37 at different level reveals area of nonfilling in outer portion of superficial lobe. *Sarcoid granulomas in gland and intraparotid lymph nodes.*

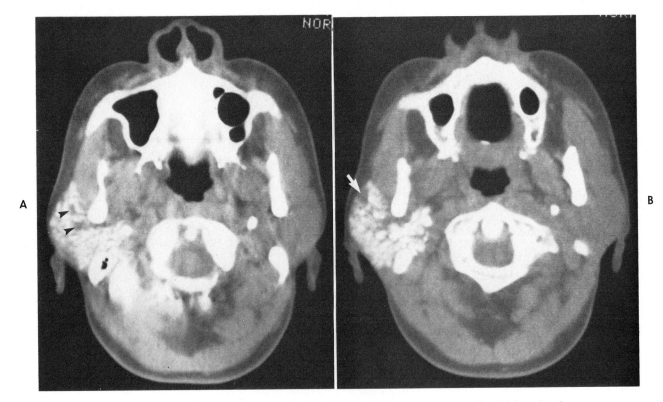

Fig. 4-40. A, Axial CT sialogram reveals two small filling defects in superficial lobe of right parotid gland *(arrowheads).* **B,** Axial CT sialogram just caudal to **A** reveals another filling defect in right superficial parotid lobe *(arrow). Sarcoid.*

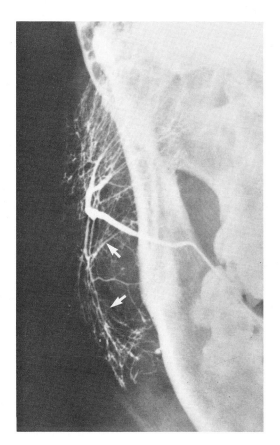

Fig. 4-41. Frontal sialogram reveals benign-appearing mass in parotid gland displacing ducts around it *(arrows).*

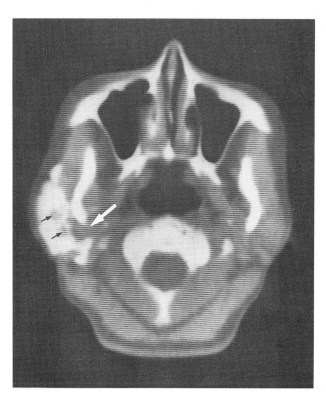

Fig. 4-42. CT sialogram reveals retromandibular node *(white arrow)*, which is mass seen on sialogram in Fig. 4-41. There are also two 5 mm areas of nonfilling in gland *(black arrows). Sarcoid.*

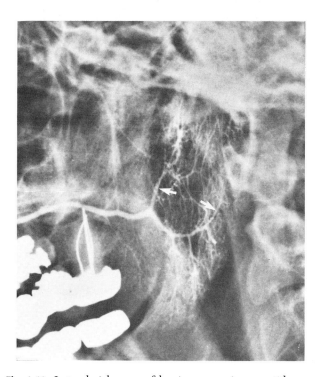

Fig. 4-43. Lateral sialogram of benign-appearing parotid mass *(arrows). Mucous cyst.*

□ Cysts and mucoceles

As a group cysts and mucoceles comprise less than 5% of all salivary gland masses. The majority of these lesions are unilateral and may simulate benign tumors (Figs. 4-43 to 4-45).[1]

True cysts are rare and occur most often in the parotid gland. They can have a variety of different epithelial linings and they all look like benign tumors on sialograms; that is, they displace the intact parotid ducts around them.

The congenital cystic lesions of the parotid gland include dermoid cysts, branchial cleft and pouch cysts, and ductal cysts.

The congenital ductal cysts that occur in infancy are probably true congenital retention cysts. They appear clinically as parotid gland enlargement. Therapy is not suggested in infancy unless an infection occurs. At a later age surgery is curative.

Dermoid cysts occur as isolated masses that lie either deep within the gland or near its surface. They appear as benign parotid masses and are cured by complete surgical removal.

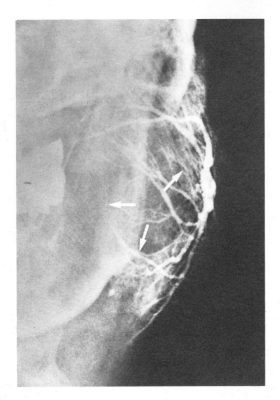

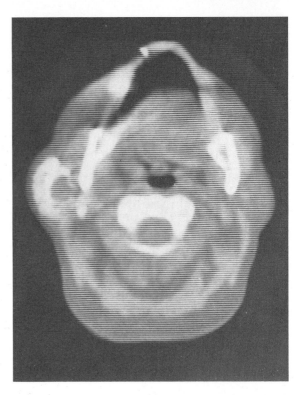

Fig. 4-44. Frontal film of benign-appearing mass *(arrows)*. *Mucous cyst*. This cannot be differentiated from benign mixed tumor.

Fig. 4-45. CT sialogram of benign-appearing mass with sharp mass-parotid interface. *Mucous cyst.*

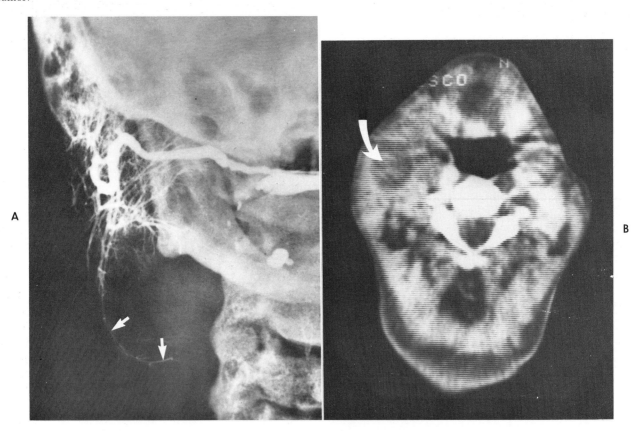

A

B

Fig. 4-46. A, Frontal sialogram reveals large benign-appearing mass in lower portion of superficial parotid lobe *(arrows)*. **B,** CT scan of same patient as in **A** reveals isodense mass *(arrow)* surrounded by thick rim of enhancement. *Infected branchial cleft cyst of parotid gland extending into neck.*

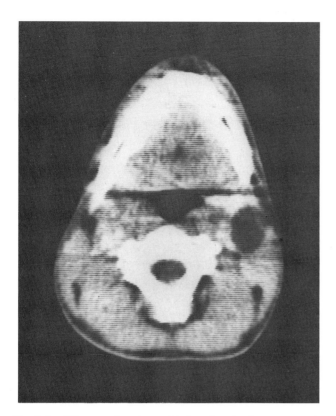

Fig. 4-47. CT scan of patient with low-density lesion in neck. *Branchial cleft cyst.*

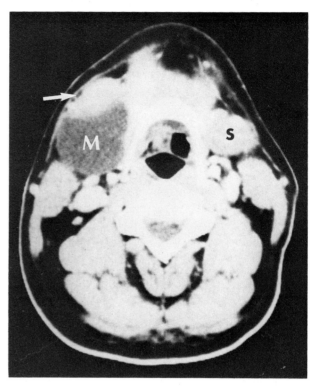

Fig. 4-48. Axial CT scan reveals large low-density mass at posterior margin of right submandibular gland *(M)*. Mass has no tissue plane separating it from gland but mass is separate from adjacent neck structures. Gland itself has been pushed anteriorly *(arrow)*. S, Left submandibular gland. *Mucocele.*

Branchial cleft cysts in the parotid gland are rare. Those arising from the first cleft can appear as preauricular parotid masses, whereas those arising from the second cleft may appear as masses in the lower pole of the parotid gland. An infected cyst often appears clinically as a neck abscess or a parotid gland abscess. Sialographically, they smoothly displace the parotid ducts around them. On CT scans the fluid-filled contents may be either isodense or of low density, depending on the specific contents (Figs. 4-46 and 4-47). If infected, a rim of enhancement will be seen in the wall of the cyst and the immediately adjacent tissues. Clinically, these infected cysts are often followed as recurrent attacks of neck or parotid abscesses that often require multiple incisions and drainage procedures before the actual diagnosis is established.[48]

Branchial pouch cysts can rarely occur in the region of the parotid gland. They usually are located deep in the retromandibular area of the gland, near the middle ear and eustachian tube.[48]

Fibrocystic and polycystic disease rarely can affect the parotid glands, and when they do there usually is bilateral involvement.[21]

A mucous retention cyst results from intermittent ductal obstruction, which leads to a dilatation of the proximal duct. Thus a mucous retention cyst has an epithelial lining. If complete ductal obstruction occurs, salivary gland atrophy follows without the formation of a mucous cyst.[38] Mucoceles represent an extravasation of mucous into the surrounding salivary gland tissues and as such have no epithelial lining. They result from mechanical trauma to minor excretory ducts, which results in a severance of the duct. Surgery is the treatment of choice; however, if the mucocele's contents escape at operation, a recurrence will result (Fig. 4-48).

The ranula is a retention-type phenomenon and most commonly involves the sublingual glands. The simple ranula results from obstruction of the salivary ducts in the submucosal layers of the lining of the oral cavity and is a form of retention cyst. The plunging or deep ranula extends beyond the mucous membranes into the floor of the mouth and most probably results from mucous extravasation.[1] Thus it is a pseudocyst that clinically appears as a mass in the floor of the mouth and usually is an obvious indication of the diagnosis.

All of these intrasalivary gland cysts and mucoceles smoothly displace the adjacent salivary ducts.

■ Trauma, fistulae, and sialoceles

The salivary glands may be injured by blunt trauma, contusions, lacerations, or penetrating injuries. The injury may involve the main salivary duct, the gland parenchyma, the facial and lingual nerves, the external carotid artery, the facial artery and vein, and the masseter muscle.[24] The main duct is lacerated in about 50% of the cases as an isolated incident.[16]

If the laceration goes undetected, a fistula almost always will develop. It communicates primarily with the skin but also can drain to the mouth or into surrounding structures.[26] A fistula may also occur as a postoperative complication. This is especially true with an attempted stone removal from either Stensen's or Wharton's duct.

If a sialogram can be performed, the contrast material will extravasate through the fistulous tract, usually to the overlying skin, or a blindly ending main duct will be demonstrated (Fig. 4-49). Because extravasation may occur into the adjacent soft tissues, a water-soluble contrast agent is suggested in these cases.

Obstruction at Stensen's duct orifice can occur from trauma to the papilla. This is related primarily to faulty dentures or buccal mucosal ulcerations with edema. Such repeated trauma can result in an orifice stenosis. Clinically, the parotid gland swells, especially at mealtimes. Sialography may be impossible in these cases because of inability to cannulate the obstructed orifice.

Ductal obstruction can also occur from a stricture secondary to ductal epithelial damage resulting from a stone. This is especially true with Wharton's duct stones.

Lacerations of the cheek can lead to a suture being placed across Stensen's duct and causing an obstruction. In these instances the sialogram will locate the level and degree of the obstruction.

Injury to the gland parenchyma can result in either a parenchymal laceration or an intracapsular hematoma. These lesions appear as areas of lack of parenchymal filling, with splaying of the ducts around the region.

Saliva can accumulate within a cystic collection, which occurs because of interruption of the excretory ducts draining the area. This sialocele usually appears as a benign lesion smoothly displacing the adjacent ducts around it. If the region of glandular laceration maintains a communication with the distal ductal sys-

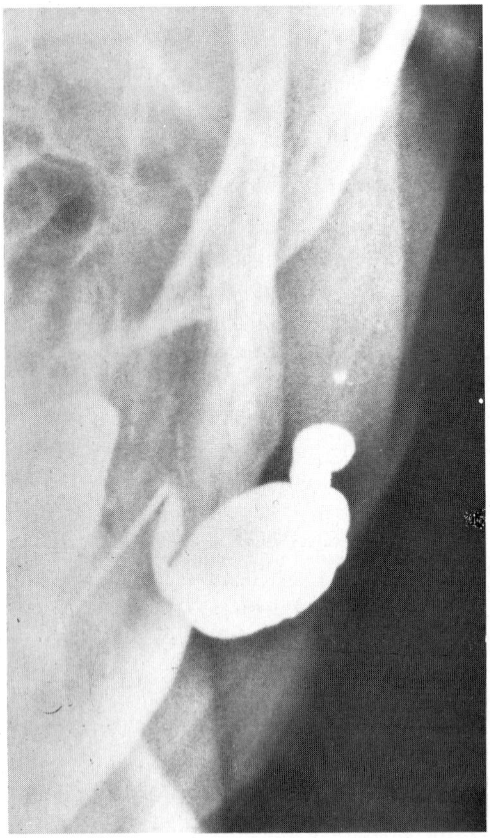

Fig. 4-49. Frontal sialogram of cystic-appearing duct and gland caused by traumatic stricture near Stensen's duct orifice. No identifiable peripheral ducts were demonstrated.

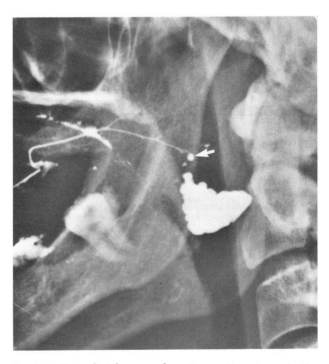

Fig. 4-50. Lateral sialogram of posttraumatic communicating sialocele. Droplets of contrast material (*arrow*) filled cystic cavity.

tem, then a sialogram will reveal the contrast material dripping into a cystic parenchymal cavity (Fig. 4-50). A sialocele or laceration can also communicate with the skin by way of a fistula.[33]

Frey's syndrome results from an injury to the auriculotemporal nerve and clinically appears as sweating and flushing of the skin over the distribution of this nerve following the stimulus to salivate. It most probably results from a communication between the postganglionic parasympathetic fibers from the otic ganglion and the sympathetic nerves from the superior cervical ganglion. It is a difficult disease to treat, is extremely trying for the patient, and has a normal sialogram.

□ Masseter hypertrophy

Masseter hypertrophy is an uncommon condition that usually occurs bilaterally but can be unilateral. The masseter muscle enlargement can be related to abnormal mastication or can have a congenital cause. The muscle hypertrophy can cause bony overgrowths, or exostoses, on the outer surface of the angle of the mandible where the muscle attaches to this bone. The masseter enlarges when the teeth are clenched. A sialogram reveals a smooth lateral bowing of Stensen's duct around the muscle. This is also well seen on an axial CT scan (Figs. 4-51 to 4-53).

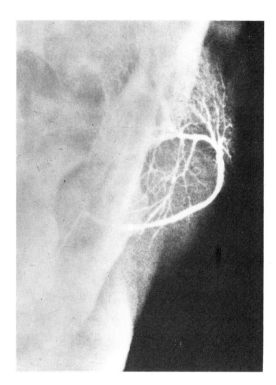

Fig. 4-51. Frontal sialogram reveals wide lateral bowing of Stensen's duct. Hilum of parotid gland is greater than 20 mm from mandible.

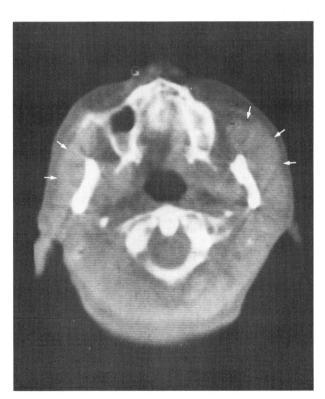

Fig. 4-52. CT scan reveals masseter muscle to be almost twice as large on left side *(three arrows)* as it is on normal right side *(two arrows)*.

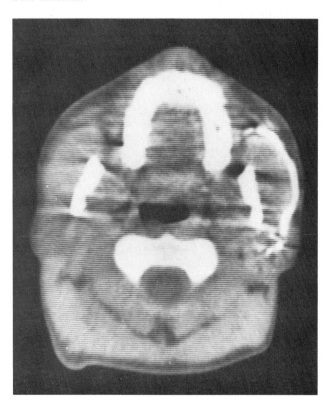

Fig. 4-53. CT sialogram reveals displacement of Stensen's duct around hypertrophied masseter muscle.

If the muscle becomes large enough, it can interfere with salivary flow in Stensen's duct and eventually result in stone formation and inflammatory ductal changes.

■ Postirradiation sialadenitis

Radiation therapy directed at oral and pharyngeal carcinomas often includes the parotid glands within its portals. Although considerable variation in radiosensitivity exists between individual patients, all salivary glands will exhibit some postirradiation changes if a sufficient dose is given. The degree of these changes is dose dependent.

Acute changes are extremely rare and occur usually after single doses of 1000 R or more.[35] Initially, there is acute parotid swelling caused primarily by interstitial edema. This tender enlargement occurs within 24 hours of the initial treatment. The gland decreases in size 3 to 4 days later, and within 1 month after a cancericidal dose parotid degeneration is present and may continue to progress for about 3 months. With lower doses some regeneration may occur.

Finally, 4 or more months after initial treatment the later changes of acinar degeneration and fibrosis are established. If these glands are examined radiographically the sialogram reveals patchy areas of lack of acinar filling and focal areas of ductal pruning.[18,33]

□ **Tumors**

Salivary gland tumors represent less than 3% of all tumors.[7] Of those neoplasms that occur, 95.4% are parenchymal in origin and only 4.6% originate from interstitial tissues (blood vessels, lymph nodes, and nerves).[33] Nearly 80% of the tumors occur in the parotid gland, less than 10% in the submandibular gland, less than 1% in the sublingual gland, and 10% to 15% in the minor salivary glands.[8] Thus the parotid lesions far outnumber the tumors in all of the other salivary glands combined.

The incidence of malignancy increases as the size of the salivary gland decreases. That is, about 50% of minor salivary gland lesions are malignant, whereas only 20% of parotid tumors are malignant.[33]

Many different classifications of salivary gland neoplasms exist. They are based on the cell of origin, clinical presentation, or personal experience of the physician.[1,33]

The classification of the World Health Organization (see box) presents a good working background on which a brief discussion of tumors of the salivary glands can be based.[46]

■ Epithelial tumors

Pleomorphic adenomas (mixed tumors) are the most common epithelial tumors, representing about 70% of

---

WORLD HEALTH ORGANIZATION CLASSIFICATION OF SALIVARY GLAND TUMORS

I. Epithelial tumors
   A. Adenomas
      1. Pleomorphic adenoma (mixed tumor)
      2. Monomorphic adenomas
         a. Adenolymphoma
         b. Oxyphilic adenoma
         c. Other types
   B. Mucoepidermoid tumor
   C. Acinic cell tumor
   D. Carcinomas
      1. Adenoid cystic carcinoma
      2. Adenocarcinoma
      3. Epidermoid carcinoma
      4. Undifferentiated carcinoma
      5. Carcinoma in pleomorphic adenoma (malignant mixed tumor)
II. Nonepithelial tumors
III. Unclassified tumors
IV. Allied conditions
   A. Benign lymphoepithelial lesion
   B. Sialosis
   C. Oncocytosis

---

all benign neoplasms of the salivary glands and 70% of all parotid tumors. They are solitary, slow-growing, painless encapsulated lesions (Figs. 4-54 to 4-59) (see Chapter 5). Simultaneous occurrences of these tumors in multiple salivary glands have been rarely described and there is an estimated bilateral occurrence rate of 1 in 40,000 cases.[33] Recurrences occur and are related to rupture of the tumor's capsule and seeding of the operative site. Malignant changes occur in only 3% to 15% of the cases and the treatment of choice is complete surgical resection.

Monomorphic adenomas as a group are characterized by the regularity of their cellular structure and pattern, in contradistinction to the pleomorphic adenomas, which have a varied cellular composition.

Adenolymphoma (Warthin's tumor, papillary cystadenoma lymphomatosum) is a tumor occurring in salivary ductal tissue that is embryologically included within lymph nodes. This unusual situation develops only in the region of the parotid gland and thus this tumor only occurs within the intraparotid and paraparotid lymph nodes. It does not occur in the other salivary glands. It is a bicellular tumor and requires a lymphoreticular and an oncocytic component for definitive diagnosis. Failure to require both components has led to erroneous diagnoses of this tumor in the larynx, trachea, and nasal and oral cavities.[1]

These lesions occur primarily in the tail of the parotid gland (posteroinferior margin of the superficial lobe)

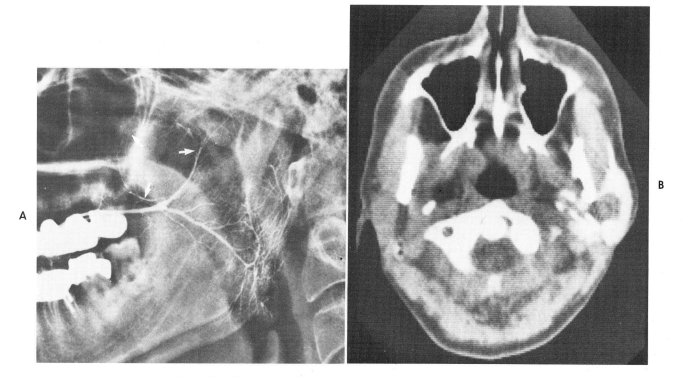

Fig. 4-54. A, Lateral sialogram reveals benign-appearing mass in parotid accessary gland. Ducts are smoothly displaced around lesion *(arrows). Benign mixed tumor.* **B,** CT sialogram reveals superficial lobe round lesion with sharp mass-parotid interface. *Benign mixed tumor.*

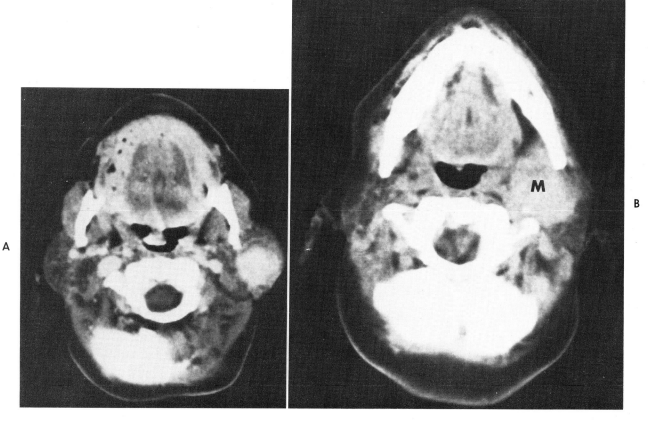

Fig. 4-55. A, Axial CT scan reveals an enhanced benign-appearing left superficial lobe parotid mixed tumor. **B,** Axial CT scan reveals large enhanced deep lobe tumor *(M)* of left parotid gland. *Mixed tumor.*

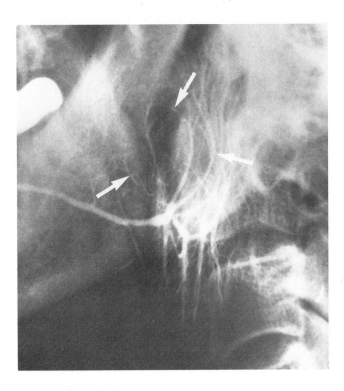

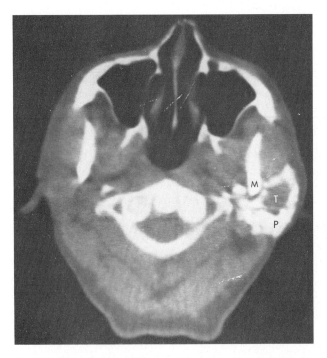

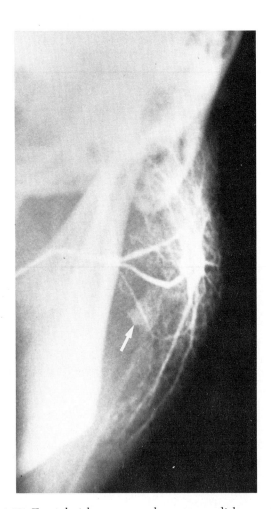

Fig. 4-56. Lateral sialogram reveals benign-appearing mass (*arrows*) that is only faintly seen. (Reprinted from Som, P.M., and Biller, N.R.: Radiology **135:**387-390, 1980.)

Fig. 4-57. CT sialogram of same patient as in Fig. 4-56. Tumor (*t*) is clearly seen in contrast-filled parotid gland (*P*). *M,* mandible. *Benign mixed tumor.* (Reprinted from Som, P.M., and Biller, N.R.: Radiology **135:**387-390, 1980.)

Fig. 4-58. Frontal sialogram reveals vague medial mass that displaces parotid gland outward (ball-in-glove appearance). Calcification (*arrow*) is seen in mass. *Deep lobe benign mixed tumor.*

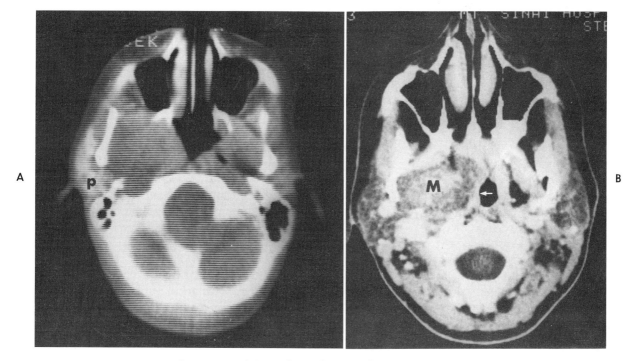

Fig. 4-59. A, CT sialogram reveals large deep lobe parotid mass extending into parapharyngeal space and pushing lateral pharyngeal wall toward midline. *P,* Contrast-filled parotid gland. **B,** Axial CT scan reveals large deep lobe mixed tumor of right parotid gland *(M).* Mass enhances slightly and pushes right pharyngeal lateral wall toward midline *(arrow).*

Fig. 4-60. A, Lateral sialogram reveals mass effect in tail of parotid gland *(arrow). Warthin's tumor.* **B,** CT sialogram reveals benign-appearing mass in tail of left parotid gland *(arrow). M,* Mandible; *P,* contrast material–filled parotid gland. *Warthin's tumor.* (Courtesy D. Beekler, M.D.)

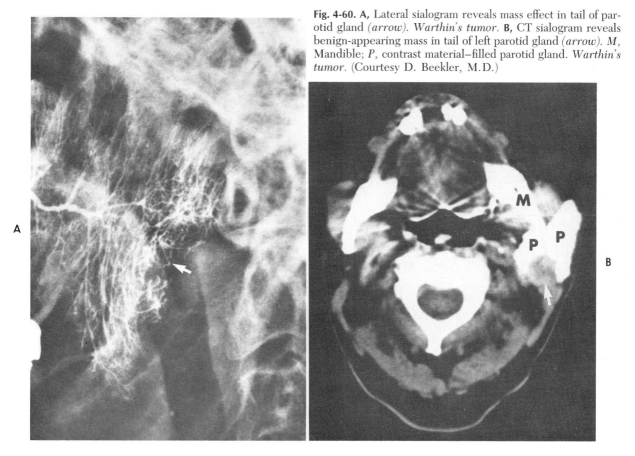

(Fig. 4-60). They rarely are seen in the deep lobe. They are the most common tumor to occur bilaterally, with a reported incidence of 6%.[12] However, the true multicentric nature of this tumor may be closer to 30%.[29] Adenolymphomas are thus the most common parotid neoplasms to occur as either unilateral multiple tumors or as bilateral lesions (Figs. 4-61 and 4-62). They are benign lesions, with malignant transformation being extremely rare. They occur primarily in males (a 5:1 ratio), and facial nerve involvement is rare. They accumulate technetium Tc-99m sodium pertechnetate or radioactive iodine on nuclear scans. It is the oncocytic component that is responsible for this phenomenon.

Oxyphilic adenomas (oncocytomas) are uncommon tumors representing less than 1% of all salivary neoplasms. Almost all patients are over the age of 50 years, a statistic that may correlate with the increase in salivary oncocytes that occurs normally with age. These tumors occur primarily as solitary parotid lesions although there are rare reports of bilateral occurences. They are almost always cured by surgical excision, and malignancy is very rare. The tumors involving the nasal cavity appear to be more resistant to treatment and local

recurrences in this region have been reported.[33] Oncocytomas accumulate isotopes on nuclear scans, as do Warthin's tumors. It is the oncocytic cell, common to both these lesions, that accounts for this phenomenon. These are the only salivary tumors that intensely accumulate radionuclides.

Other types of monomorphic adenomas comprise less than 2% of all salivary gland tumors. They are characterized by a uniform epithelial pattern throughout the tumor and an absence of a myxochondroid stroma. This distinguishes them from the mixed tumors. They are benign, encapsulated lesions that usually occur in the sixth to seventh decades. The basal cell and clear cell adenomas occur primarily in the parotid gland, as do the unusual sebaceous adenomas.

Mucoepidermoid tumors represent 6% to 9% of all salivary tumors and about 30% of malignant lesions. Sixty percent to 70% occur in the parotid gland and 15% to 20% occur in the oral cavity, primarily in the palatal region. They are the most common parotid malignancy in all age groups. They are classified as well-differentiated or low-grade carcinomas, intermediate types, and finally high-grade or poorly differentiated carcinomas that have considerable anaplasia. The 5-year survival rates vary from 90% to 100% for the low-grade lesions to 65% for the intermediate tumors and only 10% for the high-grade neoplasms.[1] Most of these lesions are circumscribed and poorly encapsulated. The more malignant forms have obvious infiltrative margins (Figs. 4-63 to 4-66).

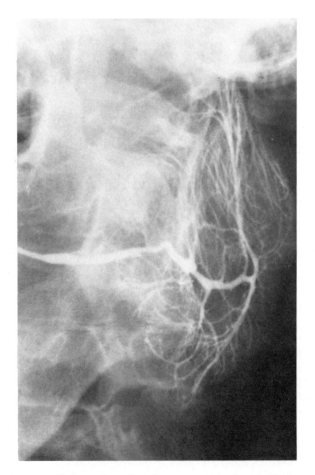

Fig. 4-61. Oblique frontal sialogram reveals ductal displacement around several benign-appearing masses.

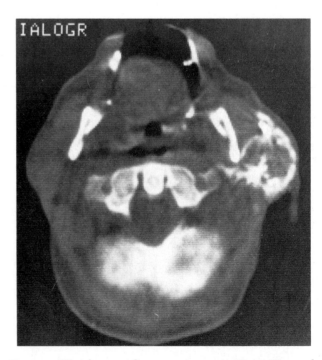

Fig. 4-62. CT sialogram of same patient as in Fig. 4-61 reveals two adjacent benign-appearing masses. *Warthin's tumors.*

Fig. 4-63. CT sialogram reveals benign-appearing mass *(t)* in superficial lobe of contrast-filled parotid gland *(P)*. *M,* Mandible; *Ph,* pharynx. *Low-grade mucoepidermoid carcinoma.* (Reprinted from Som, P.M., and Biller, N.R.: Ann. Otol. Rhinol. Laryngol. **88**:590-595, 1979.)

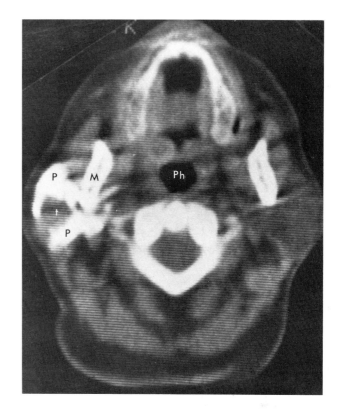

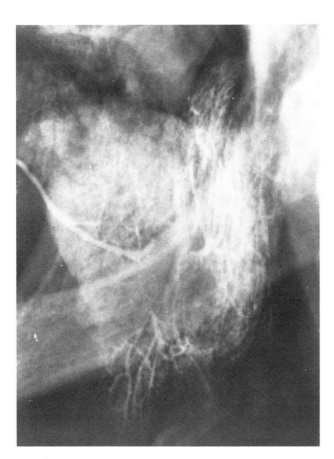

Fig. 4-64. Lateral sialogram reveals malignant-appearing mass with lack of parenchymal filling and areas of main ductal cutoff. *High-grade mucoepidermoid carcinoma.* (Reprinted from Som, P.M., and Biller, N.R.: Ann. Otol. Rhinol. Laryngol. **88**:590-595, 1979.)

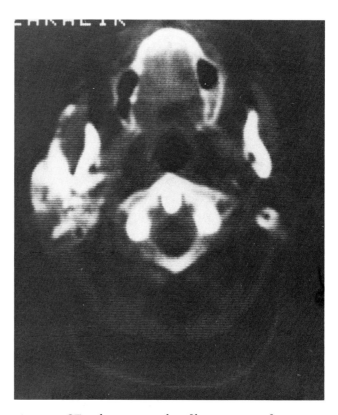

Fig. 4-65. CT sialogram reveals infiltrative type of tumor in posterior parotid margin. *High-grade mucoepidermoid carcinoma.*

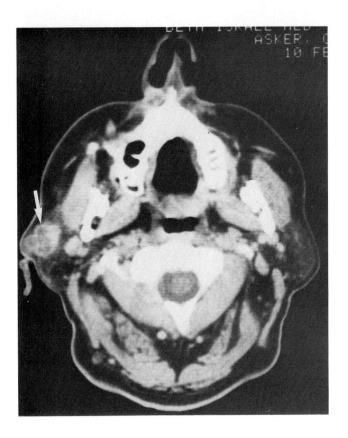

Acinic cell tumors account for between 2.5% and 4% of all parotid tumors. They are almost exclusively reported in the parotid glands and only rarely occur in the oral cavity minor salivary glands (Fig. 4-67).

Their incidence of bilateral involvement is estimated to be 3%, which is second only to Warthin's tumor.[1] They also may be second to Warthin's tumor in having a multifocal origin; acinic cell tumors can arise in ductal or acinar inclusions in the intraparotid or paraparotid lymph nodes. They are the second most common salivary gland malignancy in children. The tumors appear as well-defined solitary masses with a thin capsule. As with mixed tumors, simple enucleation with capsular spillage is associated with a high recurrence rate, and complete surgical excision is the treatment of choice. Patients with these tumors have a 5-year survival rate

Fig. 4-66. Axial CT scan reveals large nodular mass in superficial lobe of right parotid gland *(arrow).* Mass has several low attenuation areas within it and an unevenly enhanced outer margin. *Mucoepidermoid carcinoma.*

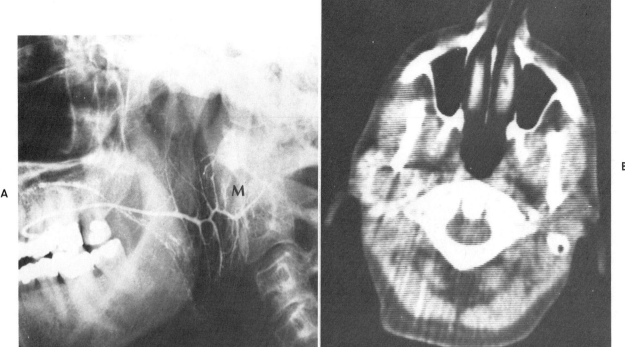

Fig. 4-67. A, Lateral sialogram reveals posterior mass *(M)* that appears benign and displaces ducts around it. **B,** CT sialogram of same patient as in Fig. 4-66 reveals benign-appearing retromandibular parotid mass. *Acinic cell carcinoma.*

of 90%; however, the 20-year rate is only 56%. They metastasize in 20% of the cases to the lungs or peripheral skeleton, especially to the spinal column.[1,33]

Adenoid cystic carcinomas (cylindromas) represent from 4% to 8% of all salivary gland tumors. They rarely occur in the parotid gland but are the most common malignancy in the submandibular and minor salivary glands.[18] The prognosis is poor and overall only 10% to 20% of patients are alive at 15 years.[33] Usually, the carcinomas are well-circumscribed lesions with microscopic marginal involvement and perineural skip metastases.

Adenocarcinomas are highly malignant tumors that metastasize widely to regional lymph nodes and distant viscera. They actually represent all those glandular malignancies that cannot be placed into the other more definable classes, such as acinic cell, mucoepidermoid, or adenoid cystic tumors. They represent probably less than 3% of parotid neoplasms.[1] The 5- and 20-year sur-

vival rates for patients with adenocarcinomas are 78% and 41% respectively for low-grade tumors and 70% and 20% for high-grade lesions.

Epidermoid carcinomas are rare, highly malignant carcinomas that presumably arise from metaplastic salivary duct epithelium. About two thirds occur in the parotid gland and one third in the submandibular gland. They often appear as masses that are fixed to the skin or adjacent underlying structures. There is a five-year survival rate of 25%.[33]

Undifferentiated carcinomas are rare and highly malignant carcinomas. They represent less than 3% of all major salivary gland tumors and between 1% and 4.5% of all parotid malignancies. Undifferentiated tumors have been grouped into solid, trabecular, and salivary duct varieties (Fig. 4-68).[1]

Carcinomas in pleomorphic adenoma (malignant mixed tumors) represent tumors with invasive malignancy and histologic areas of typical pleomorphic ade-

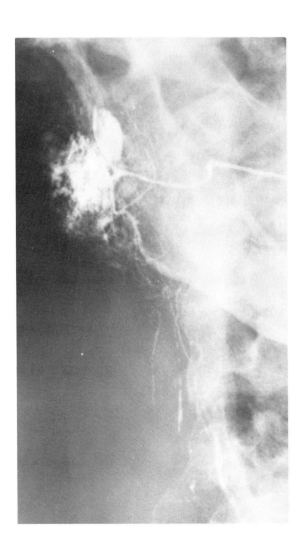

Fig. 4-68. Frontal sialogram reveals amorphous pooling of contrast material within undifferentiated carcinoma. This aggressive appearance is unusual. Parotolymphatic backflow is also seen in neck. (Reprinted from Som, P.M., and Shugar, J.M.A.: Ann. Otol. Rhinol. Laryngol. **90:**64-66, 1981.)

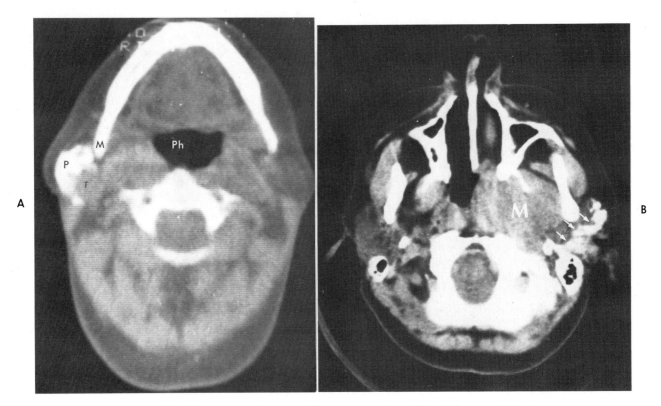

Fig. 4-69. A, CT sialogram reveals tumor *(T)* in posterior deep lobe. It has invaded adjacent tissue planes. *P,* Contrast-filled parotid gland; *M,* mandible; *Ph,* pharynx. *Malignant mixed tumor extending into adjacent soft tissues.* **B,** CT sialogram reveals large left deep lobe parotid tumor *(M).* Lesion has unsharp infiltrative margin with contrast material–filled parotid gland *(arrows).*

noma (Fig. 4-69). Often the malignancy is an undifferentiated carcinoma and its occurrence is signaled clinically by a sudden enlargement of a long-standing, slow-growing lesion. Pain or facial nerve paralysis may also be present.

■ Nonepithelial tumors

Nonepithelial tumors are uncommon as a group; the only lesions of any statistical consequence are the hemangiomas and lymphangiomas. In adults they represent less than 5% of the salivary gland tumors; however, in children they comprise over 50% of the lesions.

The *hemangioma* is the only common tumor in this group and, in fact, it is the most common nonepithelial tumor in children. Parotid gland enlargement is noticeable within the first few days of life and slowly progresses over the next several months. Almost all the patients are females. There is a bluish discoloration of the overlying skin and other hemangiomas or tetangiectasias may or may not be present on the skin. The lesion may enlarge when the child cries. Most often the mass is located at the angle of the jaw and displaces the

adjacent ear lobe. The tumor is confined to the gland itself, and multiple phleboliths may be present. These phleboliths are best seen on plain films and they characteristically have a lucent center that distinguishes them from calculi (Figs. 4-70 and 4-71).

Lymphangiomas are unusual tumors that involve the parotid gland and infiltrate the surrounding structures. About 50% occur in the neck and are often referred to as cystic hygromas when in this location.

All of the remaining nonepithelial tumors, such as neuromas, lipomas, and sarcomas, are very rare (Figs. 4-72 to 4-74).[33]

Lymph node hyperplasia can rarely occur as an isolated finding in the intraparotid lymph nodes. It is indistinguishable from other benign appearing masses (Fig. 4-75).

Primary lymphoma of the parotid gland is also very rare. In order to make this diagnosis, there must be no extra salivary gland lymphoma at the time of diagnosis, there must be histologic proof that the lymphoma involves the salivary parenchyma and that it is not secondary to intraparotid lymph node involvement, and lastly, there must be histologic evidence of the malig-

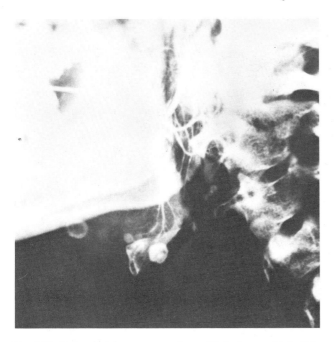

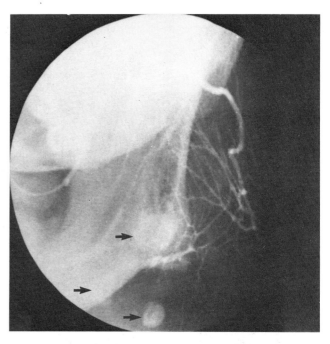

Fig. 4-70. Lateral sialogram reveals multiple large phleboliths in lower margin of parotid gland. *Hemangioma.*

Fig. 4-71. Frontal sialogram reveals several large phlebolith-type calcifications *(arrows)* in parotid mass. *Arteriovenous malformation.* Hemangioma is radiographically indistinguishable (see Fig. 4-70).

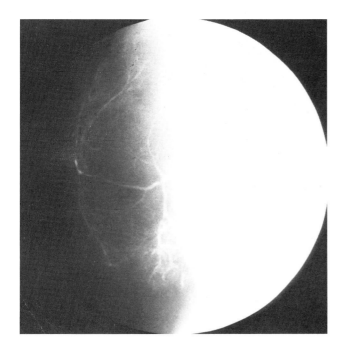

Fig. 4-72. Frontal sialogram reveals lateral displacement of parotid ducts by benign-appearing mass. Note that lipoma is not noticeably of fat density.

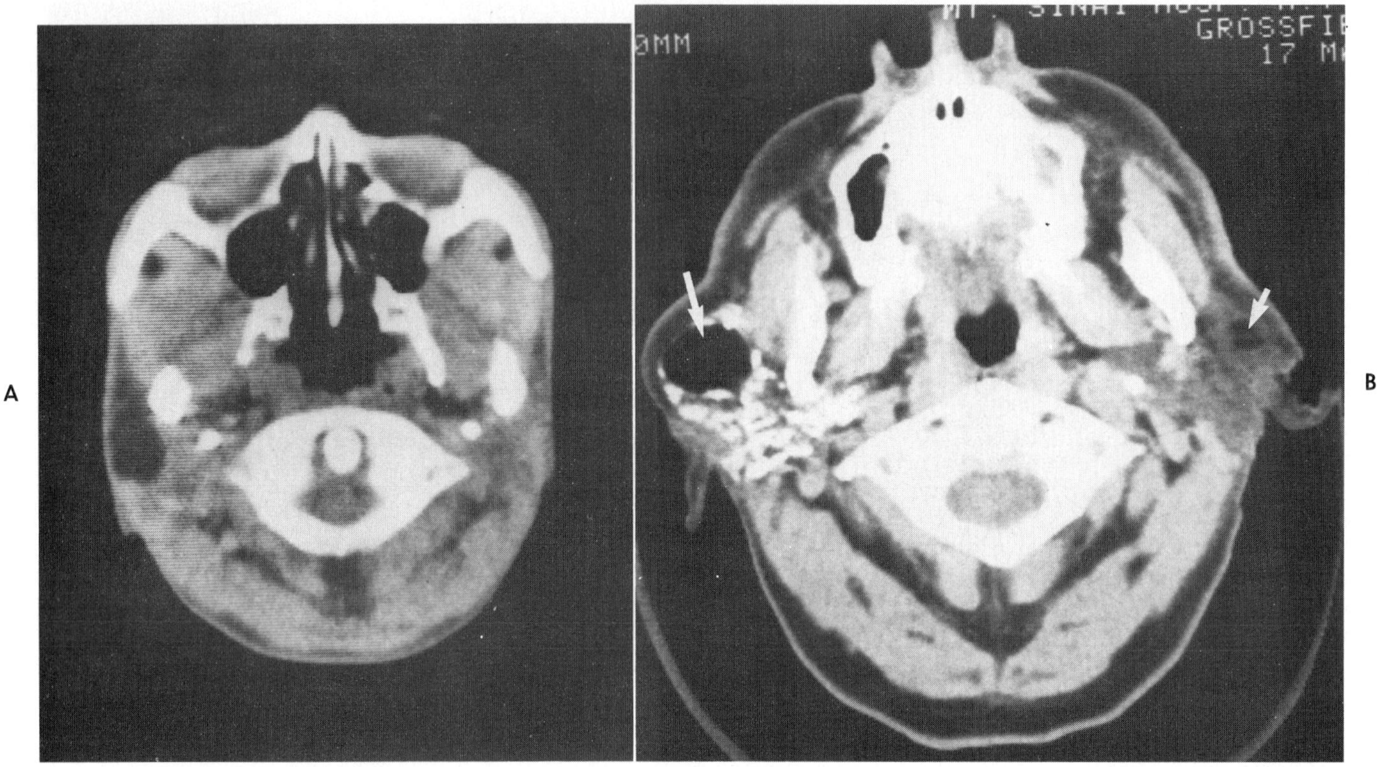

A

B

Fig. 4-73. A, CT scan reveals lipoma in right parotid gland. **B,** Right parotid CT sialogram reveals fatty benign-appearing mass in superficial lobe of right parotid gland *(arrow).* Smaller, less obvious lesion is seen in left parotid gland *(small arrow). Bilateral parotid lipomas.* (**A** Courtesy Dr. Charles Slatz.)

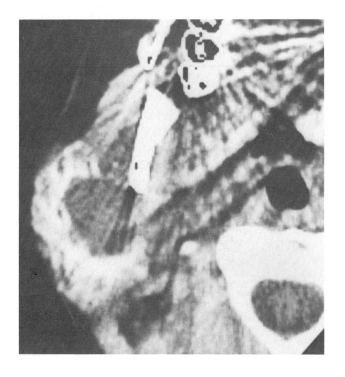

Fig. 4-74. CT sialogram reveals benign-appearing lesion in parotid gland. *Neuroma of facial nerve.* (Courtesy Dr. William Hanafee.)

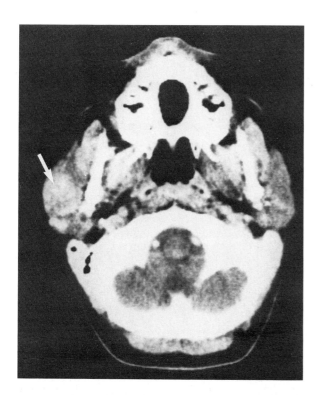

Fig. 4-75. Axial CT scan reveals enhanced benign-appearing mass in superficial lobe of right parotid gland *(arrow) Hyperplastic lymph node.* (From Som, P.M., and Biller, H.R.: Radiology **135**:387-390, 1980.)

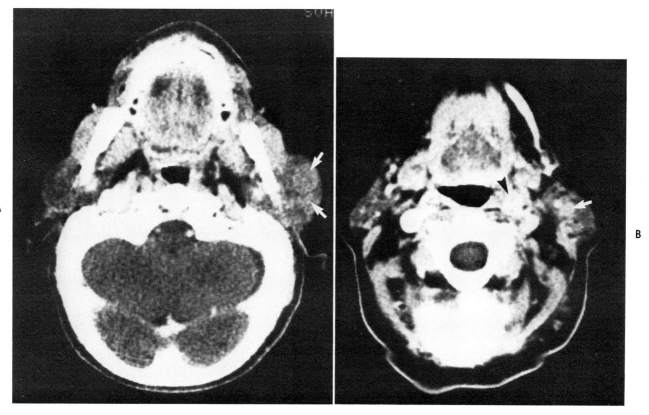

Fig. 4-76. A, Axial CT scan reveals two adjacent minimally enhanced left superficial lobe parotid masses *(arrows).* **B,** Axial CT scan more caudal than **A** reveals small third parotid mass *(arrow).* In addition, there is a fullness in left anterior parapharyngeal space secondary to nodal mass *(arrowhead). Lymphoma.* (From Som, P.M., and Biller, H.R.: Radiology **135**:387-390, 1980.)

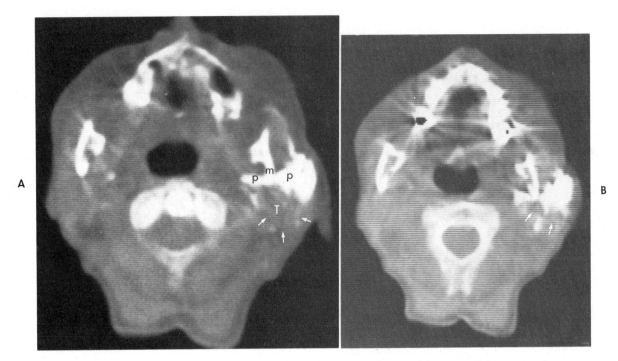

Fig. 4-77. A, CT sialogram of same case as in Fig. 4-75 reveals mass *(T)* to extend from parotid gland *(P)* into adjacent soft tissues *(arrows).* M, Mandible. *Malignant lymphoma.* **B,** CT sialogram reveals two posterior parotid masses *(arrows)* that are invading adjacent soft tissue planes. *Lymphoma.* (**A** Reprinted from Som, P.M., and Biller, N.R.: Radiology **135:**387-390, 1980.)

nant nature of the lesion. Secondary salivary gland involvement is also rare and the parotid gland is far more commonly involved than the submandibular gland by both primary and secondary lymphomas (Figs. 4-76 and 4-77).

There is a relationship between lymphoma and the autoimmune salivary diseases. Patients with Sjögren's syndrome have an increased incidence of both intra- and extraglandular lymphomas. In addition, these lymphomas have a much graver prognosis than similar disorders occurring in patients without Sjögren's syndrome.[1]

■ Unclassified tumors

Unclassified tumors comprise those benign and malignant tumors that cannot be included in the other described groups.[18] *Metastases* to the salivary glands are rare and usually involve the lymph nodes or invade the salivary glands by direct extension. The most common primary lesions are melanomas and carcinomas of the skin of the scalp and face. Next in order are primary lesions of the lung, kidney, pancreas, and stomach; lymphomas; and distal genitourinary tract (Figs. 4-78 to 4-80).

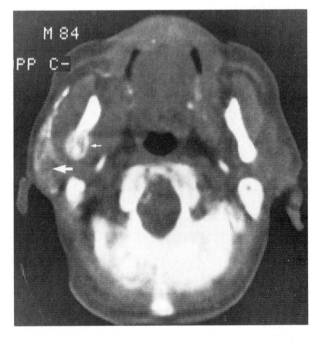

Fig. 4-78. CT sialogram reveals invasive tumor of parotid gland *(large arrow)* and destructive lesion of mandible *(small arrow). Metastasis to parotid gland and mandible.*

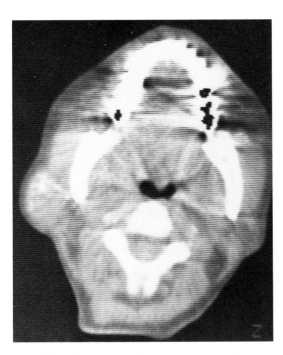

Fig. 4-79. CT sialogram reveals posterior parotid tumor extending into adjacent soft tissues. *Metastasis to parotid gland and adjacent nodes.*

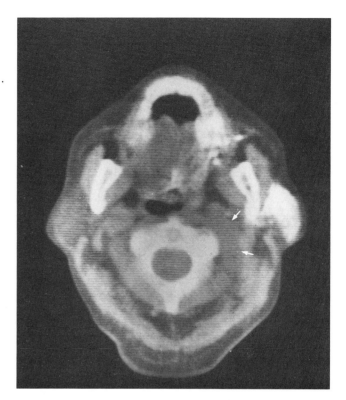

Fig. 4-80. CT sialogram reveals parotid gland to be laterally displaced by deep nodular mass of metastatic nodes *(arrows).*

■ Tumors in children

Tumors in children are uncommon. The most common epithelial lesion is the pleomorphic adenoma. However, unlike those tumors in adults that occur primarily in the parotid gland, in children they occur mainly in the submandibular and minor salivary glands. The most common malignancy is the mucoepidermoid tumor, which has a local recurrence or metastatic rate of 30% to 50%. The second most common malignancy is the acinic cell tumor.

Rarely, adenoid cystic, adenocarcinomas, or undifferentiated carcinomas occur. When these neoplasms are present they are highly malignant and often metastasize early. In general, children have a malignancy rate of 25% to 30%, which is higher than that seen in adults.[1,18]

The most common nonepithelial tumor in children is the hemangioma, which comprises over 50% of all salivary tumors. The second most common nonepithelial tumor is the lymphangioma.

Nontumorous parotid swelling in children can be caused acutely by viral parotitis. Mumps is the major cause; however, rarely other viruses (parainfluenzavirus 1 and 3, coxackievirus A, etc.) can be the cause. Acute suppurative sialadenitis and chronic sialadenitis are un-

usual lesions in childhood; however, the autoimmune disease of recurrent parotitis is not uncommon and can at times simulate a tumor mass.

□ **Sialography of masses**

The conventional sialogram, the CT scan, and the CT sialogram can accurately identify the location and number of mass lesions within a salivary gland.[3] In the vast majority of cases the relationship of the mass to the facial nerve can be established.[44] A more difficult distinction is the differentiation between a peripherally placed intrinsic lesion and an extrinsic mass that is indenting the peripheral salivary gland contour. The CT scan and the CT-sialogram has been of particular help in making this distinction.[39,40]

The differentiation between a benign and a malignant tumor is the most difficult aspect of sialography. This reflects the fact that both benign lesions and many malignant tumors have a benign appearance on sialography and CT. It is only when a tumor has aggressive sialographic changes that a diagnosis of malignancy can be made. If cavitation or low attenuation areas are seen within a mass, the lesion is more likely to be a malignancy (Fig. 4-66).

Distinction between a solitary interstitial lesion (pri-

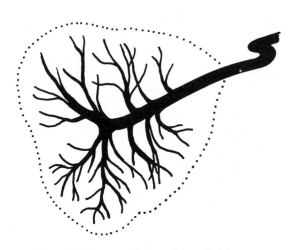

Fig. 4-81. Diagram of normal lateral sialogram.

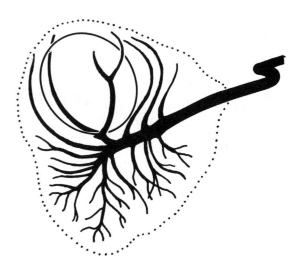

Fig. 4-82. Diagram of lateral sialogram with parotid mass well within gland. Ducts encircle mass. Some pruning or nonvisualization of adjacent minor side ducts is caused by pressure from mass.

marily lymph nodes) and a parenchymal lesion is extremely difficult, if not impossible, and clinically may have little significance. Multiple nodes or masses are usually easy to identify; however, multiple small lymph nodes can go undetected on the conventional study. These occult nodes can be demonstrated on the CT scan and the CT sialogram.

Extension of disease either from the salivary gland into the adjacent tissues or vise versa is also better evaluated on the CT scans.[39,44]

No matter how accurate sialographic detection may become, especially in evaluating subclinical disease or in differentiating clinical entities that are otherwise indistinguishable, the quality of the interpretation will always be improved if the clinical appearance of the patient is considered.

All patients sent for sialography come from a preselected population with some form of salivary gland pathology. Each lesion has a specific clinical history. A slow-growing, painless, freely movable mass is clinically benign. A rapidly growing, tender or painful mass with fixation to the adjacent tissues is clinically malignant. Facial nerve paralysis, if present, strongly suggests a malignancy. If any of these more aggressive findings occur in a previously clinically benign mass, the possibility of a malignant tumoral transformation or coexistence must be considered. It is with this background that the sialographic findings should be viewed.

Benign-appearing masses smoothly displace the adjacent parotid ducts around them. There is no abrupt

ductal cutoff or irregular ductal narrowing. There may be some pruning of the minor ducts in the immediately adjacent region, which reflects a pressure effect from the mass. If acinar filling is achieved, a region of lack of parenchymal filling will be visualized that corresponds precisely with the size of the mass seen on the filling phase films. The contours of the defect have a sharp interface with the adjacent parenchyma. This is also confirmed on the CT scan.

If the mass is centrally located or well within the gland parenchyma, the salivary ducts will encircle more than 50% of its circumference. When this is seen, the mass can confidently be said to be intraglandular in origin (Figs. 4-81 and 4-82).

If the ducts go only halfway or less around the circumference of the mass, then a definite distinction between an intraglandular and an extraglandular lesion cannot be made (Figs. 4-83 and 4-84). This sialographic finding has been described as a "ball in hand" appearance and reflects a mild, essentially unilateral pressure effect from a peripherally located mass. CT scans and CT sialograms have been very helpful in differentiating between such a deep lobe parotid tumor and an adjacent parapharyngeal space extraparotid lesion[41] (see Chapter 5).

As previously mentioned, differentiation between a parenchymal and interstitial mass may be very difficult. The parenchymal lesions are described as having a delayed emptying phase on sialography because some of the glandular tissue is directly involved by the mass and

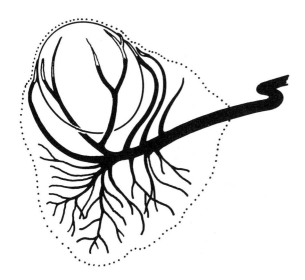

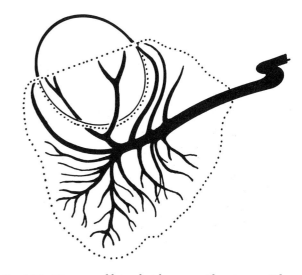

Fig. 4-83. Diagram of lateral sialogram with peripherally placed mass. Although ducts encircle mass, white portions of these ducts are not visualized because of pressure created between mass and capsule of gland.

Fig. 4-84. Diagram of lateral sialogram with extraparotid mass indenting gland. Ducts only go halfway around mass; however, sialographically this is same appearance as in Fig. 4-83.

thus there is some decreased salivary function. An interstitial lesion, on the other hand, only displaces the adjacent parenchyma and thus is not related to decreased function and a delayed emptying phase. This latter distinction is often a question of degree and is not a reliable enough sign to use confidently in making a distinction between parenchymal and interstitial masses.[33]

Aggressive malignant-appearing masses cause abrupt ductal cutoff, irregular ductal narrowing, irregular areas of lack of parenchymal filling, and pooling of contrast material within the confines of the tumor. These changes are usually seen with aggressive neoplasms such as epidermoid, undifferentiated, or adenocarcinomas. Less often, high-grade mucoepidermoid and acinic cell tumors give this aggressive appearance. Rapid tumor erosion into an intraparotid lymph node can result in parotolymphatic backflow during sialography with visualization of contrast material within the cervical nodal chain.[41]

The tumor-parotid interface is unsharp and irregular on CT sialography and CT scans.

Rarely, an abscess may show irregular pooling of the contrast material within its necrotic center or abrupt ductal cutoff. However, in this rare circumstance the clinical picture suggests an inflammatory process.

A primary lymphoma may appear as either a discrete mass or as a focal area of peripheral punctate sialectasis. This latter appearance is secondary to a cellular infiltration that accumulates at the peripheral branch points of the ducts and causes a luminal narrowing and eventual obstruction. A patchy region of lack of parenchymal filling may reflect local extension of the disease.

The secondary lymphomas usually reveal multiple discrete benign-appearing masses that represent intraglandular adenopathy. If these nodes are small, they may only be detectable on a CT sialogram. The CT scan can also detect other cervical adenopathy that might suggest the diagnosis.

■ Summary of sialographic and regional patterns of disease

The pattern of disease seen on the sialogram can in general give a good impression as to the actual underlying pathology. If there is any dilatation of Stensen's or Wharton's duct, an inflammatory process is almost always the cause. The possibility of a partial obstruction resulting from a stone or stricture should come to mind.

Punctate or globular collections of contrast material, if focal and only in one portion of the gland, are the result of an infectious disease with small abscess formation. This is especially true if there is associated main duct dilatation. On the other hand, if the punctate and globular changes are uniformly distributed throughout the gland, an autoimmune disease is the cause. Usually, the main ducts are normal in caliber. Combinations of infection and autoimmune disease can also occur.

If multiple nodular benign-appearing masses are seen, the granulomatous diseases must be considered. This is especially true of sarcoid. Less often, Warthin's tumor and lymphomas are the cause. Very rarely, acinic cell tumors, oncocytomas, mixed tumors, von Recklinghausen's disease, and metastases are in the differential diagnosis.

A technetium scan will differentiate the Warthin's tumors and oncocytomas by showing intense accumulation of the radionuclide.

A solitary benign-appearing mass will usually be a benign mixed tumor. If the mass is in the posterior portion of the superficial lobe, Warthin's tumor is probable. If it is in the inferior portion of the gland and an inflammatory history is present, the possibility of a rare infected second branchial cleft cyst should be entertained.

Solitary masses in the submandibular gland are very unlikely to be Warthin's, acinic cell, or oncocytic tumor because they almost exclusively involve the parotid gland.

About 11% to 12% of all parotid tumors occur in the deep lobe and of these nearly 80% are benign mixed tumors.[1] The remaining lesions are primarily mucoepidermoid or acinic cell carcinomas.

It is extremely important to remember that only a few malignant lesions actually appear malignant on sialography. An unsharp tumor-parenchymal interface on CT or abrupt ductal cutoff, irregular tumor pooling, and lack of parenchymal filling on the sialogram are unusual albeit diagnostic findings. Most malignant tumors have a benign radiologic appearance. Differentiation between a sialocele, an adenopathy, and a neoplasm may be impossible without history. Trauma should at least suggest the possibility of a sialocele, whether or not a fistula was present. If local or coarse calcifications are present within a mass, a mixed tumor should be considered. If phleboliths are present, a hemangioma is most likely.

□ Adjunctive studies

As a group these procedures are less specific and less often used than sialography and CT. Each provides limited but valuable information that helps contribute to the overall evaluation of the salivary glands.

■ Radionuclide salivary studies

The salivary glands normally concentrate technetium Tc-99m sodium pertechnetate. Originally this was considered a nuisance on brain scans; however, today it has developed into its own subspecialty. After the patient is given an intravenous injection of 10 mCi of Tc-99m sodium pertechnetate, gamma camera exposures are taken at 2-minute intervals from 2 to 16 minutes and then at 10-minute intervals until 60 to 80 minutes after injection.[33]

There is a normal vascular phase that occurs immediately after injection of the radionuclide. The concentration phase runs from 5 to 15 minutes after the injection and represents active parenchymal accumulation. The secretory phase runs from 15 to 60 minutes after injection. During this time there is a progressive accumulation of radionuclide in the saliva, and the activity steadily increases in the mouth as the glandular activity decreases.

Hyperfunction is seen in acute sialadenitis, granulomatous diseases, lymphoma, and the sialoses. In acute purulent sialadenitis, a cold area within the increased glandular activity may suggest an abscess. Decreased

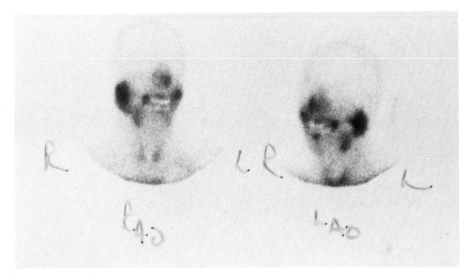

Fig. 4-85. Oblique technetium sialograms reveal intense bilateral parotid uptake. *Bilateral Warthin's tumors.*

activity is seen with Sjögren's syndrome and most primary and metastatic tumors. The major exceptions are Warthin's tumors and oncocytomas, which intensely accumulate the radionuclide (Fig. 4-85).

Viral sialadenitis gives a decreased uptake, as does the normal atrophic aging process. The function of the salivary glands behind a ductal obstruction can be estimated by the activity of the gland. Prolonged glandular activity on the secretory phase indicates ductal obstruction. Increased glandular activity indicates acute sialadenitis, whereas patchy or decreased uptake relates to chronic and atrophic disease.[36,37]

■ Angiography

Interventional vascular studies are for the most part unnecessary in the salivary glands. Most hemangiomas are clinically diagnosable, and because they are usually microfistulous or capillary in nature they tend to appear as avascular masses. The angiogram can diagnose a very rare salivary arteriovenous malformation (AVM). The remaining salivary tumors are all essentially avascular lesions.

■ Ultrasonography

The main applicability of ultrasonography is differentiating between solid and cystic salivary gland masses, the most classic example being a sialocele (echo-free mass) versus a benign mixed tumor (multiple echoes).[22]

□ References

1. Batsakis, J.G.: Tumors of the head and neck: clinical and pathological considerations, ed. 2, Baltimore, 1979, The Williams & Wilkins Co.
2. Blatt, I.M.: Chronic and recurrent inflammations about the salivary glands with special reference to children: a report of 25 cases, Laryngoscope 76:917-933, 1966.
3. Carter, B.L. Karmody, C.S., Blickman, J.R., and Panders, A.K.: Computed tomography and sialography. 2. Pathology, J. Comput. Assist. Tomogr. 5(1):46-53, 1981.
4. David, R.B., and O'Connell, E.J.: Suppurative parotitis in children, Am. J. Dis. Child 119:332-335, 1970.
5. Davis, R.A., Anson, B.J., Budlinger, J.M., and Kurth, L.E.: Surgical anatomy of the facial nerve and parotid gland based upon a study of 350 cervico-facial halves, Surg. Gynecol. Obstet. 102:384, 1956.
6. Deegan, M.J.: Immunologic diseases of the salivary glands, Otolaryngol. Clin. North Am. 10:351-361, 1977.
7. Eneroth, C.M.: Histological and clinical aspects of parotid tumors, Acta Otolaryngol. (Suppl) 191:1-99, 1964.
8. Eneroth, C.M.: Salivary gland tumors in the parotid gland, submandibular gland and the palate region, Cancer 27:1415-1418, 1971.
9. Ericson, S.: The parotid gland in subjects with and without rheumatoid arthritis, Acta Radiol. (Suppl) 275:1-67, 1968.
10. Godwin, J.: Benign lymphoepithelial lesion of the parotid gland, Cancer 5:1089-1103, 1952.
11. Goss, C.M.: Gray's anatomy of the human body, ed. 27, Philadelphia, 1963, Lea & Febiger.
12. Hales, B., and Hansen, J.E.: Bilateral simultaneous Warthin's tumor in a woman, South Med. J. 70:157-158, 1977.
13. Hemenway, W.G.: Chronic punctate parotitis, Boulder, Colo., 1971 Colorado Associated University Press.
14. Johns, M.E.: The salivary glands: anatomy and embryology, Otolaryngol. Clin. North Am. 10(2):261-271, 1977.
15. Kushner, D.C., and Weber, A.L.: Sialography of salivary gland tumor with fluoroscopy and tomography, AJR 130:940, 1978.
16. Manashil, G.B.: Clinical sialography, Springfield, Ill., 1978, Charles C Thomas, Publisher.
17. Mancuso, A., Rice, D., and Hanafee, W.: Computed tomography of the parotid gland during contrast sialography, Radiology 132:211-213, 1979.
18. Mason, D.K., and Chisholm, D.M.: Salivary glands in health and disease, London, 1975, W.B. Saunders Co., Ltd.
19. Maxwell, J.H.: Chronic lymphoepithelial sialadenopathy with sialodochiectasis, Trans. Am. Acad. Ophthalmol. Otolaryngol. 64:225-234, 1960.
20. Maynard, J.D.: Recurrent parotid enlargement, Br. J. Surg. 52:784-789, 1965.
21. Mihalyka, E.E.: Congenital bilateral polycystic parotid glands, JAMA 181:634, 1962.
22. Neiman, H.L., Phillips, J.F., Darrel, J.A., and Brown, T.L.: Ultrasound of the parotid gland, J. Clin. Ultrasound 4:11-13, 1976.
23. Ollerenshaw, R, and Ross, S.S.: Radiological diagnosis of salivary gland disease, Br. J. Radiol. 24:538-548, 1951.
24. Olson, N.R.: Traumatic lesions of the salivary glands, Otolaryngol. Clin. North Am. 10(2):345-350, 1977.
25. Osmer, J.C., and Pleasants, J.E.: Distention sialography, Radiology 87:116-118, 1966.
26. Pallin, J., and Trail, M.: Trauma to parotid region, South Med. J. 63(12):1389-1392, 1969.
27. Patey, D.H.: Inflammation of the salivary glands with particular reference to chronic and recurrent parotitis, Ann. R. Coll. Surg. Engl. 36:26-44, 1965.
28. Patey, D.H., and Thackray, A.C.: Chronic "sialectatic" parotitis in the light of pathological studies on parotidectomy material, Br. J. Surg. 43:43-50, 1955.
29. Patey, D.H., and Thackray, A.C.: The treatment of parotid tumors in the light of a pathological study of parotid material. Br. J. Surg. 45:477-487, 1958.
30. Potter, G.D.: Sialography and the salivary glands, Otolaryngol. Clin. North Am. 6(2):509-522, 1973.
31. Rabinov, K.R., and Joffe, N.: A blunt-tip side injecting cannula for sialography, Radiology 92:1438, 1969.
32. Ranger, I.: An experimental study of sialography, and its correlation with histological appearances, in normal parotid and submandibular glands, Br. J. Surg. 44:415-418, 1957.
33. Rankow, R.M., and Polayes, I.M.: Diseases of the salivary glands, Philadelphia, 1976, W.B. Saunders Co.
34. Rauch S., and Gorlin, R.J.: Diseases of the salivary glands. In Gorlin, R.J., and Goldman, H.M., editors: Thoma's Oral pathology, St. Louis, 1970, The C.V. Mosby Co.
35. Rubin, P., and Casarett, G.W.: Clinical radiation pathology, vol. 1, Philadelphia, 1968, W.B. Saunders Co.
36. Schall, G.L.: The role of radionuclide scanning in the evaluation of neoplasms in the salivary glands: a review, J. Surg. Oncol. 3:701-716, 1971.
37. Schall, G.L., Smith, R.R., and Barsocchini, L.M.: Radionuclide salivary imaging usefulness in a private otolaryngology practice, Arch. Otolaryngol. 107:40-44, 1981.
38. Sela J., and Ulmansky, M.: Mucous retention cyst of salivary glands, J. Oral Surg. 27:619, 1969.
39. Som, P.M., and Biller, H.F.: The combined computerized tomography-sialogram: a technique to differentiate deep lobe pa-

rotid tumors from extraparotid pharyngomaxillary space tumors, Ann. Otol. Rhinol. Laryngol. **88**(5):590-595, 1979.

40. Som, P.M., and Biller, H.R.: The combined CT-sialogram, Radiology **135**(2):387-397, 1980.

41. Som, P.M., Biller, H.F., and Lawson, W.: Tumors of the parapharyngeal space: preoperative evaluation, diagnosis and surgical approaches, Ann. Otol. Rhinol. Laryngol. **90**(suppl. 80):1-15, 1981.

42. Som, P.M., Shugar, J.M.A., and Biller, H.F.: Parotid gland sarcoidosis and the CT sialogram, J. Comput. Assist. Tomogr. **5**(5):674-677, 1981.

43. Stafne, E.C.: Bone cavities situated near the angle of the mandible, J. Am. Dent. Assoc. **29**:1969-1972, 1942.

44. Stone, D.N., Mancuso, A.A., Rice, D., and Hanafee, W.N.: parotid CT-sialography, Radiology **138**:393-397, 1981.

45. Tandler, B.: Ultrastructure of chronically inflammed human submandibular gland, Arch. Pathol. Lab. Med. **101**:425-431, 1977.

46. Thackray, A.C., and Sobin, L.H.: Histological typing of salivary gland tumors. In International histological classification of tumors, no. 7, Geneva, 1972, World Health Organization.

47. Travis, L.W., and Hecht, D.W.: Acute and chronic inflammatory diseases of the salivary glands: diagnosis and management, Otolaryngol. Clin. North Am. **10**(2):329-338, 1977.

48. Work, W.P., and Hecht, D.W.: Inflammatory diseases of the major salivary glands. In Paparella, M.M., and Shumrick, D.A., editors: Otolaryngology, Philadelphia, 1973, W.B. Saunders Co.

49. Yoel, J.: Pathology and surgery of the salivary glands, Springfield, Ill., 1975, Charles C Thomas, Publisher.

5 □ The parapharyngeal space

PETER M. SOM

Until a few years ago the radiologist offered little significant help toward the preoperative diagnosis of parapharyngeal space tumors. Angiograms were performed in almost all cases, and if the lesion was avascular, further differentiation was not possible. Recent advances have allowed a far more accurate radiographic preoperative assessment of the lesions involving this space. By using the technique of contrast enhanced CT scanning and CT sialography the physician can avoid resorting to an angiogram in about 60% of patients. A histologic preoperative diagnosis is now possible in many cases, and in addition, the tumor's extent can be accurately mapped as to size, shape, and region of involvement. Based on this information, an appropriate surgical approach for tumor removal can be planned.

□ Anatomy

A familiarity with the anatomy of the parapharyngeal space is mandatory for an appreciation of the roentgenographic findings.

The parapharyngeal space is shaped like an inverted pyramid whose base is the base of the skull and whose apex is the greater cornu of the hyoid bone. The pyramid can be thought of as having three sides. The medial wall is formed by the superior pharyngeal constrictor muscle and the tonsillar fossa. As such, it contains no bony elements and is the only entirely pliable border. The lateral wall, or second side of the pyramid, is formed anteriorly by the internal pterygoid muscle and the inner surface of the ramus of the mandible. More posteriorly, the deep lobe of the parotid gland and the posterior belly of the digastric muscle and sternocleidomastoid muscle (SCM) form the lateral boundary. Below the level of the mandible the lateral wall is composed of the muscles and soft tissues of the neck. Thus it is only in its lower half that this margin is completely pliable; the upper half is rigid because of the presence of the mandibular ramus, with only the region of the deep lobe of the parotid gland being pliable (Fig. 5-1).

The posterior, or third wall, is formed by the paravertebral muscles and the rigid vertebral column. Traversing the parapharyngeal space are the internal carotid artery, internal jugular vein, cranial nerves IX, X, XI, and XII, the cervical sympathetic chain, the styloid muscles, and numerous lymph nodes. All of these structures are embedded within and supported by a fibrofatty matrix.[2,4,7]

From the preceding discussion, it is not surprising that masses arising within the parapharyngeal space will bow its medial wall toward the midline. Clinically this is appreciated as a bulging in of the lateral pharyngeal wall and tonsillar fossa, and if the mass attains sufficient size, eventual medial and downward displacement of the palate. If the tumor extends inferiorly, a mass can be seen in the neck just below the angle of the mandible and lying above the hyoid bone.

□ Clinical aspects

Clinically, most patients with parapharyngeal space masses are asymptomatic and the presence of their mass is usually discovered as an incidental finding by the patient or an examining physician. The most common finding is a bulging inward of the lateral pharyngeal wall. Many patients will also have a visible or palpable mass near the angle of the mandible, and a vague fullness in the parotid region is also common. Symptoms vary with both size of the tumor as well as its histology. They include sore throat, dysphagia, change in voice, nasal obstruction, and the sensation of aural fullness. Symptoms may also be related to involvement of the last four cranial nerves.[3,5,7]

□ Objectives

The first major objective for the radiologist is to determine whether the parapharyngeal mass is intraparotid or extraparotid in origin. This is of more than pure

235

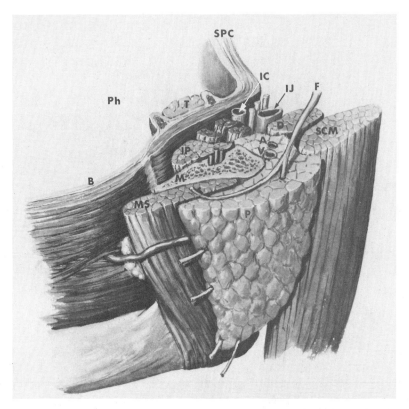

Fig. 5-1. Normal anatomic relationship of left parotid gland and parapharyngeal space is viewed obliquely and from above. *Ph*, Pharynx; *SPC*, superior pharyngeal constrictor muscle; *T*, tonsil; *B*, buccinator muscle; *MS*, masseter muscle; *SCM*, sternocleidomastoid muscle; *D*, posterior belly of the digastric muscle; *IP*, internal pterygoid muscle; *M*, mandible; *IC*, internal carotid artery; *IJ*, internal jugular vein; *P*, parotid gland; *F*, facial nerve; *A*, external carotid artery; *V*, posterior facial vein. (From Som, P.M., and Biller, H.F.: Radiology **135:**387-390, 1980.)

academic interest because it will be the major determinant of the surgical approach. If the lesion is in the parotid deep lobe, then a transparotid approach will be used with isolation of the facial nerve. Although there is some recognized morbidity with such a procedure, it is the only approach for such a deep lobe mass. On the other hand, if the parapharyngeal mass is extraparotid in origin, a transcervical approach, with or without partial mandibulotomy, is performed. This surgery avoids manipulation of the facial nerve and its associated morbidity and provides a better field for tumor removal.[8] This first objective is accomplished with CT scanning and the CT sialogram.

Once an extraparotid origin is established, further differentiation of the various lesions involving this space is accomplished by evaluating the tumor's response to intravenous contrast material. In those cases in which enhancement occurs, an angiogram may at times be performed to provide further differentiation. This approach limits the number of patients requiring an invasive procedure to about 40% of the cases. Overall,

with the use of this technique a preoperative diagnosis can be established in the majority of patients.

□ Technique

A contrast enhanced CT scan is performed. The scans are taken as contiguous 5 mm scans from the level of the TMJ to the angle of the mandible. The physician should monitor the study to ensure that both the cephalad and caudal margins of the lesion are seen. If not, further scans must be taken so that all of the lesion is included in the study. Coronal scans can be obtained as indicated on in individual case basis. This is especially true when the skull base is thought to be involved.

The CT sialogram may also be obtained by first performing a sialogram (see Chapter 4) and then a CT scan. This study probably has to be performed only in those cases in which the decisive diagnostic information cannot be obtained from the contrast enhanced CT study.[6-8]

A bolus injection of 50 ml of contrast material (Renographin-60) should be given. The patient can also then be given a drip infusion of additional contrast material.

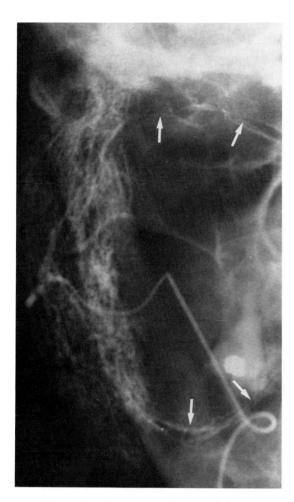

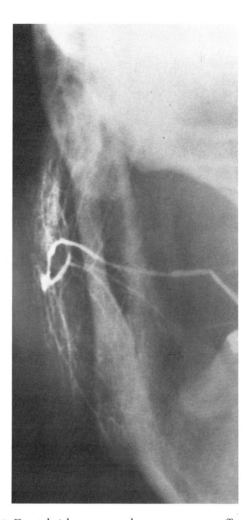

Fig. 5-2. Oblique frontal sialogram film reveals large deep lobe parotid mass smoothly displacing ducts around it *(arrows)*. Ducts almost encircle entire mass, indicating its parotid origin.

Fig. 5-3. Frontal sialogram reveals vague pressure effect on inner aspect of parotid gland. This could be from either intra- or extraparotid mass.

It is important to scan immediately after the bolus of intravenous contrast material is given in order to appreciate the maximal enhancement of a lesion. Delayed scanning may miss the true enhancement and lead to an erroneous conclusion.

■ Rationale of the technique

The main purpose of the technique is to reliably differentiate between an intraparotid and an extraparotid tumor. On the basis of a conventional sialogram, this can be accomplished only if the mass displaces the parotid ducts around it in such a way as to allow the ducts to encircle more than 50% of the mass's circumference. When this appearance is evident, the lesion can reliably be said to be intraparotid in origin (Fig. 5-2). If, however, the mass displaces the ducts so that they encircle less than 50% of its diameter (as is far more often the

case), then two possibilities exist: first, that the mass is parotid in origin but very peripherally placed in the gland or, second, that the mass is extraparotid in origin but pressing into the adjacent parotid gland. The conventional sialographic appearance is that of a mild pressure effect on the deep lobe ducts that has been described as a ball in hand appearance (Fig. 5-3). When this is seen, a reliable distinction between a peripherally placed intraparotid mass and an adjacent extraparotid mass can not be made.

The purpose of the CT scan and the CT sialogram is to allow further differentiation in these cases. The supporting tissue of the parapharyngeal space is composed of a loose fibrofatty matrix. This becomes displaced as a parapharyngeal space mass enlarges and eventually becomes compressed between the periphery of the tumor and the adjacent structures. If the tumor is extraparo-

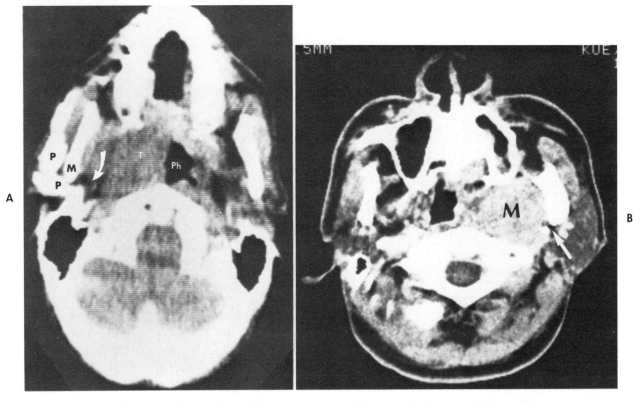

Fig. 5-4. A, CT sialogram of nonenhancing, extraparotid benign mixed tumor of minor salivary gland origin *(T)*. Note lucent zone *(arrow)* between mass and contrast-filled parotid gland *(P). M*, Mandible; *Ph*, pharynx. **B,** Axial CT scan reveals enhanced extraparotid left parapharyngeal space mass *(M)*. Narrow fat zone is seen *(arrow)* between tumor and parotid gland. *Schwannoma.* (**A** From Som, P.M., et al.: Ann. Otol. Rhinol. Laryngol., **90**[suppl. 80, 1 pt. 4]:1-15, 1981.)

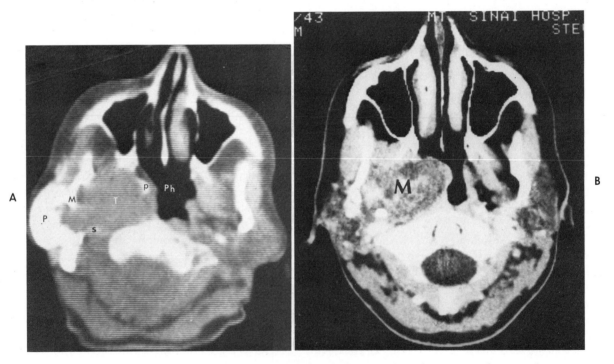

Fig. 5-5. A, CT sialogram of same patient as Fig. 5-2. There is a large benign mixed tumor of parotid deep lobe. *P*, Parotid gland; *M*, mandible; *T*, tumor; *p*, medially displaced, contrast-filled parotid duct; *Ph*, pharynx; *S*, styloid tip. **B,** Axial CT scan of another patient reveals large right deep lobe parotid tumor *(M)*. Mass has nonhomogeneous enhancement. *Mixed tumor.*

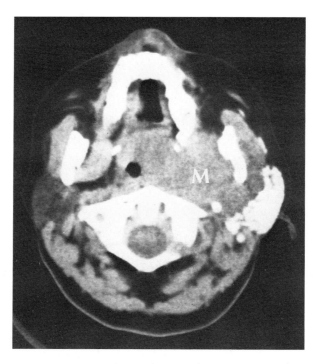

Fig. 5-6. CT sialogram reveals large left parapharyngeal space mass *(M)* that has invaded deep lobe of parotid gland, obliterating fat line. *Malignant lymphoma.*

tid, this compressed fibrofatty tissue can be seen lying between the posterolateral tumor margin and the contrast-filled parotid gland (Fig. 5-4). In order to be so identified, it must have an attenuation number consistent with fat density. Override artifacts from the posterior edge of the mandible can often give linear lucent lines that may be mistaken for the fat zone if the observer is not careful.

If the mass is intraparotid in origin, the mass compresses the fat medially, against the lateral pharyngeal wall. On occasion a thin lucent zone can be seen just outside the superior pharyngeal constrictor muscle. This, however, is of no consequence. The important thing is that no lucent fat zone will be present between the posterolateral tumor margin and the deep lobe of the parotid gland (Fig. 5-5). This lucent zone sign has so far proved to be reliable. If the fat zone is seen, the lesion is definitely extraparotid in origin. However, if the fat zone is not seen, the lesion is probably intraparotid, the complicating factors being extraparotid aggressive tumors that can infiltrate and obliterate the fat zone, simulating an intraparotid lesion (Fig. 5-6).

Because the parotid gland usually is a low attenuation number organ, the visualization of a fat zone adjacent to it can prove arbitrary at times. If the fat zone is not seen, a CT sialogram will be a more sensitive method of detecting this finding. Because the presence of this fat zone will determine the surgical approach, a CT sial-

ogram can be resorted to in difficult cases. The important thing to remember is that clinically, a deep lobe lesion almost always cannot be ruled out of the differential diagnosis. Because this fact bears heavily on the choice of the operative approach, the combined study offers more information about the parotid gland itself and the intraparotid or extraparotid nature of the lesion[7,8] if this distinction cannot be made on routine CT scanning. With the high-resolution CT machines of today, only rarely does one have to resort to the CT sialogram.

Few parotid masses are enhanced significantly, and whether or not they do will not influence the surgical approach or operative technique. However, if the tumor is extraparotid in origin, further differentiation is possible, depending on whether or not the lesion is enhanced and the homogeneous or nonhomogeneous nature of the enhancement.

□ **Nonenhancing parapharyngeal space masses**

Deep lobe parotid tumors represent about one fifth of all the parapharyngeal space lesions and about 10% of all parotid tumors. Of these lesions, 80% to 90% are benign mixed tumors.[1] Virtually all the remaining lesions are either adenoid cystic, acinic cell, or mucoepidermoid carcinomas. Other tumors occur as isolated case reports. None of the these lesions enhance to any significant degree and minimal enhancement does not characterize a particular tumor.

Conventional sialography often does not identify the malignant nature of the tumor. A pseudocapsule may be present or foci of malignancy may be located within the confines of the neoplasm. Thus a benign-appearing lesion will probably, but by no means definitely, be benign (Fig. 5-7). Detection of early malignant ductal changes is more reliably accomplished at the present time on the conventional sialogram rather than on the combined CT-sialogram study.

The deep lobe benign mixed tumors have two configurations, spherical and dumbbell-shaped (Figs. 5-5 and 5-8). It is the stylomandibular tunnel that is the determining factor. This tunnel is best appreciated by looking at the skull laterally. The tunnel is triangular in shape and is defined by the styloid process and stylomandibular ligament posteriorly, the base of the skull superiorly, and the posterior margin of the mandible anteriorly. If the deep lobe tumor arises adjacent to this tunnel, as it grows through the tunnel its shape becomes constricted by the tunnel; thus the dumbbell configuration. If the mass arises deep to the plane of the tunnel, it enlarges unrestricted as a spherical tumor. This latter form is more easily confused with an extraparotid, spherically shaped tumor. Rarely, a spherical parotid mass is seen lying lateral to this liga-

ment and it represents a laterally placed deep lobe tumor (Fig. 5-8, C).

The minor salivary glands of the pharynx can also give rise to salivary gland tumors. These lesions arise from the medial wall of the parapharyngeal space and enlarge laterally as well as medially into the space to cause a midline bulge of the lateral pharynx in a way similar to that caused by deep lobe parotid tumors. These minor salivary gland tumors cannot be clinically differentiated from the parotid lesions.[8] As a group the minor salivary gland lesions are less frequent than the major salivary gland tumors by a ratio of 1:5.[1] Slightly more than half of the minor salivary gland tumors are malignant and most of these are adenoid cystic carcinomas. Almost all the benign lesions are benign mixed tumors. These minor salivary gland lesions grow either as spherical or ovoid masses, they do not enhance, and they will have a lucent zone between their posterolateral margin and the parotid gland (Fig. 5-4).

Parapharyngeal nodal enlargement may occur from lymphomatous, carcinomatous, or rarely, inflammatory involvement. The nodes usually are nonenhancing or minimally enhancing masses that have a lobulated or nodular configuration rather than a smooth ovoid or spherical appearance (Fig. 5-9). Inflammatory nodes

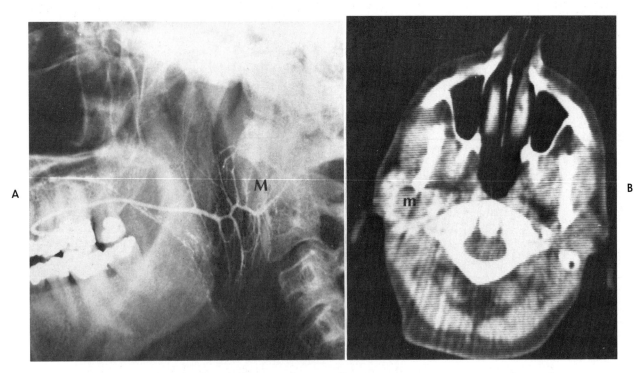

Fig. 5-7. A, Lateral sialogram film reveals mass effect in upper posterior portion of parotid gland with smooth displacement of ducts around lesion *(M).* **B,** CT sialogram of same patient reveals retromandibular parotid mass *(m)* that has smooth benign-appearing interface with adjacent contrast-filled parotid gland. *Acinic cell carcinoma.*

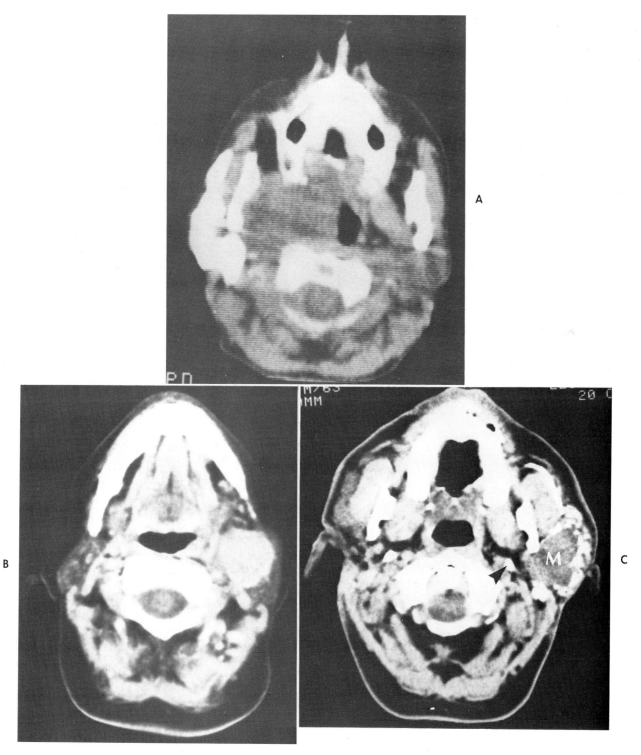

Fig. 5-8. A, CT sialogram reveals round, deep lobe parotid benign mixed tumor. Compare this tumor shape to dumbbell configuration of lesion in Fig. 5-5. **B,** Axial CT scan reveals large ovoid enhanced left deep lobe mixed tumor. **C,** CT sialogram reveals large ovoid deep lobe parotid tumor *(M)* that is lateral to stylomandibular ligament. Arrowhead points to styloid process. *Mixed tumor.*

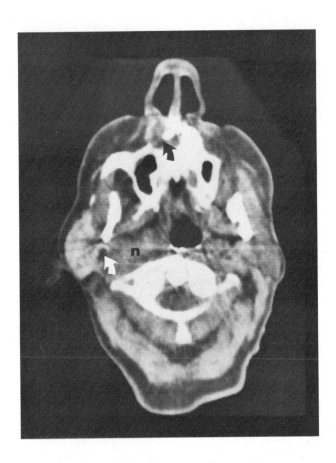

Fig. 5-9. CT sialogram reveals nonenhancing, nodular contoured, extraparotid parapharyngeal space mass *(n)*. Lucent zone separates mass and parotid gland *(white arrow)*. Bone metastasis is present in maxilla *(black arrow)*. *Metastatic squamous cell carcinoma.* (From Som, P.M. et al.: Ann. Otol. Rhinol. Laryngol. **90**[suppl. 80, 1 pt. 4]:1-15, 1981.)

may be enhanced homogeneously or rarely can have a rim of enhancement around a low-density necrotic center. Metastatic carcinoma nodes often have a necrotic center whereas lymphomatous nodes may enhance uniformly, simulating reactive nodes. The majority of nodes, however, are nonenhancing tumor masses that are best characterized by their overall nodular configuration.

A variety of miscellaneous extraparotid lesions have been reported. Among them is the branchial cleft cyst, which can be either isodense or hypodense, depending on the cyst's contents. If these extraparotid cysts become infected, a rim of enhancement can be seen on CT scans after the administration of intravenous contrast material.

□ Low-density parapharyngeal masses

Fat density is usually fairly easy to identify on the CT scan (Fig. 5-10). There are three tumors that are primarily composed of fatty tissues. The lipoma and liposarcoma are the two most common such lesions. The very rare hibernoma, a fetal fat tumor, also will appear as a low-density mass. Dermoids and teratomas may have fatty tissues scattered within their confines, but they are not primarily lipid tumors. Lipomas of the parotid gland occur, are very rare, and usually are clinically suspected. Some neurofibromas may have suffi-

cient fat content to appear on CT scans as low-density lesions and as mentioned above, branchial cleft cysts often have a low-density central portion with a thin enhanced rim (Fig. 5-10, *D*).

□ Enhancing parapharyngeal masses

The only intraparotid lesion of consequence that is intensely enhanced is the hemangioma. However, this lesion is usually clinically suspected. Most parotid tumors are enhanced mildly, but their enhancement characteristics are not diagnostic and the parotid surgery performed is the same for all of these solitary masses. Thus the enhancing lesions of interest diagnostically are the extraparotid tumors. One of the most common of these is the schwannoma, which accounts for about 20% of all parapharyngeal space tumors.[3]

These neoplasms usually originate in the vagus nerve and along the cervical sympathetic chain. They usually occur as solitary tumors and symptoms may be referable to the involved nerve, or as is more common, referable to adjacent nerves that are stretched around the tumor mass. Virtually all the neoplasms are benign and are nonhomogeneously enhanced with intravenous contrast material. Most of these tumors have areas of cystic degeneration and hemorrhage that appear as nonenhanced regions within the otherwise enhanced mass (Fig. 5-11).

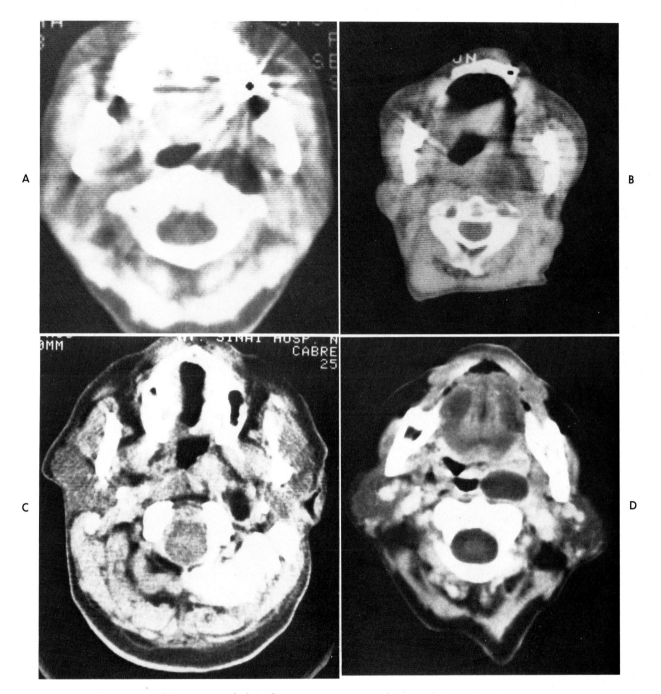

Fig. 5-10. A, CT scan reveals low density posterior parapharyngeal space mass. *Lipoma.* **B,** CT scan reveals vague low-density mass involving most of left parapharyngeal space liposarcoma. **C,** Axial CT scan reveals low-density left parapharyngeal space mass. Neurofibroma. **D,** Axial CT scan reveals low-density ovoid left parapharyngeal space mass with thin rim of enhancement. *Branchial cleft cyst.* (**A** From Som, P.M., et al.: Ann. Otol. Rhinol. Laryngol. **90**[suppl. 80, 1 pt. 4]:1-15, 1981.)

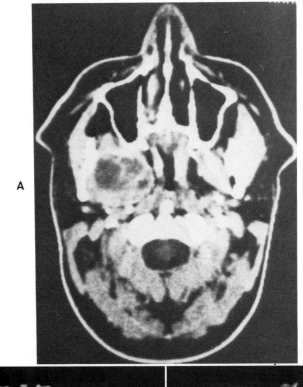

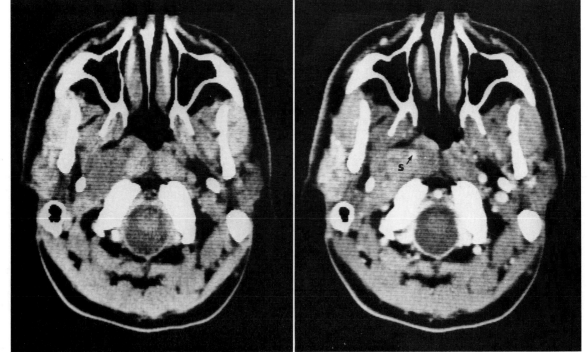

Fig. 5-11. A, CT scan reveals nonhomogeneously enhanced parapharyngeal space ovoid mass. *Schwannoma with areas of cystic degeneration.* **B,** CT sialogram of an extraparotid slightly decreased density (cystic region) parapharyngeal space mass. *Schwannoma.* **C,** CT sialogram of same patient reveals lesion to be nonhomogeneously enhancing *(s)* with anteromedial displacement of internal carotid artery *(arrow).* (**B** and **C** From Som, P.M., et al.: Ann. Otol. Rhinol. Laryngol. **90**[suppl. 80, 1 pt. 4]:1-15, 1981.)

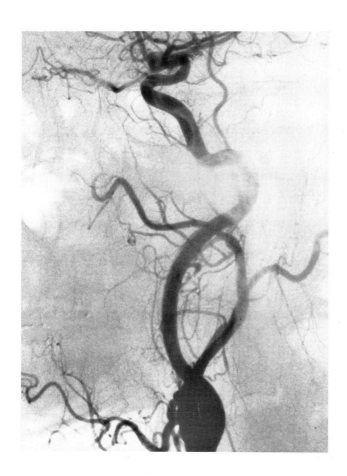

Fig. 5-12. Lateral subtraction film of carotid angiogram reveals avascular mass bowing carotid arteries. *Schwannoma.* (From Som, P.M., et al.: Ann. Otol. Rhinol. Laryngol. **90**[suppl. 80, 1 pt. 4]:1-15, 1981.)

A carotid angiogram usually, but not always, reveals anteromedial displacement of the internal carotid artery around an essentially avascular mass (Figs. 5-11, *C* and 5-12). The vascular displacement may vary with the size and location of the lesion. The enhancement seen on CT scanning appears to be the result of extravascular accumulation of the contrast material. Rare neurofibromas may occur as multiple lesions and they may at times be radiographically indistinguishable from schwannomas.

The paragangliomas, or glomus tumors, compose the next most common group of enhancing extraparotid parapharyngeal space lesions. They also account for nearly 20% of all tumors involving this space. Most of these tumors are glomus vagale lesions, with nearly two thirds of these tumors involving the parapharyngeal space. The majority of carotid body tumors are lower in the neck; however, about 8% extend upwards to significantly involve the parapharyngeal space. Glomus jugulare tumors rarely extend sufficiently downward to effectively involve this space[1,3,8] and usually extend laterally in the skull base.

The CT scan reveals a uniformly enhanced extrapa-

rotid tumor (Fig. 5-13). The angiogram reveals a characteristic, highly vascular tumor (Fig. 5-14). It is thus the angiogram that allows a definite differentiation between the paragangliomas and schwannomas, although their CT enhancing pattern is sufficient for differentiation in most cases. In the past several years, digital venous angiography has been employed very successfully in the evaluation of vascular lesions in the neck.[5a,9] It is most probable that this study will replace angiography in the diagnostic workup of these patients.

Finally, very rare meningiomas or metastases can extend from the skull base downward into the parapharyngeal space. The meningiomas may also have calcifications scattered within the enhancing tumor mass (Fig. 5-15). Whenever a lesion is seen to extend upwards towards the skull base, the CT scan should include the base of the skull in order to evaluate any possible bone erosion or intracranial extension.

The preceding preoperative scheme allows several things to be established, such as (1) which cases require an angiogram and which cases do not, (2) the exact extent and size of the tumor, and (3) the differentiation between intraparotid and extraparotid lesions. In

Text continued on p. 250.

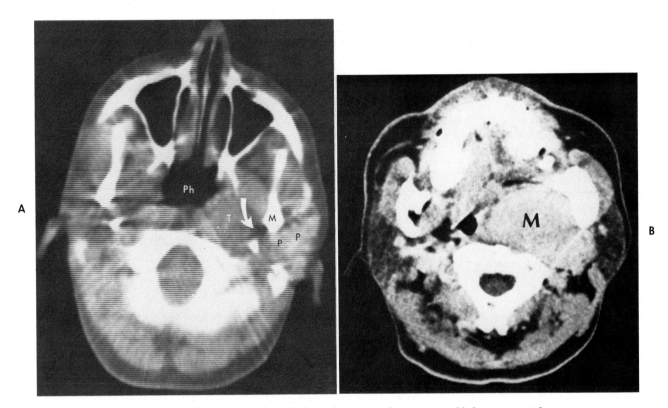

Fig. 5-13. A, CT sialogram reveals slight homogeneous enhancement of left extraparotid parapharyngeal space mass *(T)*. Lucent zone *(arrow)* separates parotid gland *(p)* and mass. *Ph,* Pharynx, *M,* mandible. *Glomus vagale.* **B,** Axial CT scan reveals large uniformly enhanced left parapharyngeal space mass *(M)*. *Glomus vagale.* (**A** From Som, P.M., et al.: Ann. Otol. Rhinol. Laryngol. **90**[suppl. 80, 1 pt. 4]:1-15, 1981.)

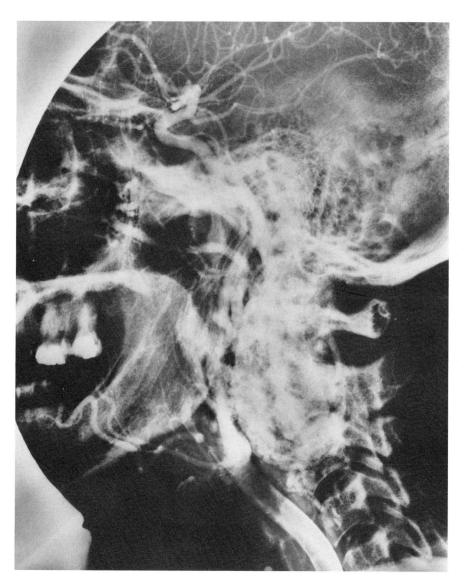

Fig. 5-14. Lateral carotid angiogram reveals typical vascular stain of paraganglioma (glomus tumor). (From Som, P.M., et al. Ann. Otol. Rhinol. Laryngol. **90**[suppl. 80, 1 pt. 4]:1-15, 1981.)

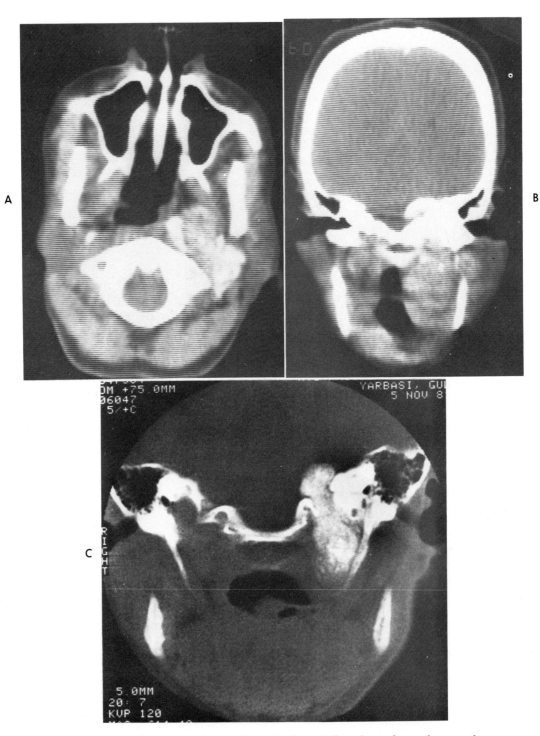

Fig. 5-15. A, Axial CT scan reveals partially calcified, partially enhanced parapharyngeal space mass. **B,** Coronal CT scan of same patient reveals mass extension through skull base from posterior cranial fossa meningioma. **C,** Coronal CT scan of another patient reveals partially calcified dumbell-shaped intracranial-extracranial enhanced meningioma. (**A** and **B** From Som, P.M., et al.: Ann. Otol. Rhinol. Laryngol. **90**[suppl. 80, 1 pt. 4]:1-15, 1981.)

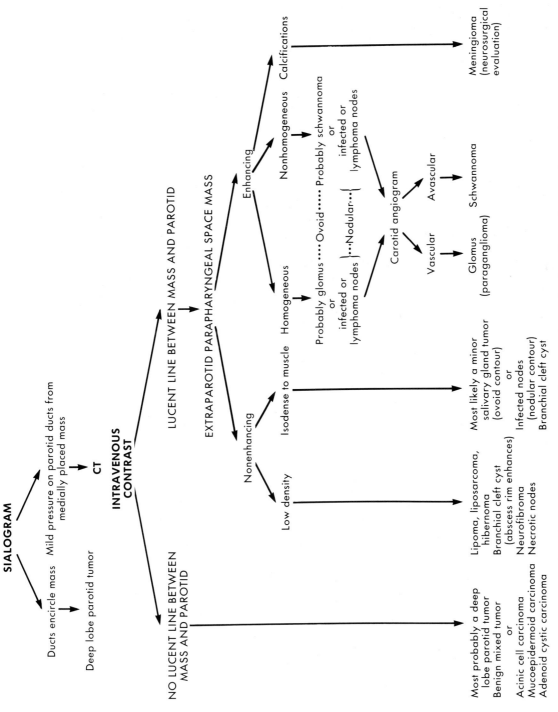

Fig. 5-16. Flow chart summarizing suggested preoperative evaluation of parapharyngeal space tumors.

addition, this scheme in many cases suggests the probable histology and directs the surgeon to choose the best surgical approach. This scheme is summarized in Fig. 5-16.

The ability to provide the surgeon with all this information was unheard of only a few years ago. It is expected that as future technological advances continue and further experience is gained an even more accurate preoperative diagnosis will be possible.

☐ **References**

1. Batsakis, J.: Tumors of the head and neck: clinical and pathological considerations, ed. 2, Baltimore, 1979, The Williams & Wilkins Co.
2. Goss, C.M.: Gray's Anatomy of the human body, ed. 27, Philadelphia, 1963, Lea & Febiger.
3. Heeneman, H., Gilbert, J.J., and Rood, S.R.: The parapharyngeal space: anatomy and pathologic conditions with emphasis on neurogenous tumors, 1980, American Academy of Otolaryngology.
4. Johns, M.E.: The salivary glands: anatomy and embryology, Otolaryngol. Clin. North Am. **10**(2):261-271, 1977.
5. Lederman, M.: Cancer of the nasopharynx: its natural history and treatment, Springfield Ill., 1961, Charles C Thomas, Publisher.
5a. Seeger, J.F., Weinstein, P.R., Carmody, R.F., et al.: Digital video subtraction angiography of the cervical and cerebral vasculature, J. Neurosurg. **56**:173-179, 1982.
6. Som, P.M., and Biller, H.F.: The combined computerized tomography–sialogram: a technique to differentiate deep lobe parotid tumors from extraparotid pharyngomaxillary space tumors, Ann. Otol. **88**(5):590-595, 1979.
7. Som, P.M., and Biller, H.F.: The combined CT-sialogram, Radiology **135**(2):387-390, 1980.
8. Som, P.M., Biller, H.F., and Lawson, W.: Tumors of the parapharyngeal space: preoperative evaluation, diagnosis and surgical approaches, Ann Otol. Rhinol. Laryngol. **90**(suppl. 80, 1 pt. 4):1-15, 1981.
9. Turski, P.A., Strother, C.M., Turnipseed, W.D., et al.: Evaluation of extracranial occlusive disease by digital subtraction angiography, Surg. Neurol. **16**:394-398, 1981.

6 □ The temporomandibular joint

DONALD P. BLASCHKE

Optimal radiographic visualization of the temporomandibular joint (TMJ) is increasingly important to medical and dental specialists. With the advent of TMJ arthrography and routine application of complex motion tomography, radiologists can detect early, subtle changes that affect the articulating surfaces of the TMJ and comment on the position of the joint bony structures in various phases of joint function. Both osseous and soft tissue components of the joint can now be evaluated. Radiographic procedures not only contribute to diagnosis but also assist in understanding TMJ structure and function in both health and disease.

This chapter will describe general aspects of temporomandibular joint radiology, including the broad topics of radiographic techniques and film interpretation. Conventional and tomographic techniques are presented, along with the relative advantages and disadvantages of various plain film projections. The normal radiographic appearance of the TMJ is described. The principal radiographic features associated with various abnormal and pathologic conditions are also discussed. It will not be possible to provide in-depth descriptions of clinical and pathologic features, a task appropriately left to texts on joint disorders and the TMJ in particular.

□ Gross anatomy

The two bony constituents of the TMJ are the condylar process of the mandible and the articular component of the temporal bone. The former is ordinarily divided into the condyle and the neck of the condyle, and the latter into the articular fossa and the articular eminence.

■ Mandibular component

The *mandibular condyle* is a bony ellipsoid connected to the ramus of the mandible by a bony isthmus or *neck* (Fig. 6-1). The condyle is longer from lateral to medial poles than in other dimensions (Fig. 6-2, *A*). The average lateral to medial condylar dimension is 20.0 mm, and the anteroposterior diameter of the condyle is about 8 to 10 mm.[34] The typical condyle has a convex superior surface, a convex posterior surface, and a convex, concave, or flat anterior surface. On many condyles there is a pronounced ridge that runs from lateral to medial along the anterior surface near the articulating area. This ridge is the upper limit of the pterygoid fovea, a small depression in the anterior condylar surface where the superior head of the lateral pterygoid muscle attaches.

Angulation of the condylar long axis in the transverse plane has been studied by several authors. Median angulation varied from just over 15°[34] between the long axis and the intermeatal or coronal axis to 22.5° (Fig.

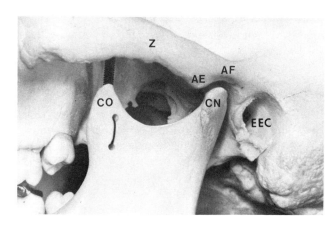

Fig. 6-1. Lateral view of TMJ of dried skull. *CN,* Mandibular condyle; *CO,* coronoid process; *AE,* articular eminence; *EEC,* external ear canal. Z, Zygomatic arch. Radiographic joint space is represented here by space between condyle and articular fossa *(AF).*

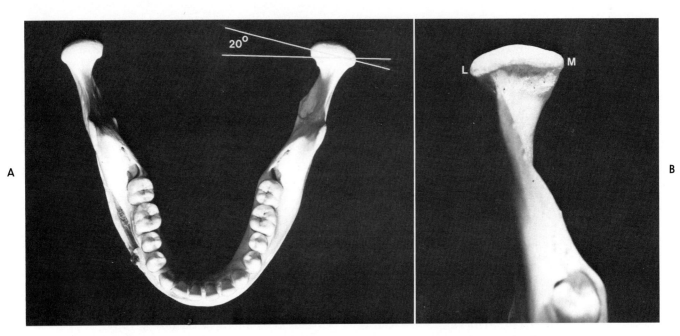

Fig. 6-2. Dried mandible showing both mandibular condyles. **A,** Frontal view of right mandibular process. Notice slight convexity of superior surface. *L,* Lateral pole; *M,* medial pole. **B,** Superior view showing both mandibular condyles. Notice angulation of longitudinal axes of condyles, obliqued approximately 20° to coronal plane. (**A** From Blaschke, D.D. In Goaz, P.W., and White, S.C.: Oral radiology: principles and interpretation, St. Louis, 1982, The C.V. Mosby Co.)

6-2, *B*).[27] This information is necessary in selecting a standard head correction angle for TMJ tomography.

■ Temporal component

The temporal component of the TMJ is comprised of the *articular fossa* and the *articular eminence* (Fig. 6-1). The most lateral aspect of the eminence displays a protuberance called the *articular tubercle.* The articular tubercle is principally a source of ligamentous attachments. In addition, it serves as the anatomic junction where the root of the zygomatic process joins the temporal squama.

There is considerable variation in the depth of the articular fossa, resulting from differences in the development of the articular eminence. The fossa is shallow in some individuals, but in others a sharp concavity behind the eminence leads to a deep fossa. Very young infants do not have a definite articular eminence and therefore may not have a demonstrable fossa.

The posterior limit of the TMJ is formed by the squamotympanic fissure and its more medial extension, the petrotympanic fissure. The superoanterior border of this bony suture often forms a ledge that laterally becomes the *postglenoid tubercle.* Below the squamotympanic fissure, the tympanic segment of the temporal bone forms the major portion of the external auditory canal's anterior wall. The articular fossa is the opposite surface of the same temporal bone that forms a portion of the middle cranial fossa floor. In essence, this thin oval layer of cortical bone is all that separates the upper TMJ space from the intracranial subdural space. The temporal component may be pneumatized, with many small air cells derived from the mastoid air cell complex.

■ Soft tissues

The TMJ is a double-compartmented joint, with distinct upper and lower joint spaces that are separated by an intervening fibrocartilaginous disc that itself is capable of motion in concert with the moving bony structures. This fibrocartilaginous *disc* (meniscus) and its ligamentous *posterior attachment* (sometimes called the retrodiscal pad) are located between the two bony articular components of the TMJ (Fig. 6-3, *A*). The disc is anchored anteriorly by the insertion of the superior head of the lateral pterygoid muscle. The inferior head of the same muscle inserts lower, on the anterior aspect of the condyle. The disc therefore is biconcave, with its thinnest, central portion normally positioned between the articulating convexities of the condyle and the articular eminence (Fig. 6-3, *B*).

■ Joint space and bony relationships

Average joint space widths are 1.5 mm between the anterior aspect of the condyle and the eminence and 2.5 mm between the condyle and the roof of the fossa.[22]

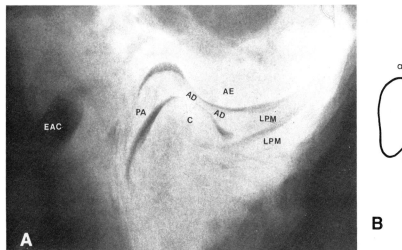
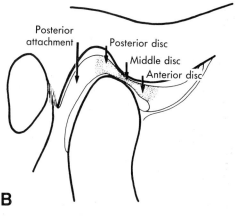

Fig. 6-3. **A,** Decalcified temporomandibular joint of autopsy specimen, seen radiographically. Between condyle *(C)* and articular eminence *(AE)* is shadow of soft tissue component of joint. On this specimen, from anterior to posterior, are seen lateral pterygoid muscle *(LPM),* including superior and inferior components; biconcave articular disc *(AD);* and posterior attachment of disc *(PA).* External ear canal *(EAC)* is seen posteriorly. Upper and lower joint spaces are seen as radiolucent slivers between bony surfaces and soft tissue component. Note that joint spaces are not distended as they are during contrast radiography. **B,** Diagram of same autopsy specimen with pertinent portions of soft tissue component labeled. Disc itself is graphically rendered as stippled area of soft tissue component. (From Blaschke, D.D., Solberg, K.K., and Sanders, R.: JADA **100:**388, 1980. Copyright by the American Dental Association. Reprinted by permission.)

In normal joint relationships, the condyle should be juxtaposed to the posterior slope of the eminence when the teeth are in occlusion. Using *area* measurements of specified regions of the joint space, Blaschke has found that the joint spaces between the condyle and temporal component in 25 normal subjects were virtually equal in anterior and posterior sectors.[3] This study demonstrated that the average condyle is thus normally centered in its fossa. Condylar *concentricity* is the term that has been proposed for condylar positioning in which the anterior and posterior aspects of the radiolucent joint space are uniform in width.[31] The condyle is said to be in *retrusion* when the posterior joint space width is less than the anterior and in *protrusion* when the posterior joint space is larger than the anterior. However, Blaschke's study has also revealed a large standard deviation in normal condylar positions. Moderate posteriorly and anteriorly positioned condyles may therefore be variants of normal TMJ anatomy and function.[23]

■ Dynamic relationships

The TMJ is classified as a ginglymoarthrodial joint; i.e., it undergoes a sliding movement between the bony surfaces in addition to the hinge movement common to diarthrodial joints. The range of motion that the mandible undergoes while a person is chewing, swallowing, or talking is extremely complex. The joint provides a sliding movement in its upper compartment, allowing the lower jaw to protrude forward or to swing to either side. In addition, the joint can make a simple hinge movement in the lower compartment to allow pure opening and closing jaw motions. The radiologist can evaluate whether the bony parts of the joint are participating in a comination of both hinge and sliding movements, purely hinge (rotatory) movement, or no movement at all. A key aspect of TMJ radiologic interpretation is therefore concerned with joint *function* in addition to morphology.

With the jaws closed, articulation occurs between the anterosuperior aspect of the condyle and the posterior slope of the articular eminence. As the condyle slides anteriorly from its closed position during jaw opening, it is said to *translate* anteriorly. With closing, the condyle *translates* posteriorly.

As the lower jaw opens, the condyle moves anteriorly and inferiorly down the posterior slope of the articular crest. In many cases, the condyle goes on to move slightly up the anterior face of the eminence. The actual extent of anterior translation of the condyle in normal persons is highly variable. Normal subjects are occasionally observed in which the condyle does not reach the eminence crest with the jaws wide open. In other cases, the condyle may appear to move completely into the infratemporal fossa. In an effort to provide some limits of normal variation, Rickets established that if one locates a static point just below the center of the condyle, the most anterior movement of this point in normal individuals ranges from 2 to 5 mm posterior to 5 to 8 mm anterior to the crest of the eminence.[22]

The mandibular condyle and articular disc both translate forward during jaw opening, moving in concert. The precise position of the articular disc at any given degree of jaw opening is determined by complex forces that are not totally understood. It is thought that an equilibrium normally exists between muscle tension anteriorly and elasticity of the posterior attachment. An understanding of disc positioning and movement during joint function is essential for the intelligent application of TMJ arthrography.

□ Radiographic anatomy
■ Plain films

The two temporomandibular joints (TMJs) are only part of the total articulation between the mandible and facial bones. The other important contribution is made by interdigitization of the mandibular and maxillary teeth. Thus the status of the TMJ is directly related to that of the dental arches. If several teeth are missing on one side of the mouth, or if there are premature or defective contacts between the teeth in occlusion, abnormal stresses may be transferred to the TMJs. The radiologic examination of the TMJ is therefore most productive when the patients' dentition is also considered.[23]

Certain anatomic constraints make the TMJ itself difficult to examine radiographically. First, the longitudinal axis of the condyle from lateral to medial poles is not parallel to the intermeatal axis (i.e., perpendicular to the skull midsagittal axis). Instead, both TMJ longitudinal axes are angled about 20° to the intermeatal axis, so that if a line were drawn pole to pole through the condyles and extended medially, these lines would intersect near the anterior margin of the foramen magnum.

Secondly, the TMJs are located at the skull base, directly beneath the petrous ridges. They are thus also in the same coronal plane as a major portion of the petrous temporal bone. The lateral portions of the petrous ridges, as well as the mastoid processes, overlie the TMJs. On routine lateral views, the TMJ of interest is thus obscured by superimposition of the petrous ridges and contralateral TMJ. Simple skull rotation separates the two joints but superimposes the mastoid process, occipital condyles, or pterygoid structures. A number of special lateral projections have been devised to overcome these limitations, but two, the transcranial and infracranial views, are particularly useful.

The *transcranial projection* is essentially identical to the reverse Schüller projection familiar to head and neck radiologists. Though many variations of the transcranial technique have been described, the postauricular approach of Lindblom best projects the longitudinal joint axis. The x-ray film cassette is positioned against the face on the side of interest, parallel to the sagittal plane. The x-ray tubehead is brought into position on the contralateral side of the skull so that the central beam projects 25° caudally (Fig. 6-4, *A*). The central beam is thus projected across the cranium, passing just above the filmside petrous ridge to the TMJ of interest (Fig. 6-4, *B* and *C*).

A routine *transcranial* TMJ series examines the joint in both closed and wide-open jaw positions on both left and right sides.[1] Some clinicians also request a third projection on each side, a slightly open, "resting" jaw position. Determinations can be made of the closed-mouth TMJ bone spatial relationships (i.e., between the condyle and the temporal component) as well as the degree of anterior condylar translation as the mouth is opened. For the closed-mouth projection, the patient bites firmly on his back teeth in his usual, most comfortable bite (a registration known in dentistry as *centric occlusion*). The open-mouth view is made with the patient's jaws opened as widely as possible without straining the muscles or ligaments.

An example of a normal closed-mouth transcranial radiograph is shown in Fig. 6-5. This view provides essentially unobstructed visualization of the articulating surface, though it is compromised by the almost universal crossing of the condylar neck by the contralateral petrous ridge. Abnormal changes in the condylar neck, such as fracture lines or tumors, may therefore at times be obscured by the petrous ridge. The transcranial projection is most helpful in detecting articulating surface changes such as those caused by the various types of arthritis. In addition, when tomographic capability is not available, the closed-mouth transcranial view can provide a fairly reliable evaluation of bony spatial relationships in the joint (Fig. 6-6). Note that the transcranial view displays only the lateral aspects of the condyle and articular fossa silhouetted against the joint space, a result of the caudal angulation of the x-ray beam (Fig. 6-7). Thus transcranial radiography may show minute, subtle irregularities on the lateral bony surfaces but will be much less sensitive to similar changes that occur on the central and medial joint surfaces. In addition, many TMJs have changing bony relationships from lateral to medial poles of the joints.

Stereoscopic TMJ views provide depth perception that is particularly helpful in differentiating superim-

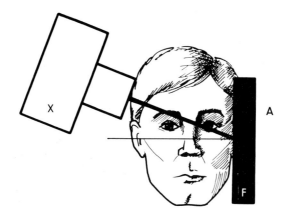

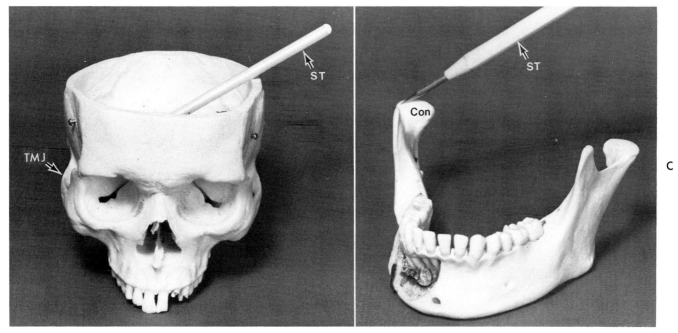

Fig. 6-4. Transcranial TMJ radiographic technique. **A,** Drawing illustrates frontal view. X-ray beam passes through cranium from contralateral (tubeside) parietal bone. *X,* X-ray tubehead; *F,* film holder. **B,** Pencil-like stylus *(ST)* indicates approximate path of central x-ray beam used in transcranial radiography of TMJ. X-ray beam is directed caudally approximately 25° in order to pass above intracranial petrous ridge (not seen) on side of condyle in question. **C,** Same stylus indicating that x-ray beam captures *lateral* surface of condyle in profile on resultant radiographic image. (**A** From Blaschke, D.D., and White, S.C. In Sarnat, B.G., and Laskin, D.M.: The temporomandibular joint: a biologic basis for clinical practice, ed. 3, 1980. Courtesy of Charles C Thomas, Publisher, Springfield, Illinois.)

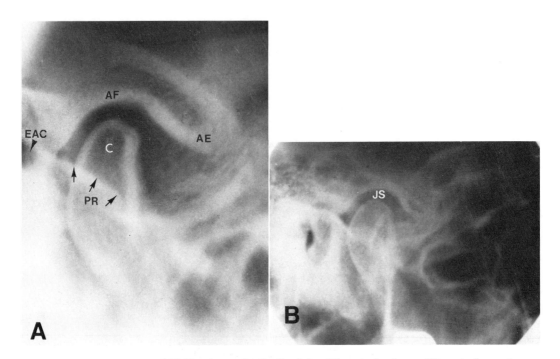

Fig. 6-5. A, Transcranial TMJ radiograph. *C,* Condyle; *AF,* articular fossa; *AE,* articular eminence; *PR,* temporal bone petrous ridge on same side as condyle and crossing condyle obliquely. Latter is a constant feature of transcranial TMJ radiography. *EAC,* External ear canal. **B,** Another example of transcranial radiography. *JS,* Radiolucent joint space between the condyle and fossa. This view is typically made with teeth in maximum intercuspation (patient biting on back teeth). In both examples notice smooth, rounded, well-defined cortices of bony articulating surfaces. (**A** From Blaschke, D.D., and White, S.C. In Sarnat, B.G. and Laskin, D.M.: The temporomandibular joint: a biologic basis for clinical practice, ed. 3, 1980. Courtesy of Charles C Thomas, Publisher, Springfield, Illinois.)

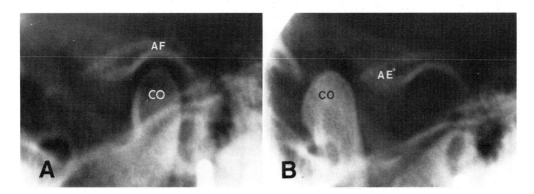

Fig. 6-6. Closed- and open-mouth transcranial radiographs. **A,** Patient biting on posterior teeth, with condyle *(CO)* seated normally in articular fossa *(AF).* **B,** Patient with jaws wide open, showing condyle *(CO)* translated anterior to articular eminence *(AE).* This is normal degree of joint function as seen on transcranial films.

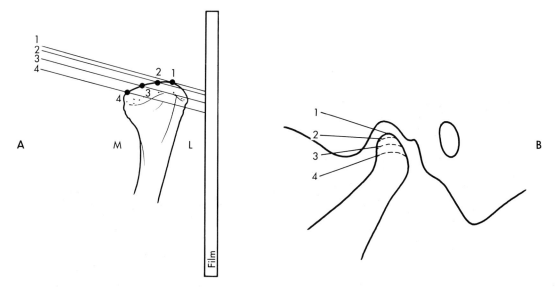

Fig. 6-7. Drawings illustrate that the lateral aspect of condylar articulating surface is portrayed in profile against radiolucent joint space. **A,** Frontal view of left condyle. Oblique lines represent parallel hypothetical transcranial central x-ray beams crossing cortical landmarks *1* to *4* on superior surface of condyle. **B,** As seen on transcranial radiography, landmark *1* (on lateral one third of condyle superior surface) forms profile image of condylar against joint space. (Modified from Weinberg, L.A.: J. Prosthet. Dent. **30:**898, 1973.)

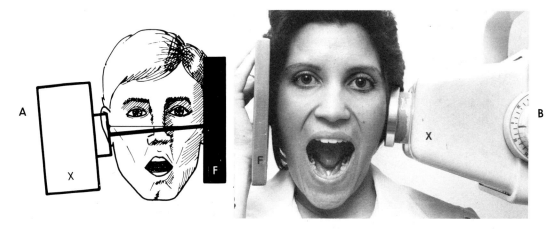

Fig. 6-8. Infracranial radiographic technique for TMJ. **A,** Drawing illustrating view of radiographic projection. Notice that projection is made with patient's mouth opened as widely as possible. *X,* X-ray tubehead; *F,* film holder. **B,** Clinical photography of technique. Cone of x-ray tubehead has been removed in order to accentuate distortion of ipsilateral condyle and enhance, by comparison, distinction of contralateral condyle. (From Blaschke, D.D., and White, S.C. In Sarnat, B.G., and Laskin, D.M.: The temporomandibular joint: a biologic basis for clinical practice, ed. 3, 1980. Courtesy of Charles C Thomas, Publisher, Springfield, Illinois.)

posed bony shadows in this area. With stereoscopic views of the TMJ, for example, the crest of the ipsilateral petrous ridge can more clearly be distinguished from the condylar neck. Magnified TMJ views are also advocated by some authors.[1]

The *infracranial TMJ projection* is not routinely used by head and neck radiologists. The procedure is more common in oral radiology clinics and oral surgery clinics, where TMJ trauma is often diagnosed and treated.

An x-ray film cassette is placed against the side of the patient's head adjacent to the TMJ of interest. The x-ray tubehead is positioned on the opposite side of the skull with the central beam centered on the TMJ of interest (Fig. 6-8, *A*). The tubehead is angled so that the central beam is directed cranially 5 to 10° and posteriorly approximately 10° (Fig. 6-8, *B*). The central x-ray beam ideally passes through the tubeside mandibular notch (i.e., the "window" between the condylar and coronoid processes of the mandible and below the zy-gomatic arch), crosses beneath the skull base (through the oropharynx), and centers on the contralateral con-dylar process.

Prior to film exposure, the patient opens his mouth widely. Mouth opening moves the condyle of interest away from the superimposed skull base and into a soft tissue region, providing far greater radiographic con-trast. It also increases the tubeside "window" between the mandibular notch and zygomatic process through which the central x-ray beam should pass. If the patient is unable to open his mouth widely (e.g., as a result of fracture, ankylosis, or other abnormality), the intracra-nial projection may still be useful but the superior por-tion of the condylar head is often superimposed on the articular eminence.

The infracranial view is designed to provide gross vi-sualization of the condylar process, from the midman-dibular ramus to the condylar apex (Fig. 6-9). The tech-nique is helpful in diagnosing fractures of the condylar head and neck and in detecting gross alterations in con-dylar form. The condyle is seen obliquely in this pro-jection, in contrast to the predominantly longitudinal, end-on view provided by the transcranial technique. Subtle bony alterations on the anterior condylar surface are not projected in profile and may consequently be missed. The infracranial projection also provides little or no diagnostic information on the temporal compo-nent of the TMJ.

The *transorbital projection* is the conventional an-teroposterior view that best delineates the TMJs. The TMJs are not visible in a straight frontal projection, but come into view only when the head is rotated about 15° to 20° toward the side of interest. Separate transorbital projections must be made for each joint.

An x-ray cassette is placed behind the patient's head and the tube-head at the front. The central x-ray beam is projected through the ipsilateral orbit to the TMJ of interest, exiting the skull behind the mastoid process. Fig. 6-10, *A*, shows proper TMJ transorbital head po-sitioning. The patient's head is tilted slightly caudally from a neutral head posture. The patient opens his mouth widely, moving the condyle out of the articular fossa and closer to the articular eminence (Fig. 6-10, *B*). This allows en face visualization of the entire laterome-dial articulating surfaces of both the condyle and the articular eminence. If the patient cannot open his mouth widely, the condylar neck is seen but the joint articulating surfaces are lost as a result of mutual super-impositions.

The transorbital view depicts the convex articulating surface of the condyle and the slightly concave, broad ridge of the articular eminence (Fig. 6-11). This is therefore the best frontal view to correlate with the transcranial projection when the presence and extent of arthritic changes need to be defined.

Anteroposterior (AP) facial projections are less con-sistent than the transorbital projection in adequately displaying the TMJ. Nevertheless, the Waters and Towne views may provide some useful information. If such projections are made to evaluate facial bone ab-normalities (e.g., multiple facial fractures or develop-mental facial asymmetries), the Waters and Towne pro-jections may be advantageously screened for TMJ pathology.

The two facial projections provide fundamentally dif-ferent information on the TMJ. The Towne projection does not display the TMJs per se but visualizes much of the condylar processes. It is particularly helpful in determining the presence of condylar fractures. If frac-

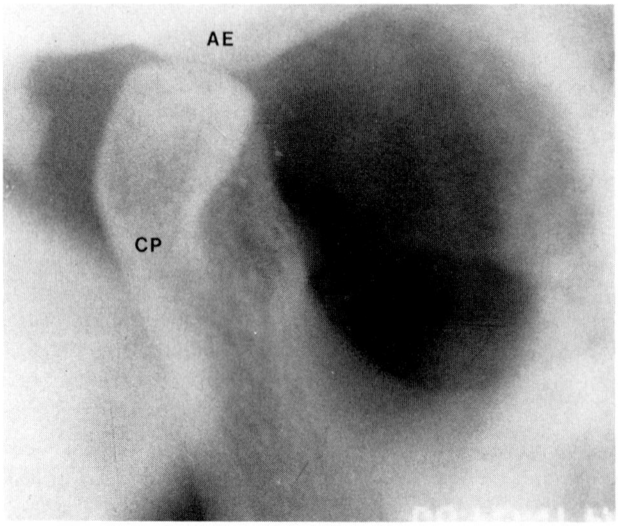

Fig. 6-9. Radiograph of TMJ by infracranial technique. Large portion of condylar process *(CP)* is seen without superimpo-sition of filmside petrous ridge. Cortices of temporal compo-nent of joint are not well seen in this projection. *AE,* Articular eminence. (From Blaschke, D.D., and White, S.C. In Sarnat, B.G., and Laskin, D.M.: The temporomandibular joint: a bi-ologic basis for clinical practice, ed. 3, 1980. Courtesy of Charles C Thomas, Publisher, Springfield, Illinois.)

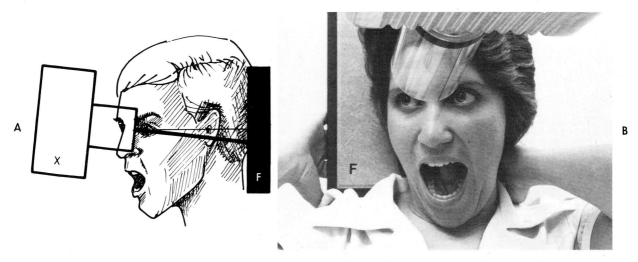

Fig. 6-10. Transorbital radiographic technique for TMJ. **A,** Drawing illustrating proper radiographic angulations. *X,* X-ray tubehead; *F,* film holder. **B,** Clinical photograph of the patient. Notice that patient's mouth is again opened as widely as possible. Beam is projected through ipsilateral orbit, centered on condylar process. (From Blaschke, D.D., and White, S.C. In Sarnat, B.G., and Laskin, D.M.: The temporomandibular joint: a biologic basis for clinical practice, ed. 3, 1980. Courtesy of Charles C Thomas, Publisher, Springfield, Illinois.)

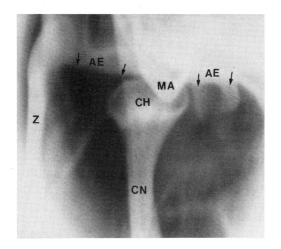

Fig. 6-11. Example of radiograph of right condylar process by transorbital technique. *CH,* Head of condyle; *CN,* neck of condyle; *AE,* articular eminence; *MA,* mastoid process superimposing over articular eminence; *Z,* zygomatic arch. (From Blaschke, D.D., and White, S.C. In Sarnat, B.G., and Laskin, D.M.: The temporomandibular joint: a biologic basis for clinical practice, ed. 3, 1980. Courtesy of Charles C Thomas, Publisher, Springfield, Illinois.)

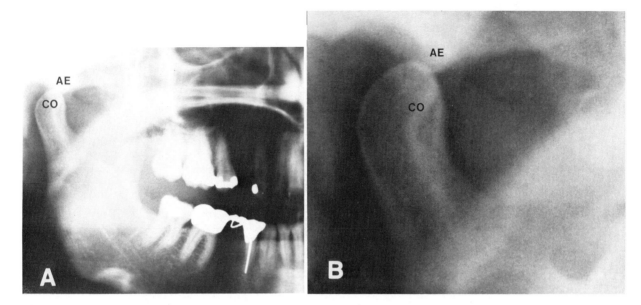

Fig. 6-12. Example of panoramic radiography of jaws. **A,** On typical panoramic radiograph (cropped to posterior mandible), mandibular condyle *(CO)* is fairly well represented in slightly oblique view. Again, temporal component of joint is not well seen. *AE,* Articular eminence. **B,** Close-up of condylar process as it appears on panoramic projection. Integrity of condylar process *(CO)* can be seen, as well as presence of any gross abnormalities. *AE,* Articular eminence. (From Blaschke, D.D., and White, S.C. In Sarnat, B.G., and Laskin, D.M.: The temporomandibular joint: a biologic basis for clinical practice, ed. 3, 1980. Courtesy of Charles C Thomas, Publisher, Springfield, Illinois.)

tures are present, the usual superomedial displacement of condylar fragments may be seen optimally on this conventional projection. The Waters projection sometimes projects the TMJ articulating surfaces bilaterally with few compromising superimpositions. However, the bulk of the condyles are superimposed by the petrous ridges, and the medial joint surfaces are often obscured by the teeth.

The *submentovertex (SMV) projection* is occasionally useful in TMJ radiography. TMJ erosions from a nasopharyngeal carcinoma near the base of the skull can sometimes be identified on this view. The submentovertex projection is also used in many radiology departments to define precisely the condylar angles for positioning for "corrected" TMJ tomographic procedures (see next section).

The increasing availability of *panoramic radiography* (see Chapter 7) has reduced the need for obtaining infracranial views (Fig. 6-12). The panoramic projection covers virtually the same condylar anatomy and simultaneously displays both TMJs. The posterior mandibular and condylar anatomy, as displayed in panoramic radiography, are seen in Fig. 6-12.

■ Tomography

Currently, tomography provides the most definitive radiologic information on TMJ bony anatomy (Fig. 6-

13). Complex motion tomography, particularly hypocycloidal tomography, is the most effective TMJ radiographic examination for two reasons: (1) the structures of the joint are relatively small, and (2) maximal blurring motion is necessary to eliminate dense superimpositions from the petrous ridges and skull base.[8] Complex motion tomography can also be potentially the most reliable method for determining joint bony spatial relationships.

When complex motion tomographic equipment is not available, linear tomography of the TMJ can often be performed with adequate results. When bony relationships of the TMJs are evaluated, linear tomography usually compares favorably with the complex motion variety if proper patient head position is carefully established. When determining the position of the condyle in relation to the articular fossa, producing the thinnest possible focal "cut" is generally not as important as producing optimal projection geometry, i.e., precisely aligning the central x-ray beam with the joint long axis.

The concept of correcting the patient's head position to align the long axis of the joint with the central x-ray beam is critical to modern, sophisticated TMJ radiographic technique.[6] It is usually necessary to rotate the patient's head approximately 20° toward the side of interest, a maneuver that provides corrected TMJ tomography (Fig. 6-14). This correction or orientation of the

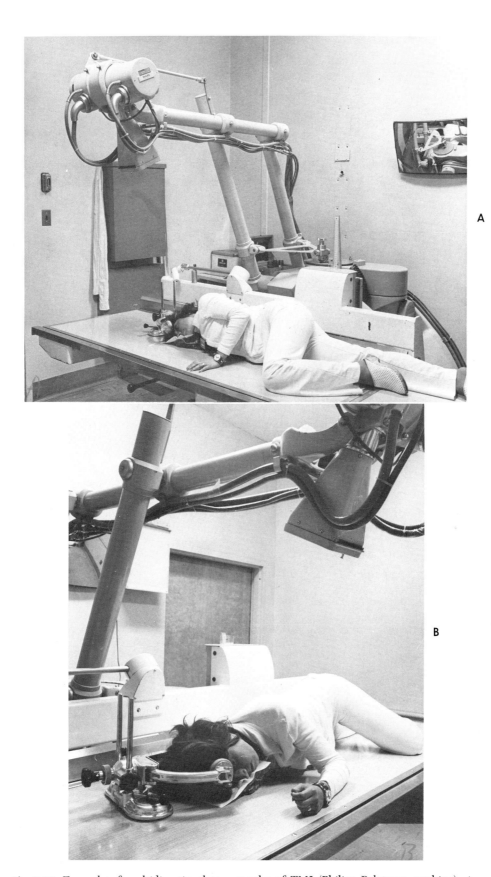

Fig. 6-13. Example of multidirectional tomography of TMJ (Philips Polytome machine). **A,** Clinical technique photograph showing patient properly positioned on Polytome table for radiograph of right TMJ. **B,** Another view of same patient. Head is stabilized with head clamp. Patient's head is slightly rotated (approximately 20°) toward side of involvement (tabletop). (From Blaschke, D.D., and White, S.C. In Sarnat, B.G., and Laskin, D.M.: The temporomandibular joint: a biologic basis for clinical practice, ed. 3, 1980. Courtesy of Charles C Thomas, Publisher, Springfield, Illinois.)

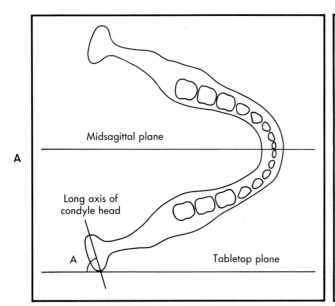
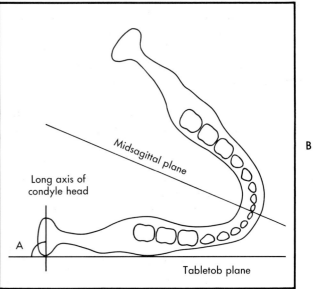

Fig. 6-14. Drawings illustrate principle behind 20° rotation of patient's head toward tabletop. **A,** Long axis of condyle forms an acute (approximately 70°) angle (*A*) with tabletop, i.e., film surface. **B,** By rotation of patient's head 20° toward tabletop, long axis of patient's head is brought perpendicular to tabletop, allowing end-on, long axis, radiographic projection of joint. This maneuver better permits subtle cortical irregularities to be visualized. (From Coin, C.G.: Dent. Radiogr. Photogr. **47:**23, 1974.)

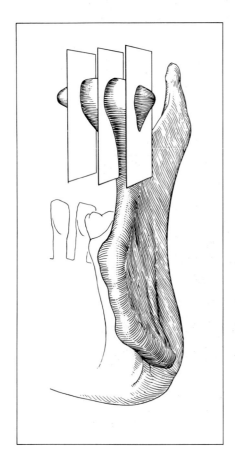

Fig. 6-15. Drawing of right mandibular ramus from posteroinferior aspect. Hypothetical thin-section tomographic planes are illustrated through lateral, central, and medial portions of condyle. Tomographic planes are perpendicular to long axis of condyle. (From Coin, C.G.: Dent. Radiogr. Photogr. **47:**23, 1974.)

patient's head should be performed before either lateral or frontal TMJ tomography. For the lateral projection, the correction provides an essentially longitudinal or end-on view of the joint; for frontal tomography, the correction orients the joint en face, i.e., with the broad frontal joint surface squared to the oncoming x-ray beam.

With *complex motion* tomography, several focal cuts through the condyle–articular fossa joint region should be obtained in precise focus. Although the extreme medial and lateral poles of the condylar head are not usually well visualized, the remaining portions of the condylar head, articular fossa, and articular eminence can be examined for minute bony defects (Figs. 6-15 and 6-16, *A*). On the other hand, if *linear* tomography is performed, only one or possibly two focal cuts through the thickest portions will be adequately focused for detailed interpretation (Fig. 6-16, *B*). When complex motion tomography is performed, it is recommended that the focal cuts be obtained 2 to 4 mm apart from each other, with the initial cut being taken 2 cm medial to the skin surface and progressing laterally. With linear tomography, the cuts are more practically spaced 4 to 5 mm apart from each other.

As with conventional views of the joint, prior to making exposures the patient is asked to bite down firmly on his posterior teeth (Fig. 6-17). When open-mouth projections are desired, the patient should open his

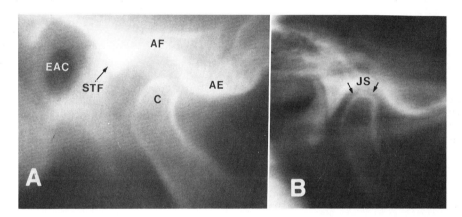

Fig. 6-16. A, Radiographic example of multidirectional tomography of TMJ, with patient's mouth slightly open. Cortical structures are well seen. *C,* Condyle; *AF,* articular fossa; *AE,* articular eminence; *EAC,* external ear canal; *STF,* squamotympanic fissure. **B,** Another tomographic example of TMJ, this time by linear tomography. Condyle is seated normally in fossa with patient's jaw closed. Joint space *(JS)* is relatively even between bony articulating surfaces.

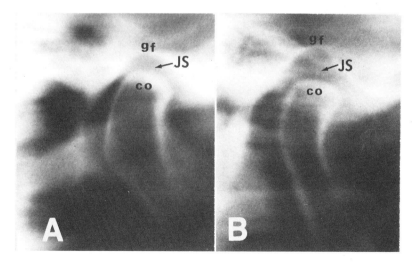

Fig. 6-17. Closed-mouth views of varying shapes of two different articular fossae, producing varying depths of radiolucent joint spaces. **A,** TMJ tomogram of relatively shallow joint space. **B,** Different example of greater depth of joint space caused by relatively deep glenoid fossa. *JS,* Joint space; *CO,* condyle; *gf,* glenoid (articular fossa).

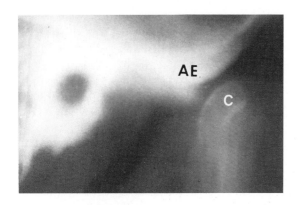

Fig. 6-18. Wide open-mouth position of condyle *(C)* here seen well anterior to articular eminence *(AE)*.

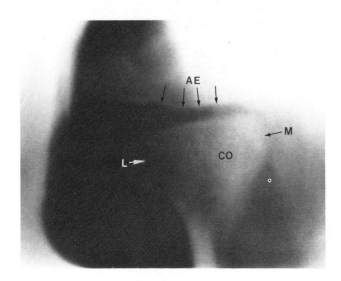

Fig. 6-19. Frontal tomogram of right TMJ with patient's mouth open. Superior surface of condyle *(CO)* is opposed to inferior surface of articular eminence *(AE)*. Lateral pole *(L)* of condyle is overpenetrated, "burned out" on this example. *M,* Medial pole of condyle.

mouth as widely as possible without straining the masticatory muscles and hold this opening posture for the length of the exposure (Fig. 6-18). Because of the rather long interval of many tomographic exposures (up to 6 seconds), a stepped bite block may be inserted between the patient's anterior teeth to aid in preventing jaw motion.

Frontal tomograms of the TMJ are ideally made with the x-ray beam tightly collimated to expose only the joint of interest unilaterally, with no attempt to obtain both joints on the same radiographic exposure (Fig. 6-19). It is often necessary to obtain only closed projections for the purpose of defining bony relationships made with the patient's teeth in occlusion. On the other hand, if the examination is primarily oriented to producing a detailed view of the articulating surfaces, the patient must be encouraged to open his mouth as widely as possible.

Submentovertex (axial) tomograms may be obtained for the temporomandibular joints with the patient in either the supine or prone positions. The submentovertex tomogram is most useful for supplying information

on the medial and lateral poles of the mandibular condyle.

■ Computed tomography

CT has recently been used to delineate the soft tissues of the TMJ.[15a] Direct sagittal scans have detected anterior meniscal displacement without the use of TMJ arthrography. Although CT is noninvasive, the routine use of this procedure in patients with temporomandibular joint dysfunction is not widespread. CT is also particularly helpful in delineating those osseous and soft tissue lesions that involve the mandible proper[20a] (see Chapter 7).

■ Arthrography

Arthrography is performed to provide evidence of TMJ disc displacement, disc perforation, or both.[12,14,18] It supplies information on TMJ soft tissue status. Specifically, the morphology and position of the disc and its posterior attachment may be evaluated. The examination is most helpful diagnostically in those cases in which little or no bony damage is seen on prearthro-

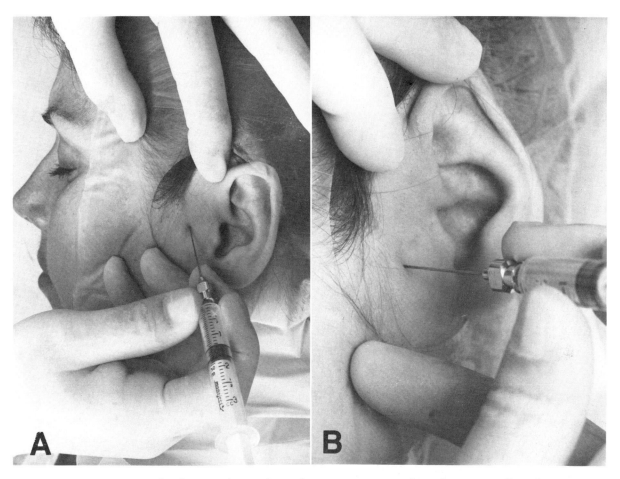

Fig. 6-20. Example of TMJ arthrographic technique. **A,** Position of anesthetizing needle and syringe, showing proper angle for penetration of upper joint space. Prior to insertion of needle, patient should open mouth in order to translate condyle and disc forward. **B,** For injection of lower joint space, syringe is directed more perpendicular to preauricular skin surface. Notice sterile drape isolating operative area.

graphic tomograms and in which clinical findings (e.g., joint clicking or popping, painful limitation of opening, or joint locking) suggest a diagnosis of disc derangement caused by nonbony joint problems such as capsulitis, myofascitis, and temporomandibular pain-dysfunction syndrome. Contraindications to the procedure include allergy to radiographic contrast media and TMJ or para-articular infection (including otitis media and parotiditis).

Technique

There are two important anatomic differences that distinguish the technique of the TMJ arthrographic examination from the more commonly performed procedure on the knee, hip, and shoulder. First, the TMJs are small (approximately the size of a metacarpophalangeal joint) and therefore require very precise needle or catheter placement. In addition, the TMJs each contain two separate, noncommunicating joint spaces, both of which should be opacified in order to obtain maximum diagnostic information. It must be said, however, that a perfectly acceptable TMJ arthrogram may be accomplished with only lower-space opacification.

Conversely, TMJ arthrography is *similar* to knee arthrography in two principal respects. First, arthrographic radiography must include various images of the functioning joint so that movement of the joint soft tissues can be ascertained; and second, the radiographic examination must be expedited following the injection of contrast. The water-soluble contrast agent disperses into the synovium and ligamentous attachments within a very short period of time, producing indistinct images of internal soft tissues. There is noticeable degradation of the TMJ arthrographic image if radiographs are not made within 10 minutes following contrast injection. Although a brief explanation of TMJ arthrography is provided below, detailed information regarding the technique is found in the recent literature.[3,32]

TMJ arthrography is performed as follows. A radiographic room equipped with fluoroscopic and tomographic capabilities is required. The patient is placed with the side of interest up, facing the operator. The preauricular area is disinfected and draped. The operator locally anesthetizes the preauricular soft tissues and catheterizes the joint spaces (Fig. 6-20). Two 20 or 22 gauge angiocatheters are used for puncture of the upper and lower joint spaces (Fig. 6-21, A). These in turn are connected by polyethylene tubing to small syringes containing a water-soluble contrast medium (Figure 6-21, B). Following the administration of local anesthesia, the operator must periodically observe the patient's eye blink reflex on the side of interest; if it is greatly diminished in activity as a result of the action of the local anesthetic, the eyelid should be taped down. This diminished activity is transitory, however; if it occurs, the patient should be reassured.

The operator injects a very small amount (0.1 to 0.2 ml) of contrast medium while fluoroscopically observing the joint (Fig. 6-22). If the injected contrast medium appears to be confined to a well-defined joint space, further increments may be injected. Following injection of the lower and then both joint spaces, tomograms are obtained in a serial fashion with the patient's mouth closed and in various stages of jaw opening. At this point, it would be desirable to videotape the fluoroscopic image of the joint in function if the appropriate equipment is available. Following successful radiography of the opacified joint spaces, the operator attempts to aspirate or passively drain the injected contrast medium during opening and closing jaw movements. The angiocatheters are removed from the joint surfaces and inspected to be certain they are intact. Firm pressure with gauze is placed over the TMJ area for 10 minutes and the examination is terminated. An ice bag should also be held over the TMJ area intermittently for the remainder of the day.

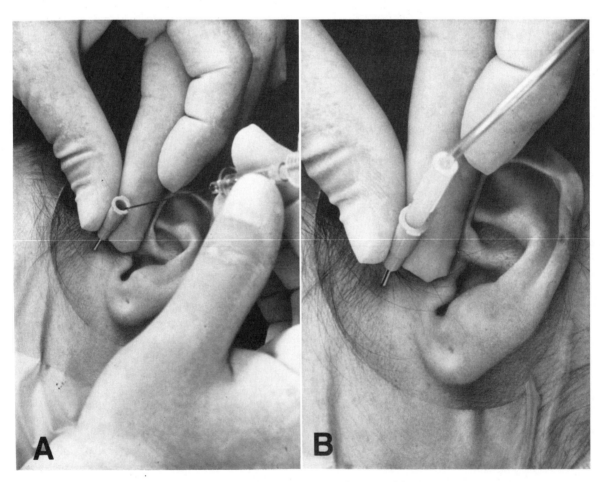

Fig. 6-21. Close-up views of angiocatheter used in TMJ arthrography. **A,** Catheter has been inserted into lower joint space and inner (needle) stylet is being withdrawn. **B,** Attached to catheter hub is adapter for connecting tubing. Joint can now be injected and flexible catheter can remain in place during fluoroscopy and radiography of joint function.

Normal TMJ arthrogram: radiographic anatomy

The articular disc is a fibrocartilaginous wafer that fills most of the space between the condylar head and temporal component and divides the joint into two compartments (actually, potential spaces), one above the other. The disc itself normally occupies only the anterior half of the joint space, with its posterior attachment filling the posterior half (Fig. 6-3). The disc and its posterior attachment are generally referred to as the soft tissue component of the TMJ.

If the disc were to be sectioned sagittally through its center portion and the medial half viewed from the side, it would appear as the biconcave structure seen in Fig. 6-3, *B*. The thin portion in the middle is the area of the disc that normally serves as the articulating cushion between the condylar head and the articular eminence. As the condyle translates forward, the disc also moves forward so that the thin central portion remains between the condylar head and articular eminence. Tension in the elastic posterior attachment is thought to be responsible for the smooth recoil of the disc posteriorly as the jaw closes. The thick posterior portion of the disc merges imperceptibly with the posterior ligamentous attachment and fills the entire space between the superior condylar convexity and the deepest concavity of the articular fossa.

The disc and its posterior attachment provide absolute separation of the upper and lower joint spaces in normal subjects. There is no known normal situation or developmental abnormality in which a communication exists between the two TMJ spaces.[12] The joint spaces as they appear on a normal TMJ arthrogram are shown in Fig. 6-23. (Joint space appearances at arthrography

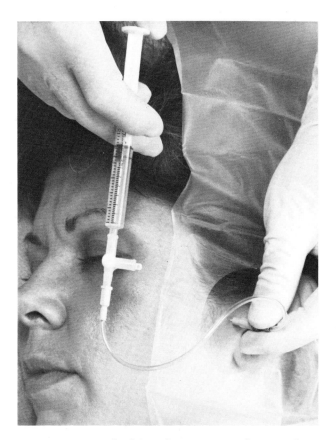

Fig. 6-22. Injection of radiographic contrast medium into lower joint space. As seen here, it is helpful to use connecting tubing and stopcock between indwelling catheter and contrast syringe.

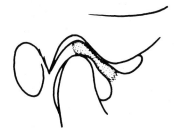
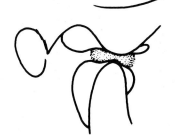
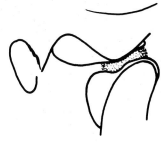

Closed   Partial   Maximum

Fig. 6-23. Normal TMJ arthrographic interpretation represented by drawings. *Left,* With mouth closed, disc (stippled) is positioned between posterior slope of articular eminence and anterior aspect of condylar articulating surface. *Middle,* At partial jaw opening, thin, central portion of disc remains positioned between articulating bony surfaces. *Right,* At maximum jaw opening, disc is still interposed between bony articulation. Notice in all three drawings that distention of recesses of joint spaces is dependent on condyle position. As condyle translates forward, hydraulic pressure moves contrast medium to posterior recesses. (From Blaschke, D.D., Solberg, W.K., and Sanders, B.: JADA **100:**388, 1980. Copyright by the American Dental Association. Reprinted by permission.)

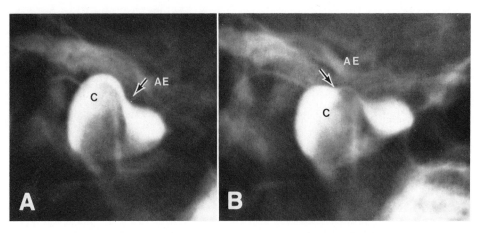

Fig. 6-24. Abnormal TMJ arthrogram, clicking joint. **A,** closed-mouth view. Lower joint space only has been opacified on this plain radiograph. Posterior part of disc is represented by radiolucent convexity *(arrow)* just anterior to condyle head *(C).* This is an abnormal relationship. *AE,* Articular eminence. **B,** Same case at partial mouth opening. Condyle has assumed normal relationship with disc. Notice that thick posterior part of disc *(arrow)* is now in its normal position, just posterior to condyle articulating surface. See also Figs. 6-32 and 6-33.

are somewhat artificial to the extent that such spaces are predominantly potential spaces in the nonarthrographic state). Optimal joint space distension with water-soluble contrast solution during arthrography is not synonymous with the normal physiologic state of the joint spaces. However, arthrography has not yet been shown to alter the morphology of the disc or its posterior attachment nor to alter or unduly influence the anteroposterior position of the disc vis a vis the condyle.

Fig. 6-23 reveals the change in shapes that the joint spaces assume in the normal arthrogram as the condyle and disc translate forward. Notice that on anterior movement of the condyle the contrast medium is forced hydraulically from the anterior recesses to the characteristically shaped posterior recesses. This obliteration of the anterior recesses at full opening is one of the most characteristic findings of the normal arthrogram. The other significant diagnostic feature of the normal arthrogram is the maintenance of the thin portion of the disc between the articulating bony convexities during joint function. A typical abnormal arthrogram is illustrated in Fig. 6-24.

□ Pathologic conditions
■ Developmental

Developmental defects of the TMJ can be broadly categorized as anomalies of either underdevelopment or overdevelopment. In both conditions, the most striking radiographic changes in the TMJ are usually seen in the condylar process, although the opposing articular surface of the temporal bone may also be deformed. Be-

cause the condylar articular cartilage is roughly the equivalent of an epiphyseal plate in the mandible, developmental abnormalities at this site may additionally be manifested by altered growth patterns of the mandibular ramus, body, and even the alveolar processes on the affected side.

Underdevelopment (hypoplasia) of the condyle is generally manifested radiographically by a reduction in size of the condylar process but with substantial preservation of its normal shape (Fig. 6-25). Mandibular growth deficiencies usually closely parallel the degree of condylar hypoplasia. Such cases are typically associated with decreased mandibular height and length. The radiographic appearance of the condyle and mandible is dependent not only on the severity and duration of the cause but also on the age of the patient at the time of involvement.

In certain prenatal conditions manifesting condylar underdevelopment, such as hemifacial microsomia and Treacher Collins syndrome, aural and zygomatic anomalies may also be radiographically apparent. Ossicular defects may even be appreciated if complex motion tomography is used. Antegonial notching of the mandible may be seen in certain of these developmental abnormalities, such as Treacher Collins syndrome, hemifacial microsomia, and congenital deformity of the condyle.[2]

Overdevelopment (hyperplasia) of the mandibular condyle (Fig. 6-26) may be local or systemic in origin and may occur either as a solitary event or as part of a larger growth abnormality. Overgrowth not associated with systemic causes, such as hyperpituitarism (giant-

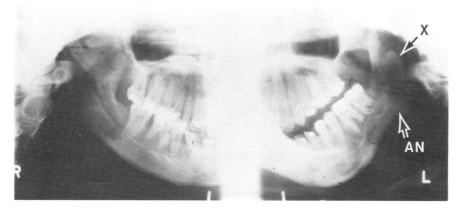

Fig. 6-25. Aplasia of left condyle, leading to left mandibular hypoplasia and marked left mandibular antegonial notching *(AN)*. X marks area of missing left condyle. (Courtesy B. Sarnat, M.D., Los Angeles).

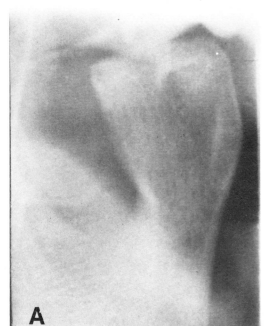

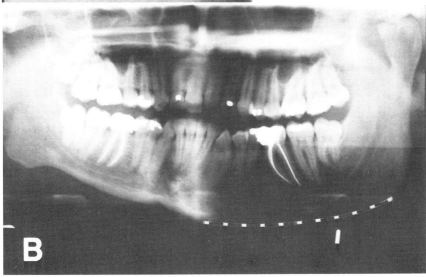

Fig. 6-26. Hyperplasia of the left condylar process. **A,** Notice altered, box-like shape of condyle. **B,** Panoramic view of same case. Hemimandibular hypertrophy (right side of illustration) has been caused by increased condylar growth. Dashes indicate inferior mandibular border.

ism in children, acromegaly in adults) is virtually always unilateral.

The diagnostic differentiation between hyperplasia and neoplasm (e.g., osteochondroma) of the condyle may be impossible to make without critical radiographic evaluation. Osteochondroma usually appears as a focal growth or mass without other associated abnormality. Radiographically, hyperplasia appears as a generalized enlargement of the condylar process, with or without some distortion in the shape of the process itself. Although it is common for the hyperplastic condyle to have an abnormal contour, normal cortical thickness and trabecular pattern are usually present. The hyperplastic abnormality may be confined to the condyle, but it is more common for the condylar neck to also be enlarged because of bone remodeling. Lengthening of the mandibular ramus is typically associated with condylar hyperplasia.

■ Trauma

Trauma to the TMJ may, as with other joints, result in a joint *effusion*. No definitive correlation of such a clinical diagnosis with an increase in the radiographically visualized TMJ space has been documented.

Dislocation results when the condyle is forcefully displaced out of the articular fossa but remains within the capsular confines of the joint. It is important to recognize that in some normal patients the mandibular condyle may be situated well forward of the eminence in the open-mouth position. On the other hand, clinical dislocation is sometimes present when the condyle is situated only slightly anterior to the eminence. Wide variation in the normal degree of movement during jaw-opening maneuvers makes the diagnosis of dislocation on the basis of radiographic findings alone inherently hazardous.

Unilateral condylar *fracture* is much more common than the bilateral fracture (Fig. 6-27). If a condylar fracture is diagnosed, appropriate radiographs must be carefully evaluated to rule out coexisting occult fractures of the skull base or other portions of the mandible.

Condylar fractures are often clinically described as intra- or extracapsular. The former are quite infrequent. Because the joint capsule cannot be identified on plain films, the radiologist should not describe condylar fractures as intra- or extracapsular. Although this differentiation is definitely of clinical importance, the

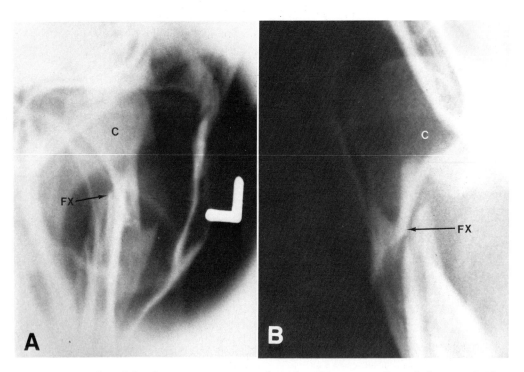

Fig. 6-27. Subcondylar fractures as seen on frontal radiogram. **A,** Typical fracture *(FX)* through condylar neck, caused by severe, direct blow to chin point. *C*, Condyle. **B,** Different case, showing essentially the same finding of oblique fracture line *(FX)* through condylar neck. (From Blaschke, D.D., and White, S.C. In Sarnat, B.G., and Laskin, D.M.: The temporomandibular joint: a biologic basis for clinical practice, ed. 3, 1980. Courtesy of Charles C Thomas, Publisher, Springfield, Illinois.)

defects are best described radiographically as either (1) condylar and high condylar neck fractures or (2) fractures of the low condylar neck. Some condylar fractures are seen only with high quality tomography. Rarely, a condyle may be split in the sagittal plane, with the defect seen only on frontal projections.

Approximately 60% of condylar fractures show some evidence of fragment angulation and a variable degree of displacement.[25] If displacement is present, it is characteristically seen as anterior and medial deviation of the condylar fragment, produced by contraction of the lateral pterygoid muscle (see Chapter 7).

■ Arthritis

Degenerative joint disease (DJD, osteoarthritis, arthrosis) increases in incidence with advancing age. Early degenerative arthritis may either have no radio-graphic manifestations or appear as mild joint space narrowing.

Autopsy studies on young TMJs have revealed that the normal condylar articulating surfaces are very smooth and regular in form. A tendency toward articular surface flattening is indicative of a prearthrotic lesion and is often associated with stressful loading of the TMJ secondary to lost posterior tooth support or increasing age. Recent studies also indicate that internal joint derangements related to meniscal dysfunction may be an important causative factor in TMJ arthritis.[14a]

Small bony outgrowths (osteophytes or spurs) are the radiographic hallmark of degenerative disease (Fig. 6-28). They are most obvious when seen protruding from the anterior or superior aspect of the condyle into the joint space. They are not as easily appreciated when they occur on the articular fossa side of the joint space.

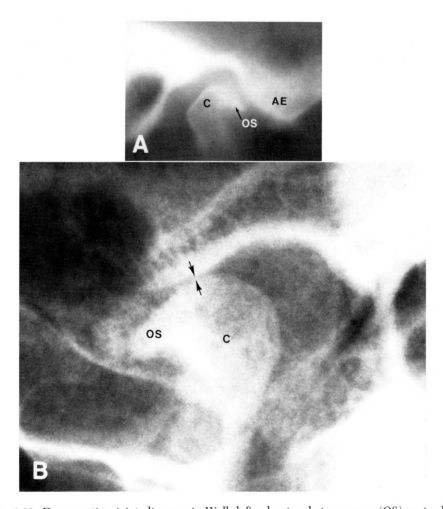

Fig. 6-28. Degenerative joint disease. **A,** Well-defined osteophyte or spur *(OS)* protrudes from anterior surface of condyle *(C)*. Notice also slight flattening of posterior surface of articular eminence *(AE)*. **B,** Another example of large osteophyte *(OS)* on anterior condyle *(C)* surface, here seen on transcranial radiography. Notice considerable narrowing of joint space with articulating bony surfaces almost touching at arrows.

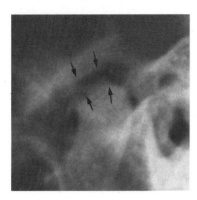

Fig. 6-29. Degenerative joint disease of TMJ. Marked subchondral sclerosis *(arrows)* is apparent at condylar and temporal components of joint. There is also severe flattening of posterior articular eminence slope.

As the articular surface becomes worn and thinned, the condyle becomes flattened (Fig. 6-29). Flattening is most obvious along its anterosuperior surface. The posterior aspect of the articular eminence may also flatten, appearing reduced in height with the articular fossa considerably shallowed. The density of the bony surfaces becomes noticeably increased because of sclerosis of subchondral bone. With disease progression, further narrowing or complete obliteration of the joint space may be seen, as may minimal to severe limitation of motion. Worth[33] notes that bony ankylosis does not complicate this form of arthritis. Minute areas of fibrous tissue near the bony surface (pseudocysts) may occasionally be identified.

Rheumatoid arthritis has almost always been diagnosed in the small joints of the hand and feet by the time any temporomandibular involvement is detected. The radiologist may be asked to confirm the presence of TMJ disease and determine the degree of involvement. Several investigators have recently noted that the TMJ is affected by this disease more often than generally suspected.[5,10,11,20] In an unselected population of patients with confirmed rheumatoid arthritis, over three fourths showed some TMJ changes.[5]

The most common radiographic manifestation of rheumatoid arthritis involving the TMJ is flattening of the condylar head. The next most common finding is frank erosion, followed by reduced mobility of the condyle. The latter feature is related to the duration of joint disease. Condylar erosions are present in about two thirds of those cases showing radiographic abnormalities. They are most common on the antero-superior surface although they may also be seen on both the superior and posterior surfaces. Spurlike proliferations of bone (osteophytes) are less commonly identified, although they are also a well-known finding. These entities represent a degenerative element complicating the inflammatory process, identical to those seen in degenerative arthritis. Spurs are more evident in severe or long-standing rheumatoid disease.

As rheumatoid destruction progresses, the condylar cortex becomes increasingly irregular and ragged. Advanced disease has been described as the "sharpened pencil deformity"[26] or likened to the "mouthpiece of a flute."[30] This characteristic radiographic picture is a result of extensive erosions on the anterior and posterior condylar surfaces at the synovial lining attachments. The situation is analogous to preferential rheumatoid erosion of the metacarpal heads at their synovial attachments. Anterior positioning of the condyle within the articular fossa becomes increasingly prominent. In the most severe cases, the condyle may be completely resorbed, although function can remain surprisingly satisfactory. Rheumatoid arthritis typically affects both TMJs relatively symmetrically.

According to Chalmers and Blair,[5] several radiographic findings, which in the past have been popularly associated with rheumatoid arthritis of the TMJ, are actually quite rare. These authors found TMJ space narrowing in only 0.5% of confirmed rheumatoid arthritis patients. Ankylosis was not seen in any of the joints.

Juvenile rheumatoid arthritis (Still's disease) produces radiographic TMJ changes similar to those identified with the adult variety. In addition, the juvenile disease form may cause interference with normal condylar growth, leading to a characteristic micrognathia. Restricted mandibular movement may also develop, with little or no condylar translation noted on opening. Still's disease with TMJ involvement has been reported, in which persistent and gradual deterioration of jaw movements culminated in complete TMJ ankylosis.[16]

Ankylosing spondylitis of the TMJ has been described by Resnick.[24] When present, both TMJs are usually affected. Davidson and associates[7] have noted that this disease produced TMJ abnormalities less often and at a later stage than rheumatoid arthritis.[7] Joint space narrowing, erosions (especially at the anterosuperior aspect), and restricted anterior movement of the condyle are the radiographic features most often cited.

Infectious arthritis of the TMJ occurs less frequently than degenerative and rheumatoid arthritis. This disease may be caused by direct spread of organisms from an infected mastoid process or tympanic cavity or (more commonly) by way of the blood from a distant nidus.[17] Early stages of the disease may lack radiographic manifestations. Some authors contend that the joint space may be increased by the inflammatory exudate in the early infective period.[33] Bony changes are seen later, usually no sooner than 7 to 10 days following the onset of the clinical symptoms.

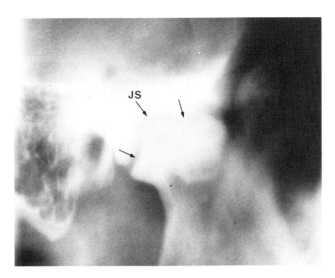

Fig. 6-30. Ankylosis of TMJ resulting from trauma sustained during childhood. Florid overgrowth of bone on both sides of joint has caused obliteration of joint space in segments. There was complete restriction of movement at this joint. Patient could open mouth approximately 4 mm between front teeth. *JS*, Remnants of radiolucent joint space. (From Blaschke, D.D., and White, S.C. In Sarnat, B.G., and Laskin, D.M.: The temporomandibular joint: a biologic basis for clinical practice, ed. 3, 1980. Courtesy of Charles C Thomas, Publisher, Springfield, Illinois.)

Because of the osteolytic effects of infection, the condylar articular cortex may appear slightly radiolucent. Discontinuities or subtle irregularities of the anterior cortical surface are important radiographic findings. Osteoporosis of the adjacent parts of the condyloid process or mandibular ramus may be seen in the acute phase. Later radiographic features include peripheral condensing osteitis and approximation of the joint surface as the articular cartilage is eroded.

■ Ankylosis

TMJ ankylosis is a relatively rare disability. True joint ankylosis is intra-articular in nature; false ankylosis is extra-articular, usually secondary to fibrous or bony union between the coronoid process and either the posterior maxilla or the zygomatic arch. In false ankylosis the radiographic appearance of the TMJ is normal.

True ankylosis may be caused by a *fibrous* union of joint parts resulting from previous arthritis or traumatic injury. Such fibrous adhesions cannot be detected radiographically. A true *bony* ankylosis within the joint may be present, with the joint space itself either partially or completely obliterated (Fig. 6-30). A large mass of new bone obscuring the condyle as well as the joint space can sometimes be seen. Occasionally, it extends into the region of the condylar neck. Free movement of the affected condyle is impossible in such cases, al-

though the patient may be able to produce several millimeters of interincisal opening.

TMJ ankylosis is a disturbance primarily of young persons. El-Mofty[9] studied 39 cases of TMJ ankylosis and noted that 50% occurred in patients between 1 and 10 years of age, a finding in general agreement with other investigators. Most cases in this study were caused by trauma, some were a result of infectious arthritis, and only two were secondary to rheumatoid arthritis. Significantly, no radiographic differences could be detected between those cases caused by trauma and those resulting from infection. The most common cause of bilateral TMJ ankylosis is rheumatoid arthritis, although bilateral fractures may also produce this result. Worth[33] contends that most, if not all, cases of TMJ ankylosis in infancy are secondary to birth injury.

If TMJ ankylosis occurs before the completion of mandibular growth, development of the affected side of the jaw is inhibited. Some degree of mandibular asymmetry is present, with the severity depending on the patient's age at the onset of the condylar damage. An important and consistent radiographic finding in these cases is the presence of a prominent antegonial notch on the affected side of the mandible.

■ Tumors

Benign and malignant neoplastic lesions originating in or involving the TMJ are rare. Most case reports of tumors in this region give only perfunctory descriptions of the radiographic findings. The possibility for more definitive radiographic criteria of TMJ tumors has become enhanced recently because of the wider availability and use of tomographic equipment and standardized techniques.

Benign tumors involving the TMJ include osteoma, osteochondroma, chondroma, chondroblastoma, fibromyxoma, giant cell reparative granuloma, and synovial chondromatosis. Such tumors in this location are indeed rare. Out of 3200 head and neck tumors seen during a 20-year period, Nwoku and Koch[19] reported only seven confirmed cases of tumor of the condyle, of which three were osteomas and three were reported as benign giant cell tumors.[19]

As discussed previously, the differentiation between condylar osteoma or osteochondroma (Fig. 6-31) and condylar hyperplasia is occasionally difficult. Thoma delineates two possible areas of differentiation: (1) osteochondroma is not as common an abnormality as hyperplasia, and (2) osteochondroma usually appears radiographically as a bulbous, globular enlargement of the condyle, whereas condylar hyperplasia better preserves the characteristic condylar shape and proportions.[23] The radiographic distinction between these two entities is important because different treatment and follow-up considerations may apply.

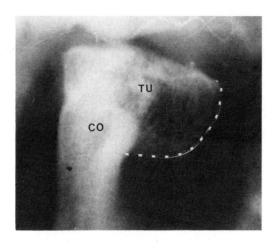

Fig. 6-31. Osteochondroma of right condyle. Bony tumor *(TU)* is seen as lobular mass protruding anteriorly from condyle head *(CO).* (From Blaschke, D.D., and White, S.C. In Sarnat, B.G., and Laskin, D.M.: The temporomandibular joint: a biologic basis for clinical practice, ed. 3, 1980. Courtesy of Charles C Thomas, Publisher, Springfield, Illinois.)

Worth[33] states that osteochondroma of the coronoid process is probably the most common tumor in the region of the TMJ, although he concedes that it too is rare. James et al.[13] could find only 16 reported cases of this coronoid tumor in the literature and added one case of their own. The deformity may be seen as a bulbous, mushroom-shaped enlargement of the coronoid process. The lesions usually cause a progressive limitation of mandibular opening. Such a tumor is typically nonpainful and should be considered in cases of false ankylosis in which the TMJs appear radiographically normal.

Benign tumors and cysts of the mandible proper may cause considerable destruction of the ramus. It is striking to note, however, that they so infrequently involve the condyle. For example, ameloblastoma may involve the entire mandibular ramus and yet generally spares the condylar process.

Primary intrinsic *malignant tumors* of the TMJ, which are extremely rare, include chondrosarcoma, synovial sarcoma, and fibrosarcoma of the joint capsule. Richter et al. reviewed the English literature from 1934 to 1973 and found only 38 cases of mandibular chondrosarcoma. Only two of these lesions arose in the TMJ.[21] Primary malignant tumors extrinsic to the joint are generally direct extensions of parotid salivary gland, nasopharyngeal, or other regional carcinomas.

Although malignant processes in this region as a rule destroy bony margins, benign lesions typically do not (with the exception of the rather characteristic erosions of rheumatoid arthritis). Chondrosarcoma may be seen as an indistinct, somewhat radiolucent enlargement of the condyle. These tumors in other skeletal sites are often associated with a characteristic speckled, punctate

type of intrinsic calcification. This particular type of tumor calcification has not been seen in the few reported cases of TMJ chondrosarcoma.[21]

■ Temporomandibular pain and dysfunction

Pain and impaired function are the two predominant characteristics seen in an array of TMJ disorders of unknown cause. Characteristic symptoms include one or more of the following: (1) pain and tenderness in the muscles of mastication and the TMJs, (2) sounds emanating from the joint during condylar movement, and (3) limitation of mandibular movement. The vast majority (70% to 90%) of patients with TMJ pain and dysfunction are women between the ages of 20 and 40 years. Individuals manifesting these clinical features and falling into these age and sex profiles have commonly been grouped together as "TMJ patients." Too often they have been subjected to one-track modes of therapy. Unfortunately, the one disease–one treatment philosophy for the management of TMJ disorders has frequently led to clinical failures. Patients with TMJ-related conditions of diverse causes but with similar symptoms have understandably not all responded favorably to a single form of treatment. Careful clinical examination and analysis of patients with TMJ pain and dysfunction usually permits the differentiation of such cases into the following areas: (1) abnormalities within the TMJs, (2) abnormalities within the muscles of mastication, and (3) abnormalities of the neck (i.e., referred pain).

Patients manifesting symptoms of TMJ pain and limited function are often referred for radiographic evaluation. Knowing the clinician's impression as to whether the problem is primarily centered within the joints, within the muscles of mastication, or within the neck is helpful. Audible TMJ sounds such as clicking or crepitus (a grinding sound), a popping sensation, and palpable TMJ pain (by way of the ear canal) are probably the most reliable indications of intrinsic TMJ alterations.

The two most important subgroups of temporomandibular pain and dysfunction abnormalities are (1) *intrinsic disc derangements within the TMJ*, in which either macro- or microtrauma is assumed to be a prime causal factor, and (2) the so-called *myofascial pain-dysfunction syndrome*, in which muscle spasm, resulting from muscle fatigue that is in turn produced by chronic clenching or nervous grinding of the teeth, is the foremost cause.

Intrinsic disc derangements can be a significant cause of TMJ dysfunction. The basic premise of the internal derangement hypothesis for TMJ pain and dysfunction is that an intracapsular mechanical obstruction prevents the condyle from fully translating anteriorly in the joint, and the consequent pressure of the condyle against the obstruction produces inflammation and pain. The source of such an obstruction is an anteriorly displaced disc, i.e., a disc prolapsed anterior to the condyle. Much less commonly, the disc may be dislocated posterior to the condylar head. The patient is then unable to close his mouth completely because of the posterior obstruction. The precise cause for anterior disc dislocation is not known but it is thought that either a defective posterior attachment or a disequilibrium between the superior and inferior heads of the lateral pterygoid muscle or both are of potential importance.

The normal TMJ arthrographic findings have been described previously. The abnormal arthrographic findings associated with pain-dysfunction cases will be described next, followed by a correlation with the findings seen on prearthrographic lateral tomograms of the TMJ.

The principal findings of TMJ arthrography that indicate internal disc derangement are (1) anterior displacement of the disc in relation to the condyle, (2) communication of the joint spaces as evidenced by the upper-space filling following contrast medium injection into only the lower space, (3) deformation or alteration in the shape of the disc, and (4) thinning of the posterior attachment of the disc.

Fluoroscopic observation and videotape recording of the actual joint space filling and jaw movement sequences may provide as much as or more diagnostic information than arthrographic tomograms. There are two main reasons: (1) the operator may, by seeing both spaces filling on a lower space injection, estimate the degree of soft tissue perforation by the speed of contrast spread into the noninjected upper space; and (2) the operator may be able to evaluate the behavior of the disc at the precise instant the patient experiences a TMJ click during jaw opening. The movement of the disc just before and after a click often happens so quickly that static radiographs cannot supply such dynamic information. The TMJ arthrogram is therefore as much a study of joint function as it is a portrayal of joint morphology.

The articular disc as seen on lateral projection is a biconcave structure. With the jaws closed, the critical posterior thick portion of the disc is normally positioned directly above the vertex of the condyle. The posterior thick portion can usually be identified, even in abnormal states, by arthrography as the thick portion of the disc immediately posterior to the thin portion of the biconcave disc. In persons having pain-dysfunction problems, the thick posterior portion of the disc is positioned anteriorly or anterosuperiorly to the articulating surface of the condyle. In such situations, the condyle does not articulate through the disc (as would be normal) but rather rides the junction between the disc and its posterior attachment.

In such a deranged state of jaw opening, the shearing force of the condylar head against the posterior thick part of the disc may force the latter anteriorly ahead of the former during translation. It is postulated that often there is associated tearing or pathologic stretching of the posterior attachment. The articulating portion of the condylar head may also pop under the posterior thick part of the disc in order to reassume a normal, physiologic articulating relationship between the two. For this latter situation to prevail, the disc presumably remains relatively static while the condylar head negotiates (passes beneath) the bump of the posterior thick rim of the disc. This occurs each time a patient feels a pop and hears a click; the pop and click indicate the precise instant that the condyle passes beneath the rubbery posterior rim of the disc (Figs. 6-32 and 6-33). Fluoroscopically, the disc appears to "squirt" or "slither" posteriorly over the approaching anterosuperior surface of the condylar head, rather than the condyle popping anteriorly under the disc.

If this process of condyle-disc repositioning does not take place early during translation, a limit is soon reached in the shearing or pushing force of the condyle moving the disc increasingly anterior. This point is reached prior to the normal maximal translation position of the condyle because the dislocated disc serves as a mechanical obstruction. At this point, the patient experiences a closed lock* of the condyle and further anterior movement is impossible. On the arthrogram, this occurrence is identified as a partially translated condyle blocked in its path by a radiolucent mass representing the prolapsed disc (Figs. 6-34 and 6-35). Abutment of the condyle against the posterior part of the disc usually produces a visible deformity in the latter. Any degree of deformity, from a pronounced abnormal thickening of the posterior rim to an amorphous rounded mass representing the entire disc, may be seen.

Whereas the changes of internal TMJ disc derangement may progress to frank degenerative changes in both the hard and soft components of the joint, bony changes are usually not seen on prearthrographic tomograms and transcranial radiographs. Careful examination of the lateral and frontal tomograms of these typically young female patients generally shows intact, well-corticated, normally contoured TMJ bony margins with no evidence of intraosseous changes such as reactive sclerosis.

Myofascial pain-dysfunction (MPD) syndrome was described by Laskin in 1969.[15] MPD syndrome has been characterized by unilateral preauricular pain that radiates to the mandibular angle, the temporal area, or the lateral cervical region. Tenderness in the masticatory muscles is a common sign of the condition, presumably caused by muscle spasm. The third most common symptom is a clicking or popping noise in the

---

*Some TMJ clinicians refer to this state of affairs as an "opening lock."

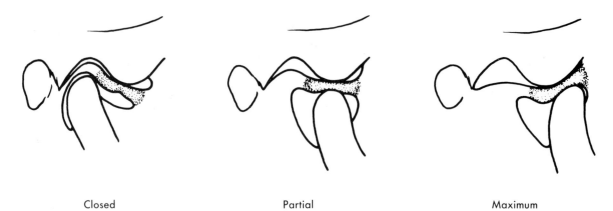

Closed   Partial   Maximum

Fig. 6-32. Drawings of abnormal TMJ arthrography illustrating internal derangement of TMJ, clinically apparent as click during opening condyle movement. Notice that biconcave disc is completely anterior to the condyle *(left)*. At partial opening *(middle)*, condyle assumes normal relationship with disc, at precise time that click is heard clinically. From this point on (right), arthrogram is normal. (From Blaschke, D.D., Solberg, W.K., and Sanders, B.: JADA **100:**388, 1980. Copyright by the American Dental Association. Reprinted by permission.)

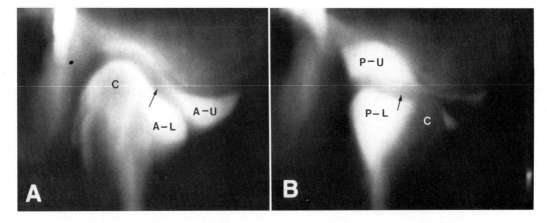

Fig. 6-33. TMJ arthrotomograms, showing mild internal disc derangement. **A,** Tomogram of TMJ showing both upper and lower joint spaces optimally opacified. Radiolucent structure between two pools of contrast is joint soft tissue component, comprised of biconcave articular disc (here slightly displaced anterior to condyle) and posterior attachment. *Arrow,* Posterior part of disc; *AU,* anterior recess of the upper joint space; *AL,* anterior recess of the lower joint space. The two joint spaces do not communicate. **B,** On opening jaws to approximately one finger-breadth interincisal distance, condyle becomes situated beneath thin part of the disc, i.e., normal condyle-disc relationship. By this point in time there has been a clinically evident click but no locking of joint. Posterior part of disc *(arrow)* is now just posterior to actual bony articulation. *PU,* Posterior recess of upper joint space; *PL,* posterior recess of lower joint space. (From Blaschke, D.D., Solberg, W.K., and Sanders, B.: JADA **100:**388, 1980. Copyright by the American Dental Association. Reprinted by permission.)

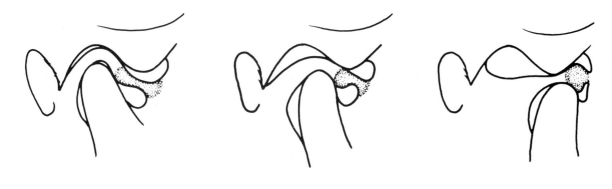

Closed   Partial   Maximum

Fig. 6-34. Abnormal TMJ arthrogram, showing severe internal derangement of TMJ. In this situation, disc *(left)* is severely displaced anteriorly to condyle and remains so *(center* and *right)* during attempts at condyle anterior movement. Clinically, this is manifested as opening lock of condyle (obstruction of its anterior movement) at about one half of normal jaw opening. Notice thick posterior part of disc anterior to condyle articulating surface in all joint positions. This indicates anterior displacement of disc. Contrast medium is not normally extended from anterior joint space recesses. (From Blaschke, D.D., Solberg, W.K., and Sanders, B.: JADA **100:**388, 1980. Copyright by the American Dental Association. Reprinted by permission.)

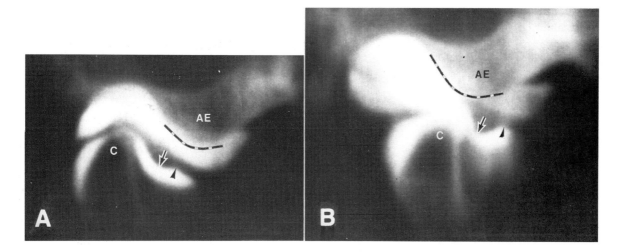

Fig. 6-35. TMJ arthrotomograms, showing severe internal TMJ derangement as evidenced clinically by complete locking of joint at one third normal degree of jaw opening. **A,** Arthrogram shows biconcave disc severely displaced anterior to the condyle *(C),* here with patient's jaws closed. Notice thick posterior part of disc *(arrow)* completely forward of condyle. Condyle normally is situated beneath thin portion *(arrowhead)* of disc. *AE,* articular eminence. **B,** On opening, further condyle *(C)* anterior movement is prevented by mechanical obstruction on part of posterior lip of disc. This radiograph is made at point of patient's maximum (but restricted) mouth opening. Delineation of biconcave shape of disc by contrast pools on its upper and lower surfaces is all-important in determination of anteroposterior position of disc. Shapes of joint spaces themselves provide only secondary information. *AE,* Articular eminence.

TMJ. These patients often have limitation of jaw function evidenced by inability to open the mouth widely or by deviation of the lower jaw on opening. The inclusion of these four cardinal symptoms and signs in the MPD syndrome is primarily of interest to the clinician.

Of importance to the radiologist is the fact that the diagnosis of MPD syndrome is also made by the *exclusion* of radiographic abnormalities in the TMJ. (This latter point is cited by Laskin as support for the belief that the primary site of the problem in MPD syndrome is in the mandibular musculature as opposed to the actual joint structures.) The radiographic examination in such cases is intended to rule out organic TMJ conditions such as degenerative arthritis and to support, by the absence of bony changes, the clinical impression of the psychomuscular abnormality, MPD syndrome.

Although MPD syndrome may eventually lead to degenerative changes within the joint, it probably begins as a functional problem. Proponents of the MPD syndrome believe that masticatory muscle spasm is the primary factor responsible for the clinical features exhibited. The muscle spasm in this region is thought to be most commonly caused by muscle fatigue produced by chronic oral habits such as clenching or grinding of the teeth.

The validity of the MPD syndrome is being questioned with the emergence of TMJ arthrography. The clinical presentation of the typical patient suspected of having the MPD syndrome has recently been shown to be virtually identical to the typical patient manifesting an anteriorly displaced disc at arthrography.[14a,32] It may be that true MPD syndrome exists without TMJ disc displacements in some patients but this is a controversial point at the present time.

□ References

1. Adams, R.J., Murphy, W.A., and Gilula, L.A.: Magnification radiography of the temporomandibular joints, Scientific exhibit, Sixty-fourth scientific assembly and meeting, Radiologic Society of North America, Chicago, November 26-December 1, 1978.
2. Becker, M.H., Coccaro, P.J., and Converse, J.M.: Antegonial notching of the mandible: an often overlooked mandibular deformity in congenital and acquired disorders, Radiology **121**:149-151, 1976.
3. Blaschke, D.D., Solberg, W.K., and Sanders, B.: Arthrography of the temporomandibular joint: review of current status, JADA **100**:388-395, 1980.
4. Blaschke, D.D., and Blaschke, T.J.: Normal TMJ bony relationships in centric occlusion, J. Dent. Res. **60**:98-104, 1981.
5. Chalmers, I.M., and Blair, G.S.: Rheumatoid arthritis of the temporomandibular joint, Q. J. Med. **42**(166):369-386, 1973.
6. Coin, C.G.: Tomography of the temporomandibular joint, Med. Radiogr. Photogr. **50**:26-39, 1974.
7. Davidson, C., Wojtulewski, J.A., Bacon, P.A., and Winstock, D.: Temporomandibular joint disease in ankylosing spondylitis, Ann. Rheum. Dis. **34**:87-91, 1975.
8. Eckerdal, O.: Tomography of the temporomandibular joint, Acta Radiol. (Suppl.) **329**:11, 44-47, 102-104, 1973.
9. El-Mofty, S.: Ankylosis of temporomandibular joint, Oral Surg. **33**:650-660, 1972.

10. Ericson, S., and Lundberg, M.: Alterations in the temporomandibular joint at various stages of rheumatoid arthritis, Acta Rheum. Scand. **13**:257-274, 1967.
11. Franks, A.S.T.: Temporomandibular joint in adult rheumatoid arthritis, Ann. Rheum. Dis. **28**:139-145, 1969.
12. Helms, C.A., Katzberg, R.W., Dolwick, M.F., and Bales, D.J.: Arthrotomographic diagnosis of meniscus perforations in the temporomandibular joint, Br. J. Radiol. **53**:283-285, 1980.
13. James, R.B., Alexander, R.W., and Traver, J.G.: Osteochondroma of the mandibular coronoid process, Oral Surg. **37**:189-195, 1974.
14. Katzberg, R.W., Dolwich, M.F., Helms, C.A., et al.: Arthrotomography of the temporomandibular joint, AJR **134**:995-1003, 1980.
14a. Katzberg, R.W., Kieth, D.A., and Guralnick, W.C.: Internal derangements of the temporomandibular joint, Radiology **146**:170-172, 1983.
15. Laskin, D.M.: Etiology of the pain-dysfunction syndrome, JADA **79**:147-153, 1969.
15a. Manzione, J.V., Seltzer, S.E., and Katzberg, R.W.: Direct sagittal computed tomography of the temporomandibular joint, AJR **140**:165-167, 1983.
16. Martis, C.S., and Karakasis, D.T.: Ankylosis of the temporomandibular joint caused by Still's disease, Oral Surg. **35**:462-466, 1973.
17. Mayne, J.G., and Hatch, G.S.: Arthritis of the temporomandibular joint, JADA **79**:125-130, 1969.
18. Murphy, W.A.: Arthrography of the temporomandibular joint, Radiol. Clin. North Am. **19**:365-378, 1981.
19. Nwoku, A.L.N., and Koch, H.: The temporomandibular joint: a rare localization for bone tumors, J. Maxillofac. Surg. **2**:113-119, 1974.
20. Ogus, H.: Rheumatoid arthritis of the temporomandibular joint, Br. J. Oral Surg. **12**:275-284, 1975.
20a. Osborn, A.G., Hanafee, W.H., and Mancuso, A.A.: Normal and pathologic CT anatomy of the mandible, AJR **139**:555-559, 1982.
21. Richter, K.J., Freeman, N.S., and Quick, C.A.: Chondrosarcoma of the temporomandibular joint: report of case, J. Oral Surg. **32**:777-781, 1974.
22. Ricketts, R.M.: Variations of the temporomandibular joint as revealed by cephalometric laminagraphy, Am. J. Orthod. **36**:877-898, 1950.
23. Reiter, D.: Concepts of dental occlusion, Am. J. Otolaryngol. **1**:245-255, 1980.
24. Resnick, I.: Temporomandibular joint involvement in ankylosing spondylitis, Radiology **112**:587-591, 1974.
25. Rowe, N.L., and Killey, H.C.: Fractures of the facial skeleton, ed. 2, Edinburgh, 1970, E. & S. Livingstone.
26. Simon, G.: Principles of bone x-ray diagnosis, ed. 2, London, 1965, Butterworth & Co. (Publishers), Ltd.
27. Taylor, R.C., Ware, W.H., Fowler, D., and Kobayashi, J.: A study of temporomandibular joint morphology and its relationship to the dentition, Oral Surg. **33**:1002-1013, 1972.
28. Thoma, K.H.: Tumors of the mandibular joint, J. Oral Surg. **22**:157-163, 1964.
30. Uotila, E.: The temporomandibular joint in adult rheumatoid arthritis, Acta Odontol. Scand. (Suppl. 39) **22**:50, 1964.
31. Weinberg, L.A.: What we really see on a TMJ radiograph, J. Prosthet. Dent. **30**:898-913, 1973.
32. Wilkes, C.H.: Arthrography of the temporomandibular joint in patients with the TMJ pain-dysfunction syndrome, Minn. Med. **61**:645-652, 1978.
33. Worth, H.M.: The role of radiological interpretation in disease of the temporomandibular joint, Oral Sci. Rev. **6**:3-51, 1974.
34. Yale, S.H., Allison, B.D., and Hauptfuehrer, J.D.: An epidemiological assessment of mandibular condylar morphology, Oral Surg. **21**:169-177, 1966.

7 □ The mandible and teeth

DONALD P. BLASCHKE and ANNE G. OSBORN

Because radiography of the teeth involves both the mandible and the maxilla, these two bones are subjected to more radiographic examinations than any other bones of the body. Intraoral radiography is an important method for diagnosing dental decay (caries). The jaws are also the sites of many types of developmental, traumatic, inflammatory, and pathologic abnormalities, both odontogenic (dental) and nonodontogenic in nature. Jaw abnormalities need to be critically studied in various radiologic examinations, whether the setting is a dentist's office or a medical radiology department. This chapter is intended to increase the interpretive sophistication of the medical radiologist in examining the lower jaw* and teeth.

We will address both oral and dental radiographic techniques and interpretation. Excluded from the discussion are the maxillary sinuses (see Chapter 1) and the temporomandibular joint (see Chapter 6). Only brief descriptions of the general and clinical features of pathologic entities are practical for this chapter. Authoritative oral pathology texts are available that give detailed information to the interested reader.[21,45,54]

□ Historical perspective

The first reported dental x-ray image was made by Dr. Otto Walkhoff in Germany in 1896, only 2 weeks after W.C. Roentgen announced the discovery of x-rays.[33] Early dental x-ray images were made on small plates of glass coated with photographic emulsion, wrapped in black paper and rubber sheets, and placed in the mouth. Within 6 months of Roentgen's discovery Dr. C. Edmund Kells of New Orleans made the first dental x-ray images in the United States. By 1909 Raper had established the first regular course in dental radiography.[5] Dr. Raper predicted that radiography would ultimately be used by the general dentist, an

amazing and controversial pronouncement at the time. One of the first textbooks on dental radiography, *Elementary and Dental Radiography*, appeared in 1913. By 1923 the invention of the shockproof dental x-ray machine, incorporating a Coolidge tube, had induced many dentists to purchase such a device. By 1929 one dentist in three owned radiographic equipment.[5]

Other significant milestones in oral and maxillofacial radiology include the development of cephalometric and panoramic radiography. Cephalometric radiography was introduced in 1922 by Pacini. Cephalometry provided a reproducible, accurate measure of the facial skeletal structures on lateral radiographic projections. The cephalostat, a device that permitted standardized fixation and orientation of a patient's head during radiography, was invented in 1931. Because of the reproducibility the cephalostat afforded, it became possible to superimpose serial lateral skull radiographs (or their tracings). This in turn gave dentists the ability to detect and measure true growth and development of the jaws on consecutive radiographs.

The theory of producing a curved tomographic (i.e., panoramic) radiograph of the dental arches was first proposed by Heckman in 1939, although he was never able to produce a workable panoramic radiographic machine.[36] Paatero succeeded in applying Heckman's concept to a clinical apparatus in 1951.[41] Panoramic x-ray technology has since developed to the point that the teeth and jaws can now be visualized on a single film with reasonably sharp definition.

□ Gross anatomy

A rudimentary review of bony and dental gross anatomy is presented here. A more detailed discussion of radiographic anatomy follows.

■ The mandible and teeth

The mandible or lower jaw is a horseshoe-shaped bony arch that supports a row of teeth anteriorly and

---

*Although the maxilla is also called the upper jaw, when the term *jaw* is used in this chapter it will refer to the mandible alone.

articulating processes posteriorly (Fig. 7-1, *A*). Each side of the mandible has two main components, a horizontal *body* and a vertical *ramus* (Fig. 7-1, *B*). Although the two halves of the mandible are separated at the midline by a synchondrosis until about the first year of life, it is conventional to refer to the lower jaw as a single bone. If all or some of the teeth are present, the jaw is dentulous; if no teeth are present, the jaw is edentulous. The portions of the lower and upper jaws that surround and support the teeth are called the alveolar processes. They are also sometimes referred to as the dental arches.

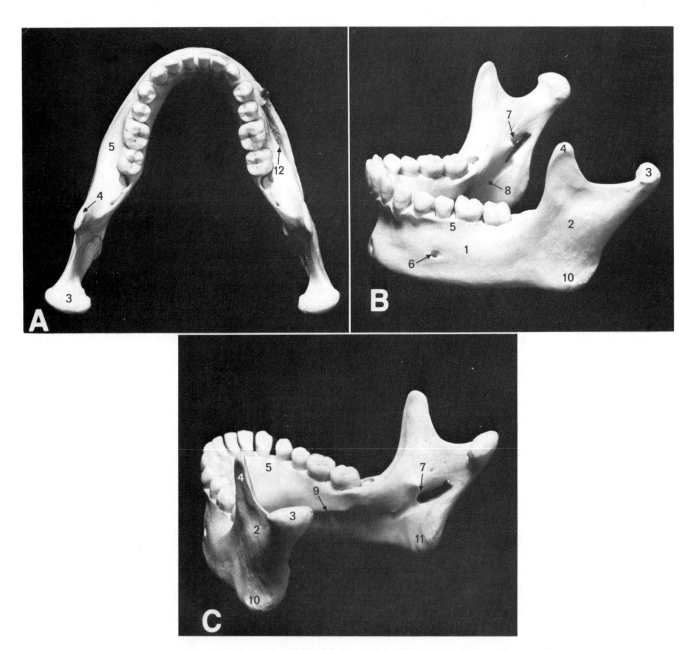

Fig. 7-1. Superior, lateral, and posterior oblique views of dried mandible with normal complement of teeth (third molars are unerupted). Mandible is horseshoe-shaped structure supporting teeth and having processes for masticatory muscle attachments and for articulation with skull base. *1*, Mandibular body; *2*, mandibular ramus; *3*, condyle; *4*, coronoid process; *5*, alveolar process; *6*, mental foramen; *7*, mandibular foramen; *8*, submandibular fossa; *9*, mylohyoid ridge; *10*, angle, masseter muscle side; *11*, angle, medial pterygoid muscle side; *12*, cut surface of bone for display purposes.

The ramus supports the *condylar process* and the *coronoid process*. The condylar process articulates with the skull base. The temporalis muscle attaches to the coronoid process. The *angle* is the posteroinferior corner of the mandible where the body joins the ramus. Two major muscles of mastication (the masseter and the medial pterygoid) attach to this portion of the bone, producing a noticeable ridging of the inferior cortex. The neurovascular bundle carrying the mandibular nerve and vasculature enters the bone at the *mandibular foramen*, which is situated approximately at the geographic center of the lingual surface of the ramus (Fig. 7-1, *C*).

The body of the mandible encloses the *mandibular canal*, which in turn houses the neurovascular bundle. The major portion of this canal terminates anteriorly at the *mental foramen*. On the lingual surface of the mandibular body there is a broad depression in the bone below the *mylohyoid line*, which accommodates the sublingual and submandibular salivary glands (Fig. 7-2).

The normal deciduous (primary) dentition of children contains 20 teeth. The mandibular and maxillary dental arches each support 10 teeth (Fig. 7-3, *A*). There are 32 teeth in the normal complement of the adult permanent (secondary) dentition, 16 in each of the two arches with eight in each division known as a *dental quadrant*. Each quadrant of permanent teeth consists of two incisors, one canine, two premolars, and three molars (Fig. 7-3, *B*). The most posterior molar in each quadrant is often called the "wisdom tooth." Anterior teeth have only a single root; posterior teeth have mul-

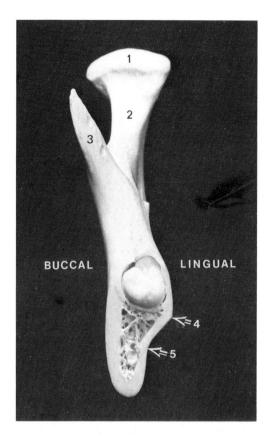

Fig. 7-2. Coronal section of right side of mandible at third molar region, seen on anterior view. *Left*, Buccal surface; *right*, lingual surface. Note varying buccal-lingual bone thickness. Concavity on lingual surface accomodates submandibular gland. Third molar is embedded in bone. *1*, Condyle; *2*, neck of condyle; *3*, coronoid process; *4*, mylohyoid ridge; *5*, submandibular fossa.

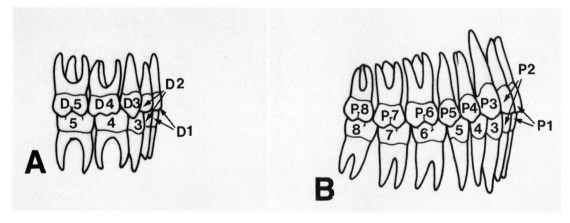

Fig. 7-3. Lateral view of teeth in occlusion, as seen without supporting bone. **A,** Deciduous (primary) dentition. *D1*, Central incisor; *D2*, lateral incisor; *D3*, canine; *D4*, first molar; *D5*, second molar. **B,** Permanent (secondary) dentition. *P1*, Central insicor; *P2*, lateral incisor; *P3*, canine; *P4*, first premolar; *P5*, second premolar; *P6*, first molar; *P7*, second molar; *P8*, third molar. (Redrawn from Massler, M., and Schour, I.: Atlas of the mouth in health and disease, ed. 2, Chicago, 1958, American Dental Association. Copyright by the American Dental Association. Reprinted by permission.)

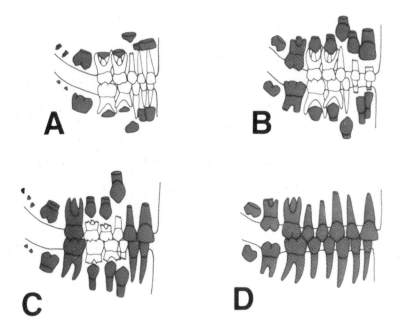

Fig. 7-4. Development and eruption sequence for deciduous and permanent dentitions. Lightly shaded teeth are deciduous; heavily shaded teeth are permanent. Ages given roughly correspond to state of dental development shown. **A,** Deciduous dentition stage (3 years ± 6 months). **B,** Beginning of mixed dentition stage (6 years ± 9 months). **C,** Middle of mixed dentition stage (9 years ± 9 months). **D,** Beginning of permanent dentition stage (12 years ± 9 months). (Redrawn from Massler, M. and Schour, I.: Atlas of the mouth in health and disease, ed. 2, Chicago, 1958, American Dental Association. Copyright by the American Dental Association. Reprinted by permission.)

tiple roots (the premolars and mandibular molars have two roots and the maxillary molars have three). The tips of the roots are referred to as the *root apices.*

■ The dental eruption sequence

A child between the approximate ages of 9 months and 6 years is in the primary dentition stage. This means that some or all of the primary (deciduous) teeth will normally have erupted into the oral cavity (Fig. 7-4, *A*). Between the ages of 6 and 12 years the child is in the mixed dentition stage and has both primary and several secondary (permanent) teeth in the oral cavity (Figs. 7-4, *B* and *C,* 7-5, and 7-6). At about age 12, the last of the primary teeth usually have been shed (exfoliated). During adolescence, the secondary dentition stage provides the individual with a full complement of 32 permanent teeth (Fig. 7-4, *D*). The latest of these, the third molars or wisdom teeth, will not normally erupt until ages 18 to 22 and then only if there is sufficient room in the dental arches. Most persons with a full complement of erupted teeth will have at least one impacted wisdom tooth because of a lack of available space in the dental arches.

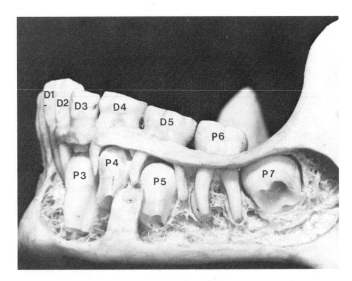

Fig. 7-5. Cutaway view of dried mandible from approximately 9-year-old child. Buccal cortex has been removed to expose roots of deciduous teeth and developing crowns of permanent teeth. Only first molar of permanent teeth has erupted. Deciduous teeth: *D1,* central incisor; *D2,* lateral incisor; *D3,* canine; *D4,* first molar; *D5,* second molar. Permanent teeth: *P3,* Canine; *P4,* first premolar; *P5,* second premolar; *P6,* first molar; *P7,* second molar.

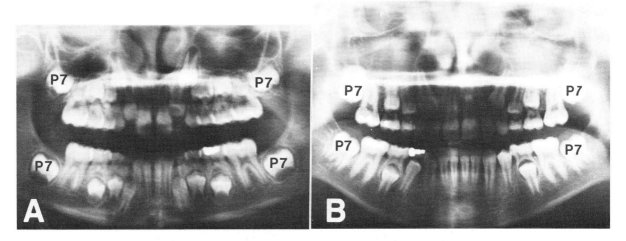

Fig. 7-6. Developing permanent dentition in panoramic view. **A,** 7-year-old child. Unerupted permanent second molar teeth *(P7)* have completed crown formation and are just beginning root formation. **B,** Eleven-year-old child. Note degree of root formation of teeth *(P7)* in comparison with **A.** Within a year these teeth will have erupted into oral cavity.

■ The maxilla

The *hard palate* is the part of the maxilla that separates the oral and nasal cavities. Three bony canals traverse parts of the maxilla and can be visualized radiographically: the midline *incisive (nasopalatine) canal* and the bilateral *nasolacrimal canals.* The incisive foramen is situated at the anterior aspect of the hard palate near the alveolar process. In the posterior maxilla, bilateral bony buttresses called the *zygomatic processes* are usually pneumatized to a slight degree by extensions of the maxillary sinuses. The *alveolar process* supports the teeth.

□ **Technical considerations**

Intra- and extraoral radiographic projections of the jaws are described here. Panoramic radiography, the single most useful radiographic projection for examining the jaws as a whole, will also be discussed. Linear and complex motion tomography are generally not as informative as panoramic and intraoral radiography in assessing changes within the mandible. The former will therefore not be covered in this section.

■ The mandibular series

Lateral oblique projection

The lateral oblique projection of the mandible is both the most common and the most useful of the conventional mandibular projections. This projection is made using a medical or dental x-ray machine and a relatively small (5 × 7 inches) film cassette. The patient holds the cassette to the side of the lower jaw, over the area of interest (Fig. 7-7, *A*). The x-ray tube is then positioned on the opposite side of the face, with the beam-directing cone at a point just below the angle of the mandible. The tube is angled 30° cranially, with the central beam directed toward the area of interest (Fig. 7-7, *B*). Cranial angulation allows the beam to pass below the ipsilateral, uninvolved side of the mandible and thereby avoid bony superimposition. Because the film cassette is directly adjacent to the side of interest, distortion and magnification are insignificant. This projection is simple to perform and provides consistently good visualization of a large area of mandible and teeth (Fig. 7-7, *C*).

Posteroanterior projection

The conventional frontal projection of the lower jaw is normally made posteroanteriorly in order to maximize image definition and minimize magnification. The PA projection of the mandible complements the lateral oblique projection. Technical factors and patient head position are similar to the standard PA skull or facial projections. When the mandible is the sole area of clinical interest, the central x-ray beam should coincide with the mandibular midline and the beam should be collimated so that extraneous bone and soft tissue areas are not exposed (Fig. 7-8, *A*). The term *PA of the mandible* basically refers to a frontal projection of the lower face (Fig. 7-8, *B*). The patient's head position should be free of rotation and the cervical spine should be straight. Even slight head rotation or lateral head tilt will make the evaluation of mandibular symmetry more difficult. As seen from the side, the PA projection of the mandible will normally be made with the head at a neutral tilt (i.e., Caldwell position). The Caldwell head

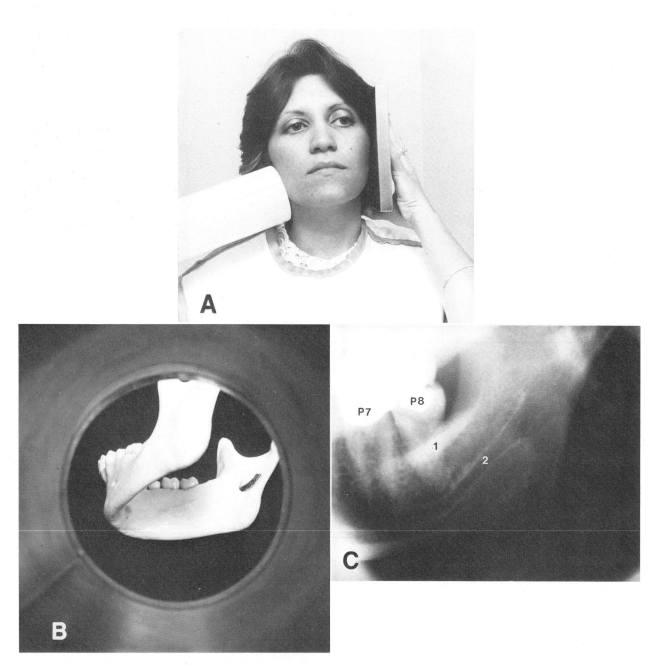

Fig. 7-7. Technique for lateral oblique projection of mandible. **A,** Patient holds 5 × 7 inch cassette against face. Central x-ray beam is angled cranially approximately 35° and enters at point just below mandibular angle. **B,** Lateral oblique projection, looking down x-ray cylinder toward object. This displays bony anatomy, which corresponds to x-ray projection. **C,** Normal lateral oblique radiograph of right mandibular ramus. Two teeth, *P7* and *P8* (second and third molars), are seen. Two bony structures, one opaque and one lucent, stand out: *1,* internal oblique line, and *2,* mandibular canal.

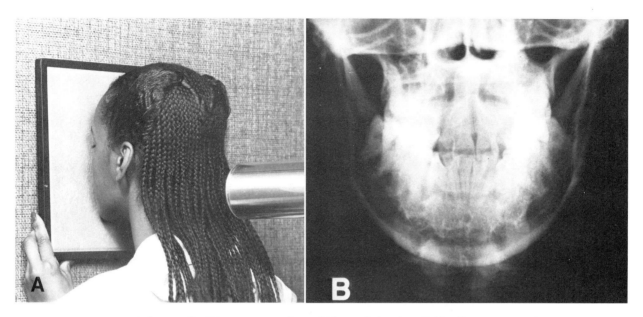

Fig. 7-8. Technique for PA projection of mandible, with head in Caldwell position. **A,** Cassette may be held by patient. PA projections are preferred over AP projections for this area. **B,** PA radiograph of mandible, with head in Caldwell position. Note upper cervical spine faintly superimposed over anterior mandible. Towne PA head positions are generally preferred for ramus and condyle visualization.

position is especially useful if fractures or bony lesions in the mandibular body or symphysis are suspected. The Towne head position better delineates changes in the rami and condylar processes. The Waters facial projection is virtually useless for mandibular and interpretation because the superimposed petrous ridges obliterate almost all mandibular detail, with the exception (occasionally) of the condylar articulating surfaces.

■ Panoramic radiography

Panoramic x-ray machines are becoming increasingly widespread in dental clinics and offices. Most hospitals now also have similar units that are often situated in the dental or oral surgery department, but that may also be found in the radiology department. The utility of the panoramic x-ray machine is highly specific: it can only make curved-plane tomograms of the middle and lower face. However, the modern machine is so proficient at this specific task that many radiologists are beginning to appreciate its value, as dentists have for many years. The panoramic x-ray machine is central to the practice of oral radiology and is heavily used by the practitioners of several dental specialties. For an in-depth discussion of the concepts, principals, and technical considerations of panoramic radiography, the reader is referred to Manson-Hing's text.[36]

On a single panoramic exposure, visualization of all the teeth in the jaws, erupted and unerupted, as well as coverage of the two jaws with virtually complete outlines is possible. The posterior portions of the jaws are seen in a lateral projection, with frontal visualization of the anterior segment. The panoramic examination thus duplicates the coverage of the conventional mandibular series but provides less image superimposition and improved bony detail. The panoramic examination can be produced in about one third the time required to produce the mandibular series.

Although several panoramic x-ray devices are designed to be used with standing patients, other models are flexible enough to accommodate sitting patients or those in wheelchairs. One model has even been designed for use with supine conscious or unconscious patients in hospital emergency rooms.*

The basic design of a typical panoramic x-ray machine (Fig. 7-9, *A* and *B*) is that of synchronous and reciprocal movement of the x-ray tube and film cassette around the lower region of the patient's head. The curved plane of focus is engineered to correspond to the size and shape of the average dental arch. The curved focal plane (or "focal trough") (Fig. 7-9, *C*) requires multiple centers or fulcrums of tomographic rotation; panoramic x-ray machines typically employ two or three such rotation centers. From the technical standpoint, it is nec-

*Tomorex panoramic x-ray machine, S.S. White Corp., Division of Pennwalt Corp., Philadelphia, Pa.

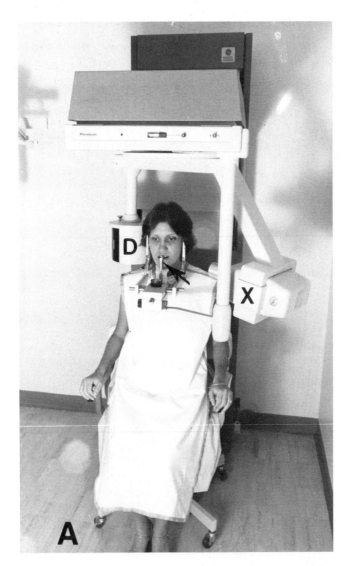

Fig. 7-9. Technique for panoramic radiography. **A,** Patient, draped with lead apron, is seated in machine chair. Patient's head is stabilized between two vertical plastic bars. Bite block (*arrow*) is inserted between front teeth to position dental arches in focal trough. X-ray tube-head (*X*) revolves around front of patient during exposure; drum containing film (*D*) revolves around back of patient's head. Machine shown is GE Panelipse.

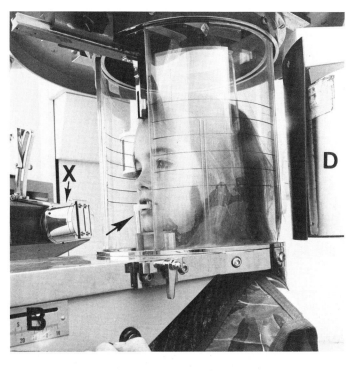

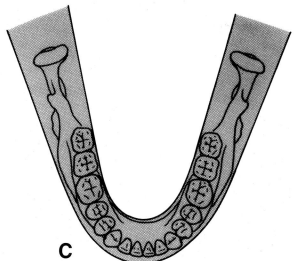

Fig. 7-9, cont'd. B, Patient standing for different type of panoramic x-ray machine. Notice small white bite block *(arrow)* held between incisor teeth. X-ray tubehead *(X)* swings around back of head during exposure; drum containing film *(D)* swings around front of patient. Machine shown is Siemens Orthopantomograph. **C,** Artist's rendition of focal trough of typical panoramic machine, projected over superior view of mandible. Structures within dark stippled area will be projected in tomographic focus. (**B** from Sanders, B.: Pediatric oral and maxillofacial surgery, St. Louis, 1979, The C.V. Mosby Co.)

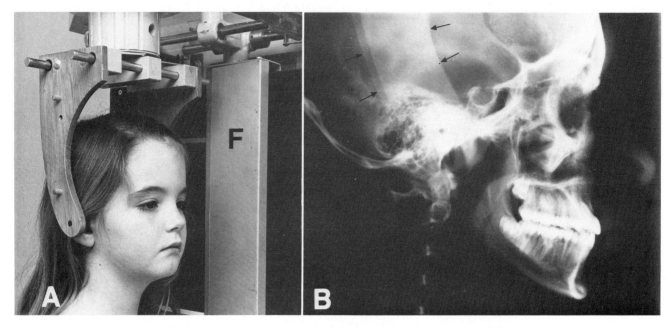

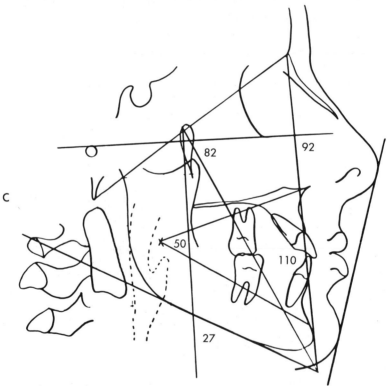

Fig. 7-10. Technique for lateral cephalometric radiography of facial bones. **A,** Patient is shown with head stabilized by cephalostat. Blunt plastic ear rods (not shown) inserted in external auditory canals prevent head rotation and lateral head tilt. Central x-ray beam is aligned to precisely pass through ear rods. Aluminum wedge filter *(F)*, placed over anterior part of the film-holding device, may be used to display soft tissue profile on image. **B,** Cephalometric lateral skull radiograph of different patient. This is essentially pure lateral projection of facial bones. Anterior soft tissue profile of nose is faintly seen. Wooden head positioning bars are projected over temporal bones *(arrows)*. Teeth must be in occlusion. For better example of soft tissue profile see Fig. 7-38. **C,** Cephalometric tracing from **B.** Growth of jaws in relation to skull and other facial bones is calculated by measuring various distances and angles between standard anthropometric landmarks. (**A** from Sanders, B.: Pediatric oral and maxillofacial surgery, St. Louis, 1979, The C.V. Mosby Co.)

essary to place the anterior parts of the jaws within the machine's manufactured focal plane; if this is done, the posterior parts on either side will automatically also be in focus. Most panoramic x-ray machines employ a small plastic bite block fixed in the anteroposterior position. When the patient bites on the bite block with the front teeth, both jaws are automatically positioned within the focal plane. Spring-loaded or movable plastic head clamps are set against the patient's head in order to prevent head rotation and lateral tilt. Such head clamps are necessary because of the relatively long exposure times (up to 22 seconds) necessary to produce a panoramic image.

Most panoramic machines use a small stationary anode. The tubehead is mounted on a fixed track allowing it to circle the patient's head. Also movable on the circular track is the film-holding device. The film cassette itself is usually manufactured in two sizes, 5 × 12 inches and 6 × 12 inches, and encloses paired intensifying screens.

No flexibility exists for controlling exposure time. The milliamperage (mA) setting is also restricted because of the use of a small dental x-ray tubehead (maximum of 12 to 15 mA). This leaves only kilovoltage peak (kVp) as the determining control for radiographic density. Some facilities use very fast film-screen combinations in panoramic procedures, allowing kilovoltage peak settings to remain fairly low (65 to 75 kVp) even for larger patients.

■ Cephalometric radiography

Cephalometric skull radiography (cephalography) is a special type of lateral and PA radiography of the facial skeleton and portions of the skull (Fig. 7-10, A). Cephalograms are highly reproducible. There are three important differences between the techniques for producing lateral cephalometric and conventional skull radiographs. In cephalography (1) the anode-patient distance is a standard 60 inches, (2) the patient's head is stabilized in a cephalostat to produce a true lateral projection (norma lateralis), and (3) the soft tissue profile of the patient's face (i.e., forehead, nose, lips, and chin) must be seen in addition to the skeletal structures.

Cephalometric radiographs (Fig. 7-10, B) are used primarily by orthodontists and oral and maxillofacial surgeons in the evaluation of facial growth and development. By marking bony landmarks on tracings of the facial skeleton and skull base and by measuring distances and angles between these landmarks (Fig. 7-10, C), the clinician can gauge the activity of jaw growth as well as the potential for future growth. Cephalometric radiography ensures that changes from one cephalogram to the next represent true anatomic changes, not

artifacts introduced by technical variables. (See Cohen[15] for identification and further discussion of cephalometric landmarks.)

Radiographic distortion obviously must be minimized in cephalometric radiography. A 60-inch distance between the anode and the midsagittal plane of the head (for lateral projections) is standard. In order to ensure that the midsagittal plane is strictly parallel to the plane of the film, the patient's head is placed in a cephalostat that is built as an integral unit with the x-ray tube positioning device and the film holder assembly. The central x-ray beam is oriented absolutely perpendicular to the plane of the x-ray film.

Most cephalostats maintain patient head position by means of short, blunt rods that can be moved into the external ear canals (Fig. 7-10, A). The application of ear rods effectively prohibits rotation and lateral tilt of the head if the patient's head, neck, and body are comfortably positioned. It should be noted that the ear rods are difficult or impossible to employ with very young children or patients with developmental anomalies in which one or both ear canals are missing, atretic, or at different horizontal levels.

Several methods have been devised to permit visualization of the soft tissue profile of the patient's face on the lateral cephalometric radiograph. An aluminum wedge filter can be placed at the cassette surface and within the anterior part of the x-ray beam to attenuate photons that would otherwise "burn out" the facial soft tissue profile. The soft tissues are then seen at a radiographic density comparable to bone and teeth. The thin, knife-edge margin of the wedge filter is placed toward the center of the beam so that the anterior beam attenuation is gradual and not obtrusive. A newer development is the production of variable-speed intensifying screens that selectively underexpose the extreme anterior portion of the radiographic film. For cephalometric work, the "slow" position of such film cassettes is set to correspond to the anterior facial profile. A typical cephalometric lateral skull radiograph and its tracing are shown in Fig. 7-10, B and C.

■ Intraoral radiography
Film

Intraoral dental radiography is performed with small paper or plastic film packets containing one or two sheets of nonscreen x-ray film and a sheet of lead foil to reduce x-ray backscatter (Fig. 7-11, A). Head cassettes and intensifying screens are not used in dental radiography. Patients do not tolerate the feel of hard cassettes in their mouths, in comparison with the traditional pliable dental film packets. More importantly, dentists require fairly exquisite radiographic definition for the di-

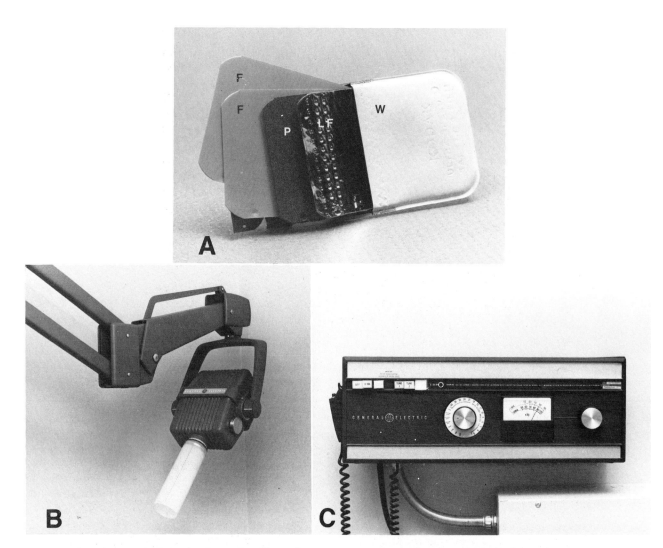

Fig. 7-11. Dental radiographic film and equipment. **A,** Opened packet of standard (no. 2) size dental x-ray film. Many dentists use double film packets so that duplicate radiograph is available. *P,* Black paper; *LF,* lead foil; *W,* outer plastic wrapper. Lead foil prevents backscatter fogging of film during exposure. Opposite side of packet would face x-ray source. **B,** Typical dental x-ray tubehead. Connection to wall mounting bracket is not shown. Highly mobile tubehead contains, among other items, transformers, stationary anode, and heat-dissipating oil jacket. **C,** Control panel for dental x-ray tube. At 15 mA, maximum kilovoltage peak possible is 90.

agnosis of interproximal ("between teeth") dental caries. Thus a tradeoff of fine definition for screen-produced radiographic speed is generally not favored in dental diagnosis. As a compromise dental practitioners employ a relatively high-speed nonscreen x-ray film.

Machines

Dental radiography is performed with a small, lightweight, highly maneuverable dental x-ray tubehead (Fig. 7-11, *B*). This device contains a stationary tungsten anode embedded in a copper bar. The cathode of the tube uses a single tungsten filament. The maximum x-ray tube current is generally 10 to 15 mA. The range of kilovolt peak available (Fig. 7-11, *C*) is generally adjustable between 65 and 100 kVp. Modern dental x-ray machines employ electronic timers that make exposures as short as 1/60 second (1 impulse). More information on dental x-ray machines can be found in Barr's[6] text and in the Kodak monograph *X-rays in Dentistry.*[32]

Projections

There are three basic intraoral radiographic projections: periapical, bitewing, and occlusal. The first two

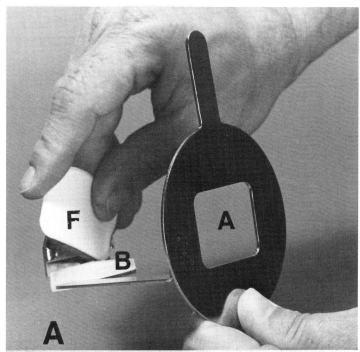

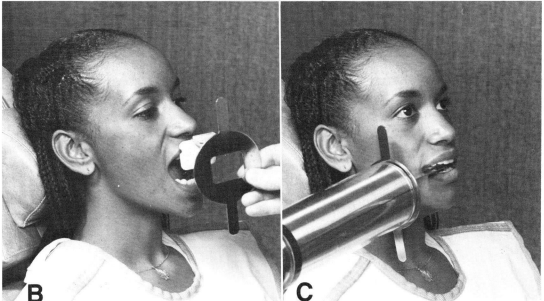

Fig. 7-12. Technique for intraoral periapical radiography using metal film-positioning devices. **A,** White dental x-ray packet is placed on combination film-positioning–beam-collimating device. *F,* Film; *B,* plastic bite block. Rectangular aperture *(A)* limits size of x-ray beam so that it only slightly exceeds dimensions of film. **B,** For mandibular molar periapical projection, device is placed in mouth, film down. Bite pressure will hold it steady. **C,** X-ray cylinder is brought flush against steel faceplate of collimating instrument. This technique ensures accurate aiming of x-ray beam, as well as proper alignment of film vis-à-vis teeth.

are made with standard size (1 ¼ × 1 ¾ inch) dental x-ray film; the last is made with a slightly larger film about the size of a credit card. The occlusal projection affords a greater area coverage of teeth and supporting bone than the other two intraoral projections.[6,32]

Periapical. As the name implies, the periapical projection is designed to visualize the periapical bone, i.e., the bone surrounding the tooth roots (Fig. 7-12). The crowns of several teeth in the area may be seen but the main purpose of this view is to detect inflammatory changes in the periapical bone. As part of a "full-mouth" adult radiographic survey, two periapical projections are normally taken in each of the four posterior dental quadrants: a molar periapical projection and a premolar periapical projection. Three to five projections are usually also made for the mandibular and maxillary anterior teeth. Thus the routine full-mouth series of periapical projections for an adult patient consists roughly of 14 to 17 individual periapical projections.

In order to reduce distortion, periapical projections are best made with precision intraoral film holders (Fig. 7-13, A). These film holders are rigid metal and plastic devices placed in the mouth by the operator (Fig. 7-13, B), with the patient's biting pressure holding them steady during the exposure. The intraoral film holding device provides a parallel relationship between the plane of the film and an imaginary plane through the long axes of the patient's teeth. The device will also align both planes perpendicular to the central x-ray beam. If precision x-ray film holders are not available, intraoral film positioning can also be performed with inexpensive plastic film holders designed to be used with intraoral film. (See Figs. 7-13 and 7-19 for examples of periapical radiographs, including the normal radiographic anatomy.)

Bitewing. Bitewing intraoral radiography visualizes the crowns of the teeth and the crest of the alveolar bone (Fig. 7-14, B) and also provides an optimal view of the pulp chamber in relationship to restorations or caries.[10] The roots of the teeth and the deeper areas of bone are not visualized. Bitewings are most useful in identifying those areas of the dental crowns that the dentist has the greatest difficulty inspecting directly, i.e., the interproximal parts of the crowns. The interproximal segments are prime regions for the initiation of dental caries. Bitewing films are placed in paper holders that have a tab or "wing" made of folded paper (Fig. 7-14, A). As the patient bites on the tab the film is held close to the lingual surfaces of the mandibular and maxillary crowns. As with the periapical procedure, several individual exposures (usually four) are necessary to cover a full complement of teeth.

Occlusal. The occlusal projection is not a part of the routine adult full-mouth intraoral radiographic examination. It is used when more extensive coverage of surrounding mandible or maxilla is required (Fig. 7-15, A). In adults the occlusal projection is valuable in cases of suspected canine tooth impaction, alveolar process fracture, or pathologic bone changes. In children and adolescents the same projection may be used to evaluate

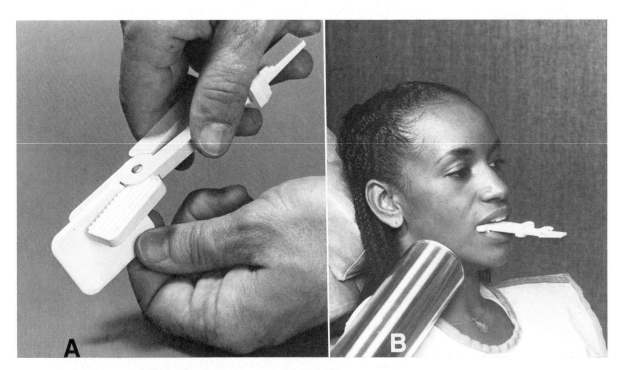

Fig. 7-13. Simpler alternative periapical film placement technique. **A,** Special plastic device grips film between two "jaws". Ridged, larger jaw serves as bite block for intraoral film stabilization. **B,** With film placed intraorally, handle of device protrudes from mouth. This device lacks beam alignment and collimating advantages of device shown in Fig. 7-12 but is simpler and less time consuming to use.

the state of the developing unerupted (permanent) dentition. Occlusal views provide coverage of 6 to 8 teeth and much of the alveolar process that supports these teeth.

The film is positioned flat across either dental arch, with the patient stabilizing the film in position by biting on it. Care must be taken to orient the correct side of the packet toward the x-ray source. Depending on the particular area of interest, one might position the film for either an anterior, left lateral, or right lateral occlusal projection. The technician positions the film in the mouth diagonally for anterior coverage or lengthwise when the posterior areas of the jaws are to be viewed. The x-ray beam is directed toward the center of the film packet at a 60° to 75° angle (Fig. 7-15, *B*). When the standard mandibular occlusal projection is made, the beam is directed perpendicular to the plane of the film packet, much like the submentovertex skull projection (Fig. 7-15, *C*). Proper angulation is essential in intraoral radiography because incorrect angulation can cause misrepresentation of tooth caries, tooth contact, restorations, pulp chambers, and interproximal crestal bone.[60a] Several correctly angled, representative occlusal radiographs of both jaws are seen in Fig. 7-16.

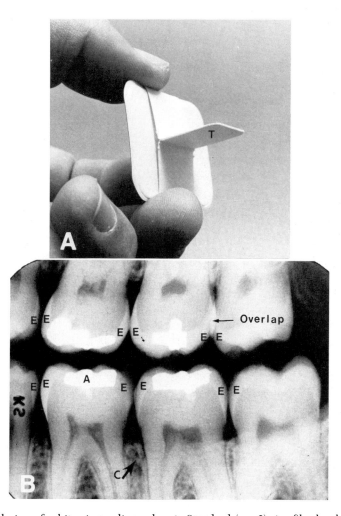

Fig. 7-14. Technique for bitewing radiography. **A,** Standard (no. 2) size film has been slipped into paper sling. Film is placed in mouth and patient bites on tab, *(T)*, or "bitewing." Properly positioned tab points toward x-ray tube. **B,** Example of molar bitewing radiograph. Goal is to visualize crowns but not necessarily roots of teeth and crests of interdental alveolar bone. It is important that beam be aligned so that adjacent enamel surfaces *(E)* do not overlap (as between maxillary second and third molars). Interproximal tooth surfaces need to be critically examined for caries *(decay)*. *A,* Amalgam restoration (filling).

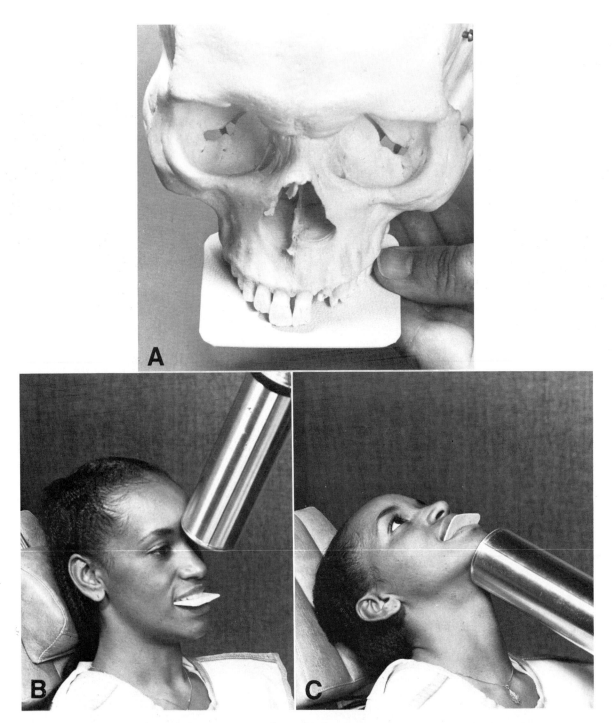

Fig. 7-15. Technique for maxillary and mandibular occlusal projections. **A,** Occlusal film packet is shown in position on dried skull for maxillary projection. Occlusal film is considerably larger than standard (no. 2) size intraoral film. Textured side of film must face x-ray source. **B,** Film in place, held steady by bite pressure. X-ray cylinder points at film center and is angled caudally about 65° to 70°. **C,** For standard mandibular occlusal projection, neck is hyperextended and beam is directed perpendicular to film plane.

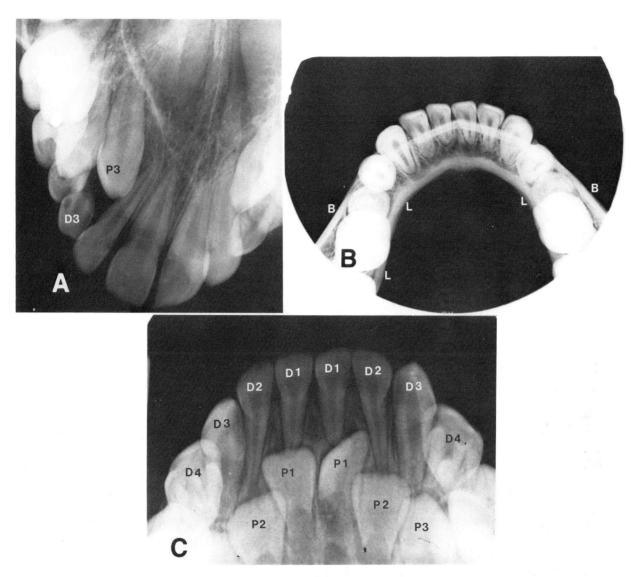

Fig. 7-16. A, Maxillary lateral occlusal radiograph. Film was deliberately positioned laterally off midline to more effectively demonstrate impacted permanent canine *(P3)*. Deciduous canine *(D3)* has still not exfoliated. This projection provides considerably more dental and bone coverage than periapical projection. **B,** Mandibular standard occlusal projection. Object is not to visualize tooth structure or internal bone anatomy per se but to demonstrate integrity of lingual *(L)* and buccal *(B)* bone cortices. Calcifications in submandibular salivary gland ducts may also be seen on this type of projection. **C,** Mandibular anterior occlusal projection, made with 65° to 70° cranial beam angulation (analogous to technique in Fig 7-15, *B*). Patient is approximately 4 years old. In general, occlusal projection is useful in demonstrating many erupted and developing teeth on one film. *D1,* Deciduous central incisors; *D2,* lateral incisors; *D3,* deciduous canines; *D4,* deciduous first molars; *P1,* permanent central incisors; *P2,* lateral incisors; *P3,* permanent canines.

■ Xeroradiography (cephalometric and dental)

In xeroradiography, images are produced not on film but rather on electrostatically charged selenium plates. For some purposes xeroradiography produces superior radiography in comparison with conventional x-ray film because of its inherently wider image latitude and higher resolution. In addition, xeroradiography affords high radiographic contrast between subtle tissue densities because of its "edge effect." The process has been used intermittently for head and neck and sialographic applications. The usefulness of xeroradiography in cephalometrics has also been investigated. Because a soft tissue profile of the patient's face is seen in addition to skeletal and dental visualization, xeroradiography was initially favorably received by many orthodontists. However, few orthodontists are actually using xeroradiography routinely because of the expense, the limited additional applications of the Xerox 125 system in the dental setting, and the unfavorable dosimetry required.

Xeroradiography of dental structures has recently undergone extensive experimentation and clinical trials. Although xeroradiography was first applied to evaluation of teeth in 1963, considerable limitations held back the process until recently. The Xerox 125 system, which has been employed in medical mammographic studies, has been shown to be inferior in several respects to conventional dental radiography.[65] A new dental Xerox (110) system has, however, shown promise in producing high-detail dental images (Fig. 7-17) with relatively low patient radiation doses.[27,64] The new xeroradiography dental system, which uses small plastic cassettes for intraoral placement, may prove to be superior to traditional radiography for imaging dental car-

ies, lamina dura changes, and alterations of apical bone trabeculae.

□ Normal radiographic anatomy

Normal radiographic anatomy, as seen on the panoramic and intraoral periapical projections, is described below. Basic knowledge of the radiographic anatomy of the teeth, bone, and soft tissue as seen on these commonly used projections can then be applied to the study of all oral and facial radiographic examinations.

■ Normal anatomy on panoramic projections
The mandible (Fig. 7-18)

On the panoramic projection the mandible is seen virtually in its entirety, from condyle to condyle and from the inferior cortex to the occlusal plane of the teeth. The most superior or articulating aspects of the condyles are superimposed over the articular eminences of the temporal bone. The condylar and the saber-shaped coronoid processes are, however, easily identified. The funnel-shaped mandibular foramen is seen at the center of the ramus, as is the proximal portion of the mandibular canal. The heavy anterior ramus line that extends inferiorly across the molar roots is the internal oblique line. It merges with the mylohyoid ridge on the lingual surface of the body. Just anterior to the mandibular angle on the inferior cortex is a gentle concavity known as the antegonial notch.

The mandibular body consists of (1) the tooth-supporting alveolar process, (2) the cancellous bone below the teeth and surrounding the mandibular canal, and (3) the thick, ribbonlike inferior cortex. The trabeculae of the mandibular cancellous bone are normally discrete

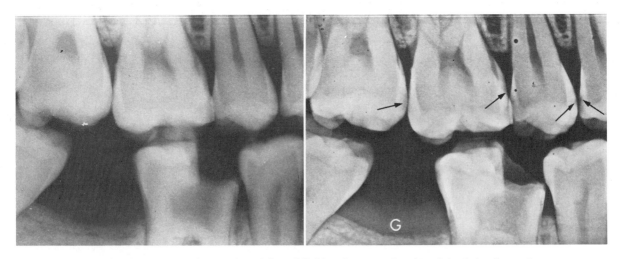

Fig. 7-17. Comparison of conventional dental *(left)* and xerographic dental *(right)* radiographs. These are bitewing projections of same dental area of same patient. Notice increased contrast of xeroradiograph image. Early, incipient dental caries *(arrows)* are better seen on xeroradiograph. *G*, Gingiva.

and lacelike. Around the posterior teeth, the bone trabeculae tend to assume a horizontal "stepladder" pattern. This portion of the jaw is subjected to maximal occlusal pressure during chewing and it is thought that the interdental trabeculae are arranged in a pattern that most effectively resists these forces. The mandibular canal can be seen coursing anteriorly below the apices of the posterior teeth. The major portion of this canal ends near the root of the first premolar tooth, at the mental foramen. On coronal section of the mandible, below the canal in the posterior body of the mandible, the bone has only about one third the thickness of the alveolar process. This inferior, relatively thin part of the

posterior mandible accommodates the submandibular gland on its lingual aspect.

The entire dentition in both jaws is clearly seen on a panoramic projection. As noted previously, the portion of each tooth embedded in the bone is called the *root;* the part protruding from the bone (i.e., erupted into the oral cavity) is the *crown.*

The maxilla

On panoramic radiographs the posterior two thirds of the left and right maxillae are seen in a basically lateral view, while the anterior portions of those bones are seen in a frontal view. Nearly all the maxilla is visual-

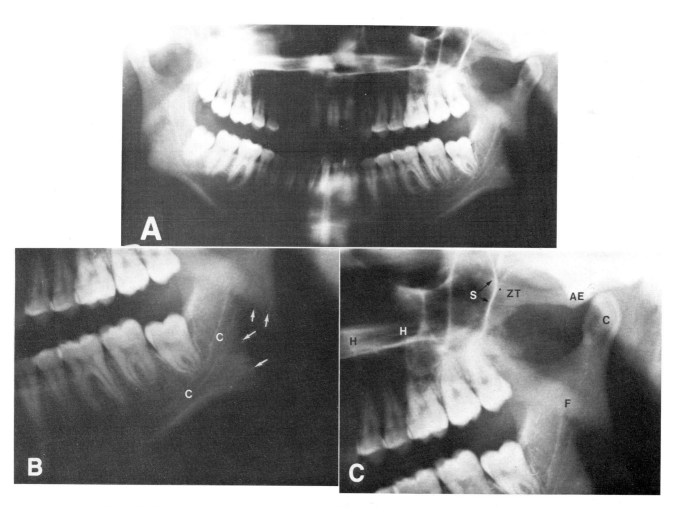

Fig. 7-18. Panoramic radiographic anatomy. **A,** Normal panoramic radiograph. On this single projection both jaws are seen in panorama from condyle to condyle and from inferior mandibular border to maxillary infraorbital rim. **B,** Close-up of **A.** Mandibular body and ramus are seen. Third molar is impacted against distal surface of second molar. Oropharyngeal airway, between dorsum of tongue and soft palate (arrows), is broad radiolucency "burning out" shadow of mandibular angle. *C,* Mandibular canal. **C,** Another close-up of **A.** *C,* Condyle. Zygomatic arch is seen between zygomaticotemporal suture area *(ZT)* and the articular eminence *(AE)*. *S,* Posterior wall of maxillary sinus; *H,* hard palate. Nasopharyngeal airway is superimposed across neck of condyle. *F,* Area of mandibular foramen.

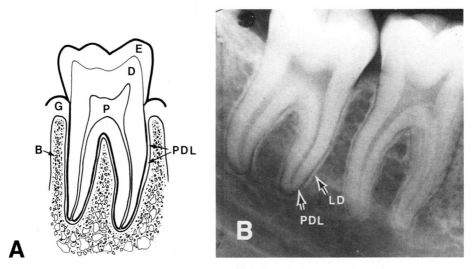

Fig. 7-19. Dental and periodontal gross anatomy. **A,** Artist's rendition of sagitally sectioned mandibular molar tooth, seen in buccal view. *E,* Enamel cap; *D,* dentin (forms bulk of tooth crown); *P,* pulp chamber, with thin pulp canals leading down to root apices; *PDL,* periodontal ligament space (exaggerated thickness); *G,* gingiva (gums), not seen radiographically; *B,* interdental alveolar bone. **B,** Portion of normal molar periapical radiograph. Around tooth roots notice thin radiolucent line, periodontal ligament *(PDL)* space, and thin radiopaque line, lamina dura *(LD)*, of the alveolar bone. Discontinuity of these periodontal structures is highly suggestive of disease, especially at root apices and when gross dental caries are apparent.

ized, from the occlusal plane of the teeth to the infraorbital rims and from one zygoma to the other. The principal areas of interest are typically the maxillary sinuses and the alveolar process.

On panoramic radiographs the maxillary sinuses are seen above the posterior teeth. The floor of each sinus dips down (evaginates) around the roots of several molar teeth. The latter almost appear to be protruding through the sinus floor into the air space; however, a thin, regular bony wall normally separates the two (Fig. 7-18, *A*). This cortical floor of the sinus represents the lamina dura of the molar teeth. This bony lining can be seen in greater detail on posterior maxillary periapical views. The panoramic projection also delineates the superior and posterolateral bony walls of the maxillary sinuses in reasonable detail. (For a more extensive discussion of the radiology of the maxillary sinuses, see Chapter 1.)

Other facial structures generally seen on the panoramic projection include the hyoid bone, the zygomatic bones, the pterygoid processes, occasionally the lateral pterygoid plates of the sphenoid bone, and sometimes a major portion of the orbits. The dorsum of the tongue is usually seen from oral cavity to epiglottis in a lateral view; above the tongue the soft palate is seen as a posterior extension of the hard palate. The nasopharynx is projected as a definite curvilinear radiolucency superior

and posterior to the soft palate and anterior to the posterior pharyngeal wall.

■ Normal anatomy on intraoral periapical projections
The teeth (Figs. 7-19 and 7-20)

The various shapes and sizes of the individual teeth within each dental quadrant are seen in Fig. 7-4. A cross-section of a lower molar tooth and its associated alveolar ridge, demonstrating the various structures that may be discerned radiographically, is seen in Fig. 7-19. Each tooth is projected as three distinct radiographic densities. The very radiopaque cap covering the entire crown is the *enamel* portion (the hardest, most radiopaque natural substance in the body) (Fig. 7-20, *A* and *B*). The central radiolucent chamber in the crown and the linear radiolucencies leading to it from the roots are, respectively, the pulp chamber and pulp canal(s). These pulp spaces are filled with connective tissue and contain neurovascular tissue and specialized tooth-forming cells. Between the enamel cap and the pulp spaces, and comprising the greatest bulk of the tooth, is the portion composed of *dentin*. Dentin is a calcified tissue of roughly equal hardness and radiographic density as cortical bone. Thinly covering the root is another specialized hard tissue called *cementum*, which provides a specialized surface for ligamentous attachment of the tooth to bone. The thin cementum

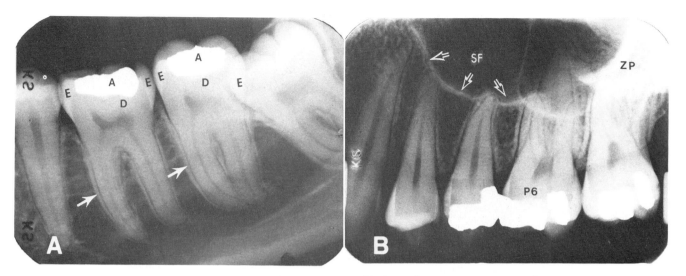

Fig. 7-20. Periapical radiographic anatomy. **A,** Mandibular molar projection. Lamina dura can be seen distinctly around most of root surfaces. Notice difference in radiographic densities between amalgam restorations *(A)*, enamel caps *(E)*, and dentin *(D)* in crowns. Broad radiolucency *(arrows)* crossing molar root apices is not mandibular canal but rather submandibular fossa on lingual bone surface. *C*, Mandibular canal; *I*, inferior border. **B,** Maxillary molar projection. First molar *(P6)* root apices appear to project into maxillary sinus, although they are separated from sinus air space by lamina dura. *SF*, Maxillary sinus floor; *ZP*, zygomatic process of maxilla.

layer cannot, however, be radiographically distinguished from the dentin of roots.

Periodontal structures

The socket *(alveolus)* for each tooth is situated within the alveolar process of the mandible and maxilla and has a thin, regular lining of the cortical bone called the *lamina dura* (Fig. 7-19). The lamina dura is essentially a continuum of the cortex from the crest of the alveolar process into each socket. Because of its relative thinness compared to the exterior cortical walls, the lamina dura is most easily seen on periapical radiographs. When optimal periapical radiography is provided the lamina dura can be traced around most tooth roots in an intact, continuous line. Only at the point adjacent to the extreme apex (tip) of the root can one occasionally see a fine discontinuity where the neurovascular bundle enters the tooth.

Interspaced between the tooth root and the lamina dura is an even, regular radiolucent lining called the periodontal ligament space (Fig. 7-19). In this space, which is normally about ½ to 1 mm thick (about the same width as the lamina dura), there are bundles of connective tissue fibers that insert into the lamina dura and attach to the cementum of the root, providing a strong ligamentous attachment for each tooth to the jaw. These connective tissue bundles are oriented precisely so that the various forces acting on the teeth during chewing can be efficiently transmitted to the supporting bone.

The crest of the alveolar bone will normally be close to the neck of each tooth (the neck is defined as the region of the inferior extention of the enamel cap). No more than 2 mm should separate the enamel cap edge (the cementoenamel junction) and the crest of the alveolar bone in a healthy periodontium.

□ Abnormalities of the mandible and teeth
■ Dental and periodontal conditions
Developmental abnormalities

Teeth, like other multiple structures in the body such as ribs and vertebral segments, occasionally vary in number.

Congenital absence. It is not uncommon for one or more teeth to be congenitally absent. The permanent third molars, mandibular premolars, and maxillary lateral incisors are most often missing. Radiographs are necessary to determine if a particular tooth is actually missing or merely unerupted (Fig. 7-21). If some or all of the teeth are missing, the term *partial* or *complete anodontia* may be employed. In the developmental condition known as ectodermal dysplasia, partial or complete anodontia of the permanent dentition is almost always found.

Supernumerary teeth. Teeth formed in excess of the normal complement of teeth are called supernumerary teeth. This situation usually involves the permanent dentition. Most supernumerary teeth are found in the maxillary arch, although many are also seen in the man-

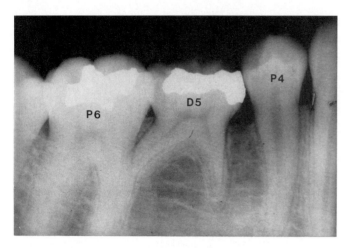

Fig. 7-21. Congenital absence of permanent second premolar tooth in an adult. *D5,* Deciduous second molar; *P4,* permanent first premolar; *P6,* permanent first molar. Notice difference in root lengths between deciduous and permanent molars.

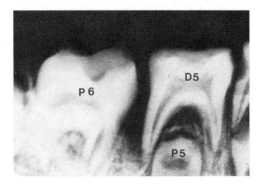

Fig. 7-22. Amelogenesis imperfecta, hypoplastic type. Enamel caps have not formed on erupted deciduous *(D5)* and permanent *(P6)* molars. Directly exposed to oral cavity is dentin of teeth, which is softer than enamel and subject to rapid attrition. Even unerupted premolar *(P5)* can be seen to be devoid of enamel coverage.

dibular premolar region. Most are discovered radiographically while they are still unerupted. These extra teeth are typically small and conical, particularly those found in the maxillary midline and molar regions. In cleidocranial dysostosis, several supernumerary teeth will generally be seen in each jaw. Cleft palate patients occasionally have supernumerary maxillary lateral incisors associated with the cleft. Partial duplication of the alveolar ridge with supernumerary teeth may also occur in complex midfacial malformations.

Supernumerary roots. Extra or additional roots may be found on any tooth. This is not an uncommon finding, especially on premolars and mandibular molars. The condition has no significance except that it should be appreciated before initiating either exodontic (extraction) or endodontic (root canal) procedures.

Amelogenesis imperfecta. Amelogenesis imperfecta is caused by a generalized developmental disturbance of ameloblasts, the cells that form the matrix for dental enamel. This abnormality affects all or most of the permanent teeth and often the primary teeth as well. Only the enamel is involved; the cementum, dentin, and pulp tissue are all normal. Two types of amelogenesis imperfecta are usually described, (1) the hypoplastic type, and (2) the hypocalcific type. The former causes decreased thickness of dental enamel. The enamel cap may in fact be completely absent (Fig. 7-22). The latter type is characterized by a normal thickness of soft, friable, easily fractured enamel.

Although the diagnosis of amelogenesis imperfecta is usually evident clinically, the radiographic features are distinctive and may confirm the clinical impression. Radiographically, one notices either a thin layer or complete absence of the normally radiopaque enamel caps of affected teeth (the hypoplastic type of disease) or a more normal thickness of enamel that has a decreased density in comparison to the adjacent dentin (the hypocalcific type of disease).

Dentinogenesis imperfecta. This condition, also referred to as hereditary opalescent dentin, is one of the most common dominantly inherited disorders of humans, affecting approximately 1 in every 8000 persons.[11] Clinically, the teeth have an unusual amber translucency. The main clinical problem is, however, a functional one. The enamel caps are ineffectively bonded to the dentin of the crowns. The teeth undergo rapid attrition once the covering enamel surfaces are fragmented and worn away.

Radiographic findings in dentinogenesis imperfecta are characteristic. The pulp spaces of the affected teeth are obliterated early (occasionally even before the teeth erupt) because of excessive, dysplastic dentin formation (Fig. 7-23). The shapes and sizes of the involved teeth are unusual. The overall length of an affected tooth is often noticeably decreased, and the root portion is particularly prone to shortening. The proximal surfaces of the crowns have accentuated curvatures, giving them a somewhat bulbous appearance. Mild cases of dentinogenesis imperfecta, those in which the opalescent appearance may go unnoticed clinically, are occasionally discovered radiographically as incidental findings.

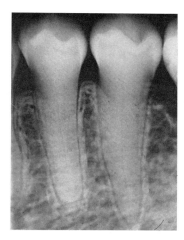

Fig. 7-23. Dentinogenesis imperfecta. Most noticeable is virtually complete obliteration (filling in) of pulp chambers and pulp canals by dysplastic dentin. Crowns are abnormally bulbous on their proximal contours. This dental defect is often present in cases of osteogenesis imperfecta.

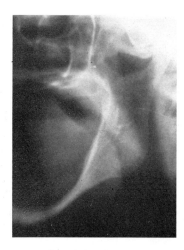

Fig. 7-24. Severe atrophy of alveolar ridges secondary to tooth loss. Structure of ramus on either side is not altered, but mandibular body has been reduced to little more than inferior cortex. Most edentulous jaws undergo far less severe alveolar process atrophy.

Congenital syphilis. Syphilis, if contracted in utero, may produce enamel hypoplasia. The hypoplasia is different from that found in amelogenesis imperfecta. With congenital syphilis, usually only a few teeth are infected by the *Treponema* organism. The tooth most commonly affected is the maxillary central incisor. Such an affected incisor (a "Hutchinson's incisor") has a peculiar "barrel" shape and a notch in the middle of its incisal edge. The peculiar shape of this tooth is occasionally seen radiographically even prior to the tooth's eruption. If so, it may confirm a clinical suspicion of congenital syphilis. "Mulberry molars" is another characteristic dental manifestation of congenital syphilis. In this condition the first molar teeth have multicusped or knobby occlusal (chewing) surfaces. These abnormal posterior teeth are not as amenable to radiographic detection as are the central incisors but are easily identified clinically.

Regressive alterations

The abnormalities presented in this section are all lesions "of a retrograde nature."[52] These abnormalities are neither developmental nor inflammatory in nature.

Pulp stones. Although calcifications of the dental pulp have been histologically identified in a large percentage of extracted teeth selected at random, only a small number of these calcifications are apparent radiographically. Most of these radiopaque pulp stones are concentric conglomerations of calcium salts. Some are small round masses of dentin. They are always of a homogeneous radiographic density, and most are found in the pulp chambers of affected teeth.

Alveolar process atrophy. Because the normal function of the alveolar process is to support the teeth, loss of one or more teeth inevitably leads to a variable degree of bone resorption from the alveolar ridge. If only one or perhaps two adjacent teeth are lost, the ridge in this area will gradually develop a smooth, regular apical concavity. Totally edentulous jaws usually undergo a slow, even, overall lowering of the alveolar ridge. In most edentulous jaws, a mild to moderate degree of resorption takes place and the altered bone height remains static for an indefinite period of time. In a few severe cases, however, this alveolar bone loss progresses to a point at which the only remaining part of the mandibular body is the inferior cortex (Fig. 7-24). Bone resorption also occurs in the alveolar ridge of the maxilla when teeth in this arch are lost.

Hypercementosis. This condition, also called cemental hyperplasia, is caused by the deposition of excessive amounts of secondary cementum on the tooth root surfaces. It is usually confined to the apical one third of the involved root (Fig. 7-25) but in some cases an entire root may be enlarged. Premolars are most commonly affected. The periodontal ligament space and the lamina dura tend to remain intact around the added cementum. The only exception to this rule occurs when the hypercementosis is stimulated by a periapical infection. In this instance the periodontal ligament space is widened and the lamina dura is obliterated. A high incidence of dental hypercementosis is seen in Paget's disease involving dentulous portions of the jaws.

Embedded and impacted teeth. Permanent teeth that should be erupted but are not and show no physical

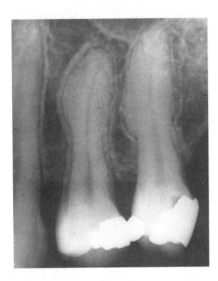

Fig. 7-25. Hypercementosis of maxillary premolar roots. These roots do not have normal conical shape, and they bulge at their apical halves because of secondary (reactive) cementum formation. Notice that periodontal ligament spaces and lamina dura remain intact around excess cementum.

obstacle to the path of eruption are called *embedded teeth*. The term should be reserved for those rare cases in which tooth eruption is long overdue. The cause is sometimes ascribed to a simple lack of eruptive force. When several or many teeth remain embedded in the jaws the cause is often related to endocrine dysfunction. Multiple embedded teeth can be seen in hypothyroidism, rickets, or cleidocranial dysostosis.

Teeth that remain embedded in bone for long periods (i.e., 2 to 5 years or more) may become pathologically altered. Dentigerous cysts may arise from the follicles (epithelium coverings) of long-embedded teeth. The long-embedded dental follicle may also give rise to the odontogenic tumor, ameloblastoma.

Developing and mature permanent teeth that cannot erupt into the oral cavity because their eruption paths are obstructed are termed *impacted teeth*. The eruption path may be blocked by other erupted or unerupted teeth or by pathologic mandibular and maxillary third molars and the maxillary canines. Such teeth usually become impacted simply because there is not sufficient room for them in the dental arches. Premolar teeth can become impacted if the deciduous molars are lost prematurely in childhood, with subsequent closure of the arch space that they were "reserving." Intraoral radiography is clearly of primary importance in the diagnosis of impacted and embedded teeth and in the planning of appropriate corrective action.

Prolonged retention of deciduous teeth

This not uncommon condition is most often caused by the congenital absence of a permanent "successor"

tooth, particularly the mandibular first or second premolar. The deciduous mandibular molar is the tooth most commonly retained into adulthood because of the absence of its successor, which during the eruptive process normally initiates the shedding phase of the deciduous tooth. Abnormal retention of primary teeth is also a common feature of two developmental abnormalities, cleidocranial dysostosis and ectodermal dysplasia.

Inflammatory conditions

Dental caries. Tooth decay is by far the most common dental abnormality. Dentists refer to decay lesions as caries and to the pathologic process as carious destruction of the teeth. Dental caries is the most common cause of loss of teeth in persons under the age of 30.

Caries is produced by microorganisms growing on a substrate tooth coating called dental plaque. It is plaque that protects and nourishes the bacteria that cause subsequent tooth decalcification and physical destruction. Cariogenic bacteria, principally *Streptococcus mutans*, produce lactic acid that slowly etches the tooth surface. Frank demineralization, i.e., loss of calcium and phosphate, ensues. Demineralization is followed in turn by outright dissolution of the enamel hydroxyapatite matrix and noticeable destruction of the crown (Fig. 7-26, *A* to *C*). Because the tooth enamel is the hardest natural substance in the body, the process of carious destruction may take months or years to penetrate the 2 to 3 mm enamel cap. If good dental hygiene is maintained and dental plaque is not allowed to reaccumulate, a carious lesion may be halted while it is still limited to the enamel layer. If the disease penetrates the enamel cap, however, gross breakdown of the bulk of the tooth crown occurs relatively quickly. This is because much of the tooth mass is composed of dentin, a considerably softer calcified substance than enamel and one far less resistant to caries. Without prompt dental treatment, invading microorganisms eventually reach the dental pulp chamber, quickly overwhelm its innately feeble inflammatory response, and cause necrosis of the entire tooth. The infection then passes through the pulp canals of the tooth roots to produce osteitis near the root apices, or in unusual circumstances, frank osteomyelitis of the medullary bone.

Early recognition of caries is highly important to preserving tooth vitality. Many areas of incipient carious destruction can be seen by direct visual inspection. However, the diagnosis of interproximal (between teeth) caries usually requires bite-wing intraoral radiographs because these regions are almost impossible to see directly. The most common site for the occurence of caries is at the interproximal surface, at or just below the contact point of two adjacent teeth.

Incipient caries limited to the enamel surfaces will

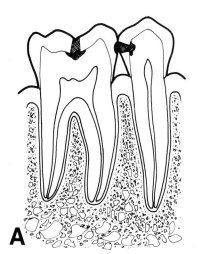
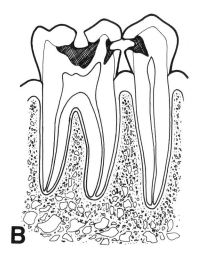
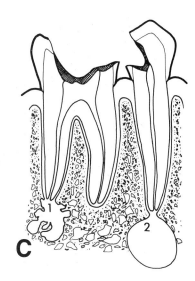

Fig. 7-26. Process of carious destruction of teeth as it would appear radiographically. **A,** Early dentinal (i.e., through enamel and into dentin) caries, represented by dark shaded area in tooth crowns. Notice that lesion becomes diffuse after it breaks through dentinoenamel junction into softer dentin. This action eventually weakens and fragments overlying enamel. Molar tooth has both occlusal (chewing surface) caries and very early interproximal caries. **B,** Lesions seen in **A** have progressed to severe dentinal caries in both teeth. Some enamel has fragmented away and is represented by voids in crown outlines. Lesions have considerably dispersed into dentin of crowns and now threaten pulp chambers, which contain vital cellular, connective tissue, and neurovascular elements. **C,** Late, gross carious destruction of crowns as represented by marked fragmenting away of undermined enamel and carious dentin. Pulp chambers have been invaded and overwhelmed by infection and disease had progressed to periapical bone. Notice discontinuity of lamina dura. At root periapices two potential inflammatory sequellae are illustrated: *1,* irregular defect, simulating appearance of periapical inflammatory granuloma or abscess, and, *2,* roundish, regular defect simulating appearance of inflammatory induced radicular cyst. Rarely, one root of such necrotic teeth may show no evidence at all of periapical bone damage.

generally not be apparent on extraoral radiographs of the jaws, regardless of the technique used. However, the more extensive dentinal caries can sometimes be detected on radiographs of the jaws if technical factors are optimal. The typical appearance of caries is a radiolucent defect in the tooth crown on a surface on which tooth contact is present (Fig. 7-27). The enamel portion of the defect is typically discrete and limited, as opposed to the more extensive destruction that occurs in the softer, internal dentinal portions of the crown. The margins of the radiolucency in the dentin are ill defined and appear to fade away from the main carious lesion. Gross caries tend to spread diffusely, undermining and weakening the enamel walls. If a large carious lesion radiographically appears to approach or actually contact the pulp chamber, the observer should inspect the periapical bone areas for signs of osteolysis, because the tooth is usually devitalized by that time.

Periodontal disease. Inflammation of the gingiva surrounding the teeth is also caused by plaque-harboring oral bacteria, including anaerobic as well as aerobic strains. This process, when limited to the soft tissue, is

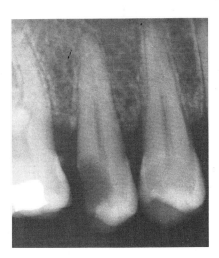

Fig. 7-27. Gross dentinal caries in distal half of second premolar tooth. Large radiolucency represents area of loss of calcified structure in crown. This lesion started at distal interproximal surface, adjoining mesial molar surface. Pulp chamber is clearly involved. At periapical bone area, part of lamina dura has been eroded but no major periapical radiolucency has yet been produced.

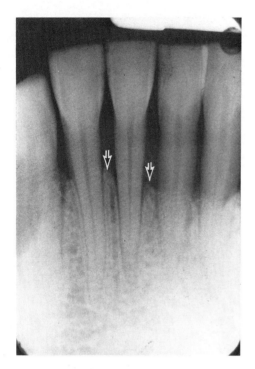

Fig. 7-28. Severe periodontal disease. Radiographically this is termed *horizontal bone loss* because horizontal level of interdental alveolar bone has been eroded from normal level, usually considered to be within 1 to 2 mm of cementoenamel junction of adjacent tooth crowns. Clinically, teeth seen here would be moderately mobile to finger pressure. Arrows indicate alveolar crest height.

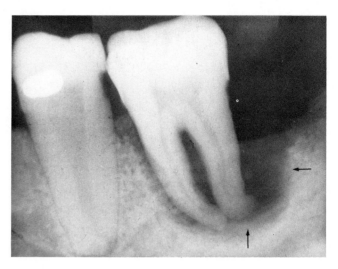

Fig. 7-29. Chronic periodontal abscess around roots of permanent first molar tooth. Tooth is essentially devoid of supporting bone. Such a lesion is characterized by vertical bone loss. Arrows show border of lesion.

called gingivitis, a common oral inflammatory condition. Progression of this disease inevitably involves the underlying supporting alveolar bone. The disease then becomes known as the more serious periodontitis, or periodontal disease. Radiographic detection of gingivitis is not possible. However, the interpretation of intraoral radiographs is one of the most fundamental and clinically important methods by which periodontal bone loss is detected and gauged.

The diagnosis and evaluation of periodontal bone loss on radiographs mainly depends on the height of the alveolar crest of bone between the teeth. The crestal bone height level normally is 1 to 2 mm apical to (i.e., below) the level of an adjacent tooth's enamel edge (the cementoenamel junction). If the crestal height level is found to be apical to this standard (for example, at the midroot level), the patient has periodontal disease. This kind of resorption of the alveolar bone, if generalized, is called horizontal bone loss (Fig. 7-28). The term *vertical bone loss* refers to a wedge of bone loss along a surface of a particular tooth. A few millimeters of generalized horizontal bone loss around the teeth in both arches is consistent with mild, chronic periodontal disease. It is also a routine effect of aging reflected in the

oral cavity. If, however, such a condition progresses to the point that only half or less of a given tooth root remains embedded in the bone, then the situation may be considered to be severe and the longevity of the affected tooth seriously compromised. Periodontal disease is responsible for most tooth loss in persons over the age of 30 years (Fig. 7-29).

Periapical rarefying osteitis. Periapical rarefying osteitis is an inflammatory lesion often identified at the apex of a nonvital tooth. The apex is the site at which dental pulp tissue communicates with the surrounding bone. The condition is almost exclusively the result of carious involvement of the pulp with subsequent necrosis. It may also follow a traumatic blow to a tooth that results in pulp ischemia secondary to strangulation or rupturing of apical blood vessels (i.e., aseptic necrosis of the tooth occurs). In both instances the pulp dies and inflammatory disease supervenes at the apex.

The radiologic term *periapical rarefying osteitis* does not signify a particular histopathologic lesion or entity, such as periapical abscess, periapical granuloma, or periapical (radicular) cyst. All three of these entities may produce an identical radiographic picture and it is generally not justifiable or even useful to differentiate between these entities solely on the basis of radiographic appearance. Even if such a distinction were possible, all three of the apical inflammatory lesions are treated identically (by either root canal filling or tooth

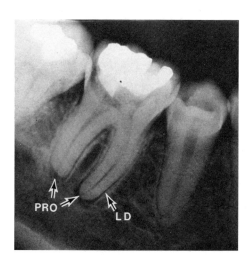

Fig. 7-30. Early periapical rarefying osteitis (PRO) at roots of molar. Notice especially periapical region of molar mesial root where radiopaque lamina dura *(LD)* has become discontinuous. Periapical radiolucency has developed. Cause is large filling and caries in crown of tooth that impinge on pulp chamber.

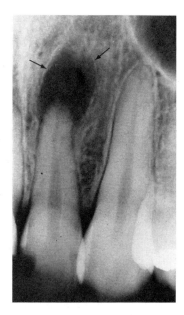

Fig. 7-31. Periapical rarefying osteitis associated with maxillary lateral incisor. Lamina dura can be seen around canine root apex but not around lateral incisor apex *(arrows)*. Histopathologically this lesion may be either granuloma, cyst, or abscess; one cannot tell which by radiographic means alone.

extraction) and all three nearly always respond favorably. Periapical rarefying osteitis is merely the most appropriate radiographic term for the round, radiolucent shadow at the apex of a nonvital tooth. Again, it is incorrect to refer to the latter as simply an abscess on the basis of the x-ray picture.

To establish the radiographic diagnosis of periapical rarefying osteitis, an actual radiolucency at a tooth apex must be present or the apical lamina dura must be discontinuous (Fig. 7-30). In most cases of chronic, longstanding periapical infections, both discontinuities of the lamina dura and a roundish radiolucency at the tooth apex are present (Fig. 7-31). In cases of very early rarefying osteitis at the apex of a nonvital tooth, however, slight widening of the apical periodontal ligament space with an intact lamina dura might be the only radiographic presentation. This early manifestation, most often observed in children, is produced by inflammatory edema in the ligament space that slightly lifts the tooth from its socket.

The lamina dura surrounding a maxillary molar root apex is the same layer of bone as the floor of the maxillary sinus itself. Pulpal infection at this site tends to destroy the lamina dura but does not usually perforate the antral floor mucoperiosteum. Instead, the inflammatory lesion elevates the mucoperiosteum, inducing periosteal new bone formation that then appears as an ossified "halo" around the apical lesion itself (Fig. 7-32).

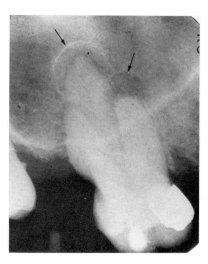

Fig. 7-32. "Halo" sign *(arrows)* at apex of palatal root of maxillary molar. This tooth was clinically nonvital. Periapical rarefying osteitis (radiolucency) is faintly seen around all three root apices. More obvious, however, is shell of reactive bone produced by sinus mucoperiosteum in attempt to "wall-off" inflammatory lesion.

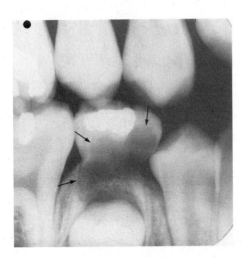

Fig. 7-33. Gross deciduous molar caries and associated periapical rarefying osteitis. With deciduous molars, periapical lesions resulting from caries localize in furcation area of bone, i.e., between roots and above developing premolar crown, not at root periapices.

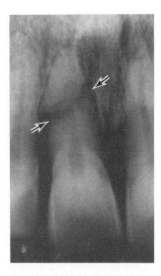

Fig. 7-34. Fractured root of central incisor, caused by traumatic blow to anterior maxilla. In such cases there is moderate chance that tooth can be saved if vascularity of tooth remains intact.

The reactive bone-forming capacity of the antral mucoperiosteum serves to maintain bony separation between dental infections and the antral air space.

With deciduous molars, caries-induced osteolytic lesions usually develop between the roots rather than at the apices (Fig. 7-33).

Traumatic injuries

Teeth. The greatest incidence of traumatic injuries to teeth occurs in childhood, especially in the 8- to 11-year age group. Maxillary incisors are the teeth most likely to be injured at any age.

A traumatized tooth that is only loosened in its socket may still retain its vitality. In such circumstances early radiographs of the affected tooth may reveal uniform widening of the periodontal ligament space around the entire root. A traumatized tooth can also remain physically intact but may become devitalized because of a disruption of its vascular supply. In such an event, periapical rarefying osteitis will eventually occur. Trauma may also fracture a tooth. Dental fractures are usually easily seen on periapical and occlusal radiographs (Fig. 7-34). A traumatized tooth may also be completely avulsed from its socket or forcefully pushed into the alveolar bone.

If traumatic injury to teeth is evident or suspected, thorough radiographic examination of the involved dental area is indicated. A radiograph of the traumatized tooth should also be made in about 3 to 6 months in order to assess the possible occurrence of interval tooth

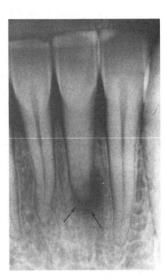

Fig. 7-35. Periapical rarefying osteitis of mandibular central incisor secondary to devitalization of tooth from traumatic blow. Aseptic necrosis of tooth was preceded by pulpal stimulation, as evidenced by obliteration of pulp spaces by secondary dentin formation. Arrows indicate periapical rarefying osteitis.

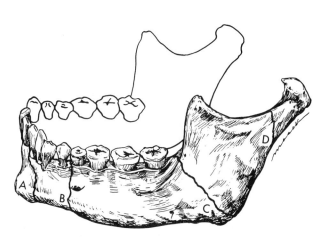

Fig. 7-36. Anatomic drawing of common site of mandibular fractures. (Modified from Rowe, N.L. and Killey, H.C.: Fractures of the facial skeleton, Baltimore, 1968, The Williams & Wilkins Co.)

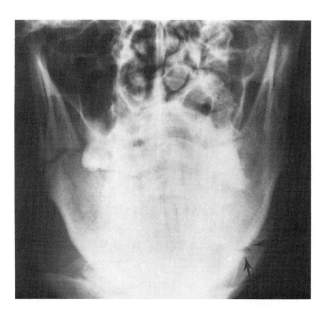

Fig. 7-37. Unilateral angle fracture *(arrows)*.

death, periapical rarefying osteitis (Fig. 7-35), or the failure of continued root formation. In many cases of tooth fractures a radiograph of the lips should be made as well to rule out the presence of embedded fractured tooth fragments. This is easily accomplished by placing a standing dental x-ray film packet behind the lip in question and exposing it at half the normal dental exposure.

Most dental roots fracture through their midportion. Because union of fractured root segments is not the rule, a visualized dental fracture line does not necessarily indicate a recent fracture. A noticeable dental fracture line might in fact be several years old. If the tooth remains vital, root fracture lines generally become somewhat less radiolucent and slightly rounded at their margins.

Mandible. The mandible is a prominent, exposed segment of the facial skeleton and is therefore a common site for both intentional and accidental trauma. Fractures of the alveolar ridge or teeth may occur independently (see previous discussion). Fractures of the mandible proper can be divided into several distinct categories.[50]

Simple. These are linear fractures that do not communicate with the oral cavity. Typical examples include fractures of the condyle, coronoid process, ascending ramus, or edentulous mandible.

Compound. By definition, this includes all fractures through the alveolar ridge that involve the roots of erupted teeth. Also included are those instances in

which an external or intraoral wound is present involving the fracture.

Comminuted. Gunshot wounds, high-velocity missiles, and other forceful impacts produce this type of injury.

Complicated. These are fractures that involve the inferior alveolar artery and nerve, etc.

Impacted. These fractures are uncommon in the mandible.

Pathologic. Structural weakness predisposing to fracture following minimal trauma can be caused by systemic disorders such as osteogenesis imperfecta or hyperparathyroidism. Focal disease such as mandibular cysts, tumors, and radionecrosis may also predispose to such fractures.

Although maxillary fractures most often occur in the horizontal plane, trauma to the mandibular arch tends to follow the long axis of the teeth (Fig. 7-36). An angle fracture is the most common with regard to site. (Fig. 7-37). Forces applied to the mandible may also be transmitted to the condylar region, and a condylar neck fracture is often found opposite the point of impact. These fractures often occur with medial and anterior displacement of the condylar process (Fig. 7-38). Isolated fractures of the coronoid process are uncommon. Displacement is the exception and occurs when the temporalis tendon is ruptured.

Because the mandible functions essentially as a bony ring, bilateral fractures are common (Fig. 7-39). The most frequent combinations are an oblique fracture of

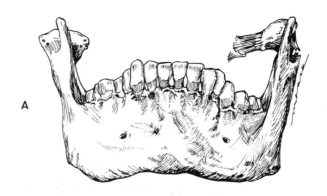

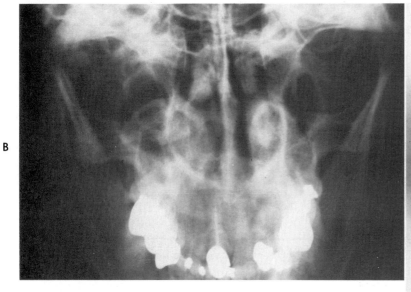

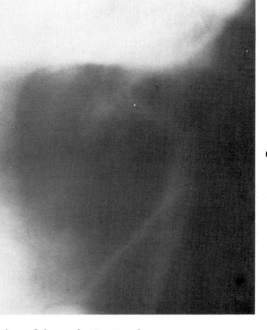

Fig. 7-38. **A,** Anatomic drawing of unilateral fracture through left condylar neck. Traction from lateral pterygoid muscle displaces condylar neck anteromedially. **B,** PA radiograph of patient with fracture through right condylar neck. Compare abnormal angle produced by fracture with normal left side. **C,** AP hypocycloidal tomogram of patient with left subcondylar fracture. Note typical medial displacement of condyle *(arrows).* (**A** modified from Rowe, N.L., and Killey, H.C.: Fractures of the facial skeleton, Baltimore, 1968, The Williams & Wilkins Co.)

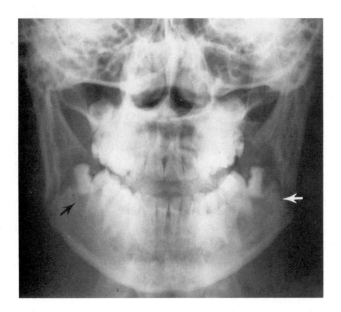

Fig. 7-39. Bilateral angle fractures *(arrows).*

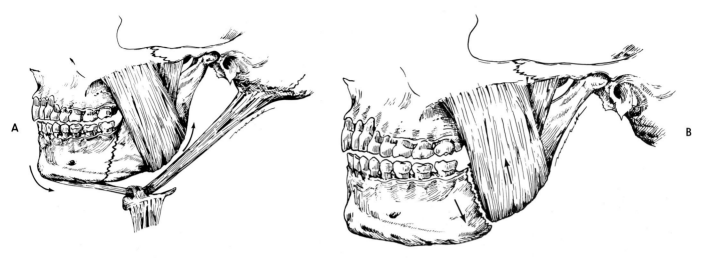

Fig. 7-40. A, Stable angle fracture. Pull of suprahyoid and masseter muscles against fracture line stabilizes it. **B,** Unstable angle fracture. Posterior fracture fragment is elevated while anterior segment is depressed by traction from suprahyoid musculature. In mandibular fractures, displacement of fragments almost always results from muscle pull and is rarely caused by force and direction of traumatic blow. (Modified from Rowe, N.L., and Killey, H.C.: Fractures of the facial skeleton, Baltimore, 1968, The Williams & Wilkins Co.)

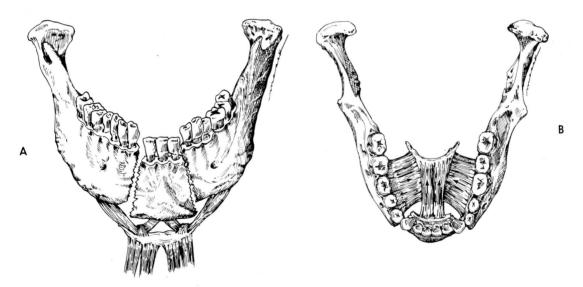

Fig. 7-41. Bilateral parasymphyseal fractures with posteroinferior displacement of symphysis caused by pull of suprahyoid (i.e., mylohyoid and digastric) muscles. (Modified from Rowe, N.L. and Killey, H.C.: Fractures of the facial skeleton, Baltimore, 1968, The Williams & Wilkins Co.)

the parasymphysis region associated with fracture of the opposite angle or occasionally the condyle.

Displacement of mandibular fractures depends on three factors: (1) the site of the fracture, (2) the direction in which the fracture line runs, and (3) the pull of powerful muscles that are attached to the mandible.[50] Midline symphyseal fractures usually have little or no displacement. Depending on the fracture line, bilateral angle fracture may be stable (Fig. 7-40, A) or unstable. Upward and medial displacement of the posterior fragments resulting from traction by the masticatory muscles may occur (Fig. 7-40, B). Bilateral parasymphyseal fractures often are associated with posteroinferior displacement of the symphysis, produced by the pull of the mylohyoid, geniohyoid, genioglossus, and anterior digastric muscles (Fig. 7-41).

Complications resulting from mandibular fractures include potential deformity, malocclusion and malunion if incorrectly treated, osteomyelitis (particularly if the host defenses are compromised), and rarely, facial nerve paralysis.[23] Multiple mandibular fractures can produce acute airway obstruction by allowing retrodisplacement of the tongue.[1] Undiagnosed, untreated intra-articular condylar fractures in children can be an unsuspected cause of growth disturbance.[46]

■ Bony conditions
Developmental abnormalities

Cleft palate. Occurring in approximately 1 in every 1500 live births in Caucasian populations, cleft palate is by far the most prevalent congenital anomaly to involve the maxillofacial skeleton. Cleft palate apparently results from a failure of fusion of the mesodermal masses that form the secondary palate in the embryo.[39] The cleft appears clinically as a midline palatal defect (except anteriorly, where it deviates to either side), usually between the lateral incisor and the canine teeth. Rarely, the cleft may occur between the central and lateral incisors. The alveolar ridge is also discontinuous in most cases of cleft palate.

Associated dental disturbances in the alveolar portion of the cleft are common. Absence of the lateral incisor tooth or the presence of an unerupted supernumerary tooth or both are frequently associated anomalies. Both findings are best evaluated on occlusal radiographs. In about half of cases of cleft palate the lateral incisor in the region of the cleft is missing.[68] The lateral incisor may also lie free within the bony gap. Supernumerary teeth can be found within the cleft or embedded on either side of it. If a normal lateral incisor is present

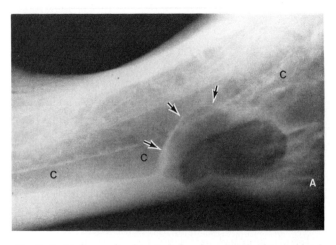

Fig. 7-42. Radiograph of typical developmental salivary gland defect. This defect is always seen below mandibular canal *(C)* and usually is located just anterior to angle *(A)* of bone. Notice corticated border *(arrows)* around defect.

along with a supernumerary tooth, the cleft usually passes between them. Some authors suggest the cleft is responsible for the presence of the supernumerary tooth by splitting the developing lateral incisor tooth bud.[68]

Developmental salivary gland defect. This entity is also known as static bone cyst, latent bone cyst, and Stafne bone cyst, none of which is as appropriate as the term *developmental salivary gland defect.* This defect is caused by embryonic inclusion of a small lobe of submandibular gland tissue in the lingual surface of the developing mandible.

Radiographically this bone defect has a distinctive, virtually pathognomonic appearance. It appears as a round or elliptical radiolucency with a regular, corticated, well defined margin. It lies below the mandibular canal, just anterior to the angle of the mandible (Fig. 7-42). The inferior mandibular border may or may not be intact.

Biopsies are usually not needed in these cases. Submandibular sialography with frontal projections may, however, be employed to confirm the presence of salivary gland tissue within the bone defect.[3] These salivary gland defects in the mandible are asymptomatic and clinically unimportant. Their presence is almost always discovered incidentally during radiography performed for an unrelated purpose. No treatment is required.

Hemifacial microsomia. Also referred to in the literature as the first and second branchial arch syndrome, this condition consists of asymmetric ear, facial, and mandibular defects. Gorlin and associates[23a] coined the term *hemifacial microsomia.* The principal radiographic feature of this condition is asymmetry of the mandible secondary to hypoplasia or agenesis of an affected condyle. With increasing severity, the condylar process and superior portions of the ramus become less recognizable and the gonial angle of the mandible becomes very obtuse. With time, hemimandibular hypoplasia is apparent as the affected side of the mandible loses its ability to grow in concert with the normal, contralateral side. The maxilla and zygomatic bones on the affected side of the face are also proportionately hypoplastic.

There is a definite correlation between the occurrence of ear defects and mandibular ramus changes in patients with this condition. Petrous ridge radiographs typically reveal otic abnormalities such as hypoplasia or atresia of the external auditory canal and ossicular deformities. About 50% of patients manifesting microtia (hypoplasia of the external ear) have mandibular ramal agenesis as well.[15]

Mandibulofacial dysostosis. Also called Treacher-Collins syndrome, mandibulofacial dysostosis is another of the heterogeneous branchial arch malformation syndromes. In contrast to hemifacial microsomia, there is fairly symmetric bilateral facial involvement. The most remarkable radiographic findings are underdeveloped or absent zygomatic bones and hypoplasia of the mandible. Micrognathia is almost always present in this condition and is one of the most notable characteristics.

Peculiar broad concave curvatures of the lower borders of the mandibular bodies have been noted in this condition (Fig. 7-43). Such inverted mandibular lower borders should not be mistakenly referred to as "antegonial notching".[47] True antegonial notching of the mandible, which is a more localized concavity near the angle, may be seen in several craniofacial developmental abnormalities, including mandibulofacial dysostosis, hemifacial microsomia, and congenital underdevelopment of the condyle.[7] Both signs, i.e., true antegonial notching and inverted (concave) lower borders of the mandible, are consistent with a radiographic impression of Treacher Collins' syndrome.

Underdevelopment of the zygomatic bones is the principal associated midfacial abnormality. The zygomatic processes of the maxillae are also hypoplastic. The maxillary and other paranasal air sinuses are usually small and in severe cases may be entirely absent. As in hemifacial microsomia, dysplasia of the external and middle ear structures is fairly common. Over a third of all patients with Treacher-Collins syndrome have narrowing or atresia of the external ear canals or associated ossicular defects.[15]

Pierre Robin syndrome. Infants born with this condition manifest micrognathia, glossoptosis, and cleft palate. Gorlin and associates[23a] believe that the lesion stems from arrested intrauterine development of the mandible as a primary defect, with subsequent glossoptosis resulting from deficient mandibular support for the tongue musculature. The retruded tongue presumably prevents a normal vertical-to-horizontal movement of the palatal shelves, leading in turn to various degrees of cleft palate. Affected infants typically have feeding problems and may require treatment for respiratory distress.

The correct diagnosis is usually established on the basis of fairly straightforward clinical features: a characteristic convex facial profile caused by the diminutive mandible, feeding and respiration difficulties, and cleft palate. Radiographic evaluation of the mandibular micrognathia performed soon after birth often provides a measure of the severity of the initial problem and an estimation of the likely long-term deformity.[47] If possible, cephalometric lateral and frontal skull projections should be obtained a month or two after birth. Pavlick and Pruzansky[43] have noted that by about 10 years of age the severe neonatal recession of the Pierre Robin mandible is diminished or absent. It was also noted that, with the catch-up in growth of the mandible, feeding and respiratory difficulties resolve in all cases in which there are not extraneous complications.

Peculiarities in the shape of the mandible in Pierre Robin syndrome have been thoroughly described.[47] The gonial angle is excessively obtuse, with the condylar process often extended distally from the distorted ramus. There is also a characteristic alteration in the ramus-to-body proportions of the mandible because of excessive reduction in mandibular body length.

Craniofacial dysostosis. This inherited disease of bone, also called Crouzon's disease, produces deformities of the cranium, midfacial bones and orbits. This abnormality is often diagnosed clinically at birth or within the first six months of life. The most consistent abnormal facial feature is maxillary hypoplasia. An unusually high palatal arch and in some cases a palatal cleft are frequently present. Malpositioning and crowding of the erupted teeth and impaction of unerupted teeth are associated findings.

Cleidocranial dysostosis. Another bone disease of unknown cause, cleidocranial dysostosis produces unusual effects in the clavicles, the skull, the jaws, and other

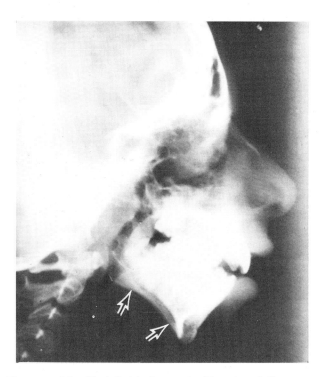

Fig. 7-43. Mandibulofacial dysostosis (Treacher-Collins syndrome). This cephalometric radiograph demonstrates typical convex facial profile, caused mainly by diminutive, retrognathic (posteriorly positioned) lower jaw. Concave contour of inferior mandibular border (*arrows*) is also evident. Aural anomalies are common in this disease.

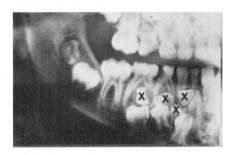

Fig. 7-44. Cleidocranial dysostosis. Four supernumerary (extra) permanent teeth *(X)* are embedded in bone along with normal complement of developing teeth. Same condition existed in other three dental quadrants of this patient.

bones. The maxilla is typically small, producing dental malocclusions and a flattened external appearance of the cheeks. The maxillary sinuses are usually poorly developed.

Dental abnormalities are almost always found in cleidocranial dysostosis. The most impressive dental manifestation is the tremendous number of embedded teeth in both jaws. The overall oral radiographic picture consists of several apparently independent conditions: (1) the presence of numerous supernumerary teeth (Fig. 7-44), (2) a failure of the deciduous teeth to exfoliate at the normal time, and (3) a simple lack of eruptive force in the developing permanent dentition. Despite the invariable loss of the relatively small deciduous teeth from the mouth by the time the patient reaches adulthood, the embedded permanent teeth usually still fail to erupt into the oral cavity.[30] All these factors produce very serious tooth crowding in the jaws. The typically underdeveloped maxilla in cleidocranial dysostosis exacerbates this problem.

Osteopetrosis. Osteopetrosis is a rare disease of bone in which there is abnormal persistence of calcified cartilage. This condition has also been called Albers-Schönberg disease and marble bone disease. An essential characteristic of the condition is increased density of the cancellous portion of all bones. There are two forms of the disease: a more severe, recessive form known as osteopetrosis congenita, which occurs in infants and young children, and a more benign, dominant form known as osteopetrosis tarda, most often initially seen in older children and young adults.

The more severe congenital form is characterized by both increased density of the bones and secondary complications resulting from bony sclerosis. Hypoplastic anemias, thrombocytopenia, splenomegaly, and hepatomegaly are common although the severity of the bone disease does not correlate well with the severity of the anemia.[19] Optic nerve atrophy may result from progres-

sive narrowing of the optic canals, ultimately leading to blindness. This severe form of the disease is usually fatal as a result of massive hemorrhage, anemia, or rampant bone infections.

Patients with the benign form of osteopetrosis tarda may be entirely asymptomatic. The disease may be discovered as an incidental finding on a dental radiographic examination or on a radiologic examination of the chest or extremities.[28] The mandible is noticeably affected in many cases of osteopetrosis, and in milder cases especially the dental radiographic examination may be the first evidence of its presence. The most common dental defect is an alteration of some root forms that may be deformed and stunted.[30] Focal areas of enamel hypoplasia on the crowns of some teeth have also been noted.[8] The normal eruptive pattern of the primary and secondary dentitions is often delayed in osteopetrosis because of the exceptional density of the alveolar bone.[52] Dental infection with secondary osteomyelitis is not uncommon.

The lamina dura surrounding the tooth roots becomes thickened, as do other cortical structures such as the borders of the mandibular canal. Osteopetrosis may be the only condition in which lamina dura thickening is associated with generalized increased density of the bone.[60] In severe cases the bone may become so dense that the tooth roots cannot be differentiated from the supporting bone.

Infantile cortical hyperostosis. A perplexing bone disease of infants, infantile cortical hyperostosis (also called Caffey's disease) remains without known cause or definite pathogenesis. Infantile cortical hyperostosis has an approximately equal incidence in males and females.[14] The average age of onset is about 9 weeks of age. It apparently never occurs after the fifth month of life.

The bones most commonly affected by infantile cortical hyperostosis are, in order of frequency, the mandible, clavicle, and ulna.[19] The high frequency of mandibular involvement is underscored by Burbank and associates,[13a] who contend that this diagnosis should probably not be made in its absence. The maxilla appears to be uninvolved. Infantile cortical hyperostosis is invariably polyostotic, except for unusual cases in which the mandible alone is involved.[14]

The mandible is affected bilaterally in almost all cases, although the two sides may demonstrate different degrees of involvement.[68] The cardinal radiographic feature is thickening of the inferior mandibular cortex. Overall enlargement of the mandibular body or thickening limited to the inferior cortex may be present. Cortical new bone is sometimes deposited in layers, producing a laminated radiographic appearance. Occasionally, the old, normal bone contour can be visualized through the dense new bone.[68]

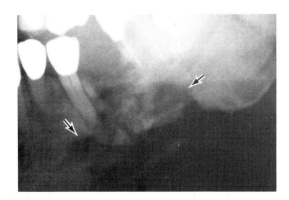

Fig. 7-45. Mandibular osteomyelitis caused by gross caries and pulpal infection of first molar tooth (previously extracted) secondarily infecting bone. Serpentine pattern of osteolysis (*arrows*) is evident.

Osteogenesis imperfecta. Osteogenesis imperfecta is an inherited skeletal disease that manifests several defects in those hard and soft tissues that have a major collagen component. These defects include, in various degrees, fragility of the bones, blue sclerae, progressive hearing loss, and dentinogenesis imperfecta. Dentinogenesis imperfecta, which was discussed earlier, usually appears as a solitary developmental abnormality limited to the teeth and without other associated skeletal lesions. However, because collagen is such a fundamental component of dentin, it is to be expected that dentinogenesis imperfecta is also often found in association with osteogenesis imperfecta.

Not all patients with osteogenesis imperfecta have perceptible dental defects, although the teeth generally are involved to some extent.[52] Heys and coworkers[26] found that 8 of 13 families with osteogenesis imperfecta also had at least one associated case of dentinogenesis imperfecta.

The radiographic features of dentinogenesis imperfecta associated with osteogenesis imperfecta are similar to those of isolated dentinogenesis imperfecta. These features include obliteration of the pulp spaces and formation of abnormal crown contours (bulbous or "dumpy" teeth). In osteogenesis imperfecta, obliteration of the pulp chambers may be confined to the permanent incisors and first molars.[30]

Osteomyelitis of the mandible

Acute and chronic osteomyelitis. The mandible is the most common bone to be affected by osteomyelitis. Carious, necrotic teeth are short, direct avenues by which infective organisms may penetrate deep within the lower jaw. By contrast, the maxilla is not often involved by osteomyelitis mainly because of its abundant collateral vasculature. Each side of the mandible receives a significant portion of its blood supply from a single source, i.e., the mandibular (inferior alveolar) artery, and is provided with minimal collateral supply. The mandible is therefore more dependent than most bones on the integrity of its major blood vessels. Therapeutic radiation of the oral cavity region, Paget's disease, and osteopetrosis all predispose the mandible to stubborn infections by compromising its blood supply. Radiation or salivary gland disorders can also diminish the production of saliva, thereby increasing the number and severity of dental caries and the chance of subsequent osteomyelitis.

No bony radiographic manifestations are present during the initial stages of infection. If osteomyelitis is of dental origin (as in the vast majority of mandibular cases) the affected side usually has a tooth with gross caries, a deep restoration, or a broken or fractured crown (Fig. 7-45). In many cases of mandibular osteomyelitis, even the early ones, dental radiographic findings are readily apparent (Fig. 7-46). Dental radiography also usually reveals periapical rarefying osteitis associated with the root apex of the responsible tooth. Here the lamina dura is discontinuous and a distinct periapical radiolucency is usually evident. If several teeth in the clinically suspicious area have carious lesions, the tooth with periapical rarefying osteitis can be incriminated as the infection source. If two or more teeth in the affected region demonstrate periapical rarefying osteitis, any or all of these teeth may cause the disease.

Radiographically, the diffuse osteolytic pattern seen in the acute inflammatory phase of mandibular osteomyelitis becomes more pronounced with time. Osteolysis follows an irregular, serpentine pattern as it borders islands of necrotic and viable bone. As larger segments or fragments of bone become separated from their blood supply, they become necrotic islands of nonvital bone (sequestra). Sequestra form in about 3 to 6 weeks

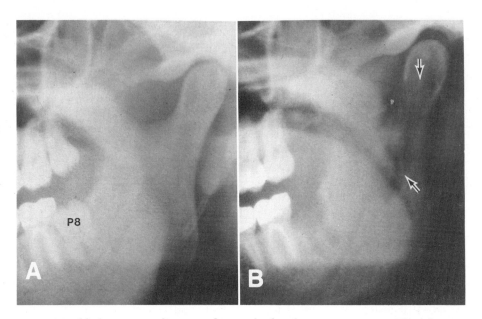

Fig. 7-46. Mandibular osteomyelitis secondary to third molar pericoronitis. **A,** Flap of gingiva covering impacted third molar *(P8)* became infected. At this time patient was febrile and oral signs of infection were obvious, but no radiographic changes of osteomyelitis were as yet evident. **B,** Same patient after 2-month interval. Notice rarefaction of condylar process *(arrows)* in comparison with **A.** This infection had been refractory to early antibiotic control.

in untreated or inadequately treated cases and are considered pathognomonic of osteomyelitis. Bone infection that spreads to the periosteum usually initiates periosteal new bone formation, producing an involucrum.

Garré's osteomyelitis. Garré's osteomyelitis occurs in response to mandibular infections secondary to necrotic teeth in children and adolescents. Though it usually occurs in response to a central bone infection, Garré's osteomyelitis can occur in response to soft tissue cellulitis near the jaw.[59] The inflammatory process is mild, chronic, and nonsuppurating. The original description of mandibular Garré's osteomyelitis notes that the condition probably occurs more frequently in the jaw than previously thought.[44] The typical picture is one of mild dental inflammation stimulating periosteal reaction out of proportion to the relatively unimpressive cancellous bone effects. This florid periosteal new bone overgrowth is similar to the involucrum formation of chronic osteomyelitis in adults.[68]

Radiographic findings include thickening of the lower mandibular border. The cortical thickening is invariably subjacent to a grossly carious tooth, usually a deciduous molar or a permanent first molar (Fig. 7-47). Other routine dental radiographic features include a periapical rarefying osteitis and often a surrounding condensing osteitis (Fig. 7-48). The degree of intraosseous bone destruction may be surprisingly minimal in Garré's osteo-

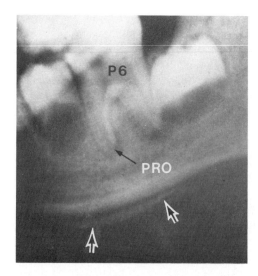

Fig. 7-47. Garré's osteomyelitis in 9-year-old child. Faint shell of subperiosteal reactive bone *(arrows)* can be seen adjacent to inferior cortex. Grossly carious first molar tooth *(P6)* was focal cause of bone disease. Except for periapical rarefying osteitis (PRO) no medullary effects are seen in bone.

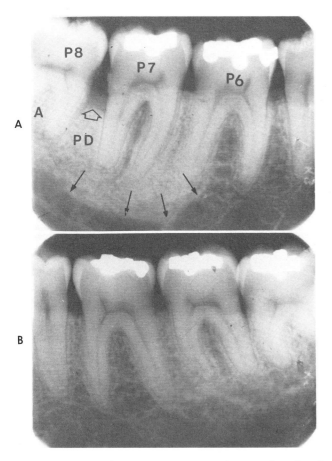

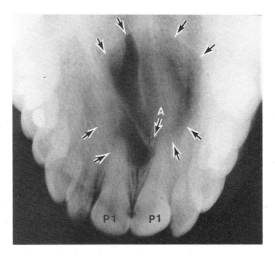

Fig. 7-49. Incisive canal (nasopalatine canal) cyst. Within confines of cyst *(arrows)*, shadow of anterior nasal spine *(A)* is superimposed. Careful inspection of lamina dura of central incisors *(P1)* is necessary in these cases to arrive at diagnosis of radicular cyst.

Fig. 7-48. **A,** Condensing osteitis, seen here as broad radiopaque area *(arrows)* surrounding roots of *P7* and distal root of *P6*. The inflammatory nidus is periodontal disease *(PD)* between *P7* and *P8*. **B,** Normal jaw side of same patient for comparison. Normal alveolar process bone density is demonstrated.

myelitis. However, the inferior mandibular cortex is often several times its normal thickness. Following treatment of the offending tooth, the cortical thickening gradually resolves although 1 or more years may pass before normal mandibular dimensions are restored.

Garré's osteomyelitis can superficially resemble infantile cortical hyperostosis (Caffey's disease) although the latter condition is a bilateral process. In Caffey's disease, increased density is present throughout the bone, not just at the inferior border. Infantile cortical hyperostosis also typically occurs in the first few months of life, while Garré's osteomyelitis in the jaw is seen in older children.

Bony cysts

True cysts are fluid-filled bony defects that are lined with epithelium. Several varieties are occasionally found in the mandible and maxilla.[38,58] With few exceptions they are derived from embedded remnants of odontogenic epithelium. In the anterior maxilla, however, true nonodontogenic bony cysts may occur. These are the *fissural cysts* that arise from epithelium trapped within lines of embryonic fissures or sutures (Fig. 7-49).

Odontogenic cysts

Radicular cyst. This entity, sometimes called a dental cyst or periodontal cyst, is the most common cystic lesion in the jaws. It occurs at the root apex of a necrotic, nonvital tooth that has typically been gutted by caries. This cyst forms from epithelial remnants or cell rests in the periodontal ligament space that proliferate when stimulated by a dental inflammation. An osmotic fluid imbalance draws tissue fluid into the cyst, which then undergoes a slow increase in size, typically reaching a maximum of 2 to 3 cm in diameter. As the cyst expands it exerts gentle expansile pressure against the surrounding bone. This pressure, equal in all directions, accounts for the tendency of these lesions to assume a regular globular configuration.

A small or moderate size radicular cyst has a radiographic appearance similar to that of routine periapical rarefying osteitis (Fig. 7-50). With both types of lesions, the thin, radiopaque lamina dura that normally surrounds the root apex is missing. Most radicular cysts, particularly those over 1 cm in diameter, have a well-defined, discrete surrounding cortex. Mandibular radicular cysts commonly displace the inferior alveolar canal inferiorly. Relatively large lesions also exert fairly uniform outward pressure on the buccal and to a lesser extent the lingual cortical plates. Radicular cysts may tilt or displace nearby teeth, and, uncommonly, may cause resorption of neighboring root apices.

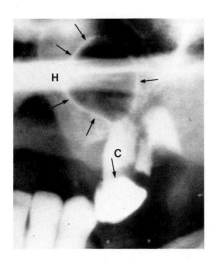

Fig. 7-50. Radicular cyst. Involved tooth has gross caries *(C)*. Shadow of hard palate *(H)* is superimposed across cyst. This lesion is typically regular in shape and well circumscribed *(arrows)*.

It takes about 10 years for the average radicular cyst to attain a size of 2 cm in greatest diameter.[3] It is unlikely that a mandibular cyst much less than 2 cm in anteroposterior diameter would produce a clinically noticeable swelling of the buccal and lingual cortical plates. Consequently, most radicular cysts are discovered as incidental findings on radiographic examinations in search of dental caries.

Dentigerous cyst. The term *dentigerous cyst* refers to a cyst that contains a tooth crown and occurs in the jaws. This lesion is also sometimes called a follicular cyst. Dentigerous cysts develop in or from some part of the follicle that surrounds the developing teeth. Specifically, dentigerous cysts develop within the enamel organ (i.e., part of the follicular epithelial lining) that surrounds the crown of a tooth still in the process of root formation. Such a lesion thus begins its development after formation of the tooth crown but before root formation is complete. Growth of the cyst occurs as tissue fluid is drawn down an osmotic gradient into the follicular sac and accumulates between the latter and the occlusal surface of the tooth.

Teeth involved with dentigerous cysts are necessarily embedded within the jaws. In most cases such teeth are impacted by an adjacent tooth or a pathologic process. Dentigerous cysts are discovered in young persons usually during routine dental radiographic survey or in a deliberate search for an unerupted permanent tooth. The teeth most likely to be involved are the third molars and the maxillary canines. Not coincidentally, these are the teeth also most commonly impacted within the jaws.

Dentigerous cysts vary in size. Most are discovered

and removed before they become greater than 4 to 5 cm in diameter. Unusual ones, however, can attain striking size. A few may enlarge to occupy a whole mandibular body or ramus. The rate of growth tends to be fairly rapid in a child, with cysts of 4 to 5 cm having developed in only 3 to 4 years. In adults, dentigerous cyst enlargement is apparently much slower.

Small dentigerous cysts are not seen on radiographs until the radiolucent pericoronal (follicular) space around the crown of an involved tooth attains a thickness noticeably larger than normal. Most normal pericoronal spaces are about 2 mm or less in thickness. A pericoronal space of 2.5 mm may thus be an early indicator of dentigerous cyst, although most experienced observers consider such a dimension equivocal. If the pericoronal space is 4 to 5 mm wide, a cyst is almost certainly present.

As the cystic lesion enlarges, the enclosed radiolucency becomes more pronounced. Eventually the involved tooth crown appears to project directly into the cyst lumen. The typical dentigerous cyst completely envelopes the tooth crown. Less commonly, dentigerous cysts arise from the side of a tooth crown. In such instances they are referred to as lateral dentigerous cysts.

With increasing size, the expansile pressure of a dentigerous cyst can displace the tooth of origin. Typically the expansile pressure of a moderate-size cyst will more than offset any eruptive force the involved tooth might still retain. In the mandible a molar tooth involved with a large dentigerous cyst may be displaced far from its developmental site, to a point near the jaw's inferior border, or even into the superior region of the ramus. In the maxilla, dentigerous cyst expansion may displace a tooth superiorly as high as the orbital floor.

Radiographically the lesion appears as a rounded, unilocular bone cavity associated with the crown of an unerupted tooth (Fig. 7-51). Lateral occlusal radiography will show that the lesion is devoid of any intrinsic structure other than the tooth crown. There are no residual trabeculae and no intrinsic septa. With very large mandibular cysts multilocularity is occasionally apparent. This is not a result of actual internal septation but merely of the formation of prominent ridges on the walls of the cavity.[31]

A distinct cortex surrounds most or all of the cystic lesion. When the buccal and lingual walls of the jaw itself are enlarged, such an expansion appears smooth, regular, and somewhat fusiform. Subperiosteal bone formation usually prevents perforation of the bony plates. The roots of adjacent teeth may be slightly resorbed by the lesion. More commonly they are intact but displaced.

Residual cyst. Continued periapical growth of a radicular cyst, after a nonvital tooth has been extracted,

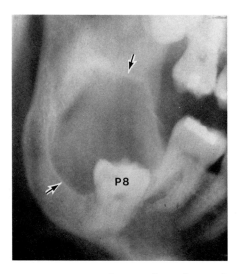

Fig. 7-51. Dentigerous cyst. This cyst formed around crown of impacted third molar (*P8*). Inertia of enlarging cyst itself, however, has pushed tooth deeper in bone.

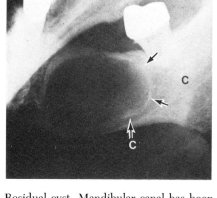

Fig. 7-52. Residual cyst. Mandibular canal has been displaced inferiorly. This lesion is residual from an earlier radicular cyst, itself having been associated with a carious, necrotic tooth (long since extracted). Mandibular canal (*C*) has been deviated toward inferior cortex.

results in a residual cyst. The typical case is that of a periapical radiolucency that is not suspected of being a cyst and consequently is not treated at the time that the causative necrotic tooth is extracted. Residual cysts nearly always are sequelae of radicular cysts, while recurrent cysts are usually remnants of dentigerous or primordial cysts.

Radiographically a residual cyst appears as a round or oval radiolucency in the alveolar process (Fig. 7-52). Most moderate-size (1 to 2 cm) residual cysts have well-delineated radiopaque margins. Occasionally, residual cysts may enlarge dramatically, completely filling the mandibular body and causing noticeable swelling of the jaw itself. The presence of a tooth extraction socket in a radiolucent cystic area strongly suggests the presence of a residual cyst.

Primordial cyst. Primordial cysts arise from special odontogenic epithelial cells that ordinarily do not participate directly in tooth development. This type of cyst develops from the tooth primordium (i.e., the undifferentiated dental lamina), not from the enamel organ of a forming tooth crown as does a dentigerous cyst. Most primordial cysts develop in the third molar region of the mandible and expand posteriorly into the ramus or superiorly toward the coronoid process.

Primordial cysts appear as purely radiolucent lesions that contain no tooth crown, unlike dentigerous cysts, which are always associated with a tooth crown (Fig. 7-53). A unilocular primordial cyst is therefore radio-

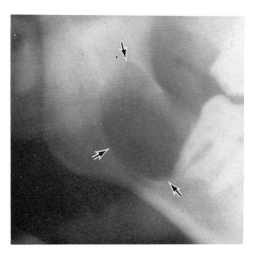

Fig. 7-53. Primordial cyst. Third molar (*P8*) is absent. This primordial cyst arose from follicle of third molar before crown had calcified. Such lesions are especially common in third molar regions but are otherwise difficult to distinguish radiographically from residual cysts.

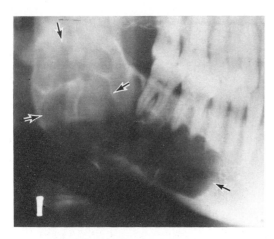

Fig. 7-54. Odontogenic keratocyst. Note multilocular internal structure. Third molar is absent.

graphically similar in morphology to a residual cyst; both are globular cystic bone defects that are not associated with teeth. There are helpful points of differentiation, however. If such a radiolucent lesion is located posterior to the dental arch, or if an entire normal complement of teeth is present, the indication is that of a primordial cyst. In contrast to most odontogenic cysts, primordial cysts can occasionally be multilocular. Actual bony septation of the cystic cavity may be present, as opposed to a simple ridging of the buccal and lingual walls. A multiloculated primordial cyst cannot easily be radiographically distinguished from other multiloculated lesions, such as an ameloblastoma.

The most significant clinical features of the primordial cysts, particularly those that contain keratin, are their high rate of recurrence (at least 40%). The need for diligent radiographic follow-up of surgically operated sites is therefore evident. Clinicians should be urged to follow up such patients radiographically for a minimum of 5 years.

ODONTOGENIC KERATOCYST. The term *odontogenic keratocyst* is often equated by dental clinicians with primordial cyst. Keratocysts (Fig. 7-54), however, are actually a subtype of primordial cyst. They usually have a keratinized layer of surface epithelium and always contain clumps of keratin within the cyst cavity. The diagnosis of a keratocyst is a *histopathologic* one, based on a particular type of epithelial lining common to many primordial cysts. Radiographic differentiation of keratocysts from other primordial cysts is probably not possible (and certainly not reliable).

GORLIN'S SYNDROME. Gorlin's syndrome, also known as multiple basal cell nevus syndrome, has as one of its principal features the occurence of multiple keratin-containing primordial cysts (i.e., keratocysts) within the mandible. This syndrome consists of multiple nevoid basal cell lesions singly or in association with basal cell carcinomas, jaw cysts, and skeletal anomalies (usually bifid, fused, or rudimentary ribs). Bilateral, unilocular or multilocular well-defined radiolucencies in one or both jaws, especially in the posterior mandible, should suggest the possibility of Gorlin's syndrome. It is the multiplicity of such jaw lesions that is most significant in establishing the diagnosis.

Gorlin's syndrome should not be confused with cherubism. The cystic lesions in Gorlin's syndrome arise in older children and adolescents, whereas cherubic cystic lesions are typically first found in much younger (less than 6 years old) children.

Nonodontogenic cysts
Traumatic bone cyst. This lesion has also been called solitary bone cyst, hemorrhagic bone cyst, unicameral cyst, and simple bone cyst. The variety of names underscores the confusion that exists about the cause of this lesion. Use of the term *cyst* may itself be inappropriate because traumatic bone cysts contain fluid but do not have an epithelial lining.

Most traumatic bone cysts are found within the mandible between the canine and third molar areas. The maxilla is rarely affected. Similar cystlike lesions are seen elsewhere in the skeleton, particularly in the long bones, and are usually called unicameral cysts.

Traumatic mandibular cysts are found in older children and adolescents. They are decidedly rare in patients over the age of 35. The lesions are usually asymptomatic and therefore are most often incidental radiographic findings. Although some lesions may destroy a considerable volume of spongy bone, bone enlargement (as evidenced by expansion of the cortical plates) is considerably less obvious than with other jaw cysts.

Radiographically, traumatic bone cyst appears as a unilocular cavity devoid of internal trabeculation but occasionally demonstrating ridging on its internal bone surfaces (Fig. 7-55, *A*). The lesion is fairly well defined at its periphery but is usually without a complete cortical border. Swelling or "bossing" of the buccal and lingual cortical plates is uncommon, and when present is not prominent.

The most characteristic radiographic feature of the mandibular traumatic bone cyst is its tendency to extend upward between the teeth toward the alveolar crest without causing splaying, movement, or erosion of the teeth. This is particularly well seen in the premolar-molar region, where the roots are fairly widely spaced. Its characteristic "scalloped" superior border seems to undulate around the roots and up into the interdental bone (Fig. 7-55, *B*). Such a scalloped border is not often seen anteriorly, where the incisor roots are packed much closer together. As a traumatic bone cyst surrounds one or more dental roots, the lamina dura is

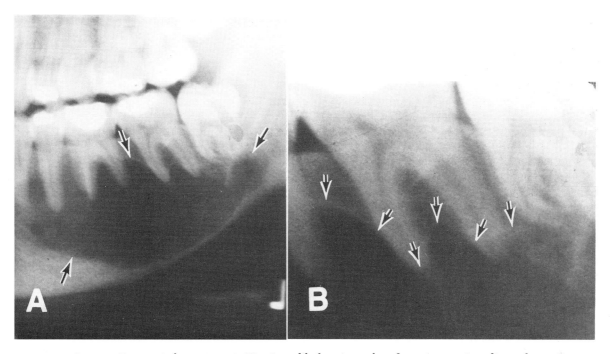

Fig. 7-55. Traumatic bone cyst. **A,** Hemimandibular view taken from panoramic radiograph. Note thinning of inferior border *(arrows).* **B,** Close-up view of same cyst. Arrows point to scalloping of superior border of lesion around roots of teeth. This finding is characteristic.

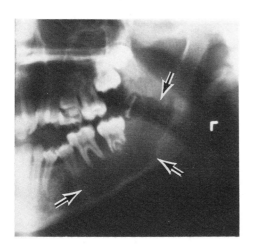

Fig. 7-56. Aneurysmal bone cyst *(arrows).* Lesion appears radiolucent and unilocular. Note adjacent root resorption.

generally preserved. In some cases the lamina dura of several teeth may be thinned to such a degree that it is not apparent radiographically although surgeons, on opening the lesion, invariably find the roots to be covered by a thin bony shell.

Aneurysmal bone cyst. Only about two dozen cases of aneurysmal bone cyst in the jaws have been reported; few of these have occurred in the maxilla. They are usually found in female patients under 20 years of age and are only discovered when the patient notices lower facial asymmetry caused by underlying bony expansion.

The radiographic features of a mandibular aneurysmal bone cyst resemble those of a giant cell granuloma. Aneurysmal bone cyst is a radiolucent lesion that can be either unilocular or divided into faint locules. Frank multilocularity, as evidenced by a "honeycomb" internal structure, has been seen in some lesions. The bony cortices are typically expanded and thinned as the cyst enlarges. It may reach a size of several centimeters or more. Displacement of the roots of erupted teeth or the follicles of developing teeth is commonly seen. Minimal root resorption may also be present (Fig. 7-56).

Tumors

Ameloblastoma. Ameloblastoma is the most common benign tumor of the jaws.[68] The lesion has also been called adamantinoma. *Ameloblastoma* is the more appropriate term because the mass is principally composed of ameloblasts, the cells that lay down the enamel matrix for tooth crowns. The ameloblastoma is derived from epithelial cells that occur in (1) the enamel organ of developing tooth crowns, (2) the follicles that line embedded teeth, (3) the periodontal ligament spaces surrounding erupted tooth roots, or (4) the linings of dentigerous cysts. Ameloblastoma is strictly a soft tissue tumor; it produces no enamel or other calcified tissue and therefore appears radiolucent. Because it develops from odontogenic epithelium, the ameloblastoma is found only in the jaws.

An ameloblastoma grows relatively slowly, often taking years to double its size. However, while the ameloblastoma is benign and does not metastasize, it is very persistent, is locally aggressive, and tends to recur unless completely eradicated. Nontreated or inadequately treated cases that recur may eventually destroy an entire hemimandible, from midline to condylar process. (Ameloblastomas occurring in the ramus tend to spare the condylar process itself.) The lesion can in time attain grossly disfiguring size.

The radiographic picture of ameloblastoma is usually nonspecific for small lesions but quite characteristic for the large ones. Small lesions are seen as rounded, unilocular cavities in the interdental or periapical bone and as such are virtually indistinguishable from a small residual or primordial cyst. With increasing size, however, the ameloblastoma takes on a characteristic mul-

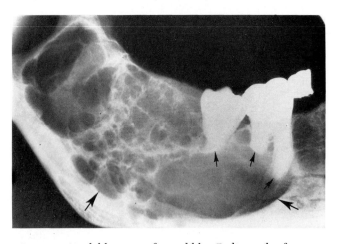

Fig. 7-57. Ameloblastoma of mandible. Radiograph of an excised surgical specimen. Lesion extends from molar region to superior portion of ramus *(upper left)*. Notice particularly (1) multilocularity of lesion, (2) heterogeneity in size of various loculations, (3) well-defined margins *(large arrows)*, and (4) resorption of tooth roots *(small arrows)*.

tiloculated pattern. Typically, the well-established lesion consists of multiple round cystic cavities with curved septa (Fig. 7-57). The typical large (greater than 5 cm) lesion contains one or two larger central cavities and numerous smaller "daughter cysts" surrounding them. Ameloblastoma can often be reliably differentiated from other multilocular mandibular lesions on the basis of its rounded loculations.

Because ameloblastomas grow slowly, they present fairly well-defined margins. As a lesion increases in size, it expands the adjacent cortex. This bony expansion is not regular and fusiform but rather irregular and undulating. Unilateral jaw expansion is the most common complaint in affected patients.

Tooth roots in the vicinity of an ameloblastoma are rarely displaced although resorption of root apices is common (Figs. 7-58 and 7-59). Ameloblastoma produces more extensive root resorption than most benign or malignant jaw lesions.[54]

Odontomas. The term *odontoma* is ordinarily reserved for two specific lesions in which ameloblasts and other tooth-forming cells (called odontoblasts) produce hard, radiopaque dental tissues in abnormal and often bizarre patterns. These two related but distinct tumors are called the compound and the complex odontomas.

Compound odontoma. The compound variety is the more common type of odontoma. It originates from the proliferation of fetal dental lamina and therefore does not increase or decrease the number of teeth normally present in the dental arch. Compound odontomas are usually located in the canine region of either the mandible or the maxilla. These tumors ultimately become only about as large as the adjacent teeth and develop at approximately the same age as do their normal neighboring teeth. They are usually asymptomatic.

Radiographically, compound odontoma usually appears as a small bundle of dwarfed, misshapen rudimentary teeth (Fig. 7-60). An enamel cap and pulp chamber can sometimes be identified in one or more of the little teeth. The number of teeth in the lesion usually varies from 3 to 36. In general, the larger the number of contained teeth the smaller they appear. One extraordinary case with 2000 tiny teeth in a single compound odontoma has been reported.[68]

On histopathologic study, the calcified masses are surrounded by a fibrous capsule. Radiographically, this capsule appears as a thin radiolucent line. If a large number of teeth are present, the line encompasses the entire lesion; if only a few teeth are identified, each may have its own surrounding "capsule." The radiolucent capsular space is very much like a normal tooth's periodontal ligament space.

Complex odontoma. The complex odontoma is generally a single tumor mass composed of two or more

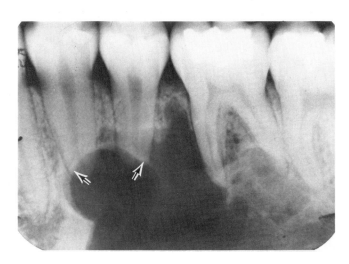

Fig. 7-58. Ameloblastoma of mandible. Periapical radiograph shows portion of lesion in posterior interdental area. Arrows indicate characteristic roundness of one anterior locule. Root apices have been slightly blunted.

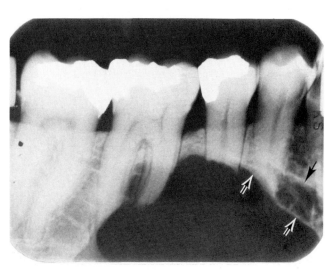

Fig. 7-59. Ameloblastoma of mandible. Lesion has resorbed roots of two premolars and first molar with almost surgical decisiveness. Notice that anterosuperior lesion margin *(black arrow)* extends past greatly radiolucent part *(outlined arrows)*.

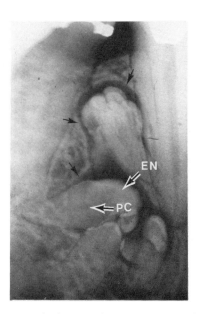

Fig. 7-60. Compound odontoma between two mandibular tooth roots. Tumor is composed of tiny vestigial teeth, clumped together and surrounded by radiolucent capsule *(arrows)*. In one larger tooth form enamel cap *(EN)* and pulp canal *(PC)* can be discerned.

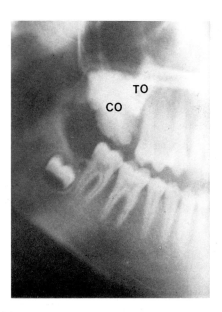

Fig. 7-61. Complex odontoma *(CO)* of posterior maxilla. This tumor of hard dental tissues appears as amorphous radiopacity rather than as small, distinct teeth (see Fig. 7-54). Notice two characteristic features: one normally occurring tooth in region is missing, and another tooth *(TO)* is impacted deep under lesion. Radiolucent capsule around lesion is not apparent on this view.

hard dental tissues (enamel, dentin, or cementum) in varying proportions. As this lesion develops, the dental substances are laid down in a totally disorganized and haphazard fashion without any semblance of normal tooth arrangement. The entire mass is surrounded by a fibrous capsule.

Complex odontoma develops from the germ of a normally occurring tooth prior to crown formation; the affected tooth therefore never develops. The complex odontoma is thus found in lieu of a normally occurring tooth and the number of teeth present in the dental arch is reduced by one.

Complex odontomas develop in generally the same time frame as the neighboring teeth and are therefore not often seen in teenagers or young adults. They usually occur in the molar regions. Complex odontomas are rarely more than two or three times larger than an adjacent tooth and are usually asymptomatic. They may be discovered incidentally during a child's first full-mouth radiographic examination.

Radiographically, complex odontoma appears as a uniformly opaque but irregular mass surrounded by a thin but intact radiolucent line. The crown of an impacted molar is usually found under the odontoma (Fig. 7-61).

The main difference between compound and complex odontomas is that in the compound variety the radiopaque structures bear at least a superficial resemblance to teeth. The irregular, jumbled radiopaque masses of the complex type do not even remotely resemble normal teeth. In addition, in the compound type several distinct dental masses will be present, whereas the complex lesion consists of only a solitary radiopaque mass.

Osteoma

Jaw osteoma. Osteoma is only one of a variety of nonodontogenic bony overgrowths that may affect the jaws. Others include (1) osteochondroma of the mandibular condyle, (2) hyperplasia of the condyle, and (3) tori of the mandible and maxilla. Only osteoma and osteochondroma are true neoplasms. In addition to these external overgrowths, the mandible often contains internal central islands of dense bone. These are appropriately called enostoses or areas of osteosclerosis, depending on their relationship to the bony endosteal surface.

Osteomas are mostly found in and around the skull, especially at the outer table. The various paranasal air sinuses are commonly affected. The jaws are also frequent sites for osteoma. Most mandibular osteomas are located below the lower molars and protrude inferiorly (Fig. 7-62).

Osteomas may occur at any age. In the jaw they tend to grow very slowly and do not produce symptoms or signs until their size causes noticeable deformity.

Osteomas are composed of dense, hard, compact bone. Histologically they are identical to normal cortical bone. Unusual osteomas may be mainly composed of cancellous bone with a covering cortex. Jaw osteomas may have a wide-based, sessile appearance or they may appear pedunculated, with a broad stalk.

Gardner's syndrome. Multiple osteomas of the skull, facial, or jaw bones with multiple colonic polyps are found in Gardner's syndrome.[63] Histologically these are identical to solitary osteomas. Multiple impacted supernumerary and permanent teeth are other oral radiographic features of this syndrome.

Tori. The term *torus* (pl. *tori*) is used to designate a

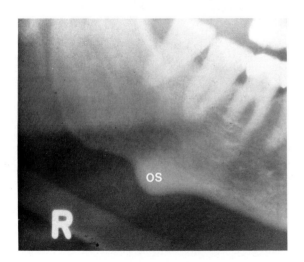

Fig. 7-62. Osteoma. Typical osteoma *(OS)* of mandible is shown. Location is usually at inferior mandibular border just anterior to angle. This sessile type of osteoma is seen as bulging of cortex inferiorly.

particular type of exostosis or bony protruberance that occurs along the midline of the palate or along the lingual surfaces of the mandible. Such bony growths generally occur bilaterally and are widely referred to as palatine and mandibular tori. These are hereditary lesions and are not true bony tumors.

TORUS PALATINUS. Palatine torus represents a bilateral enlargement of both midline margins of the palatal processes of the maxilla. These growths coalesce and appear clinically as a single dense midline palatal protuberance. The lesion is generally first noticed on clinical inspection. On periapical or maxillary occlusal radiographic projections, this entity produces a distinctive radiopaque oblong midline shadow.

TORUS MANDIBULARIS. These bony masses occur on the lingual surfaces of both sides of the mandible above the mylohyoid ridge, primarily in the canine-premolar region. They are almost always bilateral and are usually symmetric. Mandibular tori are quite radiopaque when seen on periapical, mandibular occlusal, or panoramic radiographs. Their density, location, and bilaterality make the radiographic appearance pathognomonic (Fig. 7-63).

Palatine and mandibular tori have no pathologic importance because they are benign, static growths that do not become malignant. They are only of any clinical significance if denture construction is contemplated.

Epidermoid (squamous cell) carcinoma. Oral carcinoma is the most common malignant lesion involving the jaws, surpassing primary bone malignancies such as osteogenic sarcoma and multiple myeloma. Over 90% of oral epidermoid carcinomas are of the squamous cell variety, with adenocarcinoma (principally from minor salivary glands) accounting for most of the remainder.

Squamous cell carcinoma arises (in order of frequency) from the lateral border of the tongue, floor of the mouth, tonsillar area, gingiva and alveolar mucosa, buccal mucosa, soft palate, hard palate, and oropharynx. Ninety percent of all oral malignancies occur in patients over the age of 45; the average age at diagnosis is 60 years.

Oral carcinoma involves the jaws by direct extension from contiguous mucous membranes. Because the maxilla is not in direct contiguity with the tongue or the floor of the mouth, involvement of the maxilla by oral carcinoma is much less common than involvement of the mandible. The lingual surface of the mandibular alveolar process is the site most frequently affected.

Radiographically, a concave or "dished out" osteolytic defect is usually seen at the crest of the alveolar ridge (Fig. 7-64). The term *saucerization* is occasionally used to describe a broad area of alveolar involvement. If there are teeth in the area, the tumor tends preferentially to destroy their bony support. The teeth then appear to be "standing in space" or "floating" (Fig. 7-65). Occasionally, carcinoma resorbs adjacent tooth roots, but such resorption is mild compared to the striking

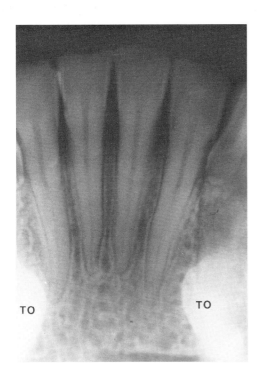

TO   TO

Fig. 7-63. Mandibular tori. On periapical view of anterior teeth, tori *(TO)* are seen bilaterally as convex radiopaque protuberances pointing medially from sides of film. These bony exostoses would be easily seen and palpated intraorally.

alveolar bone loss. Involved teeth are usually not greatly displaced even if their bony support has been entirely depleted.

The radiographic margins of any jaw erosion merit the most exacting scrutiny. Periapical and occlusal projections are particularly helpful. Permeative, destructive carcinoma produces an irregular, poorly marginated osteolytic appearance.

Radiographically, certain severe cases of periodontitis may mimic mucosal carcinoma. Both diseases may produce an ill-defined bone destruction at the alveolar crest. However, the character of infiltrating carcinoma is usually more aggressive and this entity thus appears more irregular and destructive (Fig. 7-66). Periodontitis tends to be more localized around the involved teeth. If the teeth are completely devoid of supporting bone, periodontal disease can usually be excluded because even in severe cases the root apices remain embedded in bone.

Osteogenic sarcoma. Osteogenic sarcoma of the jaws represents between 6.5% and 7.4% of all osteosarcomas. Mean patient age for mandibular osteosarcoma is 28 to 30 years, significantly higher than similar lesions in other locations.[18] The most common symptoms of mandibular osteosarcoma are swelling of the bone (pos-

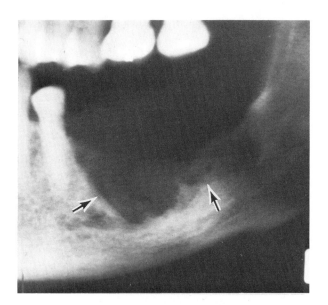

Fig. 7-64. Oral carcinoma. Shown is panoramic view of mandibular alveolar process destruction caused by large squamous cell carcinoma from lateral tongue border. Area of osteolysis has poorly defined, irregular borders *(arrows)*.

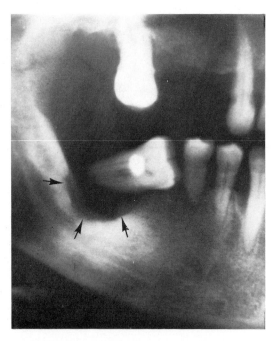

Fig. 7-65. Oral carcinoma. These tumors typically are seen radiographically as erosions into alveolar process, especially at ridge crest. Teeth in area are slowly eroded, if at all, even when completely devoid of bony support; hence classic "teeth standing in space" appearance, represented here by tilted molar tooth. Arrows show extent of bone erosion.

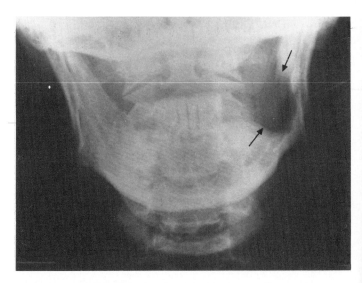

Fig. 7-66. Mandibular alveolar process erosion *(arrows)* produced by large carcinoma on left border of tongue. This AP view of mandible indicates that tumor was lingual in origin, a finding not apparent on panoramic radiography.

sibly with pain or loose teeth in the involved area) and bleeding around the necks of the teeth.

Jaw osteosarcoma may be either osteoblastic or osteolytic. Radiographically the principal features of this lesion are similar to those observed in the long bones. A central, ill-defined area of bone destruction with fluffy, coalescent radiopacities is seen. A typical osteoblastic osteosarcoma resembles a mass of cotton wool (Fig. 7-67).

As an early event in the jaws, incipient jaw osteosarcomas may invade the periodontal ligament spaces of one or more teeth.[22] Even prior to manifesting alterations in the cortical or trabecular bone, these lesions may cause a noticeable destruction in the periodontal tissues. Widening of the periodontal ligament space and erosion of the lamina dura become apparent. Such early changes are best delineated by periapical radiography (Fig. 7-68). Several other conditions may produce widening of the periodontal ligament space. These conditions include orthodontic banding of the teeth, progressive systemic sclerosis, and bruxism (grinding of the teeth).

Other radiographic signs of osteosarcoma, including "sunray spiculation" (Fig. 7-69) and "Codman's triangles," are occasionally seen at the mandibular periph-

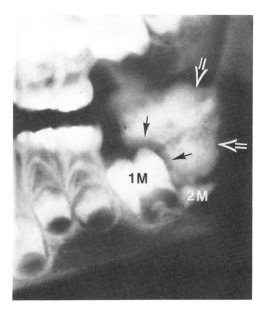

Fig. 7-67. Osteogenic sarcoma of mandible in 5½-year-old child. Outlined arrows indicate superior and posterior limits of tumor. Lesion has fluffy radiopaque character. Superiorly, lesion had extended past occlusal surfaces of teeth and had perforated oral mucosa. Notice that lesion has not yet eroded through radiolucent follicle *(black arrows)* of unerupted first molar tooth *(1M)*. *2M*, Second molar.

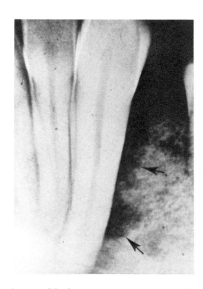

Fig. 7-68. Early mandibular osteogenic sarcoma. Lesion, which originated in interdental alveolar bone, has preferentially resorbed distal periodontal ligament space of canine tooth. Irregular, poorly contained nature of destructive process is obvious. Arrows show pathologic PDL space enlargement.

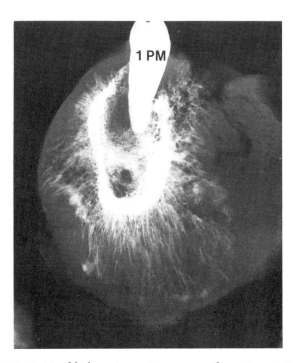

Fig. 7-69. Mandibular osteogenic sarcoma. Shown is anterior view of coronally sectioned mandibulectomy specimen completely infiltrated by osteogenic sarcoma. Level of section is at first premolar tooth *(1PM)*. On close inspection, fine "sunray" spicules can be seen emanating from bone at near-90° angles. This type of bone spiculation is caused by aggressive and rapid periosteal expansion of central bone tumor.

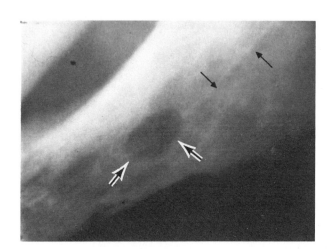

Fig. 7-70. Metastases to mandible from breast carcinoma. Multiple round to oval radiolucencies are seen in posterior body of mandible. Largest of these lesions is indicated by outlined arrows and is centered in bone, directly over mandibular canal *(black arrows)*. Clinically, this patient had right side lower jaw pain and right mental nerve paresthesia.

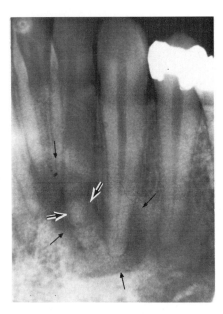

Fig. 7-71. Periapical cemental dysplasia. Lesion is seen as mixed density lesion. Black arrows delimit extent of radiolucency while outlined arrows point to intrinsic radiopaque nodules. Location of lesion in this case is characteristic: periapical area of several mandibular anterior teeth. Teeth themselves are not involved and are perfectly sound.

ery. With large tumors such periosteal signs are apparent on panoramic radiography at the inferior border of the jaw. In cases of smaller, less extensive tumors, occlusal radiographs of the suspicious mandibular area are helpful. Inconspicuous sunray spicules may sometimes be seen at the lingual or buccal cortical surfaces or both on this projection.

Metastases. Metastases to the mandible are relatively uncommon. Most appear as radiolucent lesions with ill-defined borders (Fig. 7-70).

Diseases of bone manifested in the jaws

Odontogenic conditions

Periapical cemental dysplasia. Periapical cemental dysplasia is one of the more commonly encountered noninflammatory jaw lesions. Many older dental texts have referred to this entity as cementoma, but most contemporary oral pathologists think that the name *periapical cemental dysplasia* (PCD) more accurately reflects the pathologic character of the lesion. PCD is a reactive fibro-osseous type of bone lesion that originates from odontogenic cells in the periodontal ligament spaces.

The typical patient is a middle-aged adult (mean age 40 years), female (9:1 ratio over males), and black (2:1 ratio over whites).[24] PCD has a predilection for the periapical bone of the anterior mandibular teeth. Two or more lesions simultaneously involving separate teeth apices are common.

Periapical radiographs of involved teeth demonstrate small ovoid bony defects at or near the root apices (Fig. 7-71). In its early stages, the lesion is mainly fibrous and therefore appears entirely radiolucent and virtually indistinguishable from periapical rarefying osteitis. In contrast to periapical rarefying osteitis, the involved teeth are not carious and their vitality and function are not compromised.

As these lesions mature, they elaborate minute calcific foci of a bone-cementum-like substance within the fibrous mass (Fig. 7-72). These depositions later appear as minute radiopacities within the periapical radiolucent lesion. As this stage progresses, the small opacities coalesce. Some PCD lesions become mostly filled with cementum and are substantially or completely radiopaque. A radiolucent capsule always surrounds the radiopaque mass and separates it from the surrounding normal bone. The lesion's usual occurrence in middle-aged black women, its typical involvement of the mandibular periapical bone, its tendency toward multiplicity, its course of development, and its radiographic appearance are all characteristic. Biopsies are rarely needed. Treatment is not required because the condition is harmless and self limiting.

Florid osseous dysplasia. This condition is probably the most common cause of multiple mandibular radiopacities.[20] Florid osseous dysplasia (FOD) appears to be a widespread form of PCD. Age, sex, and racial pro-

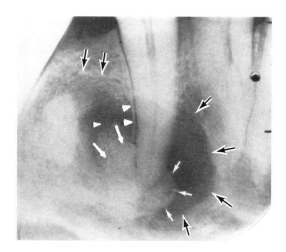

Fig. 7-72. Periapical cemental dysplasia in mandibular posterior region. Fibrous part is outlined by black arrows, calcific part by white (smaller) arrows. Notice that lamina dura *(arrowheads)* is present only at distal aspect of premolar tooth.

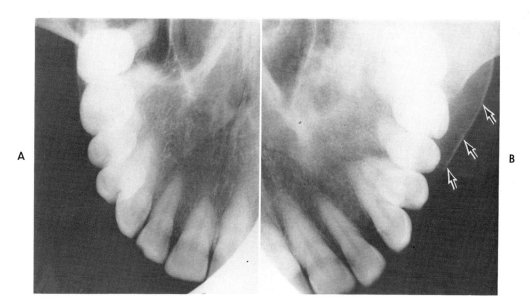

Fig. 7-73. Fibrous dysplasia of maxilla. **A,** Normal right side of maxilla seen in occlusal view. **B,** Dysplastic left side of bone. Notice that in comparison to normal side, buccal cortex *(arrows)* has been expanded by intrinsic bone enlargement. Structure of bone has also been altered. Normal lacelike trabeculae have been replaced by fine, ground-glass type of bone.

files of patients, as well as radiographic and histopathologic appearances, are similar for the two lesions. Like PCD, it is probably a reactive type of fibroosseous bone disease derived from cells in or near the periodontal ligament spaces. Prior to 1976, FOD was called gigantiform cementoma and diffuse chronic sclerosing osteomyelitis.[37]

Radiographically, florid osseous dysplasia appears as a radiolucent cavity partially filled with one or more dense, radiopaque masses. Such masses have a fluffy, soft radiopaque character that resembles the "cotton wool" opacity seen in Paget's disease. The encompassing radiolucent spaces are fairly regular and well marginated. In more mature and extensive FOD lesions the surrounding radiolucent cavity is less prominent and the internal radiopaque masses are more conspicuous.

Multiple lesions are found in one or both jaws, usually in all four alveolar quadrants. The alveolar processes of the jaws are mainly affected, although some lesions may extend into the mandibular body or into the maxillary sinuses. Individual lesions typically do not exceed 2 to 3 cm in diameter. As individual lesions enlarge, neighboring ones often coalesce.

Nonodontogenic conditions

Fibrous dysplasia. Jaw involvement occurs in less than 10% of all cases of fibrous dysplasia, though the propensity for jaw involvement increases in the polyostotic forms. The maxilla is more commonly affected than the mandible, with most of the changes occurring in the posterior regions. Fibrous dysplasia is predominantly unilateral in its distribution and, especially in the maxilla, rarely crosses the midline.

The affected portion of mandible or maxilla is usually enlarged though the asymmetry may be subtle. The buccal cortex typically shows more expansion than the palatal or lingual surface.

Definitive radiographic diagnosis of fibrous dysplasia is often difficult because the degree of bone involvement varies, as do the differing radiographic densities and lesion margins. Radiographically, fibrous dysplasia may be either devoid of bone trabeculae or composed of altered, dysplastic trabeculae (Fig. 7-73). In the former, a single unilocular radiolucent cavity may be observed; more often, bony septa are present. A preponderance of altered trabeculae may also give the lesion a radiopaque appearance.

Fibrous dysplasia of the jaws may displace the teeth (Fig. 7-74). Resorption of the roots is occasionally observed. The lamina dura and periodontal ligament spaces are rarely obliterated in this condition. If the diseases occurs in early childhood, developing tooth germs may be displaced or destroyed. Maxillary fibrous dysplasia of moderate to large size usually obliterates the sinus on the involved side. Occasionally, rapid advancement of the lesion may lead to the clinical suspicion of malignancy. In such cases, careful radiographic evaluation can lead to the correct diagnosis of pseudotumoral fibrous dysplasia.[62]

Cherubism. Cherubism is a rare, inherited fibro-osseous bone disease that affects only the jaws. It typically is found in patients between the ages of 2 and 5 years as a bilateral enlargement of the mandible. The abnormality may not be appreciated until there is obvious progression of the mandibular swellings. In many cases, bilateral enlargement of the maxilla follows.

The radiographic picture of cherubism is characterized by well-marginated, cystlike multilocular cavities found in the mandible and less often in the maxilla (Fig. 7-75). Cortical discontinuity is uncommon. Size and growth patterns of the lesions are fairly symmetric. Also typical of the disease is the initiation of bone destruction near the mandibular angles, with later expansion of the lesions superiorly into the rami and anteriorly into the body. If the maxilla becomes involved, it typically lags behind the mandible in its degree of involvement. Expansion of the buccal and lingual cortical plates is convincingly demonstrated on occlusal and frontal skull radiographs.

The destructive jaw lesions have a profound effect on the developing permanent dentition. Displacement of numerous developing tooth buds and dental follicles is the rule. The cystlike lesions may destroy one or more tooth buds prior to enamel calcification. The teeth most commonly affected are the mandibular second and third molars. This loss of permanent teeth constitutes the

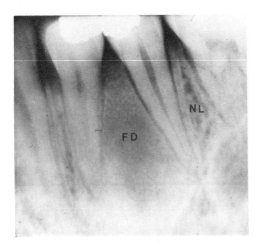

Fig. 7-74. Fibrous dysplasia, monostotic and highly localized in mandible. Lesion is confined to interdental bone between two premolar teeth. Internal structure of fibrous dysplasia lesion *(FD)* can be contrasted to normal interdental bone *(NL)*. Notice also that fibrous dysplasia has obliterated lamina dura from around involved root surfaces.

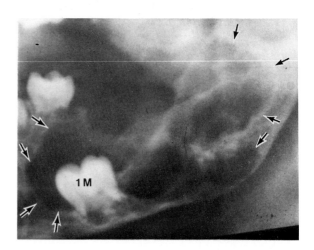

Fig. 7-75. Cherubism. Extensive, cystlike multilocular radiolucency involves all of mandibular body and ramus, seen in this cropped panoramic view. On frontal view this lesion was seen to involve both mandibular sides equally and produced comparable expansion of bone cortices. First molar *(1M)* has been impacted by expansile lesion, whereas second molar is missing. Latter has been destroyed by lesion prior to enamel formation. Notice margin of lesion *(arrows)*.

most important complication of the disease. Deciduous teeth in the involved areas are often shed prematurely because of their lost bony support.

Giant cell granuloma. The possible relationship of giant cell granuloma of the jaws to benign giant cell tumor of the skeleton is controversial. Many authorities contend that giant cell granuloma is found only in the jaws and is a separate entity. Others argue that giant cell granuloma of the jaws and benign giant cell tumor of the long bones are the same clinicopathologic entity.[52] Central giant cell granuloma of the jaws may be a nonneoplastic reactive type of bone disease initiated by some unknown stimulus. The histopathologic appearance of the two entities is virtually identical.

Giant cell granuloma of the jaws is a lesion of adolescents and young adults. At least 60% of the cases occur in persons 30 years of age or younger. The mandible is involved twice as frequently as the maxilla, with the anterior mandible showing the greatest incidence of involvement. Most mandibular lesions occur anterior to the first molars, and 20% cross the symphysis. Giant cell granuloma does not produce significant pain.

Radiographic findings in central giant cell granuloma are nonspecific. The size of the lesion has little role in radiographic differentiation. Large giant cell granulomas can occupy the whole of one mandibular body and extend past the midline. Incipient lesions may be no larger than a centimeter, simulating a small odonto-

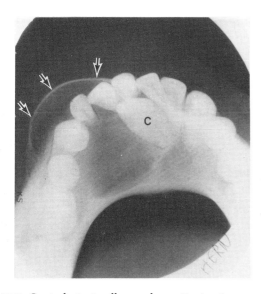

Fig. 7-76. Central giant cell granuloma. Lesion is seen on occlusal view as expansile radiolucency in anterior mandible, causing even, regular swelling of buccal cortical plate *(arrows)* and intrusion of canine tooth *(C)*.

genic cyst. The character of the cortical bulging seen may be helpful in evaluating the larger lesions. A regular, gently expanded contour is usually present although an uneven, variable bulging of the buccal cortex can sometimes be seen (Fig. 7-76).

Giant cell granuloma usually has fairly distinct margins and may even show areas of cortication. Many lesions appear devoid of internal trabecular structure. Most show remodeled curvilinear septa that give the lesion a more or less multilocular appearance. Giant cell granuloma generates sufficient expansile pressure as it enlarges to displace adjacent tooth roots and tooth follicles. Resorption of neighboring tooth roots is a common finding.

Paget's disease. The incidence of jaw involvement in Paget's disease is moderately high, occurring in approximately one case out of six.[55] Between the two jaws there is a distinct predilection for the maxilla over the mandible. In nearly every case in which the jaws are involved the skull is also affected.

The entire mandible is usually involved[68] (Fig. 7-77). Thus Paget's disease may be differentiated from fibrous dysplasia, which in all but the more severe polyostotic cases is strictly a unilateral disease and is often focused in a specific mandibular site. Paget's disease within the jaw is generally diffuse; however, asymmetric involvement is occasionally seen. The affected bone is expanded. This change is clinically manifested in dentulous patients by malocclusion and tooth migration and in edentulous patients by poorly fitting dentures.

The early or radiolucent (osteoporosis circumscripta) stage of Paget's disease is infrequently seen in the jaws. If the disease is noticed in the mandible during this stage, the inferior cortex may be osteoporotic and may appear laminated. Such cortical lamination may also be seen at alveolar crest areas of edentulous jaws. In early mandibular Paget's disease the altered internal bone pattern is one in which trabeculae, though reduced in number, run linearly in the direction of the length of the bone, with few intersections between them.[68]

In the more commonly observed later states, rounded, radiopaque foci of abnormal bone are often seen within individual lesions, giving an appearance of "cotton wool." As the fluffy, opacified areas enlarge and become more numerous they tend to coalesce.

Hypercementosis (root hyperplasia) of one or more tooth roots may be present. In long-standing or advanced cases most of the teeth have some degree of hypercementosis. Because this change is not associated with other bone or metabolic diseases, it is a helpful diagnosic sign when present. Paget's disease may obliterate areas of lamina dura and the periodontal ligament space around both normal and hyperplastic roots, but this is an inconsistent finding.

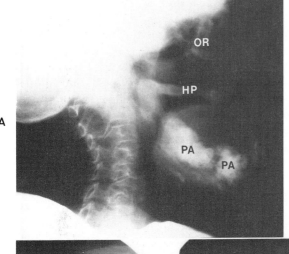

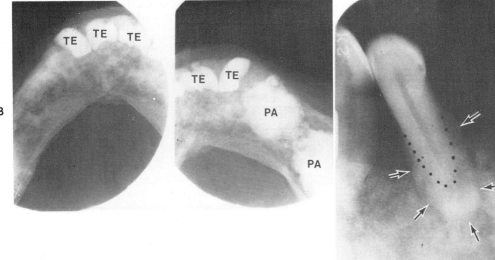

Fig. 7-77. **A,** Paget's disease of mandible, lateral view. Lower jaw is grossly enlarged and demonstrates mottled radiopacities *(PA).* Paget's disease also involves skull base. *HP,* Hard palate; *OR,* orbital rim. **B,** Occlusal views of same case. Disease involved bone bilaterally but was more pronounced in right side. Two large pagetoid lesions *(PA)* are indicated in photograph on right. *TE,* Teeth. **C,** Periapical view of same case. Characteristic hypercementosis in such cases is seen at root of canine tooth. Normal root outline is indicated by dotted lines while arrows demarcate hypercementosis. Notice that lamina dura and periodontal ligament space have been obliterated by pagetoid bone.

Potential serious complications of Paget's disease include osteogenic sarcoma. Osteomyelitis can also develop in the relatively avascular pagetoid bone. Osteomyelitis can spread throughout the involved bone and is often refractory to antibiotic therapy.

Systemic diseases manifested in the jaws

Histiocytosis X. The term *histiocytosis X* includes eosinophilic granuloma of bone, Hand-Schüller-Christian disease, and Letterer-Siwe disease as related expressions of a single disease process. In eosinophilic granuloma, the disease is localized almost exclusively to bone. The other two involve soft tissues routinely as well as bone. Hand-Schüller-Christian disease is the chronic disseminated form of the disease complex, and the jaws and oral cavity are often involved.[53] Occasionally, the oral changes are the most prominent clinical feature of the disease.

Loosening and sloughing of teeth often occur following the destruction of underlying tooth-supporting bone

by one or more eosinophilic granulomas. The sockets of teeth lost to the disease generally fail to heal normally. Multiple eosinophilic granulomas are often present in the mandible. Lesions may also be found on the gingiva and palate in addition to their usual location in bone.

Radiographically, eosinophilic granuloma is usually seen as areas of pure osteolysis that occur in or near the alveolar processes (Fig. 7-78). These lesions characteristically destroy the bone support of one or more teeth, especially in the posterior alveolar ridge, while leaving tooth structures themselves absolutely intact. The result is a distinctive "teeth standing in space" or "floating teeth" appearance. Mandibular lesions rarely if ever arise inferior to the mandibular canal. Lesions of eosinophilic granuloma typically have fairly discrete borders, although they rarely appear corticated or otherwise circumscribed.[35]

Rickets. Rickets results from failure of new bone to calcify properly. Rickets occurs in infants and children,

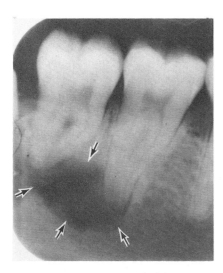

Fig. 7-78. Eosinophilic granuloma. Lesion is seen as radiolucency in periapical portion of alveolar process. Arrows outline lesion. When occurring in jaw, these lesions characteristically involve alveolar bone. As they enlarge they destroy tooth-supporting bone but not teeth, leaving them "standing in space."

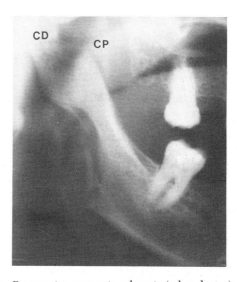

Fig. 7-79. Progressive systemic sclerosis (scleroderma). Posterior part of ramus near mandibular angle has been extensively resorbed. In similar cases, before such osseous change has taken place, many tooth roots will be surrounded by abnormally thick periodontal ligament spaces, best seen on periapical projections. *CD*, Condyle; *CP*, coronoid process.

while its counterpart, osteomalacia, is found in older persons, i.e., those in whom linear bone growth can no longer occur. Both abnormalities are caused by vitamin D deficiency.

Defects in the teeth and jaws are uncommon with rickets. A thinning of cortical structures such as the inferior mandibular border, the mandibular canal, the lamina dura, and the follicular walls of developing teeth can be seen in the jaws of rachitic children. Such changes usually arise later and are less striking than the classic epiphyseal changes seen in the ribs and long bones. Within the cancellous portion of the mandible, the fine trabeculae are reduced in number. In severe cases the mandible appears abnormally radiolucent. Rickets has also been linked with hypoplasia of developing tooth enamel. Prior to the age of 3 years, rickets-induced enamel hypoplasia of both erupted and unerupted teeth is fairly common. Tooth development and eruption can also be retarded. Dental abnormalities are not a part of the clinical profile of osteomalacia because mature teeth are not subjected to the systemic alterations of calcification processes.

Vitamin D–resistant rickets. Vitamin D–resistant rickets is also called hypophosphatemia. It may produce dental and periodontal changes in addition to the more common skeletal defects. There is a high incidence of periapical and periodontal infections associated with this disease. When periodontal infections occur in children, they tend to spread diffusely through the bone rather than remain localized around an involved tooth. Periapical and periodontal rarefying osteitis often occur

in the absence of caries. The pulp chambers of affected deciduous teeth are unusually large and the enamel caps are in some places hypoplastic. The enlarged pulp chambers near the dentinoenamel junction may be invaded by microorganisms. Pulpal necrosis can then occur long before typical caries are recognized.

Progressive systemic sclerosis (scleroderma). Progressive systemic sclerosis (PSS) is a generalized connective tissue disease that causes sclerosis of the skin and other tissues. The term *scleroderma*, previously used to describe what was once thought to be mainly a cutaneous disease, has recently been supplanted by the term *progressive systemic sclerosis*.

The periodontal ligament spaces around the teeth are widened in approximately one third of all patients with PSS. Radiographically this appears as a uniform thickening of the space around the entire root of a tooth. Most patients with PSS demonstrate this thickening around several teeth, although on occasion a solitary periodontal ligament space is enlarged. There is a strong tendency for such lesions to form around the posterior teeth. The lamina dura around affected teeth remains intact.

An unusual pattern of erosions found near the mandibular angles has been identified in some cases of PSS.[60] White and coworkers described such changes in 6 of 35 confirmed PSS patients. When present, the mandibular angle resorption typically occurs bilaterally and is fairly symmetric. The erosive borders are smooth and sharply defined (Fig. 7-79). Resorption or amputation of the coronoid process has also been noted.

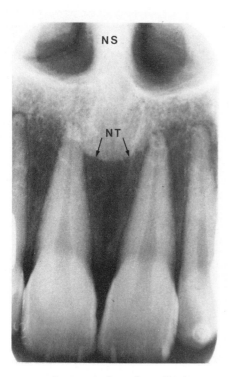

Fig. 7-80. Primary hyperparathyroidism. In this periapical radiograph, exposed for normal density of teeth, two abnormalities may be discerned: (1) Lamina dura has been lost from around roots and (2) the overall bone density between teeth is overly radiolucent, indicative of severe demineralization. Roots appear to have an accentuated taper, an optical effect of diminished lamina dura. *NT,* Tip of nose; *NS,* nasal septum.

Hyperparathyroidism. Radiographic changes in the jaws of patients with primary hyperparathyroidism include (1) bone demineralization, (2) osteitis fibrosis cystica affecting jaw cortic structures, and (3) "brown tumors." Teeth do not lose calcium and phosphate, even with high serum parathyroid hormone levels. Hard dental tissues may be destroyed by carious erosion but they are unresponsive to demineralization by systemic conditions. Changes in bone radiographic density can therefore be estimated relative to that of the teeth in cases of suspected parathyroid disease. Hyperparathyroidism may be inferred if the teeth are of normal radiogaphic density but the surrounding bone appears abnormally radiolucent (Fig. 7-80).

Resorption of the lamina dura, although basically analogous to subperiosteal cortical resorption of the phalanges, is a much less sensitive radiographic indicator of hyperparathyroidism.[57] Loss of the lamina dura is also a nonspecific finding and can be seen in Paget's disease, fibrous dysplasia, and osteomalacia. Oral radiographic diagnosis of hyperparathyroidism is improved when careful evaluation is given to other cortical structures such as the mandibular canal, the floor of the maxillary sinus, and the inferior border of the mandible itself. Diminution or outright loss of cortical structures may be consistent with a diagnosis of hyperparathyroidism, but it is not by itself pathognomonic of the disease.

Brown tumors of hyperparathyroidism may appear in any bone. In long-standing disease, they are frequently found in the facial bones and jaws. Radiographically these cystic defects appear as well-delineated, round radiolucencies that may or may not expand the affected bone. They are often multiple. If solitary, a brown tumor may be indistinguishable radiographically from giant cell granuloma of the jaws.

Hyperpituitarism (gigantism, acromegaly). Excessive pituitary growth hormone causes overgrowth of all tissues in the body retaining the capacity for growth. If the abnormality occurs in childhood, generalized overgrowth of most tissues outside the central nervous system ensues and results in gigantism. Oral soft tissues and the jaws in general respond by enlarging, with the notable exception of the teeth.

Several radiographic abnormalities do occur in the jaws of the pituitary giant. The roots of several or all teeth may be enlarged by hypercementosis (i.e., hyperplasia of the roots). The roots, which develop later than the crowns, may also appear abnormally elongated. The process is basically one of furthering tooth eruption in order to maintain occlusion during chewing as the jaws grow further apart. As normal-size teeth are present in abnormally large jaws, spaces between the teeth inevitably develop.

The articulating surface of the mandibular condyle is covered with cartilage. When stimulated by excess growth hormone in acromegaly, endochondral-like bone growth is produced. Pronounced downward and forward growth of the mandible results and is often one of the most prominent clinical and radiographic features of acromegaly.

In acromegaly, spaces develop between the mandibular anterior teeth as the lower arch lengthens. The anterior mandibular teeth are pushed forward so that they appear to fan or flare out. This is in part a result of the macroglossia that is typically prominent in acromegaly. The anterior dental fanning is also produced by overgrowth of the posterior dental segments, resulting in an anterior open bite.

Sickle cell anemia. Sickle cell disease is a chronic hemolytic anemia characterized by the formation of the abnormal hemoglobin and sickle-shaped red blood cells. The radiographic manifestations of this disease in the mandible are principally a result of marrow hyperplasia. Generalized osteoporosis is common.[49] To a lesser extent, thinning of the cortices also occurs. In the interdental alveolar portions of the jaws the trabeculae appear unusually coarse and form an accentuated stepladder pattern. This stepladder pattern in the jaws represents the greatest occlusal stresses to which the trabeculae are subjected and consequently the least resorption by the enlarging marrow.

Significant alveolar bone loss, along with severe bone porosis, is particulary common in children.[51] Mandibular bone infarcts are rare.

Diabetes mellitus. Diabetes mellitus produces no clinical or radiographic effects within the jaws except for periodontal alterations. Uncontrolled diabetes predisposes to inflammatory conditions, but diabetes does not directly cause periodontal disease. Once present, periodontal infections are more difficult to treat. From the radiographic standpoint, periodontal disease associated with diabetes is qualitatively indistinguishable from periodontal disease in nondiabetic patients. Radiographic manifestations therefore range from a slight discontinuity or blurring of the alveolar crest cortex to wide destruction of the lamina dura and surrounding alveolar bone. These changes are occasionally characteristic of rampant periodontal abscesses.

☐ Systematic radiologic approach to central mandibular lesions

The following discussion is not an exhaustive set of criteria for mandibular differential diagnosis but rather an organizational scheme that for a given mandibular lesion, allows the medical radiologist to consider systematically the various diagnostic possibilities.

■ Odontogenic vs. nonodontogenic conditions

Because of the unique character of the jaws as teeth-supporting bones, there are certain difficulties in radiographic interpretation that do not occur with other parts of the skeleton. For example, developing teeth that are normally present in the jaws of children and adolescents could be confused by inexperienced observers with certain calcifying lesions. More importantly, the developing teeth may obscure pathologic conditions that might be present in the jaws of young people. This problem is especially important in children 6 to 12 years of age (i.e., in the mixed dentition stage). At this age, the lower jaw is primarily a shell of a cortical bone containing embedded and erupted teeth and little else. Osteomyelitis is easily obscured in pediatric mandibles because there is so little cancellous bone structure to manifest the typical osteolytic changes.

Probably the most important consideration for radiologists in dealing with jaw pathology is that the odontogenic (tooth-forming) apparatus itself may give rise to a variety of pathologic lesions, many of which vary tremendously in incidence, appearance, and significance. The medical radiologist should therefore attempt to differentiate suspected lesions into two categories, those that appear to be nonodontogenic and that can appear elsewhere in the skeleton and those that are likely odontogenic and are confined to the jaws. The radiographic characteristics of a mandibular odontogenic lesion include the following.

1. Odontogenic lesions are located either near the root of an erupted tooth or the crown of an unerupted tooth.
2. The lesion is above the mandibular canal, i.e., in or near the alveolar process of the jaw.
3. If radiolucent (e.g., primordial cyst or ameloblastoma), the lesion is generally well-defined at its periphery and has a complete or at least a partial cortical border.
4. If partially or almost completely radiopaque (e.g., periapical cemental dysplasia or odontoma), the radiopaque portion of the lesion is separated from normal bone by a surrounding radiolucent capsule and a partial or a complete bony cortex.

■ Patient age

The following generalizations apply both to odontogenic and nonodontogenic conditions.

1. Developmental conditions or anomalies, such as odontomas and dentigerous or primordial cysts, tend to arise in young persons, at about the same or at a slightly later age as the normally developing teeth near that site.
2. Tumors and inflammatory conditions, including ameloblastoma and radicular and residual cysts, typically occur in adults, especially those over the age of 30.

■ Mandibular radiolucencies

Ninety-two percent of all radiographically observable jaw lesions (excluding periodontal disease) are radiolucent.[9]

Lesions occuring near the root apices of erupted teeth

Eighty-five percent of all central jaw lesions occur near the apices of teeth.[9] If a radiograph shows a radiolucency at a tooth apex, information about the vitality of the tooth is essential. If the tooth is nonvital (dead), the appropriate radiographic diagnosis is periapical rarefying osteitis; if the tooth is vital (alive), the lesion most likely represents an early stage of periapical cemental dysplasia. If the radiolucency is of moderate to large size (more than 1 cm in diameter) and the tooth is nonvital, the most likely diagnosis is radicular cyst.

Lesions occuring in the interdental alveolar bone but not related to the tooth apices

If peridontal disease can be eliminated from consideration based on clinical examination, an eroding lesion of the alveolar crestal bone is probably a peripheral benign soft tissue tumor, a squamous cell carcinoma, or a central eosinophilic granuloma. If the superior alveolar crest is intact, carcinoma can usually be excluded but other osteolytic lesions appropriate to the patient's age, such as ameloblastoma or giant cell granuloma, must then be considered. Carcinoma and the lesions of histiocytosis X, such as eosinophilic granuloma, are generally easily differentiated from each other on the basis of patient age. A multiplicity of lesions usually effectively eliminates squamous cell carcinoma from further consideration.

Lesions occuring near the crowns of unerupted (impacted) teeth

The principal lesion in this category is the dentigerous cyst. This lesion is seen as an expanding radiolucent area around a tooth crown, with the lucency itself bounded by a smooth, regular cortex. The impacted tooth crown may have been pushed far from its normal location by cyst expansion. These types of lesions definitely require biopsy. The bulk of the pathologic tissue may be that of an ameloblastoma because about 17% of these tumors originate in dentigerous cyst linings. Nevertheless, the great majority of crown-related radiolucencies are uncomplicated dentigerous cysts. Unless true radiographic multilocularity is apparent, ameloblastoma is unlikely.

Lesions occuring in deeper regions of the mandibular body and in the ramus

Lesions that originate below the mandibular canal, either in the body or in the ramus posterosuperior to the canal, are almost always nonodontogenic. The whole range of odontogenic lesions can thus be essentially excluded. For example, an asymptomatic, well-circumscribed radiolucency near the angle of the mandible at the inferior border is probably a developmental salivary gland defect. A well defined erosion at the posterior border of the ramus, particularly if bilateral, indicates progressive systemic sclerosis (scleroderma) bone involvement. Multiple deep-seated radiolucencies in the mandible are most consistent with metastases or multiple myeloma.

True odontogenic processes can enlarge and extend below the mandibular canal and into the superior ramus. For example, ameloblastoma and dentigerous cysts commonly involve the mandibular ramus and occasionally destroy large areas of it. The important consideration is that these lesions have arisen from the odontogenic bone areas, i.e., the alveolar bone or the third molar region of the anterior ramus, and have extended into the nonodontogenic bone areas.

Unilocularity vs. multilocularity

Most radiolucent mandibular cysts, tumors, and tumorlike conditions are unilocular. This group also includes most cases of giant cell granuloma, traumatic bone cysts, and small ameloblastomas. These unilocular entities should be separated into two categories on the basis of shape: (1) odontogenic cysts and (2) "others." Cysts tend to be round or at least globular in shape, with a smooth regular contour outline. Primordial and residual cysts are good examples. On the other hand, other unilocular lesions, such as traumatic bone cysts, are not particularly globular but appear more variable or lobulated in outline. A traumatic bone cyst, for example, characteristically has a scalloped superior border around the tooth roots. In most cases, only a biopsy will further differentiate the myriad possibilities in the "other" category. Regularity and smoothness of a true cyst's outline becomes a distinguishing characteristic only after a moderate size (at least 1 cm in diameter) has been obtained. Most very small jaw radiolucencies will be unilocular and thus could be produced by a half a dozen or more pathologic entities.

True multiloculated radiolucent lesions are less common. This appearance is the radiographic hallmark of the moderate-size to large ameloblastoma (smaller ameloblastomas often appear unilocular). Aneurysmal bone cyst, hemangioma, and odontogenic myxoma in the mandible might also appear multilocular but ameloblastoma can usually be distinguished from these entities in two ways: (1) the many locules in ameloblastoma very greatly in size, typically with smaller daughter cysts around the larger central cavities, and (2) the septa in ameloblastoma are characteristically curved. A true honeycomb structure (uniformly sized locules, straight septa) would be more suggestive of odontogenic myxoma than ameloblastoma.

Anterior vs. posterior

Ameloblastoma has a marked tendency to occur in the posterior tooth-forming regions of the mandible, whereas giant cell granuloma and traumatic bone cysts are more likely to be found anterior to the roots of the first molar tooth. Primordial cysts and odontogenic keratocysts are also more posteriorly localized radiolucencies. Of the radiopacities, mature periapical cemental dysplasia occurs at the anterior mandible in 90% of cases. Compound odontoma favors the canine area although the complex odontoma is more often seen in the posterior region, near the third molar.

Buccal and lingual cortical expansion

Enlarging central mandibular lesions produce expansile pressure on the adjacent bony cortical plates. With the exception of traumatic bone cyst, almost any mandibular central lesion measuring at least 2 to 3 cm in greatest dimension on a panoramic or lateral oblique projection will produce clinically and radiographically noticeable cortical plate expansion. Lesions located in the body of the mandible are best evaluated with regard to cortical expansion on the standard intraoral occlusal projection or on the submentovertex projection. Ramus lesions are best delineated on PA Towne facial radiographs.

Traumatic bone cyst produces surprisingly minimal cortical expansion. On the other hand, true fluid-filled cysts, such as the dentigerous or primordial variety, cause uniform expansion. Internal mandibular expanding soft tissue masses, such as the central giant cell granuloma, produce undulating cortical expansion, often described as bossing. The buccal and lingual cortical margins are usually intact, although thinned.

Fibrosarcoma and osteogenic sarcomas typically invade and perforate adjacent cortical surfaces, although some degree of expansion may also be present. Sunray spiculation or Codman's triangles or both are often seen at the periosteal surfaces of the affected bone. Pathologic fractures may be present.

■ Mandibular radiopacities

Only 7% of all jaw lesions are radiopaque.[9] Fibrous dysplasia, Paget's disease, Caffey's disease, osteopetrosis, and Garre's osteomyelitis are examples of conditions that impart a generalized or regionalized radiopacity to the mandible.

Odontogenic vs. nonodontogenic

Odontogenic radiopacities are usually characterized by a radiolucent capsule of varying thickness and a surrounding cortex of bone. Compound and complex odontomas and late-stage or mature periapical cemental dysplasia are common examples. With the exception of ossifying fibroma, nonodontogenic radiopacities are usually less well delineated, particularly by a capsule. Osteoblastic osteosarcoma is an example of a nonodontogenic process lacking a surrounding radiolucent capsule. The clinically insignificant "bone island," i.e., osteosclerosis, is another example of the nonencapsulated radiopacity. The latter is typically seen as a small, localized radiodense area, usually quite well-defined where it merges with the surrounding normal bone (Figs. 7-81 and 7-82).

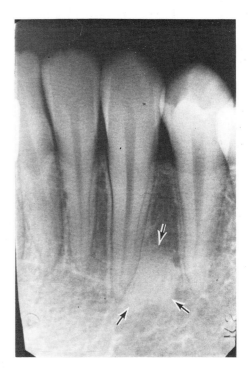

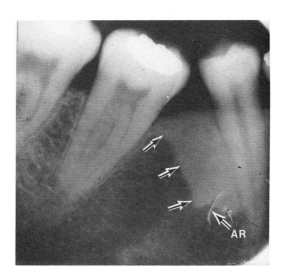

Fig. 7-81. Osteosclerosis (bone island) within alveolar process. Area of sclerotic bone is situated between arrows and premolar tooth. This dense bony area is well defined in comparison with surrounding cancellous bone. Notice that there is no apparent inflammatory cause for bone sclerosis; this fact helps to distinguish this entity from sclerosing osteitis. *AR*, Artifact on film.

Fig. 7-82. Osteosclerosis. Well-defined area of pronounced radiopacity is seen (*arrows*), associated with periapical bone of healthy teeth. Notice that osteosclerosis blends with lamina dura of canine root but does not affect thin radiolucent periodontal ligament space.

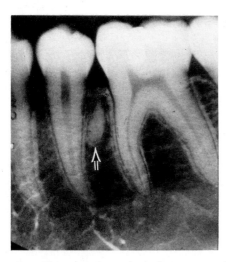

Fig. 7-83. Retained root tip *(arrow).* In this case root fragment came from deciduous molar, having been amputated by eruptive force of second premolar. This location for retained root fragment is highly characteristic. On careful inspection, thin periodontal ligament space can be seen around distal aspect of root tip.

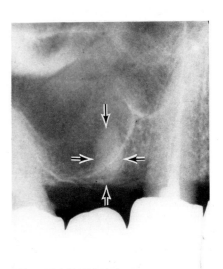

Fig. 7-84. Retained root fragment from previously extracted maxillary molar *(arrows).* Root tip, which superimposes over sinus floor, is diagnosed radiographically on basis of its conical shape, radiographic density, position in alveolar bone, and thin periodontal ligament space surrounding it.

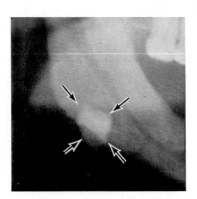

Fig. 7-85. Submandibular gland sialolith. Arrows outline large (2 × 2 cm) stone found to lie in hilum of submandibular gland. Sialoliths in hilum and parenchyma of gland are far less common than those in main (Wharton's) duct.

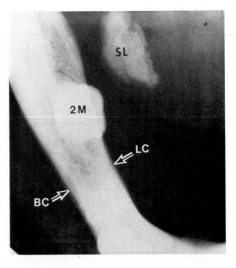

Fig. 7-86. Submandibular gland sialolith, with a radiopaque stone *(SL)* at gland hilum as seen on standard mandibular occlusal projection. These projections are often deliberately underexposed (with regard to bone structure) so as to not "burn out" image of stone. *2M,* Second molar tooth; *BC,* buccal cortex; *LC,* lingual cortex.

Retained root fragments

Broken, retained fragments in the alveolar bone of the mandible or maxilla may be seen as radiopacities on jaw or facial radiographs (Figs. 7-83 and 7-84). Retained root fragments are relatively uncommon in any patient group, although they are usually seen as incidental findings in middle-aged or older individuals in whom there are many broken down, necrotic teeth. Root tips or root fragments can easily be differentiated from other jaw radiopacities on the basis of the following radiographic criteria.

1. Root fragments are found in the tooth-bearing area of the jaws, where a tooth socket is either seen or presumed to have been.
2. Root fragments typically have a conical shape.
3. Root fragments have a homogeneous radiodensity common to other roots in the dental area.
4. Root fragments often but not always retain recognizable remnants of the internal pulp canal and are often surrounded by an intact periodontal ligament space and lamina dura.

Sialoliths

Occasionally, radiopaque concretions in one of the salivary gland ducts may overlie the mandible (Fig. 7-85). Oblique or occlusal films are often helpful in delineating their exact nature and location (Fig. 7-86).

□ Computed tomography

While many if not most uncomplicated intrinsic lesions of the mandible are best (and least expensively) examined by routine plain films, panoramic tomography, or intraoral radiography (see earlier discussion), computed tomography (CT) is of unique value in delineating those lesions that have both osseous and soft tissue extension. Involvement of the infratemporal and parapharyngeal spaces, oral cavity, skull case, and other adjacent structures can be readily determined. In such cases, CT may provide crucial information unobtainable by any other diagnostic modality and alter subsequent treatment planning.[40] CT is also helpful in excluding involvement by primary osseous or soft tissue lesions adjacent to the mandible. CT is probably of little value in examining most congenital anomalies, uncomplicated trauma, and abnormalities limited to the dentition or cancellous bone of the mandible.

■ Normal CT anatomy

The mandible is sometimes difficult to view with CT imaging because of its complex, curving surfaces and the presence of artifact-producing amalgam fillings or restorations. Because of its irregular configuration, only segments of the mandible are contained within a given CT section (Fig. 7-87). Axial scans at the level of the temporomandibular joint demonstrate the ovoid, somewhat obliquely oriented mandibular condyles lying within the articular fossae. At this level, the articular eminence is seen as a slightly curvilinear structure lying just anterior to the condyle. The condyle is separated from the external auditory canal by the tympanic portion of the temporal bone (Fig. 7-88, A).

CT scans 1 cm below the mandibular condyles include the triangular mandibular neck. It is separated from the smaller, elongated coronoid process by a hiatus, the mandibular notch (Fig. 7-88, B). Scans through the body of the mandibular ramus demonstrate a thin, flat bony plate with a slight medial concavity (Fig. 7-88, C). The middle of the mandibular ramus is perforated on its inner surface by the obliquely oriented mandibular foramen (Fig. 7-88, D). The mandibular foramen is overlapped by a thin bony lamella, the lingula. CT scans through the alveolar process include the partially

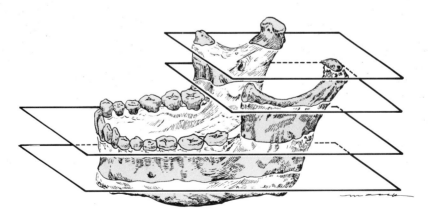

Fig. 7-87. Diagrammatic sketch of several representative CT planes through disarticulated mandible. (From Osborn, A.G., Hanafee, W.H., and Mancuso, A.A.: AJR **139**:555-559, 1982.

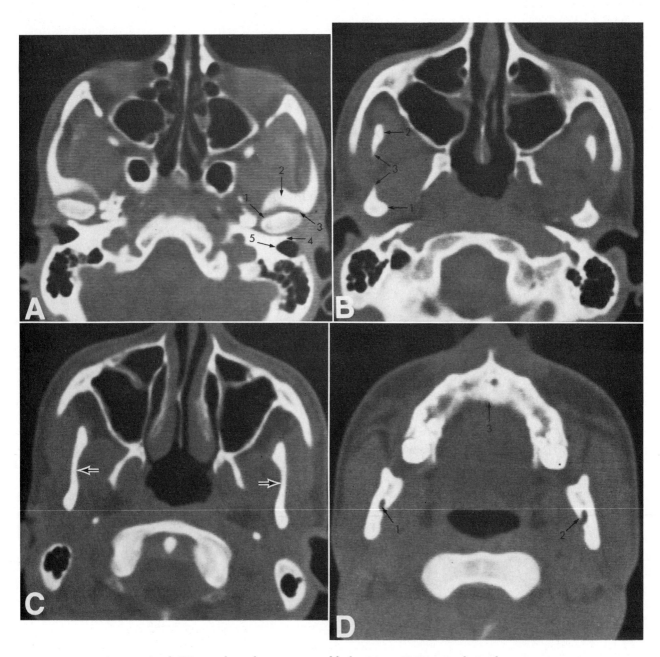

Fig. 7-88. Axial CT scan through temporomandibular joints. Notice angulation between true coronal plane and axis of mandibular condyles. **A,** *1,* Mandibular condyle; *2,* articular eminence; *3,* temporomandibular joint space; *4,* tympanic portion of temporal bone; *5,* external auditory canal. **B,** Axial CT scan 1 cm below **A.** *1,* Neck of mandibular condyle; *2,* coronoid process; *3,* mandibular notch. **C,** Axial CT scan through mandibular rami (arrows). **D,** Axial CT scan 1 cm below **C.** *1,* Mandibular foramen; *2,* lingula; *3,* maxillary alveolar process.

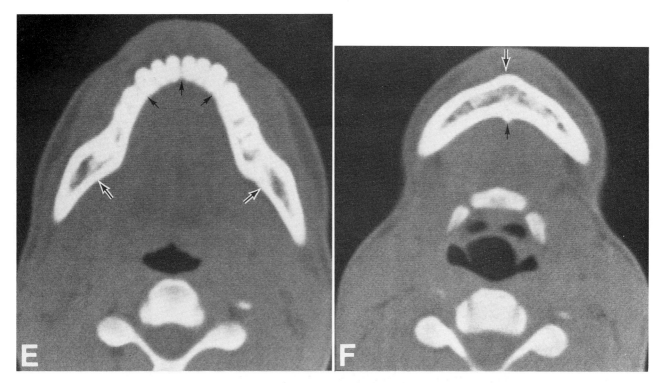

Fig. 7-88, cont'd. E, Axial CT scan through mandibular body *(outlined arrows)* and alveolar ridge *(black arrows)*. **F,** Axial CT scan 1 cm below **E.** Mental protuberance is indicated by outlined arrow. Genial tubercle (attachment of genioglossus muscle) is indicated by black arrow. (From Osborn, A.G., Hanafee, W.H., and Mancuso, A.A.: AJR **139:**555-559, 1982.)

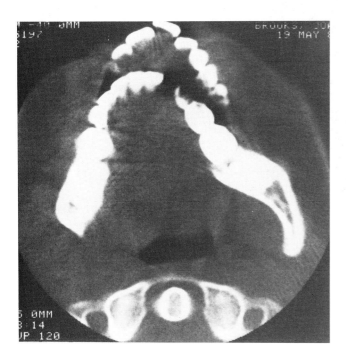

Fig. 7-89. CT scan in patient with mandibular hypoplasia. Note marked overbite.

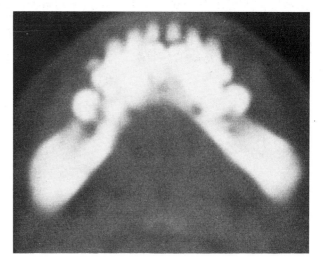

Fig. 7-90. Axial CT scan through mandibular symphysis of patient with diffuse eosinophilic granuloma demonstrated multiple lytic lesions at roots of teeth.

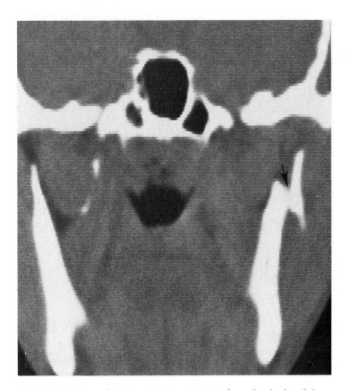

Fig. 7-91. Coronal CT scans in patient with multiple facial fractures. Fracture through left mandibular ramus and coronoid process was present *(arrow)*.

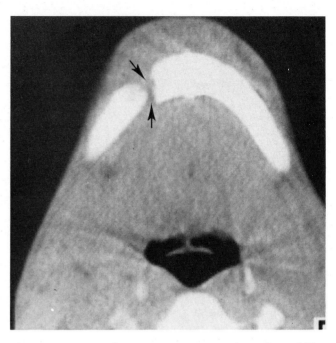

Fig. 7-92. CT scan demonstrating osteomyelitis of mandible secondary to previous compound fracture *(arrows)*. (Courtesy W. Hanafee and A.A. Mancuso, U.C.L.A. Center for Health Sciences.)

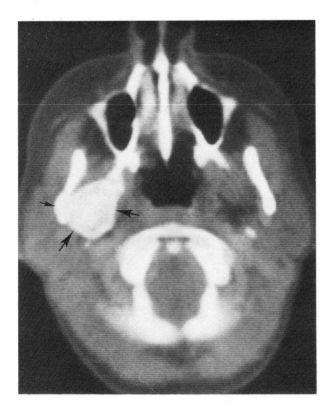

Fig. 7-93. CT scan without contrast demonstrates osteoma arising from skull base *(large arrows)*. Right mandibular ramus is bowed around lesion *(small arrow)*. Note pseudoarticulation with adjacent pterygoid plates. (From Osborn, A.G., Hanafee, W.H., and Mancuso, A.A.: AJR **139**:555-559, 1982.)

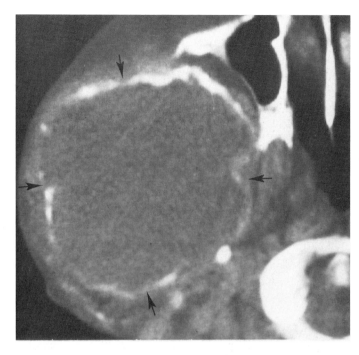

Fig. 7-94. Unenhanced CT scan in patient with cystic ameloblastoma of mandible *(arrows)*. Note discontinuity of osseous rim and pressure deformity of adjacent maxillary sinus. (Courtesy W. Hanafee and A.A. Mancuso, U.C.L.A. Center for Health Sciences.) (From Osborn, A.G., Hanafee, W.H., and Mancuso, A.A.: AJR **139**:555-559, 1982.)

sectioned teeth (Fig. 7-88, *E*). The mental protuberance and symphysis are seen on slightly lower sections (Fig. 7-88, *F*). The mental foramina are frequently not well visualized.

Pathologic CT anatomy

A variety of congenital traumatic inflammatory and neoplastic conditions involving the mandible are illustrated in Figs. 7-89 to 7-95.

□ **References**

1. Adams, G., and Nelms, C.T.: Complicated mandibular fractures, Otolaryngol. Clin. North Am. **9**:453-464, 1976.
2. Adams, R.J., Murphy, W.A., and Gilula, L.A.: Magnification radiography of the temporo-mandibular joints, Scientific exhibit, Sixty-fourth Scientific Assembly and Meeting, Radiologic Society of North America, Chicago, November 26–December 1, 1978.
3. Adra, N.A., Barakat, N., and Melhem, R.E.: Salivary gland inclusions in the mandible: Stafne's idiopathic bone cavity, AJR **134**:1082-1083, 1980.
4. Albers-Schonberg, H.: Roentgenbilder einer selenen Knochenerkrankung, MMW **51**:365, 1904.
5. American Academy of Dental Radiology: History of the American Academy of Dental Radiology, 1974, The Academy.
6. Barr, J.H., and Stephens, R.G.: Dental radiology: pertinent basic concepts and their applications in clinical practice, Philadelphia, 1980. W.B. Saunders Co.
7. Becker, M.H., Coccaro, P.J., and Converse, J.M.: Antegonial notching of the mandible: an often overlooked deformity in congenital and acquired disorders, Radiology **121**:149, 1976.
8. Bergman, G., Borggren, M.B., and Engfeldt, B.: Studies on mineralized dental tissues: osteopetrosis, Acta Odontol. Scand. **14**:81, 1956.
9. Bhaskar, S.N., Bernier, J.L., and Godby, F.: Aneurysmal bone cysts and other giant cell lesions of the jaws: report of 104 cases, J. Oral Surg. **17**:30, 1959.

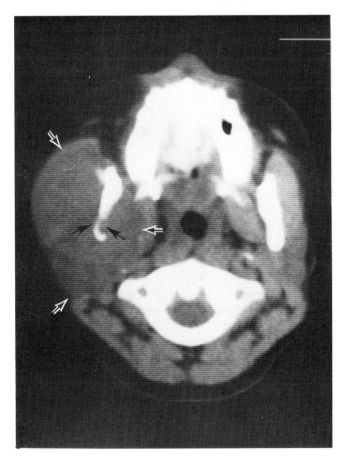

Fig. 7-95. CT scan demonstrating large fibrosarcoma of right mandible *(outlined arrows)*. Note erosion and destruction of ramus *(black arrows)*. (From Osborn, A.G., Hanafee, W.H., and Mancuso, A.A.: AJR **139**:555-559, 1982.)

10. Biesterfeld, R.C., Taintor, J.F., and Alcox, R.W.: Diagnostic radiographic aspects in endodontics, Dent. Radiogr. Photogr. **53**:21-25, 1980.

11. Bixler, D.: Heritable disorders affecting dentin. In Stewart, R.E., and Prescott, G.H., editors: Oral facial genetics, St. Louis, 1976, The C.V. Mosby Co.

12. Blaschke, D.D., Solberg, W.K., and Sanders, B.: Arthrography of the temporomandibular joint: review of current status, J. Am. Dent. Assoc. **100**:388-395, 1980.

13. Broadbent, B.H.: A new x-ray technique and its application to orthodentia, Angle Orthol. **1**:45, 1931.

13a. Burbank, T.M., Lovested, S.A., and Kennedy, R.L.: The dental aspects of infantile cortical hyperostosis, Oral Surg. **11**:1126-1137, 1958.

14. Caffey, J.: Pediatric x-ray diagnosis, ed. 7, vol. 1, Chicago, 1978, Year Book Medical Publishers, Inc.

15. Cohen, M.M.: Dysmorphic syndromes with craniofacial manifestations. In Stewart, R.E., and Prescott, G.H., editors: Oral facial genetics, St. Louis, 1976, The C.V. Mosby Co.

16. Coin, C.G.: Tomography of the temporomandibular joint, Med. Rad. Photogr. **50**:26-39, 1974.

17. Conklin, W.W., and Stafne, E.C.: A study of odontogenic epithelium in the dental follicle, J. Am. Dent. Assoc. **39**:143, 1949.

18. Dahlin, D.C.: Bone tumors: general aspects and data on 6,221 cases, ed. 3, Springfield, Ill., 1978, Charles C Thomas, Publisher.

19. Edeiken, J., and Hodes, P.J.: Roentgen diagnosis of diseases of the bone, ed. 2, vols. 1 and 2, Baltimore, 1973, The Williams & Wilkins Co.

20. Emmering, T.E.: Generalized radiopacities. In Wood, N.K., and Goaz, P.W., editors: Differential diagnosis of oral lesions, ed. 2, St. Louis, 1980, The C.V. Mosby Co.

21. Eversole, L.R.: Clinical outline of oral pathology: diagnosis and treatment, Philadelphia, 1978, Lea & Febiger.

22. Garrington, G.E., Scofield, H.H., Cornyn, J., and Hooker, S.P.: Osteosarcoma of the jaws: analysis of 56 cases, Cancer **20**:377, 1967.

23. Goin, D.W.: Facial nerve paralysis secondary to mandibular fracture, Laryngoscope **90**:1777-1785, 1980.

23a. Gorlin, R.J., Pindborg, J.J., and Cohen, M.M., Jr.: Syndromes of the head and neck, ed. 2, New York, 1976, McGraw-Hill Book Co.

24. Hamner, J.E., III, Scofield, H.H., and Cornyn, J.: Benign fibro-osseous jaw lesions of periodontal membrane origin: an analysis of 249 cases, Cancer **22**:861, 1968.

25. Helms, C.A., Katzberg, R.W., Colwick, M.F., and Bales, D.J.: Arthrotomographic diagnosis of meniscus perforations in the temporomandibular joint, Br. J. Radiol. **53**:283-285, 1980.

26. Heys, R.M., Blattner, R.J., and Robinson, H.B.: Osteogenesis imperfecta and odontogenesis imperfecta: clinical and genetic aspects in eighteen families, J. Pediatr. **56**:234, 1960.

27. Jeromin, L.S., Geddes, G.F., White, S.C., and Gratt, B.M.: Xeroradiography for intraoral radiology: a process description, Oral Surg. **49**:178, 1980.

28. Johnston, C.C., et al.: Osteopetrosis: a clinical, genetic, metabolic and morphologic study of the dominantly inherited, benign form, Medicine **47**:149, 1968.

29. Katzberg, T.W., Dolwick, M.F., Helms, C.A., et al.: Arthrotomography of the temporomandibular joint, **134**:995-1003, 1978.

30. Keller, E.E., and Stafne, E.C.: Oral roentgenographic manifestations of systemic disease. In Stafne, E.C., and Gibilisco, J.A., editors: Oral roentgenographic diagnosis, ed. 4, Philadelphia, 1975, W.B. Saunders Co.

31. Killey, H.C., Kay, L.W., and Seward, G.R.: Benign cystic lesions of the jaws, their diagnosis and treatment. ed. 3, London, 1977, Churchill Livingstone.

32. Kodak: X-rays in dentistry, Rochester, N.Y., 1977, Eastman Kodak Co.

33. Langland, O.E., and Sippy, F.H.: Textbook of dental radiography, Springfield, Ill., 1973, Charles C Thomas, Publisher.

34. Lichtenstein, L.: Histiocytosis X: integration of eosinophilic granuloma of bone, "Letterer-Siwe disease" and "Schüller-Christian disease" as related manifestations of a single nosologic entity, A.M.A. Arch. Pathol. **56**:84, 1953.

35. Lovestedt, S.A.: Radiology of the jaws: manifestations of systemic disease, Semin. Roentgenol. **6**:441-448, 1971.

36. Manson-Hing, L.R.: Panoramic dental radiography, Springfield, Ill., 1976, Charles C Thomas, Publisher.

37. Melrose, R.J., Abrams, A.M., and Mills, B.G.: Florid osseous dysplasia: a clinical-pathologic study of 34 cases, Oral Surg. **41**:62, 1976.

38. Merwin, G.E., Tilsner, T., Boies, L.R., Jr., and Shrewsbury, S.: Treatment of maxillary cysts, Ann Otol. Rhinol. Laryngol. **89**:225-228, 1980.

39. Moore, K.L.: The developing human, Philadelphia, 1977, W.B. Saunders Co.

40. Osborn, A.G., Hanafee, W.H., and Mancuso, A.A.: CT of the mandible: normal and pathologic anatomy, AJR **139**:555-559, 1982.

41. Paatero, Y.V.: Pantomography and orthopantomography, Oral Surg. **14**:947, 1961.

42. Pacini, A.J.: Roentgen ray anthropmetry of the skull, J. Radiol. **3**:231, 1922.

43. Pavlick, C.T., and Pruzansky, S.: Size, shape, posture and growth of the mandible in the Pierre Robin syndrome. Unpublished data cited in Pruzansky, S.: Not all dwarfed mandibles are alike, Birth Defects **5**:120, 1969.

44. Pell, G.J., et al.: Garre's osteomyelitis of the mandible, J. Oral Surg. **13**:248, 1955.

45. Pindborg, J.J., and Hjorting-Hansen, E.: Atlas of diseases of the jaws, Philadelphia, 1974, W.B. Saunders Co.

46. Proffit, W.R., Vig, K.W.L., and Turvey, T.A.: Early fracture of the mandibular condyles: frequently an unsuspected cause of growth disturbances, Am. J. Ortho. **78**:1-24, 1980.

47. Pruzansky, S.: Not all dwarfed mandibles are alike, Birth Defects **5**:120, 1969.

48. Reiter, D.: Concepts of dental occlusion, Am. J. Otolaryngol. **1**:245-255, 1980.

49. Robinson, I.B., and Sarnat, B.G.: Roentgen studies of the maxillae and mandible in sickle-cell anemia, Radiology **58**:517, 1952.

50. Rowe, N.L., and Killey, H.C.: Fractures of the facial skeleton, Baltimore, 1968, The Williams & Wilkins Co.

51. Sanger, R.G., and Bytron, E.B.: Radiographic bone changes in sickle-cell anemia, J. Oral Med. **32**:32, 1977.

52. Shafer, W.G., Hine, M.K., and Levy, B.M.: A textbook of oral pathology, ed. 3, Philadelphia, 1974, W.B. Saunders Co.

53. Sleeper, E.L.: Eosinophilic granuloma of bone: its relationships to Hand-Schüller-Christian and Letterer-Siwe diseases, with emphasis on oral findings, Oral Surg. **4**:896, 1951.

54. Stafne, E.C.: Value of roentgenograms in diagnosis of tumors of the jaws, Oral Surg. **6**:82, 1953.

55. Stafne, E.C., and Austin, L.T.: A study of dental roentgenograms in cases of Paget's disease (osteitis deformans), osteitis fibrosa cyctica, and osteoma, J. Am. Dent. Assoc. **25**:1202, 1938.

56. Stafne, E.C., and Austin, L.T.: A characteristic dental finding in acrosclerosis and diffuse scleroderma, Am. J. Orthod. **30**:25, 1944.

57. Steinbach, H.L., et al.: Primary hyperparathyroidism: a correlation of roentgen, clinical and pathologic features, AJR **86**:329, 1961.

58. Summers, G.W.: Jaw cysts: diagnosis and treatment, Head Neck Surg. **1**:243-256, 1979.

59. Suydam, M.J., and Mikity, V.G.: Cellulitis with underlying inflammatory periostitis of the mandible, AJR **106:**133, 1969.

60. Taveras, J.M.: The interpretation of radiographs. In Schwartz, L., editor: Disorders of the temporomandibular joint, Philadelphia, 1959, W.B. Saunders Co.

60a. Thunty, K.A.: Radiographic illusions, Dent. Radiogr. Photogr. **53:**1-12, 1980.

61. Trapnell, D.H., and Bowerman, J.E.: Dental manifestations of systemic disease, London, 1973, Butterworth & Co.

62. Vanel, D., Cauanet, D., Micheau, C., et al.: Pseudotumoral fibrous dysplasia of the maxilla: radiological studies and computed tomography contribution, Skeletal Radiol. **5:**99-103, 1980.

63. Waldron, C.A.: Nonodontogenic neoplasms, cysts, and allied conditions of the jaws, Semin. Roentgenol. **6:**414-425, 1971.

64. White, S.C., and Gratt, B.M.: Intraoral dental xeroradiography: clinical trials, J. Am. Dent. Assoc. **99:**810, 1979.

65. White, S.C., Stafford, M.L., and Beeninga, L.R.: Intraoral xeroradiography, Oral Surg. **46:**862, 1978.

66. White, S.C., et al.: Oral radiographic changes in patients with progressive systemic sclerosis (scleroderma), J. Am. Dent. Assoc. **94:**1178, 1977.

67. Wilkes, C.H.: Arthrography of the temporomandibular joint in patients with the TMJ pain-dysfunction syndrome, Minn. Med. **61:**645-652, 1978.

68. Worth, H.M.: Principles and practice of oral radiologic interpretation, Chicago, 1963, Year Book Medical Publishers.

69. Worth, H.M.: The role of radiological interpretation in disease of the temporomandibular joint, Oral Sci. Rev. **6:**3-51, 1974.

70. Yune, H.Y., Hall, J.R., Hutton, C.E., and Klatte, E.C.: Roentgenologic diagnosis in chronic temporomandibular joint dysfunction syndrome, AJR **110:**401-414, 1973.

8 □ Arteriography of the head and neck: normal functional anatomy of the external carotid artery

PIERRE L. LASJAUNIAS

The major vascular supply to the head and neck is derived from the external carotid system. Although the external carotid artery (ECA) and its branches have been the subject of numerous studies,[1,2] understanding of this arterial system remains imperfect. Recent developments in therapeutic angiography have demonstrated that the most appropriate approach to this system requires consideration of two distinct types of functions, (1) the vascular territories themselves and (2) the arterial anastomotic patterns. Thorough knowledge of these two important functions is an absolute prerequisite for safe, accurate vascular mapping and subsequent therapeutic embolization. This functional approach to external carotid angiography is briefly outlined in this chapter, along with the rationale for clinical problem solving. For a more exhaustive treatment of this subject, the reader is referred to previous work of Lasjaunias.[3]

Phylogenetically and ontogenetically, the ECA is comprised of three different anatomic groups: (1) internal maxillary, (2) pharyngo-occipital, and (3) facial-lingual.

□ Internal maxillary system

The internal maxillary artery (Fig. 8-1) is the main anastomotic channel between the external and internal carotid systems. The internal maxillary system provides the major vascular supply to the deep facial structures as well as to the orbit and the infratemporal fossa. It also supplies the peripheral segments of the trigeminal and oculomotor nerves (cranial nerves III and V) and has numerous anastomoses with the other two major

divisions of the external carotid artery. Prior to therapeutic embolization, the precise anatomy of the internal maxillary artery should be determined, the anastomoses with other facial branches delineated, and the hemodynamic balance between the major subdivisions of the ECA and the internal carotid artery outlined. Potential hazards of embolization can thus be recognized and a functional approach to therapy determined.

□ Pharyngo-occipital system

The pharyngo-occipital system (Fig. 8-2) comprises the major link between the vertebral artery and the ipsilateral (internal and external) carotid system. The pharyngo-occipital artery has an anastomotic role greater than either of the other two major ECA divisions. This complex arterial system may be compared to a metameric (intercostal) arterial pedicle. It vascularizes the skin and musculature of the occipital and suboccipital regions and supplies the peripheral segments of cranial nerves IX, X, XI, and XII as well as the posterior fossa meninges. The occipital artery represents the nutrient vessel for the musculocutaneous elements, while the ascending pharyngeal artery is responsible for the meningeal and neural territory. In some anatomic variations the pharyngo-occipital system may also supply the brainstem and cerebellum by way of anastomoses with hypoglossal, proatlantal, intersegmental, or pharyngocerebellar arteries.

□ Facial-lingual system

The facial-lingual system (Fig. 8-3) arises from the embryonic ventral pharyngeal artery. Its distribution is

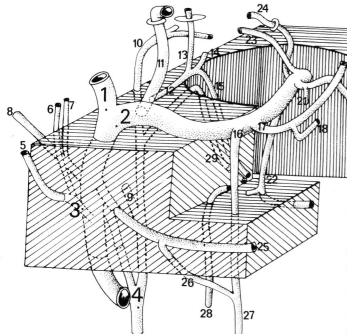

Fig. 8-1. Schematic representation of distal external carotid artery and its vascular anastomoses at level of cavernous sinus. *1,* Superficial temporal artery; *2,* internal maxillary artery; *3,* posterior auricular artery; *4,* pharyngo-occipital trunk; *5,* auricular branch, posterior auricular artery; *6,* stylomastoid branch, posterior auricular artery; *7,* stylomastoid branch, occipital artery; *8,* cutaneous branch, occipital artery; *9,* neuromeningeal trunk, ascending pharyngeal artery; *10,* superior pharyngeal branch, ascending pharyngeal artery; *11,* middle meningeal artery; *12,* meningeal artery with its intracranial *(13),* eustachian *(14),* and palatine *(15)* branches; *16,* buccal artery (branch of internal maxillary artery); *17,* deep temporal artery with its orbital branch *(18); 19,* infraorbital artery with its orbital branch *(20); 21,* antral-alveolar artery; *22,* descending palatine artery; *23,* pterygopalatine artery; *24,* artery of the foramen rotundum; *25,* transverse facial artery; *26,* superior masseteric artery; *27,* buccal branch of facial artery; *28,* ascending palatine artery; *29,* palatine branch of ascending pharyngeal artery.

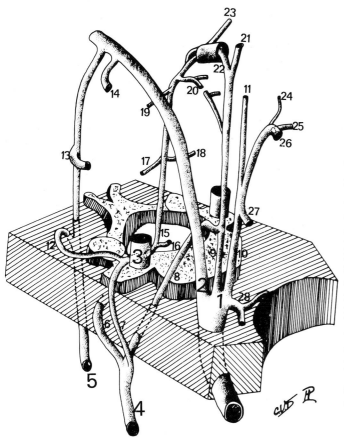

Fig. 8-2. Schematic representation of upper cervical arteries. C3 is represented, along with adjacent arterial anastomoses. *1,* Ascending pharyngeal artery; *2,* occipital artery; *3,* vertebral artery (sectioned); *4,* thyrocervical trunk; *5,* costocervical trunk; *6,* anterior radicular anastomotic artery, fourth interspace; *7,* anterior radicular anastomotic artery, third interspace; *8,* musculospinal artery; *9,* neuromeningeal trunk; *10,* pharyngeal trunk; *11,* inferior tympanic artery; *12,* posterior radicular anastomotic branch of third interspace; *13,* posterior radicular anastomotic branch of second interspace; *14,* posterior radicular anastomotic branch of first interspace; *15,* arterial arch of odontoid artery; *16,* anterior epidural branch; *17,* radicular branch of second interspace; *18,* anterior epidural branch; *19,* radicular branch of first interspace; *10,* apical arterial branch of odontoid artery; *21,* jugular branch of neuromeningeal trunk; *22,* hypoglossal branch of neuromeningeal trunk; *23,* clival branch of hypoglossal artery; *24,* carotid branch; *25,* transmedian anastomosis; *26,* superior pharyngeal artery; *27,* middle pharyngeal artery; *28,* inferior pharyngeal artery.

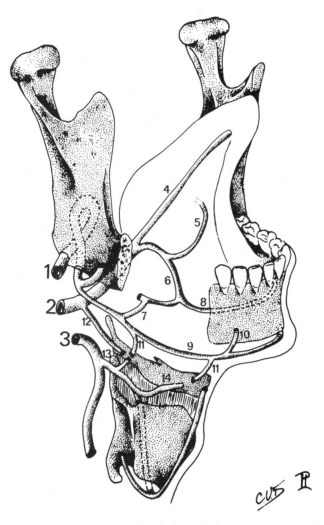

Fig. 8-3. Schematic representation of arterial pedicles and their anastomosis at floor of mouth. Ramus of mandible has been resected and tongue retracted superiorly. *1,* Facial artery; *2,* lingual artery; *3,* superior thyroidal artery; *4,* lingual artery; *5,* artery of frenulum of tongue; *6,* sublingual artery; *7,* submental-sublingual anastomosis; *8,* internal mandibular artery; *9,* submental artery; *10,* mental branch, submental artery; *11,* subhyoidal branch, submental artery; *12,* hyoid branch, lingual artery; *13,* hyoidal branches of superior laryngeal artery.

primarily musculocutaneous and does not include peripheral (cranial) nervous territory or any transcranial vascularization. On the basis of this territorial function it is comparable to other tegumentary arterial systems of the scalp, such as the superficial temporal, posterior auricular, and transverse facial arteries. All these vessels anastomose freely and their territories therefore can be supplied by other ipsilateral and contralateral cutaneous vessels.

The sublingual territory is common to both the lingual and the facial trunks. A hemodynamic equilibrium therefore exists in the floor of the mouth, providing the basis for collateral circulation between these two segments of the facial-lingual pedicle.

□ Functional anatomy of the external carotid system: theoretical and practical considerations

Each of the three major ECA divisions is in equilibrium with an adjacent vascular system: the internal carotid artery with the internal maxillary artery, the pharyngo-occipital artery with the vertebral and cervical arteries, and the facial-lingual artery with the thyroid artery. A functional approach to ECA anatomy allows the conceptualization of territorial angiographic protocols (Figs. 8-1 to 8-6) rather than lesional ones; hence a diseased territory is explored rather than the lesion alone.

Angiographic mapping cannot be delineated adequately by a nonselective external carotid study; rather,

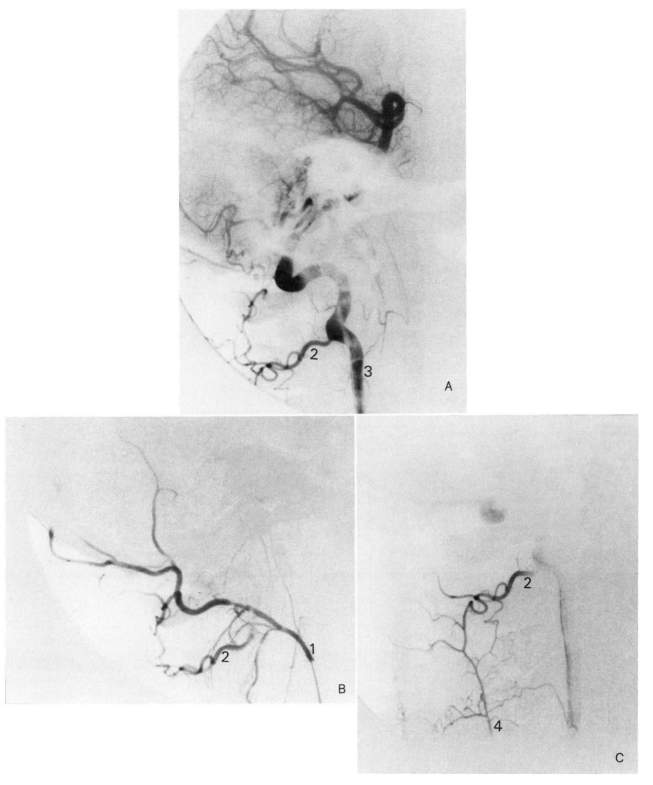

Fig. 8-4. Normal angiographic study of suboccipital region. Injected successively are, **A,** vertebral artery; **B,** occipital artery; and **C,** costocervical artery. Note on this study extent to which same vessel in given region can be opacified by injection of several different arterial pedicles. For example, posterior radicular anastomotic artery of second interspace *(2)* is seen despite its apparent origin from vertebral artery *(3)* during injection of either costocervical trunk *(4)* or occipital artery *(1)*. Vascular branch for any given region can frequently be opacified by way of different arterial pedicles.

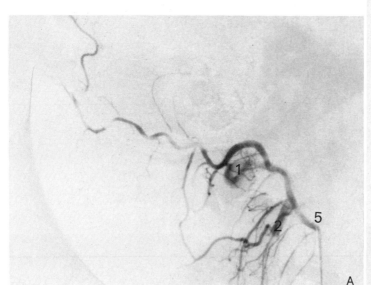

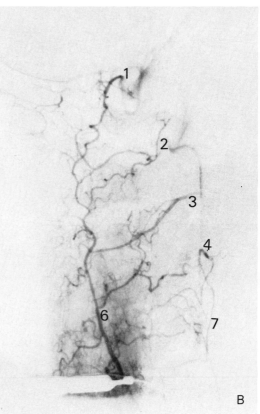

Fig. 8-5. Normal angiographic study of upper cervical area. Successively injected are, **A,** occipital artery and, **B,** costocervical trunk. On this angiogram only retrotransverse territories of upper cervical branch were examined. In this particular anatomic situation, metameric distribution of "muscular" arteries is well seen in first *(1)*, second *(2)*, third *(3)*, and fourth *(4)* interspaces. Injection of occipital artery *(5)* only delineates first two interspaces well where they opacify vertebral artery. In this case costocervical artery *(6)* is dominant vessel in supplying upper cervical region. Injection of costocervical trunk opacifies all posterior radicular anastomotic arteries and even refluxes thyrocervical artery *(7)*. This example illustrates metameric or segmental nature of these "muscular" vessels and demonstrates how two well-chosen, selective injections can delineate entire vascular supply of given region.

Fig. 8-6. **A** and **B,** Normal selective arteriography of two middle cerebral arteries, and, **C,** distal external carotid artery in three different patients. **A,** Middle meningeal artery supplies supratentorial convexity meninges by way of its parieto-occipital *(single arrow)* and frontal *(double arrows)* branches. Also note emissary arterial system in parieto-occipital region near midline *(large arrow)*. In this example virtually entire ipsilateral supratentorial vascular supply to meninges can be regarded as monopedicular. **B,** Two major pedicles of convexity meninges have separate origins. Middle meningeal artery gives origin to parieto-occipital branch *(arrow)*. Frontal branch *(double arrow)* arises from intraorbital lacrimal artery and, after recurrent course, vascularizes frontoparietal meninges. This vessel is visualized in retrograde manner by way of anastomoses at level of vault between two parieto-occipital and frontoparietal trunks. **C,** Middle meningeal artery has course opposite that depicted in **B.** It has annexed additional territory to its usual area of supply, i.e., giving rise to ipsilateral ophthalmic artery. Its transphenoidal segment is frequently seen poorly but is well visualized in this example because of choroidal crescent *(open arrows)*. These three variations illustrate an existing balance between two adjacent vascular systems (here meningeal and ophthalmic systems) and show extremes between complete annexation of part of meningeal territory by ophthalmic artery as well as obverse (annexation of ophthalmic supply by meningeal system). However, these two anatomic extremes are not equally frequent; origination of ophthalmic artery from middle meningeal artery is less common than anterior meningeal artery origination from ophthalmic artery.

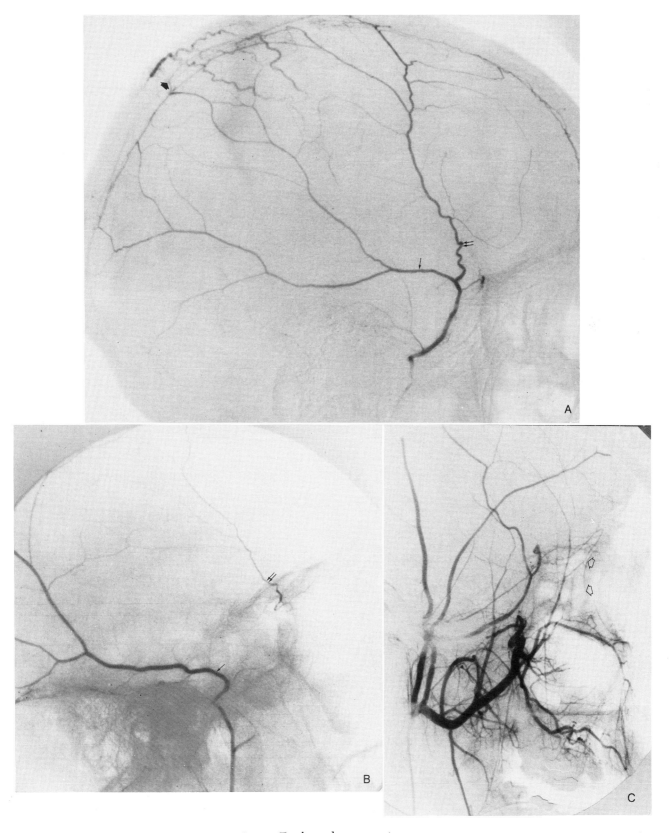

Fig. 8-6. For legend see opposite page.

painstaking reconstruction, territory by territory, of the abnormal region may be accomplished only after meticulous, selective angiography. Superselective injection of an arterial pedicle usually allows delineation of adjacent arteries and the relative size of their vascular territories. These arterial pairs exist in known patterns and varying degrees of hemodynamic balance, ranging from an extreme monopedicular form to a variety of intermediate patterns (Figs. 8-6 to 8-9).

A hierarchy also exists in the potential arterial patterns. This hierarchy is determined not by the relative importance of the territory supplied (e.g., brain vs. muscle) but by embryologic development. Thus the internal maxillary artery, a phylogenetically more "ancient" system, can more often vascularize the brain than intracranial vessels can supply the face.

The vascular territory common to two adjacent arterial systems, such as the cavernous sinus and orbit, comprises potential regions of collateral circulation should hemodynamic compromise (such as thrombosis, embolization, or surgical occlusion) occur. The major hemodynamic pairings in the head and neck are as follows.

1. Maxillo-ophthalmic (through the orbit)
2. Maxillocarotid (through the cavernous sinus)
3. Pharyngomaxillofacial (through the palate)
4. Maxillofacial (through the cheek or jugal area)
5. Occipitovertebral (C1 and C2)
6. Pharyngovertebral (condyloid canal and C3)
7. Pharyngo-occipitocervical (nape of the neck)

Each of these vascular anastomoses can be examined from either side or pedicle; failure to visualize an anastomosis during an isolated injection does not preclude its existence nor predict the direction of its circulation. The anastomosis can sometimes be seen by injecting its counterpart. Failure to visualize an anastomosis by injecting both sides usually means it is merely infra-angiographic (i.e., smaller than 200 μm). From the neu-

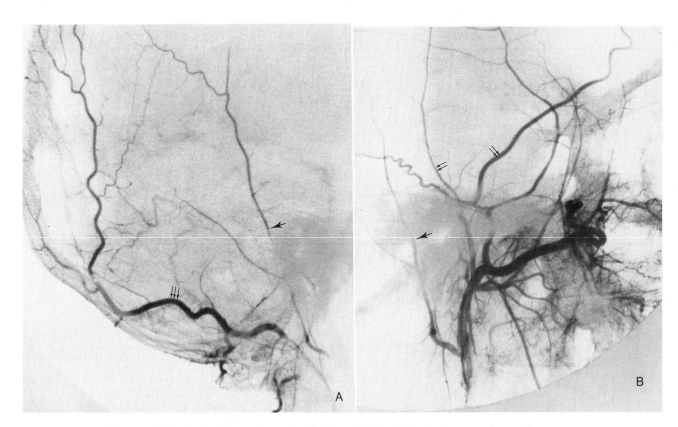

Fig. 8-7. Normal selective angiography of **(A)** occipital and **(B)** distal external carotid artery. All pedicles supplying cutaneous and subcutaneous tissues of cranial vault are well seen. Cutaneous branch of posterior auricular artery *(arrow)* is visualized during both injections. Balanced vascularization throughout cutaneous branch is achieved anteriorly by way of two branches of superficial temporal artery *(double arrows)* and posteriorly by cutaneous branch of occipital artery *(triple arrows)*. Therefore these two studies show that three sources of supply to scalp exist. From back to front these are occipital, posterior auricular, and superficial temporal arteries.

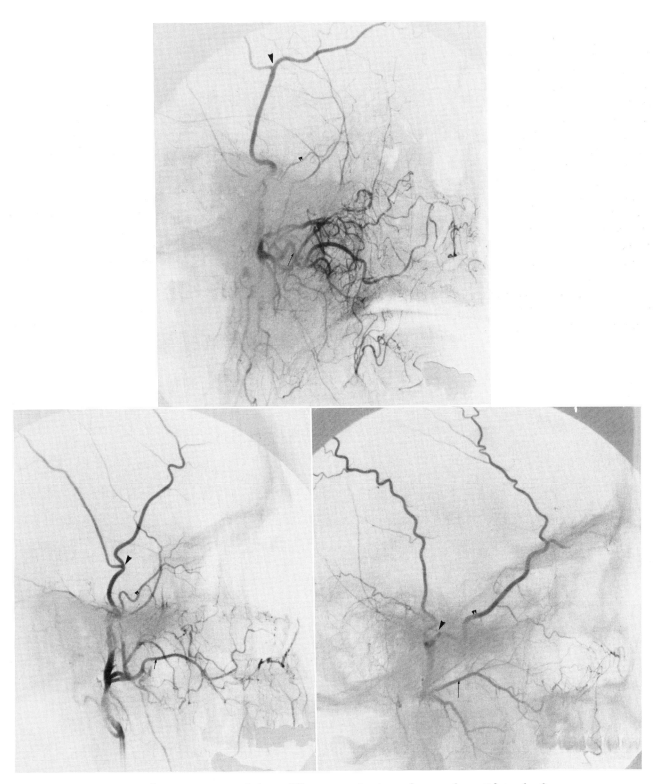

Fig. 8-8. Selective injection of three different terminations of external carotid trunk after internal maxillary artery had been embolized for epistaxis (all three patients had Rendu-Osler-Weber disease). Transverse facial *(arrow)* and superficial temporal arteries were angiographically normal. These three different cases have in common an identical appearance of transverse facial artery *(arrow)* although superficial temporal *(arrowhead)* and zygomatico-orbital arteries *(double arrowheads)* vary widely in size. These three variations illustrate that other vessels arising from superficial temporal system do not share hemodynamic balance with transverse facial artery. Regardless of branching pattern of superficial temporal artery, transverse facial artery retains same position and appearance. Zygomatico-orbital and frontal branches of artery thus do not share hemodynamic balance, in contrast to previous example in which superficial temporal artery is in equilibrium with other cutaneous pedicles of scalp.

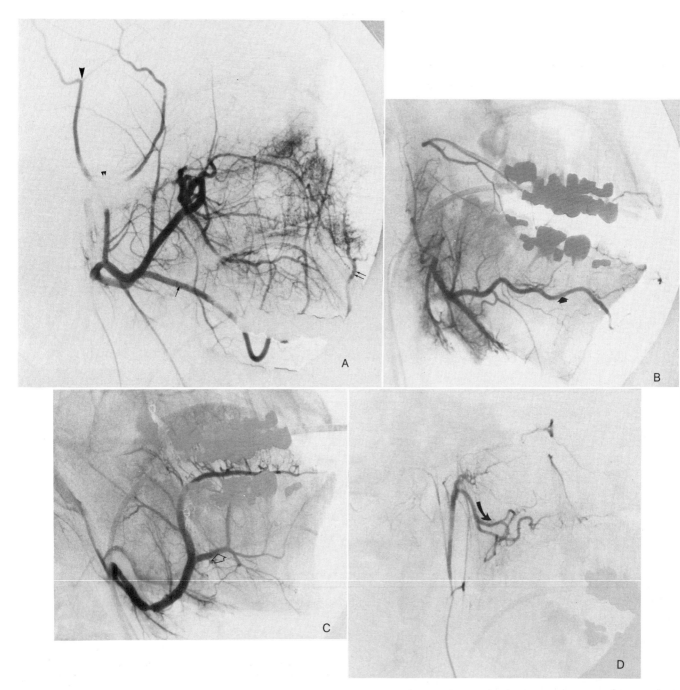

Fig. 8-9. Normal selective examination of **(A)** external carotid, **(B)** facial, **(C)** lingual, and **(D)** ascending pharyngeal artery in same patient as in Fig. 8-8. In this variation, transverse facial artery *(arrow)* has annexed supply to soft tissues of cheek and nasal alae *(double arrow).* Here superficial temporal artery has high division *(arrowhead)* and small zygomatico-orbital branch *(double arrowhead).* Facial artery is hypoplastic and its terminal branch corresponds to coronal or inferior labial artery *(large arrow).* In this particular case lingual artery is dominant arterial pedicle, supplying entire floor of mouth, frenulum, and lingual surface of mandible *(open arrow).* Ascending pharyngeal artery is also in predominant position because, besides its usual branches, it also supplies soft palate *(curved arrow).* This variation illustrates role played by transverse facial artery, which participates in supplying cutaneous territory of hypoplastic facial artery. Therefore transverse facial artery can supply the cutaneous territory of the facial artery, lingual artery can annex endobuccal and submental territories, and ascending pharyngeal artery can encompass arterial supply to soft palate in absence of ascending palatine branch of facial artery.

Table 8-1. Angiographic protocol for the orbital region

Arterial system to be explored	Region to examine*	
	Orbital	Periorbital
Internal carotid	+	+
Distal internal maxillary	+	+
Proximal internal maxillary (middle and accessory meningeal)	+	±
Superficial temporal	+	−
Facial		−
Transverse facial		−
		± other side

*±, Depending on the type.

rologic point of view the most important anastomoses are those that can potentially contribute vascular supply to the peripheral nervous system and those that communicate between the extracranial vessels and arterial pedicles of the central nervous system (Fig. 8-7). Anatomically these represent a significant hazard in endovascular occlusive procedures. Accurate delineation of their position and interrelationships through precise vascular mapping is an absolute prerequisite for safe therapeutic angiography.

A functional approach to arteriographic examination of facial lesions is based on sound anatomic principles and provides a logical basis for analysis of a broad spectrum of vascular abnormalities affecting this region. Tables 8-1 to 8-7 summarize these principles and suggest specific examinations as well as briefly outline the hazards of endovascular procedures involving each major pedicle.

Table 8-2. Angiographic protocol of the skull base

Arterial system to be explored	Region to examine		
	Cavernous sinus	Cerebellopontine angle	Temporal and tympanic cavity
Internal carotid	+	+	+
Vertebral	+	+	+
Distal internal maxillary	+	−	−
Proximal internal maxillary	+	+	+
Ascending pharyngeal	+	+	+
Occipital	−	+	+
Posterior auricular	−	−	+

Table 8-3. Angiographic protocol of the upper cervical spine region

Arterial system to be explored	Region to examine*	
	Posterior fossa	High cervical spine (C₄)
Vertebral	+	+
Ascending pharyngeal	+	+
Occipital	+	+
Ascending cervical	±	+
Deep cervical	−	+
C₄ collateral branch of the external carotid	−	+
Middle meningeal	±	−

*±, Depending on the type.

Table 8-4. Angiographic protocol of the nasopharynx

Arterial system to be explored	Region to examine*	
	Nasopharynx	Nasal fossa (bilateral)
Internal carotid	+	+
Distal internal maxillary	+	+
Proximal internal maxillary	+	+
Ascending palatine	+	+
Facial	+	+
Ascending pharyngeal	+	±

*±, Depending on the type.

Table 8-5. Angiographic protocol of the scalp region

Arterial system to be explored	Region to examine	
	Scalp	Zygomaticotemporal region
Superficial temporal	+	+
Distal and proximal maxillary	+	+
Transverse facial artery	−	+
Occipital	+	−
Posterior auricular	+	−

Table 8-6. Angiographic protocol of the oral region

Arterial system to be explored	Region to examine*	
	Cheek	Palate (bilateral)
Transverse facial artery	+	−
Distal internal maxillary	+	+
Facial	+	+
Lingual	−	+
Superior laryngeal	−	+
Ascending pharyngeal	−	±

*±, Depending on the type.

Table 8-7. Principal dangerous branches of the external carotid system

Dangerous vessels	Anastomotic branch*
Orbital branch of middle meningeal artery (internal maxillary)	Anastomosis with ophthalmic artery and with cranial nerves V_1 + IV
Artery of foramen rotundum (internal maxillary)	Intracavernous anastomosis with carotid siphon
Accessory meningeal artery (internal maxillary)	Intracavernous anastomosis with carotid siphon (C_4) and with cranial nerves $V_3 + V_m \pm VII \pm III, IV, VI, V_2, V_1$
Petrous branch of middle meningeal artery (internal maxillary)	Intracavernous anastomosis with carotid siphon (C_4 branch) and with geniculate ganglion + cranial nerve VII
Carotid branch of ascending pharyngeal artery	Sympathetic pericarotid anastomosis with recurrent branch of the anterior foramen lacerum (C_5) branch of internal carotid artery
Eustachian branch of ascending pharyngeal artery	Anastomosis with mandibular artery
Jugular branch of ascending pharyngeal artery	Intracavernous anastomosis with carotid siphon (C_5 branch) and with cranial nerves IX, X, XI, VI
Hypoglossal branch of ascending pharyngeal artery	Intracavernous anastomosis with internal carotid artery (C_5 branch) and with cervical vertebral artery (third cervical space) and cranial nerve XII
C_1 branch of occipital artery	C_1 branch of vertebral artery
C_2 branch of occipital artery	C_2 branch of vertebral artery

* I, Depending on the type.

□ **References**

1. Aaron, C., Doyon, D., Fischgold, H., et al.: Arteriographie de la carotide externe, Paris, 1970, Masson Editeur.
2. Djindjian, R., and Merland, J.J.: Superselective arteriography of the external carotid artery, Berlin, 1978, Springer Verlag.
3. Lasjaunias, P.: Cranio-facial and upper cervical arteries, Baltimore, 1981, Williams & Wilkins.

9 □ Embolization techniques used in head and neck pathology

ALEX BERENSTEIN and IRVIN I. KRICHEFF

Embolization is a technique of intravascular occlusion in which catheters are selectively manipulated into a pathologic vascular territory for the purpose of injecting occlusive or embolic agents. Its aim is to obliterate the pathologic angioarchitecture of a vascular malformation, arteriovenous communication or fistula, vascular neoplasm, or bleeding vessel. Embolization may be performed (1) as an adjunct to surgical removal of the lesion, (2) as the primary form of treatment in potentially curable lesions, or (3) in lesions not accessible to surgical removal.

At the present state of the art, specific indications for and the long-term effects of embolization are not yet fully known because follow-up time in the few reported series is short. However, rapid advancements in vascular catheterization and occlusive techniques are permitting the treatment of an ever-increasing gamut of complex hemodynamic lesions, making them amenable to intravascular surgery. In this chapter we will review the techniques used for the treatment of various pathologic entities based on our experience of over 200 embolization procedures performed in the head, neck, brain, and spinal areas, with primary emphasis on embolization in the head and neck area.

□ Historical perspective

Brooks[10] reported in 1931 the successful obliteration of a carotid cavernous fistula using the intra-arterial approach. After the feeding vessel in the neck was surgically exposed, a piece of autologous muscle was introduced into the internal carotid artery and preferential blood flow was allowed to carry the embolus to occlude the fistula. Since then, scattered reports of successful use of the Brooks technique, or modifications of this

technique, have appeared. In 1960 Luessenhop[35] reported the first embolization of a cerebral arteriovenous malformation using methyl methacrylate spheres introduced into the internal carotid artery by way of an arteriotomy. The spheres were then flow-directed to the malformation. In 1970 Boulos et al.[9] reported the value of cerebral angiography in the embolization treatment of cerebral arteriovenous malformations. Kricheff et al.[29] in 1972 introduced the use of percutaneous transcatheter techniques for the delivery of barium sulfate–impregnated silicone balls to cerebral arteriovenous malformations. Cunningham and Paletta[11] in 1970 reported the first successful embolization in the external carotid territory for control of an arteriovenous fistula in a "massive" facial hemangioma by using muscle emboli. Djindjian et al.[16] reported in 1971 a successful embolization of an angioma supplied by the external carotid artery with autologous muscle. In 1972 Hekster et al.[22] reported five cases of glomus jugulare tumors embolized by a transfemoral approach, again employing autologous muscle, and pointed out the advantages of this technique for the control of the patient's symptoms in large nonresectable tumors or for preoperative devascularization.

In 1973 Djindjian et al.[17] reported their experience in a review of 60 cases embolized by the use of percutaneous catheter techniques. They are largely responsible for the introduction of superselective catheterization of distal branches of the external carotid artery, permitting the demonstration of the true vascular supply to hypervascular lesions and providing the attractive possibility of an intra-arterial approach to their management. Since then there have been many reports of different delivery systems and embolic agents for use in a variety of pathologic conditions in different parts of the body.

An important addition to intra-arterial therapy appeared in 1974 when Serbinenko reported superselective catheterization of cerebral vessels using small balloon catheters, whereby the balloon could be detached as the occlusive agent.[41] This added versatility to the intra-arterial approach by permitting occlusion of high-flow arteriovenous fistulas with preservation of the arterial lumen, a functional improvement on Brook's original intra-arterial occlusive technique. Unfortunately, Serbinenko did not reveal his technique of balloon detachment. In 1975 Debrun,[12,13] a French neuroradiologist, published the technique of balloon detachment and improved Serbinenko's detachable balloon assembly.

Kerber[25] introduced a flow-guided balloon microcatheter with a "calibrated leak" that permits superselective catheterization of 1 to 2 mm diameter vessels and the subsequent perfusion of fluid tissue adhesives for occlusion of very fine distal arteries. We use this technique primarily in the intracerebral circulation. Pevsner[37,38] also developed flow-guided and detachable balloon microcatheters, basing his work on his experience with Serbinenko.

Improvements in radiographic and fluoroscopic imaging, with magnification and subtraction techniques, permits a detailed delineation of the angioarchitecture of external carotid lesions, a demonstration of the anastomotic connections as described by Djindjian et al.[18] and a visualization of the vascular supply to the transcranial nerves described by Lasjaunias.[33] For the best therapeutic results a good understanding of these vascular relations is imperative[31a] (see Chapter 8). Lasjaunias, Berenstein, and Doyon[32] have described a functional anatomic approach in the facial territory and Lasjaunias et al.[33,43] have extended the functional approach to plan and execute intravascular occlusion in the facial territory and other areas in the head and neck.

Preembolization investigation of vascular head and neck lesions requires superselective catheterization and injection of the functional arterial pedicles involved. Common external carotid injection or other nonselective studies are insufficient for proper investigation and may fail to demonstrate the true extent of and supply to a lesion (see Chapter 8).

□ Technique of embolization and patient preparation

When deciding what technique will best ensure the desired results, the following criteria must be considered regarding the selection of catheters and occlusive agents.

1. Safety during all phases of the procedure
2. Superselectivity during catheterization
3. Occlusion of the nidus of the lesion, not merely the feeding pedicle
4. Prevention of distal migration of the emboli to the venous circulation or beyond it

■ Patient preparation

Patients are seen in consultation before the embolization procedure and a detailed explanation of the procedure is discussed with both the patient and the family. The risks of the treatment, alternatives, and expected results must be clearly understood by the patient. In complex lesions in which multiple vessels are involved, embolization is carried out in stages. The physician performing these therapeutic procedures assumes a pivotal role in the decisions and in the planning and execution of these operations and should also be intimately involved in postprocedural care.

Patients are premedicated with corticosteroids, anticonvulsants, and antibiotics. A 100 mg dose of hydrocortisone is given intravenously 12 hours before the embolization. Anticonvulsants are only given when brain lesions are treated. An antibiotic such as oxacillin, which is effective against penicillinase-producing *Staphylococcus aureus* (the most frequent hospital pathogen), is given intravenously 4 hours preoperatively and repeated just before the embolization and at meningeal doses 48 hours after the procedure. Corticosteroids are gradually tapered over 72 hours. The duration of anticonvulsant therapy is variable. The patient's blood supply is also routinely typed and cross-matched for blood.

During the procedure the anesthesiologist induces neuroleptanalgesia with intravenous droperidol, 0.1 mg/kg of body weight, and fentanyl, 0.002 mg/kg of body weight. These drugs allow immediate awakening of the patient for clinical monitoring of their neurologic status. Infants and children are treated under general anesthesia. An indwelling catheter is placed in the bladder to prevent distention and to monitor urinary output. The patient's electrocardiograms and vital signs are monitored continuously. The skin at the puncture site is prepared in the usual manner and infiltrated with bupivacaine hydrochloride (Marcaine) 0.25%, a long-lasting local anesthetic.

■ Catheterization techniques

We do most of our embolization by the femoral route; however, percutaneous puncture of the common carotid artery or external carotid artery or arteriotomy may be advantageous in infants, in cases in which a vessel has been ligated previously, or on those occasions when a shorter catheter affords better torque control.

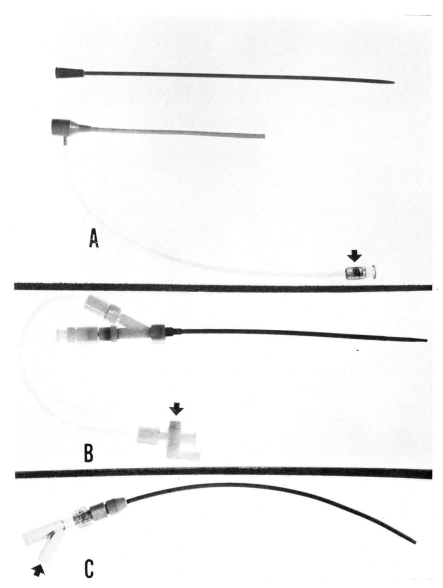

Fig. 9-1. Introducer sheaths. **A,** Cordis introducer sheath; **B,** Cook introducer sheath; **C,** Ingenor introducer sheath (note **Y** adaptor). Arrow points to side arm for continuous heparinized perfusion. (From Berenstein, A., and Kricheff, I.I.: Radiology **132:**619, 1979.)

Introducer sheaths (Fig. 9-1) are routinely employed to minimize arterial trauma during catheter changes and manipulations. The sheaths are sutured to the patient's skin to prevent accidental removal. When sheaths are used, catheters can be changed without the need of guidewires. This is of great value when liquid embolic materials harden in the catheter lumen and guidewire insertion becomes impossible. Catheters of various types and sizes can be used without pericatheter leakage of blood. A sheath also allows for a continuous perfusion of heparinized saline through its side arm. Speedy removal of the delivery system is neces-

sary if a rapidly polymerizing agent such as isobutyl-2-cyanoacrylate (IBCA) is the embolic agent. This is only possible through an introducer sheath. At the end of the procedure, compression at the puncture site for 20 minutes is necessary to ensure proper hemostasis.

Three common types of introducer sheaths are available in the United States. Each has advantages and disadvantages (Fig. 9-1).

The Cordis introducer sheath has a completely self-sealing valve at its proximal end that prevents bleeding at all times; however, one can use only a catheter one size smaller without pericatheter leakage. Small sheaths are not available, and detachable balloons cannot be used with this sheath because they may be dislodged while being withdrawn through the self-sealing valve.

The Cook introducer sheath can be used with any size catheter smaller than the introducer sheath and can be employed with detachable balloon catheters without the risk of dislodging the balloon when withdrawing the catheter. Skill and rapid maneuvering is needed to prevent blood loss unless a second catheter is wedged into the introducer sheath or the operator digitally occludes the hole or latex ring in the proximal end of the introducer sheath as it is rapidly closed.

The Ingenor introducer sheath is excellent for use with a detachable balloon catheter because the proximal end has no valve that could strip a balloon from the shaft. This introducer sheath must be coupled to a Y adaptor to prevent retrograde bleeding during balloon insertion.

□ Catheters or delivery systems
■ Conventional tapered angiographic catheters

Tapered catheters are used with a simple 0.5 cm distal curve in sizes from 7Fr to 3Fr, depending on the vessel to be catheterized. They should be wedged tightly in the artery to prevent reflux of embolic material, especially toward the end of the procedure when vascular resistance in the partially embolized lesion is markedly increased. This resistance may prevent a total obliteration of the lesion. We prefer to use tapered catheters in a coaxial manner with a double-lumen balloon catheter in the outer or coaxial position.[3] This assembly uses the balloon to prevent reflux and control flow to the lesion. It usually results in a more selective catheterization in the external carotid artery than can be accomplished by a single catheter.

TYPES OF CATHETERS

Conventional tapered catheters
Conventional nontapered catheters
Conventional nontapered catheters in coaxial assembly
Balloon catheters
    Single-lumen flow-guided (Kerber's catheter, with a calibrated "leak" for embolic agent deposition)
    Double-lumen balloon catheters
    Modified double-lumen balloon catheters for coaxial embolization or viscous fluid embolization (Berenstein's catheter)
    Detachable balloons for arteriovenous fistulas or aneurysms (Debrun's catheter)

■ Conventional nontapered catheters

Nontapered catheters are used with solid embolic agents when a large internal diameter is required, such as when using silicone balls or compressed polyvinyl alcohol foam (PVA). They are useful in coaxial techniques as the outer catheter for superselective catheterizations with torque or flow-guided catheters.

■ Balloon catheters

Balloons must be purged of air by the use of low-viscosity contrast material and should not be manipulated once the balloon is inflated or it may cause intimal damage. After deflation, the reestablished blood flow should be allowed to wash adherent thrombi into the previously embolized territory before the catheter is moved to another site. Inflation is best accomplished with a small syringe (1 ml Luer-Lok), while deflation is easier with larger syringes (10 ml Luer-Lok).

Double-lumen balloon catheters

Double-lumen balloon catheters should be used for embolization whenever possible. They can be used to prevent reflux, produce stasis, and control flow. A preembolization high-volume, high-pressure injection angiogram should be performed to confirm the absence of reflux (Fig. 9-2). With stasis, one can accurately estimate the amount of liquid embolic agent needed to obtain the desired vascular filling by using measured amounts of contrast media. The balloon can control flow and produce stasis, allowing liquid materials to harden in the vascular tree. Balloon deflation in the early part of embolization allows the flow of blood to carry solid particles to a more distal position. Balloons are easily inflated with low-viscosity contrast material.

A single-balloon catheter in one feeding artery cannot produce stasis when multiple feeding arteries are present. In such instances a modified double-lumen balloon catheter[3] can be used. In this catheter the balloon lumen has been changed to an oval shape. This modification increases the injection lumen cross-section area by 30% without changing the outer diameter of the catheter shaft. This catheter is left in the common trunk of the feeding pedicle, such as in the main trunk of the external carotid artery, while a smaller inner catheter is then advanced through the injection lumen to one of the feeding arteries (Fig. 9-3). A 7Fr double-lumen catheter of this type can accept a 4Fr catheter.[3] Catheterization is technically more difficult with this type of balloon catheter, but most difficulties can be overcome by using heparinized jelly, silicone grease, or liquid paraffin to lubricate the tip. If catheterization is unsuccessful with a balloon catheter, it can be performed with a conventional catheter that is then exchanged for the balloon catheter over a 260 cm guidewire.

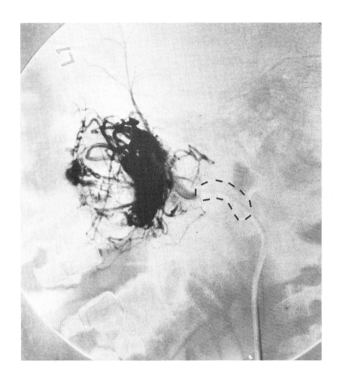

Fig. 9-2. Lateral subtraction angiogram of left internal maxillary artery supplying maxillary hemangioma. High-pressure, high-volume injection using modified double-lumen balloon catheter (dotted lines outline balloon) confirms lack of reflux. With this catheter, volume of fluid embolic agents necessary for embolization can also be measured by careful hand injection. (From Berenstein, A., and Kricheff, I.I.: Radiology **132:**619, 1979.)

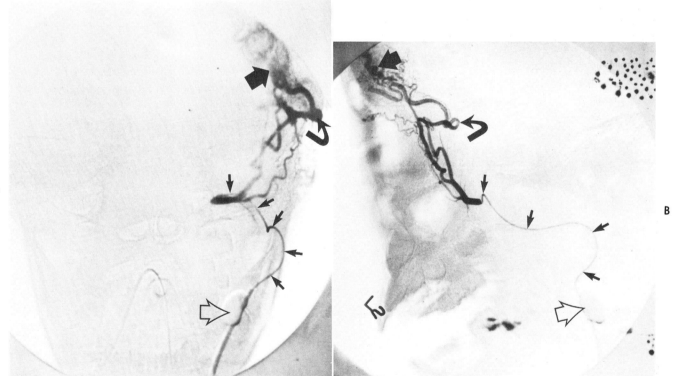

Fig. 9-3. A, Frontal and, **B,** lateral subtraction angiogram of high-flow supraorbital hemangioma *(large arrow)*. Coaxial balloon catheter *(open arrow)* is controlling flow in main external carotid artery. Smaller catheter *(small arrows)* is selectively placed in temporal artery and fills hemangioma. Note filling of frontozygomatic branch of superficial temporal artery *(curved arrow)*.

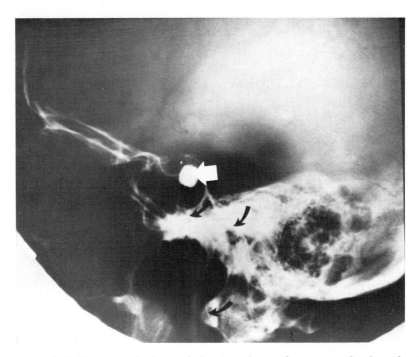

Fig. 9-4. Lateral skull radiograph after embolization of carotid cavernous fistula with single-lumen balloon catheter. Balloon *(white arrow)* is occluding internal carotid artery at fistula site. Catheter shaft *(arrows)* is bent, clipped, and anchored.

Single-lumen balloon catheters

Single-lumen balloon catheters are used for either temporary or permanent occlusion of a blood vessel. In the former instance they may be used to evaluate tolerance to occlusion of a specific vascular territory or to control bleeding until surgery can be performed.[1,45,46] They can also be used for permanent occlusion of a fistula, but this use sacrifices the normal arterial flow through the parent artery (Fig. 9-4). Unless they are flow guided, these catheters may fail to reach the selectivity desired.

Flow-guided single-lumen balloon catheters. Flow-guided single-lumen balloon catheters are used for catheterization and embolization of small distal vessels such as intracerebral arteries. They are too small (2Fr and 3Fr) to be used with particulate emboli or viscous fluids; however, cyanoacrylates will pass through them easily.

Detachable balloons

A number of different detachable balloon catheters have been introduced.[12-15,31] The balloons are made of either latex or silicone. Latex has the advantage of greater distensibility and good collapsing properties. An apparent disadvantage with latex balloons is that, if left inflated with ionic iodinated contrast material, the balloon loses the contrast agent through the balloon walls. Deflation can be partially overcome by using vulcanizing silicone fluid inside the balloon. At present the catheters are single-lumen and a dead space exists, represented by the catheter shaft, that cannot be completely purged or replaced by the silicone if first filled with contrast material. Thus a small amount of contrast material will remain in the distended balloon. With double-lumen balloon catheters this is not a problem. We have used metrizamide, 240 mg/100 ml of iodine, to inflate the latex balloons because its high viscosity retards deflation. These balloons have remained inflated and unchanged in situ for as long as 6 weeks.

Debrun's detachable balloon catheter is made by tying the sleeve of a latex balloon with latex thread to a small-diameter Teflon shaft (OD, 0.6 mm; ID, 0.4 mm), which has no elasticity and sufficient strength to permit balloon detachment without catheter fracture. An outer polyethylene catheter is passed over the inner catheter to dislodge the inflated balloon.[14] This system is ideal for large arteriovenous communications, such as carotid cavernous fistulae, where the balloon can be placed in the fistula itself in order to maintain the patency of the arterial lumen (Fig. 9-5). It is also very effective in treating vertebral artery to paravertebral venous fistulae (Fig. 9-6).

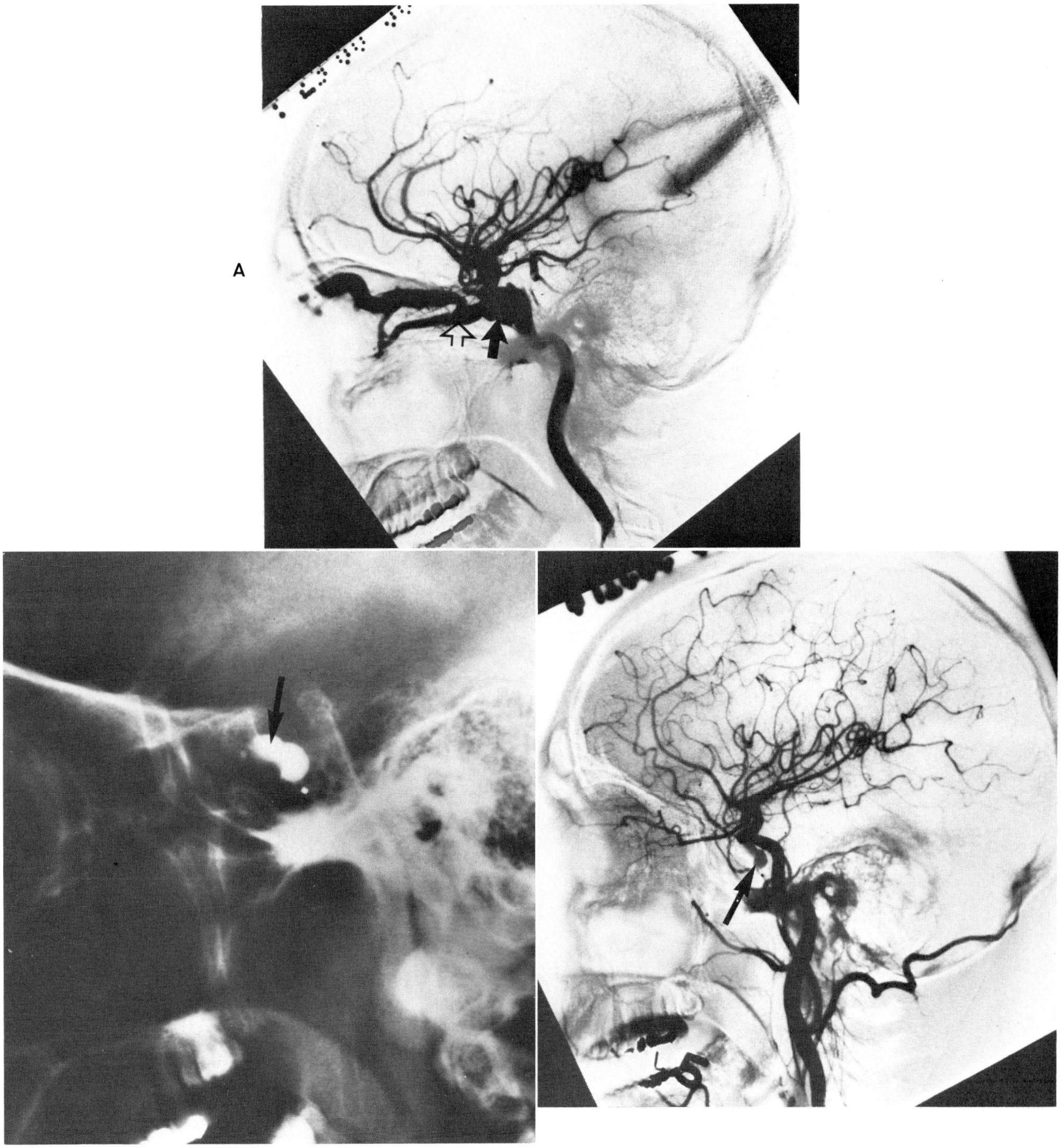

Fig. 9-5. A, Lateral subtraction angiogram of left internal carotid artery. High-flow arteriovenous fistula between internal carotid artery and anterior inferior compartment of cavernous sinus *(arrow)* drains into ophthalmic venous system *(open arrows)*. **B,** Lateral skull film after detaching balloon *(arrow)* partially filled with nonopaque silicone fluid. **C,** Lateral subtraction angiogram of left common carotid artery. Balloon *(arrow)* is occluding fistula. Internal carotid blood flow is preserved.
Continued.

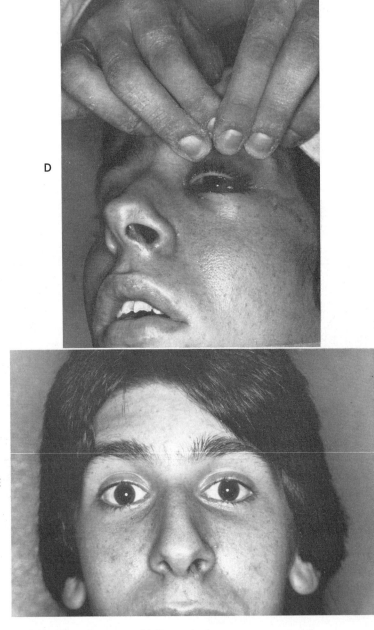

Fig. 9-5, cont'd. D, Close-up view of left eye before treatment. **E,** After treatment there is complete resolution of all patient's signs and symptoms.

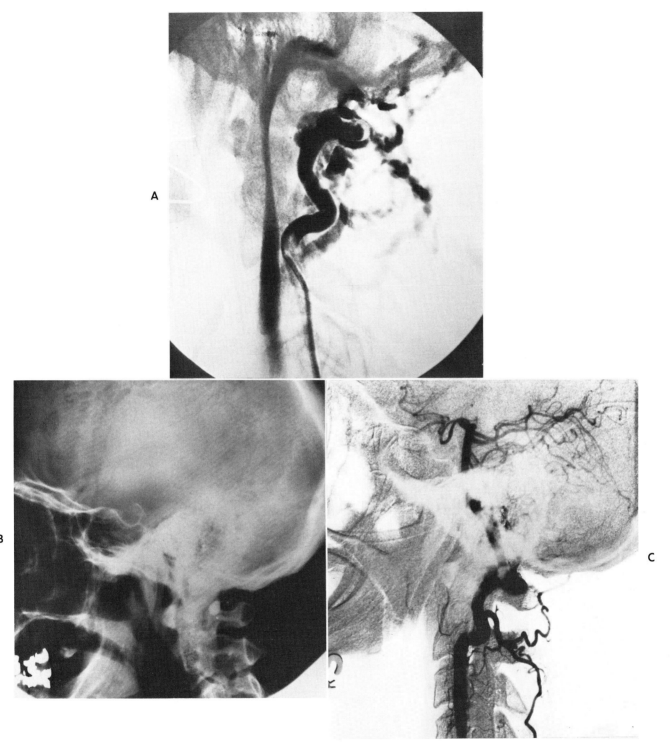

Fig. 9-6. A, Lateral subtraction angiogram of right vertebral artery, demonstrating fistula between right vertebral artery and paravertebral venous plexus. **B,** Balloon in venous side. **C,** Postembolization. There is occlusion of fistula and preservation of vertebral blood flow.

□ Embolic agents

Many embolic agents (see box) have been used for transarterial occlusion.[5,30] Differences in embolic agents because of particulate size and physical, chemical, and biologic characteristics must be carefully considered when selecting the optimal agent for each individual case. The ability of the material to be made radiopaque is important in order to monitor its course, control its placement in the nidus of the lesion, and judge the results. There is no single "ideal" or "best" agent. Instead there is a group of agents that permits dealing individually with a variety of clinical problems. Embolization materials can be divided into absorbable and nonabsorbable, solid or fluid types.

The anatomy and flow characteristics of a lesion dictate catheter selection and placement, which in turn influence the choice of embolic material. Before using an embolic agent one must consider the position of the catheter tip, the size of its lumen, and whether or not

flow can be controlled. Thorough knowledge of the advantages and limitations of the different embolic materials and the hemodynamics of the lesion will determine the embolic agent that can achieve the best and safest results.

■ Absorbable or biodegradable materials (solid)

Many biodegradable materials have been used[21] as therapeutic emboli. Gelfoam is the best known and most frequently used absorbable material[8,34] and is commercially available in sheets or powder. The sheets are cut into strips 1 mm × 2 mm in size or can be punched out with conventional catheter hand punches to make plugs of predetermined sizes. The powder consists of particles 40 to 60 μm in size. Gelfoam can be made radiopaque with tantalum powder or by adding a silver clip to a small strip, or it can be monitored as a negative shadow when injected in contrast material. It is easy to handle and can be injected through catheters when suspended in contrast material. Gelfoam particles are reabsorbable and their use is limited to temporary blockage of a vessel for protection from permanent occlusive materials or to control flow (Fig. 9-7). Here its tendency for recanalization is the advantage of allowing postoperative reestablishment of circulation to normal tissue. The powder produces occlusion at the precapillary level and can be employed in lesions such as meningiomas, making embolization superior to surgical ligation of a feeding pedicle. A point of caution: very small particles introduced into the external carotid artery may, if injected under pressure distal to a balloon, pass through the rich collateral circulation between the external carotid artery and the internal carotid circulation, producing antegrade cerebral embolization.

■ Nonabsorbable particulate material
Silicone sphere*

Silicone spheres are nonabsorbable, biocompatible, and radiopaque (impregnated with barium sulfate). They are available in a variety of sizes (0.5 mm to 3 mm in diameter) and are used primarily for cerebral angiomas.[35]

---

*Heyer-Schulte, PO Box 946, Goleta, Cal. 93017.

EMBOLIC AGENTS

Biodegradeable
  Gelfoam particles (1 × 2 mm)
  Gelfoam powder (40 to 60 μm)
Nonbiodegradeable
  Solids
    Polyvinyl alcohol foam (PVA)
      In a dry compressed form (expands 5 to 10 times its original size when wet)
      Microemboli (250 to 1000 μm) in suspension of iodinated contrast material
  Fluids
    Isobutyl-2-cyanoacrylate (IBCA *tissue adhesive*)
      1.5 g of tantalum/ml is used for radiopacity
    Silicone fluid mixtures (of varying viscosity and vulcanization time); 1 g of tantalum (nonadhesive)/ml is used for radiopacity
Opacifying agents
  Tantalum powder (1 to 2 μ) black powder
  Tantalum oxide (1 to 2 μ) white powder
  Pantopaque (used with IBCA for radiopacity and to regard polymerization time)

Fig. 9-7. A, Frontal and, **B,** lateral subtraction angiogram of right internal maxillary artery. Subselective catheterization of enlarged middle meningeal artery supplying sphenoid bone arteriovenous shunt secondary to fibrous dysplasia could not be accomplished. Note filling of maxillary artery distal to meningeal origin *(arrows)*. **C,** Frontal and, **D,** lateral subtraction angiogram. Two Gelfoam particles, each 1 × 2 mm in size, were injected into right internal maxillary artery. Note radiolucent Gelfoam *(arrow)* distal to origin of middle meningeal artery. This permitted embolization of middle meningeal artery with IBCA, a permanent fluid agent, without risks of antegrade cerebral embolization. (From Berenstein, A., and Russell, E.: Radiology **141:**105, 1981.)

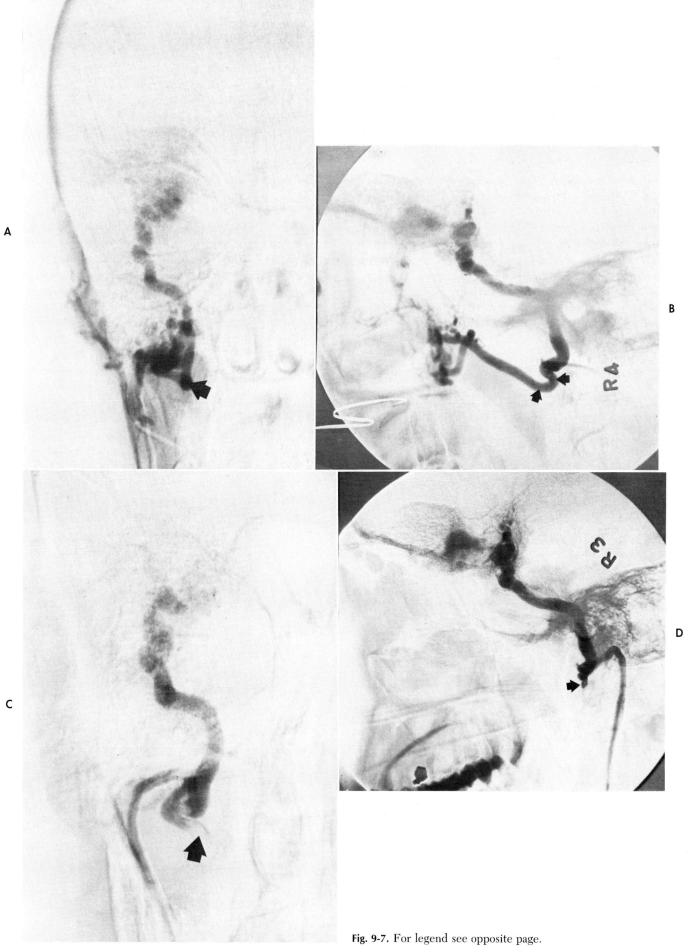

Fig. 9-7. For legend see opposite page.

These spheres are easily introduced with the aid of the NYU introducer sheath.[28] The pellets can be used for selective injection when sufficiently large catheters can be placed in the feeding vessels. Most often they are used in a flow-guided manner and there is no positive control of them once they are introduced into the circulation.

Polyvinyl alcohol foam (PVA, formerly Ivalon)*

PVA is a nonabsorbable, biocompatible sponge that is insoluble in water and has been used in a variety of situations.[6,24] In approximately 30 seconds after contact with fluids, the dry compressed sponge expands from 10 to 15 times in length, depending on its original thickness (Fig. 9-8), and is ideal for occluding medium-size to large vessels that are larger in diameter than the internal diameter of the catheter. This material is difficult to handle in the dry compressed state; however, if small discs are made from the original sheet with a catheter hand punch, the NYU introducer can be used to facilitate their delivery.[28] PVA can be made weakly radiopaque with 60% barium sulfate; however, the addition of tantalum powder may further add radiopacity to small particles. In the dry compressed form only gas sterilization should be used.

PVA can be used as a suspension of precut small particles. We have successfully simplified PVA particle delivery by using uniform hand-punched particles of 0.015 to 0.035 inches in diameter and suspending them in

*Ethicon, Inc., Somerville, N.J. 08876

contrast material which, with the particles, can be drawn into a syringe for injection. If the correct size is chosen, small vessels can be occluded (200 to 1000 μm range) while preserving the larger parent vessel (Fig. 9-9). Other permanent particulate materials, such as porcine dura mater, have been used; however, we do not see any advantages of dura over PVA.

Isobutyl-2-Cyanoacrylate (IBCA)*

IBCA is a fast-polymerization tissue adhesive of low viscosity[47] that can pass through very small catheters such as the Debrun or Kerber calibrated-leak balloon catheters.[14a] IBCA can be made radiopaque with tantalum powder. This material appears to be one of the best agents for the treatment of high-flow fistulous communications and for cerebral angiomas; it can also be used for complete occlusion of large to medium-size vessels. Because of its adhesive properties and mild inflammatory reaction, superselective catheterization is mandatory although a complete and immediate occlusion of the vessel is less critical than with silicone fluid, which is not adhesive (see below). IBCA polymerizes on contact with ionic solutions, such as normal saline, contrast material, or blood, and with the intima of vessels; therefore the delivery system must be flushed with a 5% glucose solution to prevent polymerization.[26] If maintaining patency of the catheter is necessary, the material may be followed with a 5% glucose solution. The catheter tip should be lubricated with silicone

*Unipoint Industries, Inc., High Point, N.C. 27260.

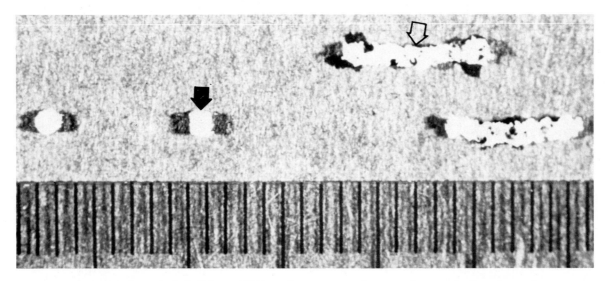

Fig. 9-8. Polyvinyl alcohol foam (PVA) in dry compressed state. The punch discs (*arrow*) expand in 30 seconds when wet (*open arrow*). (From Berenstein, A., and Kricheff, I.I.: Radiology **132**:631, 1979.)

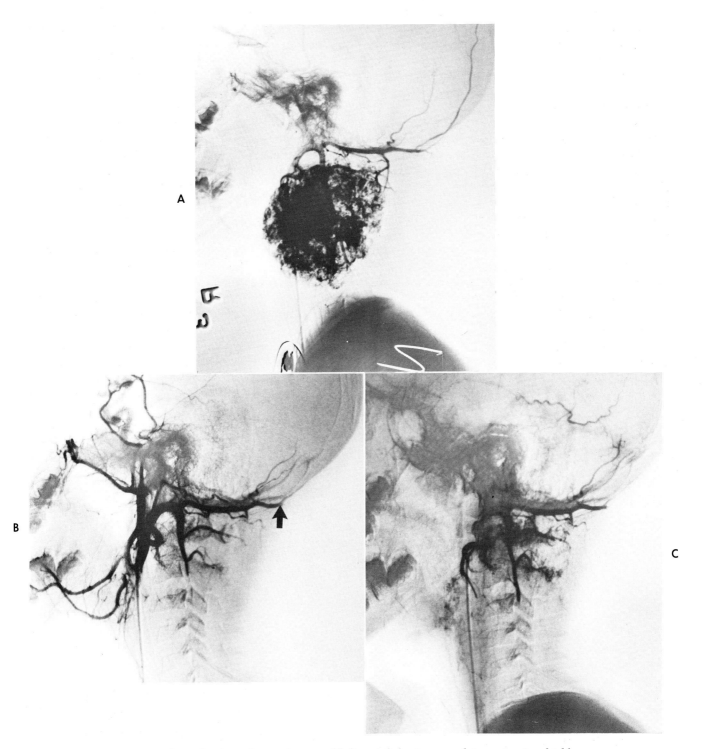

Fig. 9-9. A, Lateral subtraction angiogram of left occipital artery supplying extensive, highly vascular capillary hemangioma. **B,** Lateral subtraction angiogram after embolization, midarterial phase. Occipital artery distal to splenial branch *(arrow)* was protectively occluded with 1 × 2 mm Gelfoam particle prior to use of PVA microemboli in suspension. Note obliteration of small capillary and precapillary hemangiomatous vessels. **C,** Late phase after embolization. Note stasis in major branches of occipital artery and no filling of lesion.

grease and the catheter assembly should be removed promptly after injection to prevent the catheter from adhering to the vessel wall. Experience is required to avoid too rapid deflation of the balloon and distal migration of the liquid IBCA to the venous circulation. This material should probably not be used with a double-lumen balloon catheter when balloon deflation is slower unless dextrose and water are used to push the IBCA beyond the catheter tip.

At present there is no documentation of cancer in humans caused by any of the acrylates, although fibrosarcoma was induced in 8 of 59 cancer prone rats after a large subcutaneous injection of methymethacrylate; dogs treated similarly did not develop tumors.[36] No such data have been obtained with IBCA. At present we reserve this material for situations in which only very small flow-guided catheters can achieve the desired superselectivity such as in the intracranial circulation or with recurrent lesions when other materials have failed to produce a permanent occlusion. Considerable experience with adhesives is essential if complications are to be avoided.

Silicone fluid mixtures*

Silicone fluid is a permanent occlusive biocompatible agent easily made radiopaque with tantalum powder.[20] As with the previous liquid agent, superselectivity is mandatory. The fluid mixture consists of (1) Silastic elastomer 382, a silicone of relatively high viscosity (50,000 centistokes; C.S.P.) that contains a filler necessary for vulcanization; and (2) medical grade silicone fluid 360, a clear fluid with a lower viscosity (20 C.S.P.) that acts as the dilutant to the more viscous Silastic elastomer. These two silicones are thoroughly mixed in a 1:2 to 1:5 proportion, depending on the viscosity desired, and 1 g of opacifying tantalum powder/1 ml of mixture is added. Two catalysts are required for vulcanization: stannous octate (Dow Corning Catalyst M)* and a colinker, tetraethyl silicate, introduced by Hilal. This latter material stimulates prompt, reproducible vulcanization of fluid silicone in low-viscosity proportions and has made Silastic embolization a practical technique. We have also used tetra-N-propoxy silane as the colinker. There appears to be no practical differences in the performance of these two colinkers; however, less stannous octate is needed if the silane is used. The silicate reacts to form an ethyl alcohol, while the silane forms a propoxyl alcohol. Typically, one 21 gauge needledrop of catalyst and also of colinker per 1 ml of mixture will produce vulcanization in approximately 3 to 4 minutes depending on the age of the materials, their exposure to light, and the length of steam sterilization.

---

*Dow Corning Corp., Hemlock, Mich. 48262.

Our bacterial cultures have shown that a 10-minute, 270° F cycle is sufficient for sterilization of silicone fluid 360, both catalysts, and tantalum. The more viscous silastic elastomer 282 requires 20 minutes sterilization at 270° F. In order to assess vulcanization time accurately a sample of the mixture to be used is tested in vitro just prior to injection, and the liquid is stirred continuously to compensate for body temperature.

Complete stasis facilitates the injection of silicone fluid considerably. A double-lumen balloon catheter may be used alone or for a more distal insertion of an inner catheter. The small inner catheter is advanced to one of the main arteries feeding the lesion. Flow stasis is monitored fluoroscopically and the amount of fluid necessary to obtain the desired embolization is measured by contrast material injection.[2] Liquid silicone is injected in fluid form and can fill vessels as small as 40 μm in diameter. The balloon is deflated and the catheter assembly removed after the predetermined vulcanization time has elapsed, as judged by prior and concurrent in vitro testing of the mixture. There is no risk of catheter "gluing" with this agent and a true cast of the lesion can be obtained (Fig. 9-10).

When stasis cannot be accomplished, Silastic is injected just before vulcanization, when it has a more viscous physical consistency and creates a continuous column at the time of injection.[23] Silastic has no adhesive properties; therefore a complete cast of the vascular architecture appears necessary.

In 1975 Doppman et al.[19] reported distal migration of a silicone cast in a parathyroid adenoma. To prevent distal migration the cast should be anchored in vessels of progressively diminishing diameter. Furthermore, if the silicone is not well mixed, air bubbles may be trapped in the fluid. Such air will be reabsorbed and the cast will retract, with the possibility of subsequent distal migration.

Silastic can be used in a more viscous mixture as flow-guided globules, as originally described by Sano[40] and subsequently modified by us.[2] We make the silicone radiopaque with tantalum and use balloon catheters to control the flow. A drop of the fluid is injected with the balloon deflated and is carried by blood flow until decreasing vessel diameter terminates its movement. If the silicone does not stop, the maneuver is repeated with the balloon inflated. Deflation of the balloon causes the drop to flow distally until it reaches the desired position, where the balloon should not be deflated again until full vulcanization has occurred (Fig. 9-11). Vulcanizing globules of Silastic can also be wedged and anchored by injecting saline behind them into a vascular system occluded by a proximally inflated balloon. Low-viscosity Silastic mixtures can also be used to fill a detachable balloon and reduce late deflation.

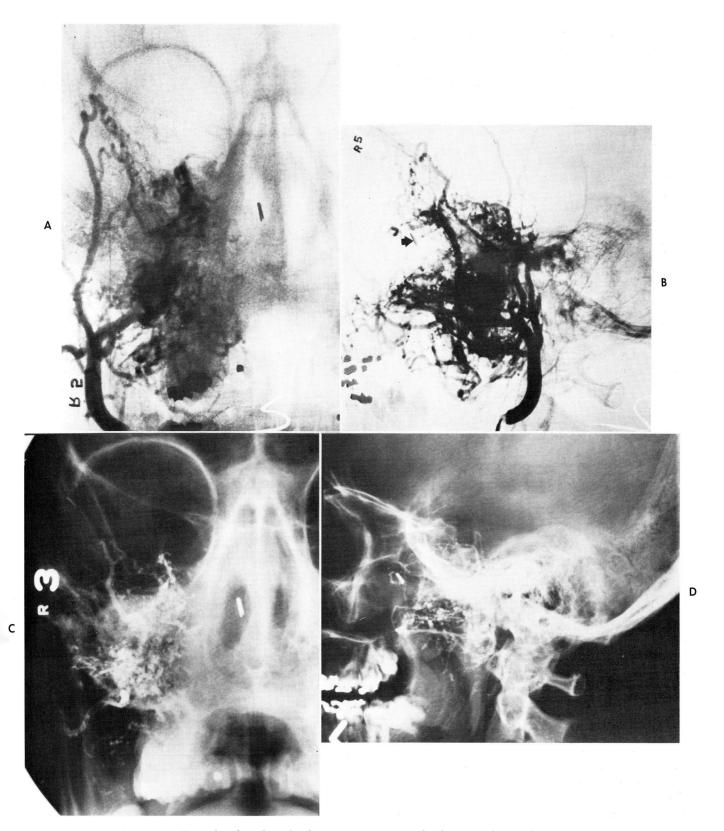

Fig. 9-10. A, Frontal and, **B,** lateral subtraction angiogram of right external carotid artery in recurrent juvenile angiofibroma. **C,** Frontal and **D,** lateral radiographs after radiopaque silicone fluid embolization. Note Silastic cast of tumor angioarchitecture (compare to **A** and **B**). (From Berenstein, A., and Russell, E.: Radiology **141:**105, 1981.)

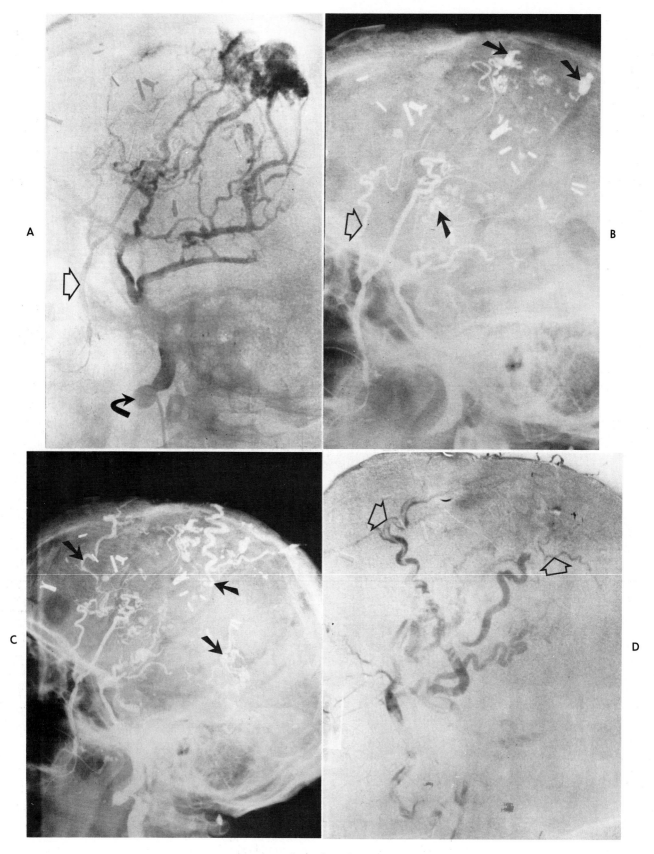

Fig. 9-11. For legend see opposite page.

Tantalum powder*

Tantalum powder is an inert, biocompatible metal that has been used in neurosurgery for many years. For embolization opacification it is used as a powder of 1 to 2 μm particles. It does not alter the chemical characteristics of the embolic agent but will increase the viscosity of the mixture. Two preparations are available: tantalum powder, which is black, should not be used in vessels supplying skin surfaces of white patients because of skin discoloration. Tantalum oxide is white and should not be used in vessels supplying skin surfaces of black patients.

*Kena Metal, Latrobe, Pa.

□ Epistaxis

The management of epistaxis has been significantly modified with the introduction of intra-arterial occlusive techniques, for the internal maxillary artery can be catheterized easily and subselective embolization of the distal maxillary branches can be easily and safely performed (Fig. 9-12). In traumatic epistaxis, embolization of the injured vessel is usually sufficient. In other cases of epistaxis, such as in the Osler-Weber-Rendu syndrome or in hemangiomas involving the nose and nasopharynx, embolization of both facial systems, in addition to the ipsilateral maxillary artery, appears best to control nasal bleeding.

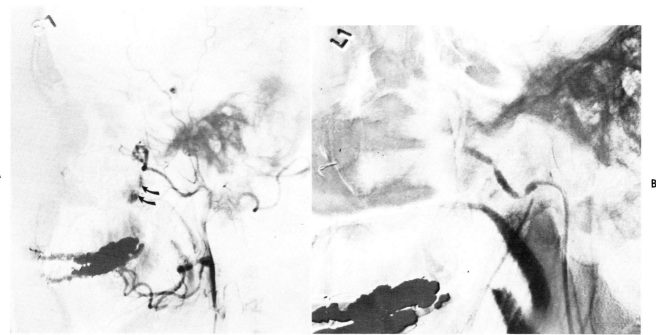

Fig. 9-12. A, Lateral subtraction angiogram of left external carotid artery. Note extravasation of contrast material from descending palatine artery *(double arrow)*. **B,** Lateral subtraction angiogram of left internal maxillary artery after Gelfoam particle embolization. Bleeding stops immediately. (From Berenstein, A., and Russell, E.: Radiology **141:**105, 1981.)

Fig. 9-11. Flow control silicone fluid embolization. **A,** Modified double-lumen balloon catheter *(curved arrow)*. Preembolization angiogram of right middle meningeal supply to dural portion of cerebral angioma. Open arrow points to previously embolized left external carotid supply. **B,** Multiple emboli have been directed by balloon flow control into meningeal arteries supplying angioma *(arrows)*. Open arrow indicates previously embolized left external carotid supply. **C,** Additional viscous Silastic emboli *(arrows)* have been introduced distally in superficial temporal artery by balloon flow control. **D,** Control arteriogram after embolization. There is no filling of angioma. Note lack of an adhesiveness of silicone. Contrast material is passing around silicone until complete cast of embolized vessel exists *(arrowheads)*. (From Berenstein, A., and Kricheff, I.I.: Radiology **132:**631, 1979.)

Table 9-1. Possible sites of anastomoses between extracerebral and intracerebral territories

Extracerebral	Intracerebral
Occipital artery	Vertebral artery
Ascending pharyngeal artery	Vertebral artery or internal carotid artery
Middle meningeal artery	Ophthalmic circulation or internal carotid artery
Internal maxillary artery	Internal carotid circulation
Superficial temporal artery	Ophthalmic artery
Ascending cervical artery	Vertebral artery
Dorsocervical artery	Vertebral artery

□ **Precautions**

An understanding of materials, vascular territories, and anastomoses is needed to minimize complications while performing these interventional therapeutic transvascular operations in a neuroradiologic practice.

One must be aware of the multiple anastomoses between the extracerebral and intracerebral vessels (Table 9-1) and of the blood supply to cranial nerves from the external carotid circulation when performing embolization using very small particles or low-viscosity liquid agents (see Chapter 8). The posterior branch of the ascending pharyngeal artery supplies cranial nerves IX, X, XI, and XII.[33] The proximal intracranial middle meningeal artery may contribute a significant blood supply to the seventh cranial nerve by way of its petrosal branch, which arises just after the middle meningeal artery enters the cranial cavity through the foramen spinosum. The use of microparticles should be avoided unless the catheter can be placed beyond these branches or the vessels are too small to be visualized. The functional importance or dominance of one vessel in its balance with others (see Chapter 8), primarily in cutaneous territories or in the supply of the transcranial nerves, must be understood to choose the safest route to reach the lesion by redistributing the flow of blood using balloon catheters or biodegradeable agents to protect normal or vital territories.

□ **Conclusions**

We have illustrated the technical possibilities in transvascular techniques and have discussed complications and their avoidance. It has become apparent that embolization may be performed with a high degree of effectiveness and safety if the lesion is reached and the normal territory is preserved. Perivascular necrosis and hemostasis prior to surgical removal can be obtained if good penetration into the lesion with microemboli is accomplished. Embolization therefore can make resection safer and more complete.

Thorough understanding of the technical possibilities and limitations will permit the physician to select the most appropriate agent in a specific instance. Knowledge of the vascular anatomy and its anastomoses will permit more distal and hence safer embolization, with preservation of vital structures. Finally, significant experience in the laboratory should precede clinical use of this procedure.[27]

□ **References**

1. Bentson, J.R., and Crandall, P.H.: Use of the Fogarty catheter in arteriovenous malformations of the spinal cord, Radiology **105**:65, 1972.
2. Berenstein, A.: Flow control silicone fluid embolization, AJNR **1**:161, 1980.
3. Berenstein, A., and Kricheff, I.I.: A new balloon catheter for coaxial embolization, Neuroradiology **18**:239, 1979.
4. Berenstein, A., and Kricheff, I.I.: Catheter and material selection for transarterial embolization: technical considerations. I. Catheters, Radiology **132**:619, 1979.
5. Berenstein, A., and Kricheff, I.I.: Catheter and material selection for transarterial embolization: technical considerations. II. Materials, Radiology **132**:631, 1979.
6. Berenstein, A., and Kricheff, I.I.: Microembolization techniques of vascular occlusion: radiologic, pathologic, and clinical correlation, AJNR **2**:261-267, 1981.
7. Berenstein A., and Lasjaunias, P.: Functional anatomy of the facial artery in the planning and execution of therapeutic transarterial embolizations, Presented at American Society of Neuroradiology, Los Angeles, 1980.
8. Berenstein, A., and Russel, E.: Gelatin sponge in therapeutic neuroradiology: a subject review, Radiology **141**:105-112, 1981.
9. Boulos, R., Kricheff, I.I., and Chase, N.E.: Value of cerebral angiography in the embolization treatment of cerebral arteriovenous malformations, Radiology **97**:65, 1970.
10. Brooks, B.: Discussion, Noland, L., and Taylor, A.S.: Pulsating exophthalmos the result of injury, Trans. South Surg. Assoc. **43**:171-77, 1931.
11. Cunningham, D.S., and Paletta, F.X.: Control of arteriovenous fistula in massive facial hemangioma by muscle emboli: case report, Plast. Reconstr. Surg. **46**:305, 1970.
12. Debrun, G., Lacour, P., Caron, J.P., et al.: Experimental approach to the treatment of carotid fistulas with an inflatable and isolated balloon, Neuroradiology **9**:9, 1975.
13. Debrun, G., Lacour, P., Caron, J.P., et al.: Inflatable and released balloon technique experimentation in dog—application in man, Neuroradiology **9**:267, 1975.
14. Debrun, G., Legre, J., Kasbarian, M., et al.: Endovascular occlusion of vertebral fistulae by detachable balloons with conservation of the vertebral blood flow, Radiology **130**:141-147, 1979.
14a. Debrun, G.M., Vinuela, F.V., Fox, A.J., and Kan, S.: Two different calibrated-leak balloons: experimental work and applications in humans, AJNR **3**:407-414, 1982.
15. DiTullo, M.V., Jr., Rand, R.W., and Frisch, E.: Detachable balloon catheter: its application in experimental arteriovenous fistual, J. Neurosurg. **48**:717, 1978.
16. Djindjian, R., Comoy, H., Hurth, N., and Houdart, R.: Embolisation par voie fémorale d'un angiome cérébral irrigue par la carotide externe, Rev. Neurol. **125**:119, 1971.
17. Djindjian, R., Cophignon, J., Theron, J., et al.: Embolization by superselective arteriography from the femoral route in neuroradiology: review of 60 cases. 1. Technique, indications, complications, Neuroradiology **6**:20, 1973.

18. Djindjian, R., and Merland J-J.: Super-selective arteriography of the external carotid artery, Berlin, 1978, Springer-Verlag.
19. Doppman, J.L., Marx, S.J., Spiegel, A.M., et al.: Treatment of hyperparathyroidism by percutaneous embolization of a mediastinal adenoma, Radiology **115:**37, 1975.
20. Doppman, J.L., Zapol, W., and Pierce, J.: Transcatheter embolization with a silicone rubber preparation: experimental observations, Invest. Radiol. **6:**304, 1971.
21. Grace, D.M., Pitt, D.F., and Gold, R.E.: Vascular embolization and occlusion by angiographic techniques as an aid or alternative to operation, Surg. Gynecol. Obstet. **143:**469, 1976.
22. Hekster, R.E.M., Luyendijk, W., and Matricalli, B.: Transfemoral catheter embolization: a method of treatment of glomus jugulare tumors, Neuroradiology **5:**208, 1972.
23. Hilal, S.K., and Michelson, W.J.: Therapeutic percutaneous embolization for extra-axial vascular lesions of the head, neck, and spine, J. Neurosurg. **43:**275, 1975.
24. Hogeman, K.E., Gustafson, G., and Bjorlin, G.: Ivalon surgical sponge used as a temporary cover of experimental skin defects in rats: a preliminary report, Acta. Chir. Scand. **121:**83, 1961.
25. Kerber, C.: Balloon catheter with a calibrated leak: a new system for superselective angiography and occlusive catheter therapy, Radiology **120:**547, 1976.
26. Kerber, C.W.: Flow controlled therapeutic embolization: a physiologic and safe technique, AJNR **1:**77-81, 1980.
27. Kerber, C.W., and Flaherty, L.W.: A teaching and research simulator for therapeutic embolization, AJNR **1:**167-169, 1980.
28. Kricheff, I.I., and Berenstein, A.: Simplified solid particle embolization with a new introducer, Radiology **131:**794, 1979.
29. Kricheff, I.I., Madayag, M., and Braunstein, P.: Transfemoral catheter embolization of cerebral and posterior fossa arteriovenous malformations, Radiology **103:**107, 1972.
30. Kunstlinger, F., Brunelle, F., Chaumont, P., and Doyon, D.: Vascular occlusive agents, AJR **136:**151-156, 1981.
31. Laitinen, L., and Servo, A.: Embolization of cerebral vessels with inflatable and detachable balloons, J. Neurosurg. **48:**307, 1978.
31a. Lasjaunias, P.: Craniofacial and upper cervical arteries: functional, chemical, and angiographic aspects, Baltimore, 1981, The Williams & Wilkins Co.
32. Lasjaunias, P., Berenstein, A., and Doyon, D.: Normal functional anatomy of the facial artery, Radiology **133:**631, 1979.
33. Lasjaunias, P., Menu, Y., Bonnel, D., and Doyon, D.: Non-chromaffin paragangliomas of the head and neck, J. Neuroradiol. **8:**281-299, 1981.
34. Light, R.U., and Prentice, H.R.: Surgical investigation of a new absorbable sponge derived from gelatin for use in hemostasis, J. Neurosurg. **2:**435, 1945.
35. Luessenhop, A.J., and Spence, W.T.: Artificial embolization of cerebral arteries: report of use in a case of arteriovenous malformation, JAMA **172:**1153, 1960.
36. Page, R.C., Larson, E.J., and Siegmund, E.: Chronic toxicity studies of metyl-2-cyanoacrylate in dogs and rats. In Healey, J.E., Jr., editor: Proceedings of the Symposium on Physiological Adhesives, University of Texas, Houston, Texas, February 3-4, 1966 (available from Ethicon Corp, Somerville, N.J. 98876).
37. Pevsner, P.H.: Micro-balloon catheter for superselective angiography and therapeutic occlusion, AJR **128:**225, 1977.
38. Pevsner, P.H., and Doppman, J.L.: Therapeutic embolization with a microballoon catheter system, AJNR **1:**171-180, 1980.
39. Portsmann, W., Wierny, L., Warnke, H., et al.: Catheter closure of patent ductus arteriosus: 62 cases treated without thoracotomy, Radiol. Clin. North Am. **9:**203, 1971.
40. Sano, K., Jimbo, M., and Saito, I.: Artificial embolization of inoperable angiomas with polymerizing substance. In Pia, H.W., Gleave, J.R.W., Grote, E., et al., editors: Cerebral angiomas: advances in diagnosis and therapy, New York, 1975, Springer-Verlag, New York, Inc.
41. Serbinenko, F.A.: Balloon catheterization and occlusion of major cerebral vessels, J. Neurosurg. **41:**125, 1974.
42. Tadavarthy, S.M., Moller, J.H., and Amplatz, K.: Polyvinyl alcohol (Ivalon)—a new embolization material, AJR **125:**609, 1975.
43. Tazi, Z., Lasjaunias, P., and Doyon, D.: Malformations vasculaires invasines de la face et du scalp, Rev. Stomatol. Chir. Maxillofac. **83:**24-35, 1982.
44. White, R.I., Ursic, T.A., Kaufman, S.L., et al.: Therapeutic embolization with detachable balloons: physical factors influencing permanent occlusion, Radiology **126:**521, 1978.
45. Wholey, M.H.: The technology of balloon catheters in interventional angiography, Radiology **125:**671, 1977.
46. Wholey, M.H., Kessler, L., and Boehnke, M.: A percutaneous balloon catheter technique for the treatment of intracranial aneurysms, Acta Radiol. (Diagn.) **13:**286, 1972.
47. Zanetti, P.H., and Sherman, F.E.: Experimental evaluation of a tissue adhesive as an agent for the treatment of aneurysms and arteriovenous anomalies, J. Neurosurg. **36:**72, 1972.

10 □ The upper aerodigestive tract (nasopharynx, oropharynx, and floor of the mouth)

ANTHONY A. MANCUSO and PETER M. SOM

Radiologic evaluation of the upper aerodigestive tract, namely the nasopharynx and oropharynx, has always been a challenge to the diagnostic radiologist. The air, bone, and soft tissue interfaces in this region have always provided a good, natural radiographic contrast; however, subtle diagnoses have been fraught with difficulties because of variations in airway contour and superimposition of the many areas of interest. Contrast nasopharyngography was introduced as a method to more critically evaluate this region. Thus far, however, the method is plagued by technical difficulties and still limits diagnosis to the air-mucosal interfaces, often failing to show the extent of deep spread of pathologic processes.

CT of the nasopharynx, on the other hand, shows not only the air-mucosal interface but also the deep tissue planes that lie beneath the mucosa. With current flexible fiberoptic and rigid nasopharyngoscopes, the head and neck surgeon can visualize the mucosa of the nasopharynx even in marginally cooperative patients. Still, because of the monocular nature of this examination, subtle asymmetries of contour escape detection because the examining physician lacks depth perception. In the absence of mucosal abnormality the head and neck surgeon might miss a lesion that is predominantly submucosal. CT, with its view of the deep tissue planes, provides the perfect complement to the clinical examination because such deep extension is the hallmark of malignancy.

The oropharynx and floor of the mouth have for the most part received little attention from diagnostic ra-diologists. Occasionally, contrast sialography, soft tissue views, and panoramic views provided useful information concerning the variety of lesions that can affect this area. Also, the region is fairly easy to evaluate clinically by inspection and palpation. CT, however, can accurately outline in their entirety a variety of processes that can occur in this region, many of which are malignant tumors.

The parapharyngeal space bridges the nasopharynx and oropharynx. It is discussed in detail in Chapter 5 and will be touched on in this chapter. Prior to the coming of CT it was difficult to get direct evidence of pathology that arose in or extended to this important region. A variety of diagnostic studies have been used to define such pathology in the past, including pluridirectional tomography, plain films, sialography, and angiography; however, for the most part CT can provide a definitive evaluation of this area by itself.

In summary, CT has greatly altered the diagnostic approach to the entire upper aerodigestive tract. It has proven itself capable of showing pathology that is undetectable by physical examination and sometimes even by biopsy. Eventually the information available from CT will alter concepts of the natural history of head and neck pathology in this region and will greatly influence the therapeutic approach to these problems. In the following chapter we hope to emphasize the role that CT now plays in the diagnosis and management of upper aerodigestive tract abnormalities and provide some insight into what may become routine uses of CT in the near future.

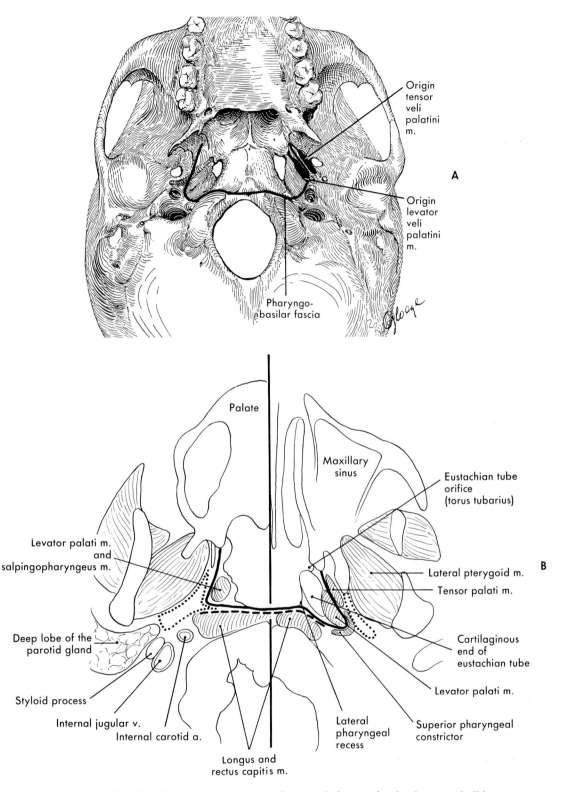

Origin
tensor
veli
palatini
m.

Origin
levator
veli
palatini
m.

A

Pharyngo-
basilar fascia

Palate

Maxillary
sinus

Eustachian tube
orifice
(torus tubarius)

Levator palati m.
and
salpingopharyngeus m.

Lateral pterygoid m.

Tensor palati m.

B

Cartilaginous
end of
eustachian tube

Deep lobe of the
parotid gland

Levator palati m.

Styloid process

Superior pharyngeal
constrictor

Internal jugular v.

Internal carotid a.

Lateral
pharyngeal
recess

Longus and
rectus capitis m.

Fig. 10-1. A, Black line shows approximate attachment of pharyngobasilar fascia to skull base. Note its relationship to origin of tensor and levator muscles of palate. **B,** Details of relationship of various muscles and tissue planes within nasopharynx. Note that left-hand side of diagram is at plane through lower nasopharynx, whereas right-hand side is through midnasopharynx. Solid black line represents course of pharyngobasilar fascia. Dotted black line shows limits of parapharyngeal space as outlined by buccopharyngeal fascia. Dashed line indicates prevertebral fascia. (From Mancuso, A.A., and Hanafee, W.N.: Computed tomography of the head and neck, Baltimore, 1982, Williams & Wilkins.)

□ Normal anatomy

■ The nasopharynx, paranasopharyngeal space, and infratemporal fossa

The nasopharynx is a relatively rigid tubular structure that forms the most superior portion of the airway. Because of its function in respiration, the anatomy is arranged so that airway patency is maintained. The pharyngobasilar fascia is a tough, fibrous membrane that supports the airway[13] (Fig. 10-1). The inner (airway) side of the pharyngobasilar fascia is lined by muscle, mucosa, and lymphoid tissue. The muscles of the infratemporal fossa, the bony structures of the base of the skull, and the fibrofatty spaces that surround the muscles lie on its deep (lateral) surface.

The nasopharynx is bounded posteriorly and superiorly by the upper clivus and sphenoid sinus. Laterally and anteriorly it is limited by the pterygoid plates. Laterally and posteriorly there are no bony limits, so the airway can remain somewhat flexible for its function during swallowing, speech, and breathing.[13] Directly posteriorly the lower clivus, upper cervical spine, and prevertebral musculature form the boundaries of the nasopharynx.

■ Superficial anatomic landmarks

The characteristic shape of the nasopharynx is nearly unmistakable on CT and closely parallels the view of the examining physician. The most prominent landmark in the upper airway is the torus tubarius, which represents a mucosal fold over the cartilaginous end of the eustachian tube (Figs. 10-1 to 10-3). Despite its cartilaginous nature, it is rarely of a density greater than the surrounding soft tissues. The paired tori are almost universally visible on CT scans of the nasopharynx although they may vary slightly in size from patient to patient.[16,17] In individual patients they are usually symmetric in appearance but may appear slightly asymmetric as a normal variant.[16,17]

The eustachian tube orifices as visualized on CT lie just anterior to the torus tubarius. At physical examination they actually lie on the anterior inferior surface of the tori. They are always seen and usually appear symmetric. In scans made during quiet respiration it is unusual to see air extending into the orifices beyond approximately 3 to 4 mm.[16,17] When the airway is distended by a variety of maneuvers, air may be forced deeper into the eustachian tubes.

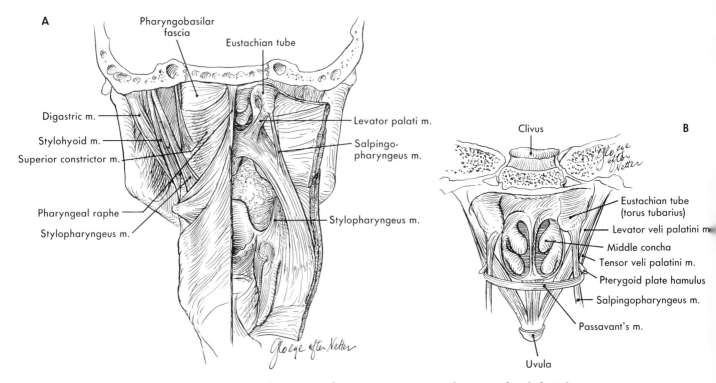

Fig. 10-2. Posterior views of upper aerodigestive tract. **A,** Nasopharynx is detailed. Relationship of various musculature to eustachian tube and to one another should be noted so that its anatomy on CT scans is better understood. **B,** Entire upper aerodigestive tract is outlined. Diagram emphasizes interrelationship of muscles surrounding this region. Note that muscles create virtual continuum between nasopharynx cephalad to skull base and caudal to tongue base and on to hypopharynx. (From Mancuso, A.A., and Hanafee, W.N.: Computed tomography of the head and neck, copyright © 1982, Williams & Wilkins Co., Baltimore.)

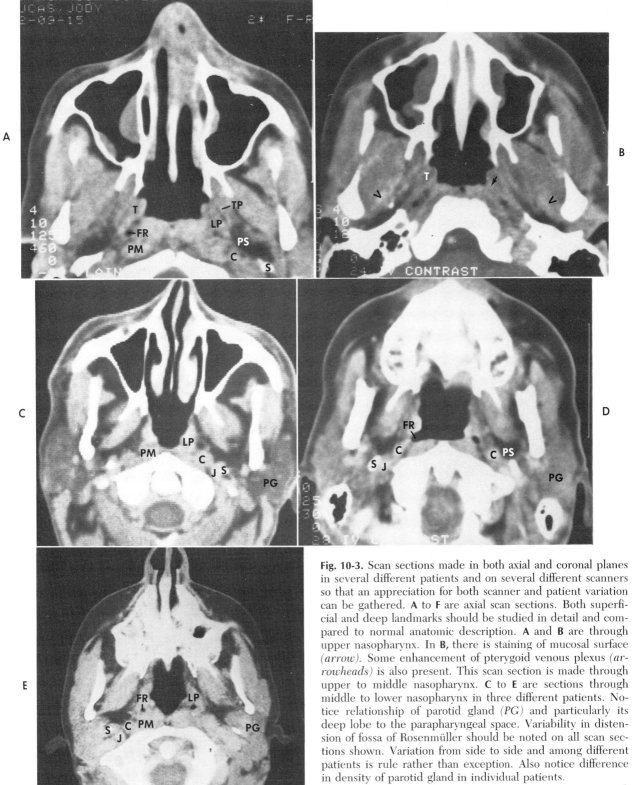

Fig. 10-3. Scan sections made in both axial and coronal planes in several different patients and on several different scanners so that an appreciation for both scanner and patient variation can be gathered. **A** to **F** are axial scan sections. Both superficial and deep landmarks should be studied in detail and compared to normal anatomic description. **A** and **B** are through upper nasopharynx. In **B**, there is staining of mucosal surface *(arrow)*. Some enhancement of pterygoid venous plexus *(arrowheads)* is also present. This scan section is made through upper to middle nasopharynx. **C** to **E** are sections through middle to lower nasopharynx in three different patients. Notice relationship of parotid gland *(PG)* and particularly its deep lobe to the parapharyngeal space. Variability in distension of fossa of Rosenmüller should be noted on all scan sections shown. Variation from side to side and among different patients is rule rather than exception. Also notice difference in density of parotid gland in individual patients.

Continued.

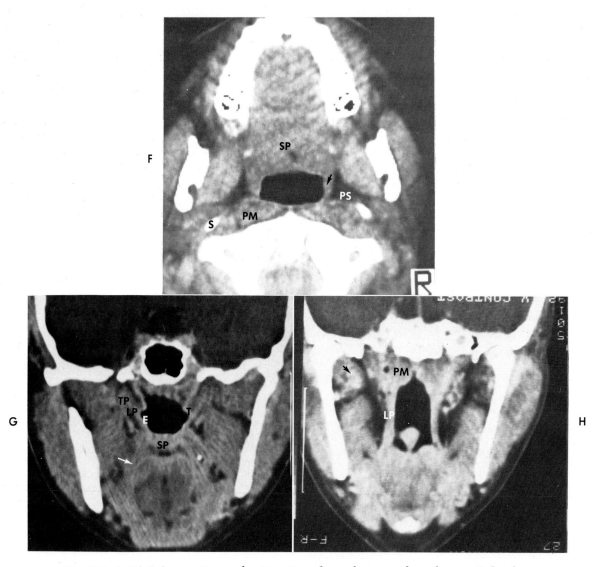

Fig. 10-3, cont'd. F, Scan section made at junction of nasopharynx and oropharynx. Soft palate *(SP)* fills most of airway anteriorly. This is level of Passavant's muscle *(arrow)*. Both **G** and **H** are coronal sections made anteriorly and posteriorly, respectively, through upper aerodigestive tract. Note that deep tissue planes surrounding nasopharynx form virtual continuum with planes surrounding tonsillar fossa. These two illustrations also show relationship of these deep tissue planes to skull base and cavernous sinus above. Entire cephalocaudal extent of levator palati muscle is shown. Notice enhancement of pterygoid plexus *(arrow)* and vessels within parapharyngeal space *(arrowhead). T,* Torus tubarius; *TP,* tensor veli palati; *LT,* levator veli palati; *FR,* fossa of Rosenmüller; *E,* eustachian tube orifice; *PS,* parapharyngeal space; *PM,* prevertebral musculature; *C,* carotid; *J,* jugular; *S,* styloid process.

Behind the torus tubarius lies the lateral pharyngeal recess (fossa of Rosenmüller). Again, these are paired, air-filled spaces (Fig. 10-3). The lateral pharyngeal recesses exist because the salpingopharyngeus muscle extends inferiorly from the cartilaginous end of the eustachian tube and inserts along the lateral wall of the nasopharynx, forming the salpingopharyngeal fold (Fig. 10-2). As the mucosa of the nasopharynx reflects over both the cartilaginous end of the tube and this muscle, a recess or gutter is created posterolaterally. The recesses tend to be slightly asymmetric in any given individual and the degree of visualization varies greatly between different people.* Generally, they tend to appear smaller in younger people because the greater content of lymphoid tissue within the nasopharynx fills the recesses. As the individual ages the lymphoid tissue involutes and the recesses tend to become air-filled and more prominent.[11,16,17]

■ Anatomy of the deep tissue planes

A large soft tissue space lies under the mucosa and submucosa of the nasopharynx. The tissue planes within this space are uniformly symmetric in the vast majority of patients.[16,18] An understanding of these deep tissue planes is essential to accurate detection and differential diagnosis of the pathologic processes that affect them.

The pharyngobasilar fascia is of particular importance because of its ability to alter the appearance of the pathology that can affect the nasopharynx and deep tissue planes.[4,14,33] Other fascial planes of interest include the prevertebral fascia, carotid sheath, and buccopharyngeal fascia (Fig. 10-1). It is very important to realize that none of the fasciae are seen as distinct entities on CT scans; however, they all have an effect on the arrangement of the tissue planes as seen on scans.

The prevertebral fascia is a fairly thick membrane that covers the prevertebral musculature, including the longus and rectus colli and the longus capitis muscles.[13,33] It extends from the base of the skull to approximately the T3 vertebral body. A loose collection of areolar tissue lies between the prevertebral fascia and the pharyngeal constrictor muscles. This allows free movement of the vascular and pharyngeal structures during swallowing and neck movements.[13]

The carotid sheath(s) lies immediately lateral and slightly posterior to the prevertebral musculature. Again, the carotid sheath is not visualized on CT scans and really only represents a condensation of a fibrous tissue around the vascular, neural, and lymphatic tissues that lie within the sheath. The carotid sheath provides an insignificant boundary to the spread of inflammatory or neoplastic processes.

The pharyngobasilar fascia creates a boundary of great significance on CT scans.[2,4,13] Intrapharyngeal structures lie to its airway side and the parapharyngeal space and infratemporal fossa lie to its deep side (Fig. 10-1). The intrapharyngeal structures visible include the levator palati and salpingopharyngeus muscles and the mucosa and lymphoid tissue of the airway surface. On the deep side lies the tensor palati and superior pharyngeal constrictor muscles (Fig. 10-3). The superior pharyngeal constrictor is rarely seen as a distinct structure on nasopharyngeal scans, even when the scans are of high quality. The densities created by the small muscles of deglutition (the tensor and levator palati muscles) are becoming much more important on high-resolution scans for picking up early deeply infiltrating lesions. These muscles will sometimes appear slightly asymmetric on scans, especially if the head is rotated or tilted.[16,17] The compartment medial to the pharyngobasilar fascia and surrounding the levator palati is a well-described pathway for the extension of tumors from the palate to the skull base.[15]

The paranasopharyngeal space is of even more diagnostic importance. Because this is bound on the airway side by the pharyngobasilar fascia, only aggressive inflammatory or infiltrating malignant processes will extend through the pharyngobasilar fascia to involve the deeper spaces. The paranasopharyngeal spaces are always symmetric in appearance on normal scans, even if the head is slightly rotated or tilted[16,17] (Fig. 10-3). Asymmetry of these fatty spaces must be taken as evidence of pathologic change, the differential diagnosis of which will be discussed subsequently. Inferiorly, the pharyngobasilar fascia thins out somewhat so that it is less of a barrier to the spread of disease.

At the level of the hard palate, a fairly thick zone of soft tissue density can be seen immediately beneath the mucosa. This is the region of Passavant's muscle ridge (Figs. 10-2 and 10-3). This muscle contracts in a sphincteric manner to separate the oropharynx and nasopharynx during swallowing.[13] Passavant's muscle marks the anatomic limit of the nasopharynx inferiorly. This band of tissue varies greatly in thickness from patient to patient. Part of the density is related to the lymphatic tissue that lines the mucosa and part of it to the density of the deeper muscles, including the tensor and levator palati and palatoglossus muscles, which interdigitate to form Passavant's muscle (Fig. 10-2).

The lateral boundary of the parapharyngeal space is formed by a very loose connective tissue layer called the buccopharyngeal fascia.[13] This is not seen on CT scans and represents no significant boundary to the spread of pathologic processes within the deep tissue planes. The medial portion of the buccopharyngeal fascia is the epimysium of the superior pharyngeal con-

*References 11, 16, 17, 24.

strictor.[13] Laterally it is formed by the reflection of the deep cervical fascia, which covers both the pterygoid musculature and the deep surfaces of the parotid glands. This layer of connective tissue must be relatively loose because its function is to allow free movement of the pharynx and jaw musculature during swallowing and chewing.[13]

Outside the parapharyngeal space lies the infratemporal fossa. This is an expansive, primarily soft tissue space that contains portions of the mandible, the lateral pterygoid plate, the pterygoid, the masseter, and portions of the temporalis muscles, and the deep lobe of the parotid gland. The tissue planes of the infratemporal fossa are always symmetric, unless there is atrophy of the muscles of mastication.

The other spaces defined by these four fasciae are important mainly because their contents are responsible for abnormalities that may affect any or all structures in the region. The retropharyngeal space lies between the pharyngobasilar and prevertebral fasciae. The high lateral and retropharyngeal lymph nodes lie to either side of this space and just medial to the structures of the carotid sheath.[15,27] This is an exceedingly important nodal group, as it provides first order drainage to the nasopharynx. Normally two to three nodes are present bilaterally in the space between the carotid and prevertebral muscles.[27] These either are not normally seen on CT scans or are seen as nonenhancing densities less than 5 mm in size.

The prevertebral muscles (longus colli and longus capitis) create most of the tissue density seen anterior to the upper cervical spine. Characteristically there are two paramedian elliptical densities separated by a midline gutter (Figs. 10-1 and 10-3). Scanning angle between ±20° (and probably greater) from the Reid baseline do not significantly alter the apparent thickness of this area[16,18,24]; however, the density of normal lymphoid tissue can blend with that of the muscle to produce the spurious notion of pathologic thickening.

The carotid sheath lies posterior and slightly lateral to the retropharyngeal space. It contains the carotid artery (more medially), the jugular vein (more posterolaterally), cranial nerves IX to XII, a sympathetic plexus, and the lymphatics. The carotid artery is usually the first structure visible as one scans caudally from the skull base (Figs. 10-1 and 10-3). It appears as a rounded density just under the lateral pharyngeal recess and about halfway between the artery and the styloid process. The jugular vein usually lies just posterior to the styloid process and is slightly larger than the carotid artery (especially on the right side). Smaller punctate densities surround the carotid artery and jugular vein and represent normal nodes, nerves, and blood vessels.

Following intravenous contrast injection the carotid artery and jugular vein can be more easily distinguished from the nonvascular structures. In addition, branches of the ascending pharyngeal artery become visible in the parapharyngeal space. The internal maxillary artery can also be seen as it winds its way through the infratemporal fossa to the retroantral fat pad and into the pterygomaxillary fossa. The pterygoid plexus of veins will also enhance and become visible as it insinuates within the pterygoid musculature. Early in the course of an intravenous bolus or rapid drip infusion a rim of nasopharyngeal mucosal enhancement may also appear. This is usually less than 2 mm thick and can be used to distinguish adenoids from more ominous mass lesions by showing that the "mass" is restricted to the mucosal surface, a very unlikely circumstance for nasopharyngeal malignancies.

□ Normal variants

The amount of adenoid (lymphoid) tissue within the nasopharynx varies greatly among individual patients. Younger patients tend to have larger amounts that often fill the lateral pharyngeal recesses and not infrequently almost the entire airway.[11,16,17] Axial scans near the roof of the nasopharynx may show a large mass that nearly fills the airway but coronal scans will show that this adenoid tissue occupies only the upper one quarter to one third of the nasopharynx (Fig. 10-4).

Hypertrophied or inflamed adenoids can produce ominous nasopharyngeal masses on both physical examinations and CT images. Adenoid masses do not alter the deep tissue plane symmetry and thus can be differentiated from malignancies and aggressive inflammatory lesions that will cross the pharyngobasilar fascia. When large amounts of lymphoid tissue are present, the levator palati muscle may not be visible on low resolution scans, but the paranasopharyngeal space should always be visible and symmetric (Fig. 10-4). Occasionally a pinched-nose modified Valsalva or open-mouth view might be necessary to distinguish adenoids from significant lesions (see section on technique of examination). This has not proven necessary with newer, high-resolution techniques.

□ Atrophy

Measuring the nasopharyngeal airway as an aid to diagnosis received some attention in the era that preceded the development of CT. This is largely a wasted exercise on both plain films and CT scans.* CT has brought us a more reliable indicator of significant pathologic deep tissue plane invasion.[16,17]

Atrophy may occur because of specific pathologic insult (e.g., fifth nerve palsy, mandibular dysfunction) or

---

*References 11, 16, 17, 27.

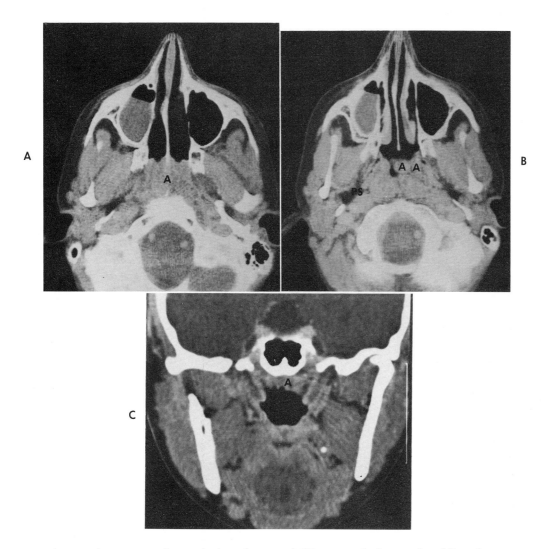

Fig. 10-4. Appearance of normal adenoids on axial CT scans in high (**A**) and middle to low (**B**) nasopharynx. High in nasopharyngeal vault, adenoidal tissue (**A**), appears to fill nasopharyngeal airway, but **C** (coronal CT scan) shows that this is only because adenoids line roof and scan is made nearly parallel to roof of nasopharynx. Most important point to recognize is that adenoid tissue, while appearing irregular and lobulated, does not obscure parapharyngeal space (*PS*). Parapharyngeal musculature as described previously (Fig. 10-3) is clearly visible.

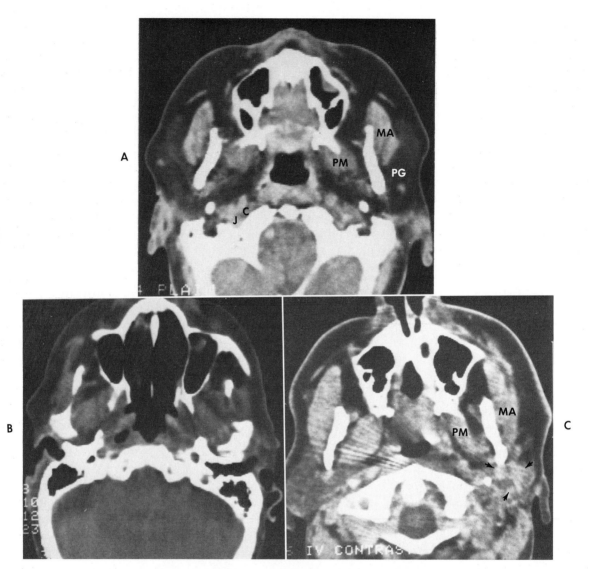

Fig. 10-5. Axial CT scans of patients with atrophy involving nasopharynx or parapharyngeal and mandibular musculature. **A,** Tissue density surrounding airway is less thick than usual and pterygoid muscles *(PM)* and masseter muscles *(M)* are smaller than usual. Fat spaces are correspondingly increased. Structures of carotid sheath are more clearly seen because of increased surrounding fat. Density of parotid glands *(PG)* is also more fatty than seen in prior scans. This diminished muscle mass and increased fat content is usually related to aging. *C,* Carotid; *J,* jugular. **B,** Mandibular and parapharyngeal musculature is atrophic on one side when compared to other. This patient had a dense fifth cranial nerve deficit on side of atrophy. This was elderly patient and involution of lymphoid tissue makes fossa of Rosen-müller and eustachian tube orifices more prominent than usual. **C,** Patient has infiltrating mass of parotid bed *(arrows)*. Adenoid cystic carcinoma causing this mass had extended to base of skull and invaded mandibular division of fifth cranial nerve, resulting in marked atrophy of pterygoid and masseter muscles on side of tumor as compared to normal side.

may be a result of the normal aging process (Fig. 10-5). It is a result of both the involution of the superficial lymphoid tissue and the loss of the deep compartment muscle mass. The result is a marked alteration of both the superficial and the deep landmarks. The lateral pharyngeal recesses appear enlarged and air filled and extend all the way to the skull base. At the extreme they may become so distended that they no longer appear as distinct structures; the airway thus assumes a uniformly distended appearance. The tori may become smaller and the eustachian tube orifices more patulous; this is also in part a result of a loss of bulk of the levator and tensor palati and salpingopharyngeus muscles. Passavant's muscle appears thinner because of a reduction in its muscle bulk and the amounts of adenoid tissue surrounding the airway at that level. A dramatic reduction in the bulk of the muscles of mastication results in a net increase in the fat spaces of the infratemporal fossa, parapharyngeal space, and carotid sheath.

Isolated lymphoid atrophy can be seen as a normal variant in the young or in patients with immunodeficiency diseases. Pathogenic muscular atrophy can have a variety of causes, some of which include mandibular dysfunction, mandibular surgery, radiation therapy, and cranial nerve deficits.

□ Oropharynx and floor of the mouth

The oropharynx is the portion of the upper aerodigestive tract visible when one looks into the mouth. The oral cavity lies anterior to it and the naso- and hypopharynx superiorly and inferiorly, respectively. Specifically, the oropharynx is bound anteriorly by the tongue and laterally by the faucial pillars. It is separated from the larynx by the epiglottis, from the hypopharynx by the pharyngoepiglottic folds, and from the nasopharynx by the soft palate.[13]

The exact superior limit of the oropharynx is Passavant's muscle.[13] On CT scans the muscle and lymphoid tissue that contribute to this density and ring the airways are inseparable (Fig. 10-3). Proceeding inferiorly, this ring of density is continued laterally by the faucial pillars and palatine tonsils and posteriorly by the middle pharyngeal constrictor. In this case the density of the palatoglossus muscle (anterior tonsillar pillar), the palatopharyngeus muscle (posterior tonsillar pillar), and the palatine tonsil (between the pillars) are indistinguishable laterally (Fig. 10-6). The middle pharyngeal constrictor is quite thin posteriorly. The bands of tissue density representing a tonsillar pillar and oropharyngeal lymphoid tissue become continuous with the tissue density that borders the airway in the glossopharyngeal sulci and the base of the tongue inferiorly.

The fibrofatty parapharyngeal space also surrounds the airway at this level. Although the superficial contours of the airway might normally appear asymmetric or irregular, the normal parapharyngeal space should not. The carotid sheaths are distinctly visible at this level, slightly posterior and lateral to the airway (Fig. 10-6).

The base of the tongue and floor of the mouth are anatomically distinct regions but will be considered together in this discussion because of the complex interrelationships of the anatomy of this region and its applications to clinical practice.

Superficially, the base (posterior one third) of the tongue extends from its junction with the anterior two thirds of the tongue at the circumvalate papillae to the valleculae. A midline flange of tissue, the median glossoepiglottic fold, separates the paired valleculae (Fig. 10-6). Two lateral pharyngoepiglottic folds separate the tongue anteriorly from the hypopharynx (pyriform sinuses) posteriorly. Two gutters, the glossopharyngeal sulci, lie between the tongue base and the lateral walls of the oropharynx.

The free margin of the anterior two thirds of the tongue has less internal architecture as seen on CT scans and is formed mainly by the intrinsic muscles. The intrinsic and extrinsic musculature of the remainder of the tongue, however, create well-defined deep tissue planes that are always visible on current scanners. The geniohyoid and genioglossus muscles form the main bulk of the extrinsic tongue musculature. They are paired and separated by the relatively low-density lingual septum. The hyoglossus and styloglossus muscles are the other extrinsic muscles of the tongue and are less easily visualized on CT scans (Fig. 10-6). These muscles interdigitate and form paired arches that extend posterolaterally from the genioglossus muscle to surround a relatively low-density intrinsic muscle group. These muscular arches are important landmarks because the lingual artery passes to their medial surface while the lingual vein, hypoglossal nerve, lingual nerve, and submandibular ducts lie lateral to them.[13] The lingual artery and vein are only visible following bolus or rapid-drip infusion of intravenous contrast.

The floor of the mouth is formed by the mylohyoid muscles. These sheetlike muscles are composed of two halves that arise from the mylohyoid ridge and from their respective mandibular rami and run an oblique inferomedial course to insert at the hyoid. The mouth lies above the mylohyoid muscle, the neck below it. The submandibular gland curves around the posterior free edge of the mylohyoid muscle and thus a small portion of the gland lies in the floor of the mouth, between the tongue and mandible, and a larger portion lies in the upper neck. The submandibular duct runs anteriorly to the floor of the mouth external to the hyoglossus muscle (Fig. 10-6).

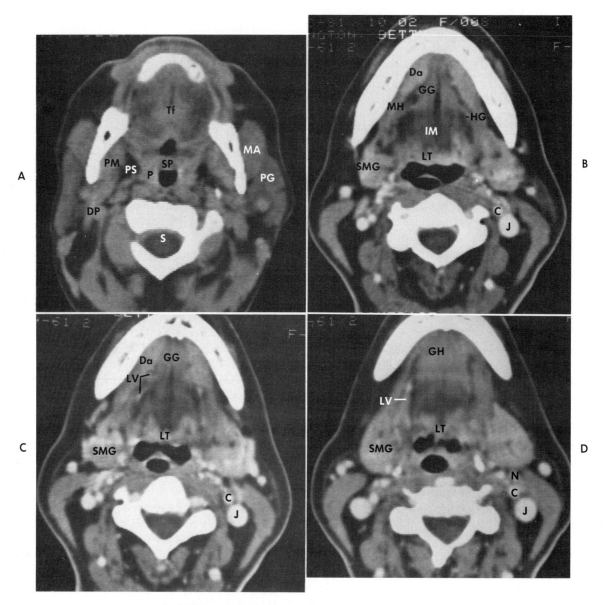

Fig. 10-6. Sections done in axial plane from midoropharynx to base of tongue and upper supraglottic larynx. In **A,** structure of tongue is not as well demarcated as on following sections through floor of mouth and tongue base. Notice that intrinsic tongue musculature *(IM)* is of lower density than surrounding extrinsic musculature. These various muscles are all separated by well-defined and consistently present low-density (fatty) planes. There is remarkable symmetry in these tissue planes in any given patient. Also notice that lingual tonsil *(LT)* may extend for variable distance from where it borders airway into intrinsic muscle mass of tongue. On infused studies, numerous branches of carotid artery and jugular vein are seen. Particular attention should be paid to course of lingual vessels as they run on either side of hyoglossus muscle *(HG)* within tongue base and floor of mouth. *Tf,* Free margin of tongue; *SP,* soft palate; *PM,* pterygoid muscles; *MA,* masseter muscles; *P,* tonsillar pillar; *Dp,* posterior belly of digastric muscle; *S,* styloid process; *PG,* parotid gland; *Da,* anterior belly of digastric muscle; *MH,* mylohyoid muscle; *GG,* genioglossus muscle; *HG,* hyoglossus muscle; *IM,* intrinsic tongue musculature; *LT,* lingual tonsil; *SMG,* submandibular gland; *C,* carotid; *J,* jugular; *LV,* lingual vessels; *GH,* geniohyoid muscle; *N,* lymph node; *H,* hyoid bone; *PES,* pre-epiglottic space; *SCM,* sternocleidomastoid muscle. **G** and **H,** Direct coronal scan sections through floor of mouth and tongue base made more anteriorly in **H** and more posteriorly in **G.** This is especially evident in comparison with axial scan sections in which muscle bundles formed by extrinsic tongue musculature are more well-defined anteriorly, whereas posteriorly scan sections are mainly through intrinsic tongue musculature.

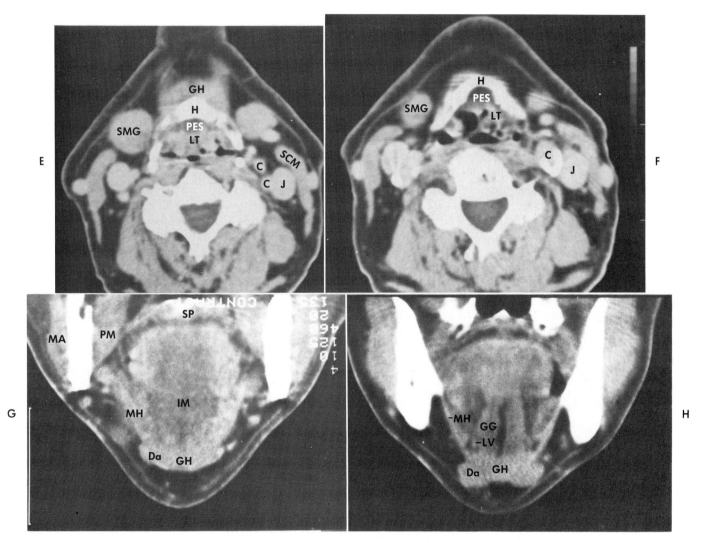

Fig. 10-6, cont'd. For legend see opposite page.

□ Technique of examination

■ Nasopharynx

It is best to study the nasopharynx with approximately 5 mm thick scan sections made at contiguous 5 mm intervals. The nasopharynx is a fairly discrete, small anatomic region and this does not result in an excessive amount of scanning. Overlapping of scan sections is almost never necessary except for adequate visualization of the base of the skull. This approach will ensure reproducibility of comparable scan sections if follow-up scans are necessary and usually ensures that subtle abnormalities are not overlooked. The scans are made with Reid's baseline perpendicular to the table-top. Angles of 20° above or below the Reid baseline do not significantly alter the appearance of the superficial contours of the airway or the deeper muscle and tissue planes. Minor tilting or skewing of the head may make interpretation slightly more tedious but does not usually cause a significantly altered appearance in the symmetry of the deep tissue planes, which is of primary importance for diagnosis.

A complete study of the nasopharynx should include scans done through the base of the skull optimized for bone detail. It is useful to obtain slightly thinner sections and process these through algorithms designed to emphasize bone detail if those capabilities are available and convenient.

Sometimes the axial views will suggest subtle abnormality near the base of the skull or in the roof of the airway. If this is the case, one should not hesitate to do a limited coronal section through the area of interest. Occasionally the superficial contours of the airways will be quite asymmetric in appearance and suggest the presence of a pathologic process. If the deep planes are intact then the process is almost surely a benign one limited to the mucosa; however, if this is still in doubt, physiologic maneuvers can be made to distend the airway and reduce the equivocation that might arise as a result of the superficial contour asymmetries. One may simply have the patient open his mouth widely. Alternatively, the patient may pinch the nares shut with either his hand or a respiratory therapy clip and the region may be rescanned. Both of these maneuvers distend the eustachian tube orifices and the lateral pharyngeal recesses. The pinched-nose modified Valsalva maneuver tends to produce more distention but also more motion artifacts (on slow scanners). This approach may also demonstrate pliability of mucosal masses, which is another indirect sign of benignity. The most practical approach is to assume that if the deep planes are normal and symmetric, any superficial change is restricted to the mucosa and physical examination with biopsy if necessary will establish the cause.

Use of intravenous contrast agents

Contrast agents should not be used routinely in investigating the nasopharynx. Many specific indications do exist, including the following.

1. If the clinical circumstances or axial scans indicate intracranial extension may be present, coronal scans with contrast infusion are necessary. If gross intracranial extension is present, the coronal scans may not be necessary; subtle changes require direct coronal scanning.

2. When a vascular lesion is suspected, such as juvenile angiofibroma or paragangliomas, contrast infusion may help in showing their full extent and in differential diagnosis.

3. Contrast enhancement will at times allow determination of whether sinus opacification represents direct extension of the tumor or is secondary to obstruction of the sinus ostium by the tumor.

4. Intravenous contrast may be required to determine the extent of the lesion in relation to the carotid sheath. This includes diagnosis of lymph node metastases as well as delineation of the primary tumor, be it benign or malignant.

5. Mucosal staining seen during contrast infusion may help distinguish benign mucosal masses (adenoids) from deeply infiltrating masses.

The most easy and efficient way to use contrast enhancement is by means of a rapid drip infusion of a solution containing about 600 mg of iodine per milliliter. We use a needle no smaller than 19 gauge and use a portable intravenous pole to put the bottle as close to the ceiling as possible. Scanning begins after approximately 25 to 50 ml of contrast medium has gone in and is usually completed by the time the entire 150 ml dose has been administered. Occasionally it will be necessary to augment this with either an additional bolus of 25 to 40 ml of the same contrast medium or up to another 150 ml by rapid drip infusion. One must pay particular attention to the timing of the study because results are most satisfactory when there is a maximal intravascular concentration of iodine. This is usually between 5 and 12 minutes after the beginning of the infusion as described. Preliminary digital radiographs of the area of interest will help to select a precise region of interest and the scan section thickness and frequency can be planned accurately so that all of the scan sections are completed before the contrast has equilibrated to the extravascular space.

■ Oropharynx

Scanning of the oropharynx, floor of the mouth, and base of the tongue may be approached in generally the same manner as scanning of the nasopharynx. Preliminary views will allow one to plan to avoid the artifacts caused by dental fillings. Also, accurate planning of the region of interest is facilitated by the views of preliminary digital radiographs done on the CT scanner. Physiologic maneuvers are not necessary in the oropharynx. Suspended respiration will sometimes help to reduce artifacts that result from swallowing and movement of the soft palate and tongue during breathing. The tongue may be held gently between the front teeth to avoid excessive motion.

The indications for intravenous contrast injection of the oropharynx are somewhat more limited than in the nasopharynx. In general they are used to define the extent of carcinomas of this region and to aid in the evaluation of the deep cervical lymph nodes. Occasionally contrast is used to aid in the differential diagnosis, especially of lesions such as carotid body tumors.

Intravenous contrast injection by the method described above also succeeds in outlining the submandibular and parotid salivary glands. It is likely that this method will replace the sialogram for the evaluation of suspected mass lesions of these glands in many cases. Routine sialography will still be necessary for demonstration of ductal pathologic and inflammatory disease and the CT sialogram may be used for demonstration of small masses (less than 1 cm) (see Chapter 4).

□ Pathology
■ Nasopharynx and paranasopharyngeal space: benign tumors and inflammation

Benign processes displace and distort the normal superficial and deep anatomy according to their site of origin, tissue type, and degree of aggressiveness. There is significant crossover in the morphology of benign and malignant lesions as seen on CT images; however, consideration of both the radiographic and clinical pictures usually leads to an accurate differential diagnosis and appropriate disposition.

In the previous anatomic discussion we emphasized the deep fasciae and compartments surrounding the nasopharynx. That normal anatomic discussion will now be used to categorize the benign lesions that affect the nasopharynx. These categories include the following.

1. Superficial lesions
2. Deeply infiltrating lesions
3. Paranasopharyngeal space lesions that distort the paranasopharyngeal space but that are separate from the carotid sheath
4. Carotid sheath lesions
5. Lesions arising outside of the nasopharynx but involving it secondarily

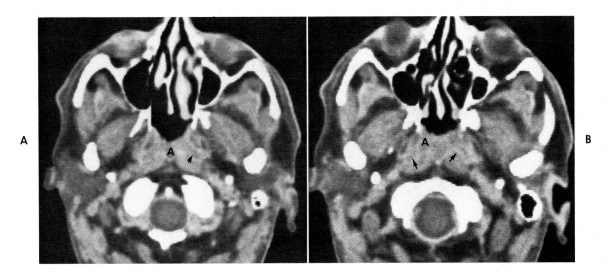

Fig. 10-7. A and **B,** Axial scans through nasopharynx of 25-year-old man who complained of severe headaches. Headaches were retro-orbital and were thought clinically to be compatible with sphenoid sinus headaches. Remainder of CT study showed that sinuses were normal. Within nasopharynx, soft tissue was filling most of airway. Soft tissue represented hyperplastic adenoid tissue *(A)*. There is no CT evidence that this is malignant mass and in fact parapharyngeal musculature is readily visible and parapharyngeal space is intact. Also, normal staining mucosa *(arrows)* can be seen between tissue within airway and deep spaces. Physical examination showed markedly hyperplastic adenoids. There was no evidence of malignancy.

Superficial lesions

Superficial lesions are confined to the mucosa and submucosa and are almost always related to very hyperplastic or inflamed adenoid tissue (Fig. 10-7). They are restricted from extending into the parapharyngeal space by the pharyngobasilar fascia. Physiologic maneuvers will demonstrate that these masses, even when intensely inflamed, are pliable and do not truly obliterate the eustachian tube orifices or the lateral pharyngeal recesses. At clinical examination these masses may look exactly like malignant exophytic tumors; however, if the appropriate CT characteristics are recognized, both the surgeon and patient can be reassured that only an adenoidectomy will be necessary.

Deep infiltrating lesions

Deeply infiltrating lesions are abnormalities in the mucosa and submucosa and are virulent enough to breach the pharyngobasilar fascia and infiltrate the parapharyngeal space. Such aggressive inflammatory and malignant lesions cannot be distinguished by their CT appearance; however, nonmalignant lesions of this nature are very unusual. A clinical history, physical examination, and biopsy are necessary for accurate differentiation. CT is the only study capable of showing the full extent of the disease.

The CT findings include widespread deep infiltration of any of the deep tissue planes. Airway encroachment and obliteration of superficial landmarks are common.

Physiologic maneuvers will show a loss of the normal pliability of the airway contour resulting from induration of the surrounding soft tissues but are rarely necessary with more current high-resolution techniques.

Invasive mucormycosis is the most common inflammatory lesion we have seen produce such findings; this in itself is a sign of how rarely an aggressive inflammatory lesion involves the paranasopharyngeal spaces. Malignant otitis externa extending medially is another "common" cause of this unusual circumstance (Fig. 10-8). Postoperative edema and postbiopsy edema and hemorrhage can produce the same CT findings as inflammatory or malignant lesions; therefore diagnostic CT scans of the nasopharynx should always be done either before or 2 to 3 weeks after surgery or biopsy to avoid equivocal interpretation.

Paranasopharyngeal space lesions

Benign lesions arising in the paranasopharyngeal space are uncommon. The detailed differential diagnosis and CT approach to the differential diagnosis of these lesions are discussed in Chapter 5. At this point it will be sufficient to realize that these lesions do arise primarily within the paranasopharyngeal space and therefore obliterate its fat density on CT scans. Clinically the nasopharyngeal mucosa over these lesions is always normal, except for bulging of the wall. The lesions are most often benign mixed tumors of accessory salivary gland origin, although other uncommon causes,

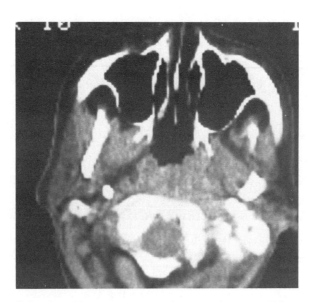

Fig. 10-8. Almost all deeply infiltrating masses within nasopharynx will be malignant tumors. Occasionally, benign aggressive inflammatory lesions present similar picture. Most common occurrence in our experience has been medial extension of malignant otitis media, as in this patient, or invasive mucormycosis.

such as cysts and mesenchymal lesions, are possible. The most important factor in the CT workup is to distinguish them from masses of parotid origin or from malignancies.*

One of the most common benign lesions involving the paranasopharyngeal spaces, infratemporal fossa, and pterygomaxillary fossa is the juvenile angiofibroma. The diagnosis is almost always made clinically by the history of a young or adolescent male with nasal stuffiness or bleeding or both and a physical examination that shows a typical nasopharyngeal mass.

The radiologic approach to juvenile angiofibroma should be tailored to the planned therapeutic approach; however, CT scanning is usually done first to determine the extent of the lesion and to confirm the clinical diagnosis if it is in question. Biopsy of these lesions by the unwary can lead to life-threatening hemorrhage. If the diagnosis is suspect, CT scanning should be done because its findings are absolutely characteristic given the proper clinical setting (Fig. 10-9). If CT scanning shows that the angiofibroma is confined to the pterygomaxillary and infratemporal fossae, then angiography may be delayed and performed as a primarily therapeutic adjunct to surgery. In such cases diagnostic angiography should be immediately followed by therapeutic embolization on the day of surgery; this will significantly reduce intraoperative bleeding.[3,6,32]

_____
*References 4, 14, 28, 29, 30.

Angiofibromas spread by growing through the naturally occurring fissures and ostia of the skull and sinus and once having gained access to a new space they continue to expand. In general they tend to displace and expand bony structures rather than erode them. This may produce the pathognomonic anterior displacement of the posterior antral wall as the lesions expand the pterygomaxillary fossa and grow from there into the infratemporal fossa. Even very extensive lesions do not obliterate the spaces around the carotid sheath.

The tumors extend into the orbit by way of the inferior and then the superior orbital fissures. From there they may continue on intracranially. They may also reach the anterior and medial portions of the middle cranial fossa by growing through the foramen lacerum or by way of the sphenoid sinus. CT scans may show a staining intracranial mass along the floor of the middle cranial fossa, even when the tumor remains extradural. Extension into the brain is unusual and is seen in only the most extensive lesions; it is a contraindication to surgical management. Careful CT scans done in the coronal and axial planes with contrast enhancement are very good at showing the full extent of the lesion. Angiography usually adds little diagnostic information in this regard but is obviously necessary to determine the blood supply and as an adjunct to surgery. Even though the tumors are extradural they may derive part of their blood supply from the cavernous branches of the internal carotid.

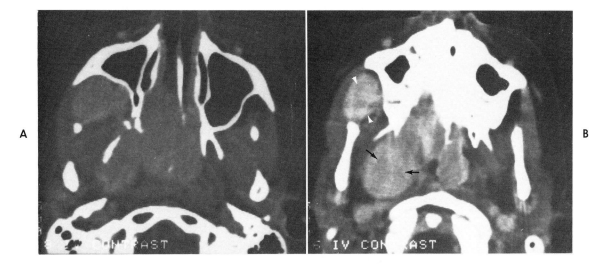

Fig. 10-9. A and **B,** Thirteen-year-old boy who complained of nasal stuffiness and bleeding. Physical examination suggested juvenile angiofibroma. CT examination revealed mass with typical displacement of posterior wall of maxillary antrum anteriorly and extension through pterygomaxillary fossa (not pictured). Erosion of pterygoid plates is seen in **A. B,** Several well-defined components of tumor extending into infratemporal fossa *(arrowheads)* and parapharyngeal space *(arrows)* and portion hanging centrally within airway.

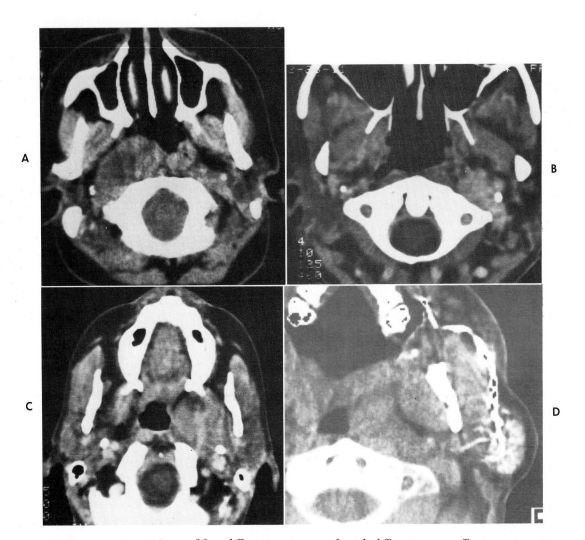

Fig. 10-10. A to **D,** Scans of four different patients, each with different tumor affecting para-pharyngeal space. Detailed approach to this problem is outlined in Chapters 4 and 5. Our approach to study and differential diagnosis is briefly outlined in text. Mass with peripheral enhancement and central low density obliterates plane surrounding carotid sheath and within infratemporal fossa. This is quite typical appearance of neuromas of nerves in carotid sheath. **B,** Slightly lobulated, intensely and homogeneously staining mass surrounds structures of carotid sheath. This is caudal extension of glomus jugulare tumor. **C,** Slightly enhancing mass with some areas of low density occupies parapharyngeal space. Mass is not arising from deep lobe of parotid gland. This was metastasis from patient with known breast carcinoma. At surgery it was very well-circumscribed mass that was easily excised from parapharyngeal space. In patient without known primary site, such an appearance would be most indicative of benign mixed tumor of salivary gland origin. **D,** Tissue planes surrounding carotid sheath are obliterated. This was result of enlarged nodes in patient with known lymphoma.

Contrast-enhanced CT images will show the mass stains intensely. Angiofibromas often extend into the nasal cavity and block the paranasal sinus ostia, raising the issue of whether a sinus is opacified because of obstruction or direct extension of the tumor. Postcontrast scans will show minimal or no enhancement of obstructed, fluid-filled sinuses.

Carotid sheath lesions

Carotid sheath lesions are unusual but not rare lesions that usually appear clinically as submucosal bulges in the nasopharynx and oropharynx or that are made evident by displacement of the parotid gland. They obliterate the carotid sheath and the parapharyngeal space. Their contrast-enhancing characteristics depend

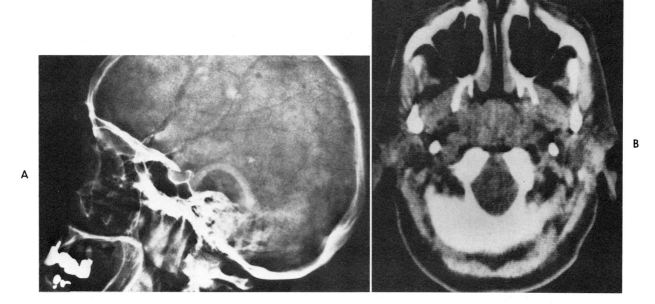

Fig. 10-11. A, Lateral view of skull showing large soft tissue mass within nasopharynx. **B,** CT scan shows very well-circumscribed mass without evidence of deep tissue plane invasion. *Thornwaldt's cyst.*

on the tissue of origin. Neuromas, neurofibromas, and paragangliomas are the most common lesions.* Neuromas can show homogeneous minimal-to-moderate staining and usually have necrotic areas within them. Paragangliomas stain intensely and uniformly (Fig. 10-10). The CT characteristics and diagnostic approach to these lesions is more fully discussed in Chapter 5.

Benign lesions arising outside of but involving the nasopharynx

Rarely, lesions involving the nasopharynx may arise from any of the surrounding epithelial, endodermal, or mesenchymal elements. The most common lesions that would have distinguishing characteristics would be enchondromas, osteochondromas, chordomas, and teratoid lesions. Chordomas will show destructive and reactive changes in the clivus and usually have calcification. Enchondromas and osteochondromas might show typical exophytic growth patterns with peripheral and central chondroid matrix calcification. The appearance of teratoid lesions varies with the dominant tissue.

Rarely, intracranial tumors such as craniopharyngiomas, invasive or recurrent pituitary adenomas, meningiomas, and dermoid (epidermoid) tumors can extend into the nasopharynx. The site and probably the tissue of origin should be apparent in a well-done CT study.

---
*References 2, 14, 21, 29.

Thornwaldt's cyst

Thornwaldt's cyst defies classification in any of the foregoing groups of benign lesions. It is an unusual lesion that has a distinctive CT appearance. It is a cyst of the pharyngeal bursa and will therefore appear as a midline, well-circumscribed round mass with internal CT values indicative of its fluid nature (Fig. 10-11). Contrast infusion is probably not necessary for diagnosis but if done should show no increase in the central attenuation values, assuming that the cyst is not inflamed or infected.

□ Nasopharynx: malignant tumors
■ Clinical considerations

CT is the most reliable imaging tool for detecting and determining the extent of nasopharyngeal carcinoma.[16,17] Most nasopharyngeal CT scans are done to discover whether or not patients appearing in one of four broad categories harbor a nasopharyngeal tumor. These clinical circumstances include:

1. Signs and symptoms related to obstruction of the eustachian tube. Serous otitis media is usually present and is often treated as the primary problem. This clinical course can be followed from several months to longer than a year before an obstructing nasopharyngeal mass is considered as a possible cause. Any middle-aged person with unilateral serous otitis media should have a careful

physical examination of the nasopharynx. If symptoms persist a CT scan is warranted, even in light of a negative clinical examination.

2. A combined neurologic and clinical picture that suggests invasion of the skull base. These usually appear as either a cavernous sinus syndrome or a jugular foramen syndrome.

3. Patients appearing with an enlarged neck node believed to be secondary to a metastasis from an unknown primary tumor of the head and neck region.

4. Nasal obstruction or bleeding. If bleeding or obstruction is a result of nasopharyngeal carcinoma, these are usually far advanced lesions.

Nasopharyngeal carcinomas are not surgical lesions. The head and neck surgeon plays a major role in diagnosis; however, the radiation oncologist is primarily responsible for treatment. At times, chemotherapy and immunotherapy are used to salvage radiation failures.

■ Pathology

Most nasopharyngeal malignancies (80%) will be either keratinizing or nonkeratinizing (lymphoepitheliomas, transitional cell) squamous cell carcinomas.[2] Another 18% will be either adenocarcinomas, adenoid cystic carcinomas, or unclassified.[2] The remaining 2% are either lymphomas or sarcomas.[2] There is really no way to distinguish various tissue types on CT scans, and this is certainly a moot point because virtually all are biopsied prior to management. The diagnostic radiologist must help diagnose the lesion, determine its extent, and follow the course of therapy.

■ CT diagnosis

The hallmark of nasopharyngeal carcinoma is deep infiltration.[17,18] Almost all deeply infiltrating lesions of the nasopharynx will prove to be primary tumors, direct extension from adjacent oropharyngeal lesions or sinus lesions, and, rarely, metastases. Invasive, inflam-

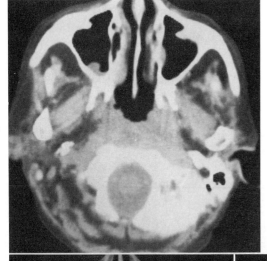

A

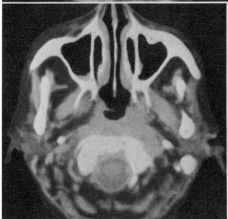

B

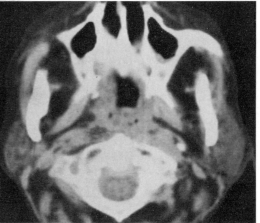

C

Fig. 10-12. Typical pattern of deep infiltration for nasopharyngeal carcinoma. Notice circumferential soft tissue thickening that is asymmetric but present bilaterally. There is encroachment on parapharyngeal spaces bilaterally, but this is worse on patient's left side. Tumor extends across midline to obliterate tissue planes surrounding prevertebral musculature. Also, patient's left carotid sheath area is grossly abnormal, most likely resulting from adenopathy, but this can also be related to direct extension of tumor.

matory lesions may have the same CT appearance; however, the clinical circumstances will usually indicate the differential diagnosis. In our experience the inflammatory lesions most likely to mimic the appearance of nasopharyngeal carcinoma are invasive mucormycosis and medial extensions of malignant otitis externa (Fig. 10-8).

Deep infiltration is manifest by obliteration (asymmetry) of the paranasopharyngeal space, carotid sheaths, and retropharyngeal space (Fig. 10-12). The tissue planes of the retropharyngeal space are not normally as distinct as the others so that its involvement may be manifest only by asymmetric thickening of the posterior wall of the nasopharynx. Subtle effacement of the planes around the levator palati may also indicate the presence of a tumor.

Obliteration of the parapharyngeal space is a sign that the pathologic process is virulent enough to breach the pharyngobasilar fascia. Once tumors have spread across

this tough membrane they have free access to spread anywhere from the base of the skull to the oropharynx within the parapharyngeal space. On CT scans such extension is evident by obliteration of the normal fatty density that surrounds the airway, deep musculature, and vessels. Extension in this space may occur without any sign of overlying mucosal abnormality, even with very careful telescopic examination of the nasopharynx. It is the ability of CT to contribute this type of information that makes it complementary to the physical examination.

Tumors may also extend from the skull base to the soft palate within the pharyngobasilar fascia and beneath the mucosa. The fascial planes that surround the levator palati provide this pathway. Findings in this compartment can be very "soft" but should be pursued by biopsy or follow-up scans if the physician has any clinical suspicion of nasopharyngeal carcinoma (Fig. 10-13).

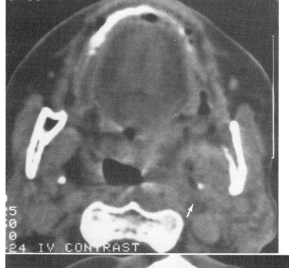

A

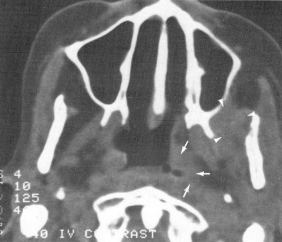

B

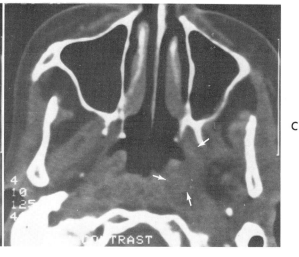

C

Fig. 10-13. Woman with recurrent carcinoma of retromolar trigone region. **A,** Recurrent mass deep to tonsillar pillar *(arrows)* is invading mandible. **B,** Extension along levator palati *(arrows)* carried tumor into nasopharynx beneath intact mucosa. There was also significant extension along pterygoid muscles into infratemporal fossa. Resulting mass *(arrowheads)* obliterates retroantral fat. **C,** Continued cephalad extension of mass beneath fossa of Rosenmüller is visible *(arrows)*. Notice encroachment on parapharyngeal space. Physical examination of nasopharynx was entirely normal. Despite CT findings this patient was operated on. All margins were positive. This case illustrates value of CT in evaluating patients with possible recurrent upper aerodigestive tract tumor. It also demonstrates natural history of spread of tumors along deep muscle bundles as detailed in text and emphasizes that tumor may have significant extension without mucosal evidence of that spread. This is especially true in setting of recurrent tumor. There was no evidence of mucosal disease within this patient's nasopharynx.

Nasopharyngeal tumors also distort the normal superficial contours of the airway. Exophytic lesions may bulge into the airway to a greater degree than they extend into the deep tissue planes. On the other hand, primarily infiltrating tumors may extensively invade and obliterate the deep tissue planes and produce little or no distortion of the airway contours. Most malignancies produce CT findings somewhere in between these extremes. Obliteration of the lateral pharyngeal recesses or eustachian tube orifices is best confirmed by scanning during physiologic maneuvers aimed at distending the upper airway (see section on technique of examination). This is usually required only in fairly subtle cases to make the distinction between normal and abnormal. These maneuvers add no useful information in obviously positive cases. A serous otitis media noted clinically might be explained either by occlusion of the eustachian tube orifice or by infiltration of the tensor and levator veli palati muscles, leading to tube dysfunction. The nerves to the tensor and levator muscles can also be infiltrated by parapharyngeal extension of a malignancy.

From the parapharyngeal space the tumors can invade or displace the parotid gland from its deep aspect and occasionally clinically mimic a parotid mass. Their deep growth also takes them to the spaces surrounding the carotid sheath and to the base of the skull by direct and lymphatic spread. The various clinical-neurologic symptom complexes seen in patients with nasopharyngeal tumors are related to these extensions and intracranial spread.

Intracranial extension of the tumor is almost always heralded by destruction of the medial aspect of the middle cranial fossa floor. The tumor may grow directly through the skull base or follow the carotid sheath.[15,17] In the latter case the epicenter of the bony defect is the foramen lacerum. Bone destruction may be seen in the absence of staining intracranial mass lesions, even on good quality coronal scans. This merely means that the tumor is either still extradural or will show minimal meningeal or microscopic spread across the dura. Therapeutically, differentiations of such subtle extensions are usually moot. Evidence of meningeal involvement may be available from analysis of the cerebrospinal fluid. Occasionally, intracranial extension will be by way of nerve roots, with enlargement of the basal foramina the only sign of such spread. This is unusual behavior for tumors other than adenoid cystic carcinomas. Gross destruction of the clivus, basisphenoid, and even upper cervical spine is usually visible on plain films.

Cranial nerve deficits are often seen as clinical symptoms in patients with nasopharyngeal malignancies.[2,15] Extension through the skull base along the carotid artery and around the foramen lacerum will produce ei-

ther a partial or complete cavernous sinus syndrome (Fig. 10-14). Posterior extension, either directly or by way of the lymphatics to the highest jugular and retropharyngeal nodes, will cause a jugular foramen syndrome by compression of cranial nerves IX to XII (Fig. 10-15). Massive tumors with extensive involvement of the skull base and posterior and middle cranial fossae will produce mixed patterns.

Carcinoma of the nasopharynx frequently metastasizes to the regional lymph nodes. The exact pattern of nodal involvement depends on the extent and focus of origin of the primary involvement. Nodal spread may be bilateral in midline tumors or a result of crossed drainage. On CT scans, lymph node extension to the highest jugular and lateral retropharyngeal nodes is manifest by obliteration of these tissue planes around the carotid sheath and just under the lateral pharyngeal recess. It is sometimes difficult to distinguish direct extension from lymphatic spread in this area. Pathologic data indicate spread to the cervical nodes occurs with the following frequencies: jugulodigastric nodes, 70%; upper deep cervical nodes, 66%; jugulomyohyoid nodes, 34%; spinal accessory nodes, 28% and inferior cervical nodes, 20%.[2] CT imaging is probably more accurate than clinical staging of cervical metastases.[17,20] False negatives can occur because of involved but not enlarged nodes and false positives can occur because of reactive nodes.

Other primary malignancies rarely produce any distinguishing characteristics. Primary lymphoma does tend to be circumferentially infiltrating following Waldeyer's ring, whereas this pattern is usually only seen in the most advanced carcinomas. Chondrosarcomas may show matrix calcification that will occur in other tumors following radiation therapy. Rhabdomyosarcomas almost always occur in very young children and will be widespread in the infratemporal fossa when they are present. Other sarcomas, plasmacytomas, and melanomas occur but are quite rare.

□ Benign conditions of the nasopharynx

Benign lesions of the nasopharyngeal region are unusual but sometimes diagnostically troublesome problems. A variety of anatomic structures surround the oropharynx and are therefore possible sources of masses that appear in the oropharynx, floor of the mouth, and base of the tongue. CT, augmented by intravenous contrast injection and sometimes by simultaneous sialography, is the single most useful diagnostic study in almost all cases. It can almost always exclude significant pathologic processes and often obviate more invasive studies. CT imaging shows the full extent of pathologic processes so that the proper surgical approach, if surgery is indicated, can be planned.

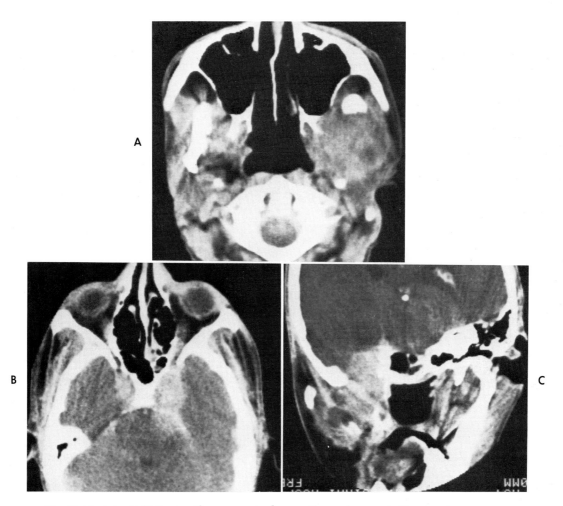

Fig. 10-14. A to **C,** Patient with recurrent adenocystic carcinoma. **A,** Recurrent mass occupies the infratemporal fossa. **B,** Widening of ipsilateral cavernous sinus is indicative of extension of tumor to this locale. **C,** Direct coronal sections are of suboptimal quality but show destruction of skull base and extension of tumor into cavernous sinus. Such spread would be likely to cause complete cavernous sinus syndrome as described in text.

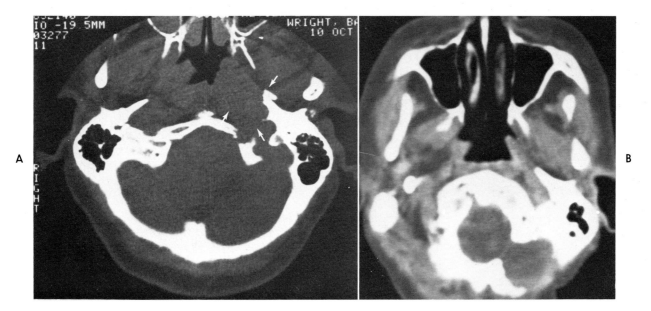

Fig. 10-15. A, Scan made through jugular fossa. Patient has nasopharyngeal carcinoma with evidence of metastases to jugular fossa *(arrows)*. **B,** Scan following radiation therapy shows remarkable return of tissue planes to normal. Patient had relief of symptoms related to compression of nerves within carotid sheath.

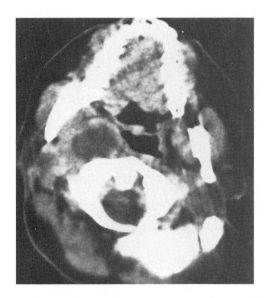

Fig. 10-16. Benign lesions that appear in parapharyngeal space adjacent to oropharynx are basically same as those present in nasopharynx. Diagnostic approach is unchanged from that described in Chapter 5. If masses also appear in lateral neck below mandible, branchial cleft cysts should be included in differential diagnosis. This figure is caudal extension of the neurilemmoma shown in Fig. 10-10, *A*.

Masses arising from the parotid and submandibular glands are best defined by CT (Chapter 4).

Paragangliomas (carotid body tumors) and neuromas or neurofibromas arise from the carotid sheath and often appear as parapharyngeal masses (Fig. 10-16). The nature and extent of these lesions is accurately demonstrated by CT with contrast infusion (see nasopharyngeal and parapharyngeal space sections of this chapter and Chapter 5).

Lingual thyroid tissue has an absolutely characteristic appearance on CT scans. Its iodine content causes it to have very high attenuation values in relation to the surrounding soft tissues. The mass of ectopic thyroid tissue usually lies in the center of the tongue base within the intrinsic muscle mass to the tongue. It is bordered laterally by the hyoglossus (extrinsic) muscles and posteriorly by the mucosa and submucosa of the tongue base. Intravenous contrast enhancement will increase the differential density between the thyroid tissue and the surrounding musculature (Fig. 10-17). Thyroglossal duct cysts may also extend through the tongue base and down into the hyoid bone and anterior midline neck. They are best shown by CT. These lesions are characteristically fluid dense, well circumscribed, and nonenhancing (Fig. 10-17). Other benign mesenchymal tumors are uncommon. Neuromas or neurofibromas are indistinguishable from malignancies except that they

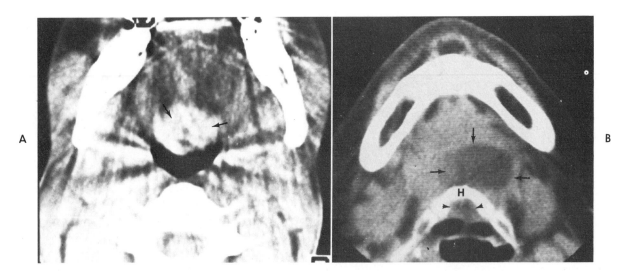

Fig. 10-17. A, Somewhat degraded image because of both motion and fillings. It does, however, show typical appearance of lingual thyroid tissue within tongue base. These are characteristically high-density lesions because of their iodine content *(arrows)*. Mass is located within intrinsic muscles of tongue base. **B,** Another of more common benign mass lesions that involve tongue base is pictured. This is cephalad extension of thyroglossal duct cyst *(arrows)*. Note that small component of cyst *(arrowheads)* lies posterior to hyoid bone *(H)*.

tend to be more circumscribed. Both are moderately enhancing lesions and may show peripheral enhancement patterns. Lucent centers in neuromas are usually a result of necrosis; in neurofibromas they may be related to the density of the tissue within the capsule.[8] Lymphangiomas and hemangiomas occur mainly in children. The diagnosis is usually apparent clinically and CT is used to define their deep extent.

Benign neck masses such as branchial cleft cysts, thyroglossal duct cysts, external laryngoceles, and pharyngeal pouches are usually diagnosed by history, clinical examination, and conventional radiographic studies. CT is reserved for the more confusing presentations of these masses and in those instances it is virtually always definitive. If the surgeon wants to know the full extent of such a lesion and its relationship to surrounding structures, CT is the imaging examination of choice.

□ Oropharynx: Malignant tumors

Tumors of the oropharynx are almost always squamous cell carcinomas.[2] In general they tend to be less well differentiated and metastasize sooner than other head and neck malignancies; this may be true as one moves more posteriorly and inferiorly.[2] Retromolar trigone and soft palate carcinomas tend to be exophytic, well-differentiated lesions that are more likely to be cured and are the least likely of the oropharnyngeal tumors to metastasize. This will vary with the degree of differentiation. Carcinomas of the tonsillar beds, posterior faucial pillars, glossopharyngeal sulci, base of the tongue, valleculae, pharyngeal walls, and pharyngoepiglottic folds seem to be more aggressive.[2]

Treatment is usually by a combination of radiation therapy and surgery but depends on the point of origin, extent of the primary involvement, and whether regional or distant metastases are present. The combination of physical examination and CT, with a newer generation of scanners, affords the opportunity to stage these lesions more accurately than ever before.*

Clinically it is of critical importance whether a carcinoma of the tongue base can be resected for cure while leaving one lingual artery intact.[10] If one lingual artery cannot be preserved, then total glossectomy as opposed to hemiglossectomy is required, and many head and neck surgeons and patients are not willing to accept the devastating morbidity that total glossectomy imposes on the patients.[31] In the past, extension of the tumor to the level of the circumvallate papillae has been used as an indication for resectability mainly because of its value as a predictor for ensuring an adequate margin of resection. With CT, however, the physician now has a

tool capable of depicting nearly the exact relationship of the tumor to the lingual arteries as well as clinically occult contralateral and regional lymphatic extensions. CT plays a definite role in providing information that can reduce the incidence of surgical failure. It can help direct more aggressive surgical therapy in appropriate cases of this disease, a malignancy that is often difficult to manage successfully.

A CT study of a malignancy in the region should demonstrate (1) the extent of local, deep infiltration, (2) whether the lesion has crossed the midline, (3) the relationship of the mass to the lingual arteries (if the tongue base is involved), (4) any spread to contiguous regions of the aerodigestive tract (e.g., preepiglottic space, hypopharynx, or nasopharynx), and (5) the extent of lymph node metastases (within the limits discussed subsequently) (Figs. 10-18 to 10-21).

While the mucosa of this region is quite accessible to inspection and palpation, clinically undetectable submucosal and parapharyngeal extension is seen on CT scans[18] (Figs. 10-19 and 10-20). This extension is manifest by obliteration of the deep tissue planes and is best appreciated following intravenous contrast injection. With the advent of digital localizing films and a tilting gantry on newer scanners, the artifacts caused by dental fillings can almost always be avoided. These amalgams now pose no difficulties except in the oral cavity. Deep spread remote from the primary tumor is not an uncommon occurrence and it might indicate that a combination of radiation therapy and surgery may be more appropriate than surgery alone in some cases, or it may completely obviate surgery in other cases.[10]

Rapid drip infusion, sometimes supplemented by 25 to 30 ml bolus injections, should be used when defining the location of the tumor in relation to the lingual artery. The course of the artery is marked by the hyoglossus muscle as it surrounds the intrinsic muscles within the tongue base (Fig. 10-6). The artery lies medial to the hyoglossus while the lingual vein lies just laterally. Approximately three or four contiguous 4 to 6 mm thick scan sections are required to show the course of the artery in relationship to the mass.

Intravenous contrast is also necessary to distinguish the numerous branching arteries and veins in the carotid sheath from enlarged nodes. Nodes may show no enhancement, thin rim enhancement, or thick rim enhancement; the last pattern is indicative of capsular or extracapsular extension.[19] Vessels show homogeneous opacification. A tumor may of course be present in normal-size nodes. Enlarged nodes may be purely reactive. Nodes greater than 2 cm in size virtually always contain a tumor. A neck with multiple nodes between 1.5 and 2.0 cm also very likely contains a tumor.[9,22] CT

*References 10, 12, 17, 23.

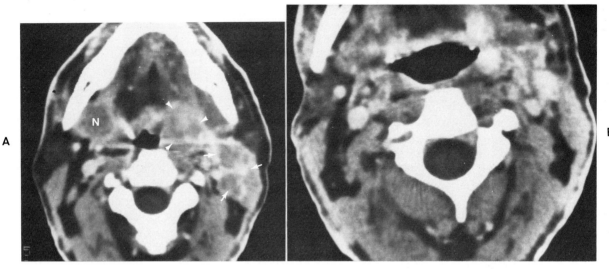

Fig. 10-18. A, Pretreatment scan of 40-year-old man with carcinoma of base of tongue. Patient had neck mass that turned out to be matted nodal mass as seen on scan *(arrows)*. Primary tumor was missed on examination by at least two head and neck surgeons. On scan it is an obviously deeply infiltrating mass that extends into intrinsic musculature on side ipsilateral to nodal mass *(arrowheads)*. Large, contralateral submandibular lymph node *(N)* was not appreciated on physical examination and advanced this patient from N-2 neck to N-3 classification. **B,** Postradiation therapy scan shows some residual asymmetry of tissue plane, but most of primary tumor has disappeared as have related ipsilateral and contralateral masses.

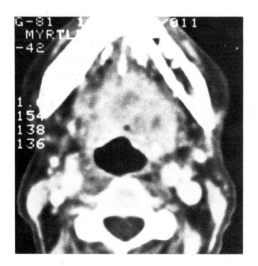

Fig. 10-19. Scan of approximately 65-year-old woman who had 1- to 2-year history of pain in throat that radiated to ear. Physical examination showed normal mucosa at tongue base. Palpation was negative. Examination under anesthesia and just prior to biopsy showed entirely normal mucosa at tongue base and only vague fullness to deep palpation. Deeply infiltrating mass obviously obliterates all tissue planes at tongue base in floor of mouth. Compare this to normal anatomy, which should be seen at this level in Fig. 10-6. High-density material just posterior to mandible is extravasated contrast material from an attempted submandibular sialogram.

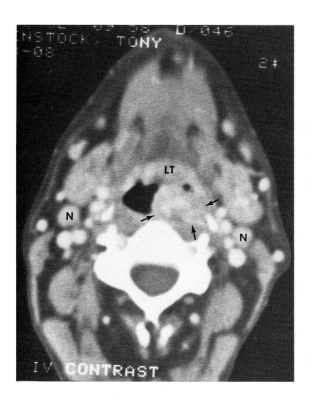

Fig. 10-20. Scan of elderly woman who complained of throat pain and an abnormal mass in lower oropharynx and upper hypopharynx. Study was done to see if tumor had invaded tongue base. Well-circumscribed, moderately enhancing mass involving posterior and lateral wall of oropharynx *(arrows)* is seen. Normal enhancing lingual tonsillar tissue *(LT)* should not be mistaken for infiltrating tumor. Small lymph nodes *(N)* in jugular digastric regions bilaterally are not definitely positive for tumor by CT criteria. These nodes measure approximately 8 mm in size and were only ones seen in neck. Surgery showed that this lesion was confined to posterior and lateral wall of oropharynx and upper hypopharynx.

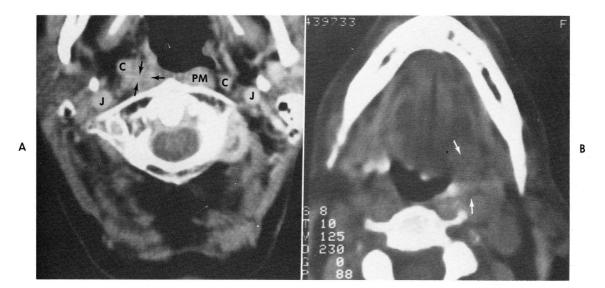

Fig. 10-21. A and **B,** Scans from two different patients with recurrent lymphoma. **A,** Patient was approximately 80 years old and had what was thought to be stage I lymphoma involving cervical nodes. On routine follow-up, vague periparotid mass was found. Scans at that level confirmed recurrent lymphoma. Scans were then continued toward patient's skull and involvement of retropharyngeal nodes was demonstrated. Mass *(arrows)* can be seen obliterating planes between prevertebral muscles *(PM)* and carotid artery *(C)*. Compare normal and abnormal sides. Subsequent scans showed regression of this mass following adjustment of radiation therapy ports. *J*, jugular vein. **B,** Patient with lymphoma of nasal cavity was studied because of findings on palpation suggestive of mass at tongue base. Contrast was not infused, but mass extending into intrinsic tongue musculature can be seen *(arrows)*. This is indicative of lymphomatous involvement of lower aspect of Waldeyer's ring. There was also marked asymmetry in carotid sheath region, indicating cervical adenopathy was probably present as well although it is difficult to be certain without contrast infusion.

is certainly capable of showing whether any nodes greater than 1.0 cm are present, and this may be critical data because evidence suggests that metastases in nodes less than 1.0 cm in size are managed with equal success rates by surgery and radiation therapy (Fig. 10-20). Whenever size criteria are used to determine whether nodal metastases are present, false positive and false negative calls are possible; however, CT has been proven more accurate than clinical staging in two limited series of patients[19,20] (Fig. 10-18).

CT is very useful for following the response of tumors to the chosen mode of therapy. It is essential to do a baseline study approximately 5 to 6 weeks after the completion of treatment. If radiation therapy has completely eradicated the tumor, the deep tissue planes in the tumor bed and lymph node–bearing regions will usually revert to a near normal appearance[10] (Figs. 10-15 and 10-18). A persistent bulky mass is unusual and should be considered evidence of persistent or recurrent tumor (Fig. 10-13). Surgery can profoundly alter the deep tissue planes; however, the mass lesion will usually be completely removed if the operation has been successful. Obliteration of the tissue planes without definite mass is not a reliable sign of recurrent tumor postoperatively because scarring and retraction can vastly alter these normal relationships. Again, it is best to get a baseline scan 5 to 6 weeks after the completion of therapy and look for one of the following as evidence of recurrent tumor.[10]

1. Persistence or enlargement of the mass in the original tumor bed
2. Direct extensions of the tumor to adjacent areas (e.g., tonsillar pillar lesion to nasopharynx)
3. Spread of the tumor to regional lymph nodes
4. Evidence of a second primary involvement in the upper aerodigestive tract

■ Occult primary tumors of the upper aerodigestive tract appearing as cervical metastatic disease

In the past, patients who had isolated cervical lymphadenopathy with no apparent cause presented very difficult diagnosis and management problems. "Skinny" needle aspiration biopsy and CT have reduced the complexity of the diagnostic approach to the patient. Excisional biopsy of a node for diagnosis (without accompanying radical neck dissection) has been shown to increase mortality rates if the primary tumor turns out to be a squamous cell carcinoma from somewhere in the upper aerodigestive tract.[2,25] Such a relationship has not been shown to be true with aspiration biopsy and current evidence suggests it will not.[2] If the aspiration biopsy shows that the tumor is squamous cell then it is most likely to be of either head and neck or lung origin if the node is low in the neck or in the supraclavicular

fossa. If the node(s) is in the posterior triangle or in the midcervical region and above, it is most likely to be from a head and neck primary origin. Adenocarcinomas are most likely to originate below the clavicles no matter where the node is found. An undifferentiated or poorly differentiated histology is of little value in locating the primary involvement site and always raises the possibility of lymphoma. Nondiagnostic aspirates require a search above and below the diaphragm, depending on the clinical situation.

Some head and neck surgeons might not be willing to do skinny needle aspiration and approach this problem more classically. Also, the aspirate might be nondiagnostic. These circumstances, taken with a negative routine examination of the upper aerodigestive tract, require further investigation. Clinically the next step is triple endoscopy and biopsy of suspicious areas or blind biopsies in the nasopharynx, oropharynx, base of the tongue, and pyriform sinuses.* Even with such a careful evaluation some primary head and neck tumors in these areas will not be discovered. Two thirds will manifest themselves over the next 18 months; others are never found.[2] Some authors contend that these lesions are tiny microscopic or macroscopic lesions, and this may be true in many instances; however, it is known that many head and neck tumors do not produce sizeable (1.5 to 2 cm) lymph node metastases until the primary mass is about 2 to 3 cm in size.[22] We have noted that head and neck tumors can grow to 2 to 3 cm in size or larger beneath intact mucosa and completely escape detection not only on routine examination by head and neck surgeons but also following triple endoscopy and biopsy.[17] For this reason we suggest that if triple endoscopy and biopsy is contemplated, it should be preceded by a CT scan of the nasopharynx, oropharynx, and base of the tongue, and perhaps a survey of the neck. This should be done during rapid drip infusion of contrast medium. CT can also reveal more extensive nodal disease than is clinically evident as well as demonstrate otherwise occult tumors (Fig. 10-19). CT should be done before or at least 2 to 3 weeks after biopsy to avoid equivocation because of postbiopsy changes. If a definite deeply infiltrating lesion is seen on scans and biopsies of the area are not positive, repeated deeper biopsies will sometimes be necessary. One should not relent in this regard, as we have personally experienced three separate unsuccessful attempts at obtaining tissue under such circumstances; the fourth biopsy was positive. Percutaneous CT-directed biopsies are also possible and have the advantage of confirming the needle placement in the area of suspicion on CT scans. This procedure is usually not nec-

*References 1, 2, 5, 26.

essary if sufficiently deep biopsies are obtained following personal communication between the head and neck surgeon and the radiologist.

□ References

1. Barrie, J.R., Knapper, W.H., and Strong, E.W.: Cervical nodal metastases of unknown origin, Am. J. Surg. **120**:466, 1970.
2. Batsakis, J.G.: Tumors of the head and neck: critical and pathologic considerations, ed. 2. Baltimore, 1979, Williams & Wilkins.
3. Biller, H.F., Sessions, D.G., and Ogura, J.H.: Angiofibroma: a treatment approach, Laryngoscope **84**:659-706, 1974.
4. Bohman, L.G., Mancuso, A.A., Thompson, J., and Hanafee, W.N.: CT approach to benign pharyngeal masses, AJR **136**: 173-180, 1981.
5. Comess, M., Behars, O., and Dockerty, M.: Cervical metastasis from occult carcinoma, Surg. Gynecol. Obstet. **104**:607, 1957.
6. Duckert, L.G., Carley, R.B., and Hilger, J.A.: Computerized axial tomography in the preoperative evaluation of an angiofibroma, Laryngoscope **88**:613-618, 1978.
7. Eller, J.L., Roberts, J.F., and Ziter, F.M.H., Jr.: Normal nasopharyngeal soft tissue in adults: a statistical study, AJR **112**(3):537-541, 1971.
8. Erlandson, R.A., and Woodruff, J.M.: Peripheral nerve sheath tumors: an electron microscopic study of 43 cases, Cancer **49**: 273-187, 1982.
9. Fletcher, G.H.: Elective irradiation of subclinical disease in cancers of the head and neck, Cancer **29**:1450, 1972.
10. Harnsberger, H.R., Mancuso, A.A., and Muraki, A.: Computed tomographic evaluation of recurrent and residual tumors of the upper aerodigestive tract and neck. Submitted for presentation to the Radiological Society of North America Sixty-eighth Scientific Assembly and Meeting, Nov. 28-Dec. 3, 1982.
11. Khoo, F.Y., Kanagasuntheram, R., and Chia, K.B.: Variations of the lateral recesses of the nasopharynx, Arch. Otolaryngol. **86**: 456-462, 1967.
12. Larsson, S.G., Mancuso, A.A., and Hanafee, W.N.: Computed tomography of the tongue and floor of the mouth, Radiology **143**:493-500, 1982.
13. Last, R.J.: Anatomy, regional and applied, ed. 6, New York, 1978, Churchill, Livingstone.
14. Lawson, V.G., LeLiever, W.C., Makerewich, L.A., et al.: Unusual parapharyngeal lesions, J. Otolaryngol. **8**(3):241-249, 1979.
15. Lederman, M.: Cancer of the nasopharynx: its natural history and treatment, Springfield, Ill., 1961, Charles C Thomas, Publishers.
16. Mancuso, A.A., Bohman, L.G., Hanafee, W.N., and Maxwell, D.: Computed tomography of the nasopharynx: normal and variants of normal. Radiology **137**:113-121, 1980.
17. Mancuso, A.A., and Hanafee, W.N.: Computed tomography of the head and neck, Baltimore, 1982, Williams & Wilkins.
18. Mancuso, A.A., and Hanafee, W.N.: Elusive carcinomas of the head and neck beneath intact mucosa. Presented at the Triologic Meeting, Palm Beach, Florida, May, 1982.
19. Mancuso, A.A., Harnsberger, H.R., Muraki, A., and Stevens, M.: CT of the cervical lymph nodes: normal, variations of normal and applications of staging head and neck malignancies. Submitted for presentation to the Radiological Society of North America Sixty-eighth Scientific Assembly and Meeting, Nov. 28-Dec. 3, 1982.
20. Mancuso, A.A., Maceri, D., Rice, D., and Hanafee, W.N.: CT of cervical lymph node cancer, AJR **136**:381-385, 1981.
21. Maniglia, A.J., Chandler, J.R., Goodwin, W.J., Jr., and Parker, J.C., Jr.: Schwannomas of the parapharyngeal space and jugular foramen, Laryngoscope **89**:1405-1414, 1979.
22. McGavran, M.H., Bauer, W.C., and Ogura, J.H.: The incidence of cervical lymph node metastases from epidermoid carcinoma of the larynx and the relationship to certain characteristics of the primary tumor, Cancer **14**:55-66, 1961.
23. Muraki, A., Mancuso, A.A., Harnsberger, H.R., and Parkin, J.: CT of the oropharynx and tongue base: normal, variations of normal and applications in staging carcinoma. Submitted for presentation to the Radiological Society of North America Sixty-eighth Scientific Assembly and Meeting, Nov. 28-Dec. 3, 1982.
24. Nicholson, R.L., and Kreel, L.: CT anatomy of the nasopharynx, nasal cavity, paranasal sinuses, and infratemporal fossa, CT **3**(1):13-22, 1979.
25. Razack, M.S., Sako, K., and Marchetta, F.C.: Influences of initial lymph node biopsy on the incidence of recurrence in the neck and survival in patients who subsequently undergo curative resectional surgery, J. Surg. Oncol. **9**:347, 1977.
26. Robinson, D.: The management of metastases in lymph nodes when the primary cannot be found, Plast. Reconstr. Surg. **113**:663, 1967.
27. Rouvier, H.: Anatomy of the human lymphatic system, Ann Arbor, Mich. 1938, Edwards Brothers, Inc.
28. Som, P.M., and Biller, H.F.: The combined CT-sialogram, Radiology **135**:387-390, 1980.
29. Som, P.M., Biller, H.F., and Lawson, W.: Tumors of the parapharyngeal space: preoperative evaluation, diagnosis and surgical approaches, Ann. Otol. Rhinol. Laryngol. **90**(suppl. 80):3-15, 1981.
30. Som, P.M., Shugar, J.M.A., and Parisier, S.C.: A clinical-radiographic classification of skull base lesions, Laryngoscope **89**:1066-1076, 1979.
31. Strong, E.W.: Carcinoma of the tongue, Otolaryngol. Clin. North Am. **12**(1):107-114, 1979.
32. Weinstein, M.A., Levine, H., Duchesneau, P.M., et al.: Diagnosis of juvenile angiofibroma by computed tomography, Radiology **126**:703-705, 1978.
33. Wong, Y.K., and Novotny, G.M.: Retropharyngeal space: a review of anatomy, pathology, and clinical presentation. J. Otolaryngol. **7**(6):528-536, 1978.

11 □ The larynx

ARNOLD NOYEK, HARRY S. SHULMAN, MARVIN I. STEINHARDT,
JUDAH ZIZMOR, and PETER M. SOM

The radiologic evaluation of the larynx has undergone considerable change in the past decade, and the single factor most responsible, for this change has been the CT scanner. For the first time the radiologist can look beneath the laryngeal mucosa and assess the submucosa and muscles as well as the cartilaginous supporting structure of the larynx.

The aim of the roentgenographic examination is to complement the clinician by revealing the anatomy that cannot be seen by clinical examination. The vocal cords or laryngeal ventricles may be hidden from the clinician's view by a bulky supraglottic mass, or the vocal cords may obscure evaluation of the subglottic region. Several different roentgenographic examinations can provide information on otherwise hidden anatomic features. The CT scanner, however, also allows some assessment of the depth of tumor infiltration and can aid detection of occult cervical adenopathy, information that can escape the clinician.

A perspective on the continued work to improve the roentgenographic evaluation of the larynx can be gained by a brief historical review of these different procedures.

Within months after its discovery, the roentgen ray was applied to the study of laryngeal anatomy. MacIntyre wrote in England in May 1896: "I have been able to photograph (radiograph) the larynx in the human subject, the picture obtained showing the base of the tongue, hyoid bone, thyroid and cricoid cartilages with epiglottis."[54] He was describing of course the radiographic appearance of the laryngeal structures and adjacent tissues on the lateral view. The same author also stated, "Experimenting on a dead subject, I have been able to obtain excellent photographs of the presence of foreign bodies in and around the region of the larynx, as well as ossification in the cartilages."[76]

In the same year, Max Scheier also described the roentgenographic examination of a cadaveric larynx and noted that the long exposure time required to make a radiograph also made films of a living patient difficult to obtain.

Within 5 years Behn[5] had made an excellent lateral radiograph of the larynx, showing a laryngeal tumor. Movements of the larynx, swallowing function at the laryngeal level, and ossification of laryngeal cartilages were studied fluoroscopically and radiographically by Scheier[90-93] Moller and Fischer, and Frankel. In 1913 Thost[100] published the first systematic roentgenographic atlas of laryngeal disease. In the United States Samuel Iglauer[35] wrote about the value of lateral radiography of the larynx in the study of laryngeal disease.

Hickey[29] described the roentgenographic appearance of the normal larynx using the lateral view and low kilovoltage soft tissue techniques. Coutard[11] also emphasized the usefulness of lateral laryngeal radiography in the study of neoplasms, and Coutard and Baclesse[12] stressed the importance of the lateral roentgenographic examination of the larynx before, during, and after radiation therapy of the larynx and hypopharynx for carcinomas.

Barton Young[103,104] recommended anteroposterior radiography of the larynx with a short 10 cm target-skin distance. This now abandoned high skin dose technique was proposed in order to diminish the obscuring effect of the bony cervical spine on the laryngeal airway and soft tissues, thus permitting better visualization of soft tissue masses or cord paralysis.

Gay and Wilkins[21] and Gay[22] commented on the poor visibility of neck structures with conventional fluoroscopy and recommended image intensification fluoroscopy, recording the study either on videotape or cine film.[44,45] Because considerably less radiation is delivered to the neck when videotape is used instead of cine film, the use of the former is preferred today.

Felix Leborgne[49-52] published the first reports of tomography of the larynx and stressed its value in the study of cancer. At about the same time, in France, Canuyt and Gunsett[7,8] wrote about tomography of the larynx, stressing that the technique required no patient preparation. In the United States Howes,[34] Young,[103] and Caulk[9] also published excellent tomographic studies of the larynx, illustrating the normal and pathologic larynx and including examples of laryngeal carcinoma, vocal cord paralysis, and laryngocele.

Iglauer[36] and Chevalier Jackson[37] studied the larynx by conventional radiography with iodized oil (Lipiodol), a radiopaque contrast material. Farinas[16] also achieved excellent laryngograms in the anesthetized larynx using a nebulized contrast medium. However, contrast laryngography was not really brought to the forefront in the United States until the work of Powers, McGee, and Seaman,[84] Ogura,[79] and Medina.[63] These investigators achieved exquisite contrast roentgenograms using oily propyliodone (Dionosil Oily) after topical anesthesia of the larynx. This represented an important improvement over iodized oil, which only coated the laryngeal mucosa irregularly.

Barium sulfate in carboxymethylcellulose water suspension has been used successfully for laryngography and pharyngography by Khoo et al.[41] The advantage of using this agent for laryngograms is its high radiodensity. This technique, however, has not enjoyed widespread use because of barium deposition in the lungs.

More recently, Zamel et al.[105] achieved excellent laryngograms using powdered tantalum insufflation with or without prior mucosal anesthesia. The ability to achieve good laryngograms without mucosal anesthesia makes powdered tantalum most useful, although its possible explosive property and its prolonged alveolar retentive property have prevented its approval by the Food and Drug Administration.

The application of CT scanning to the larynx represented a new technical breakthrough in diagnosis.[1,57-59] All of the prior techniques could only examine the mucosal surfaces and the resulting pathologic deformities. The CT scan, on the other hand, allowed for the first time visualization of tissues under the mucosa, including portions of the cartilaginous framework of the larynx. This provided the clinician with information that could not be obtained by clinical examination. It is for these reasons that CT scanning is rapidly gaining acceptance as the roentgenographic examination of choice.

□ Anatomy

The larynx can be thought of as being composed of three layers: (1) an inner mucosal layer that rests on (2) a middle zone of muscles and soft tissues, which are in

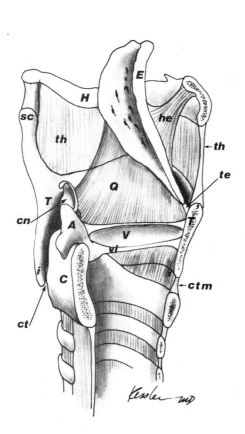

Fig. 11-1. Oblique lateral view of laryngeal cartilages and ligaments. *A*, Arytenoid cartilage; *C*, cricoid cartilage; *cn*, corniculate cartilage; *E*, epiglottic cartilage; *H*, hyoid bone; *T*, thyroid cartilage; *sc*, superior cornu of thyroid cartilage; *i*, inferior cornu of thyroid cartilage; *V*, ventricle; *Q*, quadrate membrane; *vl*, vocal ligament; *ct*, cricothyroid joint; *ctm*, cricothyroid membrane; *th*, thyrohyoid membrane; *te*, thyroepiglottic ligament; *he*, hyoepiglottic ligament.

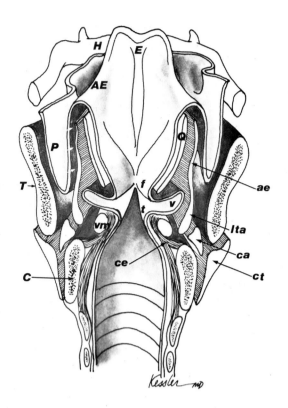

Fig. 11-2. Cut-away back view of larynx. *AE,* Aryepiglottic fold; *E,* epiglottis; *C,* cricoid cartilage; *T,* thyroid cartilage; *H,* hyoid bone; *P,* pyriform sinus; *Q,* quadrate membrane; *f,* false cord; *t,* true cord; *v,* ventricle; *vm,* vocalis muscle; *ce,* conus elasticus; *ct,* cricothyroid muscle; *ca,* cricoarytenoid muscle; *lta,* lateral thyroarytenoid muscle. Small arrows point into paraglottic space.

turn applied to (3) an outer cartilaginous framework. The cartilages of the larynx include the cricoid, thyroid, epiglottic and paired arytenoid, corniculate, and cuneiform cartilages (Figs. 11-1 and 11-2).

The *cricoid* cartilage is the main foundation of the larynx and is the only complete cartilage ring in the respiratory tract. It is shaped like a signet ring, with a thin anterior *arch* and a broad posterior *lamina,* the top of which rises cephalad to the level of the anterior arch. The upper margin of the lamina has a slanting facet on each side of the midline for articulation with the arytenoid cartilages. The joints slant downward and outward so that the arytenoid cartilages separate as they are pulled downward. On each side of the lamina there is a small facet that articulates with the inferior cornua of the thyroid cartilage. All of these cricoid joints are true synovial joints. The cricoid cartilage itself lies just above the first tracheal ring.

Each *arytenoid* cartilage is shaped roughly like a pyramid, with a slender projection anteriorly *(vocal process)* and another laterally *(muscular process).* A small corniculate cartilage articulates, by way of a synovial joint, with the top of each arytenoid cartilage and serves as a point of attachment for each aryepiglottic fold.

The *thyroid* cartilage is formed by paired alae, flattened shieldlike sections that are joined in the midline.

There is a distinctive notch at this midline junction that can extend downward nearly half the height of the larger lateral portions. The posterior edges of the lateral segments have inferior projections *(inferior cornua)* that articulate at the cricothyroid joints. There are also *superior cornua,* which are joined to the hyoid bone by the thyrohyoid ligaments.[47,57,88]

Thus a flexible mobile chain is created in the respiratory system. The hyoid bone is suspended by the suprahyoid muscles from the mandible and skull base. The thyroid cartilage is suspended from the hyoid bone by the thyrohyoid membrane and is in turn attached to the cricoid cartilage posteriorly by the cricothyroid joint. Anteriorly, the cricothyroid membrane closes the space between the undersurface of the thyroid cartilage and the downward sloping thin anterior cricoid arch. Finally, the trachea is suspended from the undersurface of the cricoid cartilage.

The *epiglottic* cartilage is a leaf-shaped structure with its slender inferior tip (petiolus) attached by way of the thyroepiglottic ligament to the midportion of the anterior midline thyroid cartilage. It is suspended from the hyoid bone's inner surface by the hyoepiglottic ligament. The space between these ligaments above, below, and between the epiglottis and thyroid cartilages anteriorly, posteriorly, and laterally is the *pre-epiglottic space,* which is normally filled with fatty fibrous tissue and lymphatics. The epiglottis can be functionally divided into two sections: the mobile or suprahyoid segment and the immobile or laryngeal portion.

The cuneiform cartilages are small, elongated cartilages in the posterior rim of the aryepiglottic folds. The epiglottis and the corniculate and cuneiform cartilages are made of yellow elastic cartilage that does not calcify; however, all of the other laryngeal cartilages are made of hyaline cartilage, which can and does calcify, albeit irregularly.

The oral pharyngeal mucosa runs down the base of the tongue and up again posteriorly to cover the upper epiglottis, creating a groove. In the midline a mucosal fold, the median glossoepiglottic fold, divides this groove into two cup-shaped areas, the *valleculae*, which rest atop the pre-epiglottic space at the base of the tongue. The mucosa then continues backward and downward over the aryepiglottic muscles to create the thin aryepiglottic folds, which run from the upper epiglottis downward to the corniculate and arytenoid cartilages. The medial surface of these folds forms the lateral and posterior boundary of the *vestibule*, which is the respiratory air space in the upper larynx extending downward to the level of the vocal cords and bounded anteriorly by the epiglottis.

The *quadrate membrane* is a fibroelastic membrane that extends from the lower lateral border of the epiglottis anteriorly to the arytenoid cartilage posteriorly. Its lower border is free and constitutes the *false cord*. The ventricle lies just below it. Thus this membrane is imbedded within the aryepiglottic fold.[47]

The *vocal ligaments* run from the vocal process of each arytenoid cartilage to the midline anterior thyroid cartilage just below the attachment of the thyroepiglottic ligament. This point on the inner surface of the thyroid cartilage is the *anterior commissure* and the triangular air space created between the edges of the *true vocal cords* defined by the vocal ligaments is called the *rima glottis*. The body of the true vocal cords is made up of the thyroarytenoideus muscles, which have a flat upper surface and a gently arched undersurface. This arch shape is best appreciated when the cords are in adduction and is referred to as the subglottic arch. The true vocal cords are thicker posteriorly (about 5 mm) and thinner anteriorly (about 1 to 2 mm) near the anterior commissure. Just above the true vocal cords are lateral air-filled outpouchings, the laryngeal *ventricles*. They lie under the inferior border of the false cords in the anterior and middle thirds of the true vocal cords. They can have small appendices that extend anteriorly and cephalad, lying medial to the thyroid cartilage.

The *conus elasticus* is a tough, fibrous membrane that originates along the undersurface of the true vocal cords, running from the anterior commissure to the vocal process of the arytenoids. As it extends inferiorly in the subglottis it divides into two sections that run to the upper and lower margins of the cricoid cartilage. In its anterior upper attachments the conus is fixed to the cricothyroid membrane where it forms a thick band, the cricothyroid ligament. The conus forms the medial submucosal border of the subglottic region.[57]

The posterolateral pharyngeal mucosa extends anteriorly to cover the inner posterior edges of the thyroid cartilage and the thyrohyoid ligament. It then bends back again over the lateral margin of the aryepiglottic fold and quadrate membrane. This creates a pharyngeal fossa, the *pyriform sinus*, that is broad and open above and narrow below. This groove is virtually obliterated during swallowing as the larynx elevates and the pharynx contracts.

The *paraglottic (paralaryngeal) space* is a potential space bounded laterally by the thyroid cartilage, medially by the quadrate membrane, inferiorly by the conus elasticus, and posteriorly by the anterior reflection of the pyriform fossa. It merges anteriorly with the pre-epiglottic space, and the ventricles extend into it.[57,88]

The muscles of the larynx are supplied by branches from the recurrent laryngeal nerve of the vagus. Sensation and secretomotor function is innervated by the internal laryngeal branch of the superior laryngeal nerve from the vagus, and the cricothyroid muscle is innervated by the external laryngeal branch of the superior laryngeal nerve.

☐ Roentgenographic techniques

There are several techniques available for the roentgenographic evaluation of the larynx.* Each has its advantages and limitations. These studies include (1) soft tissue films, (2) high-kilovolt filtration films, (3) xeroradiography, (4) tomography, (5) contrast laryngography, (6) CT scanning, (7) radionuclide scanning, (8) ultrasonography, (9) barium swallow examination, and (10) angiography.

■ Respiratory maneuvers

The dynamics of the larynx can be evaluated on all the roentgenographic modalities by having the patient perform several respiratory maneuvers. In quiet respiration the false cords, ventricles, and true cords are in complete abduction. Thus the lateral laryngeal walls are symmetrically flattened (Fig. 11-3, *A*). During phonation (EEE) the true cords completely adduct and the subglottic arches are well seen. There is a distension of all the supraglottic structures; i.e., the ventricles, the pyriform sinuses, and the pharynx are all more distended than on quiet-breathing films (Fig. 11-3, *B*).

*References 66, 69, 72, 76.

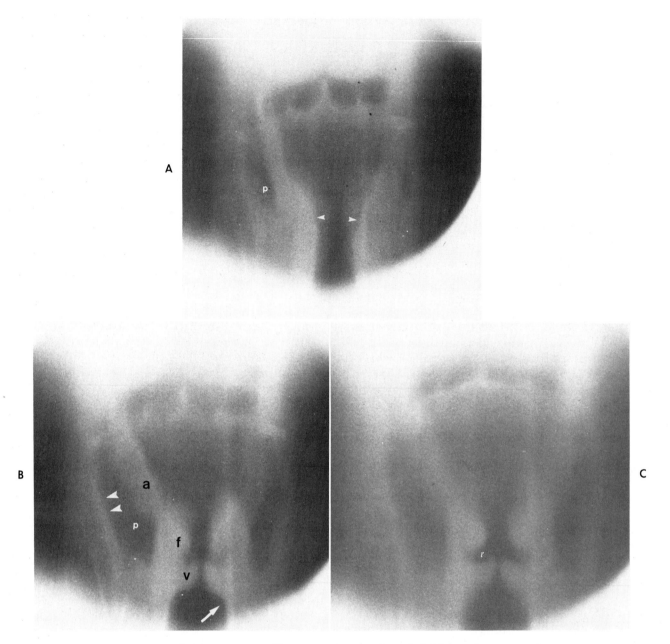

Fig. 11-3. Normal AP tomograms of larynx. *v*, True vocal cord; *f*, false cord; *a*, aryepiglottic fold; *p*, pyriform sinus. **A,** Quiet breathing; arrowheads point to abducted cord region. **B,** Phonation; arrowheads point to lateral pharyngeal wall. Arrow indicates subglottic angle. **C,** Inspiratory phonation; *r*, ventricle.

The false cords are partially adducted and are thus better visualized. If the ventricles are not seen, an inspiratory (EEE) maneuver usually distends them (Fig. 11-3, *C*).

The modified Valsalva maneuver adducts both the true and false cords and distends the supraglottic structures and pharynx even more than on phonation films. The postcricoid region is separated from the retropharyngeal soft tissues, allowing better definition of lesions in this area.

The Valsalva maneuver primarily distends the trachea and subglottis, although mild distension of the supraglottis and pharynx is also present. The true and false cords are in complete adduction.

Which of these maneuvers to employ depends on the specific case. Routinely, quiet-breathing and phonation

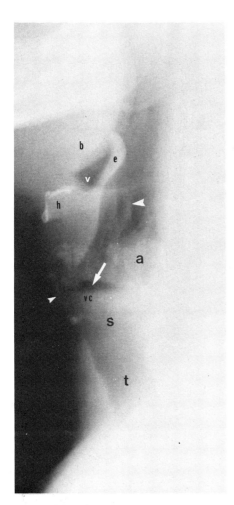

Fig. 11-4. Normal soft tissue lateral film. *b,* Base of tongue; *e,* epiglottis; *v,* vallecula; *h,* hyoid bone; *a,* arytenoid eminence; *vc,* superimposed image of both vocal cords; *s,* subglottis; *t,* trachea. Large arrowhead points to aryepiglottic fold; small arrowhead points to anterior commissure. Arrow indicates ventricles.

films are taken in the AP and lateral views. The Valsalva maneuvers are tailored to the specific patient.

■ Soft tissue films

Soft tissue films are probably the easiest and least expensive screening examinations of the larynx. The specific technique will vary with patient size, film and cassete combination, and equipment. The lateral view is usually exposed about 10 kv less than a standard lateral cervical spine film. A suggested technique uses 76 kVp, 30 mAs settings, a 72-inch focal distance, an 0.3 to 0.6 mm focal spot, a 3 mm aluminum filter with no grid, and par speed screens. The patient is placed in a straight lateral position, either sitting or standing, with the film centered vertically over the laryngeal prominence. The horizontal centering is in a coronal plane just anterior to the temporomandibular joints. The central ray is perpendicular to the midpoint of the film. This lateral soft tissue film gives good information, primarily about the midline structures (Fig. 11-4). The base of the tongue and the lingual tonsils are usually well seen. The valleculae are identified and can be followed posteriorly onto the lingual or anterior surface of the suprahyoid epiglottis. The laryngeal surface of the epiglottis can usually be followed down to the level of the anterior commissure. Some air may be seen in the ventricles, which thus identifies the upper surface of the true cords. The immediate subglottis is often not well seen. This is most evident posteriorly, where the soft tissue density of the cricoid muscles and the partially calcified thyroid and cricoid cartilages obscure detail. The tracheal air column down to the level of the thoracic inlet is well visualized, and assessment of the sagittal tracheal diameter can be made. The retropharyngeal soft tissue space is also well seen. These soft tissues should normally have a gentle lordotic curve that parallels the cervical spine curvature. At the level of the cricoid lamina in the adult the retropharyngeal space should not exceed one third the AP diameter of the body of the fourth cervical vertebra (C_4).

Calcifications of the thyroid and cricoid cartilages can partially obscure laryngeal roentgenographic detail. The thyroid cartilage tends to physiologically calcify earliest in the tips of the inferior and superior cornua and this can be seen starting about the eighth to tenth year of life. Decade by decade the calcification progresses anteriorly and superiorly until the upper rim of the thyroid alae are calcified. Eventually the midline alae junction calcifies and a figure eight shape can sometimes be seen on the lateral film. The waist of this area localizes the anterior commissure. The outer rim of the cartilage calcifies more than the central regions, creating a cortical appearance. The main problem in interpreting these cartilage findings results from the inconsistent and irregular calcifications that usually are present. Differentiating between an area of irregular cartilage calcification and destruction is impossible without secondary findings of a penetrating tumor mass. For this reason cartilage destruction in all but rare cases, should not be diagnosed radiographically. The cricoid cartilages tend to calcify more uniformly than the thyroid cartilage and usually the signet shape can be seen by the third to fourth decade of life. The arytenoid cartilages tend to densely calcify and should not be mistaken for foreign bodies.

The hyoid bone is well seen, with the body appearing as an inverted L. The greater and lesser cornua are usually less well visualized. The hyoid bone marks the level of the valleculae and the suprahyoid portion of the epiglottis. The level of the false cords, true cords, and

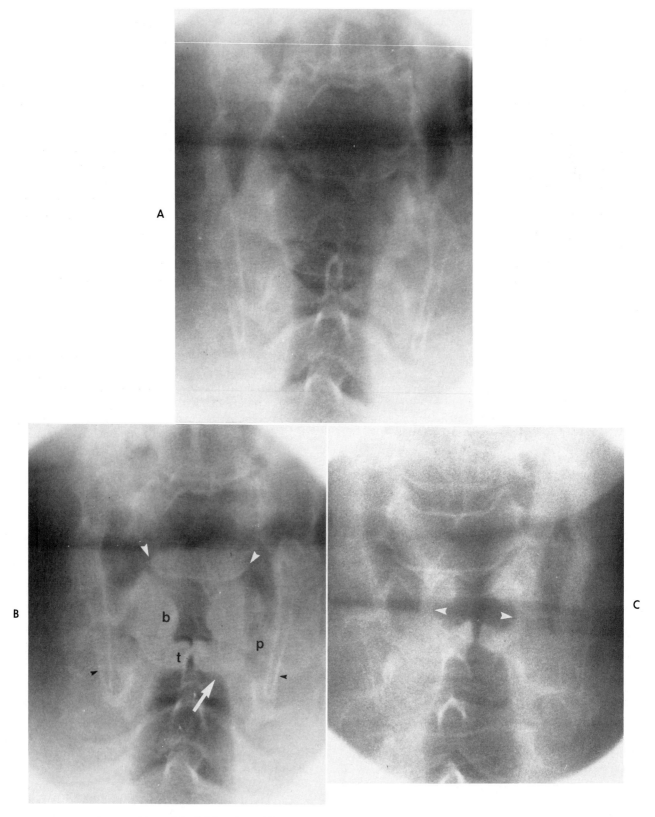

Fig. 11-5. Normal high-kilovoltage films. **A,** Quiet breathing. **B,** Phonation. *b*, False cord; *t*, true cord; *p*, pyriform sinus. Black arrowheads point to thyroid cartilage. White arrowheads point to postcricoid line. White arrow points to subglottic angle. **C,** Reverse phonation; arrows point to ventricles.

immediate subglottis often may not be adequately seen because of apposition of the right and left sides that partially displaces the air column. The aryepiglottic folds and arytenoid masses can be identified, although overlapping of the right and left sides is present. Because of this, AP films must be obtained.

■ High-kilovolt filtration

Technically the AP projection raises a problem because the dense cervical spine obscures the air–soft tissue interface of the larynx. Because of this, the high-kilovolt filtration technique was developed.

McGuire[55,56] suggested a high-kilovolt (140 kv) filtered beam (1 mm copper) for AP films of the larynx. The resulting beam has a higher average photon energy than an unfiltered low-kilovolt beam. This results in a low contrast, flatter appearing film that greatly de-emphasizes the bone density. The air–soft tissue interface, however, is still diagnostically clear. This view allows a good evaluation of the pyriform sinuses, false cords, true cords, ventricles, and subglottis (Fig. 11-5).

■ Xeroradiography

Xeroradiography has been used in mammography for the past two decades. Through a wide recording latitude and its unique property of edge enhancement, superb imaging of soft tissues and the detailing of calcifications are possible. It can produce imaging details far superior to the standard soft tissue film.*

Xeroradiography is used almost exclusively in the lateral projection, where the larynx is viewed free of the overlying cervical spine. Excellent mucosal detail is achieved, and only contrast laryngography provides a superior mucosal image (Fig. 11-6).

The main problem with xeroradiography is its high radiation dose compared to conventional filming. Because of this, it has in general fallen into disuse in laryngeal imaging.

■ Tomography

Tomography offers a method for evaluating the larynx in the AP projection that does not suffer from image degradation caused by superimposition of the cervical spine (Fig. 11-5). It is an examination easily tolerated by the patient and offers improved detail over the plain film studies. Because the thickness of the tomogram section is usually 5 mm, a series of four to six tomograms is required to fully cover the laryngeal structures. The examination is routinely performed with the patient in quiet respiration and during phonation, with the patient supine and the chin elevated so that the plane of the true vocal cords is perpendicular to the table top. Only mucosal deformity can be seen; the exact cause of this pathologic process or how deep into the laryngeal pre-epiglottic or paraglottic spaces the mass extends cannot be evaluated. However, the configuration of the mucosal surface deformity seen and the actual pathologic specimen correlate well.[80]

In effect the findings are duplicating the direct or indirect laryngoscopy findings, although subglottic or tracheal disease can often be more easily detected on tomography than by clinical examination.

Calcification within a mass can be evaluated. Cartilage destruction can still not be diagnosed with certainty, and cartilage fractures may only be seen if there is significant displacement or separation of a calcified cartilage.

Tomography in the lateral projection is not often used because it is difficult to position the patient in a true lateral projection while he is lying on the examination table.

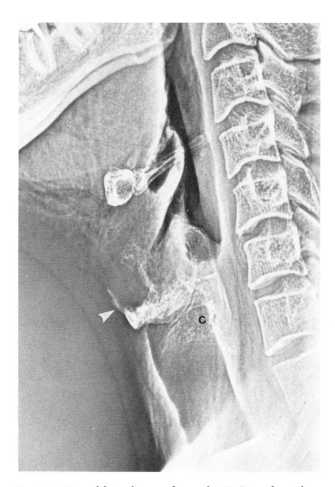

Fig. 11-6. Normal lateral xeroradiograph. *C*, Cricoid cartilage. Arrowhead points to anterior thyroid cartilage, which is incompletely calcified.

---

*References 15, 30, 35, 42, 76, 80, 95.

Another problem with tomography is that masses less than 5 mm in diameter may go undiagnosed because they are smaller than the section thickness of the tomogram and may be averaged out of the image. The accurate delineation of the air–soft tissue interface is crucial for diagnosis of small areas of mucosal abnormality. This is especially true in the region of the anterior commissure and the ventricles. Inflammatory swelling, secretions, or edema may efface the air–soft tissue interface and erroneously suggest a tumor mass.

Because of these problems, a positive contrast study was developed that does not have the limitations of dependence on positioning and delineation of the air-mucosal interface.

■ Laryngography

Laryngography can furnish all the information provided by tomography and can also more accurately demonstrate mucosal disease in the anterior commissure, the ventricles, and the postcricoid regions. Smaller lesions can be detected with laryngography than with tomography, and laryngeal function can be easily studied fluoroscopically.

The disadvantages of this technique result from the invasive nature of the procedure. Careful medical consideration must be given to the use of any premedication. In addition, airway closure as a result of a reaction to the anesthesia or contrast material must be carefully evaluated.

More specifically, atropine, employed by some as a premedication, must not be given to patients with glaucoma, an enlarged prostate, or asthma. Sensitivity to lidocaine (Xylocaine) and its relationship to any cardiac arrythmias must be questioned. Sensitivity to specific contrast agents and iodine must be elicited. Any marked airway compromise or imminent airway obstruction is an absolute contraindication to the use of contrast laryngography. Reactionary edema to either the lidocaine or the contrast material can cause unnecessary respiratory arrest.[18,46] Because the contrast agents fall into the lungs, pulmonary function must be carefully evaluated before the study is performed. Resuscitation equipment including oxygen, an airway delivery system, adrenalin, and intravenous steroids should be immediately available. If any contraindication to laryngography is present, the study should not be performed and either plain film examinations, tomography, or CT scanning should be used.

Thornbury and Latourette[99] compared high-kilovolt filtration AP films and contrast laryngography and concluded that the laryngographic procedure was more accurate in tumor delineation. However, the procedures were equal in detecting subglottic disease. Thus contrast laryngography need not be used in all cases, depending on the information desired from the study.

The technique of the procedure varies considerably. Premedication is not necessary for an excellent examination; however, atropine (0.4 mg) and codeine (60 mg) are given by some examiners. A thorough topical anesthesia with 2% lidocaine is imperative. The pharynx, pyriform sinuses, and larynx must each be anesthesized. Either spraying the pharynx or having the patient gargle the lidocaine works equally well as the initial step. A laryngeal applicator can be used to drip the lidocaine over the base of the tongue and into the larynx and pyriform sinuses. Alternately, a soft rubber tube coated with lidocaine jelly can be placed in the nose and directed over the larynx. The anesthetic can then be delivered by way of the tube. In either case the initial coughing of the patent indicates that the lidocaine is entering the larynx. When the gagging and coughing reflexes have been eliminated, the examination can proceed. With good anesthesia the laryngogram filming need only take several minutes because the patient can cooperate fully. Without good anesthesia the examination may seem endless and the quality of the study will be poor.

Contrast agents

The contrast agent most commonly used in North America is oily propyliodone (Dionosil Oily).* It has excellent radiodensity, good mucosal coating, and a slow flow. It is well tolerated by patients.[25]

Aqueous propyliodone, being water soluble, is more irritating to the mucosa and thus requires better anesthesia. It is also more quickly resorbed and does not coat the larynx as consistently well as the oily propyliodone. Because of this, the aqueous preparation is not often used.

Iopydol (Hytrast) is an excellent water-soluble, mucosal-coating, high-radiodensity contrast agent made in France by Guerbet.[25] It has been withdrawn from the United States market because of adverse pulmonary reactions (fever, pneumonia) ascribed to it during bronchography. These complications may reflect the altered composition of the product marketed in the United States from that of the French agent (0.5% [U.S.] instead of 1.5% [France] sodium carboxymethylcellulose).

Tantalum, in addition to being very radiodense, is inert and nontoxic. There is no apparant mucosal irritation, and the contrast material is not readily dislodged by coughing.[67] When delivered as a powder with a nebulizer, less than 2 ml will coat the larynx.[98] Its explosive property has been eliminated by using the oxide form[23]; however, a recent question has been raised concerning its prolonged alveolar retention. It still is not approved by the Food and Drug Administration.

---

*Glaxo Laboratories, Ltd., Greenford, Middlesex, England. Distributed in U.S. by Picker Corp., Cleveland, Ohio 44143.

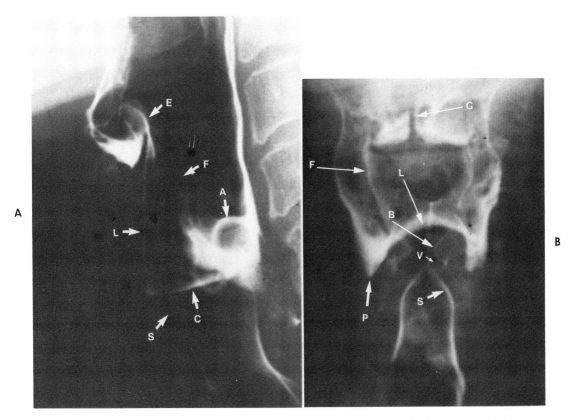

Fig. 11-7. A, Lateral view. *E,* Epiglottis; *L,* laryngeal surface of epiglottis; *F,* aryepiglottic folds; *A,* arytenoids superimposed on pyriform sinuses; *c,* ventricles; *S,* subglottis. **B,** AP view. *G,* Median glossoepiglottic fold; *F,* aryepiglottic fold; *L,* postcricoid line; *B,* false cord; *v,* ventricle; *S,* subglottic angle; *p,* floor of pyriform sinus.

The oily propyliodone should be physically well mixed, placed in a syringe, and then dripped by way of either a laryngeal cannula or a nasal tube onto the larynx and pharynx.

If possible the examination should be performed with image intensification fluoroscopy and spot filming. This allows exact positioning of the patient, spot filming when the mucosal coating is optimal, and instantaneous evaluation of laryngeal functional dynamics (Fig. 11-7). AP and lateral quiet breathing (QB) and phonation views are standard. Other views and maneuvers are tailored to the specific anatomic or functional area under examination.

Valleculae. AP and lateral views in both quiet breathing and phonation maneuvers should be used. They are distended more in the phonation and modified Valsalva maneuvers. The base of the tongue usually is slightly irregular because of the lingual tonsil; however, the floor and posterior walls of the valleculae should have smooth mucosal surfaces.

Epiglottis. AP and lateral views in both quiet breathing and phonation maneuvers should be used. The Valsalva and modified Valsalva maneuvers can deform the epiglottis, foreshortening it and bulging its laryngeal surface backward into the vestibule. This may partially obliterate the anterior commissure. Normally the laryngeal surface is smooth and almost straight. Occasionally a smooth prominence can be seen in its midportion, projecting backward into the vestibule. This is a normal variant of the epiglottic configuration; if the overlying mucosa is normal this variant should not be interpreted as a tumor mass.

Aryepiglottic folds. The folds are well seen in AP and lateral quiet breathing and phonation films. The Valsalva and modified Valsalva maneuvers distort them slightly; however, the modified Valsalva maneuver may be useful in visualizing the posterior base of these folds by displacing them forward and laterally.

True cords, ventricles, and false cords. Normally the true and false cords and the ventricles should not be visible in quiet breathing AP films. In phonation AP filming the true cords completely adduct and the subglottic arches are well seen, are symmetric, and complete almost a 90° degree curve. By comparison, the upper surface of the true cords is relatively flat. The laryngeal ventricles may be better seen on the reverse or inspiratory phonation maneuver. The false cords situated directly above the ventricles are seen as symmetric smooth prominences merging with the lower aryepiglottic folds. The Valsalva and modified Valsalva maneuvers completely adduct the true and false cords and may obliterate the ventricles. The undersurface of the cords may be better coated in the Valsalva maneuver.

Anterior commissure. The commissure should be a sharp, clean angle at the base of the epiglottis seen on the lateral views. Both quiet breathing and phonation films may be necessary for complete assessment because occasionally the normal soft tissue mass of the false and true cords can prevent contrast material from completely filling the angle. A modified Valsalva maneuver may be helpful in this instance. Normally the anterior commissure mucosa gracefully bends downward and posteriorly over the arch of the cricoid cartilage, creating a small bulge just above the anterior tracheal wall as seen on the lateral views. This must not be interpreted as a pathologic mass.

Subglottis. The true vocal cords are thicker posteriorly and thinner anteriorly. The important clinical consideration is the degree of subglottic tumor extension to or below the level of the cricoid cartilage, which is lower anteriorly (arch) and higher posteriorly (lamina) (see tumor section).

The Valsalva maneuver will distend the trachea but will make the subglottic soft tissues appear fuller, possibly simulating a mass lesion. The subglottic is best evaluated on AP and lateral quiet breathing and phonation films.

Pyriform sinuses. The pyriform sinuses are best seen on phonation and quiet breathing films. Oblique positioning may be helpful to see the medial and lateral sinus walls. The apex of the pyriform sinus usually lies at about the level of the true vocal cords. Some slight irregularity of these apices may be present because of normal small mucosal infoldings that create appendix-like structures. Irregular mucosal coating can also be caused by retained secretions. Specific attention should be paid to ensuring that both pyriform sinuses are filled with contrast material. The aryepiglottic fold–medial pyriform sinus wall thickness must be assessed in order to evaluate a subtle supraglottic mass lesion.

The lateral pyriform sinus wall is continuous with the lateral pharyngeal wall. There usually is a slight lateral bulging of this area (pharyngeal ears) that occurs between the level of the hyoid bone and the thyroid cartilage. It is best seen on the modified Valsalva maneuver. It is through this region of the thyrohyoid ligament that pharyngoceles and laryngoceles project laterally.

Postcricoid region and posterior arytenoid region. This is normally a radiologically silent area and is best evaluated on the lateral modified Valsalva film. This maneu-

ver distends the pharynx and maximally separates the postcricoid region from the posterior pharyngeal wall. On AP films, the postcricoid line is seen. It is created by contrast material collecting in the groove created by the impression of the back of the cricoid cartilage against the posterior pharyngeal wall. The line disappears on swallowing.

It must be remembered that although contrast laryngography provides the most sensitive mucosal evaluation, there are submucosal areas that cannot be evaluated well by this technique. These include the pre-epiglottic and paraglottic spaces and cartilage abnormalities. The CT scan allows further evaluation of these areas.

■ CT scanning

CT scanning adds a new dimension to laryngeal imaging. For the first time, preoperative evaluation of the submucosa and the pre-epiglottic and paraglottic spaces is possible.* In addition, a better assessment of the laryngeal cartilages can be made than ever before (Fig. 11-8). Although mucosal detail is not as good as with contrast laryngography, this information can almost always be seen by clinical examination. In fact, the main advantage of CT scanning is that it is a quick, noninvasive technique that provides information that cannot be obtained by clinical examination. The specific areas scanned help to determine whether or not conservation surgery can be performed. By way of comparison, CT scanning has been shown to be equal to or better than laryngography in evaluating laryngeal pathology in nearly 90% of cases.[57] Because respiratory motion can cause the larynx to have an excursion of 1 cm or more, thinly collimated, rapid–scanning time CT imaging is necessary in order to optimally visualize laryngeal anatomy and tumor extent. The patient lies supine with the neck extended sufficiently to bring the plane of the vocal cords perpendicular to the tabletop. Continuous 5 mm thick scan sections are obtained from the upper trachea to the base of the tongue. These 12 to 14 scans are performed while the patient is breathing quietly, and the patient is cautioned not to swallow, talk, or move during the scanning. If necessary, scans can be obtained during the phonation maneuver (cord mobility), the modified Valsalva maneuver (to distend the pyriform sinuses and supraglottic larynx),[20] or the reverse phonation maneuver (to better distend the ventricles), if clarification of these specific areas is required.[57,93]

In the supraglottic larynx the tip of the epiglottis and the uppermost aryepiglottic folds are seen at the level of the hyoid bone. Below this, the laryngeal vestibule

---

*References 60, 62, 74, 95.

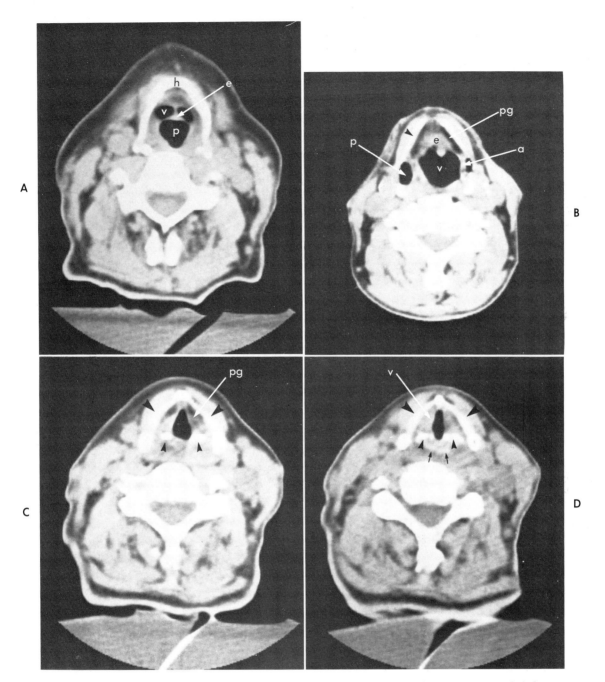

Fig. 11-8. Serial normal laryngeal CT scans from hyoid bone to trachea. **A,** Most cephalad scan. *h,* Hyoid bone; *v,* right vallecula; *p,* laryngopharyngeal junction with vestibule; *e,* tip of epiglottis. **B,** Arrowhead points to right thyroid cartilage. *p,* Pyriform sinus, with one aryepiglottic fold *(a)* separating it from vestibule *(v)*. Low-density paraglottic space *(pg)* and pre-epiglottic space can be seen lying just inside thyroid cartilage. *e,* Epiglottis. **C,** Large arrowheads point to thyroid cartilage. *pg,* Paraglottic space. Small arrowheads point to top of arytenoid cartilages. This is level of false cords. **D,** Level of true cords *(v)*; note they are of same density as muscle. Large arrowheads point to thyroid cartilage; small arrowheads point to base of arytenoid cartilages, which rest on top of cricoid lamina *(arrows)*.

Continued.

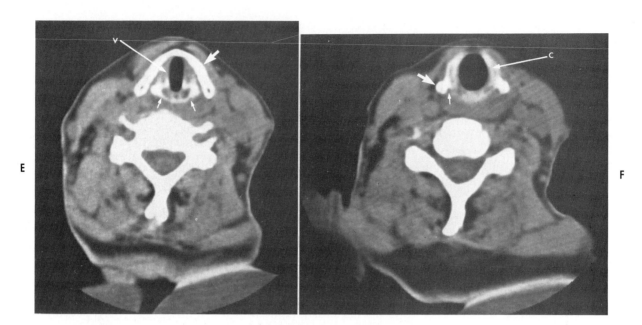

Fig. 11-8, cont'd. E, Level of undersurface of true cords (v). Small arrows point to cricoid lamina; large arrow points to thyroid cartilage. Notice normal minimal soft tissue thickness at anterior and posterior commissures. **F,** Lower cricoid cartilage level. Large arrow points to inferior cornu of thyroid cartilage; small arrow points to cricothyroid articulation. Almost entire ring of cricoid *(c)* is seen at this level.

is seen extending down to the level of the true cords. On either side the air-distended pyriform sinuses are seen to be separated from the vestibule by the aryepiglottic folds, which can be followed down to the level of the arytenoid cartilages. The pyriform sinuses extend anteriorly and bulge into the paralaryngeal space. Some asymmetry in the size and the caudal extent of the sinuses is normal.

The thyroid cartilage is seen as two paired laminae that are fused in the anterior midline at the laryngeal prominence. Above this level is the midline thyroid notch; this region should not be mistaken for an area of cartilage destruction or a fracture. The thyroid laminae calcify or ossify quite irregularly, so that segmental interruptions are seen along both the inner and outer margins of the laminae, which can simulate focal destruction. The superior and inferior thyroid cornua are well seen, and the cricothyroid articulations of the inferior cornua with the lateral cricoid lamina can be identified.

The epiglottis can be followed caudally as it narrows to a level immediately cephalad to the anterior commissure. The pre-epiglottic space is seen between the epiglottis and thyroid cartilage as a fat-containing, low-density space that is continuous laterally with the paraglottic (paralaryngeal) spaces. The paralaryngeal space is very thin near the level of the true cords and it widens as it extends cephalad to the level of the valleculae.

The true vocal cords are normally seen as soft tissue–

density structures in an abducted position during quiet breathing. The free margins may be slightly denser, possibly reflecting the vocal ligaments. At the anterior commissure only a small zone of mucosa is seen lying directly on the inner surface of the thyroid cartilage. Above this level the false cords are seen as lower density bands that may appear to cross the midline anteriorly. The true vocal cords are narrow anteriorly (2 mm) and thicker posteriorly (5 to 7 mm). The posterior margin of each true cord can be seen as it attaches to the vocal process of the arytenoid cartilage. In fact, identification of the lower arytenoid cartilages resting on the top of the cricoid lamina is an excellent way of localizing the level of the upper surface of the true vocal cords. The rima glottidis is shaped like an isosceles triangle, with the apex anteriorly at the anterior commissure and the wider base posteriorly between the vocal processes of the arytenoid cartilages. The laryngeal ventricles may occasionally be seen as air-containing spaces extending into the paralaryngeal spaces in the anterior and middle thirds of the true cords. These ventricles separate the true cords and the false cords.

The arytenoid cartilages are usually homogeneously calcified, pyramid-shaped structures that lie atop the cricoid lamina on either side of the midline. Between the arytenoid cartilages is the posterior commissure, which is similar to the anterior commissure but has a slightly thicker mucosa over it. The anterior vocal process can be identified at the level of the true cords while the superior and lateral muscular processes are seen at the level of the false cords and ventricles. These lateral muscular processes normally lie 2 mm or less from the posterior inner surface of the thyroid cartilage.[88]

The cricoid cartilage has a signet-ring shape, with its broader posterior lamina measuring 2 to 3 cm in vertical height. Calcification, as with the thyroid laminae, can be irregular and can simulate areas of destruction. Usually there is a dense cortical rim of calcification with a central area of lower density representing either noncalcified cartilage or a medullary space. The cricoarytenoid joint level can be seen on the upper surface of the lamina. The mucosa over the cricoid cartilage is thin and closely adherent to the surface of the cartilage. The cricoid cartilage demarcates the subglottic region of the larynx.

The carotid arteries lie just posterolateral to the thyroid cartilages. The larger, somewhat asymmetric jugular veins lie just posterolateral to the carotid arteries. These vessels are better seen on contrast-enhanced scans. The carotid sheath usually can be identified as a thin, low-density plane surrounding these vascular structures.

The cervical lymph nodes can also be examined on CT scans of the neck. Normal nodes may be difficult to identify; however, enlarged nodes with low attenuation centers represent either metastatic or aggressive inflammatory nodes. Clinical correlation can distinguish between these entities.

Laryngeal scanning in the sagittal plane or sagittal and coronal reconstructions can be obtained; however, they usually add little significant information to that gained in the standard axial projection.

■ Radionuclide scanning

Radionuclide scanning has limited application to laryngeal imaging but is being used by some investigators[27,70] to complement the other imaging techniques. Technetium Tc99m polyphosphate, pyrophosphate, or diphosphorate bone scanning reflects osteoblastic activity and the rate of collagen or mature osteoid production. This response can be seen in the presence of cartilage fractures, osteomyelitis, tumor invasion, or destructive arthropathy. The cartilage changes are sensitive but nonspecific, and because they reflect functional changes they can give positive uptake scans prior to detectable structural changes on tomography or CT scanning (Fig. 11-9). The cricoarytenoid and cricothyroid joints can give localized uptakes in osteoarthritis and rheumatoid, gonococcal, and gouty arthritis.

Gallium Ga 67 citrate accumulates in actively proliferating inflammatory or neoplastic cells (Fig. 11-10). It is most useful in determining whether or not a systemic component to the laryngeal disease is present. How-

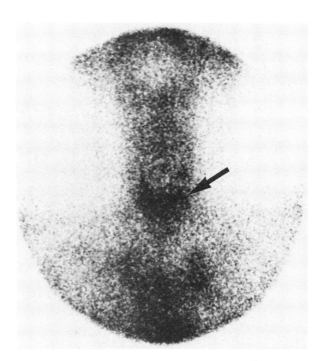

Fig. 11-9. Normal bone scan of larynx. Anterior view of delayed phase of bone scan demonstrates normal uptake of radionuclide (technetium Tc 99m methylene diphosphonate) by bone component of thyroid and cricoid cartilages *(arrow).* (From Noyek, A.M.: Laryngoscope **89**[9 pt. 2]:1-87, 1979.)

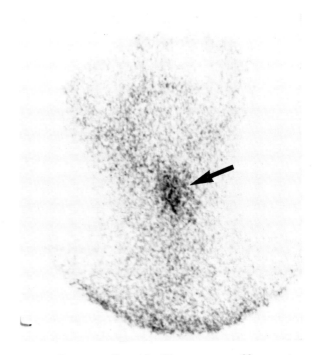

Fig. 11-10. Positive gallium Ga 67 citrate scan of larynx. Anterior view of neck demonstrates positive gallium scan with uptake of radionuclide by supraglottic carcinoma of larynx involving primarily right ventricular band. Arrow indicates area of increased uptake.

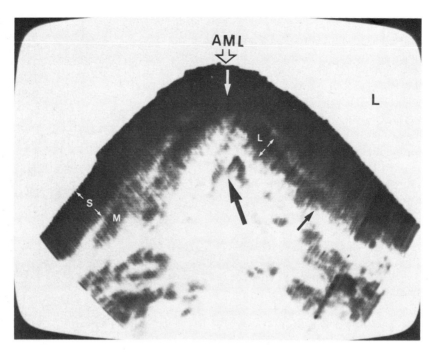

Fig. 11-11. Normal transverse B-mode ultrasonogram of larynx. Transverse B-mode cervical ultrasonogram, using contact technique at level of midthyroid cartilage, demonstrates anatomy of thyroid alae. *AML,* Anterior midline. *L* (in white) indicates position of left thyroid alae. Two small white arrows in relation to *L* indicate width of left thyroid ala. Left thyroid ala terminates posterolaterally at approximately position of small black arrow. Large black arrow in midline beneath thyroid cartilage indicates some nondescript echoes, presumably in region of attachment of epiglottis. Air-containing laryngeal lumen prevents ultrasound imaging because of impedance characteristic of air. *S,* Skin; double white arrows indicate its thickness. *M,* Strap muscle.

ever, there is no consistent correlation with its uptake within either primary or metastatic deposits. If it is picked up by the tumor in a particular patient, then it can be expected to do so persistently throughout that patient's scanning history.

Gallium and bone scanning can be used in combination in evaluating osteomyelitis and perichondritis. The gallium scan reflects activity of the primary infection, whereas the bone scan reflects the osteoblastic response. When the infection is eliminated, the gallium scan will no longer be positive; however, the bone scan may remain positive for 6 to 18 months, as cartilage and bone repair continues.

■ Ultrasonography

Ultrasonography provides a single, quick imaging technique that is free of patient irradiation. It is best applied in the larynx to study the thyroid cartilage, and the examination can easily be repeated as required (Fig. 11-11). In B-mode scanning the thyroid laminae can be seen in the axial plane, while gray scale recordings can give information about cartilage integrity and

thickness. Cartilage thickening can be detected in perichondritis, and although the images are diagnostically sensitive they are nonspecific and require close clinical correlation.[64]

■ Barium swallow examination

Barium swallow examination is not part of the normal routine assessment of the larynx, but it is a complementary study. Any swallowing difficulty automatically warrants examination of the upper digestive tract. However, because 5% to 10% of patients with carcinoma of the larynx will develop a coexisting tumor in the upper digestive tract, some people suggest that a barium swallow examination be performed on all such patients. Thus while a barium swallow examination can help define tumor extension from a laryngeal lesion into the pharynx, it is also useful in evaluating a coexisting primary lesion.[42] The barium study can also be of assistance in studying the cause of laryngeal aspiration. The effectiveness and coordination of pharyngeal peristalsis, laryngeal mobility, and cricopharyngeal function can all be well seen.

■ Angiography

Angiography is only rarely applied to laryngeal tumors.[30,31] It may play a role in evaluating hemangiomas or arteriovenous malformations of the larynx, although contrast-enhanced CT scans can localize these lesions. If intra-arterial embolization techniques become more applicable to laryngeal pathology, it is possible that subselective arteriography will become a more commonly employed procedure.

□ Laryngeal pathology
■ Congenital anomalies

Congenital lesions of the larynx are rare.[42] They may be life threatening, are often associated with severe aspiration, and are frequently associated with multiple systemic abnormalities. The laryngeal lesion requires careful clinical and radiographic evaluation in order to plan approrpiate conservative or operative treatment. The range of anomalies includes hypoplasia, stenosis, laryngomalacia, webs, clefts, and fistulae (Fig. 11-12). Conventional roentgenographic examination or CT scanning usually suffices and contrast laryngography is contraindicated because of airway compromise. Contrast esophagrams may be helpful in detecting a fistula and aspiration.

The small size of the infant airway and the rapid respiratory rate make laryngeal imaging difficult. In addition, if the airway is visualized in expiration, a more extensive airway collapse or stenosis may be suggested than is actually present.

Congenital webs or stenosis can occur at any level of the larynx and represent a failure to recannulize the larynx during the tenth fetal week.[17,94] Symptoms occur at delivery and a tracheostomy is required. The webs most commonly occur in the anterior two thirds of the vocal cords. A firm web will produce both inspiratory and expiratory stridor, and the voice will be hoarse.

The stenoses are usually subglottic, appearing as a circumferential narrowing below the vocal cords to the level of the cricoid cartilage. It is the most common congenital airway problem necessitating a tracheostomy in the first year of life.[32] The voice is normal, with both inspiratory and expiratory stridor.

Congenital vocal cord paralysis is associated with other anomalies in 50% of patients.[94] Those patients without anomalies have a better prognosis with spontaneous recovery in a few weeks. For patients in whom the paralysis is related to increased intracranial pressure related to meningomyelocele, Arnold-Chiari malformation, or hydrocephalus, the paralysis may be spontaneously reversed when the abnormal pressure is relieved. Unilateral paralysis is more common on the left side because of the longer course of the left recurrent nerve, which may be involved by cardiovascular anomalies.

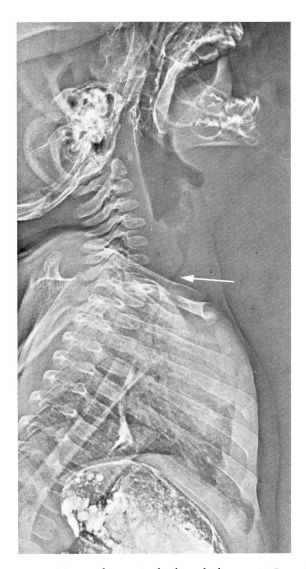

Fig. 11-12. Massive laryngotracheobronchial stenosis. Lateral xeroradiograph in infant demonstrates massive narrowing of airway from subglottic larynx inferiorly. White arrow indicates narrowed cervical trachea at level of thoracic inlet. Barium is seen in stomach from previous examination. (From Noyek, A.M., Steinhardt, M.I., and Zizmor, J.: Otolaryngol. Clin. North Am. 2[2]:445, 1978.)

Laryngomalacia is the most common congenital anomaly to cause pediatric airway obstruction.[17,94] It results from an immature cartilaginous support of the supraglottis, allowing the drawing in of the epiglottic and aryepiglottic folds on inspiration. The voice is normal and the symptoms usually appear at 3 weeks of age and resolve by 6 to 12 months as the cartilaginous framework matures.

Congenital hypoplasia of the larynx is very rare and may be suggested radiographically in the absence of the hyoid bone.[6] Congenital cysts are usually located in the supraglottis and appear with symptoms referable to this location. The diagnosis is made by laryngoscopy and definitive treatment is by endoscopic marsupialization.

The developing larynx and trachea are separated from the esophagus by the laryngotracheal septum. Incomplete fusion of this septum results in a fistula or cleft of the larynx. Aspiration occurs on swallowing, and the symptoms are manifest soon after birth. Laryngoscopy reveals a vertical defect in the posterior laryngeal wall between the artyenoids and through the posterior cricoid.

Congenital papillomas have been reported in neonates, although the vast majority appear between the ages of 3 and 12 years.[81] They occur as multiple small papillomas that primarily involve the vocal cords. Seeding of the lower tracheobronchial tree can occur and appears to be related to trauma inflicted on the respiratory mucosa by endoscopy.[86] Spontaneous involution may occur at puberty.

Congenital subglottic hemangioma is a congenital vascular malformation that can cause airway obstruction, necessitating a tracheostomy. Fifty percent of cases have associated cutaneous hemangiomas. About 90% of cases appear by the third month of life[94] and the natural history is for spontaneous involution by the eighteenth to twenty-fourth month of life. If the hemangioma is small, a tracheostomy may be avoided by systemic steroid therapy.[94]

It is important to recognize that anomalies of the nasopharynx, nasal cavity (choanal atresia), tongue, and mandible may also produce upper airway obstruction. These lesions may exist separately or may coexist with laryngeal abnormalities.

■ Inflammatory lesions

The most common causes of laryngeal airway obstruction in the pediatric patient are acute laryngotracheitis (croup) and epiglottitis.

Croup is an inflammatory process involving the subglottis and tracheobronchial tree. It is most often caused by the parainfluenza viruses. Swelling of the soft tissues at the level of the unyielding cricoid cartilage produces the airway obstruction.

Epiglottitis is an inflammatory process that affects the supraglottic larynx. Almost all cases are caused by *Haemophilus influenzae* type B bacterial infections. The onset of the disease can be extremely rapid and complete obstruction may occur in 4 to 5 hours. Symptoms include inspiratory stridor, a "hot potato" voice, and dysphagia.[94] The lateral neck films characteristically reveal a swollen epiglottis (Fig. 11-13).

Acute laryngitis may be caused rarely by diphtheria, adenoviruses, and irritant chemicals, dust, or fumes.[14] The epithelium may become edematous and necrotic,

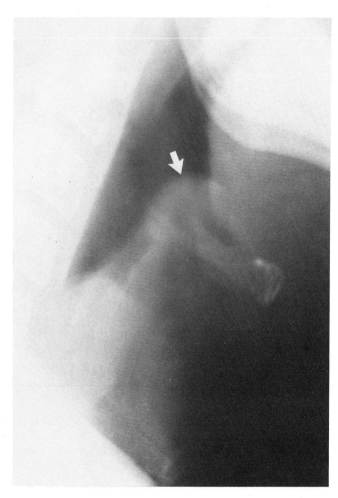

Fig. 11-13. Acute epiglottitis. Soft tissue lateral radiograph demonstrates swelling of epiglottis, obliterating its normal landmarks *(arrow)*.

leading to ulcerations that become covered by a fibrinopurulent exudate. The larynx roentgenographically appears edematous. This is a nonspecific finding. Rarely, an acute inflammatory disorder such as diphtheria can result in a cicatricial stenosis. This depends on the degree of both mucosal and submucosal involvement.[14] It most characteristically involves the junction between the cricoid cartilage and the upper trachea (Fig. 11-14).

The allergic responses of the larynx to inhaled, ingested, or injected allergens can be dramatically acute and life threatening (Fig. 11-15). Acute responses can also be seen in patients with angioneurotic edema.[14]

Specific granulomatous diseases that involve the larynx include tuberculosis, sarcoidosis, mycotic lesions, Wegener's and midline granulomatoses, rhinoscleroma, leprosy, and syphilis.[3,81]

These chronic inflammatory diseases often are clini-

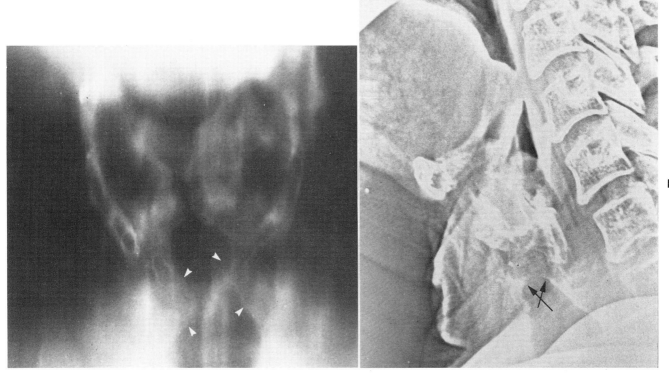

Fig. 11-14. Subglottic stenosis following diphtheria. **A**, AP tomogram demonstrates marked subglottic stenosis (arrowheads) approximately 1 cm in length, in 52-year-old woman who had diphtheria as teenager. **B**, Lateral xeroradiograph demonstrates inferior aspect of subglottic stenosis *(arrows)*. (**A** Courtesy Dr. J. Coleman, Toronto.)

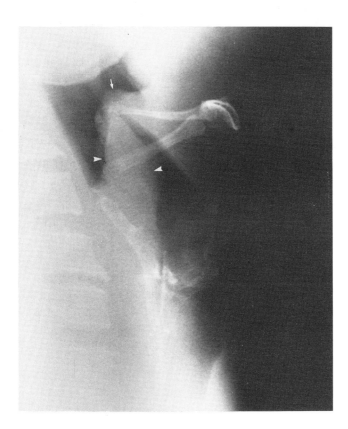

Fig. 11-15. Supraglottic edema resulting from allergy. Soft tissue lateral radiograph demonstrates marked edema of epiglottis and aryepiglottic folds. Arrowheads indicate extent of edema in aryepiglottic folds. Arrow indicates edematous free margin of epiglottis.

cally thought to be neoplastic until endoscopic biopsy. The role of the radiologic examination is to evaluate the extent of the lesion and to assess the adequacy of the airway. The laryngeal response to therapy can also be followed conveniently.[97]

The roentgenographic findings are nonspecific and may not distinguish the lesion from a neoplasm. In general, however, the larynx is seen to be more diffusely involved with these lesions than with neoplasms. There may be a circumferential involvement, and the mucosal surfaces usually appear intact and smooth, albeit widened (edematous or infiltrated). Occasionally, focal granulomas can be seen; these cannot be radiographically differentiated from a carcinoma. The diagnosis of these chronic inflammatory diseases is best established by the clinical setting in which the laryngeal changes are seen.

Tuberculosis tends to involve the supraglottic larynx, causing exposure of the underlying cartilage that in turn leads to cartilage necrosis. Less often, the true vocal cords may be diffusely involved. The larynx appears swollen in the initial stages, and scarring and stenosis can be seen in the later phases of the disease. The laryngeal involvement is almost always a complication of active pulmonary tuberculosis[81] (Figs. 11-16 to 11-18).

Sarcoidosis may affect the larynx as the only clinical manifestation of the disease. It is estimated to occur in 1% to 4% of patients with this disease. There usually is a nonspecific edematous appearance, with little loss of mucosal integrity. The laryngeal disease does not often respond to systemic steroid therapy; however, local steroid injections have produced good results, at times allowing a tracheostomy to be avoided. These changes can be followed by laryngeal imaging[97] (Fig. 11-19).

The mycotic granulomas rarely involve the larynx. The nonspecific roentgenographic findings have been reported in actinomycosis, blastomycosis, and histoplasmosis.[86]

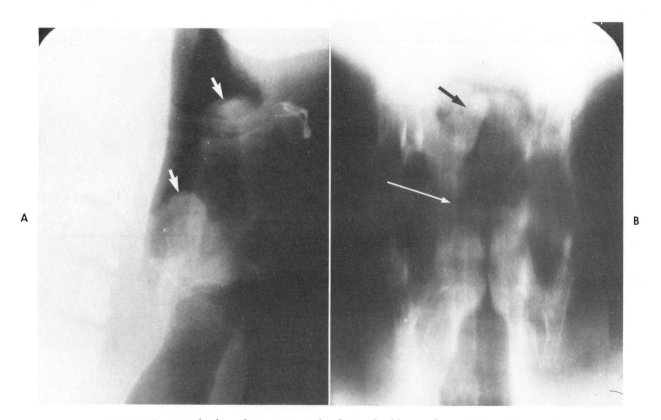

Fig. 11-16. Laryngeal tuberculosis. **A,** Lateral radiograph of larynx demonstrates diffuse nodular thickening of entire supraglottis. Upper arrow demonstrates thickened edematous epiglottis. Lower arrow indicates thickened elevated arytenoid mucosa. **B,** AP tomogram demonstrates diffuse thickening and nodularity of vocal cords and false cords bilaterally. Ventricles are obliterated. Aryepiglottic folds are thickened, especially on right *(lower arrow)*. Nodularity extends to free margin of epiglottis, more so on right *(upper arrow)* than on left. This patient had active pulmonary tuberculosis. (From Zizmor, J., and Noyek, A.M.: Semin. Roentgenol. **9**[4]:311, 1974.)

A

B

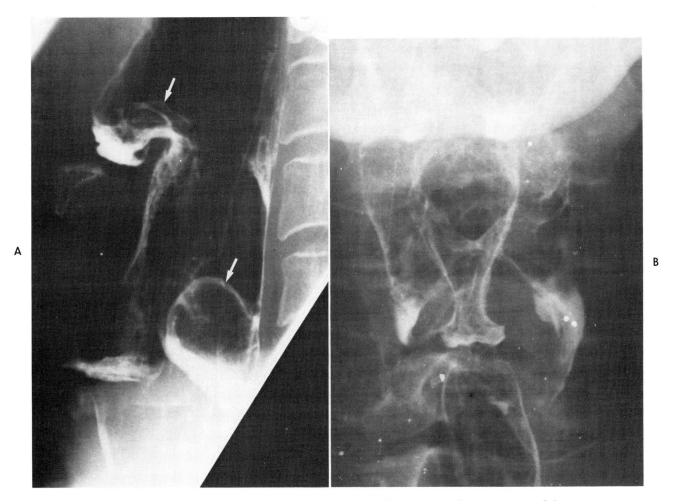

Fig. 11-17. Laryngeal tuberculosis. **A,** Lateral view of laryngogram demonstrates nodular, thickened, and shortened epiglottis *(upper arrow)*; its appearance produces typical turban configuration seen clinically. Aryepiglottic folds are thickened. Arytenoid mucosa is markedly edematous *(lower arrow).* **B,** AP view of same laryngogram demonstrates prominence of arytenoid eminences. Normal appearance of ventricular bands, ventricles, vocal cords, and subglottic larynx are well maintained. (Courtesy Dr. P. Som, New York.)

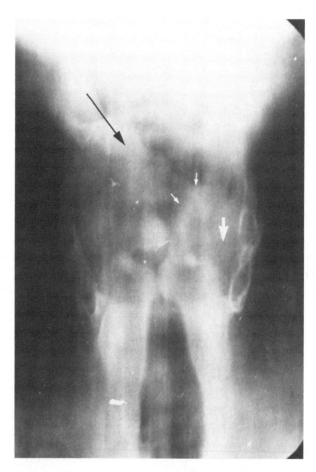

Fig. 11-18. Laryngeal tuberculosis. AP tomogram of larynx demonstrates significant mass lesion of larynx. Small white arrows indicate upper portion of confluent mass that involves left half of larynx and obliterates left pyriform sinus *(thick white arrow)*. On right side, nodular form of tuberculous involvement is noted. Black arrow indicates thickening of right free margin of epiglottis and upper portion of aryepiglottic fold, below which single ulcer crater is noted. Subglottic angles are preserved, as disease only involves supraglottic structures.

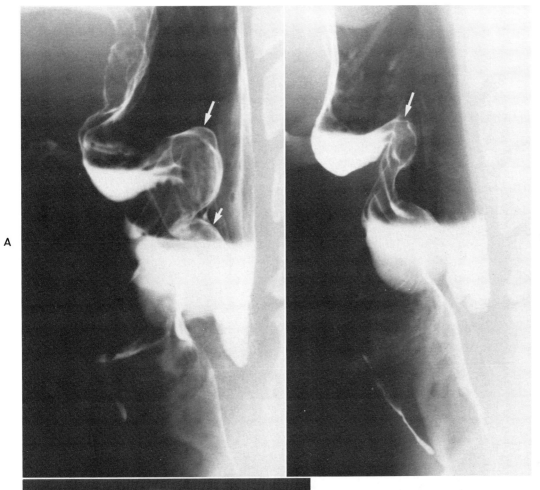

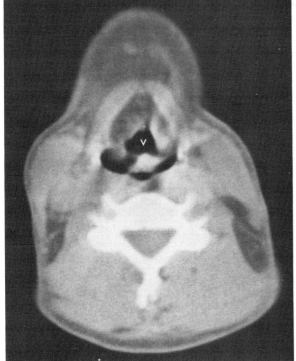

Fig. 11-19. Sarcoidosis. **A,** Lateral view of laryngogram demonstrates enlarged thickened epiglottis *(upper arrow),* as well as thickened arytenoid mucosa *(lower arrow).* **B,** Lateral view of laryngogram obtained following injection of cortisone into epiglottis indicates marked diminution in size of epiglottis *(arrow).* Arytenoid mucosal edema is only minimally reduced. **C,** CT scan reveals diffuse infiltration and thickening of supraglottic larynx with resultant narrowing of vestibule *(v).* (Courtesy Dr. P. Som, New York.)

Wegener's granulomatosis and midline granuloma are rare diseases that can involve the larynx. The diagnosis is usually considered because of the other upper airway disease present, and in the case of Wegener's granulomatosis, because of the presence of lesions in the lungs, kidneys, and skin.

Rhinoscleroma is a rare chronic granulomatous disease caused by *Klebsiella rhinoscleromatis*. It invariably involves the larynx after first affecting the nose, sinuses, and pharynx. Clinically it suggests a neoplasm, but the diffuse laryngeal disease is more indicative of a chronic inflammatory process (Fig. 11-20).[3]

Leprosy very rarely involves the larynx and invariably does so after nasal cavity disease is evident. Attention to establishing an early diagnosis is important because effective chemotherapy is now available.[81] It involves the supraglottic larynx first, primarily affecting the epiglottis.[3]

Syphilitic laryngeal involvement is very rare. Secondary syphilis can cause a diffuse erythema, which may be mistaken clinically for a diffuse laryngitis. The gummata, on the other hand, may appear as well-defined masses that simulate tumors.[3,81]

Inflammatory conditions involving the joints of the extremities can also affect the synovial joints of the larynx. The cricoarytenoid and cricothyroid joints can be involved by rheumatoid arthritis, osteoarthritis, or gout (Figs. 11-21 and 11-22).[13,14] Rarely, more acute inflammatory conditions such as gonococcal infection can cause aseptic arthritis of these joints.[66]

Relapsing polychondritis is a rare disease that affects the cartilages primarily of the nose, external ear, lar-

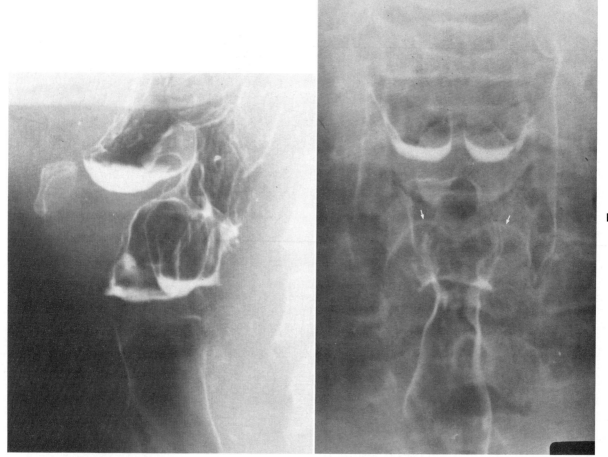

Fig. 11-20. Rhinoscleroma. **A,** Lateral view of laryngogram demonstrates thickened epiglottis in patient with rhinoscleroma. Laryngeal surface of epiglottis is polypoid. **B,** AP view of same laryngogram demonstrates shortened, thickened aryepiglottic folds as well as thickened free margin of epiglottis. On inspiration both halves of larynx abduct well. Arytenoid eminences are well shown on each side *(white arrows).* (Courtesy Dr. P. Som, New York.)

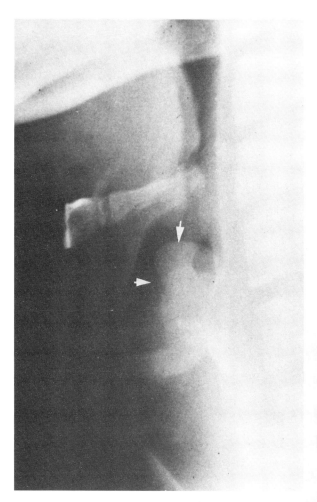

Fig. 11-21. Cricoarytenoid arthritis. Lateral radiograph of larynx demonstrates rounded, well-demarcated, soft tissue mass formed by edematous mucosa overlying arytenoid eminences (*arrows*). Patient is an adult woman with acute cricoarytenoid rheumatoid arthritis and manifestations of systemic rheumatoid arthritis. Notice sparing of epiglottis by edema, which is confined to region of cricoarytenoid joints. Radiographic findings are not specific, but localization of edema is suggestive in light of clinical picture. (From Zizmor, J., and Noyek, A.M.: Semin. Roentgenol. **9**[4]:311, 1974.)

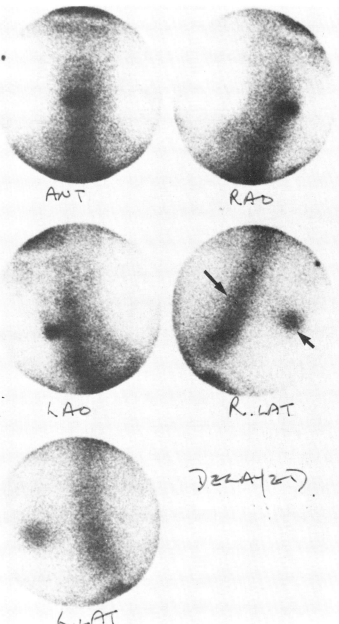

Fig. 11-22. Gout, larynx. Anterior, right and left anterior oblique, and right and left lateral views of delayed phase of bone scan imaging of neck and larynx demonstrates uptake of bone scan agent by cricoarytenoid gouty involvement (*short arrow*). Laryngeal pathologic process is shown in relationship to normal cervical spine uptake by radionuclide (*long arrow*) on right lateral view. (From Greyson, N.D., and Noyek, A.M.: J. Otolaryngol. **2**[2]:541, 1978.)

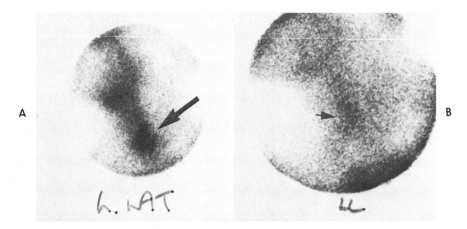

Fig. 11-23. Relapsing perichondritis. **A,** Comparative blood pool phase images of bone scan with technetium 99m methylene diphosphonate demonstrates marked hyperemia of inflammatory lesion on pretreatment bone scan. Left lateral view of neck is shown; large arrow indicates hyperemia in plane of image of larynx. **B,** Same view of blood pool phase of bone scan carried out 3 days after treatment with steroid indicates marked reduction of hyperemia (*small arrow*) as inflammatory lesion has responded dramatically to treatment. (From Noyek, A.M.: Laryngoscope **89**[9 pt. 2]:1, 1979.)

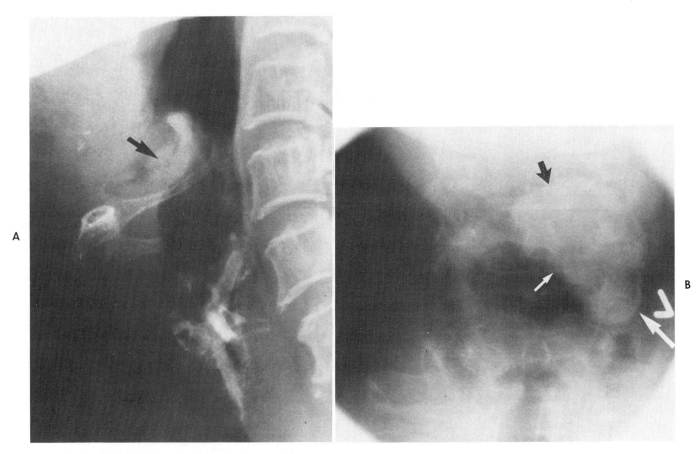

Fig. 11-24. Epiglottic abscess. **A,** Lateral radiograph demonstrates mottled appearance of epiglottic abscess (*arrow*). **B,** High-kilovoltage selective filtration AP radiograph demonstrates transverse and vertical dimension of epiglottic abscess (*arrows*).

ynx, trachea, and bronchi.[13] There are recurrent sterile, inflammatory reactions present that progressively destroy the cartilages. The perichondritis can be detected on isotope scans, which show a marked uptake during the acute phase. Steroid therapy can result in an excellent response that can be followed on the scans (Fig. 11-23).

Perichondritis, acute or chronic, with or without suppuration can occur after trauma, surgery, or irradiation. There is cartilage widening as a result of inflammatory edema of the perichondrium.[71] This is best evaluated on CT scanning although because of the irregular cartilage calcification or ossification even this technique may not detect these changes.

A laryngeal abscess is rare today. When it occurs it can be either acute or chronic. It may result from the presence of a foreign body, from injury, from a virulent infection, or may occur after irradiation.[66] It usually occurs singly (Figs. 11-24 and 11-25). If an air-fluid level is present, it can be detected on erect plain films, CT, or ultrasonography. There may be a cartilage sequestrum, and the resulting abscess mass

may necessitate a tracheostomy for maintenance of the airway.

Laryngeal foreign body aspiration is rare. Usually any ingested foreign body will pass through into the trachea and the bronchus.[3] If a foreign body does lodge in the larynx, rapid respiratory arrest often follows unless it is dislodged or a tracheostomy is performed (Fig. 11-26, *A* and *B*). Laryngeal aspiration occurs more often in infants than in adults. When it does occur in an adult, some contributing factor, such as a neurologic swallowing defect, obtunded reflexes, alcohol, or surgery, is usually present. Conventional soft tissue films are most often adequate for assessing the airway. Distinguishing between a small radiopaque laryngeal foreign body and calcified cartilage may be impossible on plain films. However, CT scans usually can resolve this problem (Fig. 11-26, *C*).

■ Trauma

The larynx may be injured by either external or internal trauma. Almost all external forces result from blunt or penetrating trauma (car accident, choking,

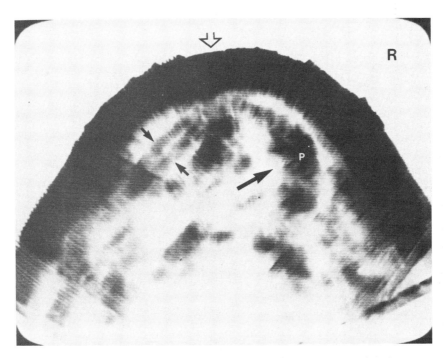

Fig. 11-25. Perichondritis with intralaryngeal abscess. Transverse B-mode ultrasonogram, taken 8 cm above sternal notch at midheight of thyroid cartilage demonstrates ultrasonic evidence of laryngeal perichondritis involving right thyroid ala. Transverse image is reversed; viewpoint is from above and behind patient. Hollow upper arrow demonstrates anterior midline of neck; *R* indicates the right side. Normal left thyroid ala is demonstrated between small black arrows. Thickened right thyroid ala *(P)* is clearly shown. Large black arrow indicates clear, echo-free zone beneath right ala. This zone represents area of abscess formation, confirmed surgically. (From Noyek, A.M., et al.: J. Otolaryngol. **6**[suppl. 3]:95, 1977.)

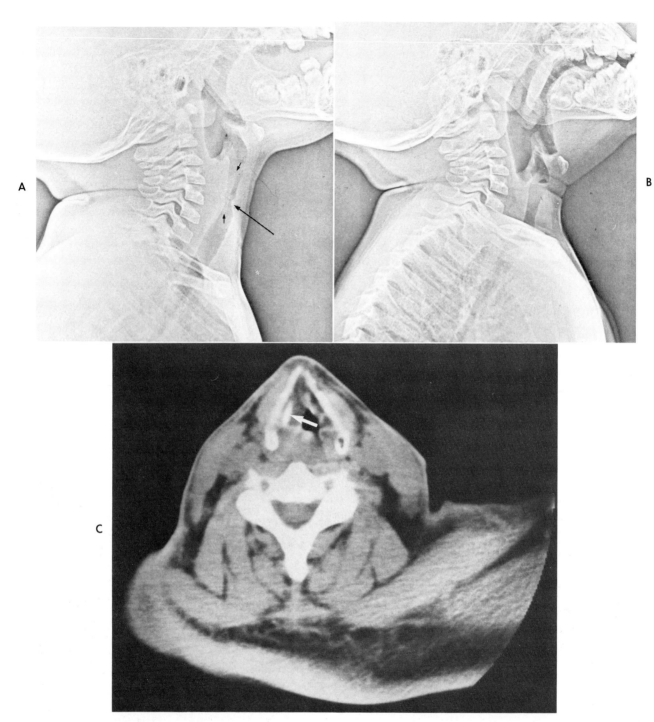

Fig. 11-26. Foreign body, larynx and trachea. **A,** Lateral xeroradiograph demonstrates longi-
tudinally positioned foreign body, piece of plastic, extending from subglottic larynx *(small
upper arrow)* along posterior wall of trachea to midpoint of cervical trachea *(lower small
arrow)*. Extent of airway compromise is well demonstrated in sagittal plane, as there is
considerable mucosal edema anteriorly *(long black arrow)*. **B,** Lateral xeroradiograph several
days following successful endoscopy shows normal larynx and trachea and demonstrates resolution of anterior tracheal mucosal edema seen in pretreatment examination. **C,** CT scan on
different patient than **A** and **B.** Adult patient swallowed chicken bone that could not be
localized on plain films and tomograms and that could not be seen on endoscopy. CT scan
reveals the bone *(arrow)* in right paraglottic space under thyroid cartilage. There is surrounding laryngeal edema. (**A** and **B** Courtesy Dr. Paul Holinger, Chicago.)

etc.) or surgery. Internal trauma is usually a result of prolonged intubation, vocal abuse, or chemical or thermal burns.

The trauma may be localized or may be complex and extensive. There can be mucosal disruption, soft tissue swelling, hemorrhage, edema, cartilage dislocation, or fracture. The vocal cords may be immobile because of scarring, fibrosis, cricoarytenoid dislocation, or recurrent laryngeal nerve trauma.[26]

The soft tissue injuries of the larynx include hemorrhage, edema, and mucosal disruption. The blood and edema fluid spread along the deep spaces of the larynx. In the subglottis the conus elasticus limits the spread circumferentially. Above the glottis the spread is primarily cephalocaudad in direction, extending along the paralaryngeal and pre-epiglottic spaces.[59] The resulting submucosal fluid narrows the airway. Localization of this compromise is essential. The plain film examination can be helpful, but the CT scan is the examination of choice. Contrast laryngography usually is contraindicated immediately after injury because of the narrowed airway. The mucosal alterations are best evaluated by contrast laryngoscopy or by direct laryngoscopy after the patient's condition has been stabilized.

Supraglottic injuries include transverse or vertical fractures of the thyroid cartilage. The epiglottis may be avulsed from the thyroid cartilage, resulting in hemorrhage into the pre-epiglottic space, with posterior displacement of the epiglottis. The arytenoid cartilages may also be dislocated.[59] These supraglottic injuries are associated with infection and granulation tissue–type healing, which if untreated results in a supraglottic stenosis.[3]

Glottic injuries occur as the thyroid cartilage is compressed against the cervical spine. The thyroid ala fractures and the support of both the true and false vocal cords can be absent.[59] Mucosal tears are common and cartilage fragments can be displaced into the larynx. The arytenoid cartilages can be avulsed or there can be recurrent nerve damage. The arytenoids most often are displaced anteriorly and superiorly, foreshortening the true vocal cords and often leaving them in the paramedian position, thus simulating a nerve paresis or paralysis.

Subglottic injuries primarily involve the cricoid cartilage. Because it forms a closed ring, cartilage separation requires at least two fracture sites, one usually involving the thin anterior arch and the second involving

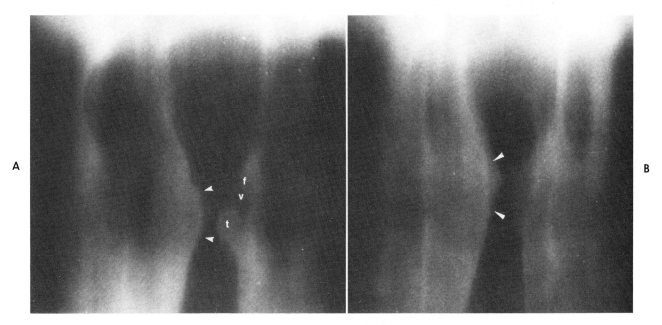

Fig. 11-27. Extensive laryngeal hematoma. **A,** Coronal tomogram at midcord level demonstrates larynx during modified Valsalva maneuver in patient with a laryngeal hematoma. Laryngeal hematoma produces confluent soft tissue mass in plane of right aryepiglottic fold, and false cord *(white arrowheads)*, ventricle, true cord, and subglottic larynx. Normal left hemilaryngeal structures are indicated. Modified Valsalva maneuver distends ventricle and pyriform sinuses. *f,* Left false cord; *t,* left true cord; *v,* left ventricle. **B,** Coronal tomogram taken during quiet breathing demonstrates abduction of left hemilarynx but preservation of outline of hematoma involving right half of larynx *(arrowheads)*. (From Zizmor, J., and Noyek, A.M.: An atlas of otolaryngologic radiology, Philadelphia, 1978, W.B. Saunders Co.)

the thicker posterior lamina. Hemorrhage and edema narrow the airway. Disruption of the cricothyroid joints can also contribute to dysfunction of the vocal cords. These fractures and soft tissue changes are best evaluated on CT scans. Conventional tomographic and contrast studies can outline the residual airway, but they rarely demonstrate the fracture site, the number of fractures, and the fracture segment displacement. The more calcified the laryngeal cartilages are and the greater the fracture displacement, the better the imaging of the laryngeal trauma (Figs. 11-27 to 11-30). Subcutaneous emphysema in the soft tissues of the neck may signal that an underlying laryngeal fracture is present (Fig. 11-31). Thyroid ala fractures can also be visualized by B-mode ultrasonography or by bone scanning (Fig. 11-32).

The major complications of trauma, after the securing of an airway, involve unfavorable healing of the displaced cartilages, with fibrosis and loss of cord function (Fig. 11-33). The immobile cord could be the result of a displaced arytenoid cartilage, recurrent laryngeal nerve damage, or simply fixation as a result of fibrosis. Early detection of the true extent of the trauma may lead to a decrease in the extent of the residual anatomic and functional deformities.

The supraglottic larynx and posterior commissure are most commonly exposed to thermal and chemical injury,[3] and resulting posterior laryngeal stenosis can occur (Fig. 11-34). Total laryngeal stenosis usually follows more extensive trauma (Fig. 11-35).

A variety of granulomas can affect the larynx. The contact ulcer and granuloma predominantly occur in adult men and are most likely the result of vocal abuse. The tips of the vocal processes of the arytenoid cartilage are traumatized during forceful speech. This results in an ulcer, and eventually cartilage is exposed. Healing occurs by granuloma formation[3] (Fig. 11-36).

Traumatic granulomas can be caused by endotracheal intubation and bronchoscopy. The lesions occur primarily in the posterior larynx and are more common in females. This probably relates to the smaller size and configuration of the female larynx and the thinner epithelium over the vocal processes of the arytenoids[3] (Fig. 11-37). Some granulomas can attain considerable size and may obstruct the airway[2] (Fig. 11-38).

Posterior granulomas can also rarely occur with gas-

Text continued on p. 440.

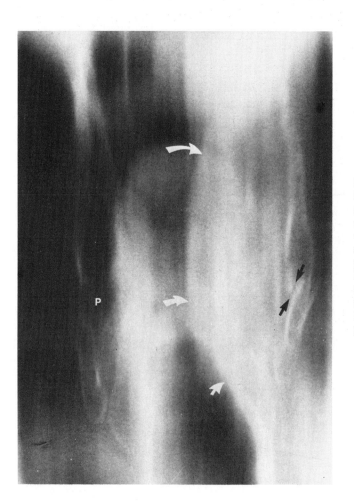

Fig. 11-28. Vertical fracture, thyroid ala. Coronal tomogram demonstrates overriding fracture line of left thyroid cartilage ala. Black arrows demonstrate overriding of internal calcified cortices on either side of fracture line. Massive hematoma involves entire left lateral laryngeal wall, from supraglottic to subglottic larynx *(white arrows)*. Hematoma extends into upper trachea, and entire left lateral pharyngeal wall is effaced by hemorrhage as well. Notice obliteration of left pyriform sinus as it is opacified by hematoma, in contrast with air-containing right pyriform sinus *(P)*. (From Zizmor, J., and Noyek, A.M.: An atlas of otolaryngologic radiology, Philadelphia, 1978, W.B. Saunders Co.)

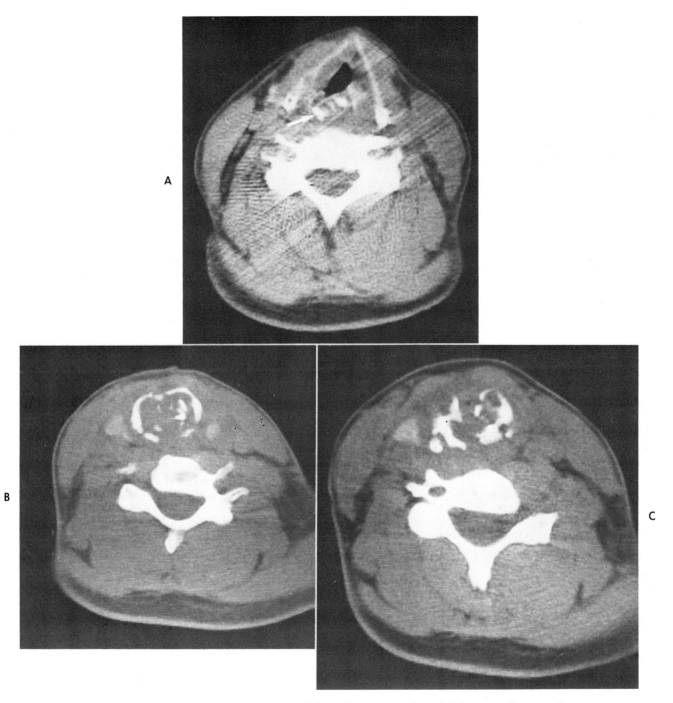

Fig. 11-29. A, CT scan reveals flattening of thyroid anterior angle and dislocation of arytenoid cartilages. Right arytenoid cartilage is displaced far posteriorly *(arrow).* **B,** CT scan on different patient than **A** reveals diffuse fragmentation of thyroid and cricoid cartilages and obliteration of airway. **C,** CT scan on another patient reveals comminuted cricoid cartilage fracture with obliteration of airway.

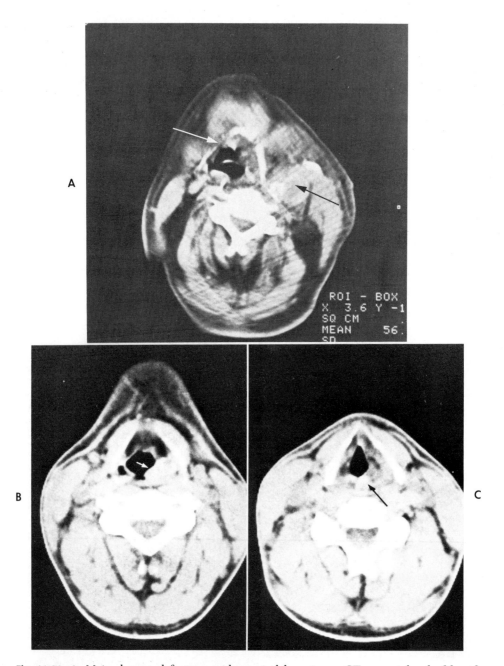

Fig. 11-30. A, Major laryngeal fracture with cervical hematoma. CT scan at level of hyoid bone indicates dysruption of hyoid arch laterally by laryngeal trauma. Body of hyoid bone has been fractured *(white arrow)* on right, at its junction with greater cornua; notice medially displaced bone fragment. Larynx is displaced from midline by huge deep cervical hematoma *(black arrow)* on left. **B,** CT scan of different patient reveals hematoma of left aryepiglottic fold *(arrow).* **C,** CT scan at lower level reveals lower margin of hematoma and medial displacement of arytenoid cartilage *(arrow).* (From Noyek, A.M., et al.: Radiologic evaluation of the larynx. In Bailey, B.J.: Surgery of the larynx, Philadelphia, W.B. Saunders Co. [in press].)

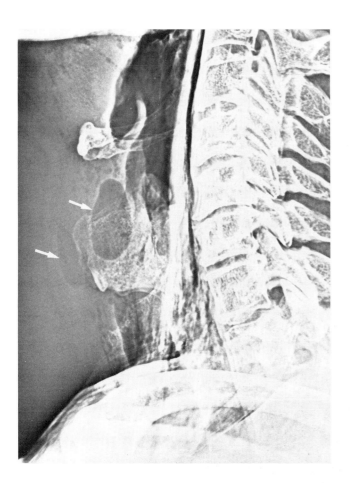

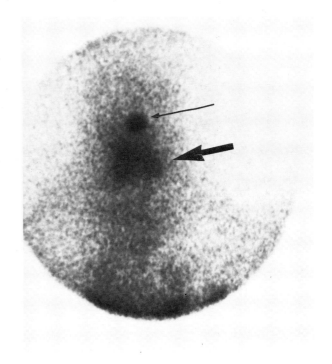

Fig. 11-31. Laryngeal fracture with cervical emphysema. Lateral xeroradiograph of larynx demonstrates two large collections of entapped air *(arrows)* following thyroid cartilage fracture. Air is also seen under prevertebral fascia and within paratracheal soft tissues. These are secondary signs of laryngeal fracture; fracture line itself is not seen. (From Noyek, A.M., Steinhardt, M.I., and Zizmor, J.: Otolaryngol. Clin. North Am. 2[2]:445, 1978.)

Fig. 11-32. Laryngeal fracture with positive bone scan image. Anterior view of delayed bone scan demonstrates increased uptake of bone scan agent by thyroid cartilage vertical fracture. Increased uptake is seen diffusely throughout entire thyroid cartilage *(heavy black arrow).* Thin black arrow indicates marker placed on thyroid prominence. (From Noyek, A.M.: Laryngoscope **89**[9 pt. 2]:1, 1979.)

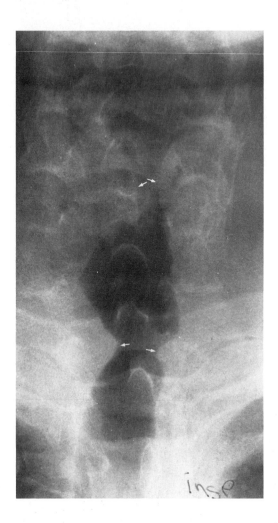

Fig. 11-33. Posttraumatic laryngeal and tracheal stenosis. AP high-kilovolt selective filtration radiograph taken during inspiration demonstrates fixation and distortion of right hemilarynx *(upper right arrow)* that resulted from previous extensive trauma and scarring. Left half of larynx moves in abduction *(upper left arrow),* while right side of larynx remains in paramedian position. There is narrow hourglass segment of transverse tracheal stenosis *(lower white arrows)* in lower cervical trachea.

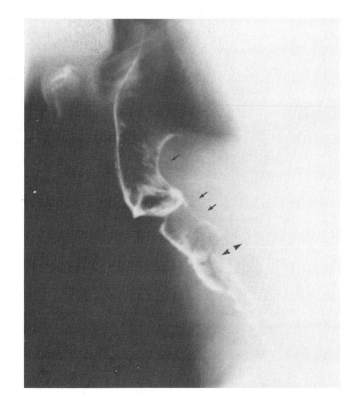

Fig. 11-34. Posterior laryngeal stenosis caused by thermal injury. Lateral view of laryngogram demonstrates great increase in soft tissues in plane of arytenoids *(upper black arrow)* extending inferiorly into subglottic larynx *(lower parallel black arrows).* Here, posterior segment of airway is narrowed by hypertrophic soft tissue response to thermal injury of larynx. Paired black arrowheads demonstrate upper limits of Montgomery T tube that had been positioned following tracheal resection for a segmental stenosis, which also resulted from same injury. (Courtesy Dr. J. Cooper, Toronto. From Zizmor, J., and Noyek, A.M.: An atlas of otolaryngologic radiology, Philadelphia, 1978, W.B. Saunders Co.)

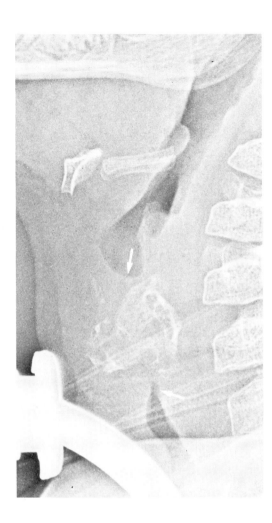

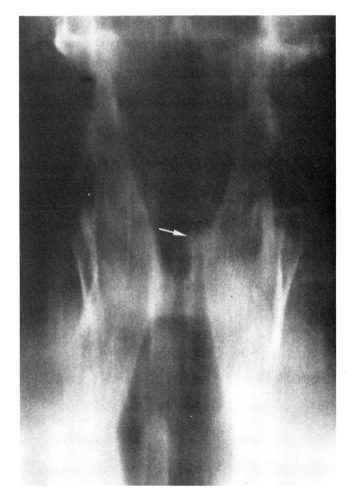

Fig. 11-35. Total laryngeal stenosis, postsurgery. Lateral xeroradiograph demonstrates total laryngeal stenosis resulting from infection that followed a tracheostomy performed through circoid cartilage. Notice excellent edge-enhancement effect of xeroradiograph in demonstrating mucous membrane at superior and inferior margins of totally obstructed air column *(upper and lower white arrows).* (From Noyek, A.M.: J. Otolaryngol. 5[6]:468, 1976.)

Fig. 11-36. Contact granuloma caused by vocal abuse. AP tomogram in region of posterior commissure of larynx demonstrates smooth, soft tissue projection *(white arrow)* profiled against left aryepiglottic fold above vocal process of arytenoid cartilage. This is well seen in inspiration and occupies classic location of contact granuloma. (From Zizmor, J., and Noyek, A.M.: An atlas of otolaryngologic radiology, Philadelphia, 1978, W.B. Saunders Co.)

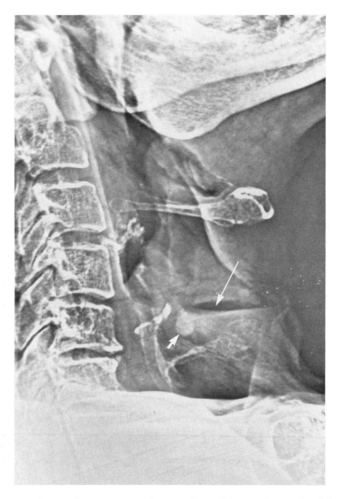

Fig. 11-37. Arytenoid granuloma, postintubation. Lateral xeroradiograph of larynx demonstrates small discrete polypoid mass projecting inferiorly from vocal process of right arytenoid cartilage. Sharp mucosal detail of granuloma as a result of edge-enhancement effect is well seen *(lower white arrow).* Superimposed air shadow of ventricles is noted *(upper white arrow).* Notice also sharp imaging of superior surface of superimposed vocal cords bordering ventricles.

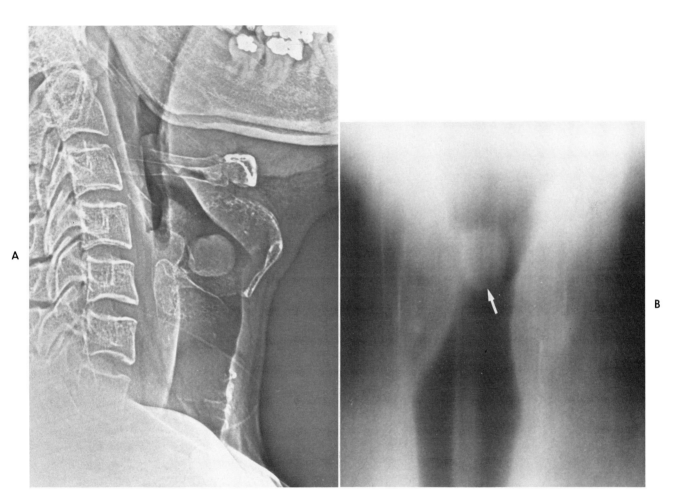

Fig. 11-38. Postintubation granuloma. **A,** Lateral xeroradiograph defines large discrete granuloma occupying major portion of airway at level of glottis. This lesion arises from vocal process of right arytenoid cartilage. **B,** Coronal tomogram of larynx taken during inspiration demonstrates abduction of both halves of larynx. Large contact granuloma *(arrow)* is visualized profiled against airway.

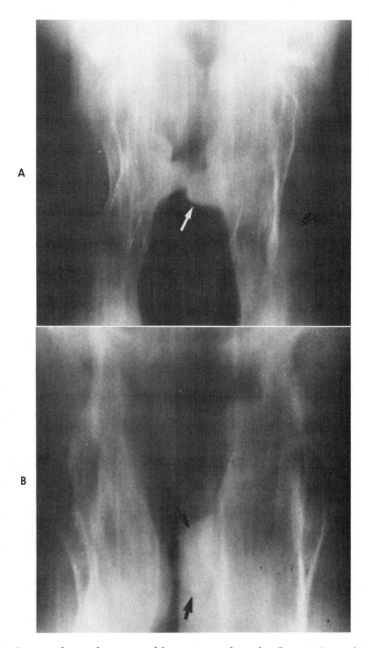

Fig. 11-39. Laryngeal granuloma caused by gastroesophageal reflux. **A,** Coronal tomogram of larynx in phonation demonstrates smoothly outlined granuloma arising from free margin and subglottic surface of left vocal cord (*arrow*). It is attached to posterior two thirds of left vocal cord. **B,** Coronal tomogram of larynx during quiet breathing profiles granuloma (*arrows*) as both vocal cords abduct. (From Goldberg, M., Noyek, A.M., and Pritzker, K.P.H.: J. Otolaryngol. 7[3]:196, 1978.)

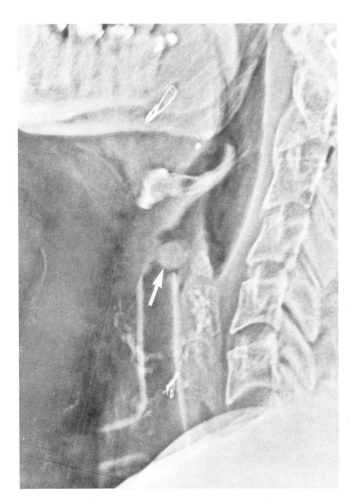

Fig. 11-40. Laryngeal granuloma caused by indwelling Montgomery T tube. Lateral xeroradiograph demonstrates discrete granuloma *(white arrow)* arising at cord level in relation to upper extent of Montgomery T tube. Anterior attachment of laryngeal granuloma is clearly seen.

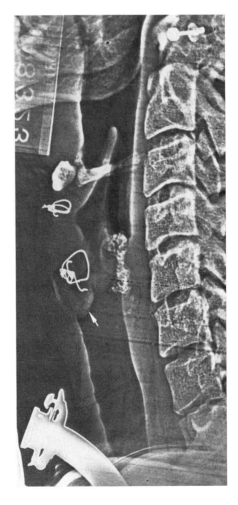

Fig. 11-41. Subglottic granuloma following laryngeal surgery. Lateral xeroradiograph demonstrates anterior subglottic granuloma *(arrow)* following extensive laryngeal surgery. (From Noyek, A.M., et al.: J. Otolaryngol. **6**[suppl. 3]:73, 1977.)

troesophageal reflux[24] (Fig. 11-39) and as the result of indwelling stents (Figs. 11-40 and 11-41).

■ Cystic lesions

There are a variety of cystic lesions that involve the larynx. True cysts (epithelial-lined, fluid-filled sacs) usually result from obstruction of a minor seromucinous gland in the supraglottis. The most common locations are in the valleculae, epiglottis, and aryepiglottic folds. These cysts may be present at birth and may be mucosal or submucosal in position. Most are small asymptomatic lesions. However, large cysts can compromise the airway[3,4] (Figs. 11-42 and 11-43).

The laryngocele develops from the normal laryngeal ventricle and saccule (appendix). The ventricles are recognized in the developing larynx by the second fetal

month and extend far laterally under the floor of the pharynx. The appendix may be related to the fourth branchial cleft. At birth the appendix is still relatively large; however, by age 6 it begins to regress in size in relation to the remaining larynx and in the normal adult it is a small rudimentary structure opening into the upper anterior ventricle. These appendixes are more common in men than women (7:1 ratio) and tend to be larger in white than in black people. Almost 90% occur clinically in whites.[3,4] Laryngoceles are very rare in children; when they occur in adults they are believed to be related to activities that increase intralaryngeal pressure, i.e., coughing, straining, glass blowing, playing a wind instrument, etc. Dilatation or herniation of the appendix beyond a range associated with the various stages of development and age represents a laryn-

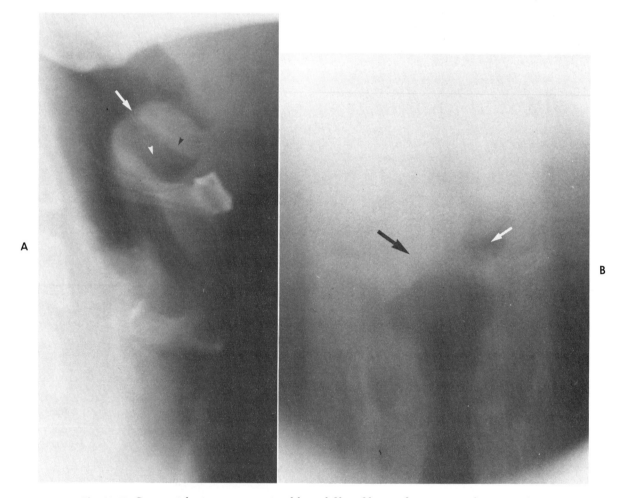

Fig. 11-42. Cyst, epiglottis. **A,** conventional lateral film of larynx demonstrates large cyst (*arrow*) arising from lingual surface of epiglottis, on its right side. Cyst is superimposed on air-containing shadow of left vallecula (*white arrowhead*). Anterior one third of cyst is superimposed on shadow of base of tongue (*black arrowhead*). **B,** AP tomogram in quiet breathing demonstrates mass lesion to right of midline in suprahyoid larynx (*black arrow*); air shadow within left vallecula is indicated by white arrow.

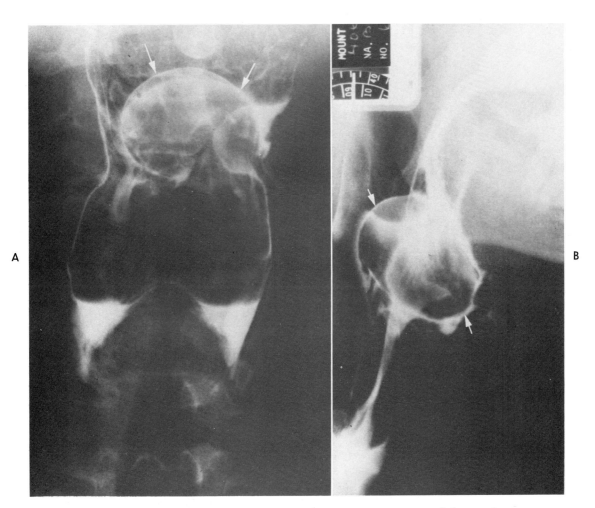

Fig. 11-43. Massive supraglottic retention cyst. **A,** Anteroposterior view with barium demonstrates massive, smooth, round mass *(arrows)* occupying valleculae and displacing epiglottis inferiorly. It arose from lingual surface of epiglottis, presumably as mucous retention cyst caused by obstruction of minor seromucinous gland. Both pyriform sinuses are well filled. **B,** Lateral view of same examination demonstrates relationship of this enormous retention cyst *(arrows)* in hypopharynx. (From Zizmor, J., and Noyek, A.M.: An atlas of otolaryngologic radiology, Philadelphia, 1978, W.B. Saunders Co.)

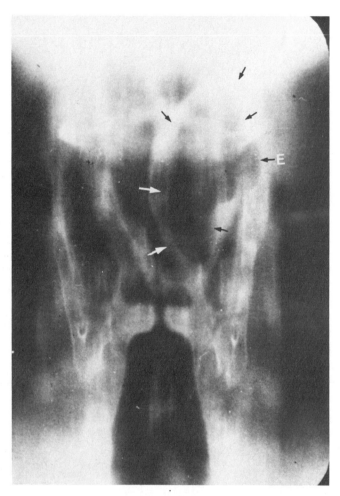

Fig. 11-44. Mixed laryngocele. Coronal tomogram during phonation demonstrates large air sac *(arrows)* displacing left aryepiglottic fold medially and encroaching on supraglottic airway. Notice small external component to laryngocele *(E)* in region of left thyrohyoid membrane. Smooth, uniform displacement of mucous membrane in this region demonstrates classic radiographic appearance of an internal laryngocele. (From Zizmor, J., and Noyek, A.M.: Semin. Roentgenol. **9**[4]:311, 1974.)

gocele. They usually are air-filled sacs communicating with the laryngeal ventricle.[4] They may be unilateral or bilateral and may be internal, external (lying in the neck lateral to the thyrohyoid membrane), or mixed (internal and external). The internal laryngoceles extend cephalad, medial to the thyroid cartilage, and appear as submucosal supraglottic masses (Fig. 11-44). The external laryngocele often appears as a mass in the lateral neck that can be easily demonstrated to be air-containing on Valsalva maneuver soft tissue films. The internal component of these laryngoceles connecting them with the laryngeal ventricle apparently collapses (Fig. 11-45). The mixed or combined laryngocele can also be demonstrated radiographically. In these cases, both components are distended (Fig. 11-46).[106]

If the orifice of the appendix becomes obstructed, the laryngocele can become filled with a sterile mucinous material, forming a mucocele (Fig. 11-47). Rarely these secretions can become infected, creating a laryngopyocele.

■ Tumors

Benign tumors of the larynx are rare when compared to the more common occurrence of laryngeal malignancies. The most common benign lesion is the papilloma, which occurs either singly or as multiple warty masses primarily of the true vocal cords, although they may rarely occur in the supraglottis and subglottis.[3] On the glottic level they often involve both true cords primarily along their superior surfaces or free margins and

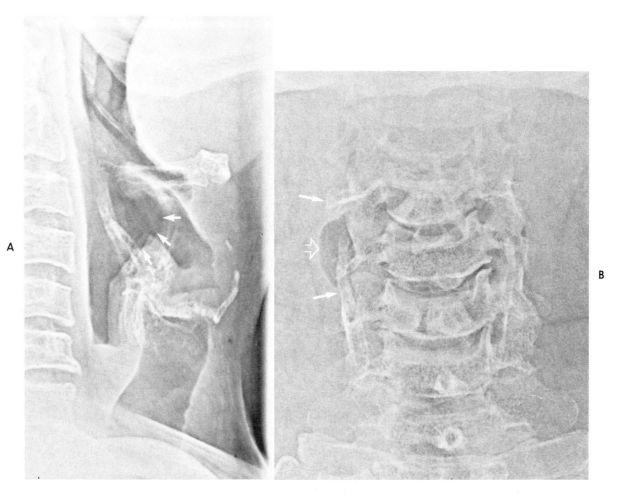

Fig. 11-45. External laryngocele. **A,** Lateral xeroradiograph of larynx demonstrates superimposed air shadow of external laryngocele *(arrows)* on laryngeal lumen. **B,** AP xeroradiograph demonstrates anatomic relationships of right external laryngocele *(hollow arrow)* herniating through thyrohyoid membrane between hyoid bone above *(upper solid arrow)* and thyroid cartilage below *(lower solid arrow).* (From Noyek, A.M., et al.: J. Otolaryngol. **6**[suppl. 3]:73, 1977.)

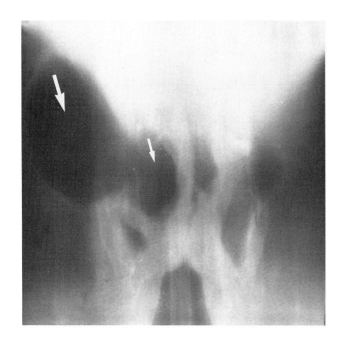

Fig. 11-46. Large combined external-internal laryngocele. AP tomogram demonstrates large dumbbell-shaped air cyst producing so-called double bubble sign. Small white arrow demonstrates internal component of laryngocele; large white arrow demonstrates external component. Supraglottic mucosa is displaced across midline, as frequently occurs, obscuring glottis to clinical examination from above. (From Noyek, A.M., et al.: Radiologic evaluation of the larynx. In Bailey, B.J.: Surgery of the larynx, Philadelphia, in W.B. Saunders Co. [in press].)

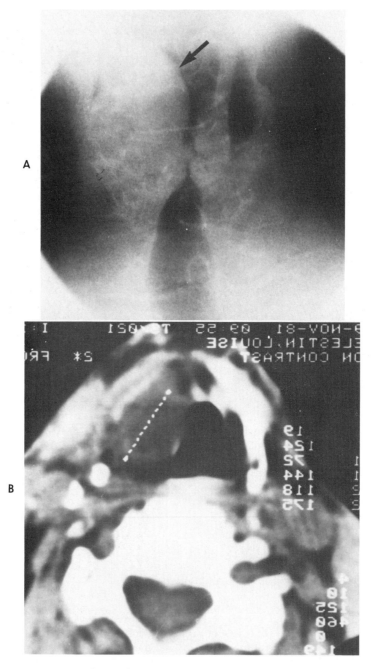

Fig. 11-47. A, Laryngopyocele. AP high-kilovolt selective filtration film of larynx demonstrates large oval, cystic, expansile soft tissue mass occupying entire right aryepiglottic fold *(arrow)* and encroaching on airway. Right pyriform sinus is effaced by lesion, as compared with air-filled left pyriform sinus. **B,** CT scan reveals ovoid low-attenuation right supraglottic mass *(dashed line). Mucocele.* (**A** From Zizmor, J., and Noyek, A.M.: An atlas of otolaryngologic radiology, Philadelphia, 1978, W.B. Saunders Co.)

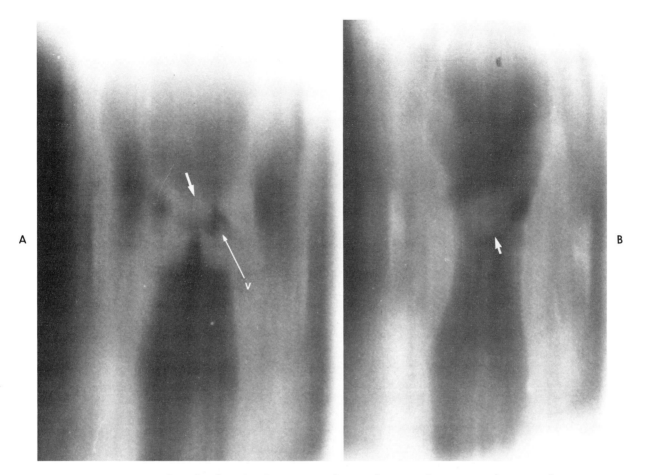

Fig. 11-48. Vocal cord polyp. **A,** AP tomogram during phonation demonstrates large round mass *(arrow)*, apparently arising from superior surface of right vocal cord. Vocal cords are seen in approximation. Polyp arises anteriorly, adjacent to anterior commissure. Left ventricle is well shown *(V)*; polyp obscures imaging of right ventricle. **B,** AP tomogram during inspiration demonstrates polyp *(arrow)* profiled against air column following abduction of both halves of larynx.

they may rarely cause glottic airway compromise. Radiographically they are impossible to distinguish from true cord carcinomas unless they are pedunculated polypoid masses (Fig. 11-48).

Multiple papillomas of the larynx (see congenital lesions, p. 418) have already been discussed. In children there is virtually no malignant potential; however, in the adult there may be some question as to whether or not malignancies can rarely occur[4] (Figs. 11-49 to 11-51).

The laryngeal chondroma is a rare tumor that arises in mature hyaline cartilage.[10] It usually arises along the cricoid lamina on its inner surface, which causes subglottic airway narrowing (Fig. 11-52).[87] Less often it arises from the thyroid, arytenoid, or epiglottic cartilages. Clinically, chondromas are firm masses with in-

tact overlying mucosa. Radiographically they have coarse areas of calcifications within the tumor mass and are indistinguishable from chondrosarcomas.[101,107,108]

Hemangiomas may be either congenital malformations or neoplasms (see p. 418). In infants they occur most frequently in the subglottis, while in adults they occur primarily at the glottic and supraglottic levels.[4] In infants there is an association with cutaneous hemangiomata (Sturge-Weber disease). As an isolated lesion it can be either pendunculated or sessile. Phleboliths may be seen and are indicative of the diagnosis (Fig. 11-53).

Neurofibromas are very rare lesions of the larynx. Most occur in the aryepiglottic folds or in the false cords[4] (Fig. 11-54).

Other rare benign tumors include fibromas, myomas, lipomas, paragangliomas, and angiofibromas. The CT

Text continued on p. 451.

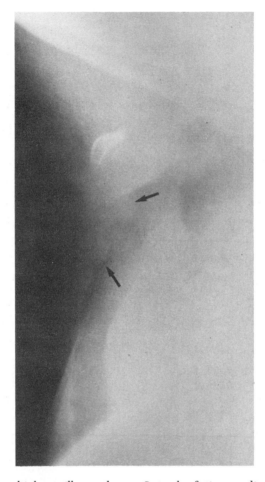

Fig. 11-49. Juvenile multiple papillomas, larynx. Lateral soft tissue radiograph of larynx demonstrates multiple, small, polypoid soft tissue densities along anterior wall of upper trachea, subglottic larynx, and anterior commissure to level of base of epiglottis *(arrows)*. (From Zizmor, J., and Noyek, A.M.: Semin. Roentgenol. **9**[4]:311, 1974.)

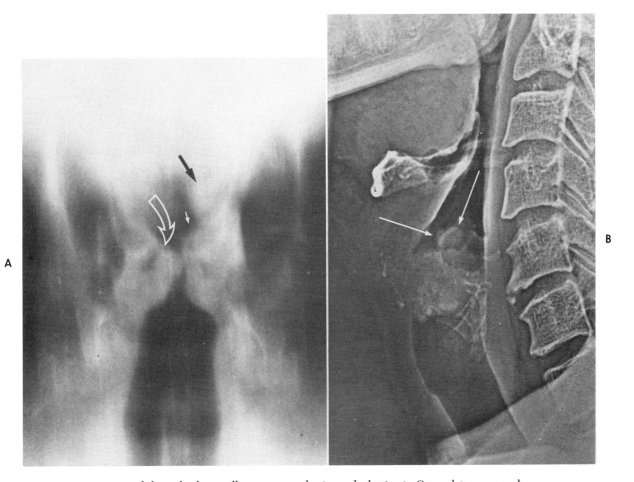

Fig. 11-50. Adult multiple papillomas, supraglottis, and glottis. **A,** Coronal tomogram demonstrates multiple papillomas involving larynx at glottic and supraglottic levels. Hollow white arrow points to large papilloma occupying superior surface of right vocal cord, abutting against opposite ventricular band during phonation. Small white arrow demonstrates papilloma of left ventricular band, and black arrow demonstrates papilloma arising from left aryepiglottic fold. **B,** Lateral xeroradiograph of the larynx profiles two discrete papillomas (*arrows*). (From Zizmor, J., and Noyek, A.M.: An atlas of otolaryngologic radiology, Philadelphia, 1978, W.B. Saunders Co.)

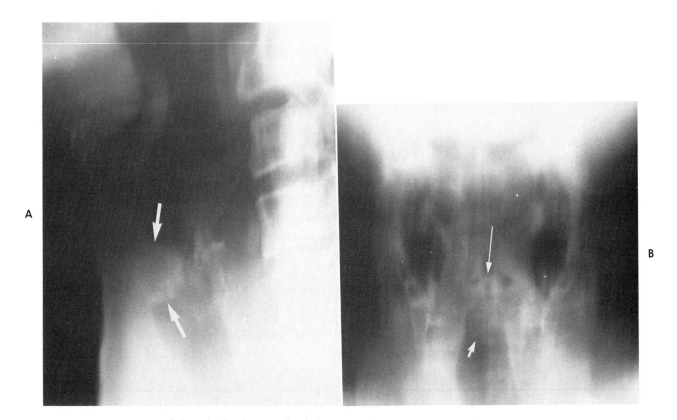

Fig. 11-51. Adult multiple glottic and subglottic papillomas. **A,** Lateral radiograph of the larynx demonstrates large mass of papillomas arising anteriorly *(arrows)* at glottic and subglottic levels. **B,** AP tomogram demonstrates mass of papillomas projecting into subglottic space *(lower arrow)*. Papilloma is also seen at level of ventricles (profiled by air) *(upper arrow)*.

Fig. 11-52. A, Chondroma. Lateral radiograph of larynx demonstrates sharply defined rounded mass *(arrow)*, chondroma, arising from posterior lamina of cricoid cartilage on its internal surface. It extends anteriorly to diminish laryngeal airway by 50%. Chondroma was impinging on right vocal cord, producing fixation. There is no radiologic evidence of macroscopic calcification or ossification, and inferior extent of lesion is at level of second tracheal ring. **B,** Chondrosarcoma, larynx. Lateral radiograph demonstrates low-grade chondrosarcoma arising from internal surface of posterior lamina of cricoid cartilage *(arrows)*. It extends upwards to level of arytenoid eminence, encroaching on laryngeal airway, diminishing it by less than 50% in anteroposterior diameter. Multiple foci of coarse calcification are present, a diagnostic feature. **C,** Chondrosarcoma. Axial CT scan reveals irregular calcifications within tumor mass involving right thyroid cartilage and cricoid lamina. Left side of larynx is normal. (**A** and **B** From Zizmor, J., Noyek, A.M., and Lewis, J.S.: Arch Otolaryngol. **101**:232, 1975. **B** Also courtesy Dr. R.D.R. Briant, Toronto.)

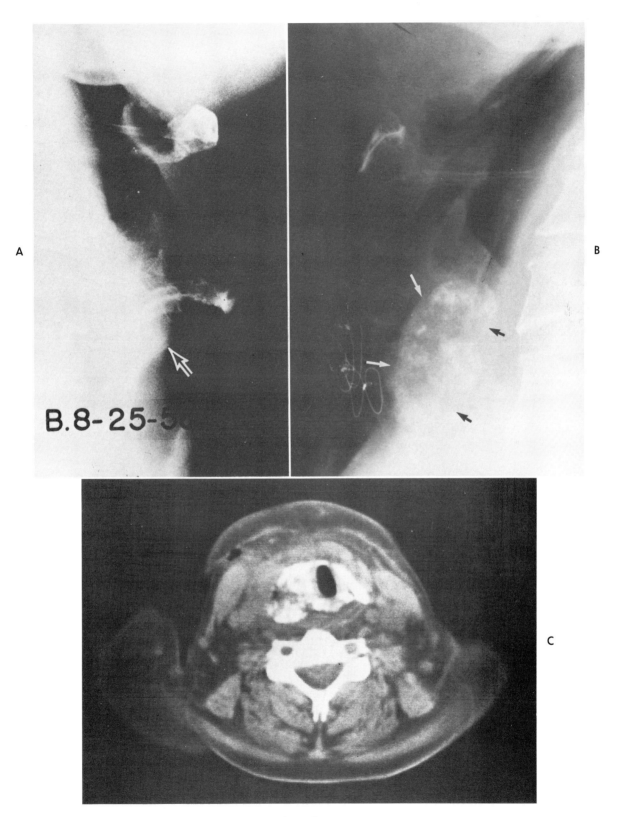

Fig. 11-52. For legend see opposite page.

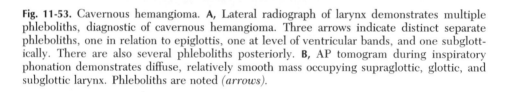

Fig. 11-53. Cavernous hemangioma. **A,** Lateral radiograph of larynx demonstrates multiple phleboliths, diagnostic of cavernous hemangioma. Three arrows indicate distinct separate phleboliths, one in relation to epiglottis, one at level of ventricular bands, and one subglottically. There are also several phleboliths posteriorly. **B,** AP tomogram during inspiratory phonation demonstrates diffuse, relatively smooth mass occupying supraglottic, glottic, and subglottic larynx. Phleboliths are noted *(arrows)*.

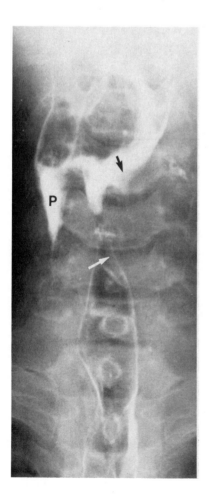

Fig. 11-54. Neuroma, pyriform sinus. AP laryngogram outlines neuroma occupying entire left pyriform sinus *(black arrow)*; notice normal configuration of right pyriform sinus *(P)*. Subglottic larynx is displaced somewhat to right *(white arrow)*. (Courtesy Dr. P. Som, New York.)

scan should help in establishing the diagnosis of lipomas, and enhancement should occur with the vascular lesions.

The subject of laryngeal malignancy deals almost exclusively with squamous cell carcinomas, which include over 90% of all laryngeal epithelial neoplasms. Only carcinoma of the lung is a more common tumor of the respiratory tract and oral cavity.[4]

Several causative factors are associated with larynx cancer. Pipe and cigar smoking are commonly implicated and studies have shown that laryngeal cancer rarely develops in men who do not smoke.[102]

Irradiation for "benign lymphomata" of the neck and thyroid disease was practiced in the 1920s through the 1950s. Nearly 10% of patients with laryngeal cancer had this type of prior irradiation with intervals of 10 to 30 years between the radiation and the development of the tumor.[4]

Alcoholism has also been associated with all oral cavity and upper respiratory tract cancers and laryngeal cancer is almost eight times more common in men than it is in women.[96]

The key to successful management of laryngeal cancer is early diagnosis and treatment. The radiologist can provide more detailed information today than ever before. The surgeon also has developed new techniques for treating larynx cancer. Conservation surgery, which aims to preserve some voice function, requires the most accurate radiologic analysis for patient selection. A total laryngectomy is now reserved only for those patients that do not meet the criteria for a conservative operation.

In order to evaluate treatment success in various institutions, a common classification had to be used so that all physicians could be confident that they were comparing similar cases. The TNM classification (see box) is the most acceptable common language that fulfills these criteria. It is a clinical classification based on the estimation of the tumor's location and extent and on the presence or absence of distant metastases. The

---

The TNM Classification

Supraglottis
TIS Carcinoma in situ
T1   Tumor confined to the site of origin with normal mobility
T2   Tumor involves adjacent supraglottic site(s) or the glottis without fixation
T3   Tumor limited to the larynx with fixation or extension to involve the postcricoid area, the medial wall of the pyriform sinuses, or the pre-epiglottic space
T4   Massive tumor extending beyond the larynx to involve the oropharynx or soft tissues of the neck or destruction of the thyroid cartilage

Glottis
TIS Carcinoma in situ
T1   Tumor is confined to the vocal cord(s) with normal mobility (includes involvement of the anterior or the posterior commissure)
T2   Supraglottic or subglottic extension of the tumor with normal or impaired cord mobility
T3   Tumor confined to the larynx with cord fixation
T4   Massive tumor with thyroid cartilage destruction or extension beyond the confines of the larynx

Subglottis
TIS Carcinoma in situ
T1   Tumor confined to the subglottic region
T2   Tumor extension to the vocal cords with normal or impaired cord mobility
T3   Tumor confined to the larynx with cord fixation
T4   Massive tumor with cartilage destruction or extension beyond the confines of the larynx

Nodal involvement
N0   No clinically positive nodes
N1   Single clinically positive ipsilateral node 3 cm or less in diameter
N2   Single clinically positive ipsilateral node more than 3 cm, but not more than 6 cm in diameter
N2b Multiple clinically positive ipsilateral nodes, none more than 6 cm in diameter
N3   Massive ipsilateral node(s), bilateral nodes, or contralateral node(s)
N3a Clinically positive ipsilateral node(s), one more than 6 cm in diameter
N3b Bilateral clinically positive nodes
N3c Contralateral clinically positive node(s) only.
Metastasis
M0   No (known) distant metastasis
M1   Distinct metastasis is present
Stages
     Stage I   T1 N0 M0
     Stage II   T2 N0 M0
     Stage III   T3 N0 M0, (T1, T2, or T3) N1 M0
     Stage IV   T4 N0 M0, T4 N1 M0
                 any T, N2 or N3, M0
                 any T, any N, M1

radiologist plays an important role in this staging process.

For the purposes of classification the anatomic boundaries of the larynx are defined as follows.

The anterior limit: the posterior surface of the suprahyoid portion of the epiglottis, the thyrohyoid membrane, and the anterior margins of the thyroid cartilage, the cricothyroid membrane and the anterior arch of the cricoid cartilage.

The posterior limit: the aryepiglottic folds, the arytenoid region, the interarytenoid space, and the respiratory mucosa covering the cricoid cartilage (posterior subglottis).

The superior limit: the tip and lateral borders of the epiglottis and the free edges of the aryepiglottic folds.

The inferior limit: a plane passing through the inferior edge of the cricoid cartilage.

Excluded from the larynx by this definition are the lateral and posterior pharyngeal walls, the pyriform sinuses, the postcricoid area, the valleculae, and the base of the tongue.

The larynx is further subdivided into the following regions.

Supraglottis: the false cords, ventricles and the laryngeal surfaces of the arytenoids, epiglottis and the aryepiglottic folds.

Glottis: the true vocal cords including the anterior commissure.

Subglottis: the area below the true cords extending to the lower limit of the larynx.

Out of all laryngeal cancers, about 60% to 70% of the lesions are glottic tumors, about 30% to 35% supraglottic tumors, and only 4% to 6% subglottic tumors.

There are several clinical and pathologic observations regarding lymph node metastases and tumor spread that should be considered while radiographically evaluating the larynx.[20] They help identify high-risk patients and those patients who may benefit more from a CT scan examination.

Tumor size, location, and histologic grading must all be considered when placing a lesion in a high-risk category for lymph node metastases. Overall, metastases are more common when the primary tumor is greater than 2 cm in diameter and is poorly differentiated. Nodal disease is more common, in descending order of frequency, in supraglottic lesions, subglottic tumors, and transglottic tumors (cancers that cross the ventricles) than in glottic cancers. The ossified portions of the laryngeal cartilages offer the least resistance to tumor spread and therefore are the most likely areas of extralaryngeal extension.[4]

Most supraglottic cancers tend to remain supraglottic, and as long as the anterior commissure is not involved clinically a supraglottic laryngectomy can be performed. Similarly, supraglottic tumors tend not to invade the thyroid cartilage unless the tumor extends below the anterior commissure. Most supraglottic lesions invade the pre-epiglottic and paraglottic spaces, where there is a higher incidence of lymph node metastases. In fact, lymph node metastases are the greatest cause of failure of supraglottic laryngectomies.

Most glottic cancers do not invade the supraglottis. If extralaryngeal spread occurs it usually is by way of anterior commissure cartilage penetration or violation of the cricoarytenoid membrane. Anterior commissure extension also allows subglottic spread and penetration of the cricothyroid membrane. Glottic tumors with cord fixation have a higher incidence of nodal disease than mobile glottic lesions. In fact, metastases may be possible in glottic cancers only when the neoplasm has spread beyond the limits of the true cords.[4] Perineural and vascular invasion are found in about 25% of glottic cancers, and most glottic lesions occur in the anterior half of the cord.

Early glottic carcinomas have the best prognosis, with a 5-year survival rate of nearly 90%. T1 and T2 lesions can be treated by either conservation surgery or radiation therapy; however, hemilaryngectomy is the treatment of choice if there is involvement of the anterior commissure. Once a T3 or T4 tumor size is reached, the 5-year survival rate drops to 50%, and nearly 25% of these patients have metastases to cervical lymph nodes. If clinically positive nodes are detected at the initial appearance of the lesion, the survival rate drops to 20%.[4] T3 and T4 lesions do best with total laryngectomies.

Subglottic cancers have 5-year survival rates of only about 40% whether treated by irradiation or surgery, and the most common cause of failure is lymph node metastases.

From the above discussion, the radiologic points of particular interest include (1) the lowermost limit of a supraglottic tumor, especially in relationship to the anterior commissure, (2) the evaluation of the lateral extent of a supraglottic mass into the pyriform sinus or the superior extent into the vallecula, (3) determining if pre-epiglottic and paraglottic space invasion has occurred, (4) the evaluation of cord fixation in glottic cancer, (5) the involvement of the anterior commissure and the degree of subglottic extension, (6) whether or not cartilage is invaded, and (7) evaluation of cervical nodal metastases.[61]

The two main laryngeal conservation operations are the supraglottic laryngectomy and the hemilaryngectomy. The former requires that no tumor extend into the glottis and the latter requires limited subglottic extension; specifically, that normal mucosa remain to cover the cricoid cartilage. If there is involvement of the cricoid cartilage or its mucosa, a hemilaryngectomy should not be performed. If it is done under these circumstances, there is an increased incidence of recurrence, and airway obstruction as a result of the loss of the supporting cartilage ring occurs.

Specific radiographic demonstration of supraglottic tumors and their margins can reveal epiglottic carcinoma and its inferior extent (Figs. 11-55 and 11-56), its surface irregularity and extent (Fig. 11-57), its extension onto the lingual surface of the epiglottis (Fig. 11-58), and any tumor involvement of the base of the tongue and pharynx (Figs. 11-59 to 11-61). The degree

of airway compromise (Fig. 11-62), tumor extension into the pyriform sinus and glottis (Figs. 11-63 and 11-65), and involvement of the false cord (Figs. 11-66 to 11-68) all can be seen.

Glottic carcinomas can be shown to extend into the laryngeal ventricle (Figs. 11-69 and 11-70), the subglottis (Figs. 11-71 and 11-72), or the anterior commissure (Fig. 11-73). The presence of a laryngocele may occasionally be seen with a glottic carcinoma extending into the ventricle (Fig. 11-74). Cord fixation can be demonstrated (Figs. 11-75 to 11-77), although it may be difficult at times to differentiate between muscular infiltration and recurrent laryngeal nerve paralysis. Dilatation

Text continued on p. 471.

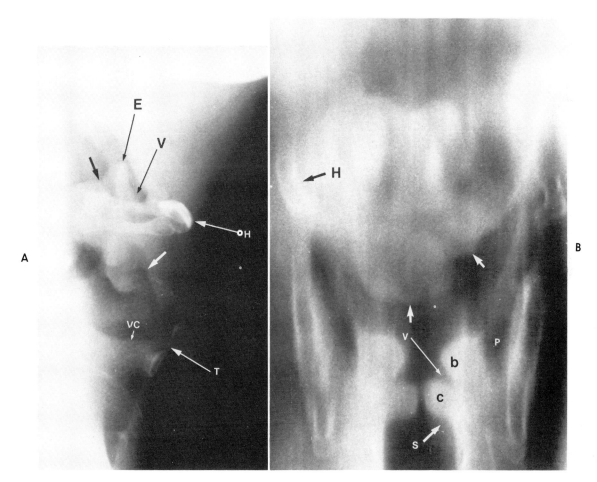

Fig. 11-55. A, Soft tissue lateral film demonstrates bulky exophytic carcinoma arising from laryngeal surface of epiglottis. Its origin is indicated by black arrow above and white arrow below. *H,* Hyoid bone; *v,* vallecula; *E,* epiglottic tip, *T,* anterior commissure region; *vc,* superimposed upper surface of vocal cords. **B,** Coronal tomogram during phonation demonstrates height and width of lesion. Inferior aspect of this lobulated tumor is indicated by two short white arrows. On right side it appears to extend laterally to hyoid bone *(H).* Coronal tomogram confirms integrity of glottic and immediate supraglottic structures. *b,* Left false cord; *c,* left vocal cord; *v,* left ventricle; *s,* left subglottic angle; *p,* left pyriform sinus. All of these structures are uninvolved by cancer extension.

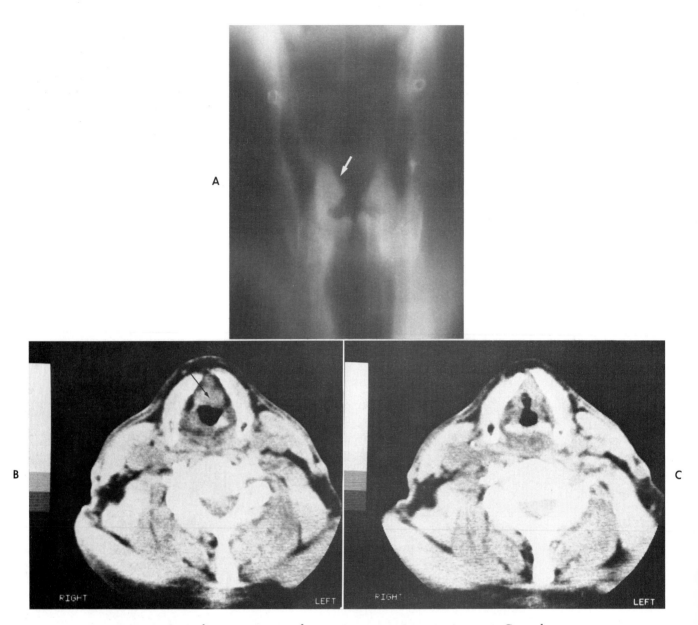

Fig. 11-56. Supraglottic carcinoma with extension to anterior commissure. **A,** Coronal tomogram during phonation demonstrates fullness of right ventricular band, with some irregularity *(arrow),* in 71-year-old man. Left ventricular band also has some measure of irregularity. Superior surfaces of both vocal cords appear clear and both ventricles are adequately seen. Notice suggestion of tumor bulging into roof of ventricle on each side. **B,** CT scan shows squamous cell carcinoma *(black arrow).* Its axial supraglottic dimension is well appreciated, as is its bilateral and anterior extension. **C,** Lower CT scan demonstrates midline anterior commissure extension of squamous cell carcinoma in relation to vocal cords. Patient was therefore unacceptable candidate for conservation surgery by partial supraglottic laryngectomy.

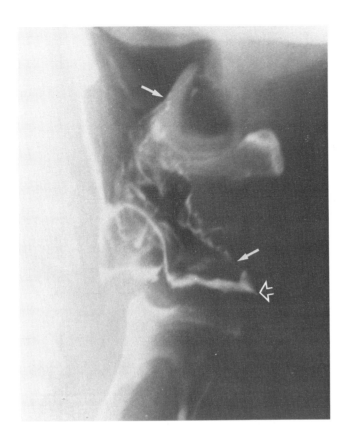

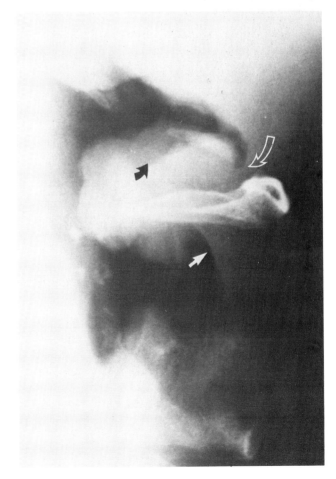

Fig. 11-57. Carcinoma, laryngeal surface of epiglottis. Lateral view of laryngogram demonstrates irregular mucosal surface of exophytic and ulcerative squamous cell carcinoma confined to laryngeal surface of epiglottis. Mucosal irregularity can be observed from immediately below free margin of tip of epiglottis *(upper solid white arrow)* to lowest portion of laryngeal surface of epiglottis *(lower solid white arrow)*, immediately above insertion of vocal cords at anterior commissure *(hollow white arrow)*. (From Zizmor, J., and Noyek, A.M.: An atlas of otolaryngologic radiology, Philadelphia, 1978, W.B. Saunders Co.)

Fig. 11-58. Bulky carcinoma, epiglottis, with vallecular extension. Lateral radiograph demonstrates bulky carcinoma involving lingual and laryngeal surfaces of epiglottis as well as its free margin. It overhangs vestibule, obstructing laryngeal airway to large measure. Curved black arrow points to area of ulceration involving superior surface of tumor. Tumor's relationship to depth of valleculae, as it involves base of tongue, is well demonstrated *(hollow white arrow)*. Notice that infrahyoid laryngeal surface of epiglottis is free of tumor *(solid white arrow)*. (From Zizmor, J., and Noyek, A.M.: An atlas of otolaryngologic radiology, Philadelphia, 1978, W.B. Saunders Co.)

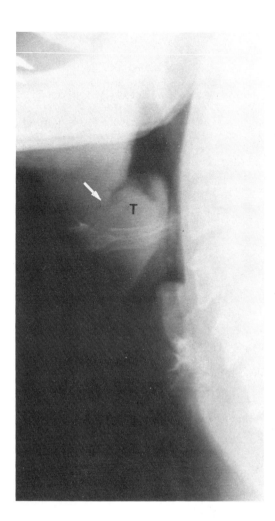

Fig. 11-59. Carcinoma, lingual surface of epiglottis and base of tongue. Soft tissue lateral radiograph demonstrates an ulcerative mass *(T)* that involves base of tongue *(white arrow)* and diffusely thickened lingual surface of epiglottis. Apparently intact laryngeal surface of epiglottis is displaced posteriorly.

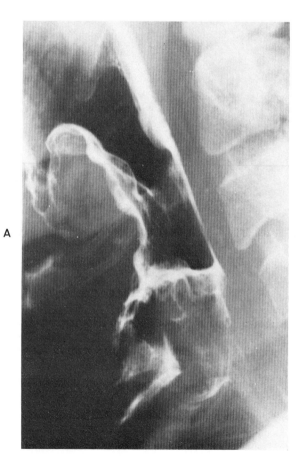

Fig. 11-60. A, Lateral view of laryngogram defines lobulated bulky epiglottic mass. Mass appears to be well clear of vocal cord level inferiorly.

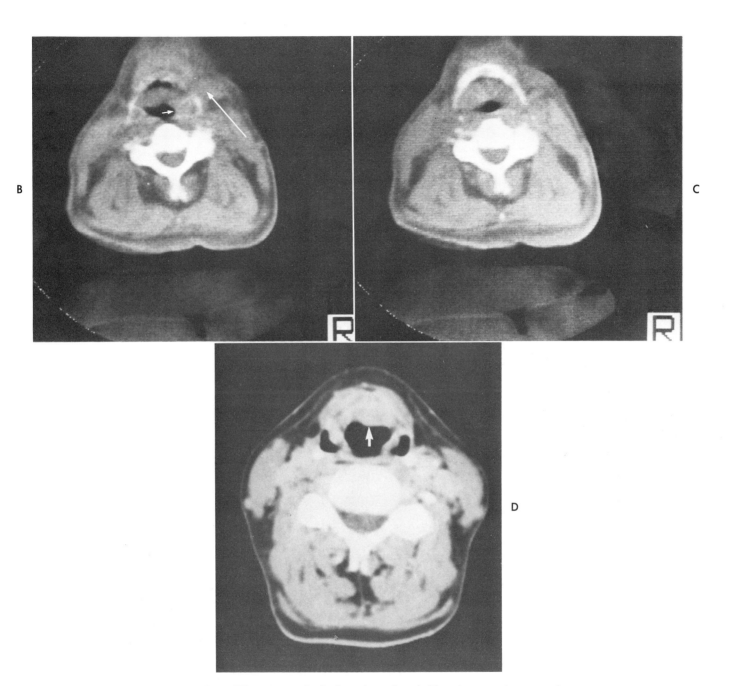

Fig. 11-60, cont'd. B, CT scan reveals thickened epiglottis. Short horizontal arrow indicates extension of tumor into upper end of left aryepiglottic fold. Long oblique arrow indicates ill-defined soft tissue density not seen on patient's left side and presumably representing tumor extension either into soft tissues of neck or into draining lymph nodes. **C,** CT scan reveals pre-epiglottic space to be of more homogeneous soft tissue density than normal. Loss of fat density indicates anterior tumor extension into pre-epiglottic and paraglottic spaces. **D,** CT scan on different patient than **A-C** reveals large midline epiglottic mass *(arrow)* that has infiltrated pre-epiglottic fat. *Carcinoma.*

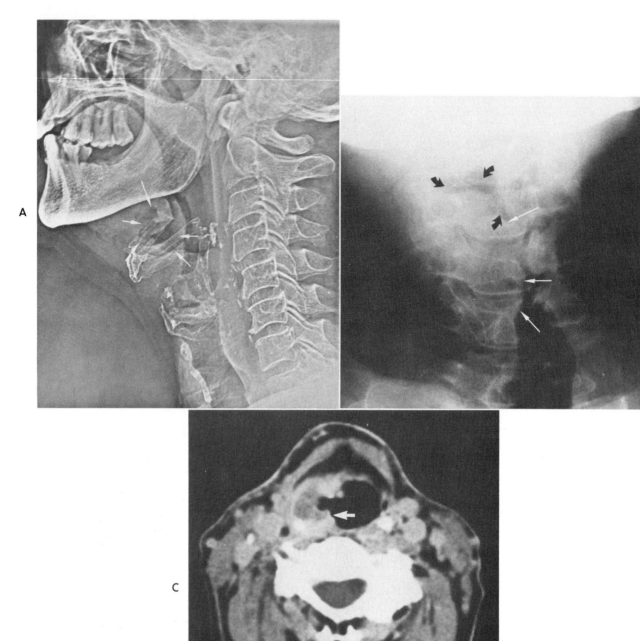

Fig. 11-61. Massive transglottic carcinoma with involvement of base of tongue and lateral pharyngeal wall. **A,** lateral xeroradiograph demonstrates extensive ulcerations *(arrows)* involving base of tongue and extending almost to level of body of hyoid bone anteriorly. **B,** Anterior-posterior high-kilovolt selective filtration film of the larynx demonstrates total replacement of right hemilarynx by infiltrating tumor. Massive ulcerative lesion is shown extending laterally into base of tongue and lateral pharyngeal wall *(curved black arrows).* White arrows demonstrate laryngeal involvement. Left side of larynx is also irregular in appearance because of tumor infiltration. **C,** CT scan reveals right supraglottic tumor that has spread from aryepiglottic fold onto pharyngeal wall *(arrow).* (**A** and **B** From Noyek, A.M., et al.: J. Otolaryngol. **6**[suppl. 3]:73, 1977.)

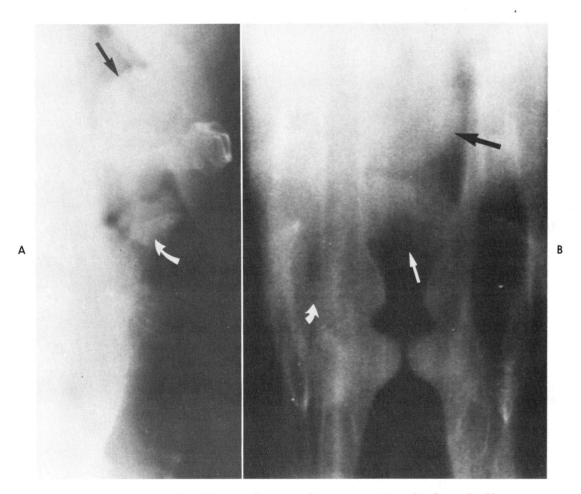

Fig. 11-62. Carcinoma of epiglottis, with airway obstruction. **A,** Lateral radiograph of larynx demonstrates large lobulated mass completely transforming normal configuration of epiglottis *(black arrow)*. Vallecula is obliterated, and deep projection of mass into laryngeal vestibule *(curved white arrow)* almost completely obstructs airway. **B,** Coronal tomogram demonstrates bulk of lobulated squamous cell carcinoma of epiglottis, arising from right side of larynx and projecting across midline at hyoid level *(black arrow)*. Another large lobulation is seen immediately above level of ventricular bands *(white arrow)*, virtually obstructing airway. Right pyriform sinus is also obliterated *(curved white arrow)*. (From Zizmor, J., and Noyek, A.M.: An atlas of otolaryngologic radiology, Philadelphia, 1978, W.B. Saunders Co.)

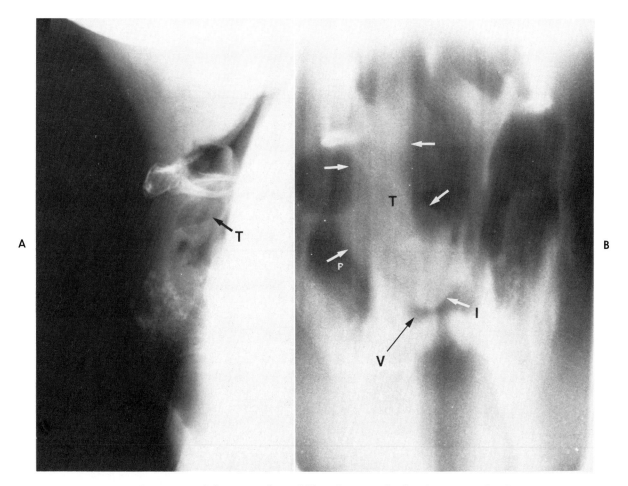

Fig. 11-63. Carcinoma of the aryepiglottic fold and ventricular band. **A,** Lateral soft tissue radiograph indicates distortion of aryepiglottic fold by tumor *(T)*. Soft tissue lateral radiograph does not allow for lateralization. Tip of epiglottis is spared. **B,** Coronal tomogram during inspiration defines extent of squamous cell carcinoma involving right aryepiglottic fold *(T)*; white arrows indicate its margination. *P,* Displacement of medial wall of right pyriform sinus laterally by tumor mass. *I,* Inferior extent of tumor as it replaces right ventricular band and bulges across midline. Roof of right ventricle *(V)* is involved but its floor and lateral extent appear uninvolved, although there is only minimal margin between supraglottic tumor above and base of ventricle itself.

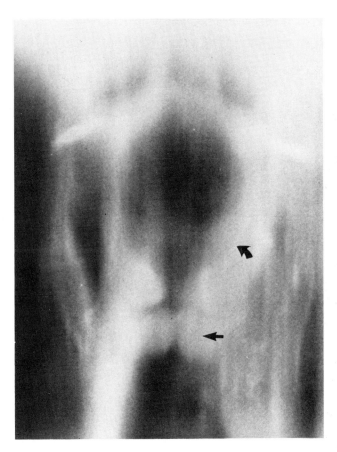

Fig. 11-64. Carcinoma, aryepiglottic fold and ventricular band. AP tomogram demonstrates diffuse swelling of lower two thirds of left aryepiglottic fold *(curved black arrow)* in continuity with swelling of left ventricular band. Left ventricle is markedly compromised, as compared with ventricular outline on normal right side. Left vocal cord *(straight black arrow)* may be minimally thickened, but no real evidence of tumor extension is noted. Subglottic angle is preserved. Adjacent left pyriform sinus outline is partially obscured by aryepiglottic fold mass. (From Zizmor, J., and Noyek, A.M.: An atlas of otolaryngologic radiology, Philadelphia, 1978, W.B. Saunders Co.)

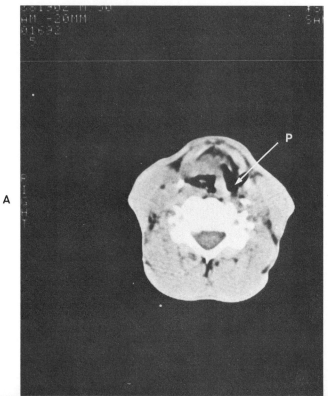

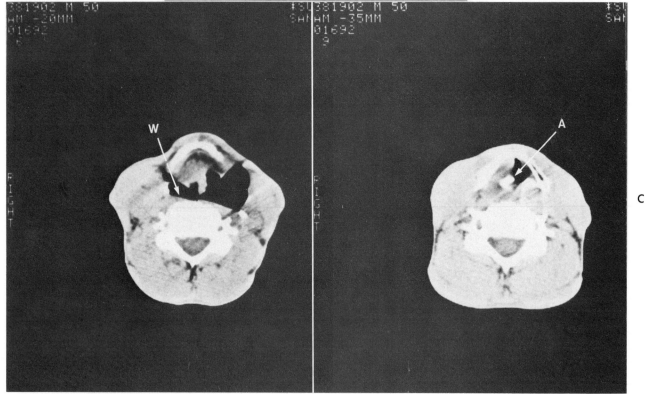

Fig. 11-65. A, CT scan shows tumor mass that appears to involve both right pyriform sinus and posterior pharyngeal wall. Left pyriform sinus *(P)* is normal. **B,** CT scan at similar level to **A** taken during constant Valsalva maneuver. This balloons out mucosa of hypopharynx, allowing demonstration of tumor relationships in axial plane. It is now clear that tumor is confined to medial aspect of right pyriform sinus, and that posterior wall of pharynx *(W)* is uninvolved. Left pyriform sinus is entirely normal. **C,** Lower CT scan at glottic level demonstrates right arytenoid cartilage *(A)* and infiltration of right vocal cord.

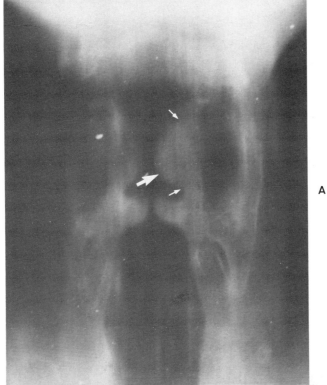

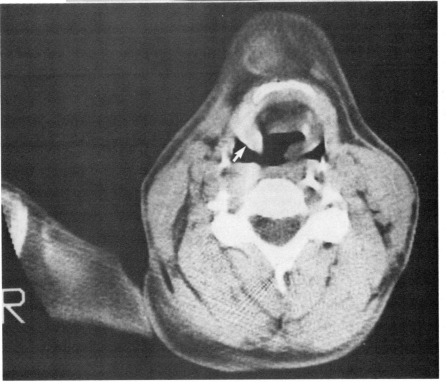

Fig. 11-66. A, Carcinoma, ventricular band. AP tomogram during phonation demonstrates discrete mass *(large white arrow)* confined primarily to left ventricular band. Its upper and lower limits are indicated by small white arrows. It extends upward into left aryepiglottic fold for approximately one third its length. Inferiorly it bulges into roof of ventricle, but base of ventricle is presumably free of tumor. Pyriform sinus is clear. **B,** CT scan of different patient reveals infiltrated right aryepiglottic fold *(arrow).* This was upper margin of carcinoma.

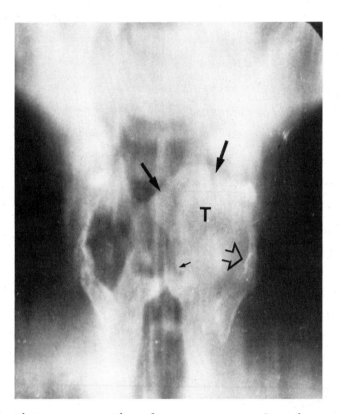

Fig. 11-67. Supraglottic carcinoma with pyriform sinus extension. Coronal tomogram demonstrates large left supraglottic tumor *(T)* whose upper level is noted by two large black arrows. Medially it encroaches on roof of left ventricle *(small black arrow)* and ventricular anatomy is largely distorted by tumor invasion. It occupies entire pyriform sinus in plane of this image and extends up to thyroid ala on left side *(open arrow)*.

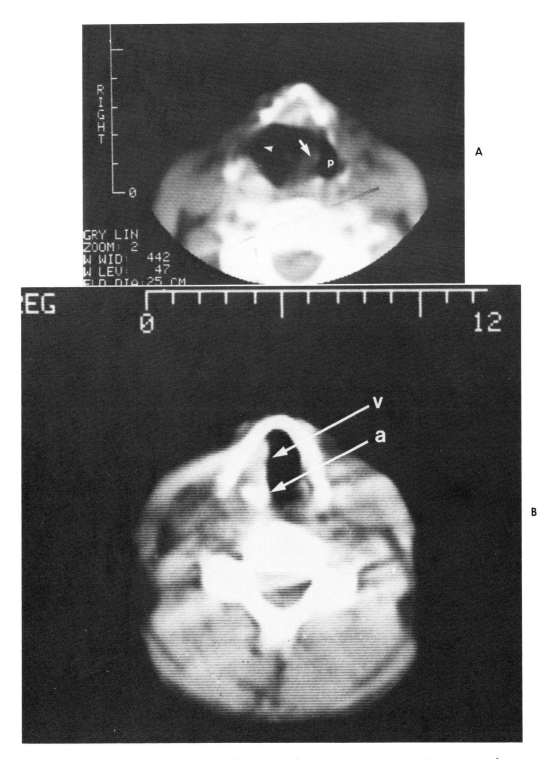

Fig. 11-68. Carcinoma, aryepiglottic fold with pyriform sinus extension. **A,** CT scan at mid-level of aryepiglottic folds demonstrates intact left aryepiglottic fold *(white arrow)*. Right aryepiglottic fold is destroyed by tumor; huge ulcer crater results in no CT image in anticipated location of right aryepiglottic fold *(white arrowhead)*. Left pyriform sinus *(p)* is normal in appearance. Ulcer appears to involve lateral margin of pyriform sinus on right, as tumor extends into lateral hypopharyngeal wall. **B,** CT scan section at level of vocal cords demonstrates fixed vocal cord *(v)*. *a,* Right arytenoid cartilage.

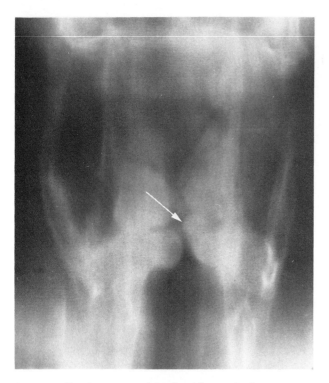

Fig. 11-69. Carcinoma, vocal cord, with ventricular extension. AP tomogram during phonation demonstrates polypoid squamous cell carcinoma involving superior surface of left vocal cord *(arrow)*. Outline of left ventricle is almost completely obliterated, and left aryepiglottic fold is thickened. Left subglottic angle is normal.

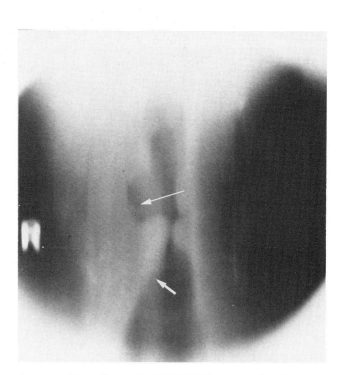

Fig. 11-70. Transglottic carcinoma, with ventricular ulceration and subglottic extension. Coronal tomogram during phonation demonstrates thickening of right vocal cord by infiltrating tumor as well as extensive ulceration of right ventricle, extending upward from its roof *(thin white arrow)*. Subglottic extension is shown by thick white arrow.

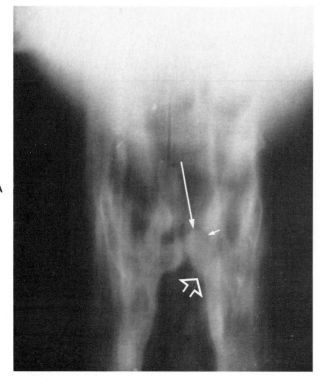

A

Fig. 11-71. A, Carcinoma, vocal cord, with subglottic extension. Coronal tomogram during phonation demonstrates involvement of left vocal cord by squamous cell carcinoma. Tumor mass elevates superior surface of left vocal cord as polypoid lesion *(long white arrow)*, but lateral outline of ventricle is preserved *(small white arrow)*. There is evidence of early subglottic extension *(open arrow)* as normal approximately 90° angle has become obtuse and flattened when compared with opposite side.

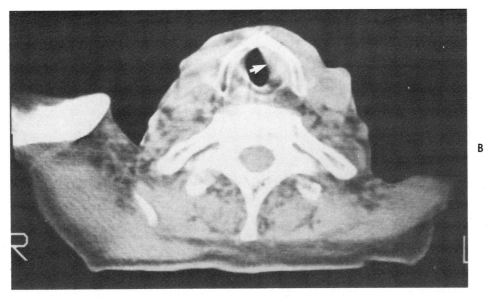

Fig. 11-71, cont'd. B, CT scan reveals subglottic extension of left vocal cord tumor *(arrow)*.

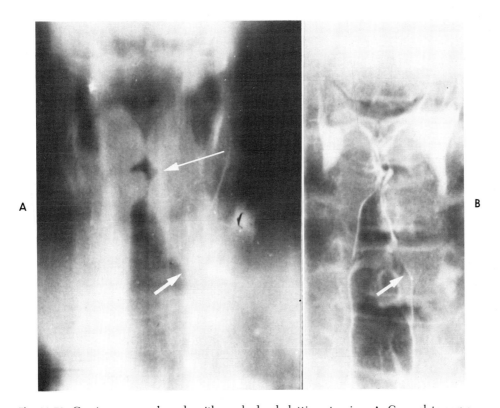

Fig. 11-72. Carcinoma, vocal cord, with marked subglottic extension. **A,** Coronal tomogram during phonation demonstrates carcinoma of left vocal cord. Depth of left ventricle is shortened *(thin arrow)*. Polypoid mass of tumor extends inferiorly into subglottic larynx; termination of its inferior extent is suggested by thick white arrow. **B,** AP view of laryngogram demonstrates subglottic extension of left glottic carcinoma. Inferior limit of cancer is shown *(white arrow)* as it merges with normal tracheal airway.

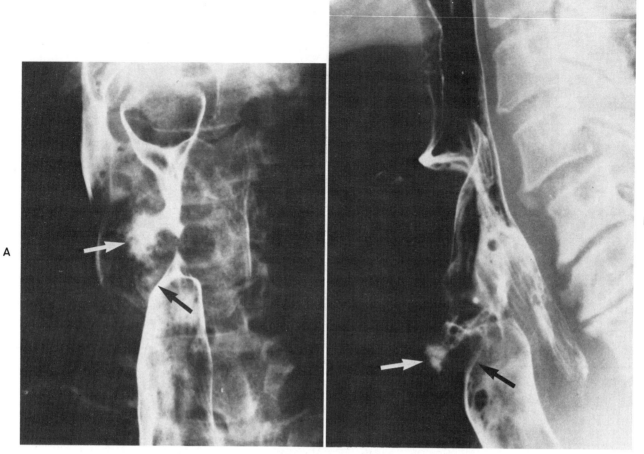

Fig. 11-73. Carcinoma, vocal cord, with ventricular anterior commissure and subglottic extension. **A,** Anterior-posterior view of laryngogram demonstrates extensive ulceration of right ventricle *(white arrow)* by carcinoma of right vocal cord. Lesion has infiltrated inferiorly to efface right subglottic angle *(black arrow).* **B,** Lateral view of laryngogram demonstrates quite clearly anterior commissure extension of ulcerative carcinoma involving vocal cords and right ventricle *(white arrow).* Subglottic extension is again evident in anterior half of subglottic larynx *(black arrow).* (From Noyek, A.M., et al. : J. Otolaryngol. **6**[5]:368-373, 1977.)

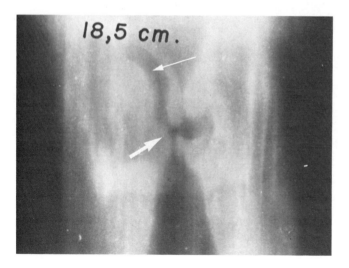

Fig. 11-74. Carcinoma, right vocal cord, with coincident internal laryngocele. AP tomogram during phonation demonstrates mass lesion involving superior surface of right vocal cord *(thick arrow)* and associated with internal laryngocele *(thin arrow).*

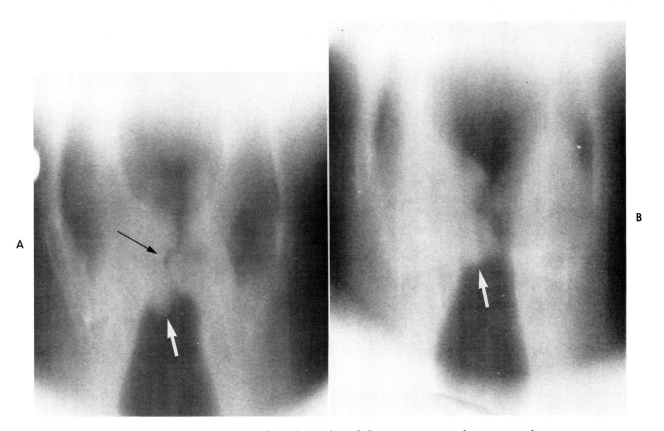

Fig. 11-75. Carcinoma, vocal cord, with vocal cord fixation. **A,** Coronal tomogram during phonation demonstrates polypoid tumor mass involving right vocal cord and hanging from its inferior surface *(white arrow)*. Right ventricular outline is obliterated *(black arrow)*. **B,** Tomographic scan section during quiet breathing demonstrates morphology of polypoid tumor *(arrow)*. Right vocal cord does not abduct although normal left vocal cord does. This indicates fixation by malignant infiltration.

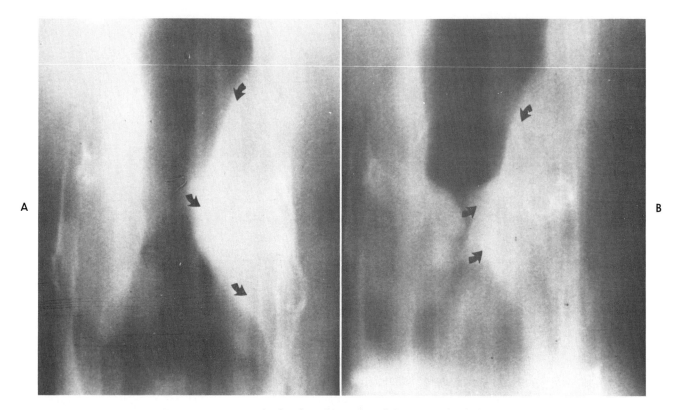

Fig. 11-76. Carcinoma, ventricular band, with vocal cord fixation and subglottic extension. **A,** Coronal tomogram during quiet breathing demonstrates relatively unchanged appearance of confluent squamous cell carcinoma involving left transglottic structures *(arrows)*. Uninvolved right side of larynx abducts during inspiration. This demonstrates left vocal cord fixation. Extension into left pyriform sinus is also suggested. **B,** Coronal tomogram in phonation demonstrates coalescent thickening of left false cord and true vocal cord along with loss of left subglottic angle *(arrows)*. (From Zizmor, J., and Noyek, A.M.: An atlas of otolaryngologic radiology, Philadelphia, 1978, W.B. Saunders Co.)

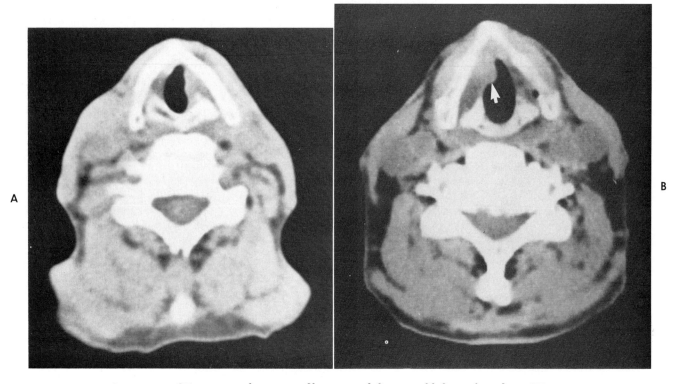

Fig. 11-77. A, CT scan reveals tumor infiltration and fixation of left vocal cord. **B,** CT scan reveals nodular tumor of right vocal cord *(arrow)* that involves anterior commissure.

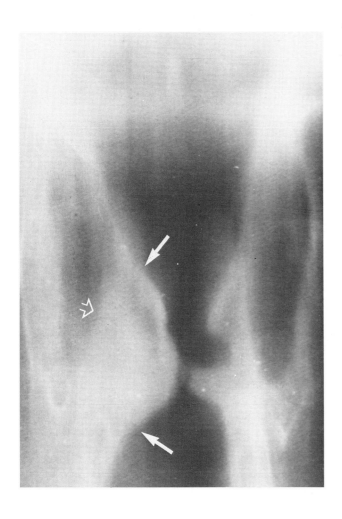

Fig. 11-78. Transglottic carcinoma. Coronal tomogram in phonation demonstrates vertical dimension of laryngeal cancer. It involves aryepiglottic fold above *(upper white arrow)*, subglottic angle below *(lower white arrow)*, and medial wall of the pyriform sinus *(open arrow)*.

of the ipsilateral pyriform sinus is a good indicator that recurrent nerve paralysis is present. Transglottic extension can also be well demonstrated (Fig. 11-78).*

Cartilage destruction can be demonstrated in several ways (Figs. 11-79 to 11-86). If the laryngeal malignancy is slow growing, cartilage displacement and destruction may be seen (Fig. 11-87). Extension outside of the larynx can also be seen (Figs. 11-88 to 11-90). Although the CT scanner probably gives the best imaging of cervical lymph node metastases, gallium scanning (Fig. 11-91) and B-mode ultrasonography (Fig. 11-92) may at times provide similar information. It appears that even with high-resolution CT scanners early cartilage invasion cannot be reliably detected. Both false positive and false negative diagnoses are made, and it is only in the more advanced, yet possibly still clinically silent cases that a more reliable diagnosis can be established.[68]

As with local cervical nodal disease, distant metastases occur more often with supraglottic tumors than with subglottic lesions, which in turn metastasize more often than glottic cancers. Three fourths of patients

with distant metastases have local involvement of the neck;[4] however, control of the regional metastases does not ensure that distant metastases will not occur. Alternately, an uncontrolled primary tumor was present in 53% to 80% of patients with distant metastases. Thus the factors of cervical nodal disease and local recurrence appear to be the most important indicators of the patient who may develop distant metastases.

The majority of infraclavicular metastases are to the lungs, most being less than 3 mm in diameter. The next most common sites of spread are the mediastinal nodes, the lumbosacral spine and ribs (lytic lesions), the liver, and the heart.

The best way of evaluating recurrent local tumor is to compare follow-up postoperative or postirradiation studies to baseline posttreatment examinations. These baseline studies are best obtained 6 to 8 weeks after treatment, when edema and hemorrhage have subsided and the altered anatomy has reached a more stable appearance. Unfortunately, differentiation between early recurrent tumor and fibrosis is impossible with present technology. It is hoped that as imaging developments

*References 38, 39, 53, 77, 83.

Text continued on p. 480.

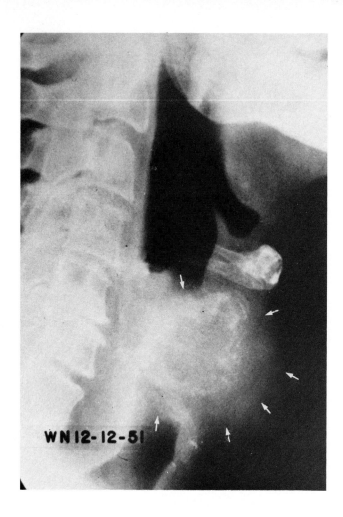

Fig. 11-79. Squamous cell transglottic carcinoma, with cartilage destruction and subcutaneous extension. Lateral film of larynx demonstrates massive extension of tumor *(arrows)* anteriorly through thyroid cartilage into subcutaneous tissues. Heavy calcification of thyroid cartilage is disrupted because of cartilage necrosis. (From Zizmor, J., and Noyek, A.M.: An atlas of otolaryngologic radiology, Philadelphia, 1978, W.B. Saunders Co.)

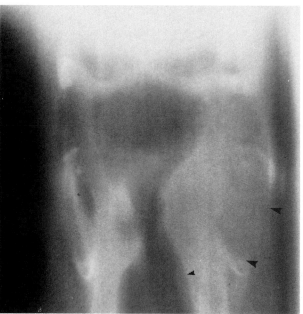

Fig. 11-80. Transglottic carcinoma, with thyroid cartilage destruction. Coronal tomogram demonstrates large squamous cell carcinoma involving supraglottic, glottic, and subglottic regions of larynx on left. Subglottic angle is effaced by tumor extension *(small arrowhead).* Left thyroid cartilage is destroyed by tumor *(between large black arrowheads),* which has advanced through pyriform sinus. Compare defect in left thyroid cartilage with uninvolved right side. (From Noyek, A.M., et al.: J. Otolaryngol. **6**(5):368-373, 1977.)

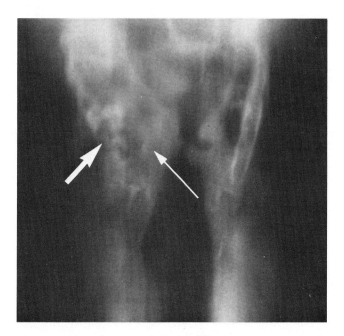

Fig. 11-81. Transglottic carcinoma with pyriform sinus and thyroid cartilage extension. Coronal tomogram demonstrates large soft tissue mass replacing right hemilarynx *(thin white arrow),* which extends subglottically. Multiple cartilage sequestrae extend subglottically. Multiple cartilage sequestrae are indicated in region of right thyroid ala *(thick white arrow).* Coalescent mass that has involved right hemilarynx has extended through pyriform sinus.

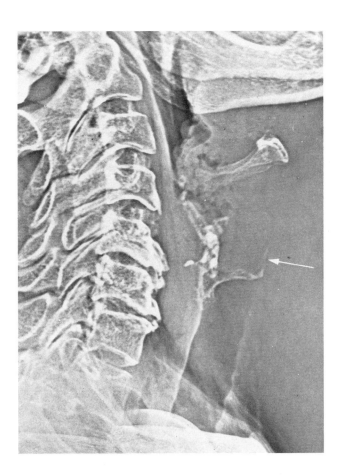

Fig. 11-82. Supraglottic carcinoma with thyroid cartilage destruction. Xeroradiograph of larynx demonstrates lobulated tumor mass replacing epiglottis. Posterior aspect of each thyroid ala is imaged by its calcification and appears intact, as does its inferior surface. Anterior three quarters of each thyroid alae is completely demineralized. Small fragment of calcified cartilage is imaged anteriorly (*arrow*) at point of union of both thyroid alae, and their inferior surfaces are still imaged. Loss of figure eight calcific image in this instance is strong evidence of cartilage destruction by tumor. (From Noyek, A.M., Steinhardt, M.I., and Zizmor, J.: Otolaryngol. Clin. North Am. **2**[2]:445, 1978.)

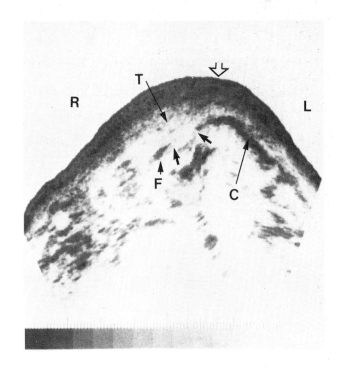

Fig. 11-83. Transglottic carcinoma with thyroid cartilage destruction and extralaryngeal extension. Transverse B-mode ultrasonogram at level of midthyroid cartilage demonstrates intact thyroid ala *(C)*. Thyroid cartilage is intact up to and slightly to right of midline. Anterior midline of neck is indicated by open arrow. Thyroid cartilage is destroyed by large tumor *(T)*, which is imaged by echoes both within and without larynx. *F*, Small fragment of posterior aspect of right thyroid ala. Cartilage dehiscence is indicated between two black arrows. *L*, Left; *R*, right. (Courtesy Dr. M. Miskin, Toronto.)

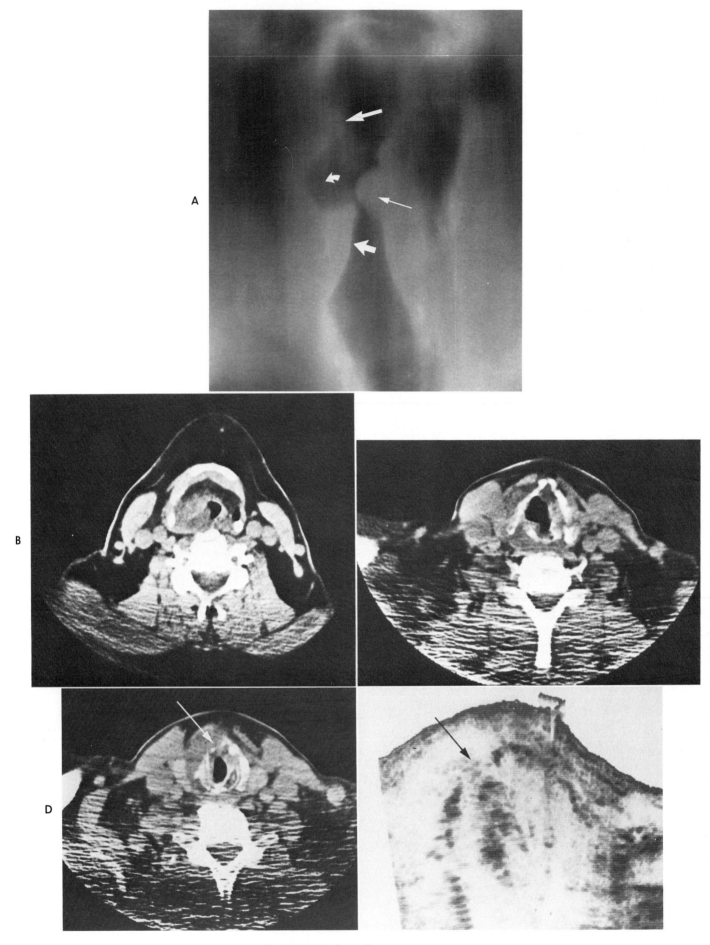

Fig. 11-84. For legend see opposite page.

Fig. 11-84. Transglottic carcinoma with cartilage destruction (with correlation of CT and ultrasonographic images). **A,** Coronal tomogram during phonation demonstrates classic transglottic carcinoma involvong right hemilarynx. Large ulcer crater has replaced region of right vocal cord and right ventricular band. It is marginated in supraglottic and subglottic regions by rolled ulcer edges caused by squamous cell carcinoma. Tumor has infiltrated anterior commissure to expand and thicken left vocal cord. Curved arrow indicates ulcer crater; long thick arrow indicates supraglottic exophytic tumor bulge; short straight thick arrow indicates subglottic extension from right hemilarynx; thin arrow indicates expanded distorted left vocal cord caused by squamous cell carcinoma infiltration. **B,** CT scan at hyoid level demonstrates extent of airway compromise. **C,** CT scan at level of false cords depicts tumor seen on coronal tomogram. Ulcer crater extends up to subjacent thyroid ala on right. Marked lymph node enlargement caused by tumor involvement is well seen. **D,** Transverse ultrasonographic image recorded with 5 MHz probe and placed at exactly same level as CT scan indicates matching cartilage destruction. Black arrow indicates echogenic appearance of tumor extending through thyroid cartilage into neck. Area of thyroid cartilage destruction matches CT image exactly *(white arrow)*. More externally placed echoes indicate tumor spread directly into anterior cervical structures, again matching CT image. (**A** to **C** From Noyek, A.M., et al.: Radiologic evaluation of the larynx. In Bailey, B.J.: Surgery of the larynx, Philadelphia, W.B. Saunders Co. [in press]. **D** Courtesy Dr. R. Rothberg, Toronto.)

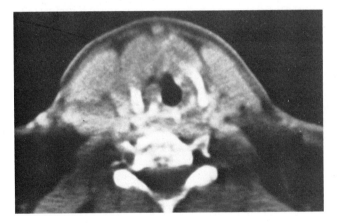

Fig. 11-85. CT scan reveals destruction of most of anterior thyroid cartilage bilaterally by supraglottic carcinoma with extension into right neck. (Courtesy Dr. N. Bryan, Houston.)

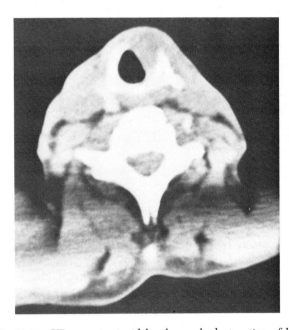

Fig. 11-86. CT scan at cricoid level reveals destruction of left arch of cricoid cartilage by glottic carcinoma with subglottic extension. (Courtesy of Dr. N. Bryan, Houston.)

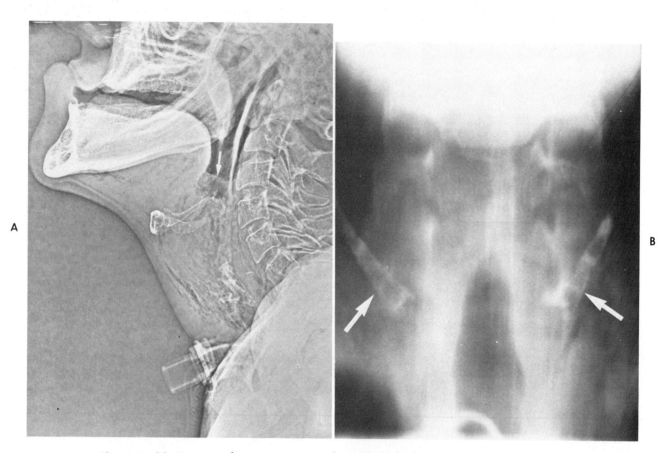

Fig. 11-87. Massive transglottic carcinoma with cartilage displacement and destruction. **A,** Lateral xeroradiograph of larynx demonstrates complete obliteration of airway and total destruction of laryngeal cartilages, except for hyoid bone, by extensive transglottic malignancy. Supraglottic extent of tumor is indicated by white arrow. Prevertebral soft tissue air and cervical emphysema are result of tracheotomy. **B,** AP tomogram demonstrates splaying of both thyroid alae and complete obliteration of airway with disappearance of all normal landmarks. Slowly progressive enlargement of anaplastic carcinoma has displaced thyroid alae (*white arrows*), but not significantly destroyed them in plane of this tomographic cut. (**A** from Noyek, A.M., et al.: J. Otolaryngol. **6**[5]:368-373, 1977. **B** from Zizmor, J., and Noyek, A.M.: An atlas of otolaryngologic radiology, Philadelphia, 1978, W.B. Saunders Co. and courtesy Dr. G. Rosen, Toronto.)

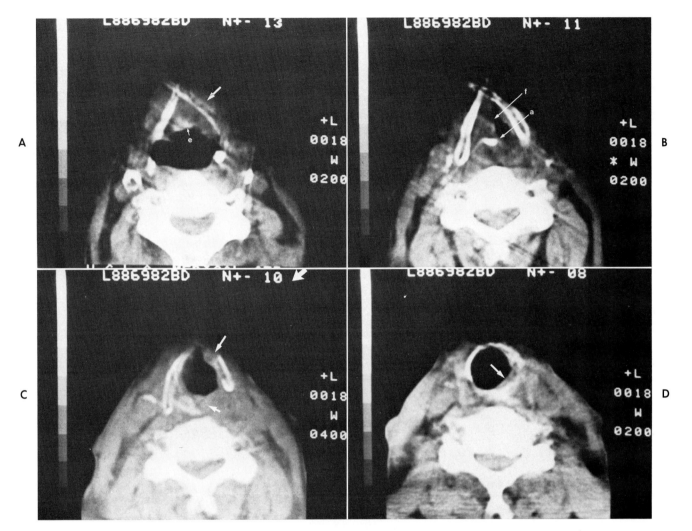

Fig. 11-88. Extensive transglottic carcinoma with pre-epiglottic space involvement and cartilage destruction. **A,** Transverse CT scan section at level of pre-epiglottic space demonstrates posterior displacement of epiglottis *(e)* and softening and buckling of left thyroid ala *(white arrow)* caused by tumor infiltration. **B,** CT scan demonstrates overlapping of right thyroid ala by left thyroid ala, which appears to be demineralized anteriorly, presumably result of tumor invasion. Right vocal cord *(f)* is infiltrated and fixed. Right arytenoid cartilage *(a)* with its vocal process appears to be pushed posteriorly. **C,** CT scan section 1 cm below image in **B** demonstrates destruction of left half of posterior lamina of cricoid cartilage *(small white arrow).* Tumor extends into adjacent soft tissues. Anterior portion of left thyroid ala is also destroyed at this level *(large white arrow).* **D,** A final CT scan section 2 cm below C demonstrates subglottic extension of tumor on left *(white arrow).* (Courtesy Dr. A. Mancuso, Salt Lake City.)

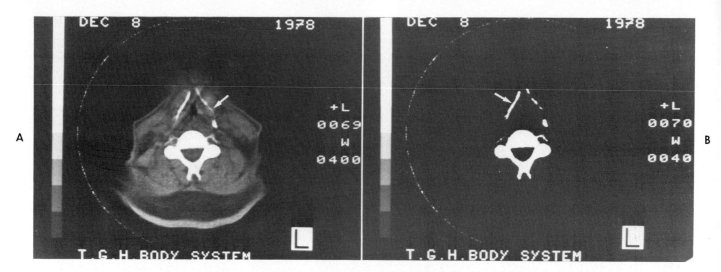

Fig. 11-89. Supraglottic carcinoma with thyroid cartilage destruction. **A,** CT scan demonstrates destruction and fragmentation of left thyroid ala *(arrow)*; there is also soft tissue thickening both within and without larynx in relation to this cartilage destruction. Right thyroid ala appears intact. **B,** CT scan at same midthyroid cartilage level using bone window clearly demonstrates intact right thyroid ala *(thick white arrow)* and fragmented left thyroid ala. Fragmented sequestered cartilage results from cancer invasion. (Courtesy Dr. G. Wortzman and Dr. M. Steinhardt, Toronto.)

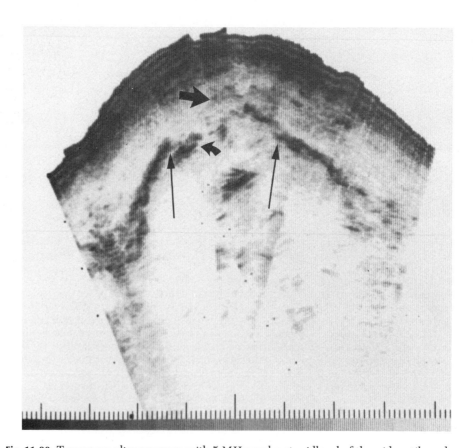

Fig. 11-90. Transverse ultrasonogram with 5 MHz probe at midlevel of thyroid cartilage demonstrates destruction of anterior aspect of thyroid cartilage. Thyroid cartilage is deficient between two long thin black arrows. Thick black arrow indicates numerous echoes representing interface produced by tumor extension through thyroid cartilage. There are areas of distorted and displaced cartilage seen within mass *(curved arrow)*. (Courtesy Drs. R. Blair, M. Steinhardt, and R. Rothberg, Toronto.)

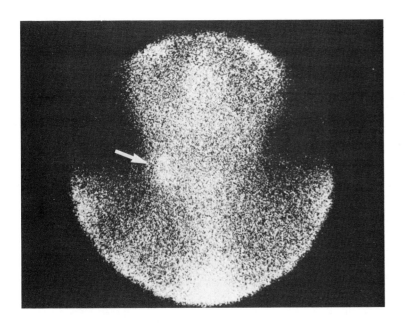

Fig. 11-91. Gallium Ga 67 citrate scan demonstrates uptake of radionuclide by metastatic squamous cell carcinoma of larynx involving right middle deep cervical lymph nodes of internal jugular chain *(arrow)*. Anterior view is shown. (From Zizmor, J., and Noyek, A.M.: An atlas of otolaryngologic radiology, Philadelphia, 1978, W.B. Saunders Co.)

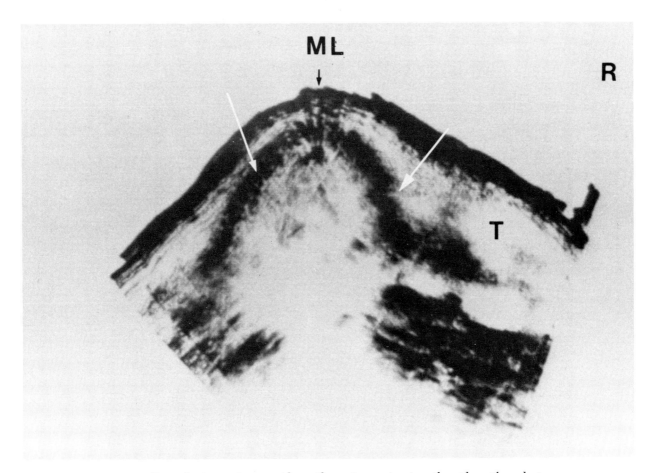

Fig. 11-92. Supraglottic carcinoma with pyriform sinus extension, thyroid cartilage destruction, and lymph node metastasis. Transverse B-mode gray scale ultrasonogram at level of vocal cords demonstrates intact left thyroid ala *(small white arrow)*. Continuity of right thyroid ala is preserved in part; it is disrupted by tumor invasion in its posterior portion *(large white arrow)*, which produces thickened irregular image. Tumor extension into adjacent cervical lymph nodes is noted. Lucent, echo-free area *(T)* represents necrotic tumor within cervical lymph nodes along right internal jugular vein. *ML*, anterior midline of neck. An ultrasonic frequency of 5 MHz was used for this study. *R*, Right. (From Zizmor, J., and Noyek, A.M.: An atlas of otolaryngologic radiology, Philadelphia, 1978, W.B. Saunders Co.)

continue to progress this problem can be overcome. Some of the criteria to examine include (1) an enlarging localized laryngeal mass, (2) progressive loss of the subglottic angle, (3) new mucosal ulcerations, (4) alteration in vocal cord mobility or cord fixation, and (5) an increase in cartilage demineralization or cartilage destruction.[85]

Postoperative strictures (Fig. 11-93) are recognized complications of surgery, as is postradiation perichondritis. Occasionally this can be a suppurative peridritis with abscess formation (see p. 421) (Fig. 11-94).

Although other malignancies can occur within the larynx, they are very rare. Most of them have nonspecific appearances and require biopsy for diagnosis. Infiltrative tumors can occur and appear as smooth masses (lymphoma, Fig. 11-95; extramedullary plasmacytoma, Fig. 11-96) or as more diffuse infiltrative lesions (lymphosarcoma, Fig. 11-97). Minor salivary gland lesions also occur; the most frequent of these is the adenoid cystic carcinoma.

Rare chondrosarcomas will be encountered, and for all practical purposes they can not be radiographically differentiated from the benign chondroma (Fig. 11-52) (see p. 445). Most occur in the cricoid cartilage.[4]

Several unusual nonneoplastic conditions can be seen in the larynx. Laryngeal amyloidois can occur as part of a systemic process or as a result of isolated local deposits of amyloid (Fig. 11-98). The mass almost always has smooth overlying mucosa. Rarely, systemic lupus erythematosus can involve the larynx (Fig. 11-99), having a nonspecific roentgenographic appearance. Oncocytic tumors are rare lesions in the larynx (Fig. 11-100).[78] They differ from Warthin's tumor in that they do not have a lymphoid stroma. Hypertrophied lymphoid tissue can rarely occur in the larynx (Fig. 11-101). This laryngeal tonsil usually involves the supraglottis and occurs as an isolated entity.[82]   *Text continued on p. 485.*

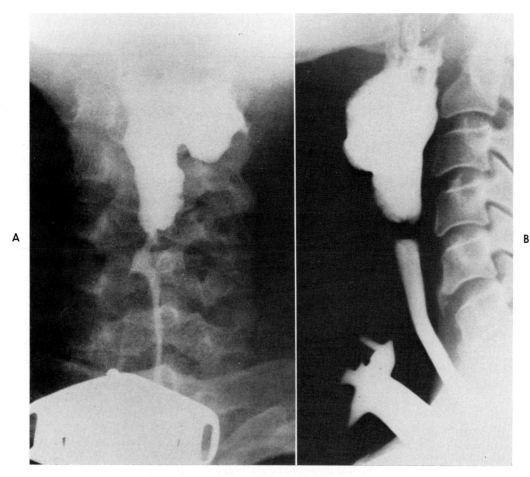

Fig. 11-93. Stricture of hypopharynx following laryngectomy. **A,** PA view of barium esophagram demonstrates stricture of hypopharymx following laryngectomy. **B,** Lateral view of barium esophagram further defines location of hypopharyngeal stricture following laryngectomy. (From Zizmor, J., and Noyek, A.M.: An atlas of otolaryngologic radiology, Philadelphia, 1978, W.B. Saunders Co.)

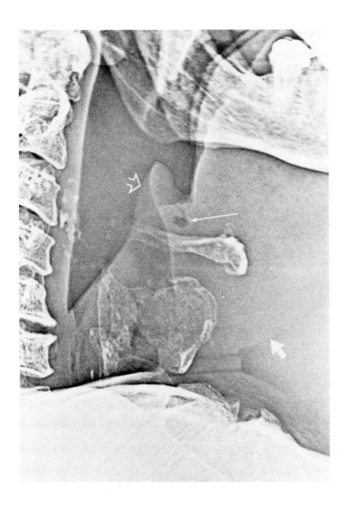

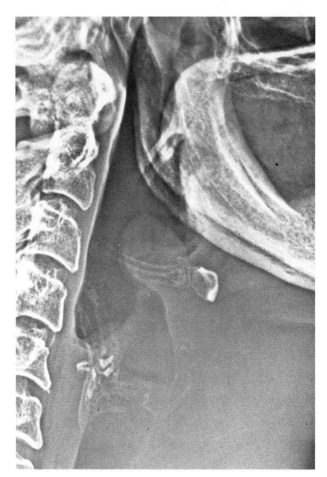

Fig. 11-94. Postradiation recurrence of supraglottic carcinoma with perichondritis and abscess formation. Lateral xeroradiograph of larynx demonstrates marked laryngeal edema involving epiglottis *(open arrow)* and aryepiglottic folds, which followed radiation therapy for large supraglottic carcinoma. There is clinical and radiologic evidence of accompanying perichondritis; thick white arrow indicates massive infrahyoid edema of cervical soft tissues, and thin white arrow indicates abscess cavity in pre-epiglottic space. Airway was severely compromised and recurrent squamous cell carcinoma was demonstrated on biopsy. (From Zizmor, J., and Noyek, A.M.: An atlas of otolaryngologic radiology, Philadelphia, 1978, W.B. Saunders Co.)

Fig. 11-95. Lymphoma, epiglottis. Isolated lymphoma involves epiglottis, producing uniform swelling of this structure as seen on lateral xeroradiograph. Definition of vallecular is preserved. (From Zizmor, J., and Noyek, A.M.: An atlas of otolaryngologic radiology, Philadelphia, 1978, W.B. Saunders Co.)

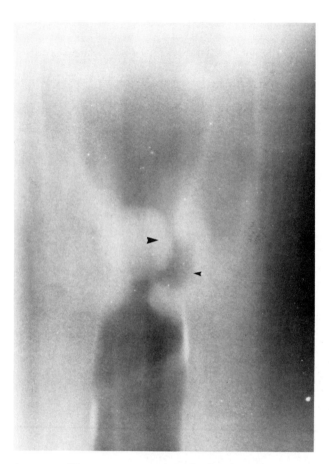

Fig. 11-96. Plasmacytoma, ventricular band. AP tomogram demonstrates large plasmacytoma *(large black arrowhead)* that appears as smooth mucosal elevation occupying entire right ventricular band and encroaching on right ventricle. It abuts against right vocal cord. Its bulk carries across midline and obscures left vocal cord to examination from above. Plasmacytoma displaces left ventricular band laterally as it encroaches on left ventricle *(small black arrowhead).* Left half of larynx is uninvolved by disease process. (From Noyek, A.M., et al.: J. Otolaryngol. **6**[5]:368-373, 1977.)

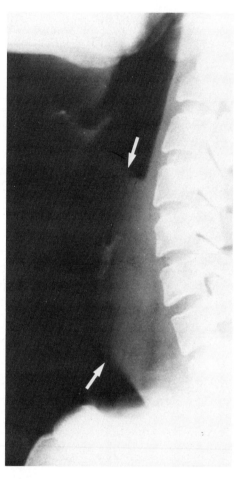

Fig. 11-97. Lymphosarcoma, larynx. Lateral soft tissue radiograph demonstrates soft tissue mass occupying the entire posterior portion of larynx, extending from arytenoid eminence above *(upper white arrow)* well into cervical trachea below *(lower white arrow).* Posterior lamina of cricoid cartilage, which is only cartilage visualized at level of tumor mass, is displaced anteriorly. Airway is reduced approximately 50% in anteroposterior diameter. (From Zizmor, J., and Noyek, A.M.: An atlas of otolaryngologic radiology, Philadelphia, 1978, W.B. Saunders Co.)

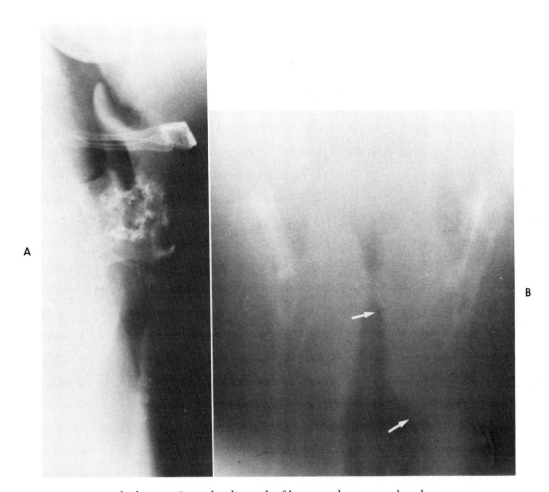

Fig. 11-98. Amyloidosis. **A,** Lateral radiograph of larynx and upper trachea demonstrates conical narrowing of upper trachea, most marked in subglottic larynx. Soft tissue thickening along posterior wall of subglottic larynx and upper trachea reduces AP dimension of airway by approximately one third. **B,** AP tomogram demonstrates subglottic component of involvement by amyloidosis between white arrows. At this level, lateral airway is reduced by almost 50%. There is coalescent involvement of both vocal cords at glottic level, with narrowing of glottic airway and obliteration of both ventricles.

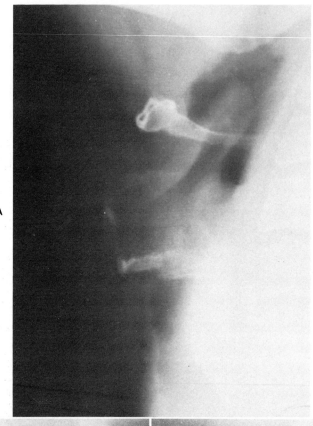

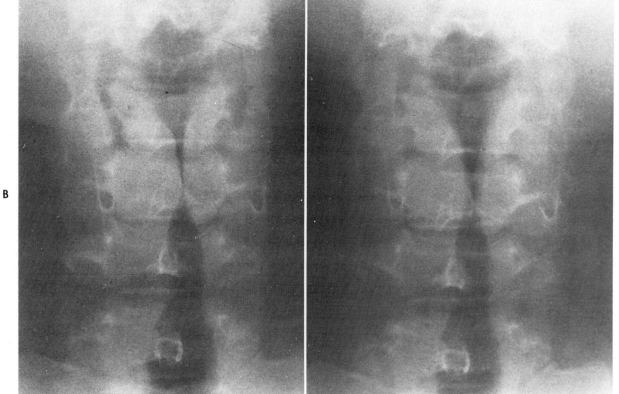

Fig. 11-99. Systemic lupus erythematosus of larynx and trachea. **A,** Lateral radiograph demonstrates almost 50% AP subglottic narrowing by inflammatory soft tissue in patient with systemic lupus erythematosus. **B,** High-kilovoltage selective filtration AP radiograph during phonation demonstrates diffuse thickening of entire endolarynx and conical narrowing of subglottic larynx and upper trachea. **C,** High-kilovolt selective filtration AP radiograph during quiet breathing shows impaired abduction of both halves of larynx, with reduced airway.

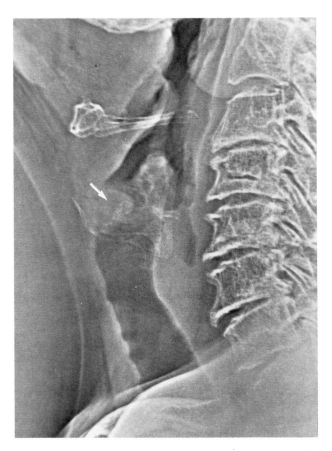

Fig. 11-100. Cystic oncocytic metaplasia. Lateral xeroradiograph demonstrates nonspecific smooth ovoid mass *(arrow)* arising anteriorly at level of glottis. (From Noyek, A.M., et al.: J. Otolaryngol. **9**[1]:90-96, 1980.)

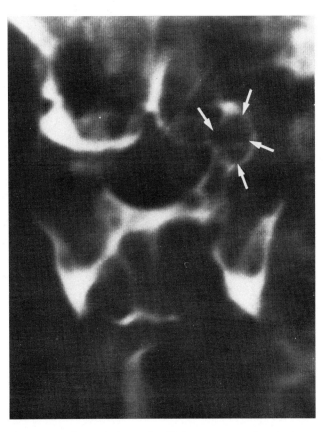

Fig. 11-101. Laryngeal tonsil. AP laryngogram demonstrates smooth polypoid mass *(arrows)* occupying left aryepiglottic fold. This proved to be normal lymphoid tissue on biopsy. Normal lymphoid elements can be found anywhere in supraglottis, including ventricle. (From Zizmor, J., and Noyek, A.M.: Semin. Roentgenol. **9**[4]:311, 1974.)

☐ Laryngeal nerves

The two main nerves supplying the larynx are the superior laryngeal and the recurrent laryngeal nerves, both of which are branches of the vagus nerve. The superior laryngeal nerve has two branches, an external and an internal division. The internal branch enters the larynx with the superior laryngeal branch of the superior thyroid artery by way of the thyrohyoid membrane. It supplies sensation to the mucosa primarily of the supraglottis. The external nerve branch runs obliquely downward across the outer thyroid alae to supply motor function to the cricothyroid muscle. Because of the superior laryngeal nerve's close proximity to the superior thyroid artery, it is prone to injury during thyroidectomy.

The recurrent laryngeal nerves supply all of the remaining motor function of the larynx and the sensory innervation to the subglottis and glottis.

The right recurrent nerve descends in the carotid sheath, bends around posteriorly under the right subclavian artery, and runs superomedially in the tracheoesophageal groove. Occasionally, the nerve can normally lie as much as 1 cm lateral to the trachea. Because of this, it is prone to surgical injury because it is erroneously assumed that it runs in the tracheoesophageal groove.

The left recurrent nerve descends in the carotid sheath, bends around posteriorly under the aortic arch, and ascends in the tracheoesophageal groove. Both recurrent nerves enter the larynx immediately posterior to the cricothyroid joint.

Because of their different courses, the left recurrent nerve is more prone to being paralyzed than is the right nerve. This is primarily because of its longer course into the upper mediastinum and its increased susceptibility to mediastinal metastatic tumors.

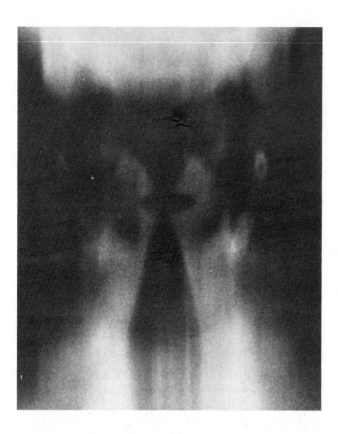

Fig. 11-102. Bilateral vocal cord paralysis. Coronal tomogram demonstrates barely adequate airway during quiet breathing. Note persistent visualization of normal laryngeal structures, which would normally be effaced in abduction. In this instance, vocal cords are paralyzed as result of trauma to both recurrent laryngeal nerves from total thyroidectomy. (From Zizmor, J., and Noyek, A.M.: An atlas of otolaryngologic radiology, Philadelphia, 1978, W.B. Saunders Co.)

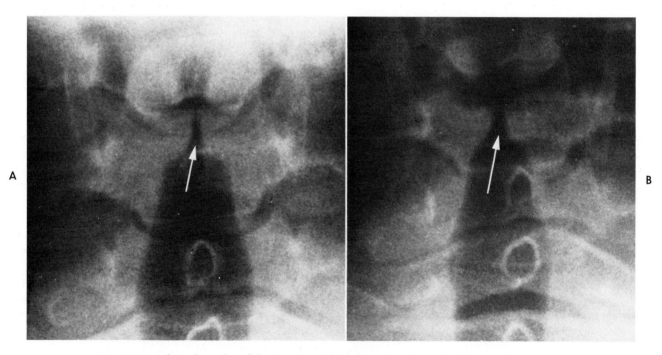

Fig. 11-103. Bilateral vocal cord fixation. **A,** AP high-kilovolt radiograph of larynx during phonation demonstrates small residual air space *(arrow)* between fixed vocal cords, resulting from trauma with secondary osteoarthritis of both cricoarytenoid joints. **B,** AP high-kilovolt radiograph of larynx during inspiration demonstrates minimal widening of airway *(arrow)* as vocal cords remain relatively adducted. (From Zizmor, J. and Noyek, A.M.: An atlas of otolaryngologic radiology, Philadelphia, 1978, W.B. Saunders Co.)

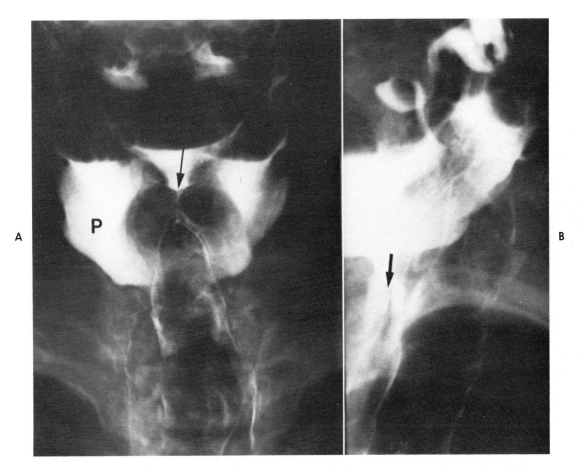

Fig. 11-104. Laryngeal anesthesia in cricopharyngeal dysfunction, postcerebrovascular accident. **A,** AP view of barium esophagram demonstrates distended, flaccid pyriform sinuses, with pooling of barium in right pyriform sinus *(P).* Barium has been aspirated into larynx and upper trachea. Vocal cords are in apposition with closed glottic airway *(arrow)*, attempting to protect airway from barium in laryngeal introitus. **B,** Oblique view of this barium esophagram demonstrates pooling of barium in distended pyriform sinuses. Some barium is seen entering cervical esophagus *(arrow)*. Some barium outlines tracheal mucosa.

With paralysis of both superior laryngeal nerves, symptoms of aspiration or difficulty with deglutition occur. When paralysis is unilateral, symptoms are minimal and compensation is rapid.[3]

Motor paralysis of the larynx may result from disease at the cortical, corticobulbar, bulbar or peripheral levels. Lastly, laryngeal nerve paralysis of unknown cause constitutes between 1% and 35% of all cases.[3] The involved vocal cord is usually in a median or paramedian position; i.e., it is incompletely abducted. Its exact position depends on factors such as which muscles retain any mobility, the presence of persistent autonomic tonus, the degree of muscle fibrosis present, and the degree of cricoarytenoid ankylosis.

Recurrent laryngeal nerve paralysis can be acute (as a result of trauma, infection, or toxicity) (Fig. 11-102) or chronic (as a result of a slowly progressive lesion ei-

ther along the course of the peripheral nerve or an advancing bulbar lesion). In the acute cases, if the cause was inflammation or was unknown, 80% of the paralyzed cords can be expected to recover.[3]

Bilateral recurrent nerve paralysis usually has an acute onset caused by trauma or acute neuritis. It may be difficult to differentiate bilateral vocal cord paralysis (Fig. 11-102) from posttraumatic cricoarytenoid joint fixation (Fig. 11-103). Laryngeal anesthesia as a result of a stroke, with concomitant disruption of the pharyngeal peristalsis and associated cricopharyngeal dysfunction, often leads to aspiration (Fig. 11-104).

Radiographically, there are several signs that indicate recurrent laryngeal paralysis (Fig. 11-105). These include incomplete abduction of the involved cord, dilatation of the ipsilateral ventricle, a flattened subglottic arch, a widened pyriform sinus on the paralyzed side, a

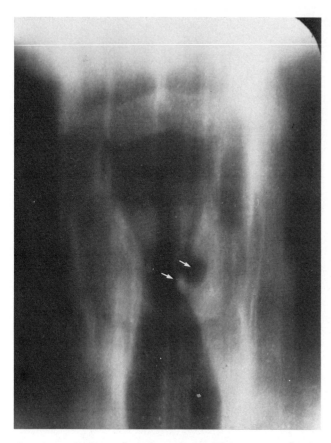

Fig. 11-105. Left vocal cord paralysis. AP tomogram during quiet breathing demonstrates normal abduction of entire right hemilarynx. Left hemilarynx remains adducted, with left vocal cord being clearly imaged in paramedian position (*lower white arrow*). Ventricular outline is widened (*upper white arrow*).

flattened false cord, and an aryepiglottic fold on the involved side. The involved arytenoid cartilage crosses the midline, and the interarytenoid line runs obliquely upward toward the uninvolved side. The edge of the paralyzed cord is thinner than normal; it lies below the normal cord in quiet breathing and above the normal cord during phonation.[44,45]

□ **References**

1. Archer, C.R., Yeager, V.L., Friedman, W.H., et al.: Computed tomography of the larynx, J. Comput. Assist. Tomogr. **2**:404-441, 1978.
2. Bachman, A.L.: Benign, non-neoplastic conditions of the larynx and pharynx, Radiol. Clin. North Am. **16**(2):273-290, 1978.
3. Ballenger, J.J.: Diseases of the nose, throat and ear, ed. 12, Philadelphia, 1977, Lea & Febiger.
4. Batsakis, J.G.: Tumors of the head and neck: clinical and pathological considerations, ed. 2, Baltimore, 1979, The Williams & Wilkins Co.
5. Behn, O.: Kehlkopf verknocherung nachgeweisen an lebenden, Fortsch geb roentgen nuklear ergean, Kiel **5**:43, 1901.
6. Caffey, J., et al.: Pediatric x-ray diagnosis, ed. 6, vol. 2, Chicago, 1972, Year Book Medical Publishers, Inc.
7. Canuyt, G., and Gunsett, A.: La tomographic ou planigraphie du larynx normal: methodé des coupes radiographiques, Ann. d'Oto-laryng. 977-986, 1937.
8. Canuyt, G., and Gunsett, A.: La tomographic ou plaingraphie du larynx pathologigue: methodé des coupes ou sections radiographiques, Ann d'Oto-laryng. 987-994, 1937.
9. Caulk, R.M.: Tomography of the larynx, AJR **46**:1-10, 1941.
10. Cocke, E.W.: Benign cartilaginous tumors of the larynx, Laryngoscope **72**:1678-1730, 1962.
11. Coutard, H.: Note preliminaire sur las radiographic du larynx normal et du larynx cancereaux, J. Belge de Radiol. **13**:287, 1922.
12. Coutard H., and Baclesse F.: Roentgen diagnosis during the course of roentgen therapy of epitheliomas of the larynx and hypopharynx, AJR **28**:293-312, 1932.
13. Decker, J.L., editor: Primer on the rheumatic diseases, New York, 1964, The Arthritis Foundation.
14. DeWeese, D.D., and Saunders, W.H.: Textbook of otolaryngology, ed. 6, St. Louis, 1982, The C.V. Mosby Co.
15. Doust, B.D., and Ting, Y.M.: Xeroradiography of the larynx, Radiology **110**:727-730, 1974.
16. Farinas, P.L.: Mucosography of respiratory tract, Radiology **39**:84-87, 1942.
17. Ferguson, C.F.: Congenital abnormalities of the infant larynx, Otolaryngol. Clin. North Am. **3**(2):185-200, 1970.
18. Fisher, M. McD.: Acute life threatening reactions to contrast media, Australas. Radiol. **22**(4):365-371, 1978.
19. Freeland, A.P.: Microfil angiography: a demonstration of the microvasculature of the larynx with reference to tumor spread, Can. J. Otolaryngol. **4**(1):111-127, 1975.
20. Gamso, G., Webb, W.R., Shallit, J.B., and Moss, A.A.: Computed tomography in carcinoma of the larynx and pyriform sinus: the value of phonation CT, AJR **136**:577-584, 1981.
21. Gay, B.B., Jr.: A roentgenographic method for evaluation of the larynx and pharynx. I. Technique of examination, AJR **79**: 301-305, 1958.
22. Gay, B.B., Jr., and Wilkins, S.A., Jr.: The fluoroscope with image amplifier in the study of the larynx and pharynx, Cancer **9**:1253-1260, 1956.
23. Goerg, R., Roeck, W.W., and Milne, E.N.C.: Tantulum oxide: a nonexplosive substitute for metallic tantalum powder, Invest. Radiol. **8**(5):333-338, 1973.
24. Goldberg, M., Noyek, A.M., and Pritzker, K.P.H.: Laryngeal granuloma secondary to gastroesophageal reflux, J. Otolaryngol. **7**(3):196-202, 1978.
25. Grainger, R.G., Castellino, R.A., Lewin, K., and Steiner, R.N.: Hytrast: experimental bronchography comparing two different formulations, Clin. Radiol. **21**(4):370-375, 1970.
26. Greene, R., and Start, P.: Trauma of the larynx and trachea, Radiol. Clin. North Am. **16**(2):309-320, 1978.
27. Greyson, N.D., and Noyek, A.M.: Nuclear medicine in otolaryngological diagnosis, J. Otolaryngol. **2**(2):541-560, 1978.
28. Hemmingsson, A., and Lofroth, P.O.: Xeroradiography and conventional radiography in examination of the larynx, Acta Radiol. (Diagn.) **17**:723-732, 1976.
29. Hickey, P.M.: Radiography of the normal larynx, Radiology **11**:409-411, 1928.
30. Holgate, R.C., Wortzman, G., Flodmark, C.O., and Noyek, A.M.: Angiography in otolaryngology: anatomy, methodology, complications and contraindications, J. Otolaryngol. **2**(2):457-475, 1978.
31. Holgate, R.C., Wortzman, G., Noyek, A.M., and Flodmark,

C.O.: Angiography in otolaryngology: indications and applications, J. Otolaryngol. 2(2):477-499, 1978.

32. Holinger, P.H.: Clinical aspects of congenital anomalies of the larynx, trachea, bronchus and esophagus, J. Laryngol. **75**:1, 1961.

33. Holinger, P.H., Lutterbeck, E.F., and Bulger, R.: Xeroradiography of the larynx, Ann. Otol. Rhinol. Laryngol. **81**:806-808, 1972.

34. Howes, W.E.: Sectional roentgenography of the larynx, Radiology **33**:586-597, 1939.

35. Iglauer, S.: Value of roentgenography in the diagnosis of the larynx and trachea, JAMA **63**:1827-1831, 1914.

36. Iglauer, S.: Use of injected iodized oil in roentgen ray diagnosis of laryngeal, tracheal and bronchopulmonary conditions, JAMA **86**:1879-1884, 1926.

37. Jackson, C.: Value of roentgenography of the neck, Trans. Am. Laryngol. **58**:112-131, 1936.

38. Jing, B.-S.: Roentgen examination of laryngeal cancer: a critical examination, Can. J. Otolaryngol. **4**(1):64-73, 1975.

39. Jing, B.-S.: Malignant tumors of the larynx, Radiol. Clin. North Am. **16**(2):147-169, 1978.

40. Johns, H.E., Plewes, D., and Fenster, A.: Electrostatic methods of imaging in diagnostic radiology, Can. J. Otolaryngol. **4**(2):102-110, 1975.

41. Khoo, F.Y., Chia, K.B., and Nalpon, M.S.R.: A new technique of contrast examination of the nasopharynx with cinefluorography and roentgenography, AJR **99**:238-248, 1967.

42. Kushner, D.C., and Harris, G.B.C.: Obstructing lesions of the larynx and trachea in infants and children, Radiol. Clin. North Am. **16**(2):181-194, 1978.

43. Landman, G.H.M.: Laryngography and cinelaryngography, Baltimore, 1970, The Williams & Wilkins Co.

44. Landman, G.H.M.: Laryngography, cinelaryngography, Amsterdam, 1970, Excerpta Medica Foundation.

45. Landman, G.H.M.: Laryngography, cinelaryngography and 70 mm intensifier fluorography in the diagnosis of laryngeal cancer, Can. J. Otolaryngol. **4**(1):74-80, 1975.

46. Lang, E.K.: A comparative study of febrile reactions to Hytrast, aqueous Dionosil and oily Dionosil, Radiology **83**:455-459, 1964.

47. Last, R.J.: Anatomy, regional and applied: ed. 6, Edinburgh, 1978, Churchill Livingstone.

48. Leborgne, F.E.: Tomography, cancer laryngotomographia, Montevideo, 1933, K. Garcia Morales.

49. Leborgne, F.E.: Tomography of the larynx, An. Ateneo Clin. Quir. 1936.

50. Leborgne, F.E.: Tomografiá laríngea, An. Oto-rino-laringol. Uruguay **8**:169-187, 1938.

51. Leborgne, F.E.: Tomography and cancer of the larynx, Arch. Otolaryngol. **31**:419-425, 1940.

52. Leborgne, F.E.: Tomographic study of cancer of the larynx, AJR **43**:493-499, 1940.

53. Lederer, F.L.: Diseases of the ear, nose and throat, ed. 6, Philadelphia, 1952, F.A. Davis Co.

54. Macintyre, J.: Note on the roentgen rays in laryngeal surgery, J. Otolaryngol. **10**:231, 1896.

55. Maguire, G.H.: The larynx: simplified radiological examination using heavy filtration and high voltage, Radiology **87**:102-109, 1966.

56. Maguire, G.H., Beique, R.A., and Rotenberg, A.D.: Selective filtration: practical approach to high-kilovoltage radiography. Radiology **85**:343-351, 1965.

57. Mancuso, A.A., Calcaterra, T.C., and Hanafee, W.N.: Computed tomography of the larynx, Radiol. Clin. North Am. **16**(2):195-208, 1978.

58. Mancuso, A.A., and Hanafee, W.N.: A comparative evaluation of computed tomography and laryngography, Radiology **133**:131-138, 1979.

59. Mancuso, A.A., and Hanafee, W.N.: Computed tomography of the injured larynx, Radiology **133**:139-144, 1979.

60. Mancuso, A.A., and Hanafee, W.N.: Computed tomography of the head and neck, Baltimore, 1982, Williams & Wilkins.

61. Mancuso, A.A., Hanafee, W.N., Juillard, J.F., et al.: The role of computed tomography in the management of cancer of the larynx, Radiology **24**:243-244, 1977.

62. Mancuso, A.A., Maccri, D., Rice, D., and Hanafee, W.N.: CT of cervical lymph node cancer, AJR **136**:381-385, 1981.

63. Medina, J., Seaman, W.B., Carbajal, P., et al.: Value of laryngology in vocal cord tumors, Radiology **77**:531-542, 1961.

64. Miskin, M., Noyek, A.M., and Kazdan, M.S.: Diagnostic ultrasound in otolaryngology, Otolaryngol. Clin. North Am. **2**(2):513-530, 1978.

65. Momose, K.J., and MacMillan, A.S., Jr.: Roentgenologic investigation of the larynx and trachea, Radiol. Clin. North Am. **16**(2):321-341, 1978.

66. Myerson, M.C.: The human larynx, Springfield, Ill., 1964, Charles C Thomas, Publisher.

67. Nadel, J.A., Wolfe, W.G., Graf, P.D., et al.: Powdered tantalum: a new contrast medium for roentgenographic examination of human airways, N. Engl. J. Med. **283**(5):281-286, 1970.

68. Nathan, M.D., El Gammal, T., and Hudson, J.H., Jr.: Computerized axial tomography in the assessment of thyroid cartilage invasions by laryngeal carcinoma: a prospective study, Otolaryngol. Head Neck Surg. **88**:726-733, 1980.

69. Noyek, A.M.: Some comments on the art of diagnosis, Otolaryngol. Clin. North Am. **2**(2):247-249, 1978.

70. Noyek, A.M.: Bone scanning in otolaryngology, Laryngoscope **89**(9 pt. 2):1-87, 1979.

71. Noyek, A.M., Friedberg, J., Steinhardt, M.I., and Crysdale, W.S.: Xeroradiography in the assessment of the pediatric larynx and trachea, J. Otolaryngol. **5**(6):468-474, 1976.

72. Noyek, A.M., Holgate, R.C., Wortzman, G., et al.: Sophisticated radiology in otolaryngology. I. Diagnostic imaging: roentgenographic (x-ray) modalities, J. Otolaryngol. **6**(suppl. 3):73-94, 1977.

73. Noyek, A.M., Holgate, R.C., Wortzman, G., et al.: Sophisticated radiology in otolaryngology. II. Diagnostic imaging: non-roentgenographic(non x-ray) modalities (ultrasound, nuclear medicine, thermography), J. Otolaryngol. **6**(suppl. 3):95-117, 1977.

74. Noyek, A.M., Shulman, H.S., and Steinhardt, M.I.: Contemporary laryngeal radiology: a clinical perspective, J. Otolaryngol. **11**(3):178-185, 1982.

75. Noyek, A.M., Steinhardt, M.I., and Zizmor, J.: Xeroradiography in otolaryngol. Clin. North Am. **2**(2):445-456, 1978.

76. Noyek, A.M., and Zizmor, J.: The evolution of diagnostic radiology of the larynx, J. Otolaryngol. **6**(suppl. 3):12-16, 1977.

77. Noyek, A.M., Zizmor, J., Sanders, D.E., et al.: The radiologic diagnosis of malignant tumors of the larynx, J. Otolaryngol. **6**(5):368-373, 1977.

78. Noyek, A.M., et al.: Familial Warthin's tumor. I. Its synchronous occurrence in mother and son. II. Its association with cystic oncocytic metaplasia of the larynx, J. Otolaryngol. **9**(1):90-96, 1980.

79. Ogura, J.H., Holtz, S., McGavran, M.H., et al.: Laryngograms: their value in the diagnosis and treatment of laryngeal lesions, Laryngoscope **70**:780-809, 1960.

80. Olofsson, J., Freeland, A.P., Sokjer, H., et al.: Radiologic-pathologic correlations in laryngeal carcinoma, Can. J. Otolaryngol. **4**(1):86-96, 1975.

81. Paparella M.M., and Shumrick, D.A.: Otolaryngology, vol. 3, Head and neck, Philadelphia, 1973, W.B. Saunders Co.

82. Pelletiere, E.V., II., Holinger, L.D., and Schild, J.A.: Lymphoid hyperplasia of larynx simulating neoplasia, Ann. Otol. **89**:65-68, 1980.

83. Pendergrass, E.P., Schaefer, J.P., and Hodes, P.J.: The head and neck in roentgen diagnosis, ed. 2, vol. 2, Springfield, Ill., 1956, Charles C Thomas, Publisher.

84. Powers, W.E., McGee, H.H., Jr., and Seaman, W.B.: Contrast examination of the larynx and pharynx, Radiology **68**:169-177, 1957.

85. Rideout, D.F.: Appearances of the larynx after radiation therapy, Can. J. Otolaryngol. 4(1):98-101, 1975.

86. Rosenbaum, H.D., Alavi, S.M., and Bryant, L.R.: Pulmonary parenchyman spread of juvenile laryngeal papillomatosis, Radiology **90**:654-660, 1968.

87. Ryan, M.D., and Zizmor, J.: Chondroma of the larynx: report of a case, AJR **62**:715-717, 1949.

88. Sagel, S.S., AufderHeide, J.F., Aronberg, D.J., et al.: High resolution computed tomography in the staging of carcinoma of the larynx, Laryngoscope **91**:292-300, 1981.

89. Samuel, E.: Xeroradiography or conventional radiography for laryngeal examination? Can. J. Otolaryngol. 4(1):59-63, 1975.

90. Scheier, M.: Ueber die ossifikation des kehlkopfes, Arch. F. Mikros. Anat. Entwicklungsgeschichte **59**, 1901.

91. Scheier, M.: Zur verknocherung des menschlichen kehlopfs, Schafer-Passow Beitr. **3**, 1909.

92. Scheier, M.: Die bereutung des rontgenverfahrens fur die physiologie der sprache und stimme, Arch. Laryngol. **22**:175-208, 1909.

93. Scheier, M.: Zur physiologie des schluckakts, Schafer-Passow Beitr. **4**, 1911.

94. Shugar, J.M.A., Biller, H.F., and Som, P.M.: Pediatric airway obstruction. Part 2, Surg. Rounds 3(9):52-69, 1980.

95. Shulman, H.S., Noyek, A.M., and Steinhardt, M.I.: CT of the larynx, J. Otolaryngol. (in press).

96. Silverberg, E., and Holleb, A.L.: Cancer statistics 1972, Cancer **22**:2, 1972.

97. Som, P.M., and Krespi, Y.P.: Laryngeal sarcoid, Radiology **133**(2):341-342, 1979.

98. Stitik, E.P., Bartelt, D., James, A.E., Jr., and Proctor, D.F.: Tantalum tracheography in upper airway obstruction: one hundred experiences in adults, AJR **130**:35-41, 1978.

99. Thornbury, J.R., and Latourette, H.B.: A comparison study of laryngography techniques, AJR **99**:555-561, 1967.

100. Thost, A.: Archiv und atlas des normalen und kranken kehlkopfes des lebenden im roentgenbild, Fortschr. Roentgenstr. **31**:1-50, 1913.

101. Weber, A.L., Shortsleeve, M., Goodman, M., et al. Cartilaginous tumors of the larynx and trachea, Radiol. Clin. North Am. **16**(2):261-271, 1978.

102. Wynder, E.L., Bross, I.J., and Day, E.: A study of environmental factors in cancer of the larynx, Cancer **9**:86, 1956.

103. Young, B.R.: Recent advances in roentgen examination of the neck: body section roentgenography (planigraphy) of the larynx, AJR **44**:519-529, 1940.

104. Young, B.R.: The value of body section roentgenography (planigraphy) for the demonstration of tumors, non-neo-plastic disease and foreign bodies of neck and chest, AJR **47**:83-88, 1942.

105. Zamel, N., Austin, J.H.M., Graf, P.D., et al.: Powdered tantalum as a medium for human laryngography, Radiology **94**(3):547-553, 1970.

106. Zizmor, J., and Noyek, A.M.: Some miscellaneous disorders of the larynx and pharynx, Semin. Roentgenol. 9(4):311-322, 1974.

107. Zizmor, J., and Noyek, A.M.: An atlas of otolaryngologic radiology, Philadelphia, 1978, W.B. Saunders Co.

108. Zizmor, J., Noyek, A.M., and Lewis, J.S.: The radiologic diagnosis of chondroma and chondrosarcoma of the larynx, Arch. Otolaryngol. **101**:232-234, 1975.

12 □ CT of the soft tissues of the neck

DEBORAH L. REEDE, R. THOMAS BERGERON, and ANNE G. OSBORN

High-resolution CT scanners permit delineation of the soft tissue structures of the neck with striking clarity. This technique is useful in defining the precise location of a lesion as well as its effect on adjacent structures; in the context of an appropriate clinical history, it is frequently possible to predict the tissue diagnosis with a high degree of accuracy. In order to make a refined diagnosis based on CT studies of the neck, however, it is critical that the normal CT anatomy be well understood. A review of the normal gross and CT anatomy of the neck will be offered prior to a discussion of pathology.

□ Normal gross anatomy

The neck spans the distance between the head and the chest. Its superior limits are the occiput posteriorly and the tip of the chin anteriorly. The inferior limit occupies a plane parallel to the first rib and is therefore higher posteriorly. The thoracic inlet is located anteriorly in this plane.

■ The muscular triangles

Traditional anatomic texts approach the soft tissue anatomy of the neck by dividing it into muscular triangles. In contradistinction, we have found it more useful

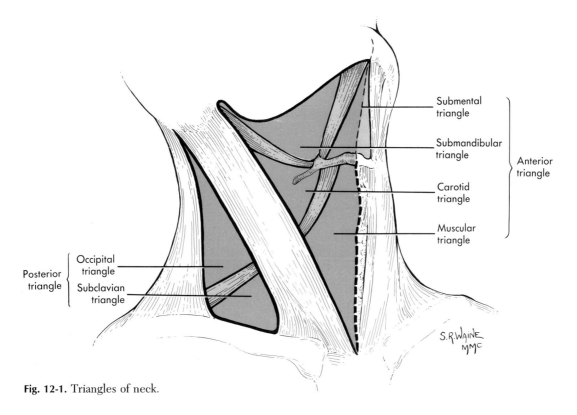

Fig. 12-1. Triangles of neck.

to approach this subject on a cross-sectional basis because of the direct application to CT analysis. One cannot ignore the traditional anatomic approach altogether, however; therefore the longitudinal and cross-sectional analysis are correlated in the following presentation.

Classically, the neck has been divided into two paired spaces, the anterior and posterior triangles (Fig. 12-1); the one of greater importance to recognize in CT analysis is the posterior triangle. It is a constant landmark visible on every section, spanning the entire length of the neck. Its boundaries are the sternocleidomastoid muscle anteriorly and the trapezius muscle

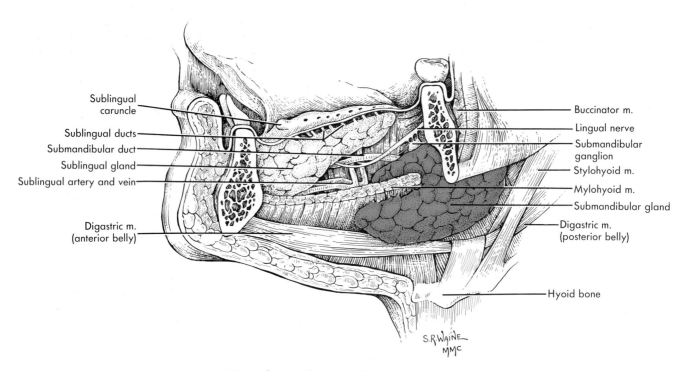

Fig. 12-2. Lateral view of suprahyoid neck and floor of mouth.

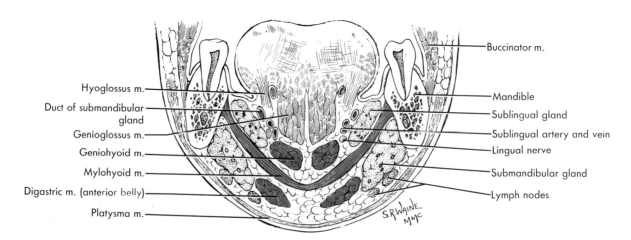

Fig. 12-3. Coronal section of floor of mouth and suprahyoid neck.

posteriorly. Its roof is composed of the superficial layer of the deep cervical fascia. Its floor is made up of the scalenes, levator scapula, and splenius muscles. More importantly from a CT point of view, the posterior triangle is filled mostly by fat.

The inferior belly of the omohyoid muscle crosses the inferior aspect of the posterior triangle and thereby subdivides it into two smaller, unequal triangles. The larger of these two subdivisions is the occipital triangle, which is located superiorly. The smaller subclavian triangle is located inferiorly (Fig. 12-1). These smaller triangles are of no importance in the interpretation of CT scans of the neck other than in the recognition of the omohyoid muscle as it makes its appearance within the inferior lateral aspect of the posterior triangle.

At approximately the midportion of the sternocleidomastoid muscle, the cutaneous branches of the cervical plexus and the spinal accessory nerve enter the posterior triangle along the posterior border of the muscle. After giving off branches to supply the sternocleidomastoid muscle, the spinal accessory nerve crosses the posterior triangle obliquely in its posterior and downward course to supply the trapezius muscle.

The cervical portion of the brachial plexus, the third portion of the subclavian artery, and the transverse cervical vessels are located in the subclavian portion of the posterior triangle.

The anterior triangles are congruent, sharing a common side as they abut against one another in the midline; their borders are defined by the sternocleidomastoid muscle posterolaterally, the mandible superiorly, and the midline medially (Fig. 12-1). The hyoid bone divides the anterior triangle into a supra-hyoid and infrahyoid portion, each of which has two subdivisions.

Below the hyoid bone the superior belly of the omohyoid muscle divides the anterior triangle into two parts, forming the carotid triangles superolaterally and the muscular triangles inferolaterally. Understanding these further subdivisions is of no importance in the CT evaluation of the neck.

Major structures situated within the anterior triangle in its infrahyoid portion are the larynx and hypopharynx, the cervical trachea and esophagus, and the thyroid and parathyroid glands. The structures of the carotid sheath traverse the entire length of the anterior triangle in both the supra-hyoid and infrahyoid portions. Also, numerous nerves and lymph nodes lie within the space of the anterior triangle.

The suprahyoid region represents the superior aspect of the anterior triangle. This area is divided into the submandibular and submental triangles. The sides of the submandibular triangles are formed by the anterior and posterior bellies of the digastric muscles, with the inferior margin of the mandible forming its base. Superiorly this triangle is limited by the mylohyoid muscle anteriorly and the hyoglossus muscle posteriorly. Superomedially it is limited in part by the styloglossus and middle constrictor muscles.

The submandibular gland and numerous small lymph nodes are the major structures located in the submandibular triangle. Both the deep portion of the submandibular gland and its duct leave the submandibular triangle by passing above the mylohyoid muscle to enter the sublingual space (Fig. 12-2). The submandibular duct then runs lateral to the genioglossus muscle. The sublingual salivary glands lie lateral to the anterior portion of the submandibular duct.

The submental triangle is formed by the anterior bellies of the digastric muscles, which attach to the lower anterior border of the mandible (digastric fossa) and the hyoid bone, which forms the base of the triangle. This triangle is also limited superiorly by the mylohyoid muscle. No major structures are located in the submental triangle, with the exception of a few small lymph nodes and small branches of the facial artery and vein.

On coronal scan sections the course of the mylohyoid muscle and its various muscular, neural, and vascular relationships can be appreciated to best advantage (Fig. 12-3). It forms a muscular sling between the two sides of the mandible and serves as the dividing line between the neck (below) and the mouth (above). It also divides the submandibular space into its two components, the submylohyoid space below and the sublingual space above.

■ Thoracic inlet

At the root of the neck is the thoracic inlet, which serves as a junction between the neck and the superior mediastinum. It occupies an oblique plane, parallel to the first rib. A knowledge of the anatomy in this area is essential to understanding the modes of disease spread from the neck into the superior mediastinum.

It is important to know the major neural-vascular relationships at this level. Although complex, these relationships are constant: the anterior scalenus muscle attaches to the superior border of the first rib; the subclavian vein lies anterior to it and the subclavian artery posterior to it. Three major neural structures are present at the level of the thoracic inlet: the inferior trunk of the brachial plexus lies posterior to the subclavian artery, and the vagus and phrenic nerves lie side by side between the subclavian artery posteriorly and the anteror scalenus muscle anteriorly. The vagus nerve is positioned medially and the phrenic nerve laterally as they cross the thoracic inlet. Because of their constant anatomic relationships, their location, in the neck, can be identified on CT. The phrenic nerve arises in

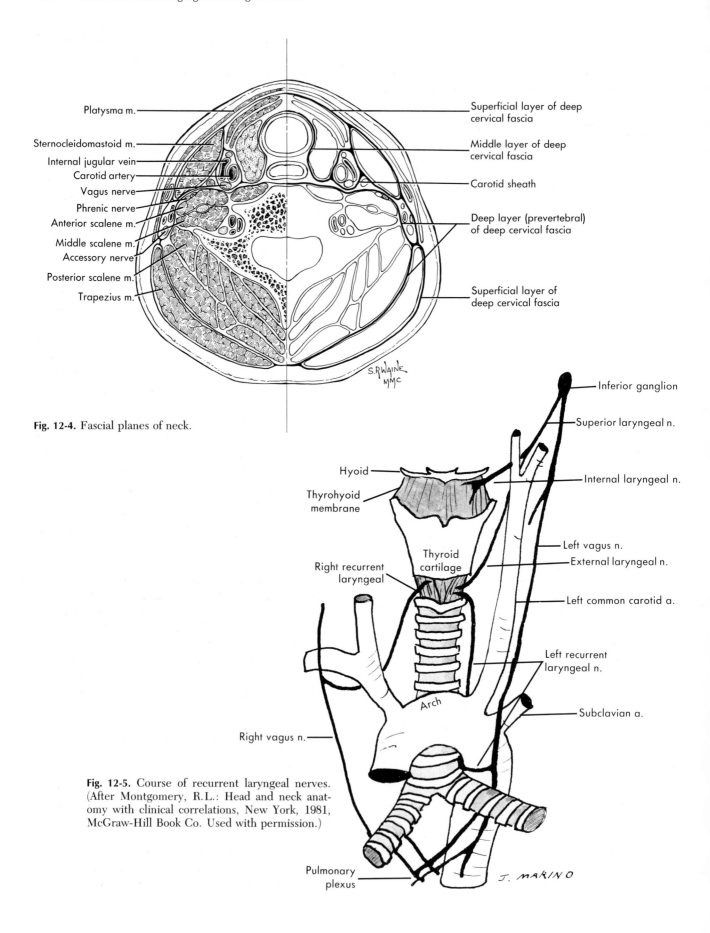

Fig. 12-4. Fascial planes of neck.

Fig. 12-5. Course of recurrent laryngeal nerves. (After Montgomery, R.L.: Head and neck anatomy with clinical correlations, New York, 1981, McGraw-Hill Book Co. Used with permission.)

the neck from the third, fourth, and fifth cervical nerves. It has an inferior and slightly medial course, lying on the anterior surface of the anterior scalenus muscle between the muscle and the prevertebral fascia (Fig. 12-4). In the neck the vagus nerve is located in the posterior aspect of the carotid sheath and is therefore anterior and medial to the phrenic nerve (Fig. 12-4).

The vagus nerves give rise to the recurrent laryngeal nerves bilaterally, but their points of origin and courses are not identical. At the level of the right subclavian artery the right recurrent laryngeal nerve takes its origin; it loops under the subclavian artery and then travels cephalad. The left recurrent laryngeal nerve takes its origin from the left vagus nerve at the level of the aortic arch and loops around under the arch in the region of the aortic-pulmonic window before traveling cephalad (Fig. 12-5). In their recurrent courses both nerves travel in the tracheal-esophageal groove. Both nerves terminate in the larynx by passing beneath the cricopharyngeal muscle and posterior to the cricothyroid joint.

■ Fascial planes

The fascial planes of the neck are divided into superficial and deep cervical layers (Fig. 12-4). The superficial cervical fascia is a fatty layer of subcutaneous tissue enclosing the platysma. The platysma divides the superficial space into two potential compartments—one above and one beneath the platysma.

Although the superficial fascia has only one layer, the deep cervical fascia is divided into three layers—superficial, middle, and deep. The superficial layer is a continuous sheet of fibrous tissue around the neck that encloses two glands, the parotid and the submandibular; two muscles, the trapezius and the sternocleidomastoid; and two spaces, the posterior triangle and the suprasternal space of Burns.[29] The carotid sheath is enclosed within the superficial layer of the deep cervical fascia.

The middle layer of the deep cervical fascia is sometimes referred to as the buccopharyngeal fascia, or visceral fascial layer, because it encloses the visceral structures of the neck and the strap muscles. Anteriorly it extends to the level of the hyoid bone and posteriorly it is situated behind the esophagus and constrictor muscles, where it forms the anterior border of the retropharyngeal space. Superiorly it attaches to the base of the skull.

The deep or posterior layer of the deep cervical fascia can be divided again into two parts, the alar and prevertebral layers. The alar layer forms the posterior wall of the retropharyngeal space, while the prevertebral layer encloses all of the deep muscles in the posterior triangle.

Understanding the anatomy of each of these cervical fascia layers is not essential in CT analysis of the neck in most circumstances but is useful in understanding the spread of infection and confinement of inflammatory processes in the neck (see section on inflammatory disease).

■ The carotid sheath

Portions of all the deep cervical fascial layers contribute to the formation of the carotid sheath. The carotid sheath begins at the base of the skull, where it attaches to the periosteum around the periphery of the jugular foramen and the carotid canal. It follows the course of these vessels in the anterior triangle of the neck, extending inferiorly into the thoracic inlet. Within the carotid sheath are located the common carotid artery medially, the internal jugular vein laterally, and the vagus nerve posteriorly, situated between the two vessels (Fig. 12-4). In the upper neck the internal carotid artery remains within the carotid sheath, but the external carotid artery exists from it. The cervical sympathetic plexus is located posterior to, and sometimes embedded within, the fascia of the carotid sheath.

□ **Normal CT anatomy**

All patients without allergic history are given contrast material intravenously. This enables one to distinguish blood vessels from other soft tissue structures. A 300 ml dose of meglumine diatrizoate (Reno-M-Drip) is infused over a 15-minute period. Scanning commences after approximately 150 ml is infused. The patient is positioned supine, with the chin extended so that the horizontal ramus of the mandible is parallel to the x-ray beam. The gantry angle is positioned at zero (0°) and 5 mm overlapping scan sections are obtained through the area of interest. During the actual scanning process the patient is asked not to swallow because this maneuver decreases the amount of motion artifacts.

For ease of discussion the normal anatomy and pathology of the suprahyoid and infrahyoid neck are addressed separately. Major anatomic structures are used as reference points in this cross-sectional analysis.

■ Suprahyoid neck CT anatomy

Because of the anatomic orientation of the suprahyoid neck structures, portions of the mouth and oropharynx are included on scans of this area.

The suprahyoid neck can be divided into three levels based on their location in reference to the mandible.

Body of the mandible

At the level of the body of the mandible (Fig. 12-6) one can identify the mylohyoid muscle medial to the mandible. In the midline are the paired genioglossus

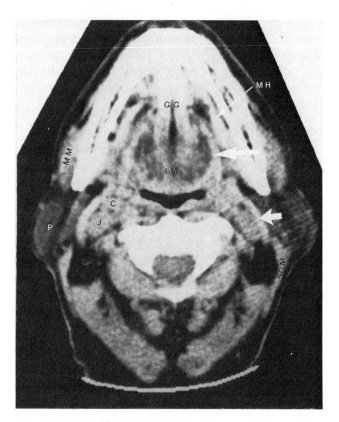

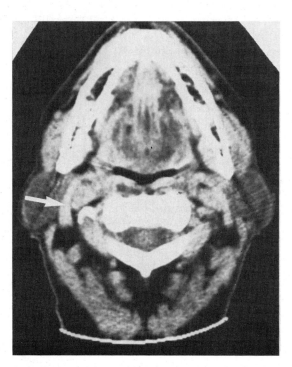

Fig. 12-6. Section through body of mandible. *GG*, Genioglossus muscle; *MH*, mylohyoid muscle; *MM*, masseter muscle; *SCM*, sternocleidomastoid muscle; *IM*, intrinsic muscles of tongue; *large arrow*, hypoglossus and styloglossus muscles; *small arrow*, posterior belly of digastric muscle; *P*, parotid gland; *C*, internal carotid artery; *J*, internal jugular vein.

Fig. 12-7. Image at level slightly higher than in Fig. 12-6, demonstrating posterior belly of digastric muscle *(arrow)*.

muscles, with a fascial plane dividing the two. Lateral to the genioglossus muscles is a curvilinear soft tissue density that represents a composite shadow formed by the hyoglossus muscle laterally and the styloglossus muscle medially. Medial to these muscles is a low-density area that surrounds the intrinsic muscles of the tongue, which are located posterior to the genioglossus muscles. The posterior belly of the digastric muscle travels obliquely in a medial to lateral direction between the parotid gland laterally and the major vascular structures medially. At a slightly higher level they can be seen to even better advantage (Fig. 12-7).

Lower border of the mandible

The anterior bellies of the digastric muscles are seen lateral to the midline geniohyoid muscles (Fig. 12-8). Posterolaterally the superior aspect of the submandibular gland can be identified. If the neck is not sufficiently extended, the same soft tissue structures will be demonstrated below the level of the mandibular symphysis (Fig. 12-9).

Mandibular symphysis

The anterior bellies of the digastric muscle are seen as they cross above the mylohyoid muscle (Fig. 12-10). Also, at this level the hyoid bone can be identified with the submandibular glands lateral to it. A cut directly above this shows the mylohyoid muscle extending between the mandible and the hyoid bone (Fig. 12-11).

■ Infrahyoid neck CT anatomy

We have divided this portion of the neck from the level of the hyoid bone to the thoracic inlet into six levels (Fig. 12-12).

The hyoid level

The hyoid bone is readily identified as the semicircular bony structures located anteriorly in the neck (Fig. 12-13). At this level, varying amounts of the submandibular salivary glands may be visualized anterolateral to the hyoid bone, depending on the degree of extension or flexion of the neck during the scan. If the neck is extended sufficiently, the submandibular glands

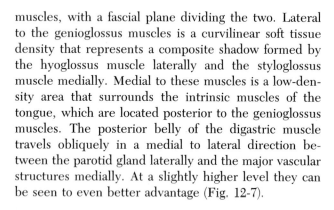

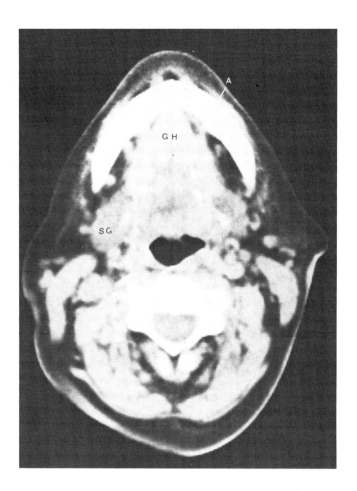

Fig. 12-8. Section through inferior portion of mandible. *GH,* Geniohyoid muscle; *A,* anterior belly of digastric muscle; *SG,* submandibular gland.

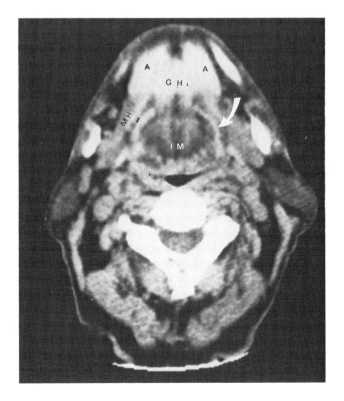

Fig. 12-9. Variation in relationship of floor of mouth and tongue structures, with suboptimal positioning. *A,* Anterior belly of digastric muscles; *GH,* geniohyoid muscle; *MH,* mylohyoid muscle; *IM,* intrinsic muscles of tongue; *large arrow,* hypoglossus and styloglossus muscles.

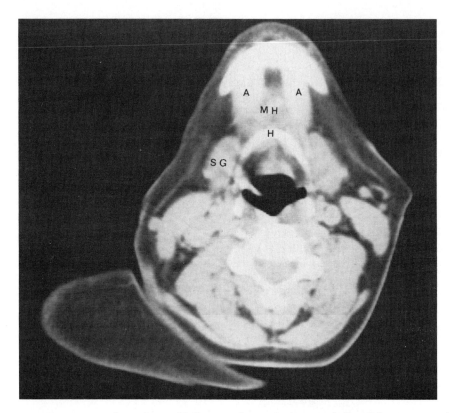

Fig. 12-10. Scan section through mandibular symphysis. *A,* Anterior belly of digastric muscle; *MH,* mylohyoid muscle; *H,* hyoid bone; *SG,* submandibular gland.

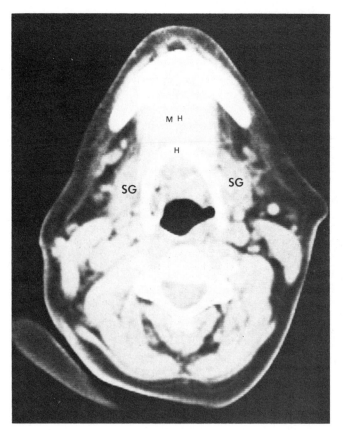

Fig. 12-11. Scan section at level just above that in Fig. 12-10 shows mylohyoid muscle *(MH)* between mandible anteriorly and hyoid bone *(H)* posteriorly. *SG,* Submandibular gland.

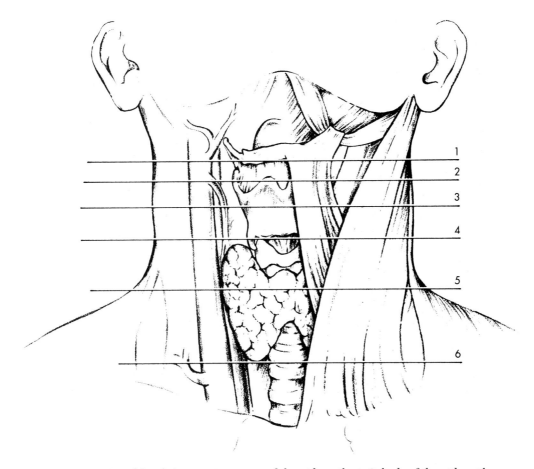

Fig. 12-12. *1,* Hyoid level; *2,* superior cornua of thyroid cartilage; *3,* body of thyroid cartilage; *4,* cricoid cartilage; *5,* body of thyroid gland; *6,* infrathyroid level. (From Reede, D.L.: Radiology **145**[2]:389-395, 1982.)

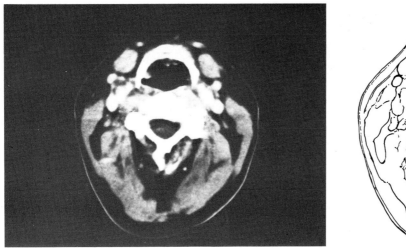
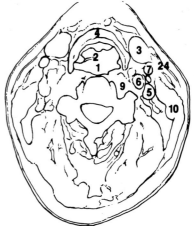

Fig. 12-13. Hyoid level. *1,* larynx; *2,* vallecula; *3,* submandibular gland; *4,* hyoid bone; *5,* internal jugular vein; *6,* internal carotid artery; *7,* external carotid artery; *9,* longus colli muscle; *10,* sternocleidomastoid muscle; *24,* platysma. (From Reede, D.L.: Radiology **145**[2]:389-395, 1982.)

will not be seen because these are suprahyoid structures. Posterior to the hyoid bone, portions of the upper airway are seen—the vallecula, the base of the tongue, the epiglottis, and the superior portions of the pyriform sinuses. Posterolateral to the hyoid bone are the major vascular structures: the internal carotid artery medially, the external carotid artery and its branches anterolaterally, and the internal jugular vein posterolaterally.

The external jugular vein usually can be seen lying on the superficial surface of the sternocleidomastoid muscle. It should be recalled that the sternocleidomastoid muscle spans the entire length of the neck, serving as the anterior margin of the posterior triangle and the posterolateral margin of the anterior triangle. It is therefore a consistent landmark and is probably the first structure that the CT analyst should identify. In the superior portion of the neck it is located rather laterally; but inferiorly it assumes a more anterior location as it comes to join the sternum.

Superior cornua of the thyroid cartilage

The superior cornua of the thyroid cartilage (Fig. 12-14) are paired, calcified structures located posteriorly on either side of the anterior neck, lying just lateral to the longus colli muscles. The longus colli are paired prevertebral muscle bundles that lie immediately anterior to the vertebral column. Lateral to the superior cornua lie the major vascular structures within the carotid sheath. The pyriform sinuses are situated anteriorly, on either side, between the thyroid cartilage cornu and the vestibule of the larynx. The most anteriorly placed structures at this level are the strap

muscles: sternohyoid, sternothyroid, thyrohyoid, and omohyoid (superior belly).

Body of the thyroid cartilage

The body of the thyroid cartilage (Fig. 12-15) is readily identified as a calcified, archlike structure, resembling a triangle without a base. At its superiormost aspect, at the level of the thyroid notch, the two halves of the cartilage fail to meet. Anterior to the cartilage are the strap muscles; lateral to it are the structures in the carotid sheath. Lying within the arch, between the two halves of the cartilage, are the vestibule of the larynx centrally and the pyriform sinuses laterally.

The cricoid cartilage

The cricoid cartilage (Fig. 12-16) forms the base of the larynx and is the only completely circular cartilaginous structure in the neck. It has a characteristic lucent medullary center with a thin rim of calcification. Shaped like an asymmetric signet ring, the posteriorly positioned "signet" or lamina portion of the ring extends to a higher level than the ring itself. At that level the cricoid cartilage is not ringlike at all but still retains its basic character of a lucent medullary center surrounded by a calcified rim.

The inferior cornua of the thyroid cartilage are just posterior and lateral to the ring. Usually at about this level the superior pole of the thyroid gland comes into view, located between the cricoid cartilage medially and common carotid artery posterolaterally. The strap muscles lie anteriorly, with the anterior jugular veins superficial to them. Posteriorly the trapezius muscle is

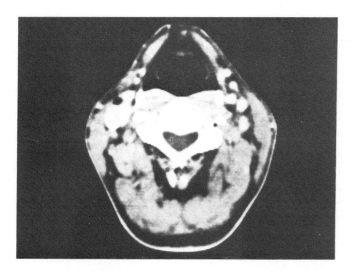 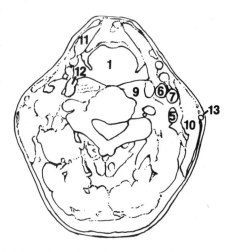

Fig. 12-14. Superior cornua of thyroid cartilage. *1*, Larynx; *5*, internal jugular vein; *6*, internal carotid artery; *7*, external carotid artery; *9*, longus colli muscle; *10*, sternocleidomastoid muscle; *11*, infrahyoid strap muscle; *12*, superior cornua of thyroid cartilage; *13*, external jugular vein. (From Reede, D.L.: Radiology **145**[2]:389-395, 1982.)

visualized and the scalenus muscles lie on either side of the vertebral body. (The sternocleidomastoid muscle assumes a more anterior position at this level in the neck than at higher levels.)

The body of the thyroid gland

The body of the thyroid gland (Fig. 12-17), which is approximately the same density as the major vessels, is seen on either side of the trachea. The normal thyroid gland in a young person, even without the intravenous infusion of iodine-bearing contrast medium, has sufficient iodine within it to appear "enhanced," appearing as two pyramid-shaped structures embracing the lateral margins of the cervical trachea. With advancing age the gland stores less iodine and thus is not as obvious without intravenous iodine infusion.

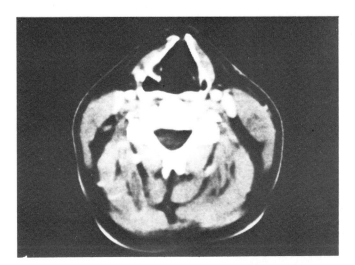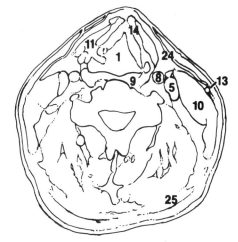

Fig. 12-15. Body of thyroid cartilage. *1,* Larynx; *5,* internal jugular vein; *8,* common carotid artery; *9,* longus colli muscle; *10,* sternocleidomastoid muscle; *11,* infrahyoid strap muscle; *13,* external jugular vein; *14,* thyroid cartilage; *24,* platysma; *25,* trapezius muscle. (From Reede, D.L.: Radiology **145**[2]:389-395, 1982.)

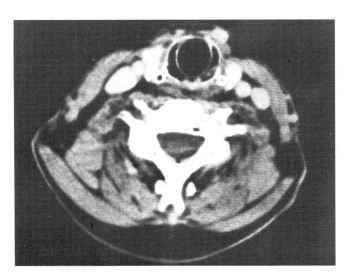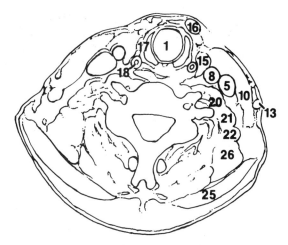

Fig. 12-16. Cricoid cartilage. *1,* Larynx; *5,* internal jugular vein; *8,* common carotid artery; *10,* sternocleidomastoid muscle; *13,* external jugular vein; *15,* thyroid gland; *16,* anterior jugular vein; *17,* cricoid cartilage; *18,* inferior cornua of thyroid cartilage; *20,* anterior scalenus muscle; *21,* middle scalenus muscle; *22,* posterior scalenus muscle; *25,* trapezius muscle; *26,* levator scapulae muscle. (From Reede, D.L.: Radiology **145**[2]:389-395, 1982.)

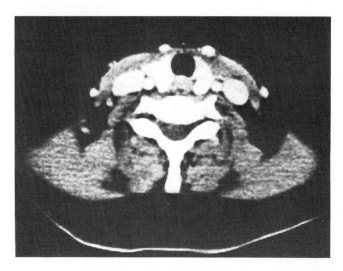

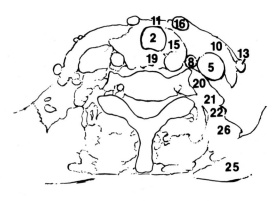

Fig. 12-17. Body of thyroid gland. *2*, Vallecula; *5*, internal jugular vein; *8*, common carotid artery; *10*, sternocleidomastoid muscle; *11*, infrahyoid strap muscle; *13*, external jugular vein; *15*, thyroid gland; *16*, anterior jugular vein; *19*, esophagus; *20*, anterior scalenus muscle; *21*, middle scalenus muscle; *22*, posterior scalenus muscle; *25*, trapezius muscle; *26*, levator scapulae muscle. (From Reede, D.L.: Radiology **145**[2]:389-395, 1982.)

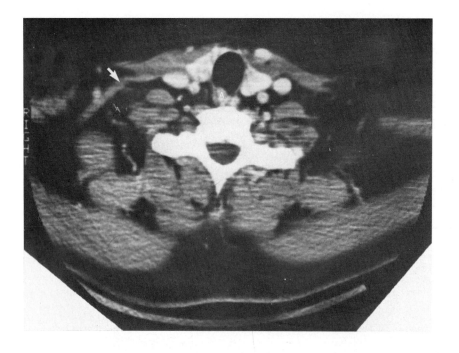

Fig. 12-18. Scan section at level of thyroid isthmus shows esophagus *(A)* partially collapsed, with figure eight appearance. Inferior belly of omohyoid muscle *(arrow)* is seen crossing inferior aspect of posterior triangle. (From Reede, D.L.: Radiology **145**[2]:389-395, 1982.)

Sometimes the isthmus of the thyroid gland joining the two laterally positioned lobes can be identified anteriorly, interposed between the trachea and the strap muscles. The recurrent laryngeal nerve and inferior thyroid artery can be identified occasionally in the space directly posterior to the lower pole of the thyroid gland, within the tracheoesophageal sulcus. The esophagus lies between the trachea and the vertebral body. It may appear as a rounded soft tissue density with a central lucency; if the lumen is collapsed, it may have

a figure eight appearance (Fig. 12-18). Often the esophagus is positioned eccentrically, slightly off toward the left side.

Occasionally the posterior belly of the omohyoid muscle can be identified crossing through the inferior aspect of the posterior triangle of the neck (Fig. 12-18).

The infrathyroid level

Below the level of the thyroid gland (Fig. 12-19) the internal jugular vein and common carotid artery assume

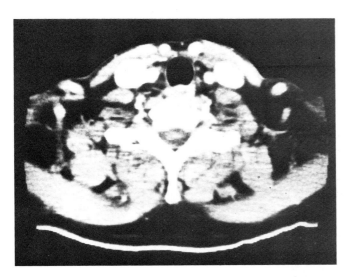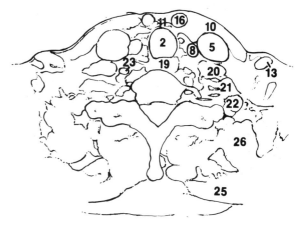

Fig. 12-19. Infrathyroid level. *2*, Vallecula; *5*, internal jugular vein; *8*, common carotid artery; *10*, sternocleidomastoid muscle; *11*, infrahyoid strap muscle; *13*, external jugular vein; *16*, anterior jugular vein; *19*, esophagus; *20*, anterior scalenus muscle; *21*, middle scalenus muscle; *22*, posterior scalenus muscle; *23*, vertebral artery; *25*, trapezius muscle; *26*, levator scapulae muscle. (From Reede, D.L.: Radiology **145**[2]:389-395, 1982.)

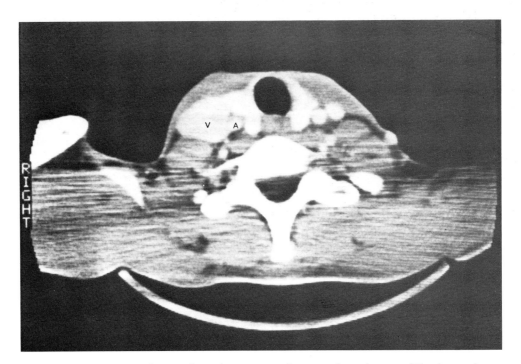

Fig. 12-20. Asymmetry of internal jugular veins. Right internal jugular vein *(V)* is larger than left. Right common carotid artery *(A)* is causing extrinsic compression of right lobe of thyroid gland. (From Reede, D.L.: Radiology **145**[2]:389-395, 1982.)

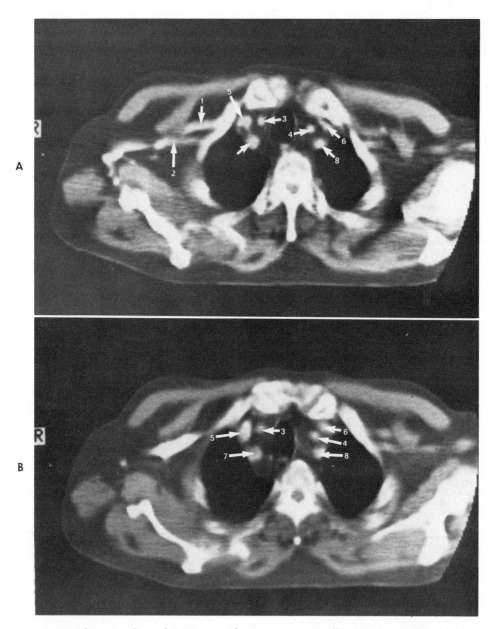

Fig. 12-21. Thoracic inlet and superior mediastinum. **A,** *1,* Axillary vein; *2,* axillary artery; *3,* right carotid artery; *4,* left carotid artery; *5,* right innominate vein; *6,* left innominate vein; *8,* left subclavian artery. **B,** *3,* Right carotid artery; *4,* left carotid artery; *5,* right innominate vein; *6,* left innominate vein; *7,* right subclavian artery; *8,* left subclavian artery. **C,** *4,* Left carotid artery; *5,* right innominate vein; *6,* left innominate vein; *8,* left subclavian artery; *9,* right innominate artery. This shows right carotid and subclavian arteries joining to form right innominate artery. **D,** *4,* Left carotid artery; *6,* left innominate vein; *8,* left subclavian artery; *9,* right innominate artery; *10,* superior vena cava. **E,** *10,* Superior vena cava; *11,* aortic arch.

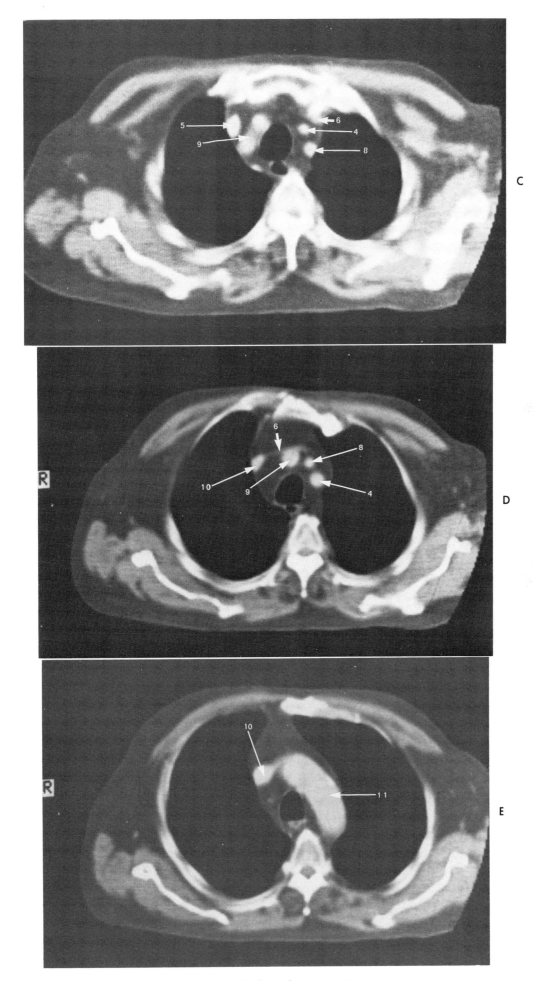

Fig. 12-21, cont'd. For legend see opposite page.

a more medial position. The jugular veins are frequently asymmetric, one sometimes appearing surprisingly large, even in the absence of disease (Fig. 12-20). The internal jugular vein occupies a more anterior position in relation to the carotid artery than it does higher in the neck. The anterior jugular vein is seen superficial to the strap muscles. The sternocleidomastoid muscles lie medially, compared to higher levels. The scalenus muscles show greater mass at this level, as does the trapezius muscle. The vertebral arteries are positioned outside the foramina transversaria, positioned between the vertebral body and the scalenus muscles.

■ The thoracic inlet and superior mediastinum

Knowledge of the CT anatomy of the superior mediastinum is necessary in order to evaluate and describe lesions that have a component in both the neck and the mediastinum. Labeled CT scans of the area are provided for anatomic reference (Fig. 12-21, *A* to *E*).

■ Suprahyoid neck
Pathology

Most of the masses encountered in the suprahyoid neck represent diseases involving the salivary glands or lymphoid tissue, or both. Occasionally, congenital and vascular lesions occur. Salivary gland pathology is discussed in detail in Chapter 4.

A mass in the submandibular area usually can be located on CT scans without the use of contrast material in the ductal system. Combined sialography is helpful (Figs. 12-22 to 12-24). Occasionally, the attenuation characteristics of the lesion may enable one to differentiate lesions such as lipomas (Fig. 12-25) and cysts (Fig. 12-26) from other lesions.

Lesions that involve the lymph nodes in this region and in the infrahyoid region of the neck will be discussed at the end of this chapter.

Congenital lesions

Congenital lesions encountered in the suprahyoid neck are related to the embryologic development of the thyroid gland, i.e., thyroglossal duct cysts and lingual or ectopic thyroid tissue.

The thyroid gland arises as a midline outgrowth from the floor of the pharynx in the region that gives rise to the tongue. This site of origin is the *foramen cecum*. It is situated at the junction between the anterior two thirds and posterior one third of the tongue.[6] Once the thyroid gland develops, it penetrates the underlying mesoderm, enlarges, and descends in front of the pharynx as a bilobed diverticulum. During this migration

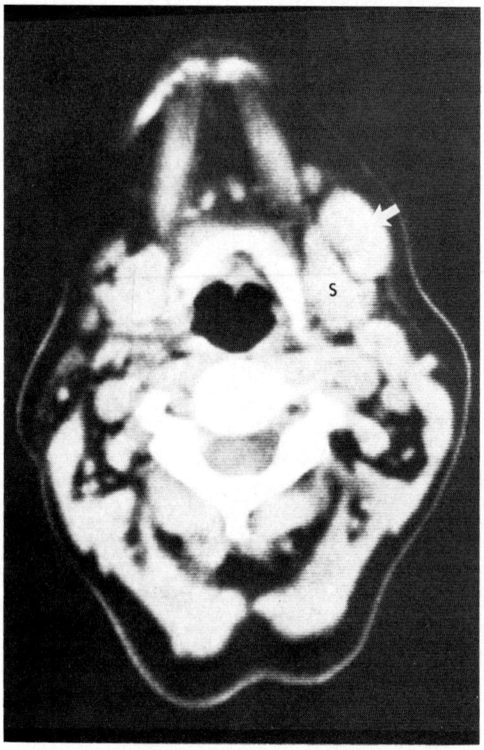

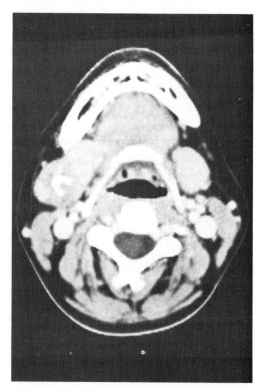

Fig. 12-22. Reactive lymph node. Mass *(arrow)* is seen lateral to left submandibular gland *(S)*. Notice cleavage plane between mass and gland.

Fig. 12-23. Benign mixed tumor. CT scan demonstrates mass in right submandibular gland, with amorphous calcification.

Fig. 12-24. Benign mixed tumor. **A,** Submandibular gland sialogram shows splaying of distal ducts *(arrow)*, which is consistent with intraglandular mass. **B,** CT scan confirms presence of mass *(M)*.

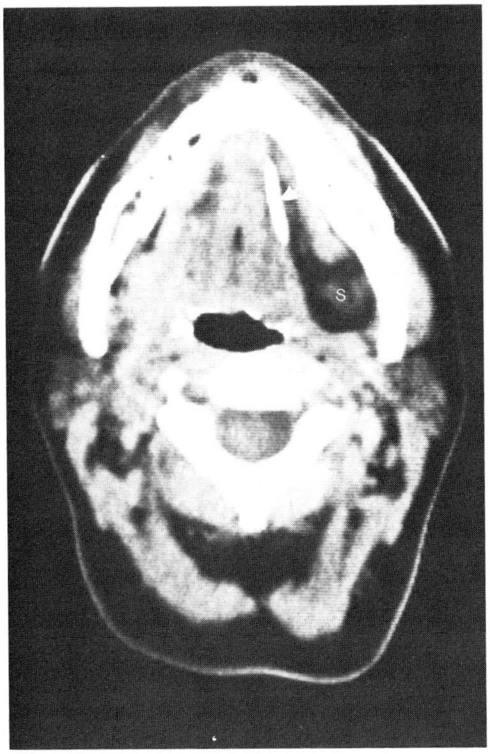

Fig. 12-25. Lipoma. Contrast material is seen in obstructed Warthon's duct *(arrow)*. Low-density lesion is seen that involves left floor of mouth and area around superior aspect of submandibular gland *(S)*.

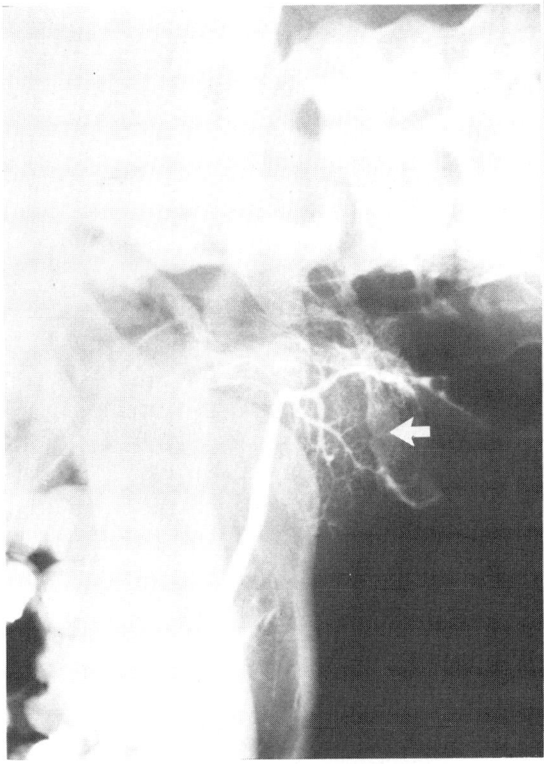

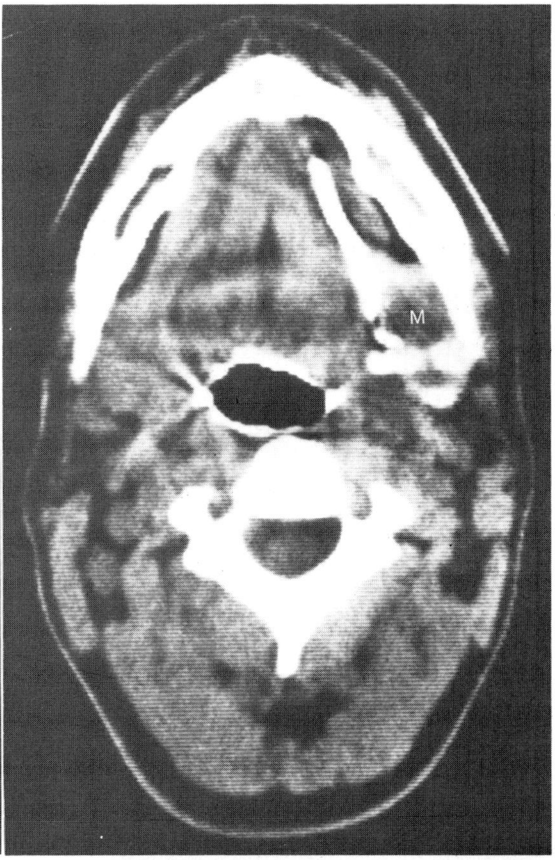

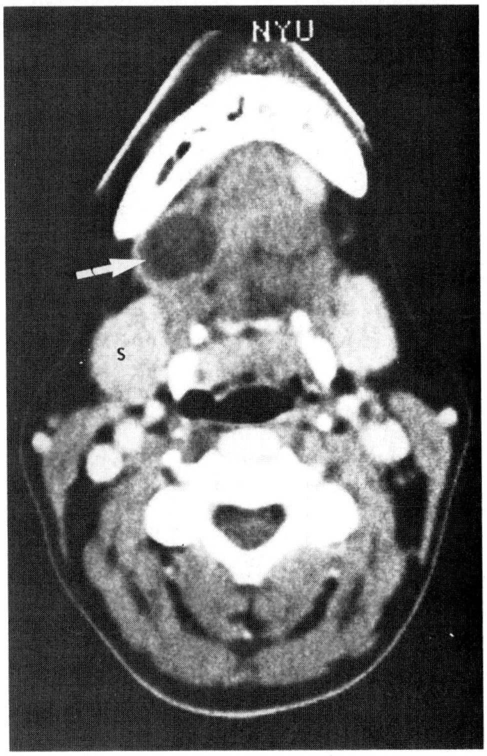

Fig. 12-26. Ranula. Well-circumscribed cystic lesion *(arrow)* is seen anterior to submandibular gland *(S)*.

the diverticulum remains patent and is known as the *thyroglossal duct*. After the thyroid gland reaches its final position in front of the trachea, the duct normally atrophies, dissolves, and disappears. If any portion of the duct persists, however, a cyst will occur as a result of secretion from its epithelial lining.[15,28,40]

These cysts can arise anywhere along the course of the thyroglossal duct and are usually located in the midline. The hyoid bone is intimately associated with the thyroglossal duct during its development. Thyroglossal duct cysts may be located anterior to, posterior to, or even within the substance of the hyoid bone.[40] Most of the cysts are located below the level of the hyoid bone in the region of the thyrohyoid membrane. They can be classified according to their location: (1) suprahyoid (20%), (2) at the level of the hyoid bone (15%), and (3) infrahyoid (65%).[2] Fistulae are not usually associated with these lesions unless the cyst has been infected or the patient has had previous surgery.

The clinical appearance of a thyroglossal duct cyst is usually that of a mass located in the midline of the neck or slightly off the center. The mass may change in size or gradually become larger over a given period of time.

These cysts appear in most patients before the age of 10 years.

The incidence of carcinoma occurring within these cysts is less than 1%; however, when it does occur, 75% to 80% are papillary carcinomas.[2]

On CT scans, thyroglossal duct cysts appear as smooth, well-circumscribed masses anywhere along the course of the thyroglossal duct. They may be midline or slightly off midline in location. The density of these lesions may be quite variable but is usually less than that of surrounding muscle (Fig. 12-27).

Ectopic thyroid tissue can be found anywhere along the course of the thyroglossal duct. These ectopic thyroid rests are commonly found above the hyoid bone in the region of the base of the tongue. They may or may not be associated with functional thyroid tissues in the lower neck. It is estimated that approximately 70% to 80% of patients with lingual thyroid tissue have no other thyroid tissue.[2] The incidence of carcinoma in lingual thyroid tissue is approximately 4% to 6%.[10] This relatively high incidence of carcinoma may be related to excessive thyroid-stimulating hormone stimulation of the gland.[43]

Lingual thyroid tissue is more common in females.

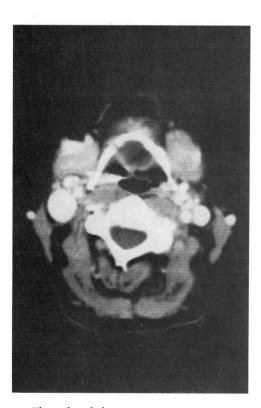

Fig. 12-27. Thyroglossal duct cyst. Contrast CT scan demonstrates well-circumscribed, low-density midline lesion posterior to hyoid bone. Valleculae are displaced posterolaterally by lesion.

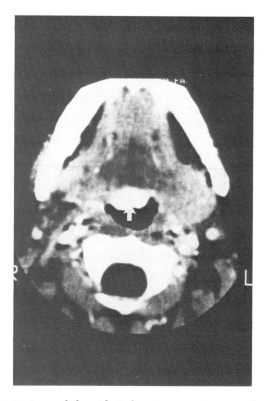

Fig. 12-28. Lingual thyroid. Enhancing mass is seen at base of tongue (*arrow*).

Clinically this may appear as a lobulated mass in the midline at the base of the tongue. Frequently, lingual thyroid tissue is not detected until there is physiologic enlargement of the gland, which usually occurs at puberty or during pregnancy.

Surgical removal of lingual thyroid tissue is not necessary unless the patient becomes symptomatic (e.g., dysphagia), although one must always be mindful of its malignant potential. Excision should be done only after a thorough search to determine if there is additional thyroid tissue present. Lingual thyroid tissue is most often identified with certainty on radionuclide scan. Plain film examination may demonstrate a mass in the region of the base of the tongue, but this finding is not specific; other lesions such as lymphoma, carcinoma, and enlarged lingual tonsils may produce similar plain film findings. The CT scan, however, usually is fairly specific. Because of the high iodine content, this tissue will appear as a highly attenuated mass at the base of the tongue on a noncontrast CT scan; after administration of contrast material it will be enhanced further because of rich blood supply (Fig. 12-28). Other nonthyroid lesions that occur in this area tend to be of the same density as muscle on CT scans (Fig. 12-29). Lym-

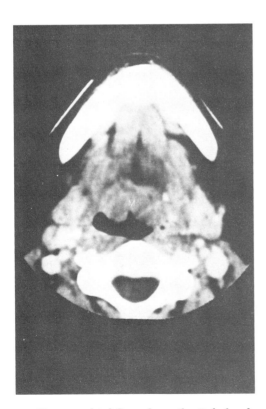

Fig. 12-29. Hypertrophied lingual tonsils. Lobulated nonenhancing soft tissue mass *(M)* is seen at base of tongue.

phoid tissue at the base of the tongue occasionally may be even less dense than the adjacent muscles.[18]

■ Infrahyoid neck
Pathology

Most neck masses are located in the infrahyoid neck. Attentiveness to several (unrelated) facts will lead to greater diagnostic accuracy. First, as a general rule neck masses in children tend to be benign and related to inflammatory disease. Congenital lesions such as thyroglossal duct cysts, branchial cleft cysts, and cystic hygromas account for a good portion of these benign lesions. Second, Lymphoma is the most common head and neck malignancy in the pediatric age group, with rhabdomyosarcoma as the second most common.[13] Third, unilateral neck masses are usually malignant lesions in young and middle-aged adults (21 to 40 years). The most common disease in this group is lymphoma. Finally, metastatic disease accounts for the majority of neck masses in patients over the age of 40.[36]

Congenital lesions

Branchial cleft cysts, cystic hygromas, and thyroglossal duct cysts are the most common congenital lesions involving the soft tissues of the neck. While these lesions may be suprahyoid, they are most commonly infrahyoid in origin.

Branchial cleft cysts. Most branchial cleft cysts arise from the second branchial apparatus. These lesions may have a fistulous tract. If so, the opening on the skin tends to appear along the lower anterior border of the sternocleidomastoid muscle. The clinical presentation is that of a painless neck mass located just below the angle of the mandible along the anterior border of the sternocleidomastoid muscle. The lesion may appear at any age but more commonly it is discovered between the ages of 10 and 40 years. The incidence of carcinoma occurring in these lesions is slight.

On CT scans branchial cleft cysts appear as well-circumscribed, low-density lesions. The fascial planes around them are usually well preserved unless the cyst is infected (Figs. 12-30 and 12-31).

Cystic hygromas. Cystic hygromas are benign, nonencapsulated lesions that arise from lymphoid tissue. These lesions are found in the neck and appear at or shortly after birth. Most cystic hygromas are located in the posterior triangle but large ones can extend into the anterior triangle.[2]

Histologically these lesions may be difficult to distinguish from lymphangiomas. Their CT appearance tends to be slightly different from that of branchial cleft cysts, but at times it may be difficult to differentiate between the two. A sometimes helpful distinction in smaller lesions is the fact that branchial cleft cysts originate as

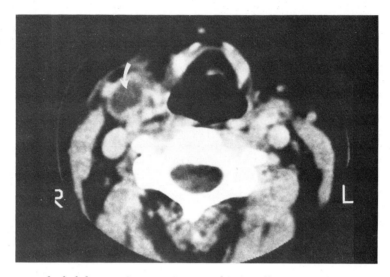

Fig. 12-30. Branchial cleft cyst. Contrast CT scan shows well-circumscribed, low-density lesion *(arrow)* anterior to carotid sheath structure. Fascial planes around lesion are well preserved.

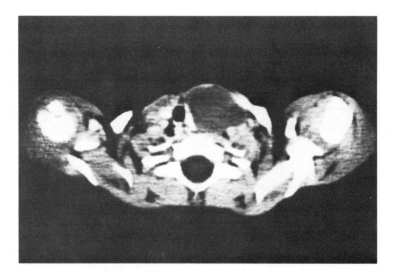

Fig. 12-31. Branchial cleft cyst. Large low-density mass is seen in left anterior triangle of neck, causing compression and displacement of trachea, left lobe of thyroid, and carotid sheath structures.

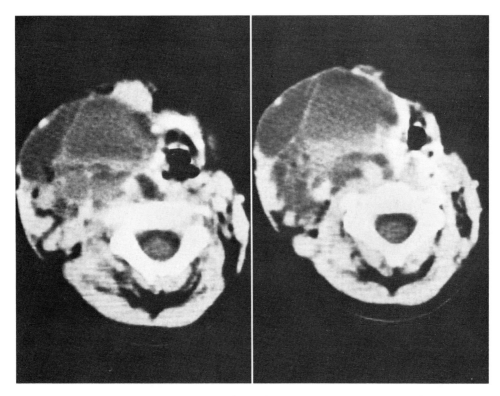

Fig. 12-32. Cystic hygroma. Multiloculated low-density mass is seen involving both anterior and posterior triangles of neck. Fascial planes around lesion are almost completely obliterated. Airway is deviated to left.

anterior triangle lesions and cystic hygromas originate as posterior triangle lesions. Large cystic hygromas tend to appear as poorly circumscribed, multiloculated, low-density lesions on CT scans. The fascial planes surrounding the lesions may not be well preserved. The tendency for these lesions to infiltrate adjacent structures may account for this finding (Fig. 12-32).

■ Inflammatory disease

The incidence of inflammatory disease processes in the neck decreased with the advent of antibiotic therapy decades ago. By and large, the majority of patients who develop abscesses or cellulitis involving the soft tissue structures of the neck are either immunosuppressed or drug abusers. Spread of infection is limited by the fascial compartments in the neck and for this reason inflammatory processes in the neck rarely cross the thoracic inlet into the superior mediastinum (Fig. 12-33).

It is worthwhile to consider the reason for this phenomenon. The fascial spaces within the neck and mediastinum are completely separate, with only two exceptions: the visceral space that surrounds the trachea, and the prevertebral space.[14,15,29] These two spaces

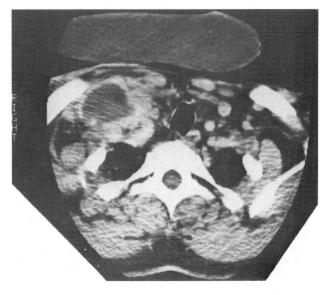

Fig. 12-33. Tuberculous adenitis. Contrast scan shows low-density mass with thick, irregular rim enhancement confined to inferior portion of right posterior triangle of neck. Fascial planes around mass are obliterated.

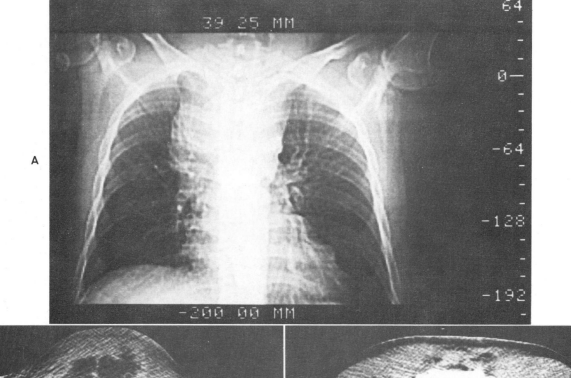

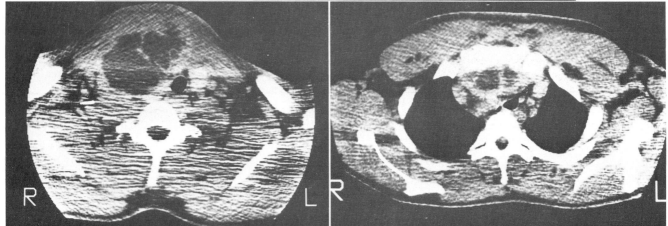

Fig. 12-34. Neck abscess with extension into mediastinum. **A,** CT scout film of chest shows evidence of mediastinal mass. **B** and **C,** Contrast CT scans demonstrate low-density masses with thick areas of rim enhancement in neck and anterior mediastinum. Fascial planes around neck mass are obliterated.

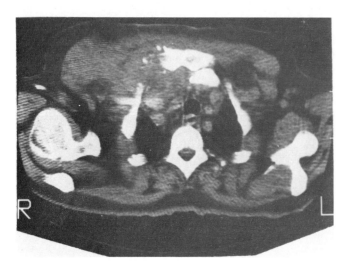

Fig. 12-35. Tuberculous osteomyelitis. Right sternoclavicular joint is destroyed. Soft tissue mass density is present on both sides of joint. Fascial planes in thoracic inlet are obliterated.

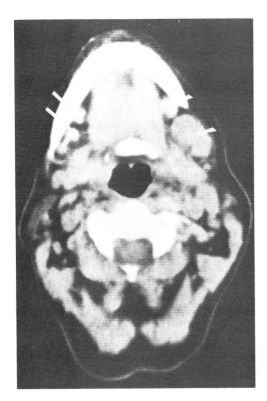

Fig. 12-36. Tuberculous adenitis. Multiple enlarged submandibular lymph nodes are demonstrated *(arrows)*.

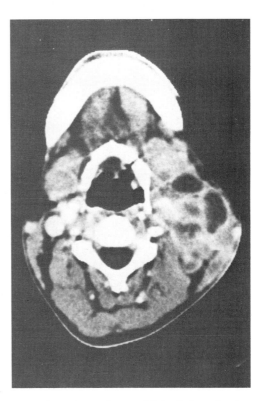

Fig. 12-37. Tuberculous adenitis. Multiple low-density masses with thick irregular rim enhancement are seen beneath left sternocleidomastoid muscle. Fascial planes around masses are obliterated and carotid sheath structures cannot be identified.

have components that cross the thoracic inlet. Infections crossing the thoracic inlet from the neck into the mediastinum therefore involve either one or both of these spaces (Fig. 12-34). Inflammatory process may also gain entrance into the thoracic inlet and upper mediastinum by way of direct extension from disease involving the chest wall (Fig 12-35).

■ Tuberculous adenitis

It is generally accepted that cervical tuberculous adenitis (scrofula) represents a manifestation of systemic disease. It may appear prior to evidence of pulmonary disease. The *Mycobacterium tuberculosis* organism is the most common cause; however, atypical mycobacteria can also be the causative agents. Posterior triangle nodes are most commonly involved in this disease. It is worth noting that those patients with cervical manifestations in the lower neck are more likely to have pulmonary disease.[45] Scrofula is seen in increasing incidence among recent immigrants to the United States from underdeveloped (Asian) countries. It is also seen in the immunosuppressed population. Most patients with scrofula have a painless enlarging neck mass with little if any constitutional symptoms.

Because the spectrum of lymph node pathology in this entity varies from mild reactive hyperplasia to frank caseation and necrosis, the CT findings are variable. Two patterns of nodal involvement are seen on CT scans. The first pattern is that of enlarged lymph nodes without central lucency or rim enhancement. Fascial planes around these nodes are usually well preserved (Fig. 12-36). These probably represent nodes that are hyperplastic. The second pattern consists of a mass comprising multiple lymph nodes that have undergone caseation and central necrosis. The capsules of the nodes tend to have thick and irregular enhancement. Fascial planes around these masses tend to be obliterated (Fig. 12-37). One or both of these patterns may be seen in any given patient.

■ Lymphomas

Lymphomas, when they occur in the head and neck region, most frequently involve the lymph nodes. The lymphoid tissue in Waldeyer's ring is the second most common site. Involvement of extranodal sites in the head and neck is rare; however, when it does occur it is more likely to be of the hystocytic or lymphocytic type. Hodgkin's and nodular lymphomas rarely occur in

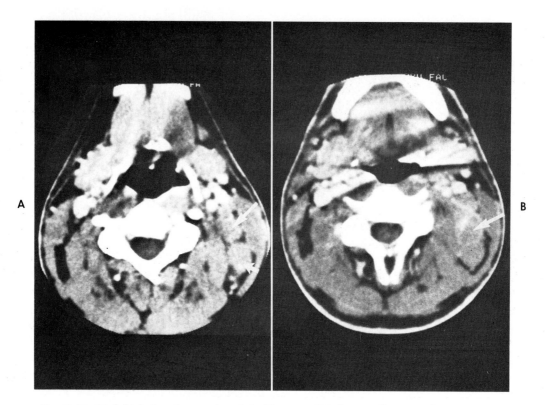

Fig. 12-38. Hodgkin's lymphoma. **A** and **B,** Contrast CT shows soft tissue density masses (*arrows*) beneath left sternocleidomastoid muscle. **B,** Streaky enhancement pattern is present. Fascial planes around masses are preserved.

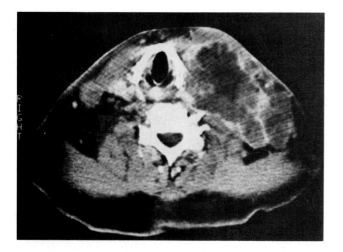

Fig. 12-39. Non-Hodgkin's lymphoma. Contrast scan demonstrates low-density mass with thin rim of enhancement beneath left sternocleidomastoid muscle. Carotid sheath structures are difficult to identify because they are engulfed by mass.

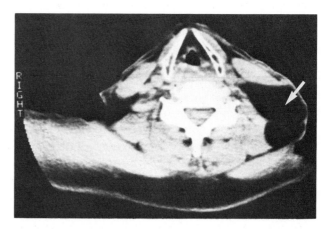

Fig. 12-40. Lipoma. Noncontrast CT shows low-density mass (*arrow*) in left posterior triangle. Mass is causing compression of paraspinal muscles and elevation of sternocleidomastoid muscle.

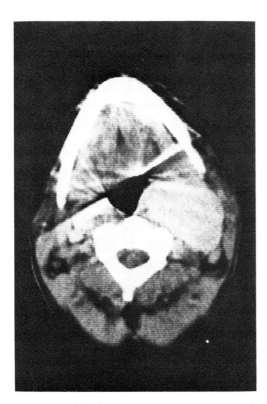

Fig. 12-41. Carotid body tumor. Homogeneous enhancing mass in left parapharyngeal area is demonstrated.

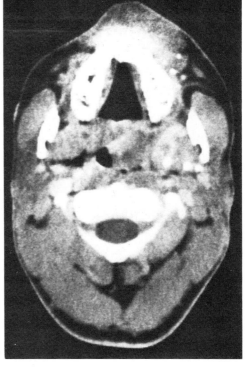

Fig. 12-42. Hemangioma. Mottled areas of enhancement are seen in region of soft palate, left pterygoid muscle, and upper lip. Multiple phleboliths are present.

extranodal sites.[2] As has been stated, lymphomas are the most common cause of a unilateral neck mass in patients between the ages of 21 and 40 years. This mass in some cases may be the sole manifestation of the disease.

The CT characteristics of lymphomas are quite variable. Based on our own limited series of patients with lymphomas of the neck (six with Hodgkin's and two with non-Hodgkin's lyphomas), there is a suggestion that the CT characteristics of Hodgkin's and non-Hodgkin's lymphomas in the neck may be different. All of the patients with Hodgkin's disease had nodes of the same density as muscle (Fig. 12-38, *A*). There was usually no enhancement. If present, the enhancement pattern was streaky (Fig. 12-38, *B*). In contradistinction, both cases of non-Hodgkin's lymphoma had nodes that were less dense than muscle. On contrast study one demonstrated no enhancement and the other showed a thin rim of peripheral enhancement (Fig. 12-39). Our present experience is obviously limited.

■ Lipomas

Lipomas are benign, well-circumscribed, encapsulated lesions. Though relatively common throughout the body, their incidence is relatively low in the head and neck region. They can be diagnosed on CT scans because of their low attenuation values (Fig. 12-40). Adjacent structures may be displaced and compressed but rarely infiltrated. Liposarcomas however, tend to infiltrate adjacent structures and on CT scans may have a density similar to that of muscle.

As a general rule, in terms of CT interpretation, a well-encapsulated mass with CT numbers below that of muscle but above that of water is a cyst; those with numbers below both muscle and water are mature fat. The fat-containing lesions include lipomas, dermoids, and epidermoids.

■ Vascular lesions

Hemangiomas, arteriovenous malformations, and chemodectomas are the major vascular lesions that can occur in the neck. These lesions are addressed in Chapters 5, 8, and 9.

Carotid body tumors (chemodectomas) have an intense homogeneous enhancement pattern on CT scans (Fig. 12-41).[39] The enhancement pattern in hemangiomas and arteriovenous malformations is nonhomogeneous, and although the demonstration of phleboliths

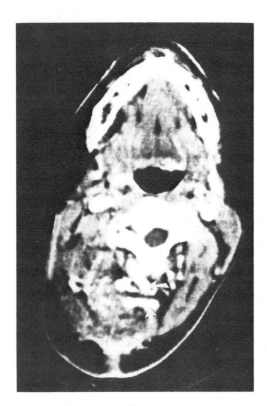

Fig. 12-43. Arterial venous malformation. Mottled areas of enhancement are seen in region of right paraspinal muscles. Large draining veins are also seen in this vicinity.

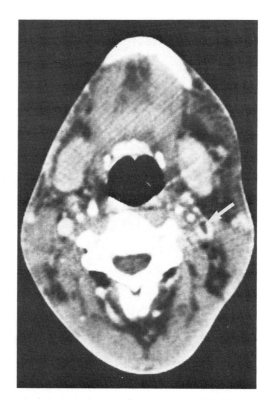

Fig. 12-44. Internal jugular vein thrombosis. Patient had multiple abscesses caused by subcutaneous drug injections demonstrated on CT scans at other levels. Left side of neck was indurated. Also noted was absence of contrast enhancement of left internal jugular vein *(arrow).* Peripheral enhancement of vessel is seen. Findings are consistent with internal jugular vein thrombosis.

in hemangiomas (Fig. 12-42), and of large-draining veins in arteriovenous malformations (Fig. 12-43), may suggest the diagnosis, an angiogram is required to make a definitive diagnosis.

■ Venous thrombosis

Venous thrombosis can be diagnosed on contrast CT scans,[30,46] thereby providing a noninvasive means of making the diagnosis. Venous thrombosis in the neck is not as common today as it was in the preantibiotic era, when it was usually associated with aerobic infections.[1] Nowadays it is seen as a complication of central venous catheterization and in patients who are intravenous drug abusers. Those who inject drugs subcutaneously may also develop venous thrombosis as a result of abscess formation (Fig. 12-44). Compression of the vein by tumor or abscess may also produce thrombosis.

The CT characteristics of venous thrombosis have been described.[30,46] The central portion of the vessel is usually less dense than the contrast-enhanced blood

(Fig. 12-45); however, a fresh thrombus may be as dense as contrast-enhanced blood and therefore escape detection. On occasion the vein may be enlarged. The wall of the vessel is usually well defined and may show enhancement confined to the wall or extending beyond it to involve the adjacent fascial planes (Fig. 12-46).

■ Neural tumors

Cervical nerve roots and peripheral portions of several of the cranial nerves pass through the connective tissue structures of the neck. Neural tumors can occur anywhere along the course of these nerves, and the location of these lesions will often help in making the right diagnosis (Fig. 12-47). Lesions located within the neural foramen may cause expansion of the foramen (Fig. 12-48). These central lesions tend to be of approximately the same density as muscle; more peripheral neuromas are more apt to be less dense than muscle (Fig. 12-47). This may be related to incomplete fatty degeneration of the neuroma. These lesions may or may

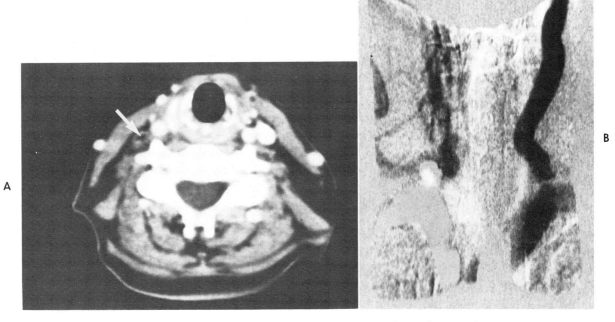

Fig. 12-45. Internal jugular vein thrombosis. **A,** Contrast scan shows absence of contrast enhancement of right internal jugular vein *(arrow)*. **B,** Digital intravenous angiography study shows normal left internal jugular vein and absence of filling of right internal jugular vein, thus confirming diagnosis of thrombosis.

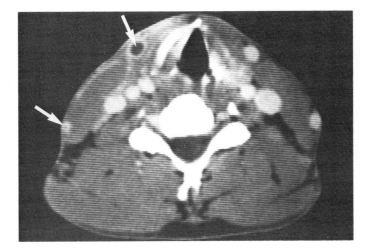

Fig. 12-46. Internal jugular vein thrombosis. Contrast CT scan shows thrombosis of right anterior jugular and superficial jugular veins *(arrows)*. Notice enhancement of fascial planes around sternocleidomastoid muscle.

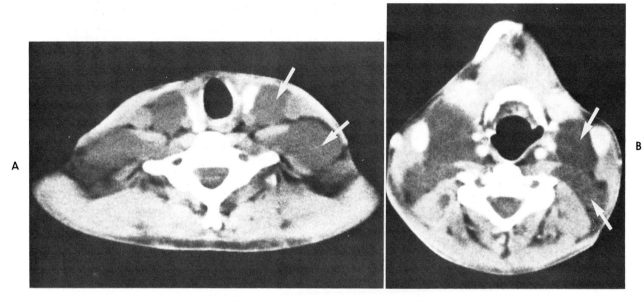

Fig. 12-47. Peripheral neurofibromas. Noncontrast and contrast CT scans show bilateral non-enhancing low-density lesions in distribution of vagus and cervical nerve roots *(arrows)*. Vagus nerve neurofibromas are causing medial deviation of carotid arteries and lateral deviation of internal jugular veins.

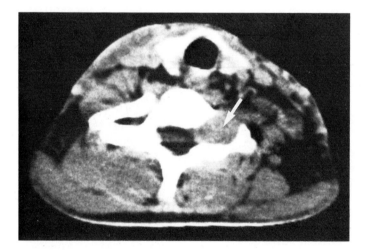

Fig. 12-48. Central neurofibroma. CT scan shows expansion of left neuroforamina by soft tissue lesion *(arrow)*.

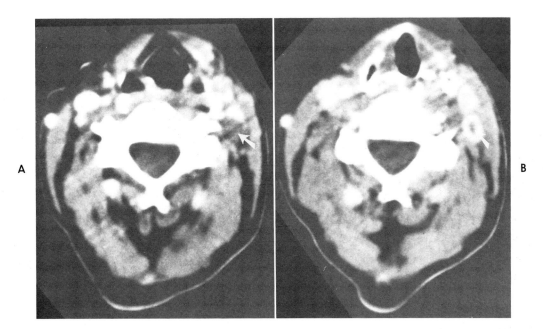

Fig. 12-49. Eleventh nerve neuroma. Nonhomogeneous enhancing mass *(arrows)* is seen beneath an atrophied sternocleidomastoid muscle.

not enhance after contrast administration. If they are enhanced, the enhancement pattern is nonhomogeneous.[39] Atrophy of the muscles supplied by the nerve involved with tumor may also be detected on CT scans (Fig. 12-49) and provides confirmatory evidence for the CT diagnosis.

□ Thyroid and parathyroid gland

■ Gross anatomy

The thyroid gland is a bilobed structure located in the anterior triangle of the neck in front of the larynx and trachea. Both lobes are joined by the thyroid isthmus. The superior pole of the thyroid gland is located just below or at the level of the inferior aspect of the thyroid cartilage. A fibroelastic *true capsule* encases the gland, giving off irregular prolongations into the gland. The true capsule is in turn surrounded by the *surgical capsule*, which comprises a portion of the middle layer of the deep cervical fascia and is also known as the *pretracheal fascia*. This fascial envelope encloses the thyroid gland and continues posteriorly, wrapping around the trachea.

Parathyroid glands are doubly paired structures located on the posterior surface of the thyroid gland in the region of the upper and lower poles. However, they may be located above or below the thyroid gland. The superior parathyroid glands enjoy a much more constant relationship to the upper poles of the thyroid than do the inferior parathyroid glands with the lower poles of the thyroid gland. The parathyroid glands may be embedded relatively deeply within the thyroid gland. Additionally, they may be located just below the pretracheal fascia, or between the pretracheal and prevertebral fasciae.[28]

■ Normal CT anatomy

As a result of its normal physiologic iodine content, the thyroid gland is visible as an "enhanced" soft tissue structure prior to intravenous contrast administration (Fig. 12-50).

On the noncontrast scan the thyroid usually has CT numbers that range between 70 and 120 Houndsfield units. Because of its rich blood supply, it is enhanced after the administration of contrast material. Patients who are hypothyroid or on thyroid replacement or suppression therapy have glands that may show less "enhanced" thyroid tissue on the noncontrast scan. Older patients may have thyroid glands that are nonhomogeneous in appearance on both pre-contrast and postcontrast scans.

The upper pole of the thyroid gland can usually be identified at or slightly below the level of the cricoid cartilage (Fig. 12-51). It is interposed between the cricoid cartilage medially and the carotid sheath structures posterolaterally. A section through the middle to lower portion of the thyroid gland will show the thyroid isth-

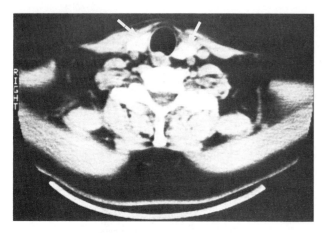

Fig. 12-50. Normal thyroid gland is enhanced *(arrows)* on noncontrast CT scan because of its physiologic iodine content.

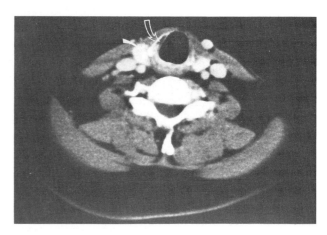

Fig. 12-51. Upper pole of thyroid gland *(arrows)* is demonstrated between cricoid cartilage *(open arrow)* and carotid sheath structures.

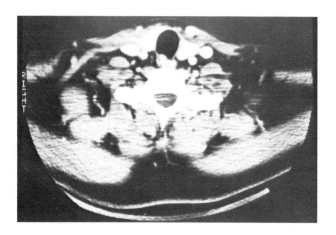

Fig. 12-52. Scan through midsection of thyroid gland shows thyroid isthmus connecting both lobes of gland.

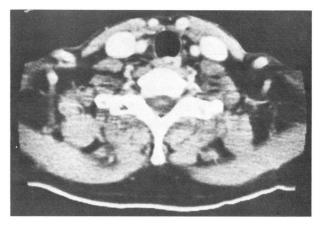

Fig. 12-53. Below level of thyroid gland, carotid sheath structures move medially to fill in space once occupied by gland.

mus connecting both lobes of the gland (Fig. 12-52). Below the level of the thyroid gland the carotid sheath structures assume a more medial position, filling the space once occupied by the thyroid gland (Fig. 12-53).

■ Thyroid gland pathology

A number of imaging modalities are available for the visualization of the thyroid gland (e.g., radionuclide scans and ultrasonography). CT may provide information that these other imaging techniques cannot; it may even detect lesions that have escaped detection on radionuclide scans or ultrasonography.

There are no CT characteristics of a thyroid lesion that are reliable indicators of benignity or malignancy

(Figs. 12-54 and 12-55). The presence of ancillary findings, e.g., nodal enlargement in the neck or mediastinum or evidence of destruction of bone or cartilage, suggests that the lesion is malignant. Also, a recurrent laryngeal nerve palsy in the presence of a thyroid mass is highly suggestive of malignancy because this is rarely seen in patients with benign thyroid disease.

Goiters have a variable appearance on CT scans, but they are all enhanced when contrast material is injected. Enhancement patterns may be either predominantly homogeneous or nonhomogeneous (Figs. 12-56 and 12-57). Occasionally, amorphous collections of calcification may be identified within the lesion; this finding has no correlation, either positive or negative, with

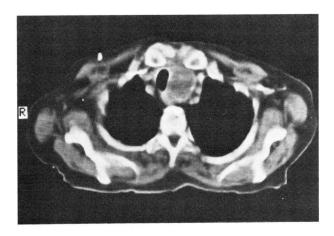

Fig. 12-54. Papillary carcinoma of thyroid gland. Contrast CT scan shows a nonhomogeneous mass in left paratracheal area that is producing tracheal deviation. This represents mass in left lower pole of thyroid gland.

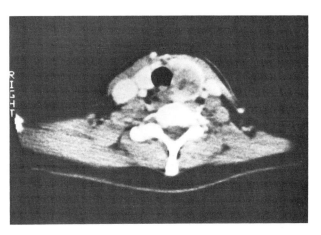

Fig. 12-55. Thyroid adenoma. Nonhomogeneous mass is seen in left lobe of thyroid gland.

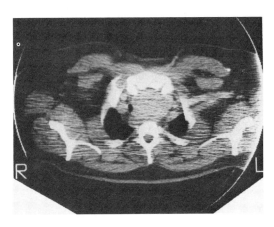

Fig. 12-56. Adenomatous goiter. Contrast CT scan demonstrates predominantly homogeneous mass in retrosternal and left paratracheal areas. Notice marked right lateral displacement of trachea.

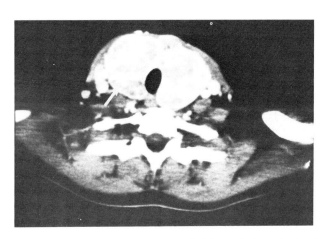

Fig. 12-57. Multinodular goiter. Both lobes of thyroid gland are enlarged and nonhomogeneous in density. Amorphous calcification *(arrow)* is seen in right lobe of thyroid gland.

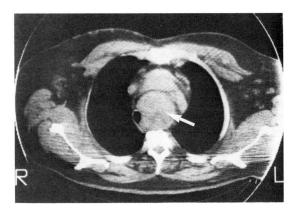

Fig. 12-58. Substernal goiter *(arrow)* located posterior to great vessels.

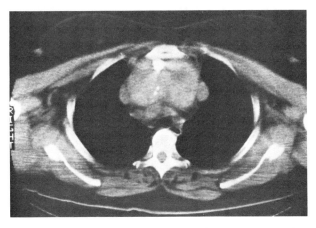

Fig. 12-59. Substernal goiter located anterior and medial to great vessels. Amorphous calcification is seen within goiter.

malignancy because calcification is identified in approximately 25% to 35% of benign and malignant thyroid lesions.[17]

CT is very useful in defining the inferior limit of a goiter. It also defines the relationship of the goiter to the great vessels and adjacent structures, and this is of considerable surgical significance.

Commonly, as the left innominate vein crosses the anterior mediastinum the vein acts as a barrier to the further downward extension of substernal goiters. Frequently, however, goiters may extend further inferiorly, posterior to the great vessels, and intrude into the middle and posterior mediastinum (Fig. 12-58). Occasionally, a goiter may extend inferiorly, anterior to the great vessels (Fig. 12-59).

The key CT findings that identify a mediastinal mass as thyroid in origin are as follows.

1. The superior portion of the lesion is usually intimately associated with the thyroid gland.
2. The lesion has CT numbers greater than surrounding muscle on the precontrast as well as the postcontrast scans, a result of the iodine content of the tissue in the former and of the vascularity of the tissue in the latter.
3. The lesion enhances after administration of contrast material. Other lesions commonly encountered in this area do not enhance, with the exception of those that are vascular.
4. The lesion is usually either located in close proximity to or intimately associated with the trachea.[12]

■ Parathyroid gland pathology

As with the thyroid gland, there are a number of competing imaging modalities used in the detection of parathyroid gland disease. Small parathyroid adenomas are notorious for their elusiveness.

Parathyroid glands can be located within either the neck or the mediastinum. In the common, "idealized" state, each of the four parathyroid glands is associated with the posterior surface of the superior and inferior poles of each lobe of the thyroid gland. However, the parathyroid gland may be located anywhere from the level of the hyoid bone to the aortic arch.

Ultrasonography is a sensitive methodology and an extremely useful technique for visualizing enlarged parathyroid glands if the glands are within the neck. However, if the lesion is small or located within the mediastinum, ultrasonography may be incapable of detecting the tumor. Under such circumstances arteriography and venous sampling have been described to be of considerable use.[7,8]

In the presence of clinical and laboratory evidence of parathyroid adenomas when ultrasonography, venous sampling, or angiography have been unsuccessful in demonstrating the lesion, CT may be helpful. This is especially true when a patient has had previous neck surgery. The distorted anatomy renders ultrasonogram interpretation extremely difficult and interrupted venous pathways may make it virtually impossible to do accurate localizing venous sampling.

CT scans should be performed both with and without intravenous contrast material for assessment of the thyroid region. Superior mediastinal evaluation may be carried out with the contrast portion of the study alone. Normally positioned, nonectopic parathyroid adenomas will reveal themselves on the noncontrast portion of the study as low-density areas embedded within or posterior to the posterior aspect of the normally "enhanced" thyroid gland (Fig. 12-60, *A*). After administration of

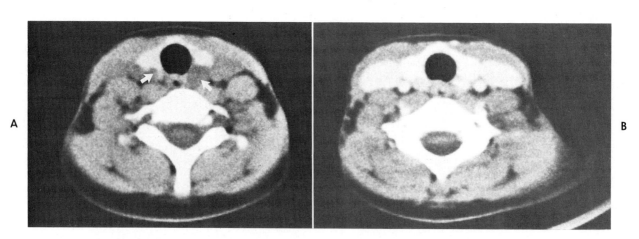

Fig. 12-60. Parathyroid adenomas. **A,** Noncontrast scan shows low-density areas (*arrows*) in posterior aspect of both thyroid lobes. **B,** After contrast infusion there is enhancement in these areas.

contrast material the degree of enhancement of the adenoma may be variable. At times it will be enhanced to the same degree as the surrounding thyroid gland (Fig. 12-60, *B*). For that reason, there must be a noncontrast study for comparison so that a small lesion does not avoid detection (Fig. 12-60, *B*).

There are no pathognomonic CT signs of a parathyroid adenoma. It is essential that the clinical and laboratory findings be correlated with the images because the pictorial aspects of these lesions may be indistinguishable from those of the thyroid lesion. Finally, it should be noted that there is a 95% chance of successfully locating and removing a parathyroid adenoma by surgical exploration alone, in the absence of any sophisticated imaging tests at all,[7,8] provided that there is good chemical evidence of the adenoma and that the operation is performed by a surgeon experienced in parathyroid adenoma removal.

□ Cervical lymph nodes

CT has improved the accuracy of staging head and neck tumors. This has been well documented, e.g., in the evaluation of laryngeal and nasopharyngeal carcinomas, and lesions of the salivary glands and parapharyngeal space.* To accurately stage lesions about the head and neck, one must recognize both the CT characteristics of the primary neoplasms as well as evidence of lymph node involvement.

A knowledge of the location of cervical lymph node chains and potential modes of disease spread is a first requisite toward successful analysis of these images. Because normal lymph nodes are not visualized commonly on CT, pathologic nodes will be used to demonstrate the locations of the various lymph node chains.

■ Normal anatomy

The French anatomist, Rouviere,[33] divided the lymph nodes of the head and neck into 10 principle groups.

1. Occipital
2. Mastoid
3. Parotid
4. Submaxillary
5. Facial
6. Submental
7. Sublingual
8. Retropharyngeal
9. Anterior cervical
10. Lateral cervical

The first six groups represent a pericervical lymphoid ring because they form a collar that may be compared

---

*References 21, 22, 34, 38, 39.

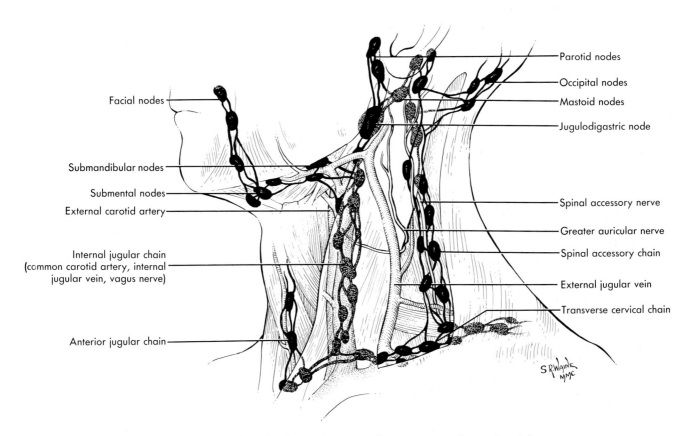

Fig. 12-61. Cervical lymph node chains. (From Reede, D.L.: J. Otolaryngol. **11**[6]:411-418, 1982.)

to a garland at the junction between the head and neck.[33] Also located within this lymphoid ring are the retropharyngeal and sublingual nodes. The anterior and lateral cervical nodes decend anteriorly and laterally, respectively, in the neck (Fig. 12-61).

For purposes of discussion these nodes may be classified as those located primarily in the suprahyoid and those in the infrahyoid regions of the neck.

Infrahyoid nodes

The *lateral cervical* and *anterior cervical* chains are the major infrahyoid nodes. Of all of the neck lymph nodes, pathologic processes are most commonly encountered in the lateral cervical chain because it serves as a common route of drainage of all major regional structures, from the nasopharynx superiorly to the thyroid gland inferiorly.

The lateral cervical chain is divided into *superficial* and *deep* portions. The deep portion has three components: *internal jugular*, *spinal accessory*, and *transverse cervical* chains. This subgroup of nodes forms a triangle of nodes; they lie within both the anterior and posterior muscular triangles (Fig. 12-61).

Lateral cervical chain. The internal jugular nodes are located in the anterior triangle, lying beneath the sternocleidomastoid muscle. They lie on the outer surface of the carotid sheath. They follow the internal jugular vein and therefore have a craniocaudal course. They may be identified in close apposition to the carotid sheath when pathologically enlarged (Fig. 12-62). If there is extension of disease outside the nodal capsule,

the fascial planes (fat planes) around the carotid sheath will be obliterated.

Following the course of the spinal accessory nerve, the spinal accessory chain crosses the posterior triangle obliquely, superior to inferior and anterior to posterior. When enlarged, these nodes appear prominently within the posterior triangle, under the sternocleidomastoid muscle (Fig. 12-63). If substantially enlarged, they may be surrounded by only a thin layer of fat and may resemble a muscle belly to the interpreter who is unfamiliar with the anatomy. It is to be emphasized that the posterior triangle will appear on CT scans as a black, fat-filled cleft spanning the entire length of the neck except as altered by a number of small structures of positive attenuation values caused by nerves, small inconsequential lymph nodes, and small nutrient vessels.

The superiormost extents of the internal jugular and spinal accessory chains join above the level of the hyoid bone. The largest node in this suprahyoid location is the *jugulodigastric* node, a node located in the upper portion of the internal jugular chain. This node is located at the junction between the posterior belly of the digastric and the internal jugular vein and may be identified with ease clinically when pathologically enlarged. It is involved primarily with lymphatic drainage of the tongue.

The transverse cervical chain joins the inferior limbs of the internal jugular and spinal accessory chains. These nodes travel along the course of the transverse cervical artery in the inferior aspect of the posterior tri-

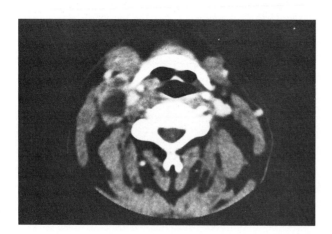

Fig. 12-62. Internal jugular nodes. Multiple low-density masses with thin rims of enhancement are seen in right posterior triangle of neck in close apposition to carotid sheath. Fascial planes around carotid sheath are obliterated.

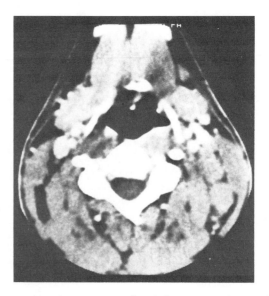

Fig. 12-63. Spinal accessory nodes. Soft tissue masses are demonstrated beneath left sternocleidomastoid muscle.

angle. On CT scans these nodes are identified in the supraclavicular location (Fig. 12-64).

The superficial lateral cervical chain follows the course of the external jugular vein. On CT scans, enlarged nodes in this group are seen above the sternocleidomastoid muscle (Fig. 12-65).

Anterior cervical chain. The anterior cervical chains are located toward the midline, between the two carotid sheaths in the infrahyoid neck. This lymph node chain has both superficial and deep components. The superficial portion lies on the outer surface of the strap muscles and follows the course of the anterior jugular veins. The deep components of the anterior cervical nodes (also known as the *juxtavisceral* nodes) take their names on the basis of their relationship to the major anterior midline structures: (1) prelaryngeal nodes (Delphian nodes), (2) prethyroid nodes, (3) pretracheal nodes, and (4) lateral tracheal (paratracheal) nodes (Fig. 12-66).

Suprahyoid nodes

The lymph node chains located in the suprahyoid region are as follows:
1. Occipital
2. Mastoid
3. Parotid
4. Submaxillary
5. Facial
6. Submental
7. Sublingual
8. Retropharyngeal
9. Superior portions of internal jugular and spinal accessory chains

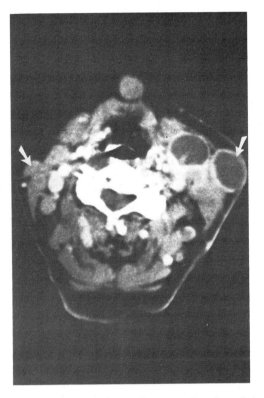

Fig. 12-65. External jugular node. Several enlarged lymph nodes are seen in various cervical lymph node chains. This scan section, however, is shown to demonstrate external jugular nodes *(arrows)*, which are located lateral to sternocleidomastoid muscle.

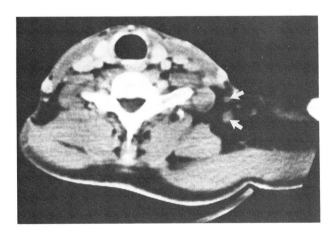

Fig. 12-64. Supraclavicular nodes. Multiple soft tissue masses *(arrows)* are seen in left supraclavicular area in patient with tuberculosis.

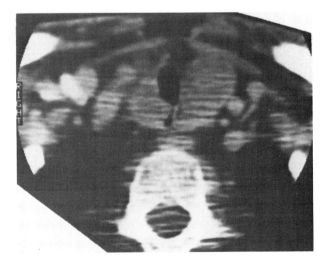

Fig. 12-66. Paratracheal nodes. Bilateral enlarged paratracheal nodes are seen in this patient with Hodgkin's lymphoma. There is extension of disease into trachea.

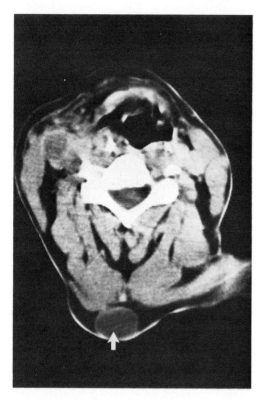

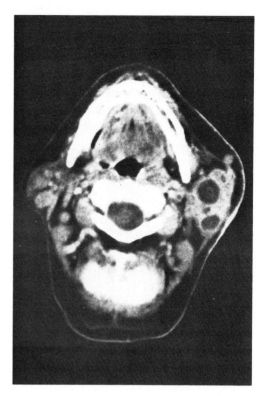

Fig. 12-67. Occipital node. Enlarged necrotic occipital node *(arrow)* is present. There is also evidence of nodal disease in right internal jugular chain.

Fig. 12-68. Parotid nodes. Multiple necrotic lymph nodes are present in left parotid gland. Several enlarged nodes are also seen in right parotid gland.

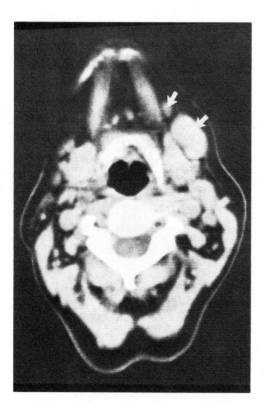

Fig. 12-69. Submandibular nodes. Noncontrast CT scan shows several enlarged left submandibular nodes *(arrows)*.

We have rarely seen enlargement of the occipital (Fig. 12-67), mastoid, and facial nodes on CT scans of patients with head and neck tumors.

The parotid group (Fig. 12-68) includes nodes located both superficial to and within the gland itself. These nodes may be enlarged in benign processes such as granulomatous disease (sarcoidosis and tuberculosis) as well as in metastatic disease and lymphomas.

The submandibular chain consists of nodes that lie along the inferior border of the mandible (Fig. 12-69). These nodes are usually located on the surface of the submandibular gland but may also be located anywhere from the insertion of the anterior belly of the digastric to the angle of the mandible.[27] These nodes may be demonstrated in the space bounded by the anterior belly of the digastric muscle medially and the horizontal ramus of the mandible laterally.

The sublingual nodes have two components, a lateral and a median group. The lateral nodes follow the course of the lingual vessels, and the median nodes are situated between the genioglossus muscles. The submental nodes lie between the anterior bellies of the digastric muscles (Fig. 12-70). Small, clinically insignificant nodes are often seen in this area on CT scans.

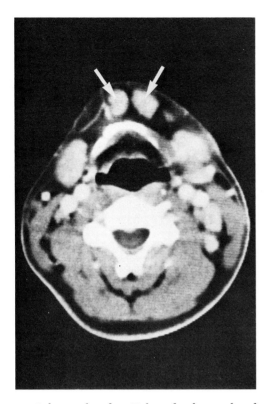

Fig. 12-70. Submental nodes. Enlarged submental nodes *(arrows)* are seen anterior to hyoid bone. Enhanced lymph nodes are also seen in left lateral deep cervical chain in this patient with tuberculosis adenitis.

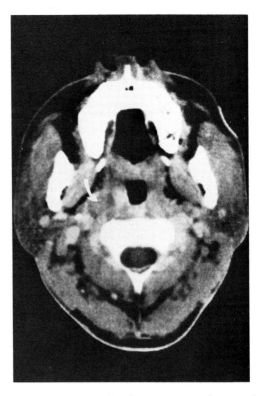

Fig. 12-71. Retropharyngeal nodes. Necrotic right retropharyngeal node *(arrow)* is demonstrated in this patient with nasopharyngeal carcinoma.

The retropharyngeal nodes are located at the level of the lateral masses of the second cervical vertebral body. These nodes consist of a median group and two lateral groups. The lateral retropharyngeal nodes are located along the lateral border of the longus capitus muscles (Fig. 12-71). These nodes lie in close proximity to the ninth, tenth, eleventh, and twelfth cranial nerves in their extracranial course. The median retropharyngeal nodes are located in the midline in direct continuity with the posterior wall of the pharynx. Both of these nodal groups are situated in the space between the fascia covering the pharynx and the prevertebral fascia.[42]

Retropharyngeal nodes are important because they receive lymphatic drainage from a host of important structures, including the nasal fossa, soft palate, paranasal sinuses, middle ear, nasopharynx, and oropharynx.

■ Lymph node pathology

A knowledge of the locations of the sites of nodal metastasis in various head and neck tumors is essential in both the clinical and CT location of these lesions. The primary and secondary locations of nodal metastasis in squamous cell carcinoma of the upper aerodigestive

tract, based on the location of the primary neoplasms, is summarized in Table 12-1. This information is taken from *Staging of Cancer of the Head and Neck Sites and of Melanoma, 1980,* published by the American Joint Committee on Cancer.

When scanned, all patients with head and neck tumors should be given intravenous contrast material unless contraindicated. This allows for better evaluation of the primary neoplasm as well as possible nodal metastasis. Because the major lymph nodes of interest, i.e., lateral deep cervical and retropharyngeal nodes, lie in close proximity to the carotid sheath structures, the use of contrast material facilitates differentiation of vascular from nodal structures.

Mancuso, et al.[23] were the first to report on the use of CT in the evaluation of cervical nodal metastases and the capability of CT to detect the clinically occult nodal metastasis. Their data and those obtained at our institution indicate that the following CT findings are suggestive of nodal disease.

1. A mass in a lymph node–bearing area with central lucency, irrespective of size, is abnormal. In metastatic disease, if there is peripheral enhancement, there is usually uniformity in the thickness

Table 12-1. Sites of nodal metastases in squamous cell carcinoma of upper digestive tract*

	Deep cervical	Jugulodigastric	Juguloomohyoid	Submental	Submaxillary	Parotid	Retropharyngeal	Parapharyngeal	Paratracheal	Paralaryngeal	Anterior mediastinal
Oral cavity lesions	X	X	X	X	X	O					
Pharynx (naso-, oro-, hypo-)	X	X	X			O	X	X			
Larynx	X	X	X						X		
Maxillary antrum (lateral and inferior)	X	X			X	X					
Maxillary antrum (superior and posterior)	X						X				
Salivary gland	X			X	X	X		(plus nodes adjacent to gland)		X	
Thyroid gland	X						X			X	

* X, Primary nodal metastasis; O, secondary nodal metastasis. From *Staging of Cancer of the Head and Neck Sites and of Melanoma,* 1980 published by the American Joint Committee on Cancer.

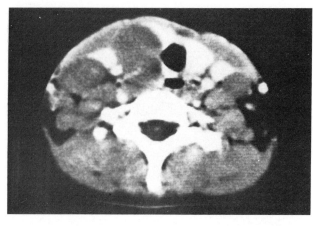

Fig. 12-72. Lymphoblastic lymphoma. Multiple nonenhancing lymph nodes are seen bilateral in lateral deep cervical chains and right anterior cervical chains.

and density of the enhanced rim (Figs. 12-62, 12-65, and 12-67). In contradistinction, the pattern of peripheral enhancement in inflammatory disease, usually tuberculosis, tends to be thick and irregular (Fig. 12-37).[32]

2. A nonenhanced mass in a lymph node–bearing area having a cross-sectional diameter greater than 1.5 cm is unequivocally abnormal (Fig. 12-72). However, both reactive and neoplastic nodes may produce this pattern. This is a potential source therefore of false positive (cancer) CT interpretations in the presence of a primary head and neck tumor.

3. Obliteration of the fascial planes around enlarged nodes in a nonoperated or nonirradiated neck is significant.[23,24] This denotes either direct extension of primary disease into adjacent tissue or extranodal extension beyond the lymph node capsule. Inflammatory as well as neoplastic processes may produce this finding. Inflammatory processes tend to cause a relatively extensive obliteration of these fascial planes; metastatic disease tends to cause a more focal disruption of the fascial planes. This is particularly well seen if the metastasis involves the jugular chain arising from the deep lateral cervical nodes. Characteristically, there is more pronounced obliteration of the fascial planes along the medial aspect of the nodes as they abut against the carotid sheath (Fig. 12-62).[32]

4. Three or more contiguous, ill-defined nodes measuring 8 to 15 mm in diameter or greater are also suggestive of neoplastic disease. Nonneoplastic processes may produce similar findings, however, and this is another potential source of false postive readings.[23,24] Obviously, correlation of the CT

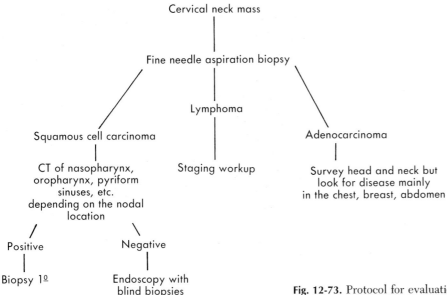

Fig. 12-73. Protocol for evaluation of patient with occult primary tumor.

findings with the history and clinical findings is helpful.

Approximately 5% of patients with cancer and 12% of patients with head and neck cancer have a cervical mass as the sole apparent symptom.[37] If thyroid neoplasms are eliminated, 90% of cervical masses in patients over the age of 40 are found to represent metastatic disease.[44]

The evaluation and treatment of patients with cervical metastasis without evidence of a primary tumor (occult primary) has been studied extensively.* A thorough history and physical examination and soft tissue films of the pharynx, neck, and paranasal sinuses should be obtained before beginning any invasive diagnostic procedures; a biopsy should then be performed. Needle biopsy is preferred over open biopsy or excision because it is less likely to produce seeding of tumor within the neck.[11] Occult neoplasms arising in the nasopharynx, pyriform sinus, and base of tongue are the common sites of primary tumors in patients with these nodal metastases.

The location of the nodal metastasis as well as the tissue type may give a clue to the location of the primary site and will also have a bearing on the prognosis. In general, the lower in the neck the nodal metastasis, the worse the prognosis. Also, patients with adenocarcinoma tend to have a poorer prognosis than those with squamous cell carcinoma.

Based on the location of the enlarged lymph nodes, the following primary sites should be suspected:

Upper cervical nodes
    Nasopharynx
    Base of tongue
    Tonsil
Middle and lower jugular nodes
    Larynx
    Pharynx
    Esophagus
    Thyroid
Midline or paratracheal nodes
    Thyroid
    Larynx
    Pulmonary
Submaxillary nodes
    Tongue
    Floor of mouth
Supraclavicular nodes
    May be metastatic from any part of body, especially bronchi, breast, stomach, and esophagus

CT may identify the primary neoplasm when other imaging modalities and physical examination have failed to do so. We have modified the protocol of Mancuso[24] and use the following work-up in the evaluation of these patients (Fig. 12-73).

□ **References**

1. Bartlett, J.G., and Gorbach, S.L.: Anaerobic infections of the head and neck, Otolaryngol. Clin. North Am. **9:**655-678, 1976.
2. Batsakis, J.G.: Tumors of the head and neck: clinical and pathological considerations, Baltimore, 1979, The Williams & Wilkins Co.
3. Byrd, R.B., Griggs, G., and Alexander, D.G.: Surgical complications of cervical and mediastinal tuberculous adenitis in an infant, Chest **70**(4):544-546, 1976.

---

*References 11, 16, 20, 37, 44.

4. Cantrell, R.W., Jensen, J.H., and Reid, D.: Diagnosis and management of tuberculous cervical adenitis, Arch. Otolaryngol. **101**:53-57, 1975.

5. Carter, B., and Karmody, C.: Computed tomography of the face and neck, Semin. Roentgenol. **13**(3):257-266, 1978.

6. Davis, J.: Embryology and anatomy of the head and neck. In Paparella, M.M., and Shumrick, D.A., editors: Otolaryngology, ed. 2, vol. 1, Philadelphia, 1980, W.B. Saunders Co.

7. Doppman, J.I., Mallette, I.E., Marx, S., et al.: Localization of abnormal mediastinal parthyroid glands, Radiology **115**:31-36, 1975.

8. Doppman, J.I.: Parathyroid localization arteriography and venous sampling, Radiol. Clin. North Am. **14**:136-188, 1976.

9. Downey, W.L., and Ward, P.H.: Branchial cleft cyst in the mediastinum, Arch. Otolaryngol. **89**:762-765, 1969.

10. Fish, J., and Moore, R.M.: Ectopic thyroid tissue and ectopic thyroid carcinoma: a review of the literature and report of a case, Ann. Surg. **157**:212-222, 1963.

11. Fried, M.P., Diehl, W.H., Brownson, R.J., et al.: Cervical metastasis from an unknown primary, Ann. Otol. **84**:153-157, 1975.

12. Glazer, G.M., Axel, L., and Moss, A.A.: CT diagnosis of mediastinal thyroid, AJR **138**:495-498, 1982.

13. Healy, G.: Malignant tumors of the head and neck in children: diagnosis and treatment, Otolaryngol. Clin. North Am. **13**(3):483-488, 1980.

14. Heitzman, E.R.: The mediastinum: radiologic correlation with anatomy and pathology, St. Louis, 1977, The C.V. Mosby Co.

15. Hollinshead, W.H.: Anatomy for surgeons. vol. 1. The head and neck, New York, 1968, Harper & Row, Publishers, Inc.

16. Jesse, R.H., Perez, C.A., and Fletcher, G.H.: Cervical lymph node metastasis: unknown primary cancer, Cancer **31**:854-859, 1973.

17. Kasai, N., and Tsuja, A.: Xeroradiography of the thyroid, Radiology **41**:439-442, 1981.

18. Larsson, S.G., Mancuso, A.A., and Hanafee, W.: Computed tomography of the tongue and floor of the mouth, Radiology **144**(2):493-499, 1982.

19. Last, R.J.: Anatomy, regional and applied, New York, 1978, Churchill Livingstone.

20. Leipzig, B., Winter, M.L., and Hokanson, J.A.: Cervical nodal metastasis of unknown origin, Laryngoscope **91**:593-598, 1981.

21. Mancuso, A.A., Calcaterra, T.C., and Hanafee, W.N.: Computed tomography of the larynx, Radiol. Clin. North Am. **16**:195-208, 1978.

22. Mancuso, A.A., and Hanafee, W.N.: A comparative evaluation of computed tomography and laryngography, Radiology **133**:131-138, 1979.

23. Mancuso, A.A., Maceri, D., Rice, D., and Hanafee, W.N.: CT of cervical lymph node cancer, AJR **136**:381-385, 1981.

24. Mancuso, A.A., and Hanafee, W.N.: The radiographic evaluation of patients with head and neck cancer. Radiological Society of North America syllabus, head and neck cancer (categorical course in radiation therapy), Chicago, Nov 15-20, 1981.

25. Miller, E.M., and Norman, D.: The role of computed tomography in the evaluation of neck masses, Radiology **133**:145-149, 1979.

26. Mitchell, S.E., and Clark, R.A.: Complications of central venous catheterizations, AJR **133**:467-476, 1979.

27. Montgomery, R.L.: Head and neck anatomy with clinical correlations, New York, 1981, McGraw-Hill Book Co.

28. Paff, G.H.: Anatomy of the head and neck, Philadelphia, 1981, W.B. Saunders Co.

29. Paonessa, D.F., and Goldstein, J.C.: Anatomy and physiology of head and neck infections (with emphasis on the fascia of the face and neck), Otolaryngol. Clin. North Am. **9**:561-580, 1976.

30. Patel, S., and Brennan, J.: Diagnosis of internal jugular vein thrombosis by computed tomography, J. Comput. Asst. Tomogr. **5**(2):197-200, 1981.

31. Reede, D.L., Whelan, M.A., and Bergeron, R.T.: Computed tomography of the infrahyoid neck: normal anatomy, Radiology **145**(2):389-395, 1982.

32. Reede, D.L., Whelan, M.A., and Bergeron, R.T.: Computed tomography of the infrahyoid neck: pathology, Radiology **145**(2):397-402, 1982.

33. Rouviere, H.: Anatomy of the human lymphatic system, Ann Arbor, 1938, Edward Brothers, Inc. (Translated by J.M. Tobias.)

34. Sagel, S.S., AufderHeide, J.F., Aronberg, D.J., et al.: High resolution computed tomography in the staging of carcinoma of the larynx, Laryngoscope **91**:292-300, 1981.

35. Shaw, H.G.: Metastatic carcinoma in cervical lymph nodes with occult primary tumor: diagnosis and treatment, J. Laryngol. Otol.: 249-265, 1970.

36. Shumrick, D.A.: Biopsy of head and neck lesions. In Paparrella, M.M., and Shumrick, D.A., editors: Otolaryngology, vol. 1, Philadelphia, 1973, W.B. Saunders Co.

37. Simpson, G.T.: The evaluation and management of neck masses of unknown etiology, Otolaryngol. Clin. North Am. **13**(3):489-498, 1980.

38. Som, P.M., and Biller, H.F.: The combined CT sialogram, Radiology **135**:387-390, 1980.

39. Som, P.M., Biller, H.F., and Lawson, W.: Tumors of the parapharyngeal space, Ann. Otol. Rhinol. Laryngol. **90**(suppl. 80, 1 pt. 4): 1981.

40. Telander, R.L., and Deane, S.A.: Thyroglossal and branchial cleft cysts and sinuses, Surg. Clin. North Am., **57**:779-791, 1977.

41. Thawley, S.E., Gado, M., and Fuller, T.R.: Computerized tomography in the evaluation of head and neck lesions, Laryngoscope **88**:451-459, 1978.

42. Warwick, R., and Williams, P.L.: Gray's anatomy, Philadelphia, 1973, W.B. Saunders Co.

43. Wertz, M.L.: Management of undescended lingual and subhyoid thyroid glands, Laryngoscope **84**:507-521, 1974.

44. Winegar, L.K., and Griffin, W.: The occult primary tumor, Arch. Otolaryngol. **98**:159-163, 1973.

45. Work, W.P.: Newer concepts of first branchial cleft defects, Laryngoscope **82**:1581-1593, 1972.

46. Zerhouni, E.A., Barth, K.H., and Siegelman, S.S.: Demonstration of venous thrombosis by computed tomography, AJR **134**:753-758, 1980.

13 □ The base of the skull

MARGARET ANNE WHELAN, DEBORAH L. REEDE, JOSEPH P. LIN, and
JON H. EDWARDS

The advent of high-resolution computed tomography has expanded the potential for radiologic diagnosis of both bony and soft tissue abnormalities of the skull base. It is the purpose of this chaper to describe the normal CT anatomy of the base of the skull and to then prescribe an orderly radiographic approach to pathologic processes in this area.

□ Embryology

Before one can adequately analyze the anatomy of any structure, it is necessary to have a working knowledge of its embryologic development. There are essentially three mesenchymal divisions in the development of the skull. The first division covers the brain and leptomeninges and later forms the dura mater, calvarium, and scalp,[54] while the second division develops into the face. The third division, the neurocranium or skull base, provides a floor for the brain and a roof for the face. It is the chondrification of this third division during the second fetal month that initiates skull development. Enchondral ossification will later transform this division into the bony chondrocranium. Thus the skull base is the only part of the skull that is preformed in cartilage; the first and second mesenchymal divisions are converted directly to bone, resulting in membranous bone formation.[4]

Multiple enchondral ossification sites develop in the chondrocranium of the embryo. They gradually enlarge and unite to form the seven bones of the adult skull base, which consists of three unpaired bones—the ethmoid, sphenoid, and occipital bones—and two paired bones, the temporal bones and the inferior turbinates.[62] Although the ethmoid and turbinates develop completely from cartilage, the other bones of the skull are partly membranous. These membranous parts are small in the sphenoid, representing the tips of the greater sphenoid wings and parts of the medial pterygoid plates, and also in the occipital bone, where membra-

nous bone forms the portion above the nuchal line. Conversely, the membranous portion of the temporal bone is large and consists of the squamousa, zygomatic process, and annulus, whereas only the petrous pyramid belongs to the chondrocranium.[21,44]

□ Normal gross anatomy

The adult chrondrocranium or skull base extends from the root of the nose to the superior nuchal line.[21] It consists of an intracranial as well as an extracranial surface. Viewed from above, the intracranial surface of the dry skull is composed of the floor of the anterior, middle, and posterior cranial fossas (Fig. 13-1). On the dry skull from below (Fig. 13-2) only the floor of the middle and posterior cranial fossas are visualized because the floor of the anterior fossa is obscured by the mandible and the facial bones.

The skull base, best demonstrated in the axial view, consists of multiple foramina and canals, through which pass the neural and vascular structures going to and from the brain. To organize analysis of this area it is useful to divide the skull base into anterior, middle, and posterior portions. The anterior division consists of the roof of the orbit and can be seen only on the endocranial surface of the skull. The middle portion, visible on both the endocranial and exocranial surfaces, is composed of the midline sella and the floor of the middle cranial fossa laterally. Within this region are the superior orbital fissures, the foramina rotundum, ovale, spinosum, vesalius, and lacerum, the pterygoid (vidian) canal, the canaliculus innominatus (Arnold's canal), and the greater and lesser palatine foramina.

The most posterior division of the skull base visible on both the endocranial and exocranial surfaces reaches from the midline clivus and lateral petrous ridges to the occiput. Contained within this area are the midline foramen magnum, the jugular foramen, the carotid canal, and the hypoglossal canal. Table 13-1 summarizes the

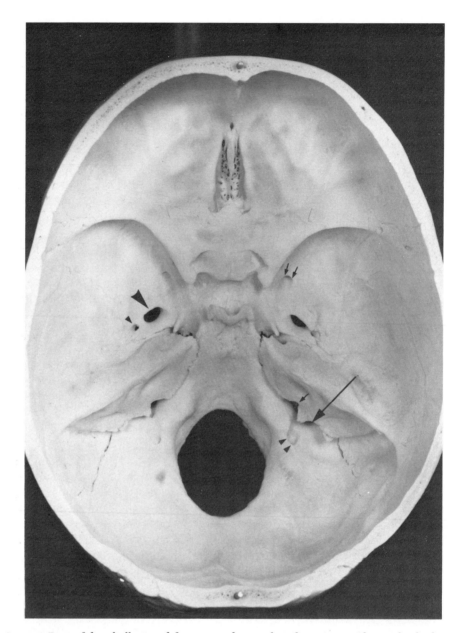

Fig. 13-1. Base of dry skull viewed from its endocranial surface. Anteriorly, roofs of orbit are visible. In middle cranial fossa, midline sella is visible with foramina ovale *(large arrowhead)* and spinosum *(small arrowhead)* laterally, and foramen rotundum *(double small arrows)* anteriorly. Posteriorly, petrous ridges are seen anterolaterally. Foramen magnum is midline, with jugular tubercle just lateral to it. Carotid *(small arrow)* and jugular *(large arrow)* canals are identified in lateral aspect of posterior fossa, with hypoglossal canal *(double arrowheads)* just medial to them.

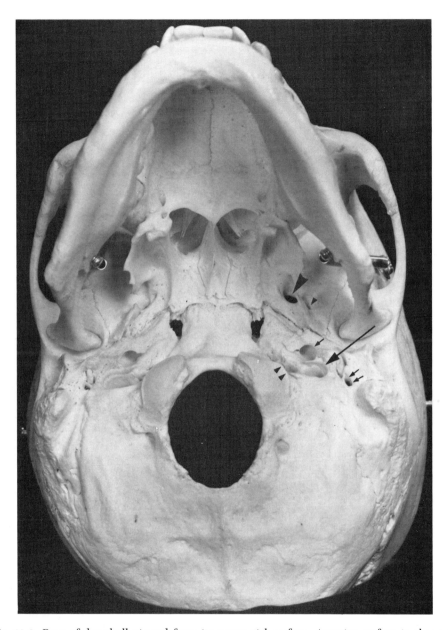

Fig. 13-2. Base of dry skull viewed from its exocranial surface. Anterior surface is obscured by overlying jaw. In middle cranial fossa, foramina ovale *(large arrowhead)* and spinosum *(small arrowhead)* are identified. In posterior fossa, carotid *(small arrow)* and jugular *(large arrow)* canals are seen, while hypoglossal canal *(double arrowheads)* is somewhat obscured by occipital condyle. On exocranial surface, facial canal *(double small arrows)* is identified posterolateral to jugular canal.

Table 13-1. Basal canals and foramina and structures contained within them

Canals and foramina	Structures contained within them
Superior orbital fissure	Cranial nerve III
	Cranial nerve IV
	Cranial nerve VI
	Cranial nerve V_1
	Superior ophthalmic vein
	Middle meningeal artery
Foramen rotundum	Cranial nerve V_2
Foramen ovale	Cranial nerve V_3
	Emissary vein or sinus
	Accessory meningeal branch of internal maxillary artery (variable)
	Middle meningeal veins (variable)
	Lesser superficial petrosal nerve (variable)
Foramen spinosum	Middle meningeal artery
	Middle meningeal vein
Foramen vesalius (variable)	Emissary sinus or vein
Foramen lacerum	Meningeal branch of ascending pharyngeal artery
	Vidian nerve
	Emissary vein (variable)
	Carotid artery
Pterygoid (vidian) canal	Vidian nerve
	Vidian artery
Canaliculus innominatus (Arnold's canal) (variable)	Lesser superficial petrosal nerve
Greater palatine foramen	Greater (descending) palatine artery
	Greater (anterior) palatine branch of the sphenopalatine nerve
Lesser palatine foramen	Lesser palatine nerve
	Branches for greater palatine artery
Carotid canal	Internal carotid artery
	Sympathetic nerve fibers
	Minor veins
Jugular foramen	Internal jugular vein
	Cranial nerve IX
	Cranial nerve X
	Cranial nerve XI
	Meningeal branches of ascending pharyngeal and occipital arteries
Hypoglossal canal	Cranial nerve XII
	Meningeal branch of ascending pharyngeal artery
	Emissary vein
Foramen magnum	Medulla oblongata
	Spinal portion of cranial nerve XI
	Vertebral arteries
	Anterior and posterior spinal arteries
	Vertebral veins

basal canals and foramina and the structures contained within them.

This chapter is primarily directed to a discussion of processes involving the floor of the middle and posterior cranial fossas; the orbit and petrous pyramids are discussed in Chapters 14 and 16. Therefore our analysis of the skull base will concentrate on the basal foramina and canals and the alterations caused by various pathologic processes.

□ Conventional radiology

The recommended projections for the skull base are the submentovertical (base) projection,[21,44] the Cald-

well and Waters projections,[71] and the modified Waters view.[78] The submentovertical view demonstrates the majority of the foramina and canals of the skull base (Fig. 13-3), while the Caldwell and Waters views better outline the foramen rotundum (Fig. 13-4). Great attention has been paid in previous articles and texts to the variable sizes and configurations of these bony canals and foramina.* Because of the limited ability of conventional radiographic technique to evaluate soft tissue changes, small degrees of variation assumed greater importance. With high-resolution computed tomography,

---

*References 5, 23-25, 34, 36, 43, 47, 67, 71, 75, 84.

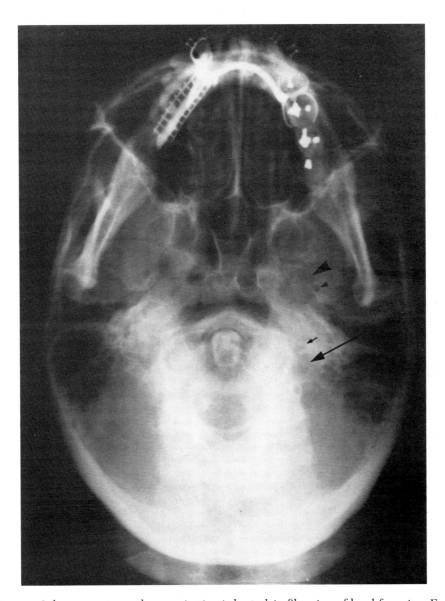

Fig. 13-3. Submentovertex or base projection is best plain film view of basal foramina. Foramina ovale *(large arrowhead)* and spinosum *(small arrowhead)* are readily identified in middle cranial fossa. Posteriorly, foramen magnum can be seen with odontoid projecting through it, while jugular *(large arrow)* and carotid *(small arrow)* canals are visible laterally.

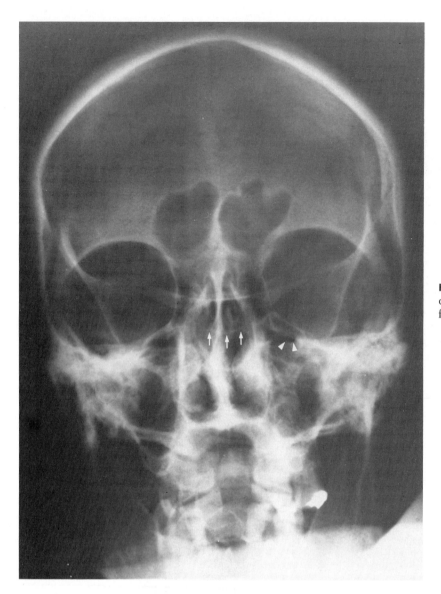

Fig. 13-4. Caldwell view provides best demonstration of sella floor *(arrows)* and foramen rotundum *(arrowheads).*

however, we can now evaluate these basal foramina and canals in the context of surrounding soft tissue changes as well as bony alterations, making CT scanning the method of choice in evaluating suspected lesions of the skull base.

At this point in time, however, the conventional skull radiograph correctly remains the first step in the evaluation of the skull base. However, now it serves a complementary role to CT scanning because it can be used to evaluate the overall integrity of the bony skull base, alerting the examiner to the general extent of disease and helping to design the most meaningful use of the CT scan in each patient. Similarly, the role of conventional tomography has now assumed a secondary but complementary role to CT scanning.

The earlier generation of scanners could provide information with regard to soft tissue changes but were unable to evaluate the bony changes as accurately as pluridirectional tomography. This limitation, however, has been largely overcome by the later generation of scanners. More sophisticated software has allowed the use of extended scale windows and target review systems, which can now match the bony detail given by pluridirectional tomography as well as visualizing the soft tissue component of lesions.

□ Normal CT anatomy

The initial CT approach to the base of the skull is the axial view, with the patient in the supine position and the gantry parallel to the skull base. This is generally accomplished by angling the CT beam cephalad, using the lateral scout of the scanner as a baseline. The scans are then done at 5 mm intervals with 5 mm thickness.

Fig. 13-5 illustrates axial scans in the dry skull. The basal canal and foramina are easily seen and correlate well with the CT scan of a normal patient (Fig. 13-6).

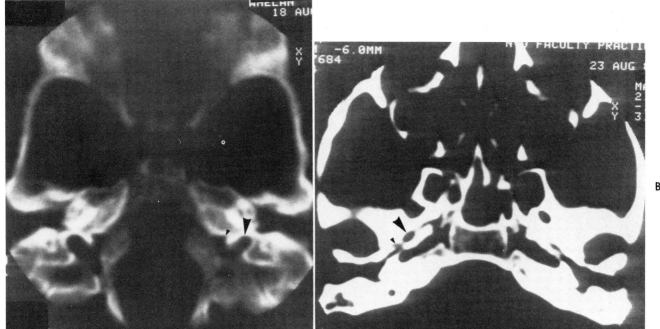

Fig. 13-5. CT of dry skull scanned in axial plane demonstrates basal foramina of the posterior fossa, **A,** and middle cranial fossa, **B. A,** In posterior fossa, foramen magnum is seen midline, with jugular *(large arrowhead)* and carotid *(small arrowhead)* canals. **B,** In middle cranial fossa, foramina ovale *(large arrowhead)* and spinosum *(small arrowhead)* are visible.

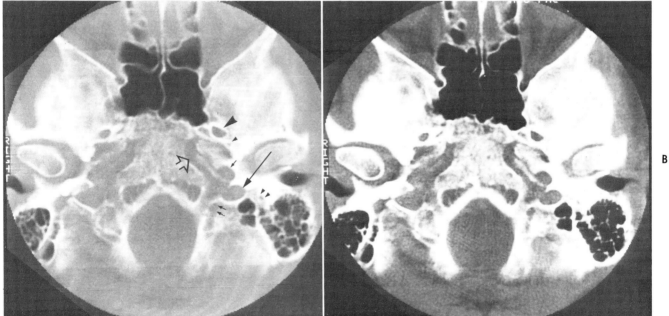

Fig. 13-6. Axial scans of skull base, done with target review and visualized at bone **(A)** and soft tissue **(B)** windows, clearly show basal foramina of middle and posterior cranial fossa. **A,** Foramina ovale *(large arrowhead)* and spinosum *(small arrowhead)* can be identified. Posteriorly, jugular *(large arrow)*, carotid *(small arrow)*, and hypoglossal *(double small arrows)* canals are visible. Groove of foramen lacerum *(open arrow)* can also be identified, coursing medially just lateral to clivus, while facial canal *(double small arrowheads)* is seen posterolateral to jugular canal.

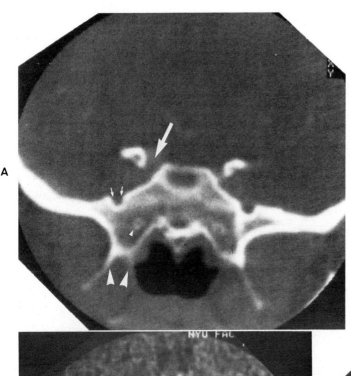

Fig. 13-7. Contrast coronal CT scans at level of anterior clinoids are made at bone (A) and soft tissue (B) windows. A, Pterygoid plates *(large arrowheads)*, vidian canal *(small arrowhead)*, foramen rotundum *(small arrows)*, and optic canal *(large arrow)* are visible. B, With soft tissue windows, cavernous sinus *(large arrow)* and carotid artery *(small arrow)* are visible as well as anterior cerebral *(small arrowhead)* and middle cerebral *(large arrowhead)* arteries. C, Coronal contrast scan at level of dorsum demonstrates foramen ovale *(large arrowhead)*. Trigeminal nerve *(small arrows)* appears as negative defect within posterior cavernous sinus. D, Coronal scan of dry skull is done at level of anterior foramen magnum. This scan shows hypoglossal canal *(small arrows)* bordered by jugular tubercle above and occipital condyle below, as well as jugular canal more laterally *(large arrow)*.

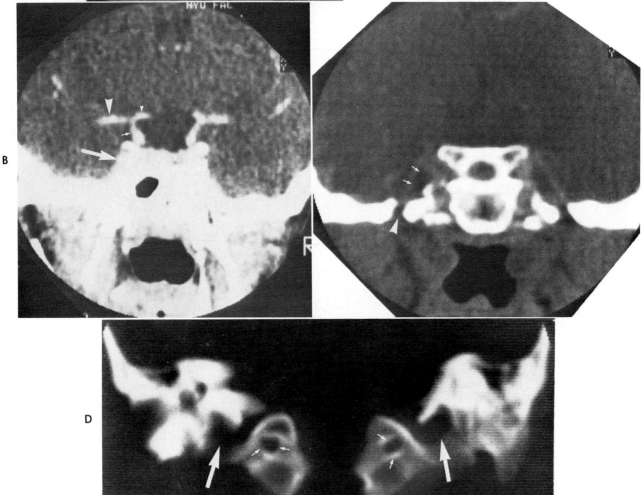

The skull base may also be demonstrated in the coronal CT plane (Fig. 13-7). This view, although valuable, poses many technical problems. It is often difficult for the patient to maintain this position for the required length of the study, and the anterior sections are often degraded by metallic artifacts from the teeth.

□ **Pathology**
■ **Congenital**

The congenital lesions affecting the skull base comprise encephaloceles, arachnoid cysts, developmental anomalies of the craniovertebral junction, and craniofacial dysostoses.

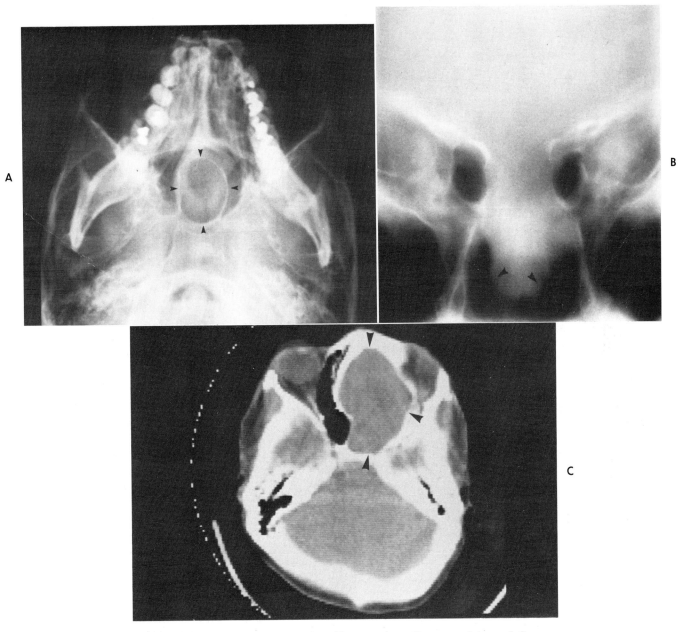

Fig. 13-8. Midline encephalocele. **A,** Plain film reveals well-corticated bony defect *arrowheads).* **B,** Coronal polytome at level of optic canals shows absence of normal midline planum sphenoidale caused by soft tissue mass extending into nasopharynx *(arrowheads).* **C,** Contrast CT scan demonstrates soft tissue mass of same density as brain extending into sphenoid and ethmoid sinuses *(arrowheads).* Bony margins are well corticated.

Encephaloceles are extracranial protrusions of meninges and brain. If externally visible, as with nasal meningoencephaloceles, they are called *sincipital*.[58] If not externally visible, they are referred to as *basal*. Approximately 12% to 15% of all encephaloceles involve the anterior cranial fossa[26,64] and characteristically occur in the midline, involving the ethmoid bone. Frontal and lateral tomography demonstrate an osseous defect in the lamina cribrosa, with an associated soft tissue mass in the nasopharynx. CT scans can outline accurately the extent of the bony defect and soft tissue mass (Fig. 13-8). Furthermore, a combined technique of water-soluble contrast material with axial and coronal CT scans, done with both bone and soft tissue windows, can delimit the margins of the dural sac. Surgically, the position of the dura with these congenital lesions is an important anatomic landmark because the surgeon prefers to have the procedure remain extradural if possible, repairing only the bony defect. Furthermore, the use of metrizamide with CT allows evaluation of ventricular communication with the encephalocele. If the encephalocele is large, an angiogram may be performed before surgery to determine if any major artery is contained within the protruding brain because it is often necessary in these cases to remove a portion of the protruding brain before closing the bony defect.

CT scanning provides a safe accurate means of diagnosing arachnoid cysts (Fig. 13-9). Depending on their size, these arachnoid cysts may result in deformity of the underlying bone as well as pressure effects on the neural structures.

The anomalies of the craniovertebral junction include platybasia, basilar invagination, atlanto-occipital fusion, and Arnold-Chiari malformation. Platybasia is a condition in which the basal angle is greater than 142° to 144°.[51] Although asymptomatic by itself, it gains more significance because of its frequent association with basilar invagination, defined as the invagination of the margins of the foramen magnum upward into the skull.[51] Although basilar invagination may occur as a congenital variant, it is often acquired from weakening of the occipital bone by primary bone processes such as Paget's disease and hyperparathyroidism (Fig. 13-10).

Various degrees of atlanto-occipital fusion are often associated with Arnold-Chiari malformation. This malformation may also be accompanied by marked concavity of the clivus, with extreme thinning of the bone near the basion.[87] This deformity is thought to be caused by transmitted pulsatile pressure from crowded posterior fossa contents and the low-lying hindbrain. High-resolution CT scans not only allow evaluation of these bony alterations but also, when combined with a water-solu-

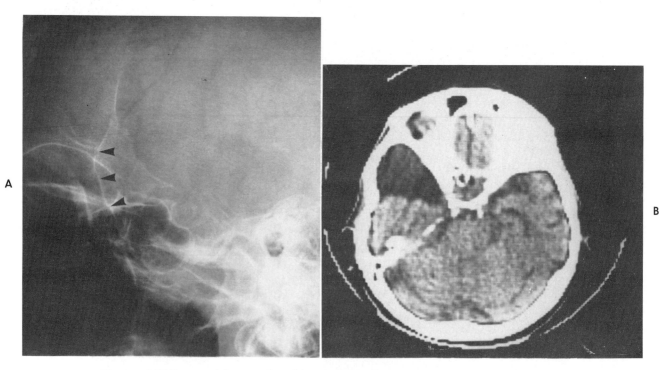

Fig. 13-9. Middle cranial fossa arachnoid cyst. **A,** Plain film reveals expansion of anterior margin of middle cranial fossa *(arrowheads)*. **B,** Axial CT scan demonstrates chronic pressure effect on sphenoid bone caused by an arachnoid cyst anterior to temporal lobe.

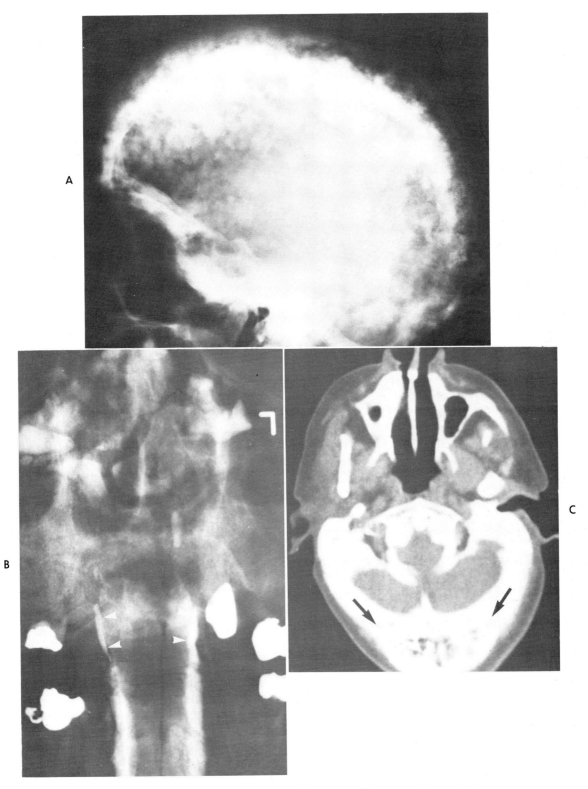

Fig. 13-10. A, Lateral skull view reveals classic "cotton wool" pattern of Paget's disease. **B,** Myelography shows widening of cord *(arrowheads)* as a result of this process. **C,** Axial CT scan demonstrates basilar invagination, with odontoid and upper cervical cord anteriorly at same level as posterior fossa. Expansile Pagetoid bone changes can be appreciated in occiput *(arrows).*

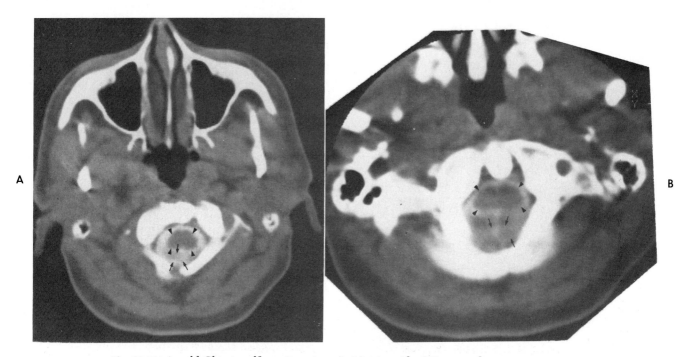

Fig. 13-11. Arnold-Chiari malformation, type I. Metrizamide CT scans, demonstrate expansion of upper cervical canal. The cord is outlined with metrizamide *(arrowheads)*. Posterior to cord, low-lying tonsils are seen with metrizamide invaginating folia *(arrows)*.

ble contrast agent such as metrizamide, allow evaluation of the low-lying tonsils and permit evaluation of the overall ventricular system (Fig. 13-11). Finally, high-resolution CT scans have also proved valuable in the evaluation of the craniofacial dysostoses and craniosynostosis.[12] The introduction of operative procedures that include basal osteotomies for the treatment of these entities has placed emphasis on the simple, noninvasive evaluation of the skull base that CT scanning provides.

■ Neoplasms
Neural origin

Tumors of neural origin affecting the skull base include neurofibromas, neuromas, neurilemmomas, neurinomas, and schwannomas; glomus tumors, neoplasms that originate from paraganglionic tissues; and chordomas, which originate from notochord remnants.

The skull base is perforated with canals and foramina containing major cranial nerves and many sympathetic fibers. Posteriorly at the base, the jugular foramen contains the ninth, tenth, and eleventh cranial nerves, while the more medial hypoglossal canal houses the twelfth cranial nerve.

Neuromas (neurilemmomas) of the jugular fossa are rare.[18] It is often difficult to determine the exact nerve of origin, and many of these lesions are associated with neurofibromatosis.[23] Similarly, neuromas of the twelfth cranial nerve occur[15,16] but are uncommon. These tumors were classically defined by conventional tomography of the skull base. They are characterized by smooth, uniform enlargement of the foramen. Although the erosion may extend beyond the foramen, the margins of the lesion remain sclerotic.[18] CT scanning, however, not only allows demonstration of this bony change but also outlines the soft tissue component of these neural tumors (Figs. 13-12 and 13-13). Thus CT provides an accurate means of separating uniform expansion of the jugular foramen caused by slow-growing neuromas from enlargement caused by jugular vein diverticulum (Fig. 13-14).

On the CT scan neural tumors are either hypodense or isodense in relation to surrounding tissue prior to intravenous administration of contrast material. After contrast material injection there is variable enhancement. The intracranial component generally demonstrates enhancement of a well-circumscribed lesion, while the exocranial component reveals little if any change after intravenous contrast material injection. These neuromas are characteristically avascular lesions. Thus the enhanced intracranial component is based primarily on the blood-brain barrier phenomenon,[3,30] while enhancement in the component below the skull base depends solely on the intrinsic vascularity of the lesion.

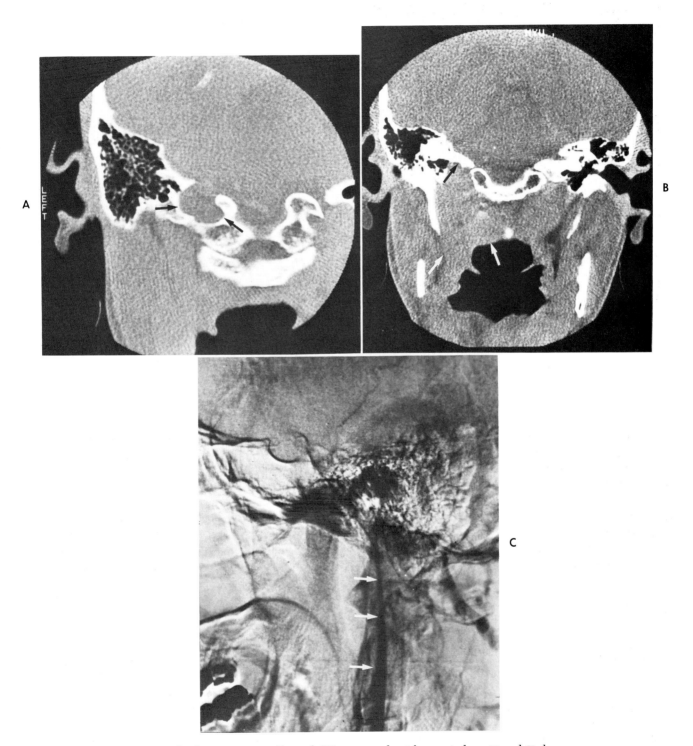

Fig. 13-12. Jugular fossa neuroma. Coronal CT scans made at bone windows **(A** and **B)** demonstrate uniform expansion of jugular foramen **(A)**, with well-corticated margins *(arrows)*. **B,** More anteriorly, bony erosion *(black arrow)* is associated with soft tissue lesion extending inferiorly to deform air column *(white arrows)*. **C,** Jugular venogram reveals extrinsic compression of vein *(arrows)* caused by neuroma. Its cranial nerve origin (9, 10, or 11) could not be definitely determined even after surgery.

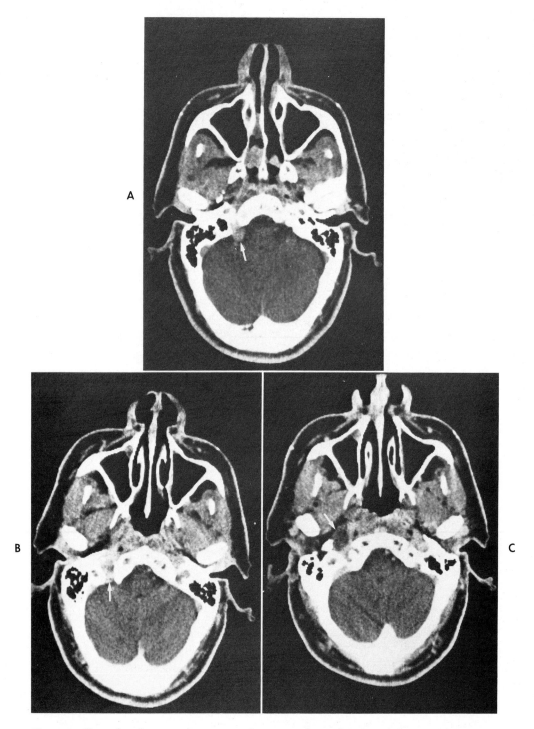

Fig. 13-13. Hypoglossal nerve schwannoma. Contrast-enhanced CT scans show a well-circum-scribed, enhanced lesion, **A,** protruding into posterior fossa *(arrow)* and, **B,** extending down through hypoglossal canal *(arrow)*. Bony margins are smooth and sclerotic. **C,** Exocranial portion is shown to be hypodense *(arrow)*.

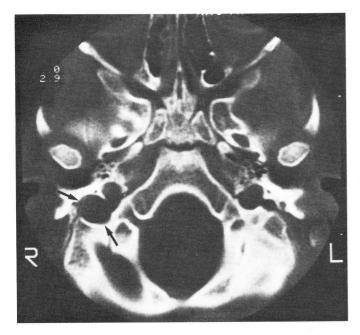

Fig. 13-14. Jugular diverticulum. Axial CT scan made at bone window reveals well-corticated expansion of right jugular canal *(arrows).*

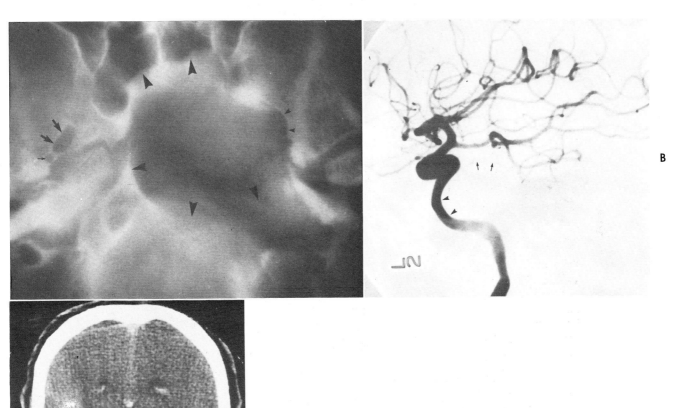

Fig. 13-15. Trigeminal neuroma. **A,** Base view demonstrates smooth erosion of skull base with well-corticated margins *(large arrowheads).* Lesion encompasses foramen ovale on left *(small arrowheads).* On right, normal foramen ovale *(large arrows)* and foramen spinosum *(small arrow)* can be seen. **B,** Left internal carotid injection outlines an avascular, extra-axial mass displacing precavernous carotid forward *(arrowheads)* and elevating temporal lobe vessels away from middle cranial fossa *(arrows).* **C,** Coronal, contrast-enhanced CT scan reveals well-circumscribed, nonhomogeneous, soft tissue mass eroding bone, deforming nasopharyngeal air column, and displacing dura upward *(arrowheads).*

In the floor of the middle cranial fossa, neuromas of the mandibular division of the fifth cranial nerve may rarely cause enlargement of the foramen ovale (Fig. 13-15) and are associated with neurofibromastosis.[75] Neuromas of the maxillary division of the fifth cranial nerve that cause enlargement of the foramen rotundum are also rare[78] and again are associated with neurofibromatosis.[75] As with neuromas involving other foramina, there is usually smooth uniform expansion of either the foramen ovale or the foramen rotundum. CT not only can demonstrate this foraminal change but also can outline the soft tissue extent of the neuroma and indicate whether the divisional nerve involvement represents only an extension of a tumor of the trigeminal ganglion itself. Additionally, the identification of a soft tissue component on the CT scan allows differentiation of foraminal enlargement caused by a small neuroma from enlargement caused either by a congenital variant in the sphenoid bone or by raised intracranial pressure.[75]

Glomus tumors (chemodectomas, nonchromaffin paragangliomas) arise from small glomus bodies that histologically are composed of many small capillaries surrounded by epithelioid cells. Although numerous locations have been reported,[31] these lesions are primarily located in the adventitia of the jugular bulb (glomus jugulare), along the course of the tympanic branch of the glossopharyngeal nerve (Jacobson's nerve), within the middle ear (glomus tympanicum), in the bony canal from the jugular foramen to the middle ear, and along the course of the auricular branch of the vagus nerve (Arnold's nerve).

The most common of these chemodectomas is the glomus jugulare. These tumors are characteristically slow growing,[37] with the incidence in women three times that in men; the average age of patients with these tumors is 49 years.[1] Most commonly these patients have hearing loss, (pulsatile) tinnitus, otorrhea, facial paralysis or pain, or palsy of the ninth, tenth, and eleventh cranial nerves.[37] Paralysis of these latter three nerves has been called the syndrome of the jugular fossa or Vernet's syndrome.

Before CT scanning the diagnosis of these lesions consisted of conventional tomography[38] followed by angiography.[19,35] Recent literature, however, emphasizes CT scanning as the best means of diagnosing these tumors because both the bony and soft tissue changes can be outlined, allowing determination of the true extent of the lesion.*

The CT appearance of the lesions as described by previous observers* agrees with our experience (Fig.

*References 9, 13, 17, 50, 57.

13-16). Before the intravenous contrast material injection these glomus tumors are isodense, with evidence of bone destruction centering around the jugular foramen. There is generally a soft tissue component above and below the skull base. After administration of the contrast material there is enhancement of these well-circumscribed tumors. The intracranial component demonstrates more marked enhancement than the exocranial portion. This differential enhancement is primarily based on the existence of a blood-brain barrier. The lack of such a barrier in the glomus tumor, combined with its vascular nature, results in a dramatic contrast to the normal brain. Below the skull base the degree of appreciable enhancement depends solely on the vascularity of the tumor as compared to normal musculature. Therefore the "actual" enhancement of the glomus tumor is similar in the endocranial and exocranial components,[17] but the enhancement in the intracranial component is more striking to the observer.

Although glomus tumors are the most common neoplasms of the jugular foramen, tumors arising in the nerves of the foramen, i.e., ninth, tenth, and eleventh cranial nerves, may in rare cases result in similar bony alteration and soft tissue changes. Such neural tumors, however, generally demonstrate less enhancement than glomus tumors and have more uniform bony margins. In order to make distinctions between these differential possibilities, however, a jugular venogram is most helpful. With glomus tumors, venography will demonstrate an intraluminal filling defect becase the glomus tumor grows from the adventitia of the jugular bulb (Fig. 13-16). With tumors arising from the foraminal nerves, however, there will be "extrinsic compression" of the jugular vein (Fig. 13-12). This venogram may be obtained by selective contrast material injection of the internal jugular vein itself or may be extracted from the venous phase of the internal carotid artery injection. Because angiography is routinely performed in these cases, the latter approach is quite helpful.

On angiograms, chemodectomas are characteristically highly vascular, while tumors of neural origin are generally avascular. The vascular chemodectomas are usually supplied by feeders from the external carotid artery, primarily the ascending pharyngeal artery.[75] Because of their vascular nature, these lesions have lent themselves to embolization techniques. Embolization has proved very successful in totally or partially obliterating these tumors, thereby either avoiding surgery or making subsequent surgery less complicated. In these instances, CT has again been useful in monitoring the results of embolization as well as serving as an easy method of follow-up care.

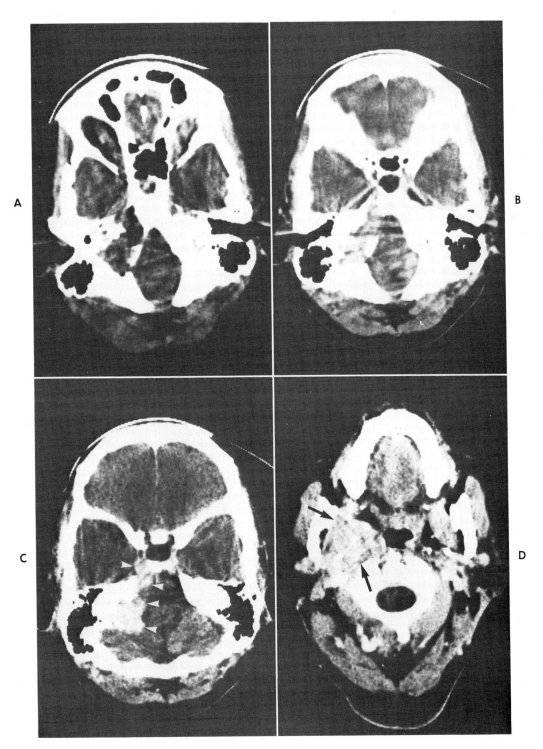

Fig. 13-16. Chemodectoma (glomus jugulare). **A,** Precontrast scan reveals area of bone destruction in region of jugular foramen. **B** to **D,** Postcontrast scans show enhancement in same region **(B),** with extension into the cerebellopontine angle and posterior cavernous sinus *(arrowheads)* **(C). D,** Exocranial, enhanced parapharyngeal component is outlined *(arrows).*

Continued.

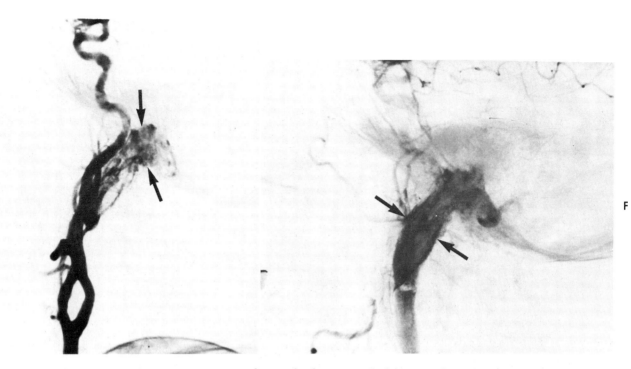

Fig. 13-16, cont'd. E, Arteriogram reveals vascular lesion supplied by ascending pharyngeal artery *(arrows)*. **F,** Late phase of arteriogram shows dilated internal jugular vein filled with tumor *(arrows)*.

Chordomas

Chordomas are rare malignancies arising from remnants of notochord. They occur primarily at either end of the vertebral column, with 35% to 40% of cases involving the skull base[20,41,86] (Fig. 13-17). These tumors are twice as common in men and generally occur in the third and fourth decades. Chordomas are slow-growing, locally invasive tumors that result in destruction of the skull base, primarily of the clivus and dorsum. The most frequent clinical symptoms are headache and cranial nerve palsies.[16] They contain calcification or fragments of bone in over one half of cases.[27,28] Before the availability of CT scanning the diagnosis was made by plain film and conventional tomography. Fifty percent of lesions reveal calcification on plain films[70] and about 60% demonstrate destruction of the clivus.[82] On angiograms these tumors are avascular, with displacement of the basilar artery posteriorly away from the region of the clivus being the most common finding (Fig. 13-17).[65]

With CT scanning both the soft tissue component and the extent of bone destruction can be evaluated (Fig. 13-17). Our CT experience with several chordomas is in agreement with previous observers.[28,55] All tumors demonstrated a nonuniformly enhanced soft tissue component at the skull base in addition to extensive destruction of the clivus. All lesions contained calcification, which was interpreted as representing fragments of bone within areas of destruction. CT accurately delineated both the superior extent of the tumor as well as any extension into the nasopharynx and prevertebral space.

Meningiomas

Meningiomas arising from the cribriform plate, planum sphenoidale, tuberculum sella, parasellar area, middle cranial fossa, cerebellopontine angle, clivus, and foramen magnum result in radiographic changes at the skull base.[32] Although most meningiomas result in hyperostosis, bone destruction may be seen, especially with sarcomatous meningiomas.[80]

Meningiomas are slow-growing tumors arising from the meninges. Three basic cell types are described, i.e., *syncytial*, *fibrous*, and *angioblastic*, with two thirds of the tumors being of the fibrous type.[80] Sarcomatous meningiomas are also encountered, but these are uncommon. They are encapsulated with a dural attachment but have a more aggressive, malignant course.[80] Meningiomas are generally a tumor of middle age, with women being affected more often than men, especially with meningiomas of the suprasellar region and the posterior fossa.[80] The symptoms are usually

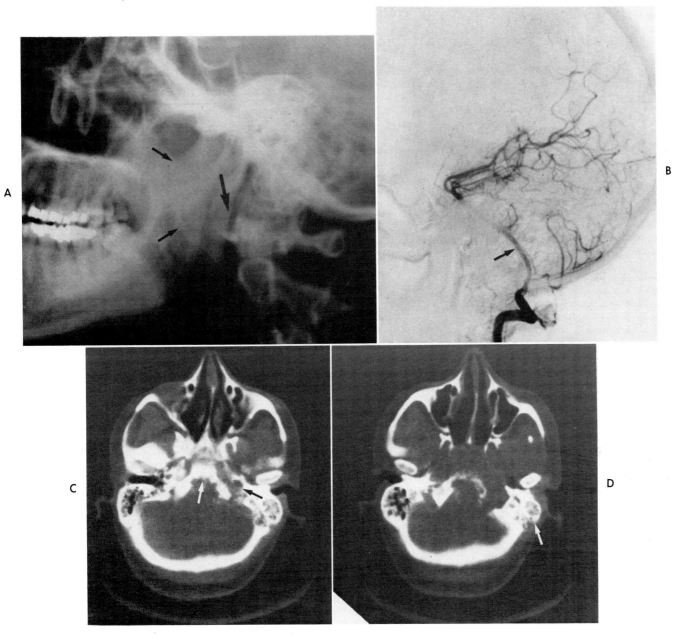

Fig. 13-17. Chordoma. **A,** Plain film reveals nasopharyngeal soft tissue mass *(small arrows)* associated with destruction of C_1 and C_2 anteriorly *(large arrow)*. **B,** Vertebral angiogram outlines avascular, extra-axial mass displacing vertebral artery away from clivus *(arrow)*. **C,** Contrast-enhanced CT scan made at bone windows demonstrates destruction of posteroinferior clivus *(white arrow)* as well as jugular foramen and carotid canal on left *(black arrow)*. More inferiorly, **D,** shows soft tissue mass occupying skull base, midline and to left. Left mastoid air cells are clouded because of blockage of eustachian tube by chordoma *(white arrow)*.   *Continued.*

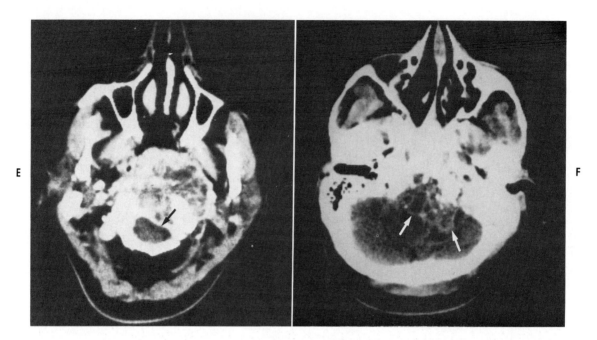

Fig. 13-17, cont'd. E and **F,** Contrast-enhanced scans made at soft tissue windows reveal nonuniformly enhanced soft tissue mass. **E,** Mass occupies nasopharynx and is destroying C_1 and C_2 and displacing dura posteriorly *(arrow)*. **F,** Enhanced soft tissue mass extends upward into posterior fossa *(arrows)*.

progressive and dependent on location. Meningiomas of the anterior and middle cranial fossa along the midline generally exhibit anosmia, visual disturbances, and headache. Lesions in the floor of the middle cranial fossa may exhibit trigeminal neuralgia or seizures, while posterior fossa meningiomas may be asymptomatic or may exhibit vertigo, dizziness, or symptoms referable to the fifth and eighth cranial nerves.[33]

With the availability of CT scanning there is much less dependence on plain film and conventional tomographic findings. Meningiomas have a characteristic CT appearance (Figs. 13-18 to 13-20). Before the use of intravenous contrast material there is a minimally hyperdense, well-circumscribed soft tissue density. After the intravenous contrast material is administered there is usually uniform, dense enhancement. These neoplasms often contain calcification (Fig. 13-21) and have a border along one of the dural surfaces.[83] Less commonly, meningiomas may demonstrate a cystic component on the CT scan.[69] Meningiomas involving the nerve sheath may result in enlargement of a neural foramen, associated with CT enhancement along the course of the nerve (Fig. 13-22).

Although the features of these lesions on CT scans are usually highly suggestive of meningioma, a vascular study, either conventional angiography or digital intravenous angiography, is still done routinely before surgery is performed.

A vascular stain is generally demonstrated. Those tumors arising along the midline in the anterior and middle cranial fossa receive supply from meningeal vessels of the internal carotid arteries (Fig. 13-23)[80]; those arising from the floor of the middle cranial fossa (Fig. 13-19), and posterior fossa receive external supply from either the middle meningeal, ascending pharyngeal, or occipital arteries.[80] Meningiomas at the cerebellopontine angle and incisura receive both internal and external carotid artery supplies.[80]

Sellar lesions

Considering the strategic importance of the sella in the skull base, special attention will be given to the lesions that can affect a change in this area. The sella is the most readily identifiable structure along the skull base on plain films. It houses the pituitary gland and is bordered by the suprasellar cistern, chiasm, and third ventricle superiorly; the cavernous carotid laterally; the sphenoid sinus inferiorly; and the clivus and brain stem posteriorly. Differential diagnosis for lesions causing alteration of the sella is dependent on the patient's age.

In the adult the most common causes of sella enlargement or erosion are pituitary adenomas, followed much less commonly by craniopharyngiomas, suprasellar or tuberculum sella meningiomas, and cavernous carotid aneurysms.[80] The sella may also be altered by metastases, increased intracranial pressure, or direct

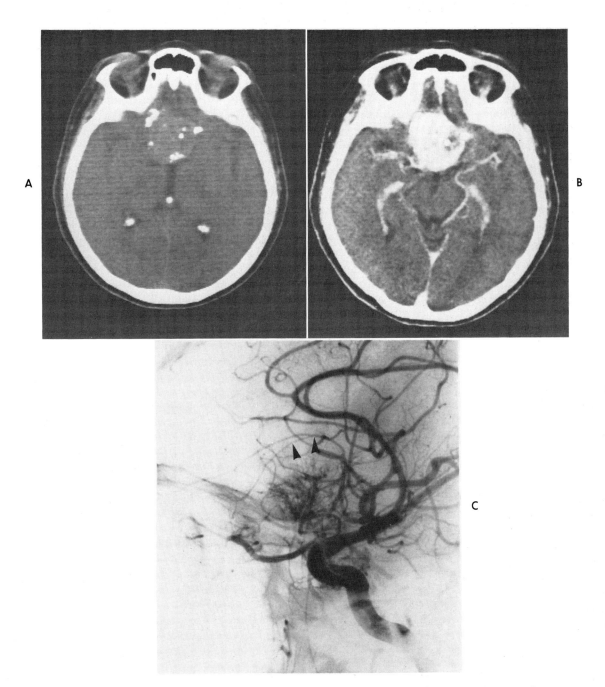

Fig. 13-18. Subfrontal meningioma. **A,** Precontrast CT scan shows midline area of increased attenuation containing calcification. **B,** Postcontrast scan demonstrates enhancement of this well-circumscribed mass. **C,** Internal carotid arteriogram reveals vascular extra-axial subfrontal mass displacing orbital frontal branches away from skull base *(arrowheads)* and anterior cerebral branches upward and posterior. Tumor is supplied by meningeal branches from internal carotid artery.

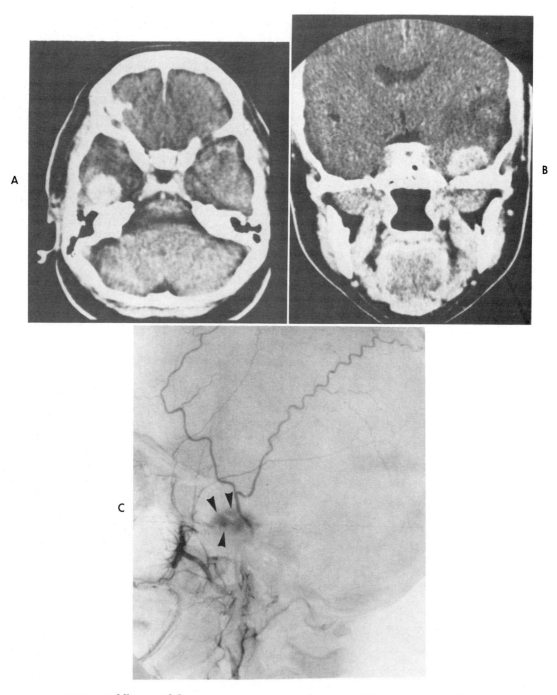

Fig. 13-19. Middle cranial fossa meningioma. **A,** Axial contrast CT scan reveals well-circum-scribed, enhanced temporal lobe lesion with surrounding edema lucency. **B,** Coronal scan demonstrates broad base along middle cranial fossa floor, which is hyperostotic. **C,** Selective external carotid injection reveals stain *(arrowheads)* supplied by posterior branch of middle meningeal artery.

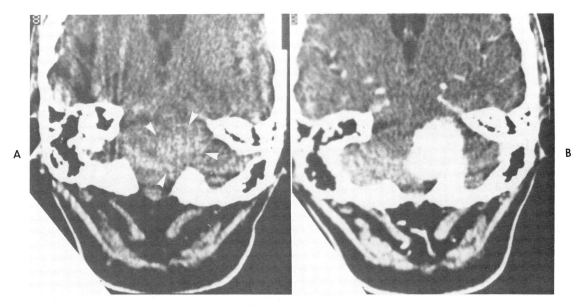

Fig. 13-20. Foramen magnum meningioma. **A,** Precontrast scan demonstrates area of increased density at foramen magnum *(arrowheads)*. **B,** Contrast scan clearly outlines well-circumscribed, densely enhanced lesion attached to lip of foramen magnum.

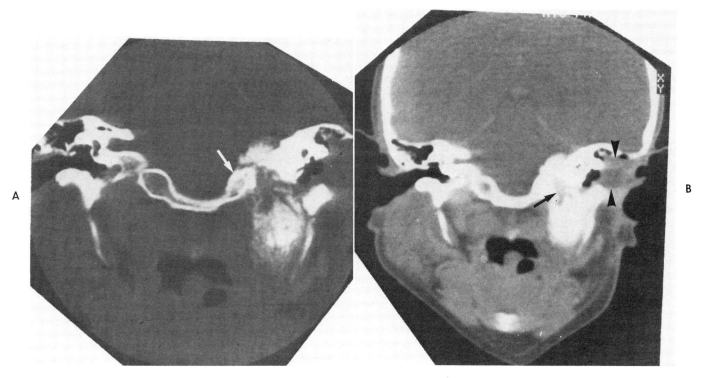

Fig. 13-21. Meningioma extending extracranially. **A,** Contrast coronal scan made at bone windows reveals calcified mass at skull base and extending through petro-occipital synchondrosis into lateral pharynx. Notice that bone is hyperostotic *(arrow)*. **B,** Contrast scan made at soft tissue settings reveals minimal enhancement *(arrow)* in this primarily calcified meningioma. There is also extension of this lesion into middle and external auditory canals *(arrowheads)*.

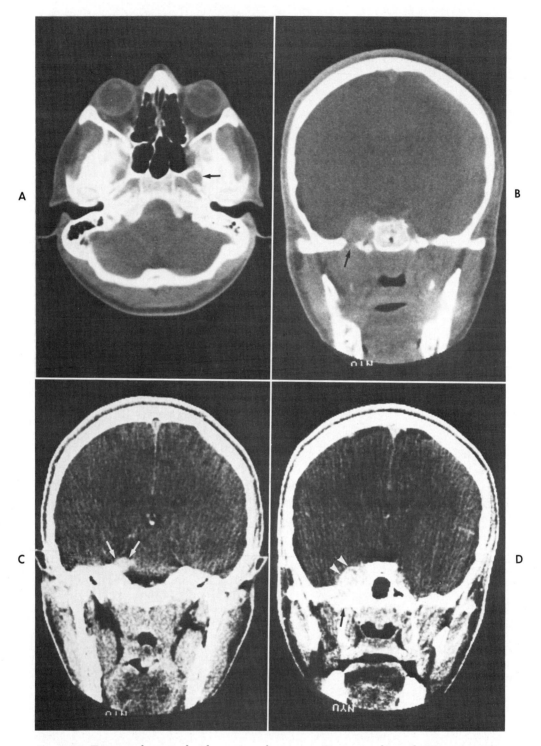

Fig. 13-22. Trigeminal nerve sheath meningeal sarcoma. Contrast-enhanced CT scans made at bone windows reveal uniform expansion of the left foramen ovale on both axial **(A)** and coronal **(B)** scans *(arrows)*. **C** and **D**, At soft tissue windows there is a well-circumscribed, uniformly enhanced lesion arising at level of Meckel's cave **(C)** *(arrows)* and extending forward **(D)** to expand cavernous sinus *(arrowheads)* and project through foramen ovale *(arrow)*.

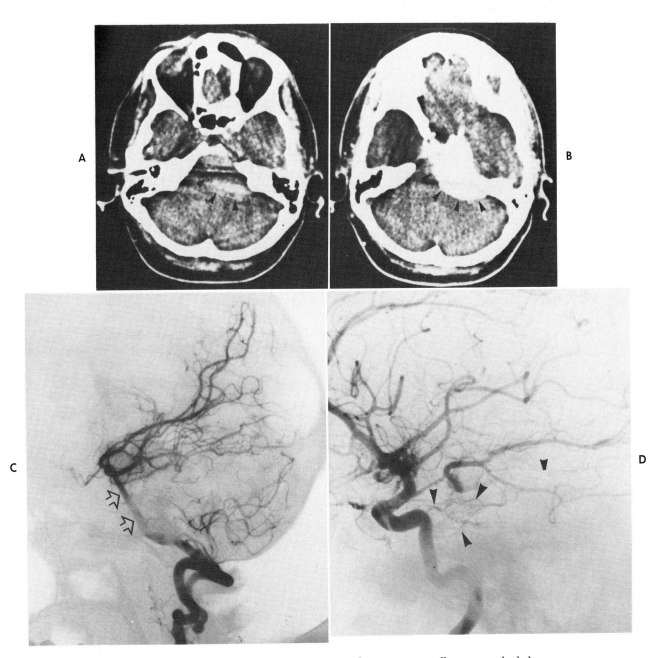

Fig. 13-23. Clival meningioma. **A,** Precontrast scan demonstrates well-circumscribed, hyper-dense area behind the clivus and along the cerebellopontine angle *(arrowheads)*. **B,** After injection of contrast material there is marked, uniform enhancement of this lesion *(arrow-heads)*. **C,** Vertebral angiogram reveals posterior displacement and stretching of basilar artery *(open arrows)* by an extra-axial mass. **D,** Internal carotid angiogram demonstrates vascular blush *(arrowheads)* supplied by meningeal branches from precavernous and cavernous ca-rotid arteries.

extension of a lesion from the sphenoid sinus, e.g., primary sinus carcinomas, nasopharyngeal carcinomas, or infections.

In the pediatric age group, pituitary adenomas are distinctly unusual. In this group the most common lesions to affect the sella are craniopharyngiomas, followed by hypothalamic-chiasmatic gliomas, histiocytosis,[52] and dilation of the third ventricle from neoplasms in other areas, especially the posterior fossa.[80] Less commonly, hamartomatous, dermoid, or arachnoid cysts may alter the sella.[52]

Although plain films remain the first step in the workup of patients suspected of harboring a sellar region mass, a high-resolution CT scan, done with and without contrast, is the diagnostic modality of choice, even in patients with negative plain films. The most common causes of pituitary enlargement in the adult are pituitary adenomas, most commonly, chromophobe adenomas. On CT scans these lesions are characteristically densely enhanced, well-circumscribed, midline lesions that rarely contain calcification (Fig. 13-24).[46,56] There is usually suprasellar extension and sometimes infrasellar extension. The use of CT scan in the purely intrasellar neoplasms or microadenomas will be addressed later in this chapter.

Craniopharyngiomas, which are tumors arising from remnants of the craniopharyngeal duct or Rathke's pouch, have three CT characteristics: calcification, cyst formation, and enhancement (Fig. 13-25).[29,52] In adult craniopharyngiomas, however, calcification and cyst formation are less commonly seen. Large cavernous carotid aneurysms may also erode the sella. Here, the CT appearance of the lesions is usually eccentric, with a thin rim of calcification around the area of enhancement (Fig. 13-26). Either conventional angiography or digital intravenous angiography is peformed before surgery for sella lesions, primarily to rule out the possibility of aneurysms but also to identify the location of the carotid arteries in relation to the pituitary tumor. Angiogaphy is also useful in distinguishing midline, noncalcified meningiomas from pituitary adenomas because these lesions may have a similar CT appearance. Generally, however, the adenoma mass grows symmetrically from the sella (Fig. 13-24), while the bulk of the meningioma is above the sella, growing down into it. Still, a distinction based solely on CT appearance, is difficult.

In the pediatric age group, CT can easily distinguish fat-containing dermoid cysts, dilated third ventricles, and arachnoid cysts filled with cerebrospinal fluid as causes of sella erosion. Furthermore, whereas CT is the most sensitive technique for detecting craniopharyngiomas and hypothalmic-chiasmatic gliomas in children, it often is necessary to perform angiography to help dif-

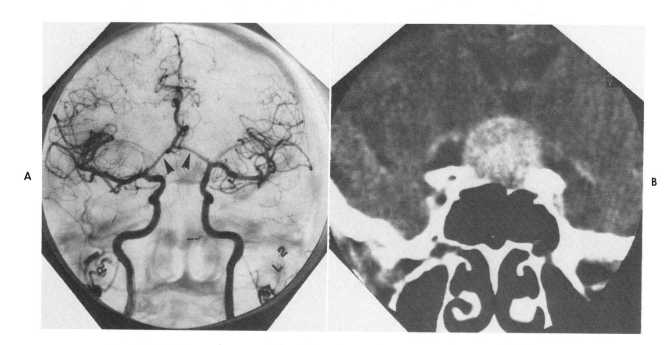

Fig. 13-24. Pituitary adenoma. **A,** Carotid angiogram demonstrates elevation of both A_1 segments by avascular mass *(arrowheads)*. **B,** Contrast coronal CT scan reveals enhanced, well-circumscribed mass arising in enlarged sella fossa and extending into suprasellar cistern.

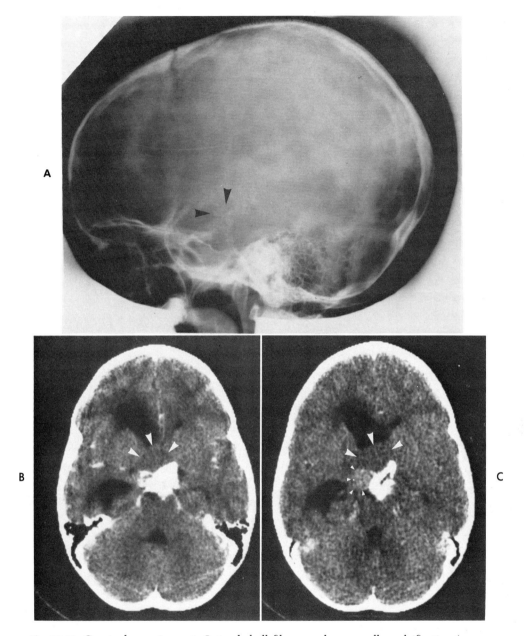

Fig. 13-25. Craniopharyngioma. **A,** Lateral skull film reveals suprasellar calcification *(arrowheads)* with split sutures. **B** and **C,** Contrast CT scans demonstrate suprasellar calcified mass with evidence of enhancement *(small arrowheads)* and cyst *(large arrowheads)*, causing obstruction at foramen of Monro.

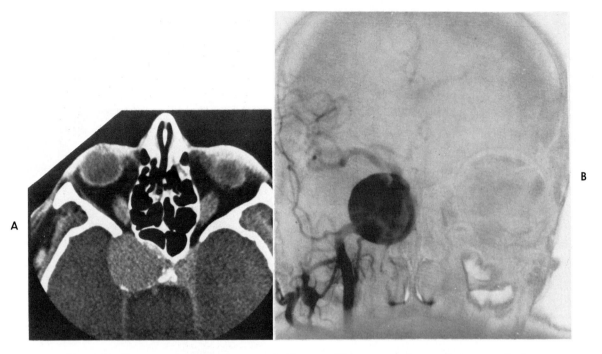

Fig. 13-26. Cavernous carotid aneurysm. **A,** Contrast CT scan reveals a well-circumscribed, enhanced lesion with rim calcification at level of cavernous sinus. **B,** Carotid angiogram confirms presence of giant cavernous carotid aneurysm.

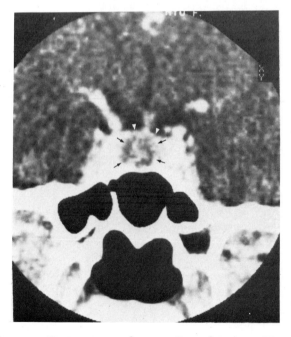

Fig. 13-27. Pituitary microadenoma. Coronal contrast CT scan reveals a relatively lucent mass *(small arrows)* occupying sella fossa with secondary elevation of diaphragma sella *(small arrowheads).*

ferentiate these variable possibilities because craniopharyngiomas are characteristically avascular, while the gliomas usually demonstrate a vascular blush.[52]

Turning now to the specific problem of the purely intrasellar mass or microadenoma, high-resolution CT scan has had a tremendous impact on the accurate diagnosis of these lesions. These totally intrasellar masses have little if any effect on the sella floor. They are suspected because of their elaborated hormonal products. Prolactin-secreting adenomas, producing galactorrhea and infertility, are the most frequently diagnosed functional pituitary neoplasms and represent 25% of all pituitary tumors.[59,60] If the tumor measures less than 10 mm, it is called a microadenoma.[46]

High-resolution CT has become the most sensitive neuroradiographic test for these tumors. Ideally, the scan should be done in the coronal plane with the use of intravenous contrast material. Microadenomas may be identified as relatively lucent areas within the sella fossa (Fig. 13-27) because they are generally enhanced to a lesser degree than the normal pituitary gland.[76,81] Other CT feaures indicating microadenomas are a convex upward diaphragma sella, a gland measuring greater than 7 mm in height, the deviation of the pituitary stalk, and the alteration of the bony floor.[81] These

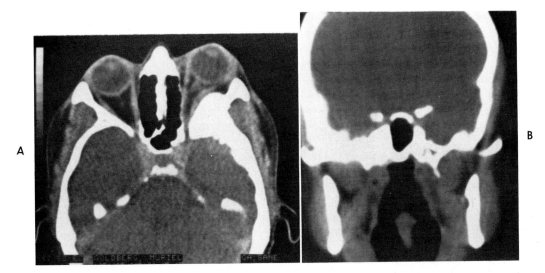

Fig. 13-28. Fibrous dysplasia. Contrast scans done in the axial (**A**) and coronal (**B**) plane reveal markedly thickened sphenoid bone impinging on the orbit causing proptosis.

last two features, however, should only be read in combination with other positive findings because the stalk may show slight deviation and the bony floor be asymmetric in normal scans.[81]

Primary bone lesions

Primary tumors of the skull base include cartilaginous neoplasms, chondromas and chondrosarcomas, epidermoids (primary cholesteatomas), osteomas, eosinophilic granulomas, fibromas, giant cell tumors, and osteogenic sarcomas.[63] The skull base may also be affected by processes such as Paget's disease (Fig. 13-10), anemias, and fibrous dysplasias (Fig. 13-28).

Although primary osseous lesions of the skull base are rare, chondromas and chondrosarcomas represent the majority of such lesions.[6] The occurrence of these neoplasms at the skull base is not surprising in light of its cartilaginous matrix. Both cartilaginous tumors are most commonly seen in the region of the spheno-occipital synchondrosis. On plain film, chondromas appear as well-defined radiolucent lesions, often with stippled calcifications. Chondrosarcomas, on the other hand, demonstrate poorly marginated bone destruction with stippled calcification.[63] These lesions occur between the second and fifth decades, with a slight female preponderance.[2] They are slow-growing tumors that are avascular angiographically.[2,53] High-resolution CT scanning provides the best method of evaluation not only of the calcific component of these tumors but also of the enhanced soft tissue component (Fig. 13-29). These lesions can be difficult to distinguish from chordomas and clival meningiomas on the CT scan; however, chordo-

mas generally show more of a bone destruction component (Fig. 13-17), while meningiomas reveal a vascular stain on angiography (Fig. 13-23).

Primary bony lesions such as epidermoids (primary cholesteatomas) and eosinophilic granulomas are rare lesions of the skull base. Their CT characteristics are similar to their plain film and conventional tomographic features, i.e., well-circumscribed lucencies in the bone, frequently with a sclerotic rim (Fig. 13-30).[63]

Metastatic lesions

The majority of metastatic lesions involving the skull base are from carcinoma of the prostate, lung, or breast.[63] Prostate metastases produce hyperostotic bone (Fig. 13-31), while breast and lung metastases are lytic processes. These lesions are best evaluated by high-resolution CT scanning after either the plain films or the clinical examination has raised the possibility of disease at the skull base (Figs. 13-32 and 13-33).

On CT scans prostate metastasis reveals hyperostotic bone that is frequently associated with a soft tissue component. This lesion may be confused with a meningioma,[45] especially when the metastasis involves the sphenoid bone (Fig. 13-32). The soft tissue components of these bony metastases are well circumscribed and are enhanced after intravenous contrast material injection. Furthermore, they may receive blood supply from the meningeal arteries (Fig. 13-34). However, these lesions are epidural and therefore displace the middle meningeal artery medially (Fig. 13-34) as opposed to the subdural location of meningiomas.

Lytic metastases, generally from the lung and breast,

Text continued on p. 567.

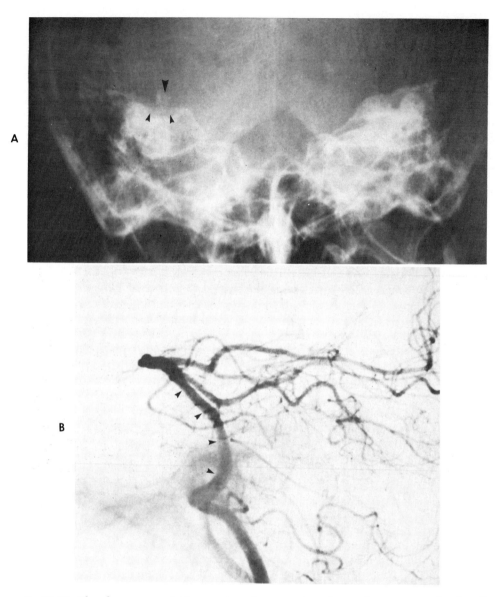

Fig. 13-29. Chondrosarcoma. **A,** Towne view shows erosion of superior petrous ridge *(small arrowheads)* associated with fluffy calcification *(large arrowhead)*. **B,** Vertebral angiogram outlines avascular extra-axial mass displacing vertebral backward *(arrowheads)*.

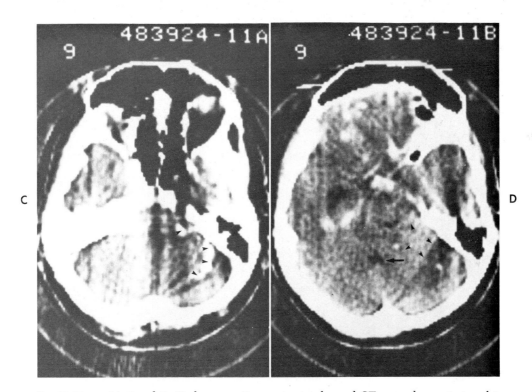

Fig. 13-29, cont'd. C and **D,** Early generation contrast-enhanced CT scans demonstrate calcification on lower section **(C)** *(arrowheads)* with enhanced lesion **(D)** at cerebellopontine angle *(arrowheads)*. This lesion is deviating fourth ventricle *(large arrow)*.

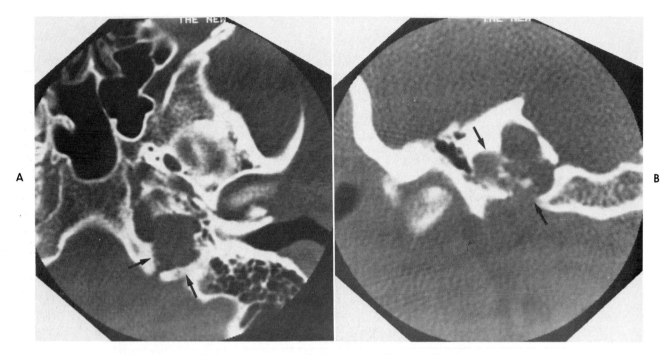

Fig 13-30. Primary cholesteatoma. **A,** Axial CT scan reveals area of bone erosion with smooth, relatively sharp borders *(arrows)*. **B,** Coronal CT scan confirms bony erosion at level of jugular canal and tubercle.

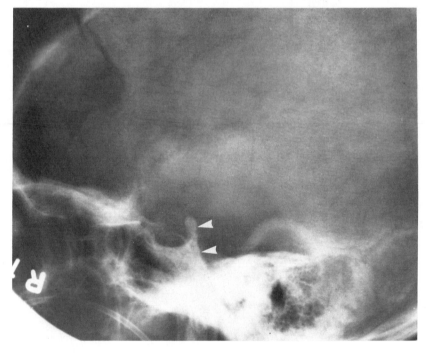

Fig. 13-31. Sella prostate metastasis. Lateral skull film demonstrates hyperostosis of sella *(arrowheads)* caused by prostate metastasis.

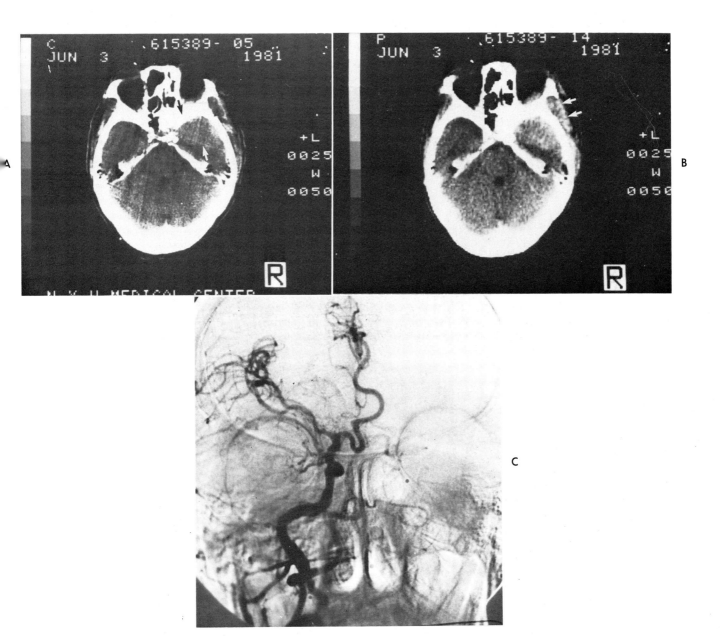

Fig. 13-32. Prostate metastasis. **A,** Precontrast CT scan demonstrates well-circumscribed area of increased density *(white arrow)* associated with hyperostosis of sphenoid wing *(black arrow)*. **B,** Postcontrast scan shows enhancement of this well-circumscribed middle cranial fossa lesion, as well as of soft tissue outside calvarium *(white arrows)*. **C,** Angiogram reveals avascular extra-axial mass displacing middle cerebral artery superiorly and medially.

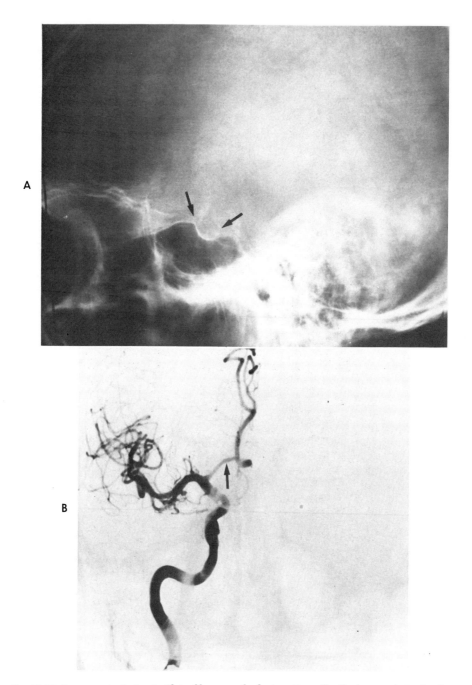

Fig. 13-33. Lung metastasis. **A,** Plain film reveals destruction of sella *(arrows)*. **B,** Angiogram shows avascular extra-axial mass elevating A₁ segment *(arrow)*.

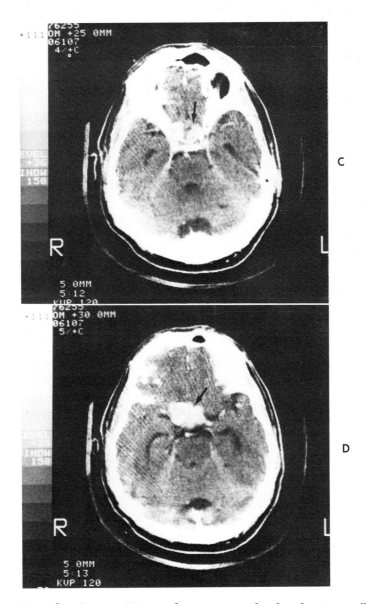

Fig. 13-33, cont'd. C and **D,** Contrast CT scans demonstrate uniformly enhancing, well-circumscribed mass occupying sella **(C)** with extension to suprasellar cistern **(D)** *(arrows).*

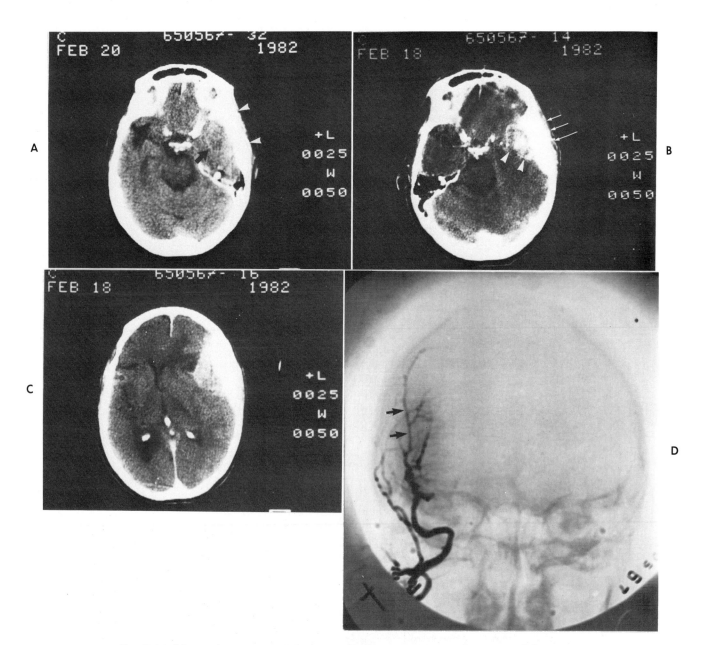

Fig. 13-34. Metastatic prostate carcinoma. **A,** Precontrast scan reveals increased density in middle cranial fossa *(black arrow)*, obliterating sylvian fissure and associated with hyperostosis of sphenoid and temporal bones *(white arrowheads)*. **B,** Postcontrast scan shows enhancement both medial *(arrowheads)* and lateral *(arrows)* to hyperostotic bone. **C,** More superiorly, postcontrast scan demonstrates well-circumscribed lesion with broad base along inner table of skull associated with edema and shift of ventricular system. **D,** External carotid contrast material injection reveals vascular blush supplied by middle meningeal artery, which is displaced medially *(arrows)*, indicating an epidural mass effect.

may also involve the skull base. As with prostate metastases, on the CT scan there is an enhanced soft tissue component associated with the lytic defect (Fig. 13-33). In these cases the age and clinical history of the patient are generally necessary to suggest the correct diagnosis.

Although multiple myeloma commonly involves the calvarium, the skull base is rarely involved. In this location, however, myeloma can result in large areas of destruction, primarily of the sella, clivus, and petrous portions of the temporal bone.[63]

Paranasal sinus and nasopharyngeal lesions

Direct extension to the skull base of processes in the paranasal sinuses and nasopharynx is not uncommon. Both malignant lesions such as carcinomas and sarcomas and benign processes such as angiofibromas and mucoceles can affect the skull base. Whereas the diagnosis was formerly based on plain films and conventional tomography, high-resolution CT scanning has now become the study of choice in outlining these disease processes.[8] In evaluating the skull base it should be noted that nasopharyngeal malignancies may cause either destruction or sclerosis, although bone destruction is far more common.[68] These tumors characteristically have a

large soft tissue component that can be clearly outlined on the CT scan (Fig. 13-35). Commonly, the CT scan will also reveal unilateral middle ear and mastoid cell fluid that is thought to be caused by obstruction of the eustachian tube from the mass. Frequently the clinical history may be helpful because nasopharyngeal carcinoma is much more common in the Chinese population.[68] Outside of the Chinese population the peak incidence occurs between the ages of 40 to 60 years, with a variably reported increased incidence in men of 2:1 to 4:1.[68] Nasopharyngeal malignancies can be seen in children as young as 3 to 4 years of age, and in this group the malignancies are usually anaplastic carcinomas (lymphoepithelioma or transitional cell carcinoma). Another helpful clinical sign is the presence of a neck mass because nasopharyngeal carcinoma commonly demonstrates metastatic neck nodes at the time of diagnosis (Fig. 13-35).[73]

The CT features of these lesions are bone destruction when the skull base has been invaded and the presence of a large soft tissue lesion. As seen in other lesions with an intracranial and extracranial component, the intracranial soft tissue component will frequently demonstrate appreciable enhancement after intravenous

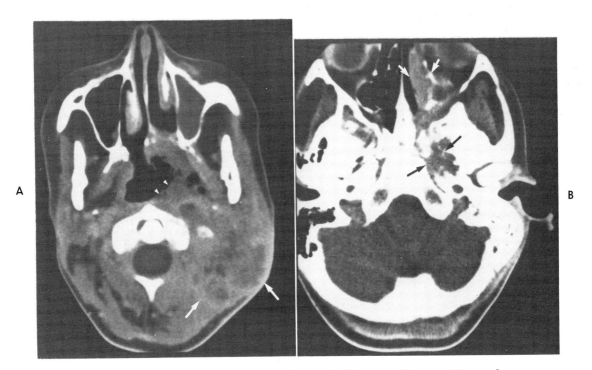

Fig. 13-35. Nasopharyngeal carcinoma extending to skull base. **A,** Contrast CT scan demonstrates nasophraryngeal soft tissue mass (*arrowheads*) destroying pterygoid plates and blocking maxillary antrum and associated with metastatic lymph nodes (*arrows*). **B,** Higher CT scan section reveals soft tissue mass extending into orbit and ethmoid sinus (*white arrows*) with bone destruction of middle cranial fossa floor (*black arrows*).

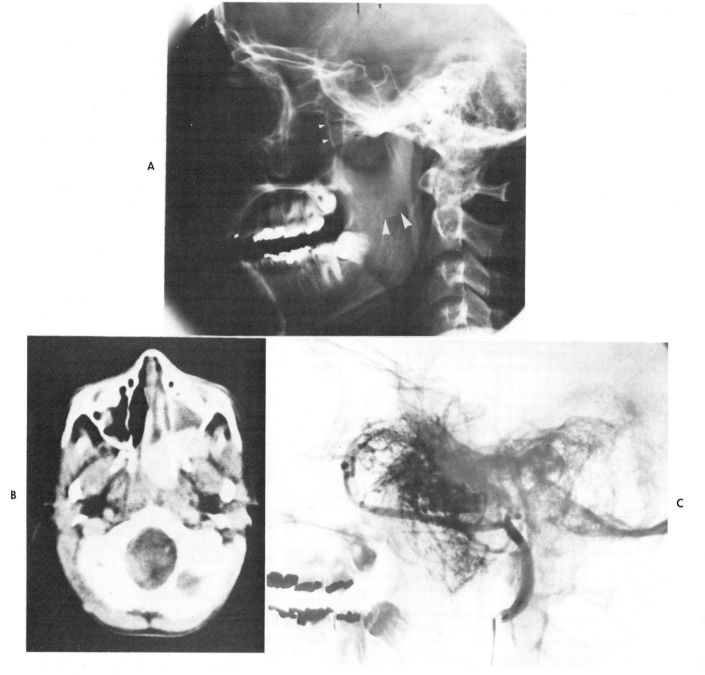

Fig. 13-36. Juvenile angiofibroma. **A,** Lateral skull film shows nasopharyngeal soft tissue mass *(large arrowheads)* as well as bowing of posterior wall of maxillary antrum *(small arrowheads).* **B,** Contrast CT scan reveals enhanced soft tissue lesion in nasopharynx and involving maxillary antrum. **C,** Angiography demonstrates vascular lesion supplied by internal maxillary artery. Notice characteristic "pallisading" of this angiofibroma blush.

contrast material injection while there will be little if any appreciable enhancement in the exocranial component. This phenomenon can be readily explained. Enhancement of the intracranial portion is dependent not only on the vascularity of the tumor itself but also on the existence of the blood-brain barrier, which blocks diffusion of iodine into the brain and therefore results in greater differential enhancement. The enhancement in the extracranial component, however, depends on vascularity alone. Here the lesion quickly equilibrates with the surrounding musculature because there is no barrier to maintain a differential iodine content.

Malignancies of the paranasal sinuses may also involve the skull base by direct extension; this topic is addressed in detail in Chapter 1. Suffice it to say that squamous cell carcinomas are the most frequent malignancies in older adults; lymphomas, in young adults; and rhabdomyosarcoma, in children. Ideally, CT scanning should be done with and without the use of intravenous contrast material injection and in the coronal and axial planes. Contrast enhancement is especially beneficial in demonstrating the intracranial extent of these lesions, which generally spread through the cribriform plate, the lateral wall of the olfactory groove, and the ethmoid and sphenoid roofs.[8]

The benign nasopharyngeal and paranasal sinus lesions affecting the skull base include juvenile angiofibromas, polyps, neurinomas, neurofibromas, and mucoceles.

The most common congenital lesions of the nasopharynx affecting the skull base are juvenile angiofibromas.

These lesions are highly vascular, noninfiltrating benign neoplasms, generally occurring in the nasopharyngeal region of pubescent males.[68] The optimum radiologic evaluation includes plain films followed by CT scanning in the axial and coronal plane, with and without contrast material injection (Fig. 13-36). These lesions are enhanced more than adjacent muscle tissue, in contradistinction to other nasopharyngeal lesions such as choanal polyps, lymphomas, and carcinomas.[1] It must be emphasized, however, that equilibration of these vascular lesions with surrounding muscle occurs rapidly; the differential enhancement of these angiofibromas may therefore be missed if scanning is delayed after the administration of intravenous contrast material. A useful anatomic classification of these lesions has been put forth, based on involvement of the sphenopalatine foramen, pterygopalatine fossa, and pterygomaxillary fissure, as well as type of extension, whether lateral or intracranial.[10] Suffice it to say that high-resolution CT scanning has provided the best means of outlining the soft tissue extent of these tumors and has allowed a more thoughtful therapeutic approach to these lesions. Although the clinical history combined with the CT findings generally lead to a presumptive diagnosis, angiography is still needed to confirm the diagnosis and plan treatment, which now generally consists of embolization, frequently followed by surgery.

The benign lesions of the sinus, such as mucoceles, cysts, and polyps, generally cause bone expansion or pressure erosion.[8] The most common benign lesion to affect the skull base is the mucocele.

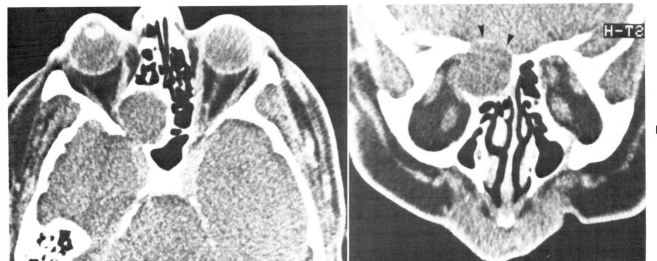

Fig. 13-37. Posterior ethmoid mucocele. **A** and **B,** Contrast CT scans reveal well-circumscribed, nonenhanced lesion causing smooth erosion of ethmoid sinuses and encroaching on orbit. **B,** Coronal scan shows enhancement of dura, which is displaced superiorly (*arrowheads*).

Mucoceles occur when the ostium of the sinus remains blocked and there is accumulation of sterile fluid, usually mucus. The most common location is the frontal sinus, followed by the ethmoid sinus. The maxillary and sphenoid sinuses may occasionally be involved. CT is the best method of demonstrating these lesions. They appear as well-marginated soft tissue densities with associated bone erosion or expansion and no enhancement (Fig. 13-37).[39,61] The finding of either calcification or enhancement associated with these lesions indicates infection.[7,39,74]

■ Inflammatory lesions

Involvement of the skull base with an inflammatory process is most commonly a result of direct extension of a suppurative process from the paranasal sinuses, mastoids, or scalp.[63] Infection, however, may be the result of contaminating trauma. Diabetics and patients taking anti-inflammatory or immunosuppressive drugs are at high risk to develop these infections.[14,48]

In patients suspected of infection, high-resolution CT scanning is not only capable of delineating the bone involved with osteomyelitis but also can outline the primary infection in the ear, sinus, or orbit (Figs. 13-38 and 13-39). Because inflammatory processes from the sinus, orbit, and ear are covered in detail in Chapters 1, 14, and 15, we will point out only the most salient features in relation to the skull base. Ethmoid sinusitis frequently occurs in children and teenagers and is the most common cause of orbital inflammation.[66,88] The usual organisms are *Staphylococcus* and *Streptococcus*. CT scans demonstrate a soft tissue density within the ethmoid and frequently the sphenoid sinus in association with a mass in the orbit. With extensive disease there may be an intracranial component causing dural enhancement. If untreated, the infection will result in either a subdural empyema or an intracranial abscess (Fig. 13-38).

Malignant otitis is generally the result of a *Pseudomonas* infection in a diabetic patient. The presence of this entity may cause extensive osteomyelitis of the temporal and occipital bone and may result in intracranial

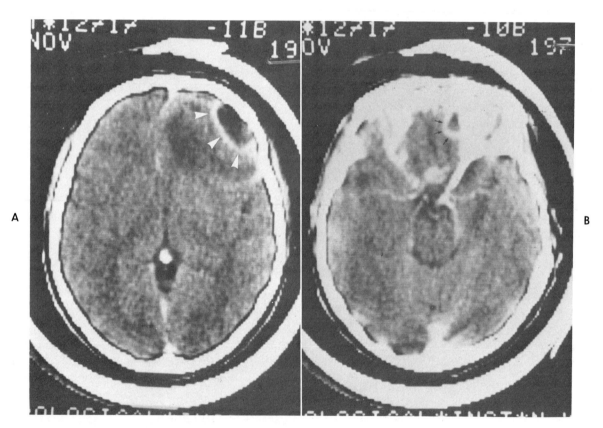

Fig. 13-38. Subdural empyema. Contrast CT scans. **A,** Ring enhanced lesion is outlined in frontal lobe *(arrowheads)*, with surrounding edema lucency and broad base along inner table. **B,** This lesion extends inferiorly where ring enhanced area is seen projecting just above ethmoid area *(small arrows)*. By history, this patient had developed fever, focal seizures, and decreased mental status after ethmoid polypectomy.

abscess. Again, high-resolution CT scanning can demonstrate the extent of bony involvement as well as demonstrate the extent of soft tissue changes (Fig. 13-39).

Whenever sinus, orbit, or ear inflammation occurs in high-risk patients, fungal disease should be considered, particularly mucormycosis in diabetic patients and as-pergillosis in immunosuppressed patients.[8] Both these lesions demonstrate a propensity for invasion of blood vessels, resulting in a purulent arteritis with rapid intracranial dissemination (Fig. 13-40).[85] CT provides an easy method of evaluating the extent of the infection as well as its response to therapy.

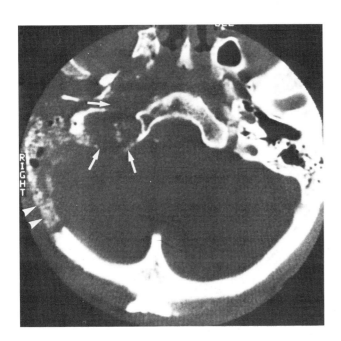

Fig. 13-39. Malignant otitis in diabetic patient. Axial CT scan made at bone window settings demonstrates extensive destruction of petrous ridge and mastoid air cells as well as osteomyelitis of occipital bone *(arrowheads)* and destruction of basal foramina *(arrows)*.

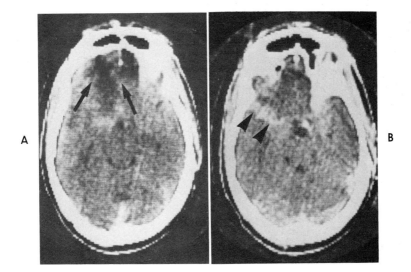

Fig. 13-40. Intracranial mucormycosis in diabetic patient. **A** and **B,** Postcontrast scans reveal diffuse frontal lobe lucency *(arrows)*. **B,** Enhancement in sylvian fissure *(arrowheads)*. Autopsy revealed fungus invading ethmoid region, subarachnoid space and brain parenchyma. Hyphae were found in anterior cerebral artery, resulting in frontal lobe infarct.

■ Trauma and cerebrospinal fluid fistulae

Fractures at the skull base are extremely difficult to demonstrate on skull radiography. Although good quality conventional tomography will improve accuracy, visualization of basal skull fractures remains a difficult problem.[63] This is especially bothersome in light of the association of cerebrospinal fluid leaks, which can serve as a pathway for the introduction of bacteria and result in intracranial infection, primarily meningitis.

Even with high-resolution CT the demonstration of a linear fracture may be difficult. However, CT has clearly enabled the accurate evaluation of associated subdural and epidural hematomas as well as the demonstration of fluid levels in the sinuses and in the mastoid area.

Cerebrospinal fluid fistulae may be sequelae of traumatic basal skull fracture or may be the result of surgery. In some cases they are spontaneous, generally associated with the so-called empty sella syndrome. In this latter instance there is an incompetent diaphragma sella that subjects the sella fossa to cerebrospinal fluid pressure. Eventually, a fistula may be established between the sella floor and the sphenoid sinus, resulting in cerebrospinal fluid rhinorrhea. Kaufman[42] reports dural defects in the middle fossa associated with cerebrospinal fluid leaks without antecedent trauma.

Accurate determination of the site of fistula may be difficult. In cases of cerebrospinal fluid rhinorrhea, the fluorescein dye technique is quite useful.[11] With this method, dilute fluorescein is instilled by lumbar puncture, and the site of the leak is determined by careful placement of cotton pledgets in strategic locations within the nasal cavity following cocainization and shrinking of the nasal mucosa. Radioactive isotopes may be used instead of fluorescein.[77]

With the availability of high-resolution scanners, the presence of fistulae may also be determined by the introduction of small amounts of a water-soluble contrast agent, such as metrizamide, into the subarachnoid space. Serial CT scanning is then used to determine the site of leakage. At this point, reports on the use of CT scanning for this purpose are limited,[20,40,49] but the possible application is promising. This is especially the case in patients with recurrent meningitis but without rhinorrhea, in which case the pledget technique is not applicable. However, it must be cautioned that if the scanning is not done in serial fashion, the metrizamide may flood the nasal cavity and sphenoid sinuses, preventing determination of the actual fistula site. It should be emphasized further that both the pledget and metrizamide techniques are most successful when the study is done during active cerebrospinal fluid leakage.

Finally, in those cases of extensive basal skull frac-

tures in association with multiple facial fractures, CT provides an easy and painless method of determining the extent of the bony fractures and their degree of displacement. Such an evaluation is often difficult by conventional techniques because of the degree of soft tissue swelling and the inability of the patient to tolerate the extensive periods of immobility necessary to obtain satisfactory conventional tomograms.

□ Conclusion

High-resolution CT scanning, performed with and without intravenous contrast material injection in both the axial and coronal plane, is the single most valuable study in the evaluation of lesions involving the skull base. Furthermore, these CT scans must be performed with both soft tissue and bone window settings.

Although CT scanning can determine accurately the presence of a lesion, the differential diagnosis is formidable. Therefore it is useful to consider each lesion as being in one of three categories intracranial, growing down to involve the skull base; primary osseous; and exocranial, growing up to involve the base. In examining these three possibilities, a variety of factors should be analyzed: location within the skull base, CT features, clinical history, and angiographic appearance. With such a combined approach a more accurate diagnosis can be rendered, leading to an effective therapeutic plan.

□ References

1. Alford, B.R., and Guilford, F.R.: A comprehensive study of the glomus jugulare, Laryngoscope **72**:765-787, 1962.
2. Acquaviva, R., Tamic, P., Thenenot, C., et al.: Los condromas intracraneales: revision de la literatura a propositio de dos casos, Rev. Esp. Otoneurooftal **24**:13-34, 1965.
3. Ambrose, J.: Computerized transverse axial scanning (tomography). II. Clinical application, Br. J. Radiol. **46**:1023-1047, 1973.
4. Arey, L.B.: Developmental anatomy, ed. 7, Philadelphia, 1965, W.B., Saunders Co.
5. Aubaniac, R.: Les variations du canal dechire posterieur, Trav. Lab. Anat. Fac. Med. Alger. :23-33, 1951.
6. Bahr, A.L., and Gayler, B.W.: Cranial chondrosarcoma, Radiology **124**:151-156, 1977.
7. Bilaniuk, L.T., and Zimmerman, R.A.: Computer-assisted tomography: sinus lesions with orbital involvement, Head Neck Surg. **2**:293, 1980.
8. Bilaniuk, L.T., and Zimmerman, R.A.: Computed tomography in evaluation of the paranasal sinuses, Radiol. Clin. North Am. **20**(suppl. 1) 51-66, 1982.
9. Bradac, G.B., Schramm, J., Grumme, T., and Simon, R.S.: CT of the base of the skull, Neuroradiology **17**:1-5, 1978.
10. Bryan, R.N., Sessions, R.B., and Horowitz, B.L.: Radiographic management of juvenile angiofibromas, AJNR **2**:157-166, 1981.
11. Calcaterra, T.C., Moseley, J.I., and Rand, R.W.: Cerebrospinal rhinorrhea: extracranial surgical repair, West J. Med. **127**:279-283, 1977.
12. Carmel, P.W., Luken, M.G., and Ascherl, G.F.: Craniosynostosis: computed tomographic evaluation of skull base and calvarial deformities and associated intracranial changes, Neurosurgery **9**(4):366-372, 1981.

13. Caughran, M., White, T.J., Gerald, B., and Gardner, G.: Computed tomography of jugulotympanic paragangliomas, J. Comput. Assist. Tomogr. 4(2):194-198, 1980.

14. Centeno, R.S., Bentson, J.R., and Mancuso, A.A.: CT scanning in rhinocerebral mucormycosis and aspergillosis, Radiology 140:383, 1981.

15. Coin, C.G., and Malkasian, D.R.: Clivus. In Newton, T.H., and Potts, D.G., editors: Radiology of the skull and brain, vol. 1, St. Louis, 1971, The C.V. Mosby Co.

16. Coin, C.G., and Malkasian, D.R.: Foramen magnum. In Newton, T.H., and Potts, D.G.: Radiology of the skull and brain, vol. 1, St. Louis, 1971, The C.V. Mosby Co.

17. Cole, J.M.: Glomus jugulare tumor, Laryngoscope 87:1244-1258, 1977.

18. Columella, F., Delzanno, G.B., and Nicola, G.C.: Les neurinomes des quatre derniers nerfs craniens, Neurochirurgie 5:280-295, 1959.

19. Conley, J.J., Chusid, J.G., and Schecter, M.M.: Angiography in head and neck surgery, Arch. Surg. 89:609-618, 1964.

20. Dahlin, D.C., and McCarthy, C.A.: Chordoma: a study of 59 cases, Cancer 5:1170-1178, 1967.

21. Dorst, John P.: Changes of the skull during childhood. In Newton, T.H., and Potts, D.R., editors: Radiology of the skull and brain, vol. 1, St. Louis, 1971, The C.V. Mosby Co.

22. Drayer, B.P., Wilkins, R.H., Boehnke, M., et al.: Cerebrospinal fluid rhinorrhea demonstrated by metrizamide CT cisternography, AJR 129:149-151, 1977.

23. Di Chiro, G., Fisher, R.L., and Nelson, K.B.: The jugular foramen, J. Neurosurg. 21:447-460, 1964.

24. du Boulay, G.H.: Principles of x-ray diagnosis of the skull, London, 1965, Butterworth & Co., Ltd.

25. Evans, T.H.: Carotid canal anomaly: other instances of absent internal carotid artery, Med. Times 84:1069-1072, 1956.

26. Fargueta, J.S., Menezo, J.L., and Bordes, M.: Posterior orbital encephalocele with anophthalmos and other brain malformations, J. Neurosurg. 38:215-217, 1973.

27. Firooznia, J., and Pinto, R.S.: Chordoma. In Dlethelm, L., et al., editors: Encyclopedia of medical radiology, Berlin, 1977, Springer-Verlag.

28. Firooznia, J., Pinto, R.S., Lin, J.P., et al.: Chordoma: radiologic evaluation of 20 cases, AJR 127:797-805, 1976.

29. Fitz, C.R., Wortzman, G., Harwood-Nash, D.C., et al.: Computed tomography in craniopharyngiomas, Radiology 127:687-691, 1978.

30. Gado, M.H., Phelps, M.E., and Coleman, R.E: An extravascular component of contrast enhancement in cranial computed tomography, Radiology 117:589-597, 1975.

31. Glenner, G.G., and Grimley, P.M.: Tumors of the extra-adrenal paraganglion system (including chemoreceptors). In Firminger, H.I.: Atlas of tumor pathology, ser. 2, fasc. 9, Washington, D.C., 1974, Armed Forces Institute of Pathology.

32. Gold, L.A., Kieffer, S.A., and Peterson, N.O.: Intracranial meningiomas: A retrospective analysis of the diagnostic value of plain skull films, Neurology 19:873-878, 1969.

33. Grand, W., and Bakay, L.: Posterior fossa meningiomas: a report of 30 cases, Acta Neurochir. 32:219-233, 1975.

34. Greig, D.M.: Congenital anomalies of the foramen spinosum, Edinburgh Med. J. 36:363-371, 1929.

35. Handel, S.F., Miller, M.H., Wallace, S., et al.: Angiographic observations on chemodectomas of the head and neck, AJR 129:477-480, 1977.

36. Hartel, F.: Roentgenographische darstellung des Foramen ovale des Schadels, Fortschr. Roentgenstr. 27:493-495, 1921.

37. Hawk, W.A., and McCormack, L.J.: Nonchromaffin paraganglioma of the glomus jugulare: review of the literature and report of six cases, Cleve. Clin. Q. 26:62-80, 1959.

38. Hawkins, T.D.: Glomus jugulare and carotid body tumors, Clin. Radiol. 12:199-213, 1961.

39. Hesselink, J.R., Weber, A.L., New, P.F.J., et al.: Evaluation of mucoceles of the paranasal sinuses with computed tomography, Radiology 133:397, 1979.

40. Hilal, S.K., Ganti, R., and Sane, P.: Evaluation of CSF leaks with CT and metrizamide cisternography. Presented at the 18th meeting of the American Society of Neuroradiology, Los Angeles, March 16-21, 1980.

41. Horowitz, T.: Chordal ectopia and its possible relation to chordoma, Arch. Path. 31:354-362, 1941.

42. Kaufman, B., Nulsen, F.E., Weiss, M.H., et al.: Acquired spontaneous, nontraumatic normal-pressure cerebrospinal fluid fistulas originating from the middle fossa, Radiology 122(2):379-387, 1977.

43. Khoo, F.Y.: Giant jugular fossa with brief notes on the anatomical variations of the jugular fossa, AJR 55:333-336, 1946.

44. Kier, E.L.: Fetal Skull. In Newton, T.H., and Potts, D.G., editors: Radiology of the skull and brain, vol, 1, St. Louis, 1971, The C.V. Mosby Co.

45. Kirkwood, J.R., Margolis, M.T., and Newton, T.H.: Prostatic metastasis to the base of the skull simulating meningioma en placque, AJR 112:774-778, 1971.

46. Kricheff, I.I.: The radiologic diagnosis of pituitary adenoma: an overview, Radiology 131:263-265, 1979.

47. Lafon, R., Gros, C., Labange, R., et al.: Tumeur du foramen ovale, confrontations anatomo-radiologiques, J. Radiol. Electr. 34:258-260, 1953.

48. Lazo, A., Wilner, H.I., and Metes, J.J.: Craniofacial mucormycosis: computed tomographic and angiographic findings in two cases, Radiology 139:623, 1981.

49. Levy, J.M., Christensen, F.K., and Nykamp, P.W.: Detection of a cerebrospinal fluid fistula by computed tomography, AJ 131:344-345, 1978.

50. Marsman, J.W.P.: Tumors of the glomus jugulare complex (chemodectomas) demonstrated by cranial computed tomography, J. Comput. Assist. Tomogr. 3(6):795-799, 1979.

51. McRae, D.L.: Craniovertebral junction. In Newton, T.H., and Potts, D.G., editors: Radiology of the skull and brain, vol. 1, St. Louis, 1971, The C.V. Mosby Co.

52. Miller, J.H., Pena, A.M., and Segall, H.D.: Radiological investigation of sella region masses in children, Radiology 134:81-87, 1980.

53. Minagi, H., and Newton, T.H.: Catilaginous tumors of the base of the skull, Am. J. Radiol. 105:308-313, 1969.

54. Moss, M.L., and Young, R.W.: A functional approach to craniology Am. J. Phys. Anthropol. 18:281-292, 1960.

55. Naidich, T.P.: Infratentorial masses. In Norman, D., Korobkin, M., and Newton, T.H.: Computed tomography 1977, St. Louis, 1977, The C.V. Mosby Co.

56. Naidich, T.P., Pinton, R.S., Kushner, M.J., et al.: Evaluation of sella and parasellar masses by computed tomography, Radiology 120:91-99, 1976.

57. Naidich, T.P., Pudlowski, R.M., Leeds, N.E., and Deck, M.D.F.: Hypoglossal palsy: computed tomography demonstration of denervation hemiatrophy of the tongue associated with glomus jugulare tumor: case report, J. Comput. Assist. Tomogr. 2:630-632, 1978.

58. Nakamura, T.P., Grant, J.A., and Hubbard, R.E.: Nasoethmoidal meningoencephalocele, Arch. Otolaryngol. 100:62-64, 1974.

59. Nasr, H., Mozaffarian, G., and Pensley, J.: Prolactin secreting pituitary tumors in women, J. Clin. Endocrinol. Metab. 35:505-512, 1972.

60. Nielson, K.D., and Clark, K.: Transphenoidal microsurgery for selectric removal of functional pituitary microadenomas, Tex. Med. 72:61-66, 1976.

61. Osborn, A.G., Johnson, L., and Robert, T.S.: Sphenoidal mucoceles with intracranial extension, J. Comput. Assist. Tomogr. 3:335, 1979.
62. Patter, B.M.: Human embryology. ed. 3, New York, 1968, McGraw-Hill Book Co.
63. Peterson, H.O., and Kieffer, S.A.: Introduction to neuroradiology, New York, 1972, Harper & Row, Publishers, Inc.
64. Pinto, R.S., George, A.E., Koslow, M., et al.: Neuroradiology of basal anterior fossa (transethmoidal) encephaloceles, Radiology 117:78-85, 1975.
65. Pinto, R.S., George, A.E., Kricheff, J.J., et al.: The base view in vertebral angiography, Radiology 124:157-164, 1977.
66. Quick, C.A., and Payne, E.: Complicated acute sinusitis, Laryngoscope, 82:1248, 1972.
67. Rischbieth, R.H.C., and Bull, J.W.D.: The significance of enlargement of the superior orbital (sphenoidal) fissure, Br. J. Radiol. 31:125-135, 1958.
68. Rizzuti, R.J., and Whalen, J.P.: Nasopharynx. In Newton, T.H., and Potts, D.G., editors: Radiology of the skull and brain, vol. 1, St. Louis, 1971, The C.V. Mosby Co.
69. Russell, E.J., George, A.E., and Kricheff, I.I.: Atypical computerized tomographic features in intracranial meningioma: radiological correlations in a series of 130 consecutive cases, Radiology 135:673-682, 1980.
70. Schecter, M., Liebeskind, A., and Azar-Kia, B.: Intracranial chordomas, Neuroradiology 8:67-82, 1974.
71. Shapiro, R., and Janzen, A.H.: The normal skull: a roentgen study, New York, 1960, Paul B. Hoeber, Inc.
72. Shapiro, R., and Robinson, F.: The foramina of the middle fossa: a phylogenetic, anatomic, and pathologic study, AJR 101:779-794, 1967.
73. Simpson, G.T.: The evaluation and management of neck masses of unknown etiology, Otolaryngol. Clin. North Am. 13(3):489-497, 1980.
74. Som, P.M., and Shugar, J.M.A.: The CT classification of ethmoid mucoceles, J. Comput. Assist. Tomogr. 4:199, 1980.
75. Sondheimer, F.K.: Basal framina and canals. In Newton, T.H., and Potts, D.G., editors: Radiology of the skull and brain, vol. 1, St. Louis, 1971, The C.V. Mosby Co.
76. Syvertsen, A., Haughton, V.M., Williams, A.L., and Cusick, J.F.: The computed tomographic appearance of the normal pituitary gland and pituitary microadenomas, Radiology 133:385-391, 1979.
77. Tamakawa, M.D., and Hanafee, W.N.: Cerebrospinal fluid rhinorrhea: the significance of an air-fluid level in the sphenoid sinus, Radiology 135:101-103, 1980.
78. Tanzer, A.: Die Veranderungen am Shadel bei der Neurofibromatosis Recklinghausen: versuch einer einteilung, Fortschr. Roentgenstr. 105:50-62, 1966.
79. Taveras, J.M., and Wood, E.H.: Diagnostic neuroradiology, Baltimore, 1964, The Williams & Wilkins Co.
80. Taveras, J.M., and Wood, E.H.: Diagnostic neuroradiology, ed. 2, vol. 1, The skull, Baltimore, 1976, The Williams & Wilkins Co.
81. Taylor, S.: High resolution computed tomography of the sella, Radiol. Clin. North Am. 20(suppl. 1):207-236, 1982.
82. Utne, J.R., and Pugh, D.H.: The roentgenological aspects of chordoma, AJR 74:593-608, 1955.
83. Vassilouthis, J., and Ambrose, J.: Computerized tomography scanning appearances of intracranial meningiomas, J. Neurosurg. 50:320-327, 1979.
84. Wheeler, P.S., and Honda, M.: Enlargement of the foramina ovale by increased intracranial pressure, Neurology 15:785-786, 1965.
85. Whelan, M.A., Stern, J., and de Napoli, R.: The CT spectrum of intracranial mycosis, Radiology 141:703-707, 1981.
86. Wood, E.H., and Himadi, G.M.: Chordomas: a roentgenological study of 16 cases previously unreported, Radiology 54:706-716, 1950.
87. Yu, H.C., and Deck, M.D.F.: The clivus deformity of the Arnold-Chiari malformation, Radiology 101:613-615, 1971.
88. Zimmerman, R.A., and Bilaniuk, L.T.: CT of orbital infection and its cerebral complications, AJR 134:45, 1980.

14 □ The eye

SECTION ONE
CT of the orbit

R. Nick Bryan and John A. Craig

The determination of mass lesions of the orbits and their localization has long been a goal of medicine, but achievement of this capability has been frustrating until the past 25 years. The importance of defining orbital lesions is obvious from their critical relationship to the eye and its related structures and subsequent effects on vision. Teleologically, because of the importance of this sensory system, the anatomy of the orbit has been developed exquisitely to protect its contents; but the protective bony and soft tissue boundaries of the orbit, while critical for protective purposes, have been a very effective barrier to the interrogating physician. Direct visualization is limited to portions of the globe and covering structures, while palpation and auscultation also have limited usefulness. These obstructions to direct physical examination have resulted in a continuous search for indirect means of evaluating the orbit and its contents. A great number of the techniques developed have involved imaging modalities to visually display the anatomy of the orbit.

Plain radiographs of the orbits proved to be of immediate and obvious usefulness, although they are helpful in less than 50% of orbital mass lesions.[96] More recently, modifications and improvements in the radiographic evaluation of the orbit have included complex motion tomography, angiography, venography, and orbitography. Each of these techniques has indeed resulted in improved detection of orbital masses, although they still suffer the disadvantages of the dominance of bone density over soft tissue or are invasive, with significant associated morbidity. Ultrasonography greatly improved the ability to visualize the soft tissues, chiefly the globe of the orbit. The combination of all these procedures results in approximately 90% accuracy in detection of orbital masses.[23] However, in many cases such diagnostic accuracy requires the use of many, if not all, of the above procedures—an expensive and time-consuming enterprise. The meritorious objective of imaging the bony as well as soft tissue components of the orbit noninvasively had not been realized until the development and refinement of CT.

The usefulness of CT in evaluating the orbit was obvious from the start. The anatomic structure of the orbit, which is a deterrent to conventional X-ray imaging, is almost ideally suited for imaging by CT. The orbit and its environs consist of structures with quite different absorption coefficients, allowing CT scanners to use their high-density resolution capabilities to the utmost. The orbit is primarily surrounded by either high-density bone or very low-density air and its contents consist of well-defined soft tissues such as sclera, muscles, and nerves, which are beautifully contrasted by the adjacent and surrounding orbital fat. Furthermore, the density of pathologic lesions also tends to be ideally contrasted against the adjacent normal tissues. The development of CT has provided a relatively noninvasive, safe technique for imaging the orbit in any plane, exquisitely demonstrating its normal anatomy as well as its pathologic processes. Without question, CT has become the prime means of evaluating possible mass lesions of the orbit.

Original CT scans of the orbit were performed on first generation EMI CT scanners as reported by Baker et al.,[5] Lampert et al.,[60] and Wright et al.[94] These early scans had sections either 8 to 13 mm in thickness and were reconstructed first on an 80 × 80 matrix and subsequently on a 160 × 160 matrix. It was recognized immediately that the anatomy of the orbit was best displayed by obtaining sections approximately parallel to the orbitomeatal line, rather than the caudally angled scans used for brain scanning. These early scanners produced only axial scans and had a spatial resolution of approximately 117 mm[3]. Even with this relatively poor spatial resolution, over 85% of orbital masses were demonstrated.[23,41] Since then, the improvement in CT scanners has resulted in spatial resolution less than 5 mm; axial as well as coronal and sagittal scan sections are possible. This has resulted in continuously improving orbital diagnostic capabilities.[47] There are few statistics analyzing the overall effectiveness of the newer scanners in detecting orbital lesions. Our experience using axial and coronal scans from a high-resolution scanner indicates that over 95% of orbital mass lesions are detected by CT. This certainly exceeds the capabilities of any other single method and in fact is greater than the combined accuracy of all previous methods.

This does not, however, mean that other techniques of orbit imaging are of no use and are never performed. Rather, they have become adjuncts to CT to further define specific pathologic characteristics of lesions. Plain radiographs remain the most useful images of disease processes that grossly distort the bony anatomy of the orbit. It is not that such information is not available from the CT scan, but rather that it is easier for most clinicians to visualize major orbital deformities on a plain film rather than having to mentally reconstruct the anatomy from multiple scan sections. Plain films of the orbits are probably of greatest use in planning surgical alterations of cosmetic deformities. Admittedly, however, three-dimensional reconstructions using CT information will likely become the premier method for that as well.

Until very recently it has generally been accepted that detail of bone architecture around the orbit is best evaluated with pluridirectional tomography, which supplements the bone and soft tissue information of the CT scan.[62] However, with higher resolution scanners and multiplanar scanning, the usefulness of pluridirectional tomography is diminishing and its use is indicated in relatively few cases.

Carotid angiography is seldom necessary for evaluation of orbital lesions. It is used primarily to diagnose a few vascular lesions such as carotid artery aneurysms and arteriovenous malformations, including carotid cavernous fistulas. Such lesions may be suggested by CT; however, angiography is still required for a definite diagnosis. Carotid angiography may also be necessary to define the vascular anatomy of lesions requiring subsequent surgery. In these cases, careful internal and external carotid angiography may be required to determine the inherent vascularity of the lesion, as well as the source of its blood supply, so that the surgeon may better evaluate the risk of surgery and plan the specific approach.

Orbital venography, which had previously been extensively used, is now relegated primarily to use in cases of suspected venous malformations, particularly varices.[26] Venography is no longer necessary for the detection of orbital masses because it is less reliable than CT scanning[23] and it is seldom useful in better characterizing the nature of a mass.

Orbitography by either positive or negative contrast agents, i.e., air or iodinated contrast agents,[64] is in our opinion no longer indicated.

In contrast to the previous techniques, ultrasonography of the orbit remains a valuable technique either as an adjunct to CT or as the primary diagnostic modality.[23] Intraocular disease is probably best evaluated with this method, although the newer scanners are improving in this area. Diseases associated with alterations of the optic nerve head, such as optic neuritis, papillitis, or papilledema, are also better evaluated by ultrasonography. Ultrasonographic information about retrobulbar lesions is most useful in cases in which there is a diffuse inflammatory change, such as pseudotumor and thyroid ophthalmopathy, in which there are alterations in the echo characteristics of the retrobulbar fat. Occasionally it is helpful with vascular lesions such as varices. Ultrasonography also is useful in localization of foreign bodies. It should also be remembered that in addition to the excellent imaging capabilities of ultrasonography that this is an imaging technique which does not require ionizing radiation. Therefore when lens dose is a significant factor and ultrasonography can yield the necessary clinical information, it should be used.

□ Scanning techniques

Because of the obvious central longitudinal relationship of the globe and optic nerve to the axis of the orbit, early CT scans of the orbit were performed parallel to the orbitomeatal line. With the early scanners that used 8 or 13 mm thick scan sections this was adequate, allowing visualization primarily of the globe, optic nerve, medial and lateral recti, and medial and lateral bony margins of the orbit. Because of the limitations of the scanners, as well as positioning restrictions, little anatomic detail beyond this level was routinely obtained. With improvements in scanners that allowed thinner sections as well as direct coronal views or coronal reconstructions, positioning of the patient became not only more important but more varied. Anatomically it was known, and subsequently confirmed by CT,[47] that the optic nerve does not parallel the orbitomeatal line but is angled 10°, being more cranially positioned in its posterior portion. Therefore optimum scans of the orbit displaying both optic nerves throughout their length are best accomplished with a 10° craniad angulation of the scan section in relation to the orbitomeatal line. With thinner scan sections and multiplanar reconstructions it has been demonstrated that the optic nerve does not run posteriorly in a direct course; rather, it is frequently buckled inferiorly near its midportion. This redundancy of the nerve permits the globe to move in all directions without stretching the nerve. Therefore with scan sections thinner than 4 mm the optic nerve will not be seen as one continuous structure on a single scan section. Orbital axis sagittal reconstructions, however, can ameliorate this problem. Relative symmetry of the two optic nerves is usually unaffected by the somewhat tortuous courses of the optic nerves, and multiplanar reconstructions may not be absolutely necessary in all cases for adequate evaluation of this structure. CT scans of the orbit in the axial projection should begin at the superior orbital ridge and be continued caudally to at least the inferior orbital ridge. Obviously, if a pathologic process is detected in these scan sections, one must continue either cranially or caudally as necessary to complete the display of the lesion.

Coronal scans of the orbit are required for an adequate study in most cases. They may be performed directly by positioning the patient within the aperture with the orbitomeatal line angled 70° to 90° to the section plane. This may be accomplished by hyperextending the neck, with the patient either in the prone position with appropriate support under the chin, or in the supine position with the shoulders elevated from the tabletop by a supportive device. Gantry or table tilt is then used to maximize the scan angle. In most patients an angle of at least 75° can be obtained; however, in a few patients with short or inflexible necks, angles of only 50° to 60° may be obtained. These latter scans can be useful; however, the anatomy is distorted from the usual coronal cross-sectional anatomy and care must be taken with interpretation.

Coronal scans of the orbit may also be obtained indirectly by computer reconstruction of data from thin axial scan sections. For this technique to be optimum, one should be able to perform scans in sections 3 mm or less. These thin scan sections then allow appropriate resolution in the coronal plane after computer reconstruction. Either the direct or indirect method of obtaining coronal sections is adequate, but the direct method has more difficulty with artifacts, particularly from metallic dental fillings. Coronal sections should begin anteriorly at the lateral orbital rim (unless a more anterior soft tissue lesion is present) and continue posteriorly through the sphenoid, including the sella turcica.

In addition to the axial and coronal scans, other scan section orientations may be helpful in particular cases. A very useful one is the section oriented parallel to the optic nerve and the long axis of the orbit. This plane is angled roughly 40° to the true sagittal plane. The long axis of the bony orbit is angled approximately 45° to the sagittal plane; the optic nerve, however, is angled only 30° to 35° to the sagittal plane. In addition, the optic nerve does not take a straight course in the horizontal plane as it proceeds posteriorly but is slightly laterally convex. Therefore one does not usually get, particularly with thin sections, a single section through the vertical equator of the globe that demonstrates the entire length of the optic nerve. This does not diminish the usefulness of this projection but merely necessitates multiple reconstructed sections. This view may be obtained directly by positioning the patient as if for a coronal scan; the head is then turned approximately 35° toward the side of interest.[43] In our experience it is usually difficult to predictably and optimally position a patient in this fashion. If possible, it is preferable to create this scan section by computer reconstruction from thin section axial scans.

Coronal scan sections at right angles to the orbital axis provide a truer anatomic cross-section of the orbit and may also be obtained either directly by patient positioning (again somewhat difficult) or by computer reconstructions. In our experience this view seldom adds useful information that has not been provided by regular coronal scan sections.

In addition to examination of the orbit proper, CT scans of this region also provide useful information concerning the optic canal. In many cases the previously described scanning techniques will adequately display the anatomy of this structure. However, for optimum demonstration of the optic canal (foramen), axial scans angled approximately −18° to the orbitomeatal line are necessary, as this is the usual projection of the optic canal. Thin (1.5 mm) axial scan sections with this angulation have been shown to demonstrate the optic nerve canal in both its axial and coronal projections after computer reconstructions.[88]

Intravenous injection of iodinated contrast agents is helpful in many cases and is suggested when there is no contraindication. However, contrast enhancement of pathologic lesions within the orbit is not as important in either demonstrating the lesion or determining its pathology as it is within the central nervous system. This is obviously because the contents of the orbit, with the exception of the optic nerve and retina, lack a blood-brain barrier; hence virtually any structure or pathologic tissue that has a blood supply will be enhanced after injection of contrast material. The degree of enhancement is primarily dependent on the vascular volume of the structure. Contrast material injection may better display orbital pathology; however, except in those lesions that are extremely hypervascular (vascular malformations) or hypovascular (cystic lesions), the presence and degree of contrast enhancement is not helpful in the differential diagnosis. In a very few cases, particularly vascular malformations such as varices, contrast material injection may be absolutely necessary to demonstrate the lesion. Reported methods of contrast material injection are quite varied both in dosage and in injection technique, varying from 0.25 to 1.0 gm/kg body weight and being infused by either rapid bolus injection or slow continuous drip. There does not appear to be an obvious advantage or disadvantage of most of these techniques, and we routinely give a bolus injection of 100 ml of 80% sodium meglumine iothalamate. We routinely perform only postcontrast agent injection scans, except in those patients in whom contrast material injection is contraindicated or in patients in whom the primary clinical diagnosis is thyroid ophthalmopathy. In the latter, one may be content to see the typical muscle enlargement that does not require contrast agent injection, which might alter subsequent thyroid studies.

An important consideration in CT scanning of the orbits is the radiation dosage, particularly to the lens. Total dosage to the orbit and lens is dependent on the scanning techniques used. The doses range from as low as 2 rads (radiation absorbed dose) for relatively thick section axial scans, with the beam directed primarily from the side or posteriorly. On the other hand, the dose may be as high as 12 rads for multiple thin axial scan sections, with the beam configuration having a large anterior component.[82,91] Direct coronal scans may add an additional 1 to 6 rads to the lens, depending on scanning parameters. Obviously these higher radiation dosage figures might reach significant levels if the patient undergoes multiple examinations. It is estimated that the cataractogenic radiation dose is approximately 200 rads.[16] For this reason one should tailor routine examinations in a fashion to appropriately examine, but not overexpose, the patient's eye. Because the orbit and its contents are radiographically high-contrast structures, it is not usually necessary to use high milliampere settings to improve low density resolution, although this may be necessary to improve statistical noise in very thin scan sections. Kilovolt selection is more a function of machine than anatomy, and most scanners are operated in the 125 kV range. When selecting scan section thickness one should probably use either the thin section multiplanar reconstruction approach, i.e., 1.5 to 2 mm axial sections, or thicker sections, i.e., 5 to 6 mm, and scan directly in both the axial and coronal projections. With low milliampere set-

tings, proper collimation, and elimination of unnecessary slice overlapping one should be able to perform a good scan of the orbit with no more than 5 to 6 rads exposure.

In summary, at the present time an adequate CT study of the orbit requires both axial and coronal scans, by either direct scanning or multiplanar computer reconstruction. We believe contrast agent injection should be performed in the majority of cases, although not all workers in this field agree. One alternative technique calls for a noncontrast study for mass detection; a second alternative technique calls for contrast study for characterization of the mass if identified. Additional views may be added as is clinically necessary.

□ Gross anatomy

In accordance with the complex function of the orbit and its visual system contents, it has a very detailed fine anatomy. However, its anatomy as resolved with even the highest resolution CT scanners is relatively gross. Basically the orbit consists of its central neural structures directly related to vision (optic nerve and eyeball), surrounding and embracing soft tissues primarily related to ocular motility, and the surrounding orbital margins, consisting mainly of bone and overlying soft tissues.

The optic nerve is a rostral continuation of the diencephalon, entering the orbit through the optic canal and continuing anteriorly within the orbit for approximately 3 cm until it pierces the sclera at the posterior aspect of the eyeball, where it relates to the optic disc and is neurally continuous with the retina. The optic nerve and its coverings are approximately 5 to 6 mm in diameter. It usually has a slight inferior and lateral convexity to its course as it passes from the eyeball to the optic canal. The central retinal artery and vein usually pierce and accompany the optic nerve in its anterior 1 to 1.5 cm. The optic nerve is surrounded by a very thin subarachnoid space, which is a direct continuation of the suprasellar cistern. The subarachnoid space ends as the nerve pierces the sclera. The dura at the base of the skull continues as the periosteal lining of the optic canal and then splits into two layers, one of which continues forward around the optic nerve to its scleral termination while the other spreads out to form the periorbital fascia, which lines the bony margins of the orbit. Anteriorly this periorbita fuses with the periosteum of the facial bones and continues into the eyelids as orbital septa.

The eyeball occupies the anterior third of the orbit and has an ovoid structure approximately 24 mm in diameter. The radius of curvature is modified anteriorly, where the cornea has a smaller radius of curvature. The eyeball is basically a hollow sphere with three coats.

The external coat is primarily fibrous and consists of the sclera posteriorly and the cornea anteriorly. The intermediate layer is vascular and includes the choroid posteriorly and the ciliary body and iris anteriorly. The internal layer is primarily the retina. The bulk of the globe wall is made up of the fibrous sclera and cornea, and these tissues dominate the radiographic image. Within these walls are three refractive media, the aqueous humor anteriorly between the cornea and the lens, the semicrystalline lens itself, and the gelatinous vitreous body that occupies the posterior two thirds of the globe. Surrounding the orbital portion of the optic nerve and the posterior half of the globe is intraconal orbital fat.

Confining these structures is a relatively continuous musculofascial sheath that begins at the orbital apex and continues anteriorly until its insertion near the anterior third of the globe. This sheath consists primarily of the extraocular muscles proper and their interconnecting fascia, all of which form a relatively closed compartment that separates the orbit into rather distinct "intraconal" and "extraconal" compartments.[58] The extraocular muscles include the medial rectus (bulkiest), lateral rectus, superior rectus and adjacent levator palpebrae superioris, inferior rectus, superior oblique (thinnest and longest), and inferior oblique (shortest). All of these muscles, except the superior and inferior oblique and levator palpebrae superioris, originate from the fibrous annulus of Zinn, which attaches the periorbita around the optic foramen. The superior orbital fissure is partially bridged by this tendinous origin. The superior oblique and levator palpebrae superioris muscles arise from the periorbita near the apex. The inferior oblique muscle originates from the periorbita just posterior to the lacrimal fossa at the anteromedial aspect of the orbit. All of these muscles (except the levator palpebrae superioris and the oblique muscles) insert directly into the sclera anterior to the coronal equator of the globe. The oblique muscles insert posterior to the equator. The medial and lateral recti pass directly from their origins to their insertions, and their actions are direct medial or lateral deviation of the gaze axis. The superior and inferior recti muscles also pass relatively directly forward to their insertions; however, because the axis of the globe is parallel to the sagittal plane while the axis of the orbit and the musculofascial sheath is angled 35° lateral to the sagittal plane, these recti tend to deviate the gaze axis medially, and angle gaze superiorly or inferiorly. The superior oblique muscle rises as a thin slip between the origins of the medial and superior recti and passes forward, very near the superior lateral orbital wall, until it becomes tendinous anteriorly as it makes a right-angle turn through the fibrous trochlea. It then proceeds posterolaterally to its insertion. This muscle deviates the gaze axis laterally and inferiorly. The inferior oblique muscle passes directly laterally and posteriorly from its origin and deviates the gaze axis laterally and superiorly. The levator palpebrae superioris muscle extends from the orbital apex along the superomedial aspect of the superior rectus to the anterior orbit, where it pierces the orbital septum to insert in the superior eyelid. Between the various extraocular muscles is a thin but relatively strong fascia that completes the muscle cone. In addition, relatively strong fibrous ligaments extend laterally from the medial and lateral recti near their insertions to the periorbita, which limit globe motion and are called check ligaments.

There is a completely separate fibrous sheath, called Tenon's capsule, around the posterior two thirds of the eyeball. This capsule is pierced by the optic nerve and the various extraocular muscles but is distinct from the latter. This sheath serves as a socket for the eyeball.

Surrounding the musculofascial cone is additional periorbital fat—both the previously described intraconal fat and the surrounding extraconal fat—which extends to the periorbita. This orbital fat extends anteriorly to the fibrous orbital septum, which is a strong fibrous band continuous with the periorbita at the orbital rims. It is related to the posterior fascia of the orbicularis oculi muscle of the eyelid. This orbital septum prevents anterior herniation of orbital fat into the eyelid and also forms a strong boundary between the orbital contents proper and the overlying facial soft tissues.

The anterior covering of the orbit is primarily the eyelid, which is basically a four-layered structure consisting of (from anterior to posterior) skin, underlying subcutaneous tissue, a muscular layer consisting primarily of the orbicularis oculi muscle, and a deep fibrous layer, including the tarsus. This last layer is related to the orbital septum and is strengthened medially and laterally to form the medial and lateral palpebral ligaments. Lining the inner surface of the eyelid is the mucous membrane of the conjunctiva, which has its anterior palpebral portion covering the eyelid and its posterior bulbar portion covering the anterior third of the eyeball with the exception of the cornea.

Superolaterally the lacrimal gland lies underneath the periorbita in the shallow bony lacrimal gland fossa. This gland is behind the orbital septum and is partially divided by the levator palpebrae superioris muscle. Its deep portion is immediately related to the superolateral aspect of the conjunctival fornix, into which its ducts open.

Inferomedially in the orbit, the lacrimal duct apparatus is dominated by the relatively large lacrimal sac within its bony fossa and also by the nasal lacrimal duct, which extends from the sac along the superomedial aspect of the maxillary sinus to its opening in the inferior meatus of the nose.

Coursing within these gross anatomic structures are the functionally critical but anatomically small vessels and nerves that have been extensively described. From the gross anatomic and radiographic aspects the largest and most consistent of these structures is the superior ophthalmic vein, which courses posterolaterally from the trochlea to pierce the muscle cone underneath the superior rectus muscle. It continues posteriorly under this structure until it leaves the muscle cone near the orbital apex to exit through the superior orbital fissure. The remainder of the vessels and nerves within the orbit are generally too small, irregular in course, or inconsistent in anatomy to be reliably defined by CT.

□ Radiographic anatomy

The gross anatomy of the orbit as reflected by CT can be simplified into a central lollipop-shaped visual portion, an intermediate conical musculofascial portion, and an outer tetrahedral bony portion. Centrally, the eyeball image is primarily made up of the outer soft tissue densities of the cornea and sclera and the inner lucent densities of the aqueous and vitreous separated by the high-density lens. The density of the normal lens in Hounsfield units is approximately 75, while the usual density of vitreous is 5 Hounsfield units. Approximately two thirds of the globe lies anterior to the most posterior portion of the lateral orbit rim, and proptosis is indicated when the cornea is more than 21 mm anterior to a line connecting the lateral orbit rims.[48] The optic nerve extends posteromedially from the globe, with a slightly inferolateral convexity. Its normal density in Hounsfield units is 30 to 35, which may increase after contrast agent injection to 36 to 40 Hounsfield units. It usually has homogeneous density, although after injection of water-soluble contrast agents such as metrizamide into the cerebrospinal fluid (CSF) spaces the small subarachnoid space about the optic nerve may become opacified, resulting in slightly higher density at the periphery of the nerve image.[67] As previously mentioned, the optic nerve is laterally angled approximately 35° to the sagittal plane and is also angled approximately 15° to the orbitomeatal line, with its anterior portion being inferior. The musculofascial sheath or "muscle cone" is radiographically dominated by the superior, inferior, medial, and lateral recti. The medial and lateral recti may be demonstrated throughout their length on axial scans through the midorbit. They tend to taper both anteriorly and posteriorly, with relatively broad bellies in their midportion. The superior and inferior recti are not shown throughout their length unless angled sagit-

tal scans are performed. They are best demonstrated in cross-section on coronal scans, on which they appear as sharply marginated, horizontal ovoid soft tissue densities, while the medial and lateral recti are vertically ovoid structures. The image of the levator palpebrae superioris muscle is inseparable from the image of the superior rectus muscle. The oblique muscles are not usually demonstrated by CT, although coronal scans may occasionally show either of these structures. With high-resolution scans the very thin fascial sheath between the major muscle bundles can also be demonstrated. These muscles have a density in Hounsfield units of 40 to 44 and they are enhanced significantly after contrast agent injection to 60 to 65 Hounsfield units. The specific size of these muscles varies from individual to individual and from one scan section to another and hence actual measurement of muscle size is of little use. More important is the relative symmetry between the two sides.

The remainder of the contents of the orbit, as demonstrated by CT, is primarily fat separated into the intraconal and extraconal compartments. Anteriorly the orbit is covered by the combined soft tissue densities of the eyelids, orbital septum, and associated soft tissues. It is important to remember that the orbital septum is included in this anterior border and is of great functional importance.

The lacrimal gland can be seen in most high-resolution scans as a crescentic soft tissue mass interposed between the superolateral aspect of the globe and the bony orbit. Normally it is just discernible; when it becomes obvious it is usually enlarged. The superior ophthalmic vein is usually seen as a sharply marginated curvilinear density just inferior to the superior rectus muscle. With proper window settings the bony margins of the orbit, including the floor of the anterior fossa, anterior wall of the middle fossa, roof of the maxillary sinus, and ethmoid and sphenoid sinus, can all be demonstrated along with their normal relationships to the orbit proper. In axial scans the inferior orbital fissure can usually be demonstrated; both the inferior and superior orbital fissures can be demonstrated on coronal scan sections. With thin scan sections and proper angulation the optic foramen can be displayed on one scan section in the axial projection, or on multiple coronal scans sections with proper reconstructions.[87] See references at the end of this section for additional references for normal orbital CT anatomy.*

The normal anatomy of the orbit, as displayed by routine CT, is shown in Figs. 14-1 to 14-6. Most of these scans were performed on a fourth generation scanner using low milliampere settings and 5 mm thick

Text continued on p. 587.

———————

*References 40, 48, 82, 90.

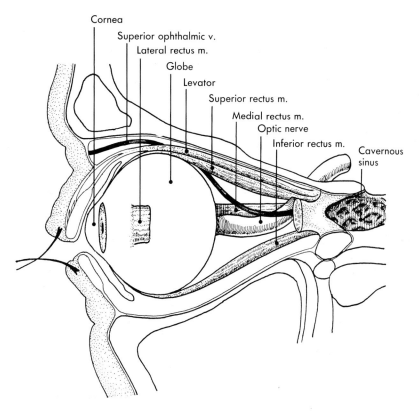

Fig. 14-1. Normal gross anatomy of orbit as seen from medial aspect.

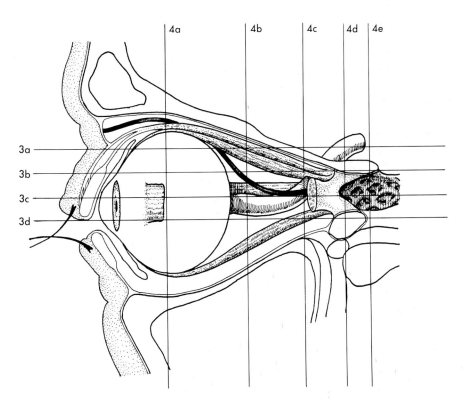

Fig. 14-2. Lateral view of orbit with superimposed lines indicating planes of axial and coronal scans that display normal anatomy in Figs. 14-3 and 14-4.

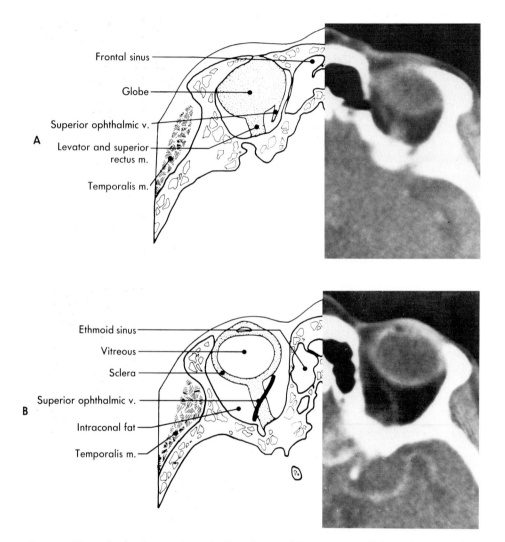

Frontal sinus

Globe

Superior ophthalmic v.

Levator and superior
rectus m.

Temporalis m.

A

Ethmoid sinus

Vitreous

Sclera

Superior ophthalmic v.

Intraconal fat

Temporalis m.

B

Fig. 14-3. Normal orbital anatomy as displayed in axial CT scans parallel to orbitomeatal line.

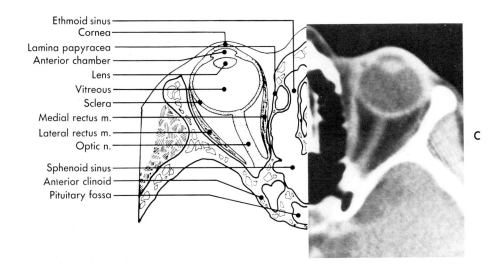

Ethmoid sinus
Cornea
Lamina papyracea
Anterior chamber
Lens
Vitreous
Sclera
Medial rectus m.
Lateral rectus m.
Optic n.
Sphenoid sinus
Anterior clinoid
Pituitary fossa

C

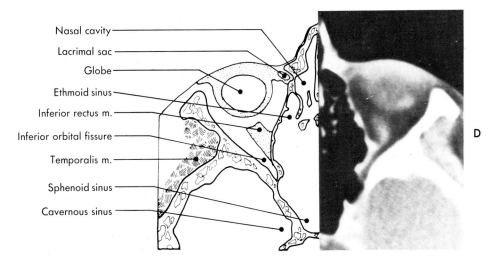

Nasal cavity
Lacrimal sac
Globe
Ethmoid sinus
Inferior rectus m.
Inferior orbital fissure
Temporalis m.
Sphenoid sinus
Cavernous sinus

D

Fig. 14-3, cont'd. For legend see opposite page.

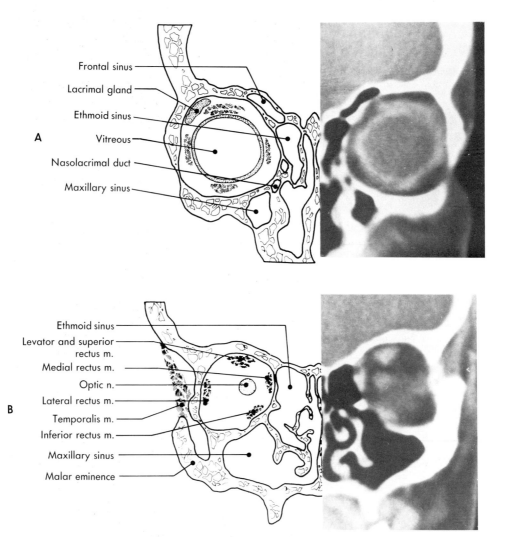

A

Frontal sinus
Lacrimal gland
Ethmoid sinus
Vitreous
Nasolacrimal duct
Maxillary sinus

B

Ethmoid sinus
Levator and superior
    rectus m.
Medial rectus m.
Optic n.
Lateral rectus m.
Temporalis m.
Inferior rectus m.
Maxillary sinus
Malar eminence

Fig. 14-4. Normal orbital anatomy as displayed in coronal scans angled approximately 75° to orbitomeatal line.

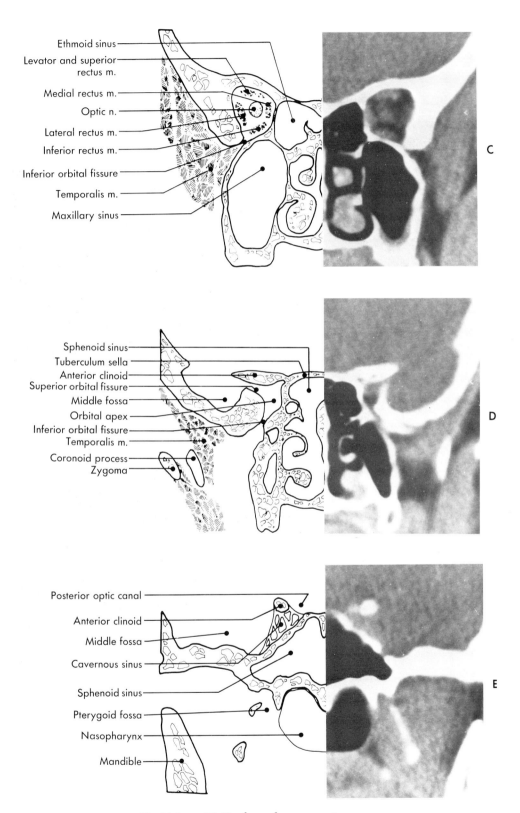

Fig. 14-4, cont'd. For legend see opposite page.

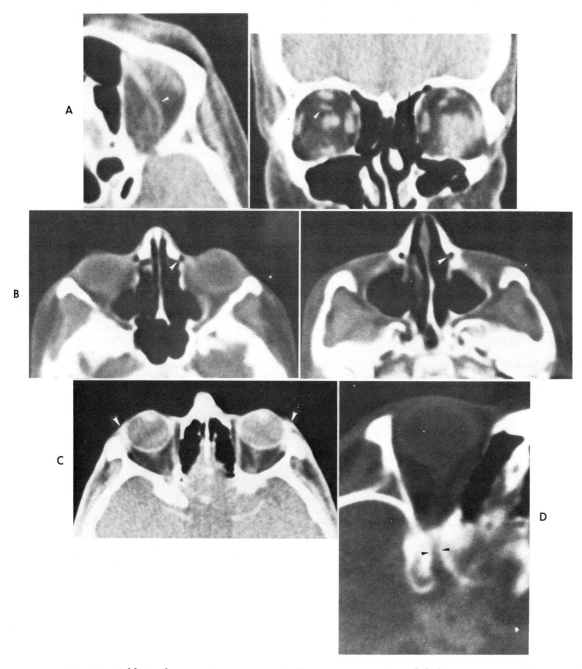

Fig. 14-5. Additional anatomic structures. **A,** Prominent superior ophthalmic vein *arrows)* courses in curvilinear fashion from anterior to posterior beneath superior rectus muscle. **B,** Nasolacrimal duct *(arrow)* originates below lacrimal sac fossa and courses along anteromedial wall of maxillary sinus. **C,** Prominent, but normal, lacrimal glands *(arrows)* embrace superolateral aspects of globe. **D,** Axial scans of optic canal *(arrows)* obtained with chin elevated approximately 15° to orbitomeatal line.

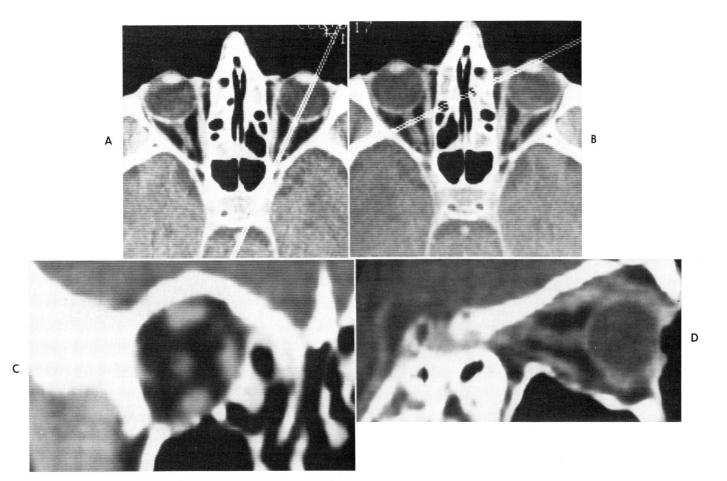

Fig. 14-6. Multiplanar reconstructions. Using thin (1.5 mm) axial scans and subsequent computer reconstructions, coronal and sagittal sections oriented to axis of orbit may be obtained. Planes of reconstructions are indicated by dotted lines. (Courtesy H. Newton and L. Yeager.)

scan sections. The axial scans are angled −10° to the orbitomeatal line and the coronal scans are angled approximately −75° to the orbitomeatal line. The individual scan sections were selected to demonstrate appropriate anatomy and are not contiguous nor equidistant apart.

Orbital CT scans should be performed with the patient in direct forward gaze. Because the location of many structures within the orbit is gaze dependent, one must take this effect into account when scanning patients with differing gaze positions. The most frequent variation is the patient scanned with eyes closed, in which case there is usually a relative downward gaze that results in a lower position of the lens image and usually a slight straightening of the inferior curvature of the optic nerve. Contracted extraocular muscles will generally be foreshortened and enlarged in the cross-sectional area. Hence patients with a right gaze prefer-

ence will show asymmetric muscles, with larger appearing right lateral and left medial rectus muscles as compared to the smaller right medial and left lateral rectus muscles (Fig. 14-7).[48]

□ Orbital pathology

Radiographic evaluation of the orbit, including CT, is primarily involved with the diagnosis of mass lesions. Although there is a very large list of possible orbital masses, there are a relatively limited number of common orbital lesions with which the radiologist should become familiar. The actual frequency of reported orbital pathologic processes varies from author to author and is primarily dependent on case source. Table 14-1 summarizes the orbital lesions seen in two series based on ophthalmologic practices and two series of patients based on radiographic referrals, including ours. As one can see there are significant differences in the individ-

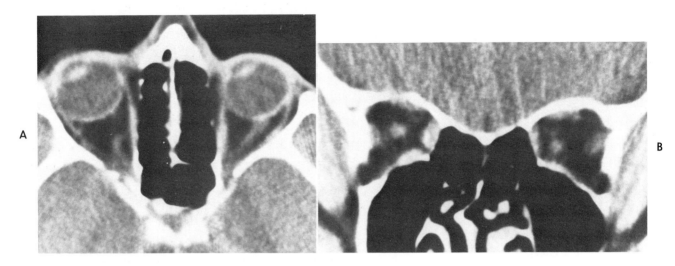

Fig. 14-7. Right lateral gaze palsy caused by extraorbital disease is indicated by corneal deviation on axial scan and by deviation of optic nerve and change in extraocular muscle caliber in both axial and coronal sections. Note prominent contraction of medial rectus of left eye.

Table 14-1. Orbital masses

Diagnosis	Series*				Total	Percent
	1	2	3	4		
Metastasis	8	84	29	28	149	20
Hemangioma	28	41	10	13	92	8
Lymphoma	22	39	8	10	79	7
Pseudotumor	18	37	9	9	73	7
Graves' disease	37		10	23	70	6
Meningioma	11	32	4	15	62	5
Lacrimal tumor	17	29		8	54	5
Trauma			10	34	44	4
Infection	3		29	10	42	4
Mucocele	3	7	30	2	42	4
Optic nerve glioma	8	14	8	11	41	4
Sarcoma	10	27	4		41	4
Primary benign bone disease	2	10	20	5	37	3
Melanoma		22		11	33	3
Dermoid	7	13	6	2	28	2
Neural tumor	7	2	8	3	20	2
Lymphangioma	10	3			13	1
Histiocytosis	2	5	6		13	1
Vascular malformation	5	2	2	3	12	1
Retinoblastoma		6	4	2	12	1
Miscellaneous	3	73	3	28	107	10
Unknown	24	1			25	2

*Series 1, data from Henderson[45]; series 2, data from Moss[72]; series 3, data from Zizmor[97]; series 4, our series.

Table 14-2. Anatomic compartmentalization of orbit lesions

Type of lesion	Cases	Total
Intraocular mass		
Retinoblastoma*	2	
Melanoma*	11	
Angioma	3	
Miscellaneous	4	
		20
Intraconal mass		
Optic nerve origin		
Optic nerve glioma*	11	
Meningioma*	10	
Miscellaneous	9	30
Extrinsic optic nerve		
Hemangioma*	5	
Pseudotumor*	9	
Miscellaneous	3	17
		47
Muscle mass		
Graves' disease*	23	
Neural tumor	3	
Lymphoma	2	
Miscellaneous	3	
		31
Extraconal mass		
Intraorbital		
Lymphoma-sarcoma*	8	
Meningioma*	5	
Dermoid-epidermoid*	2	
Lacrimal lesion*	8	
Hemangioma*	5	
Miscellaneous	5	
		33
Extraorbital mass		
Sinus origin		
Cellulitis*	10	
Mucocele	2	
Tumor*	19	31
Nonsinus origin		
Distant metastasis	4	
Skin malignancy	5	
Bone tumor	5	14
		45
Miscellaneous		
Trauma with foreign body*		12
Trauma without foreign body		22
Arteriovenous fistula		3
Anomaly		5
		42

*Most common diagnosis.

ual series, with the clinical series having a greater percentage of lesions restricted to the orbital contents while the radiographic series include more cases with disease extending beyond the orbit itself. In most series, however, the most frequent lesions are endocrine exophthalmos, hemangioma, meningioma, orbital pseudotumor, and lacrimal gland lesions. Although the analysis of orbital lesions by placing them in traditional pathologic categories such as neoplasm, inflammatory disease, etc. is helpful, subdividing the cases into anatomic compartments is more useful in radiologic differential diagnosis.

Subdivision of pathologic lesions by their occurrence in the various orbital anatomic compartments is important because different lesions tend to occur more frequently in particular compartments and also because treatment of orbital lesions is very much dependent on compartmentalization.* Table 14-2 tabulates the cases we have studied at The Methodist Hospital with a high-resolution CT scanner using coronal and axial scans over a 30-month period. The lesions are grouped on the basis of the site of their anatomic location, and one can easily perceive the relationship of the various lesions and their usual specific anatomic locale. Other published CT-oriented orbital pathology series are listed in the references at the end of this chapter.†

■ Intraocular lesions
Retinoblastoma

There are only two primary neoplasms that occur with any frequency within the eyeball: retinoblastoma and malignant melanoma. Retinoblastoma is a highly malignant neoplasm that arises from the retina in children. Most cases are diagnosed before the patient is 3 years old. Genetically there are two forms of retinoblastoma, with 60% a result of sporadic germ cell line mutations and transmitted as an autosomal dominant trait and 40% a result of a single somatic cell lesion and not heritable. The tumors may be multicentric within the same eye and are not infrequently bilateral in origin. All bilateral lesions are a result of a heritable condition.[34] The cell of origin of these tumors is still unclear; however, their pathology is very similar to that of neuroblastoma and medulloblastoma, and presumably retinoblastoma is a primitive neural cell. The tumor consists of sheets of uniform, densely staining cells with large nuclei and abundant cromatin. Rosette and pseudorosette formation is common. Necrosis within the tumor is not unusual and is frequently associated with calcification. The tumor tends to spread anteriorly into the vitreous and peripherally into the adjacent retina. Of

*References 3, 6, 48, 62.
†References 40, 41, 48, 62, 74, 79, 83, 84, 90, 91.

utmost importance is extension of the tumor beyond the globe. This most frequently occurs through the lamina cribrosa at the optic nerve head, where the tumor then extends posteriorly into the optic nerve and its surrounding meninges and subarachnoid space. The tumor may also extend beyond the globe directly into the orbit through the sclera. The tumor also quickly involves the highly vascular choroid and may gain access to vessels in this structure, which can result in adjacent orbital extension as well as generalized vascular dissemination.[28,45]

The diagnosis and subsequent treatment is highly dependent on the location and extent of the tumor. Localized intraocular retinoblastoma now has a cure rate approaching 90%, with preservation of some vision in as many as 75% of patients.[10,77] Ophthalmoscopic examination is the main means of diagnosis. Small localized lesions may be treated with photocoagulation or cryosurgery alone or in combination with local radiation therapy. Larger, more bulky neoplasms with limited extension posteriorly into the optic nerve still require enucleation with or without irradiation. Once the lesion has extended beyond the globe the prognosis becomes much worse, with cure rates below 20% despite treatment with radical surgery, extensive radiation, or chemotherapy. It is important that extraocular neoplasm be diagnosed as soon as possible for optimum therapy. Difficulty of making such a diagnosis has been a major limitation in the staging of retinoblastoma. Until recently, the diagnostic radiologist played a relatively minor role in evaluation of patients with retinoblastoma. Plain film changes were present in the minority of patients; the only direct evidence of intraocular tumor was calcification, which occurs in 15% to 20% of patients. Plain ra-

diographs yielded little additional information about the tumors until metastatic bone changes occurred. Even ultrasonography was limited in some of these cases because of the bizarre shapes of the tumors and the interference between surface, deep echoes, and tumor calcification.

CT offers a much improved method of imaging retinoblastoma and its extension (Fig. 14-8). Danziger and Price[24] evaluated 38 patients with surgically proven retinoblastoma, and tumor was identified in 36 of these patients. We have evaluated 16 patients with known retinoblastoma and have identified tumor in all those patients.[18] The tumor is seen as a faint, often lobulated mass arising from the posterolateral wall of the globe and extending into the vitreous. Calcification occurs in approximately 50% to 90% of cases.[48] With localized lesions, no further abnormality is seen. With extension of the tumor beyond the retina, choroid, and vitreous one sees thickening and increased enhancement of the sclera; with larger lesions frank intraorbital masses behind the globe are seen. Extension posteriorly into the optic nerve is indicated by enlargement of the nerve. Enhancement following intravenous infusion of contrast material has not been obvious nor has this technique been of any particular usefulness in evaluating these patients. The major difficulty in assessing these tumors is the young age of the patients and the attendant motion and positioning problems. The scans are performed with the patient premedicated with chloral hydrate (25 to 50 mg/kg).

Using the CT scan images, these tumors can be subdivided into three grades: grade I, intraocular; grade II, orbital extension; and grade III, extension beyond the orbit. The CT scan results correlate well with the sur-

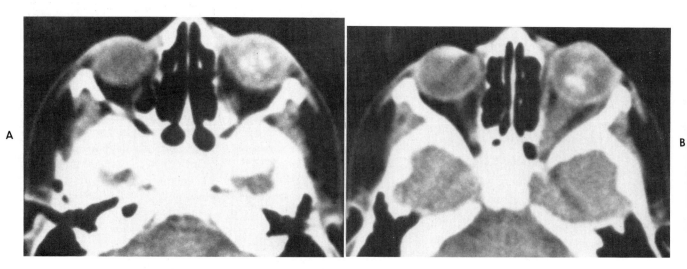

Fig. 14-8. Axial scans demonstrate large retinoblastoma with punctate calcifications filling vitreous and extending posteriorly beyond globe into an enlarged optic nerve.

gical pathologic findings. Thin section multiplanar CT scanning of patients with presumed retinoblastoma can be performed before treatment for initial staging of the tumor and may be used as one of the primary means of following the patient for possible extension and recurrence. When following these patients one should keep in mind the possibility of radiation-induced sarcoma, the location and extent of which may also be defined by CT.[33]

Melanomas

By far the most common primary intraocular neoplasms in adults are malignant melanomas. The average age of patients with melanomas is 50 years. Melanomas may arise from any portion of the uvea, but over 75% arise from the choroid, with the remainder arising from the iris, ciliary body, or optic nerve head. These tumors arise from melanocytes, which are extensively distributed throughout the pigmented uveal tract. Most tumors are first seen incidentally during ophthalmoscopic examination. The most common initial clinical symptom is loss of visual acuity, at which time a mass in the fundus is obvious by ophthalmoscopic examination. With small lesions, the pigmented lesion may be easily seen through the retina; however, with larger lesions retinal detachment, hemorrhage, and vitreous obscuration is common, and more extensive examination may be required to make the diagnosis. Although generally thought of as highly malignant tumors, the actual growth and spread of melanomas of the uvea varies greatly and is mainly a function of the histology and initial extent of the tumors. Pathologically the tumors are usually subdivided into the more benign spindle-cell varieties and the more malignant epithelioid vari-

eties. The small spindle-type A tumors have a 5-year mortality rate of less than 10%, while the large epithelioid tumors have a 5-year mortality rate of greater than 60%.[50,75] Usually the tumors are staged by ophthalmoscopic criteria and therapy is initiated, although some may be closely followed clinically for evidence of growth before treatment.[35] Small lesions may be treated by cyrosurgery, photocoagulation, or local irradiation; larger lesions are traditionally treated by enucleation. If there has been extension beyond the sclera, then the prognosis is much worse and radiotherapy or chemotherapy may be required. Five-year cure rates for tumors that have extended beyond the globe are generally less than 20%.

Radiologic evaluation of patients with melanomas has been primarily limited to ultrasonography of the orbit, nuclear medicine studies (including P32 tumor uptake), and various examinations in search of metastasis. Except for ultrasonography, none of these tests has proved to be critical in any significant number of cases. As with retinoblastomas, an important determination is extension of the tumors beyond the globe. CT scanning may offer help with this problem (Fig. 14-9). Other than random reports of cases, there is no published series of melanoma patients evaluated by CT.[7] We have evaluated 18 patients with known ocular melanomas. The tumors have been identified in 17 cases, and most importantly, extraocular extension was seen in eight cases. Extraocular extension is characterized either by distinct retro-ocular mass or by focal diffuse scleral thickening. In two cases this extension was not known before CT scanning. Obviously, very early extension into the sclera, and perhaps beyond, may not be detected by CT scanning; but further investigation into the useful-

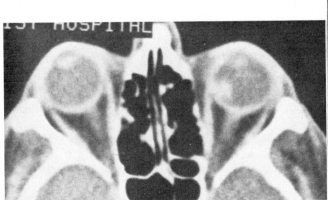
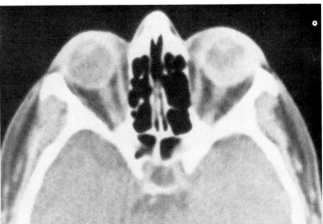

Fig. 14-9. A, Medium-sized (4 mm) bulky melanoma extending from choroid into the posterior medial vitreous. **B,** Different patient. Large infiltrating melanoma occupying posterior half of vitreous, thickening image of globe wall indicating extension into sclera, but no definite extension into optic nerve or retro-ocular space.

ness of CT scanning in investigating ocular melanomas is important.[18]

Compared to intraocular melanomas, extraocular orbital melanomas are rare.[31,92] When melanomas occur outside of the globe they may be metastases from distant primaries, a result of direct extension from facial melanomas, or rarely, primaries in the orbit. Most frequently, extraocular orbital melanomas are the result of direct extension of ocular melanomas.

■ Intraocular trauma

Another area of ocular pathology in which CT scanning is useful is trauma. By far the most common traumatic lesion to require CT scanning is the localization

of foreign bodies. Kollarits et al.[57] and Lobes et al.[63] have already reported on the usefulness of this technique in localizing not only metallic intraorbital foreign bodies but also nonmetallic foreign bodies that would not be obvious on other radiographic exams. With newer scanners and multiplanar sectioning lesions as small as 2 to 3 mm usually can be detected, and their intraocular or extraocular location identified. In addition to its accuracy in depicting foreign bodies, CT examination of the orbit is relatively painless and requires only that the patient lie still, which increases its usefulness in comparison with some of the more complicated radiographic techniques. In our opinion, when localization of a foreign body is not obvious from ultrasonog-

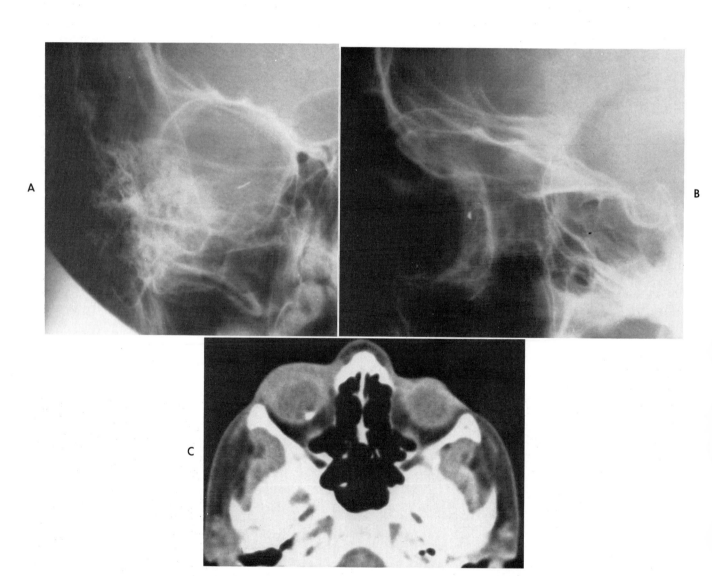

Fig. 14-10. A, PA and, **B,** lateral plain films of orbita reveal metallic foreign body triangulated near posterior globe. **C,** Axial CT scan shows thickened soft tissues covering eye caused by penetrating missile, which is clearly shown to be within globe adjacent to retina at five o'clock position.

raphy or routine plain films, CT scanning is the method of choice (Fig. 14-10).

Of course, other intraocular lesions are not uncommon in ophthalmologic practice, but most such lesions can be adequately evaluated by the ophthalmologist; hence CT scanning is seldom indicated. For this reason, there is little or no information on the CT appearance or usefulness of CT in evaluating inflammatory or degenerative lesions of the retichoroid, metastatic uveal carcinomas, retinal detachments, retinal hemorrhage, choroid hemangiomas, and other ophthalmologically common lesions. One would guess that most of these lesions will remain in the domain of the fundoscopic examination and only those lesions that tend to extend beyond the globe will require CT evaluation. An exception may be lesions with calcification, which appear very distinctly on CT scans (Fig. 14-11).

■ Intraconal lesions
Optic nerve lesions

For practical purposes, lesions producing demonstrable masses of the optic nerve are limited to optic gliomas and meningiomas.

Optic gliomas. Optic gliomas are usually benign pilocytic astrocytomas occurring in children, with the peak incidence at age 4 to 6 years. These tumors may occur within the orbital portion of the optic nerve or may involve additional portions of the visual pathway, including the optic chiasm and the intracranial portion of the optic nerve. They are predominantly unilateral lesions but may involve the entire chiasm and have been reported to involve both optic nerves.[80] Approximately 30% to 40% of the lesions will be purely intraorbital, while the remainder will be at least partially intracra-

nial. The patients usually suffer from visual loss, field defects, or proptosis, which indicates significant intraorbital tumor. Approximately 20% of patients will have a family history or other stigmata of neurofibromatosis. For such seemingly straightforward lesions, there is a remarkable amount of written material on the subject. This has not resulted in unanimity concerning certain critical questions.[20,27,51] Controversial questions remain those of growth potential, relationship to neurofibromatosis, and most importantly, treatment modality. It is generally accepted that these tumors are usually benign and very slow growing. This has perhaps been taken to the extreme by Hoyt and Baghdassarian[51] who suggest that these lesions are "congenital, non-neoplastic, self-limiting." Based on this concept, they suggest minimal if any treatment. Hoyt and Baghdassarian appear at odds with most of the rest of the authors on the subject. Most authors consider these tumors to be similar to other low-grade gliomas in the central nervous system, with a definite growth potential, and think that treatment should be based on this possibility. In general, lesions limited to the optic nerve may be treated with surgical resection by either the transorbital or transcranial approach. Lesions that extend intracranially and involve the optic chiasm or tract are generally not resectable and are usually surgically biopsied or debulked and subsequently treated by radiation.

Before the advent of CT scanning, the critical radiographic procedure was plain film optic canal views. In over 50% of cases optic gliomas resulted in a chronic expansion of the involved canal; this finding is generally considered diagnostic. The intraorbital portions of the tumor could not be well evaluated before CT, although

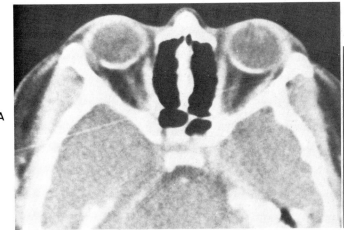
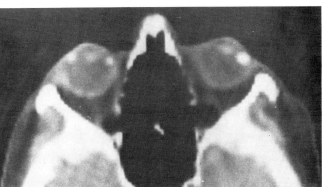

Fig. 14-11. Benign ocular calcifications. **A,** Bilateral choroid osteoma. These are benign lesions of posterior choroid. **B,** Scleral plaques. These are benign, incidental calcifications that occur in older patients near insertions of medial and lateral recti.

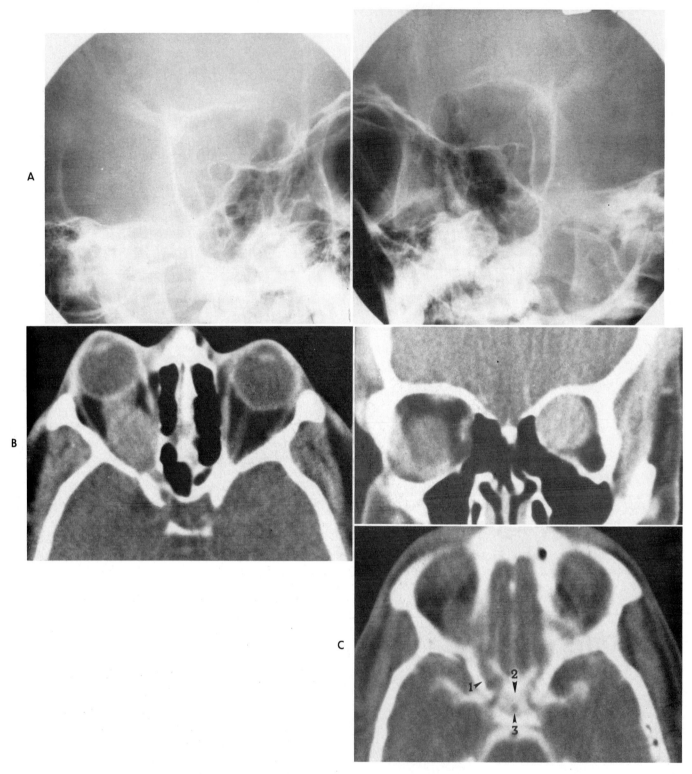

Fig. 14-12. Optic nerve glioma. **A,** PA oblique views of optic foramina reveal chronic enlargement of right optic foramen, indicating tumor within canal. **B,** Enhanced axial and coronal scans show diffuse symmetric enlargement of optic nerve from scleral junction to and within enlarged optic foramen. There is no definite posterior extension intracranially. **C,** After opacification of cerebrospinal fluid with metrizamide, an axial scan through suprasellar cistern reveals enlarged right optic canal *(1)* and normally opacified suprasellar cistern *(2),* penetrated by infundibulum *(3).* Surgical resection was performed and revealed tumor extending to posterior aspect of optic foramen, but resection cuff was without tumor proximal to optic chiasm.

the intracranial portions could be well documented by air encephalography. The CT appearance of optic nerve gliomas has been well described by numerous authors.* Gliomas involving the optic nerve characteristically enlarge the optic nerve symmetrically (Fig. 14-12). The tumors are usually inseparable from the normal nerve tissue. If strictly intraorbital, the lesions tend to be tapered on both ends. The associated proptosis is well demonstrated. The lesions are usually enhanced after intravenous contrast material injection, but not in a distinctive fashion. It is of utmost importance to evaluate possible intracranial extension. In this endeavor one may employ thin scan sections through the optic canal and thin axial and coronal scan sections through the chiasmatic region.

In many cases contrast enhancement of the suprasellar cistern fluid should be performed, either with air for encephalography or with metrizamide for CT scanning. While any enlargement of the intracranial portion of the optic nerve or asymmetry of the optic chiasm or mass in the anterior third ventricle is indicative of intracranial neoplasm, the lack of these findings does not completely exclude the possibility of subtle, early intracranial extension. This latter question can only be answered by pathologic examination of the tissue.

The relationship of optic nerve gliomas to neurofibromatosis is well documented but may be confusing.[59,86] Neurofibromatosis is associated with three distinctive lesions of the orbit that may occur separately or in any combination.[12,15,25] As previously mentioned, approximately 20% of optic nerve gliomas occur in patients with other stigmata of neurofibromatosis. There remains some question of whether or not this group of optic gliomas is different from the larger group of gliomas in patients without neurofibromatosis. From a pathologic viewpoint, there appears to be no difference. However, a larger percentage of Hoyt and Baghdassarian's[51] patients had neurofibromatosis (60%) and some authors have postulated that the relatively benign behavior of the tumors in their series was because of this relationship and the possibility that gliomas in neurofibromatosis patients are perhaps hamartomas. In addition, Hilal and Trokel[48] have suggested that on the CT scan one can separate the image of the optic nerve from the surrounding gliomatous tissue in patients with neurofibroma. While these papers are suggestive, the question remains unanswered until there is more definite pathologic information.

In addition to optic gliomas, neurofibroma patients have two other causes of exophthalmos. The first is dysplasia of the greater wing of the sphenoid which results in a defect in the posterior wall of the orbit that allows

*References 48, 62, 90, 91.

middle fossa contents to herniate anteriorly and to secondarily proptose the globe with pulsatile exophthalmos.[12,15] This bony dysplasia can occur without any other orbital abnormality. In addition, these patients may have plexiform neuromas of the orbit and overlying soft tissues. These lesions consist of wormlike structures in the subcutaneous tissue and the retro-ocular orbit that are bundles of loosely arranged collagen, through which myelinated and unmyelinated nerve fibers course. The majority of cells are Schwann cells and fibroblasts. These are usually large, disfiguring lesions most frequently occurring about the orbit.[25,36] In most reports each of these lesions is seen alone; however, they have been reported in any combination. CT scans of any of these conditions are usually diagnostic because not only the optic nerve and its pathology but also the bony anatomy of the posterior orbit are well displayed on axial views. The presence of extraconal soft tissue mass caused by plexiform neuroma is usually obvious (Fig. 14-13).

Meningiomas. Orbital meningiomas may be subdivided into three categories based on their anatomic location.[22,45] The first group of tumors arise directly from the meninges of the optic nerve sheath, the second group have no direct dural attachment, and tumors in the third group arise from the posterior bony margins of the orbit and are basically sphenoid meningiomas with secondary orbital involvement. Over 50% of orbital meningiomas are actually a result of adjacent cranial meningiomas and only 10% of orbital meningiomas do not have an obvious dural attachment. Therefore in the vast majority of cases orbital meningiomas will be either extraconal in location or intraconal with optic nerve involvement, as in the group under discussion.

Meningiomas of the orbit, as elsewhere, are most frequently seen in middle-aged women. The usual clinical complaint is proptosis followed by visual loss, although posterior lesions may manifest vision loss alone. Other early symptoms include retro-orbital pain and oculomotor palsies. The histology of orbital meningiomas is no different than these tumors elsewhere and can be subdivided into meningotheliomatous, psammomatous, fibroblastic, and angiomatous.

Meningiomas of the optic nerve sheath may occur grossly in two forms. The first, and more common, is a tumor arising eccentrically from one side of the optic nerve sheath. In the minority of cases the tumor may occur in a cufflike fashion surrounding the optic nerve. In either case the CT scan is usually diagnostic because the tumor is seen as distinct from the more lucent optic nerve (Fig. 14-14). These tumors may be enhanced (an average of 28 Hounsfield units) more than any other nonvascular lesion.[41] In the eccentric variety, these tumors are frequently seen as soft tissue masses with cal-

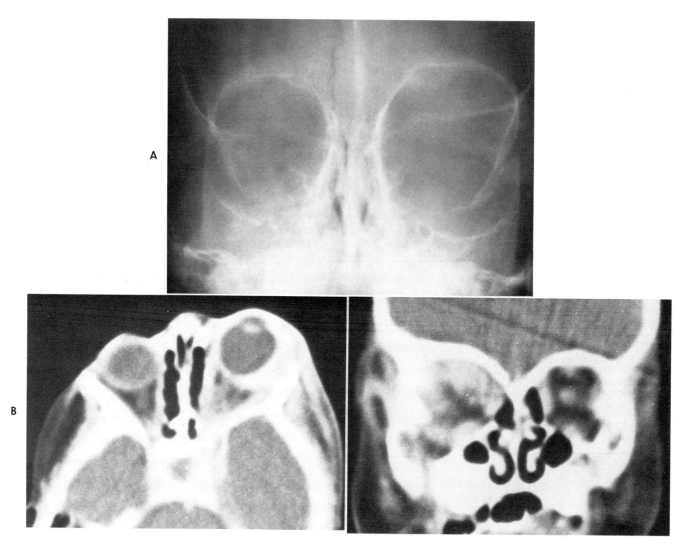

Fig. 14-13. Neurofibromatosis, plexiform neuroma. **A,** Caldwell view reveals chronic expansion of left orbit. **B,** Enhanced axial and coronal scans reveal large, diffuse, ill-defined soft tissue mass occupying superior and lateral aspect of orbit, with overlying soft tissues extending in extraconal fashion posteriorly to orbital apex, where soft tissue tumor extends through enlarged superior orbital fissure into cavernous sinus region and medial wall of middle fossa.

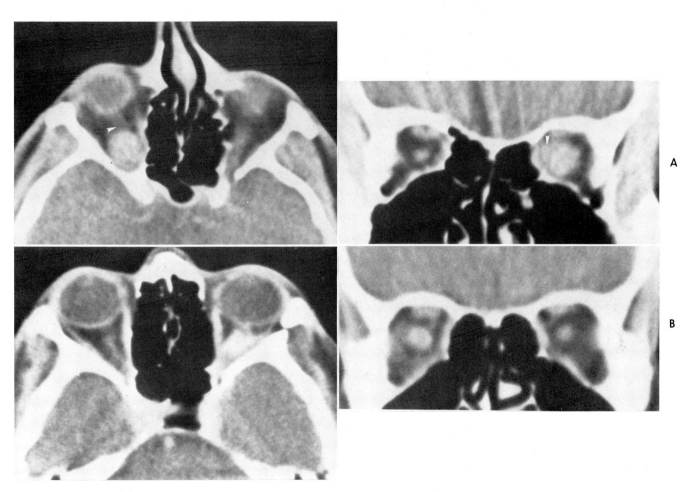

Fig. 14-14. Optic nerve meningioma. **A,** Patient 1, with globular meningioma appearing as discrete enhanced mass lateral to medially diplaced optic nerve *(arrows)*, which remains demarcated from tumor. **B,** Patient 2, with circumferential meningioma about optic nerve. Tumor appears as enhanced ring of thickened meninges about distinguishable, lucent optic nerve.

cification protruding off the side of the optic nerve, which it displaces and compresses. In the cuff variety, the usually invisible meninges of the optic nerve are seen as thickened, enhanced tissues that on coronal scan sections completely surround the central nerve. Unless very large, these tumors are usually quite distinct from the adjacent retro-orbital fat and the musculofascial sheath. It is usually easy to distinguish these optic nerve sheath meningiomas from secondary intraorbital meningiomas. This latter differentiation, however, may be difficult with small lesions at the orbital apex (Fig. 14-15). It is in this region that the CT scan should be supplemented by angiography and pluridirectional tomography to further define the bony in-

volvement of the optic foramen and the adjacent sphenoid bone. It is not unusual for lesions at the orbital apex to involve both the dura and adjacent bone of the optic canal as well as the dura extending anteriorly about the optic nerve.

Treatment of any meningioma, including orbital meningiomas, is surgical resection if possible. It is the responsibility of the radiologist to define the anatomy of these lesions as completely as possible. This includes defining their blood supply to better enable the surgeon to plan his approach. Vision can be saved in the presence of many of these lesions, particularly if they are more anteriorly located optic nerve sheath tumors. Vision preservation becomes more difficult with lesions

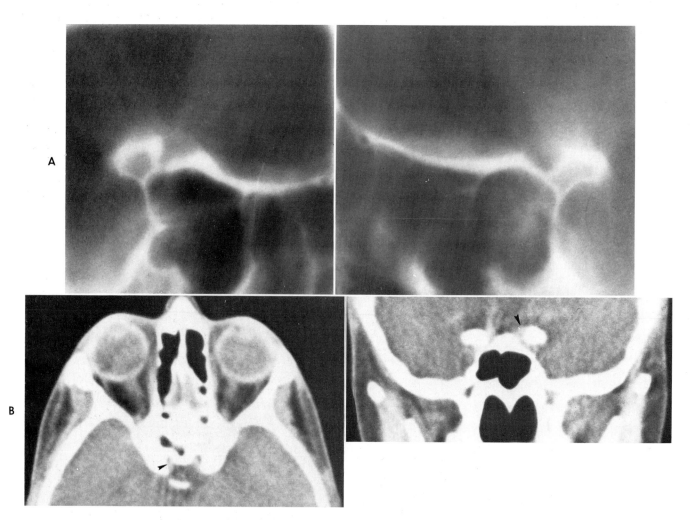

Fig. 14-15. Sphenoid, optic canal meningioma. **A,** PA oblique polytomography of posterior aspects of optic canal reveals subtle irregular sclerosis and thickening of right side of planum sphenoidale and floor and lateral wall of right optic canal. **B,** Axial and coronal enhanced CT scans reveal small soft tissue mass *(arrows)* at posteriormost aspect of optic canal on right side, indicating soft tissue as well as bony components of small meningioma. These subtle tumors may require CT and polytomography for diagnosis.

at the orbit apex and optic canal. Radiation therapy may be helpful in slowing growth in unresectable lesions.

Optic neuritis

Subtle alterations and enlargements of the optic nerve have been reported in patients with optic neuritis by Gyldensted et al.[41] and by Hilal and Trokel.[48] In these papers, as well as in other occasional references to this condition, CT changes are reported as very subtle. Because of this, when evaluating patients with visual loss and possible optic neuritis one may anticipate a normal CT scan in most circumstances. The main purpose of CT examination in these patients is not to see the subtle changes of the optic nerve and confirm the diagnosis of optic neuritis (a clinical diagnosis), but to exclude other conditions, particularly neoplasia, which may mimic this condition clinically. Likewise, subtle enlargement of the optic nerve has occasionally been reported in patients with papilledema, but again, it is probably not a definite enough finding to be of clinical usefulness. Because optic neuritis is routinely more obvious by ophthalmoscopic examination, CT is performed primarily to exclude other lesions.

■ Intraconal lesions without optic nerve involvement
Hemangiomas

Two groups of lesions, vascular and inflammatory pseudotumors, account for more than 75% of intraconal masses without optic nerve involvement.

A great variety of vascular lesions may occur in the orbit. These include tumors such as capillary hemangiomas, cavernous hemangiomas, hemangioendotheliomas, hemangioperictyomas, vascular leiomyomas, and lymphangiomas as well as vascular malformations including aneurysms, varices, and arteriovenous fistulae.* Many of these lesions are rare or have a nondistinctive CT appearance. Therefore only the more common and distinctive lesions will be discussed in this section.

In most series, hemangiomas are listed as one of the three most common masses in the orbit. The histology is usually either capillary or cavernous hemangioma. In adults, they occur most frequently as an encapsulated intraconal mass; they may or may not have phleboliths. Hemangiomas have a very slow blood flow. Patients usually have painless proptosis. Visual loss is late and complete surgical resection is usually possible. These lesions most frequently occur in the fourth decade and are more common in women.

On CT scan these lesions appear as a sharply marginated soft tissue density that may contain calcification and that are enhanced no more than adjacent muscle (Fig. 14-16). Intraconal lesions of this description in adults are most likely hemangiomas.

The other common pattern of hemangiomas is that of an extraconal mass occurring in childhood. These lesions may be associated with skin or conjunctival lesions, and the patients may have similar lesions elsewhere in the body. These are generally considered to

---

*References 8, 11, 45, 49.

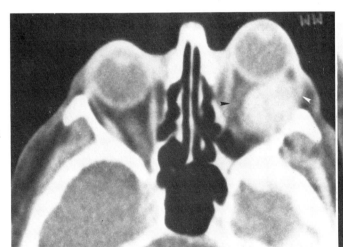
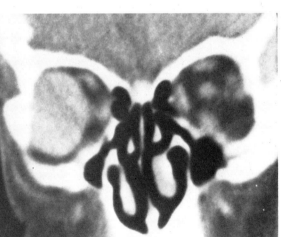

A   B

Fig. 14-16. Hemangioma. Axial and coronal CT scans reveal homogeneous, sharply demarcated intraconal mass displacing optic nerve *(horizontal arrow)* medially and lateral rectus muscle laterally *(angled arrow)*. Lesion enhanced approximately same as adjacent muscle tissue.

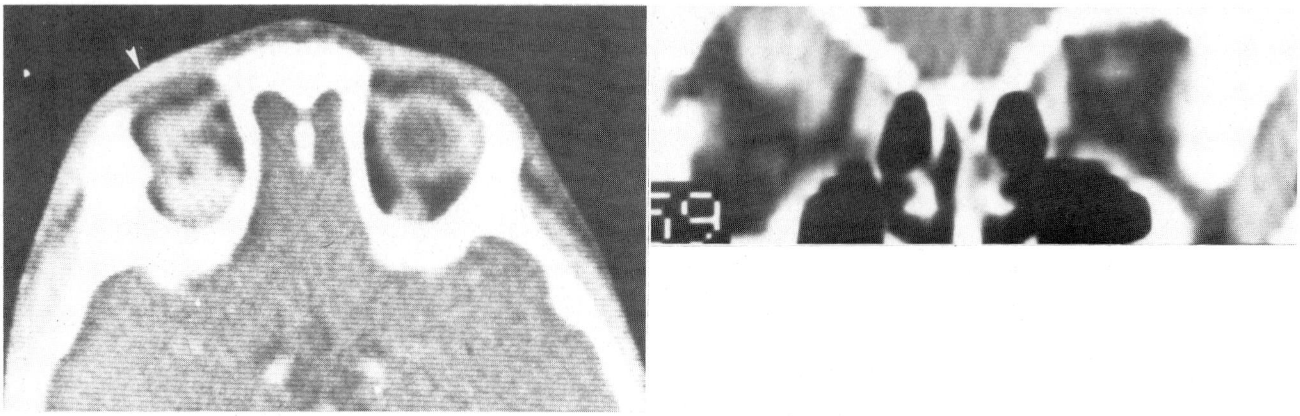

Fig. 14-17. Facial and orbital hemangioma. Eight-month-old patient with obvious facial hemangioma involving right eyelid. Axial and coronal *(reconstructed)* enhanced scans show enhanced lid soft tissues *(arrowhead),* with extraconal mass extending posteriorly into orbit.

be congenital lesions and the majority are noted within 3 months of age.[66] The patients frequently have proptosis. Visual loss is late and the primary problem is cosmetic. These lesions are prone to regress during childhood, and it is preferable to withhold any specific treatment if possible. However, during the early stages there may be compromise of vision, leading to amblyopia as well as to gross cosmetic deformity and superficial bleeding. Glaucoma may also result from distorted anterior chamber anatomy, and treatment may be necessary. Various modes of therapy have been tried and the fact that a large number are still in use suggests that none is optimum. Local excision, systemic steroid therapy, radiation therapy, cryosurgery, and other methods are all occasionally used. Fewer of these patients have been evaluated with CT because the lesions and their diagnosis are usually obvious and the CT scan is helpful only in evaluating the extent of the lesion for possible therapy. On CT scans these lesions usually appear as soft tissue swelling over and around the orbit in the obvious clinical location of the lesion. Any intraorbital extension of the tumor is usually indicated by poorly defined soft tissue mass predominantly outside of the muscle cone (Fig. 14-17). There may be irregular extensions into the muscle cone. Again, these lesions usually are not enhanced any more than adjacent muscle. Smaller subcutaneous lesions may be difficult to appreciate at all.

Less common vascular tumors of the eye are lymphangiomas, which usually occur in adults and may be indistinguishable from hemangiomas even on gross inspection, but which have the characteristic histology. Interestingly, these are the most common orbital tumors to spontaneously bleed, with resultant sudden orbital pain and proptosis. This may be reflected by high-

density, sharply marginated and possibly enhanced masses on CT scans. These lesions tend to be extraconal and frequently involve the conjunctiva.[53] Although some lymphangiomas lack sufficient vascularity to be enhanced on CT scanning, many of the lesions have sufficient vascular component to be enhanced as well as to bleed. The CT distinction is therefore not clear-cut in these lesions.

Orbital varices

Most arteriovenous malformations of the orbit are not characterized by a discrete intraconal mass, with one exception: orbital varices; these most frequently involve the superior or inferior ophthalmic vein, both of which have a large component in the muscle cone. These may be extremely difficult lesions to diagnose, as varices are only expanded intermittently and may not be obvious unless a provocative test such as venography with Valsalva's maneuver or jugular vein compression is performed. Similar provocative tests can be performed with the patient in the CT scanner. Hilal and Trokel[48] reported the correct diagnosis in such a lesion, and we have seen one similar case (Fig. 14-18). Without any effort to produce venous obstruction, the CT scan appears normal. After Valsalva's maneuver or compression of the jugular veins, varices may distend and appear as very sharply marginated masses, retro-ocular and predominantly within the muscle cone. Although some argue that these particular lesions require orbital venography for diagnosis, in our particular case the lesion involved the inferior ophthalmic vein and was not demonstrated at orbital venography and hence could only be diagnosed by CT. Orbital varices may cause proptosis on Valsalva maneuver, and this is the explanation for most cases of "voluntary exophthalmos."

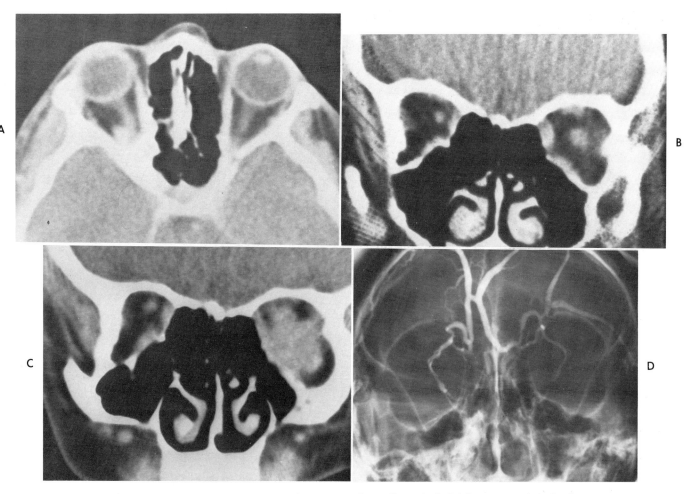

Fig. 14-18. Orbital varix. **A,** Initial axial scans reveals small poorly defined mass at right orbital apex, lateral to optic nerve. **B,** Routine enhanced coronal CT scans reveal no significant abnormalities. **C,** Enhanced coronal CT scan with jugular compression reveals large intraconal mass inferior to optic nerve. **D,** Orbital phlebogram reveals no significant abnormalities of superior ophthalamic complex; however, inferior ophthalmic vein is not visualized. Surgery confirmed large varix of inferior ophthalmic vein.

Pseudotumor

There is probably no more confusing area of orbital pathology than that of pseudotumor. For practical purposes, pseudotumor can be summarized as a nonspecific inflammatory process that mimics neoplasm or specific inflammatory lesions. Hence the definitive diagnosis of pseudotumor requires tissue, the histologic examination of which excludes neoplasia and specific inflammatory processes. At the present time pseudotumor may be diagnosed histologically on the basis of polymorphic cellular pattern, a predominance of inflammatory lymphocytes, and a nonneoplastic histology.[45] Orbital pseudotumor always involves inflammation of orbital fat, although other intraorbital structures may be affected concomitantly (e.g., muscle, Tenon's capsule). There are a variety of lesions that may have

very similar histologic patterns and clinical appearances but should be separated from this condition. Such lesions include lethal midline granuloma, cellulitis secondary to adjacent sinusitis, tissue reaction from adjacent foreign body or spilled contents of dermoid cysts, thrombophlebitis, sclerosing lymphangioma and hemangioma, various forms of lymphoma, sarcoidosis, Wegener's granulomatosis, and multiple focal fibrosclerosis. For more detailed histologic definition of this condition, one should see one of the more extensive pathologic reviews.[9,21]

Clinically, the condition occurs throughout adult life and is equally distributed between men and women. The classic signs are proptosis, soft tissue swelling, and impairment of muscle motility. The onset is usually rapid and the degree of proptosis marked, considering

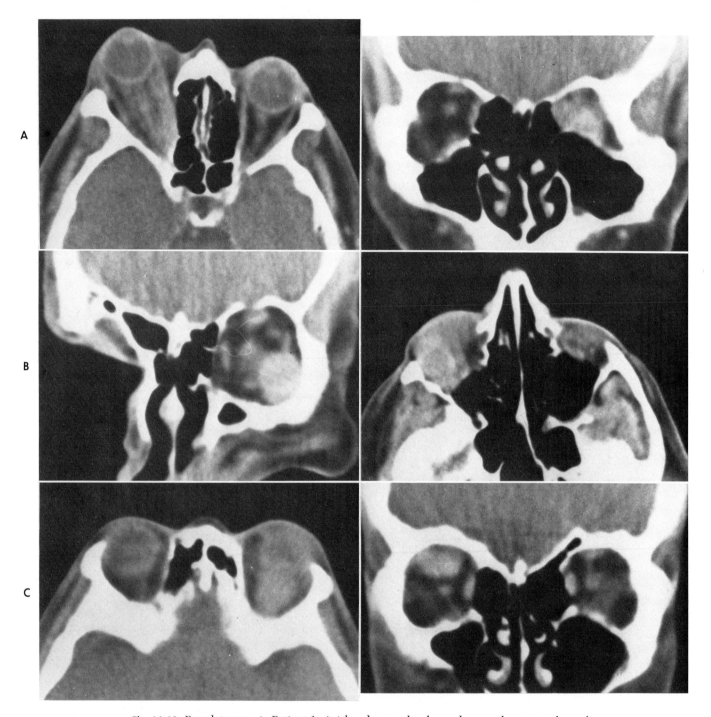

Fig. 14-19. Pseudotumor. **A,** Patient 1. Axial and coronal enhanced scans show typical poorly defined intraconal mass on right, with marked proptosis. **B,** Patient 2. Less common appearance of intraconal mass, with focal pseudotumor predominantly extraconal in inferior lateral aspect of right orbit associated with mild proptosis. **C,** Patient 3. Focal pseudotumor involving superior rectus levator complex on left, with moderately associated proptosis. This appearance is indistinguishable from lymphomatous or leukemic involvement of muscle and even thyroid ophthalmopathy. All patients had typical clinical syndromes of orbital pseudotumor and responded to steroid therapy.

the duration of symptoms. The prognosis is good, with the disease usually responding rapidly to systemic steroids. This rapid response to steroids has become one of the pivotal diagnostic criteria; the lack of response makes the diagnosis questionable.

Although the microscopic pathology of the lesion does not appear to relate directly to the CT appearance, the gross pathologic characteristics do. Orbital pseudotumor involves orbital fat, along with orbital muscles or the lacrimal gland. In concordance with this, CT reports on orbital pseudotumor by Enzmann et al.[29] and Hilal and Trokel[48] indicate that there are several basic patterns of orbital pseudotumor on CT scans (Fig. 14-19). The most common appearance is proptosis without other intraorbital abnormality, with the exception of a slight increase in fat density. The second most common appearance is that of obvious diffuse irregular increased density of the orbital soft tissues, including fat, with or without subsequent contrast enhancement. This increased density is nonfocal and tends to obliterate the usual soft tissue density differences between muscle and fat. With this pattern, there is nearly always intraconal involvement and frequently the posterior globe is involved. In some cases the contrast enhancement may be intense and appear to involve the sclera as well as retro-ocular tissues. In a smaller number of patients there may be a more sharply marginated focal mass that cannot be differentiated from true neoplasm. Such lesions may be either intraconal or extraconal. In a few patients, orbital pseudotumor is primarily reflected as a myositis and the CT image is that of an enlarged extraocular muscle or muscles. If this is the only finding, differentiation from thyroid ophthalmopathy may be difficult by CT scan alone, but the enlarged muscles in pseudotumor are usually poorly defined rather than sharply marginated as in thyroid ophthalmopathy. Finally, orbital pseudotumor may appear primarily as a lacrimal mass and is therefore extraconal. This type of lesion will be discussed in the section on lacrimal lesions.

In general, a poorly defined retro-ocular mass with intraconal and extraconal involvement in an adult is most likely to be a pseudotumor. There are a number of cases in which this diagnosis cannot be made comfortably and usually a trial of systemic steroids or biopsy is necessary. Many of the lesions that mimic orbital pseudotumor either clinically or pathologically may also mimic the CT appearance and may even respond to systemic steroids. Previous reports of CT scans on patients with orbital sarcoidosis[73] and Wegener's granulomatosis[89] show these lesions to be indistinguishable from the common appearance of orbital pseudotumor.

■ Muscle lesions
Thyroid ophthalmopathy

By far the most common cause of exophthalmos—either unilateral or bilateral—is Graves' disease. This diagnosis is the most common single diagnosis made in most clinical series as well as in series based on CT.[41,72,92] This disease is characterized by enlargement of the extraocular muscles caused by deposition of hyaluronic acid and infiltration of small round cells. Clinically, the disease may be very mild to marked; the American Thyroid Association has classified the disease into six grades of severity based on the presence and degree of proptosis, soft tissue swelling, extraocular muscle impairment, corneal involvement, and visual loss. There have been numerous articles correlating the CT findings in Graves' disease with the clinical picture.[30,85] As one would expect, the characteristic finding in patients with Graves' disease is CT evidence of muscle enlargement (Fig. 14-20). With axial scans this is primarily reflected by enlargement of the medial or lateral recti; with coronal scans, involvement of the superior and inferior recti may be appreciated. It has been found that the degree of muscle enlargement correlates well with the clinical severity of the disease and with measurable proptosis. The muscular enlargement is most prominent in their midsections, where there is a symmetric expansion with less enlargement toward the tendinous origins and insertions. Muscle involvement with ophthalmopathy has been reported to be less radiodense, i.e., 24 vs. 56 Hounsfield units.[41] In most series, over 90% of patients who were eventually diagnosed as having thyroid ophthalmopathy were found to have abnormal CT scans with muscle enlargement. The most frequently involved muscles are the inferior rectus and the medial rectus muscles. Examples of any individual muscle enlargement as well as any combination of muscle enlargement are present in the literature. It is particularly important with this condition that coronal scans be performed. Many of the early reports using axial scans and thick scan sections underestimated the involvement of the inferior rectus muscle in particular. In addition, numerous papers indicate the difficulty in differentiating enlargement of the inferior rectus muscle alone from a nonmuscle orbit mass when scanning only in the axial projection.[52,56] Although it is true that the muscles are enhanced after contrast material injection, this has not been shown to be critical in evaluating these patients. For these reasons, if the primary clinical question is whether or not the patient has thyroid ophthalmopathy, we routinely scan these patients only in the coronal projection and without contrast material injection. This not only lowers the radiation dose and speeds the examination but also obviates the contrast

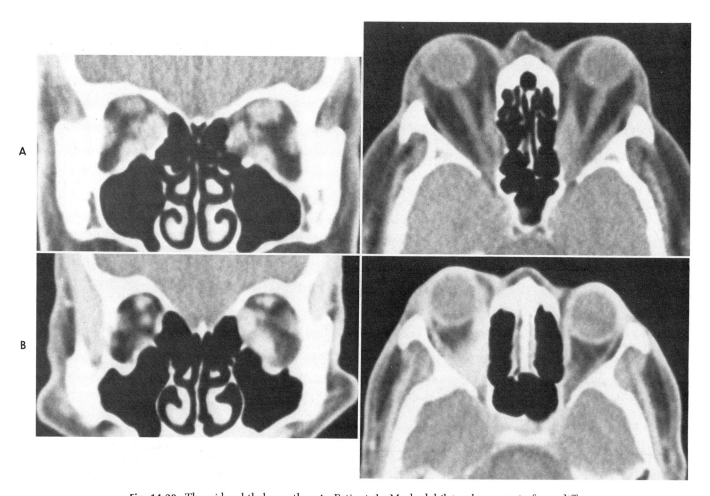

Fig. 14-20. Thyroid ophthalmopathy. **A,** Patient 1. Marked bilateral proptosis from diffuse enlargement of all extraocular muscles. Note importance of coronal scans and relative redundancy of axial scans. **B,** Patient 2. Unilateral proptosis on right side caused by enlarged medial and inferior rectus muscles. This pattern of muscle enlargement is most common in Graves' disease.

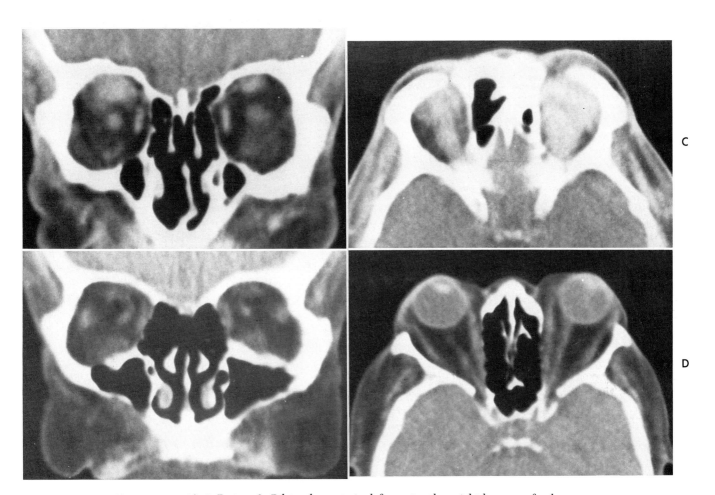

Fig. 14-20, cont'd. C, Patient 3. Bilateral proptosis, left greater than right because of enlargement primarily of superior rectus levator complex, particularly on left side. This is least common pattern of muscle enlargement. **D,** Patient 4. Bilateral proptosis with mild to moderate enlargement of medial and inferior rectus, but not sufficient to account for degree of proptosis. This patient has diffuse infiltration of orbital fat to account for much of mass effect. Note decreased contrast between fat and extraocular muscles. This is least common CT image in thyroid ophthalmopathy.

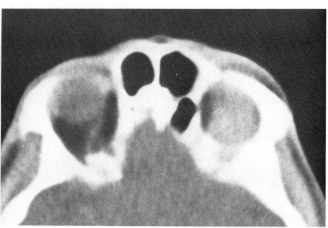

A   B

Fig. 14-21. Lymphoma. Left proptosis, with decreased inferior duction caused by lymphomatous involvement of superior rectus levator complex. This is not unusual appearance for lymphoma, which tends to primarily involve anterior orbit and extend posteriorly in extraconal or intramuscular fashion.

material injection that interferes with subsequent chemical tests.

Although thyroid ophthalmopathy accounts for over 90% of enlarged muscles on CT scans, there is an important differential diagnosis for this observation. Other lesions that have been reported to produce muscle enlargement include orbital pseudotumor, arteriovenous malformation, lesions caused by orbital trauma, and neoplasm of muscle, primarily rhabdomyosarcoma in infants and lymphoma in adults (Fig. 14-21). In most cases the clinical correlation will make this differentiation obvious, although in a few instances a biopsy may be necessary.[54] It should be emphasized that rhabdomyosarcoma is not a tumor characteristically arising from mature striated muscle of the extraocular muscles; rather it usually arises from embryonic rests within the orbit and separate from the muscles.

■ Intraorbital lesions
Lacrimal gland lesions

The lacrimal gland may become tumorous either from neoplasms or inflammatory conditions. The most common neoplasms of the lacrimal gland are benign mixed tumors, which account for almost half of lacrimal neoplasms. Approximately 5% to 10% of these lesions may be malignant. The second most common neoplasms are adenoid cystic carcinomas, which with other carcinomas account for the remaining 50% of lacrimal neoplasms.[4,45] Regardless of histology, the lesions usually appear as masses in the superolateral aspect of the orbit with proptosis and downward displacement of the globe. These lesions usually are relatively obvious on clinical examination because of their secondary effects on the eye as well as their anterior location, which allows them to be directly palpated. More benign lesions usually appear as painless masses, but the more malignant lesions may be accompanied by pain as a result of their deep involvement of the periorbita, adjacent muscle, and bone. The initial treatment of all of these lesions is surgical excision or biopsy. In cases of benign lesions, surgery is usually curative. With the more malignant lesions, more radical surgical excision and radiotherapy may be necessary.

With the earlier CT scanners a number of these lesions were not appreciated, but with high-resolution scanners that include coronal projections most of these lesions can be demonstrated. In most cases, however, one recognizes only that there is an enlarged lacrimal gland; the specific histology cannot be evaluated. With high-resolution scanning one may be able to see the well-defined, sharply marginated high-density mass typical of benign mixed tumor, as demonstrated in salivary tissue elsewhere.[14] With more malignant lesions one may see a poorly defined mass with involvement of bone and adjacent tissues, including portions of the globe and adjacent muscles (Fig. 14-22). In addition to the inability to differentiate consistently the histology of lacrimal neoplasms, the problem is further compounded by the inability to differentiate true neoplasms from the more common inflammatory lesions of the lacrimal gland.

The lacrimal gland may be involved by one of the variants of orbital pseudotumor as well as by more characteristic lacrimal inflammatory lesions reflected by lymphoid infiltrates, as in patients with Sjögren's syndrome.[32] In our experience, these inflammatory lesions

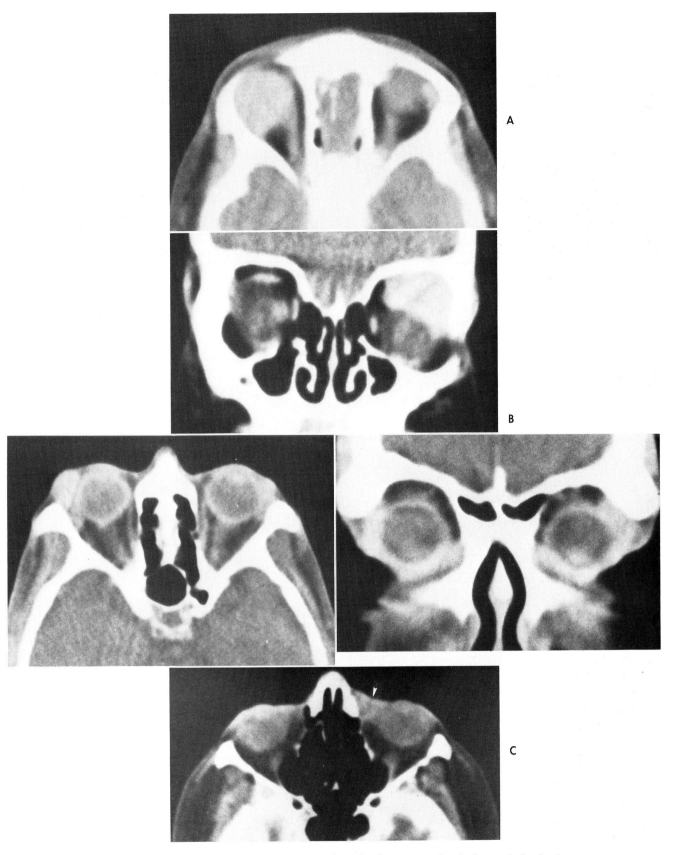

Fig. 14-22. Lacrimal lesions. **A,** Patient 1. Unilateral enlargement of right lacrimal gland seen on axial and coronal scan sections and caused by lymphoma of gland and adjacent soft tissues. **B,** Patient 2. Bilateral chronic granulomatous disease of lacrimal glands with prominent lacrimal glands, larger on right side. **C,** Patient 3. Dacryocystitis with pyogenic infection of lacrimal sac—seen on axial scans as prominent soft tissue mass *(arrows)* within lacrimal sac fossa.

are simply reflected as diffuse enlargement of the gland and are indistinguishable from neoplasms. One should also keep in mind the fact that lacrimal tissue can occur elsewhere in the orbit and this ectopic lacrimal tissue may account for masses located virtually anywhere in the ocular adnexa.[38]

Lymphomas

Histologically, lymphomas of the orbit are subdivided as elsewhere in the body. This includes Hodgkin's disease, non-Hodgkin's lymphoma, and reticulum cell sarcoma. Regardless of histology, these tumors occur primarily in the anterior orbit. This is probably related to the paucity of lymphoid tissue posterior to the orbital septum. In fact, most orbital lymphomas occur in the soft tissues of the eyelids and conjunctiva. For this reason they are characteristically easily palpable and appear early as soft tissue masses without pain or ocular findings. On CT scans they are usually poorly defined tumors in the anterior orbit; if there is no obvious skin lesion, the main differential diagnosis includes inflammatory lesions. Although they are usually restricted to the anterior orbit, they may extend more posteriorly. If so they tend to extend extraconally or, rarely, within a muscle (Fig. 14-23).[44,71]

Epidermoid and dermoid tumors

Distinctive but relatively unusual benign tumors of the orbit are dermoid or epidermoid cysts. These lesions contain a capsule that is usually well-defined, fibrous, and relatively strong except for its inferior portion. The contents of epidermoid tumors consist of keratin and epithelial debris that usually has a white

cheesy appearance. Dermoid tumors may contain in addition to the keratin and epithelial debris, sebaceous material, hair, and oily liquid. These tumors presumably arise from epithelial rests within or along the margins of the orbit. They occur most frequently in the upper orbit, either medially or laterally. They are usually located in the anterior portion of the orbit and for this reason are frequently palpable.[17] Because of the latter characteristic and the fact that they are basically congenital tumors, these lesions appear in a younger age group than many of the previously described tumors. In at least one clinical series of orbital tumors in children, dermoid and epidermoid cysts were the most common neoplasms.[94] Patients with these tumors usually have painless proptosis and a palpable mass in the upper orbit. More than half of the patients will have distinctive radiographic findings on plain films. These findings consist of a sharply marginated lucent defect in the superior bony margins of the orbit, with relatively thick sclerotic margins.[17] Such radiographic findings are almost pathognomonic of this condition. These tumors are reflected on CT scans as sharply defined, usually radiolucent, extraconal masses with adjacent bony erosion in the upper orbit (Fig. 14-24). If one can measure negative Hounsfield units confidently within the mass, the pathologic diagnosis is secure. Treatment is complete surgical excision, which is usually feasible, although occasionally recurrences do occur.

Metastasis

Metastatic disease of the eye and orbit is not unusual, particularly if one reviews the oncology literature. It may appear infrequently in the ophthalmologic litera-

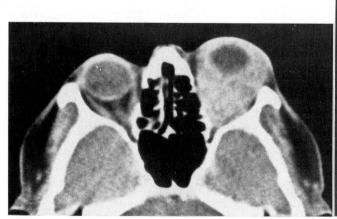

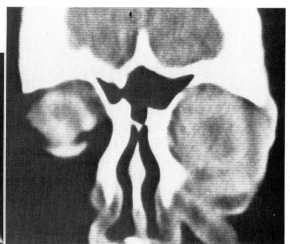

Fig. 14-23. Lymphoma. Extensive intraconal and muscle tumor with involvement of sclera and anterior orbital soft tissues. Pseudotumor may have similar appearance.

ture because many of these patients are not referred to that specialty. Albert et al.,[1] in a review of 213 patients with generalized malignancy, found a 10% orbit metastatic rate. Primary tumors that most frequently metastasize to the orbit are lung and breast tumors. Although different series vary, ocular metastases roughly equal orbital metastases.[42] Ocular metastases are usually to the posterior choroid and seldom become large tumors, while orbital tumors are usually extraconal and not infrequently involve bone. In children, by far the most common neoplasm to metastasize to the orbit is neuroblastoma, with over 50% of such cases having orbital metastasis.[2] Radiographically, ocular metastatic disease is not apparent, and orbital metastasis is usually seen as poorly defined extraconal soft tissue masses that may have associated bone destruction. Without the latter,

clinical history or biopsy is usually necessary to make the diagnosis (Fig. 14-25).

A different category of secondary involvement of the orbit by malignant disease is direct extension of neoplasm into the orbit from overlying carcinomas of the skin. This is a frequent problem in otolaryngology, ophthalmology, and plastic surgery practices. Previously, extensive evaluation of these lesions was performed with plain films and pluridirectional tomography for definition of bone destruction. Such examinations continue to play a role, but CT has added the ability to define the soft tissue extensions into the orbit and in many cases to adequately display the bony destruction (Fig. 14-26). Unfortunately, many of these tumors spread in slender strands along vascular and neural pathways; at the present time this type of dissemination is seldom defined by any radiographic method.

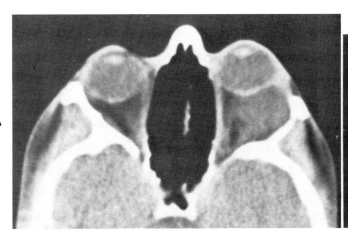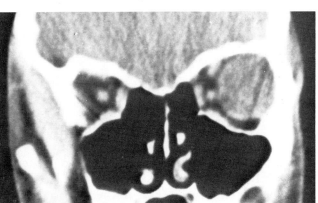

Fig. 14-24. Epidermoid. Axial and coronal scans show sharply marginated, lucent, nonenhancing extraconal mass in lateral aspect of left orbit, associated with chronic expansion of left orbital wall. CT numbers within lesions were −5 to −10, indicating fatty component and confirming diagnosis.

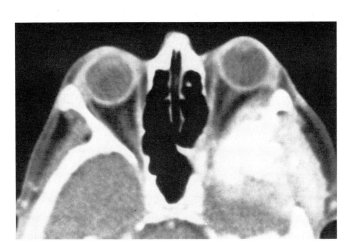

Fig. 14-25. Metastatic carcinoma of breast. Extensive soft tissue mass, with bone destruction involving greater wing of sphenoid on left side; mass extends into middle fossa, temporal fossa, and in an extraconal fashion into lateral aspect of orbit.

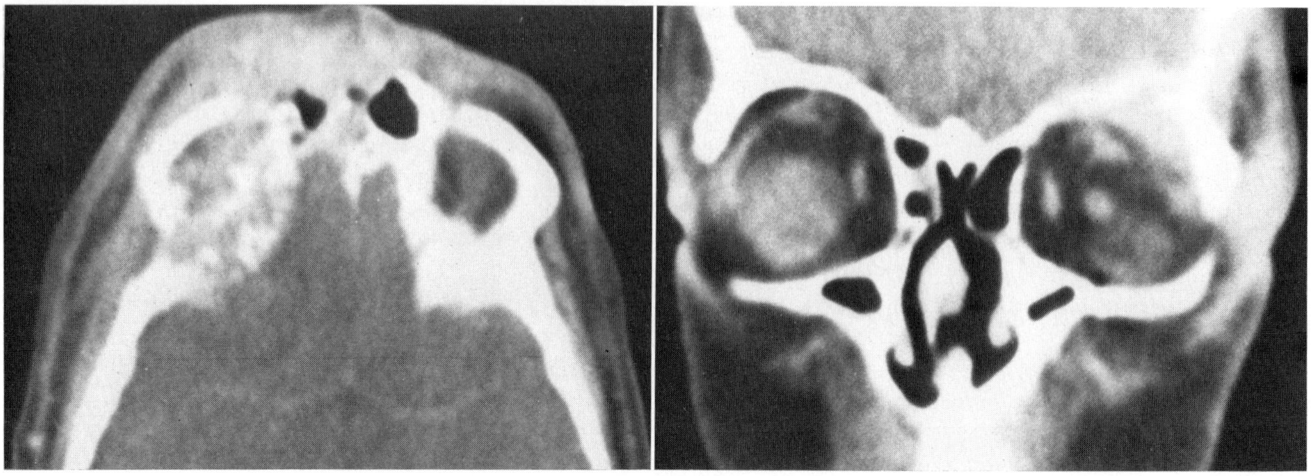

Fig. 14-26. Invasive squamous cell carcinoma. Axial and coronal scans reveal proptosis of right eye caused by extensive soft tissue mass that involves orbital rim and roof and overlying soft tissues from squamous cell carcinoma and extends in an extraconal fashion into orbit.

■ Extraorbital lesions with secondary orbital involvement

Primary bone lesions

As one would expect, virtually any pathologic process of bone can involve the margins of the orbit and secondarily involve the orbital contents. Typically, osteoblastic lesions include the previously described meningiomas, fibrous dysplasias, osteomas, infantile hyperostoses, and rarely, chronic infections.* Any of these lesions may expand bone, but meningiomas and fibrous dysplasias most characteristically do this. Any of these lesions can be displayed by CT, and although their effects on orbital contents and critical structures such as the optic canal are best displayed by this method, bony detail for differential diagnosis is probably better defined by plain films or tomography. Likewise, there is a broad list of lytic lesions of bone that involve the orbital margins, including metastases, multiple myeloma, histiocytoses, various benign bone tumors such as aneurysmal bone cysts, and osteomyelitis.† CT is useful in the detection of these lytic lesions and provides excellent definition of the extent of the pathologic process. Plain films and complex motion tomography may provide additional information concerning bone architecture and may thus be helpful in radiographic differential diagnosis (Fig. 14-27).

Sinus disease with secondary orbital involvement

At least half the orbit is normally surrounded by paranasal sinuses and in many cases it is bordered by si-

nuses on almost three quarters of its walls. The maxillary sinus is related to the floor of the orbit, while the ethmoid and sphenoid sinuses form the medial wall and the ethmoid and frontal sinuses cover varying portions of the roof of the orbit. The paranasal sinuses are separated from the orbit by bone and periorbita. Normally there are bony defects in the medial wall of the orbit that allow relatively free communication between the ethmoid sinuses and the orbit. These defects allow passage of the anterior and posterior ethmoid arteries. Primary disease of the paranasal sinuses may therefore extend into the orbit either by way of destruction of the bone and periorbita or alternatively by way of advance into the orbit by the small communications with the ethmoid sinuses along its medial wall. Direct spread is more characteristic of malignant lesions and higher grade inflammatory lesions such as osteomyelitis and granulomatous disease. Lower grade infectious diseases, particularly bacterial sinusitis, frequently involve the orbit secondarily through anatomic openings in its medial walls.

There are several natural barriers to limit the extension of sinus disease into the orbit. The bone and the periorbita are the first barrier, the musculofascial sheath is the second barrier within the orbit, and the orbital septum is an additional barrier anteriorly. It is of utmost importance for the clinician to know when these various barriers are transgressed, as the different surgical approaches affect drainage and place specific critical structures at risk.

The clinical appearance of patients obviously varies according to the particular lesion, but frequent symptoms include lacrimation, eyelid edema, episcleritis,

*References 55, 61, 68, 70.
†References 19, 45, 62, 78.

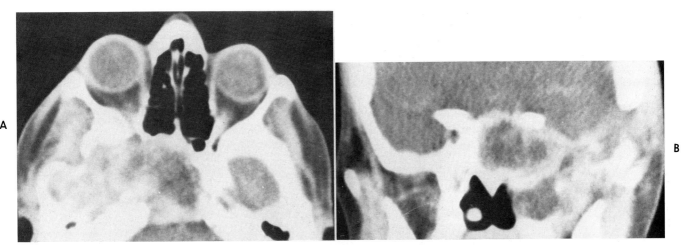

Fig. 14-27. Chondroblastoma. Axial and coronal scans reveal large, irregular, partially calcified mass involving right side of basisphenoid as well as greater wing of sphenoid. Mass involves orbital apex, with destruction of bone in this region, and also extends inferiorly into nasopharyngeal region.

proptosis, and limitation of extraocular muscle motion. In addition, patients may have a secondary optic neuritis or extraocular nerve palsies.[65,88] An important anatomic consideration is the course of the optic nerve through the optic canal, a channel in the sphenoid bone. Complete pneumatization of this canal may occur, surrounding the optic nerve with paranasal sinuses.

Orbital pathology related to sinus disease

Primary sinus disease with secondary orbital involvement can be classified in the following fashion.

Infectious lesions
    Osteomyelitis and periostitis
        Thrombophlebitis
        Cellulitis
        Abscess
    Mucocele
    Neoplasm
        Malignant
        Benign

Before CT, evaluation of secondary inflammatory processes in the orbit was a difficult problem because direct evidence was limited to identification of opacified sinuses, bone destruction, and occasional orbital emphysema. CT has been shown to be critical in the evaluation of these lesions[37,46,95] (Fig. 14-28). Focal osteomyelitis is usually indicated by local bone destruction with perhaps slight overlying periosteal thickening and contrast enhancement on CT. In the very thin bone of the lamina papyracea this may be difficult to evaluate by either CT or complex motion tomography. When

the infection breaks through the bone and into the orbit there is usually obvious involvement of the orbital fat and subsequent increased density where the inflammatory process is localized. Usually this is initially restricted to the periphery of the orbit, outside the musculofascial sheath in the extraconal space. Disease in this plane may dissect posteriorly to the orbital apex, with secondary involvement of the optic nerve and extraocular muscles and nerves. Infrequently, the infectious process may break through the musculofascial sheath into the retro-ocular fat or spread by way of the vascular channels into this region. Such extension will necessitate different surgical approaches because the intraconal region may not be adequately drained by extraconal procedures. As the intraconal or extraconal orbital cellulitis progresses it may wall off and form a well-defined abscess with a discrete and enhanced capsule. The location of such a lesion should be defined precisely for resection or drainage. CT-directed needle drainage of orbital abscesses has also been found to be feasible. Not infrequently, inflammatory disease of the frontal, anterior ethmoid, and maxillary sinuses may be associated with overlying facial soft tissue cellulitis. This is usually associated with extensive soft tissue swelling that prevents adequate orbital examination by the clinician. CT is the optimum method for determining spread posterior to the orbital septum. It should be remembered that, in addition to scanning the orbits in cases of sinus inflammatory disease, scans of the brain should be obtained to evaluate possible intracranial extension.

When the inflammatory process is associated with

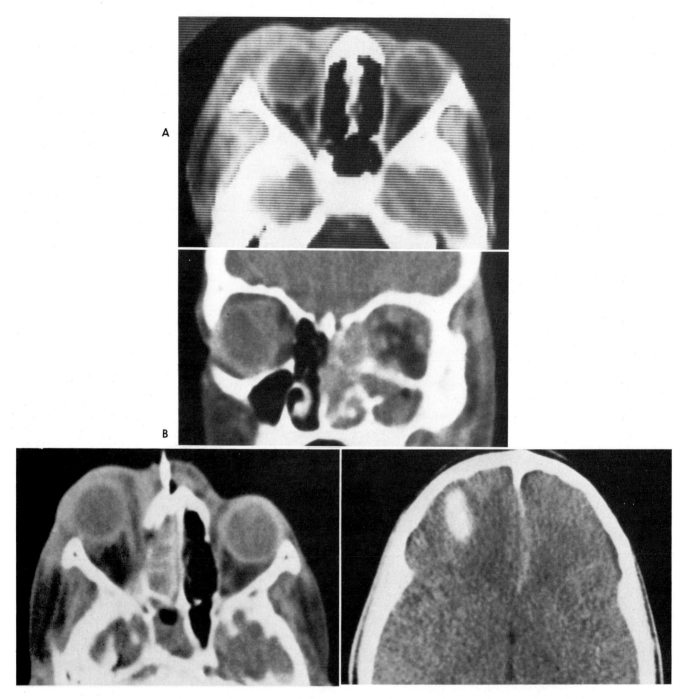

Fig. 14-28. Soft tissue inflammation. **A,** Patient 1. Anterior orbital cellulitis, with marked soft tissue swelling over right orbit prohibiting adequate clinical evaluation of orbit. Axial CT scan shows inflammatory disease to be limited to overlying soft tissues of orbit and not extending posterior to orbital septum. **B,** Patient 2. Ethmoiditis, orbital cellulitis, secondary cerebritis. Axial and coronal scans of orbit reveal soft tissue opacification of right ethmoid sinuses, with destruction of lamina papyracea and extraconal inflammatory soft tissue in medial aspect of right orbit as well as in maxillary sinus and nasal cavity. There is associated proptosis and swelling of soft tissues anterior to orbital septum. Axial CT scan through inferior frontal lobes reveals focal enhanced region, indicating clinically unsuspected cerebritis. All of inflammatory disease resolved with intensive antibiotic therapy.

thrombophlebitis, with or without thrombosis, the CT appearance may be nonspecific. There may be proptosis only or slightly increased attenuation of the retro-orbital fat. If there is involvement of the superior ophthalmic vein, this structure may be prominent, although this is an inconsistent finding. Likewise, cavernous sinus thrombosis may not be obvious by CT scanning. Angiography remains the procedure of choice when coupled with appropriate clinical history and a negative CT examination.

Mucoceles of the paranasal sinuses are a result of prior inflammatory disease. They occur most frequently in the frontal and ethmoid sinuses and usually have characteristic plain film and complex motion tomographic findings of an opacified, expanded sinus with preservation of very thin bony margins. These conventional radiographic techniques may be adequate to make the diagnosis, but CT is more accurate in fully delineating the extent of these lesions, particularly when they have broken through bone and extended intraorbitally or intracranially. The lesions usually appear as homogeneous, sharply marginated, soft tissue masses within an expanded sinus (Fig. 14-29). The lesions have approximately the same attenuation coefficients as the brain, although a few may be either more or less dense. Higher density mucoceles frequently have been found to be infected and hence "mucopyoceles."[46] The intraorbital extension of either mucocele or mucopyocele lesions is usually obvious. There may be enhancement of the capsule, but enhancement within the lesions should not occur. Enhancement of the capsule may be greater with mucopyoceles, but this is not of diagnostic

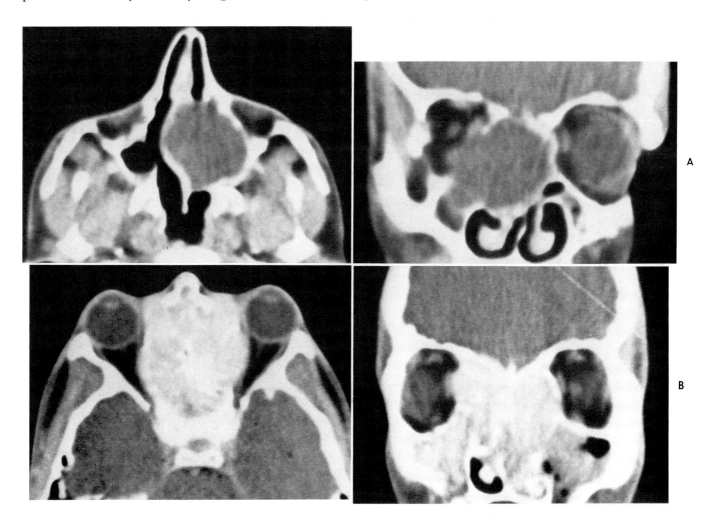

Fig. 14-29. Benign sinus masses. **A,** Patient 1. Typical ethmoid mucocele involving anterior and middle ethmoid labyrinth, with benign expansion of bone by sharply marginated, lucent, nonenhanced mass that has eroded lamina papyracea as mass extended into medial aspect of right orbit. **B,** Patient 2. Massive ethmoid inflammatory polyposis with associated hypertelorism. Scans show diffuse, chronically expanding mass in ethmoid labyrinth and upper nasal cavity, with intense enhancement typical of this disease.

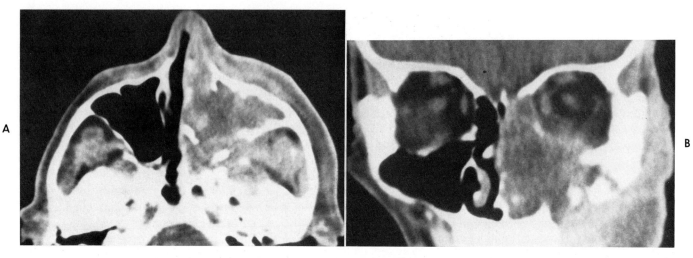

Fig. 14-30. Carcinoma of maxillary sinus. Axial and coronal scans show irregular maxillary mass of heterogeneous density extending in malignant destructive fashion through bony margins of maxillary sinus and into orbit in an extraconal fashion and occupying bulk of nasal cavity after destruction of its bony walls and ethmoid labyrinth.

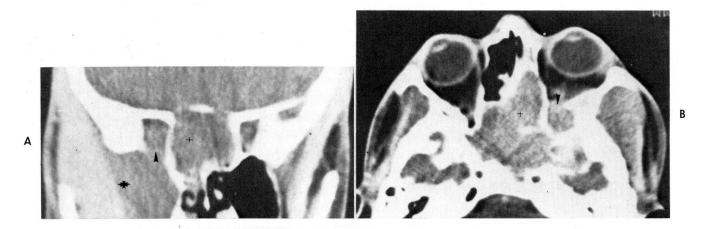

Fig. 14-31. Juvenile angiofibroma. Large juvenile angiofibroma of infratemporal fossa (*), sphenoid sinus (+), and posterior inferior orbit (*arrow*), into which it has extended by way of the expanded inferior orbital fissure.

value because it may also occur with uninfected mucoceles. Extensive sinus polyposes may mimic mucoceles because of associated expansile changes, but CT shows these lesions to be solid, and enhancement will occur throughout the substance of the lesions.

Most neoplasms of the paranasal sinuses that have orbital involvement are malignant, and these malignancies are most frequently squamous carcinomas. The patients usually complain of chronic sinus pain; they are found to have an opacified sinus with bone destruction on radiographic examination.[31] When tumor diagnosis is a clinical consideration, CT should be performed in

order to define the tumor, to demonstrate secondary obstruction of sinuses, and to define bone destruction and extension of tumor beyond the confines of the sinus. Most neoplasms of paranasal sinuses will be enhanced at least slightly after contrast material injection, while obstructed sinuses will not. This distinction may help in defining relatively small neoplasms incorporated within the mass of infected debris proximal to the obstructed ostium of the affected sinus. Malignant tumors are nearly always associated with bone destruction when they involve the orbit and usually remain extraconal until quite a late day (Fig. 14-30).

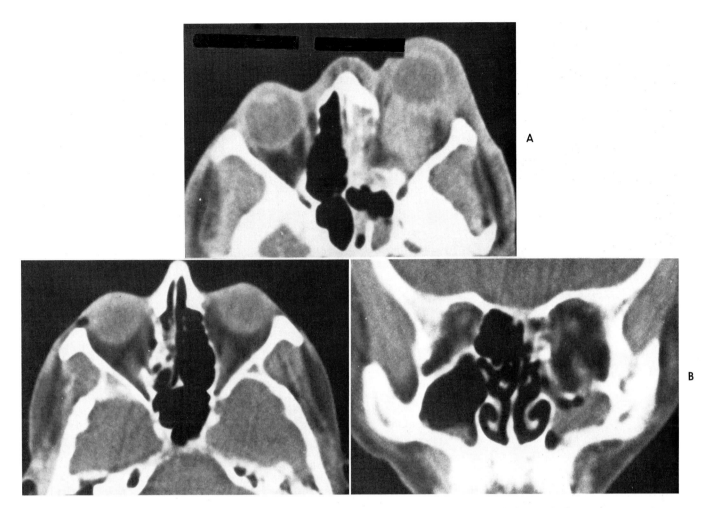

Fig. 14-32. Trauma. **A,** Patient 1. Fracture of posterior ethmoid portion of medial wall of orbit, anterior orbital soft tissue swelling, and most importantly, large hematoma of optic nerve. **B,** Patient 2. Blow-out fracture of orbit, with medial displacement of lamina papyracea seen on axial scans and inferior displacement of floor of orbit into upper maxillary sinus seen on coronal sections.

Benign neoplasms of the paranasal sinuses that involve the orbit secondarily are relatively unusual and include inverting papillomas and juvenile angiofibromas, although the latter are not true sinus neoplasms. Inverting papillomas usually occur in the region of the maxilloethmoid plate and maxillary sinus ostia. They grow into the ethmoid and maxillary sinuses in a slow, benign fashion. This growth pattern will result in erosion of the bone along the medial inferior aspect of the orbit, and more malignant neoplasms may be suspected. The true diagnosis can be suggested, however, when most of the bone changes are characterized by chronic expansion, with focal destruction limited to the area of the maxillary ostia. They are not infrequently associated with more diffuse polypoid inflammatory disease of the sinuses.[69]

Juvenile angiofibromas are benign vascular neoplasms occurring in young boys. They originate in the area of the pterygopalatine fossa and usually grow into the nasopharynx, pterygopalatine space, and infratemporal fossa. They also frequently involve the orbit by way of the inferior orbital fissure and may grow posteriorly through the foramen rotundum and superior orbital fissure to the area of the basisphenoid. This last area is the most critical in terms of treatment, and axial and coronal CT scans can define this region to best advantage (Fig. 14-31).[13] Any other tumor of the nasopharynx may involve the orbit by this same pathway, but it is not particularly common.[81]

□ Trauma

Although plain films and complex motion tomography remain the primary radiographic methods of evaluating trauma to the face and skull base, CT adds much critical information. Lacerations of critical structures as well as hematomas in important locations, e.g., in the intraconal space or even within the optic nerve sheath, can be demonstrated only by CT (Fig. 14-32). In addition, foreign bodies, including bone fragments within the orbit, can better be displayed by CT.[39] In the acute traumatized patient, CT may offer more immediately valuable information than plain films concerning damage to critical structures. Because many of these patients are initially evaluated by CT for possible intracranial pathologic processes, one should make the most of the information automatically supplied about the orbitofacial region.[76]

In addition to the direct evidence of trauma, e.g., fractures, soft tissue masses, and hematomas, indirect evidence of critical traumatic lesions such as carotid cavernous fistulae may be suggested by CT when, after contrast material injection, there is prominence of intraorbital vessels, particularly the superior ophthalmic vein.[85] Angiography remains the primary method of making this diagnosis, however.

□ Summary

CT is now without question the primary imaging method for the orbit. Ultrasonography remains the only other frequently used method, and its usefulness is largely confined to bulbar lesions. Venography and angiography supplement these other two methods only occasionally.

It should be remembered that although CT may be exquisitely sensitive in demonstrating the anatomy of an orbital lesion, in most cases it does not allow histologic diangosis. Common orbital lesions have typical CT appearances, but there is no guarantee that this will invariably be the case. In addition, there is a plethora of rare orbital lesions that may mimic any of the common tumors. For these reasons, one must interpret the CT scan with full knowledge of the patient's clinical history and physical findings; even then, histologic diagnosis may await the verdict of the pathologist. The importance of close cooperation between the radiologist and the clinician cannot be underestimated in obtaining maximal usefulness of scanning data.

□ References

1. Albert, D.M., Rubenstein, R.A., and Scheie, H.G.: Tumor metastasis to the eye. I. Incidence in 213 adult patients with generalized malignancy, Am. J. Ophthalmol. **63**:723, 1967.
2. Alfano, J.E.: Ophthalmological aspects of neurostomatosis: a study of 53 verified cases, Trans. Am. Acad. Ophthalmol. Otolarygol. **72**:830, 1968.
3. Alper, M.G.: Computed tomography in planning and evaluating orbital surgery, Ophthalmology **87**:418, 1980.
4. Ashton, N.: Epithelial tumours of the lacrimal gland. In Bleeker, G.M., Garston, J.B., Kronenberg, B., and Lyle, T.K., editors: Modern problems in ophthalmology, Basel, 1975, S. Karger, AG, Medical and Scientific Publishers.
5. Baker, H.L., Jr., Kearns, T.P., Campbell, J.K., and Henderson, J.W.: Computerized transaxial tomography in neuro-ophthalmology, Am. J. Ophthalmol. **78**:285, 1974.
6. Berke, R.N.: A modified Kronlein operation, Arch. Ophthalmol. **51**:609, 1954.
7. Bernardino, M.E., Danziger, J., Young, S.E., and Wallace, S.: Computed tomography in ocular neoplastic disease, AJR **131**:111, 1978.
8. Bisaria, K.K., Garg, K.C., and Wahal, K.M.: Calcifying orbital hemangioendothelioma, Am. J. Ophthalmol. **62**:340, 1966.
9. Blodi, F.C., and Gass, J.D.M.: Inflammatory pseudotumor of the orbit, Trans. Am. Acad. Ophthalmol. Otolaryngol. **71**:303, 1967.
10. Brown, D.H.: The clinicopathology of retinoblastoma, Am. J. Ophthalmol. **61**:508, 1966.
11. Brown, D.N., MacCarty, C.S., and Soule, E.H.: Orbital hemangiopericytoma: review of the literature and report of four cases, J. Neurosurg. **22**:354, 1965.
12. Bruwer, A.J., and Kierland, R.R.: Neurofibromatosis and congenital unilateral pulsating and nonpulsating exophthalmos, Arch. Ophthalmol. **53**:2, 1955.
13. Bryan, R.N., Sessions, R.B., and Horowitz, B.L.: Radiographic management of juvenile angiofibromas, AJNR **2**:157, 1981.
14. Bryan, R.N., Ferreyro, R.I., Miller, R.H., and Sessions, R.B.: Computerized tomography of the major salivary glands, AJR **139**:547, 1982.
15. Burrows, E.H.: Bone changes in orbital neurofibromatosis, Br. J. Radiol. **36**:549, 1963.
16. Bushong, S.C.: Pregnancy in diagnostic radiology, Appl. Radiol. **8**:63, 1976.
17. Carey, P.C.: Epidermoid and dermoid tumours of the orbit, Br. J. Ophthalmol. **42**:225, 1958.
18. Centeno, R.S., Bryan, R.N., and Cheatham, B.A.: Computerized tomography of intraocular neoplasia, Am. Soc. Head and Neck Radiology, presentation, May 1981, Los Angeles, Calif.
19. Chawla, H.B., and Cullen, J.F.: Eosinophilic granuloma of the orbit, J. Pediatr. Ophthalmol. **5**:93, 1968.
20. Chutorian, A.M., Schwartz, J.F., Evans, R.A., and Carter, S.: Optic gliomas in children, Neurology **14**:83, 1964.
21. Coop, M.E.: Pseudotumour of the orbit: a clinical and pathological study of 47 cases, Br. J. Ophthalmol. **45**:513, 1961.
22. Craig, W.McK., and Gogela, L.J.: Intraorbital meningiomas: a clinicopathologic study, Am. J. Ophthalmol. **32**:1663, 1949.
23. Dallow, R.L.: Reliability of orbital diagnostic tests: ultrasonography, computerized tomography, and radiography, Ophthalmology **85**:1218, 1978.
24. Danziger, A., and Price, H.I.: CT findings in retinoblastoma, AJR **133**:695, 1979.
25. Davis, F.A.: Plexiform neurofibromatosis (Recklinghausen's disease) of orbit and globe with associated glioma of the optic nerve and brain: report of a case, Arch. Ophthalmol. **22**:761, 1939.
26. Dayton, G.O.: Orbital venography: anatomy, technique, and diagnostic use, Trans. Am. Ophthalmol. Soc. **75**:459, 1977.
27. Dodge, H.W., Love, J.G., Craig, W.M., et al.: Gliomas of the optic nerves, Arch. Neurol. **79**:607, 1958.
28. Dunphy, E.B.: The story of retinoblastoma: the twentieth Edward Jackson memorial lecture, Am. J. Ophthalmol. **58**:539, 1964.
29. Enzmann, D., Donaldson, S.S., Marshall, W.H., and Kriss, J.P.: Computed tomography in orbital pseudotumor (idiopathic orbital inflammation), Radiology **120**:597, 1976.
30. Enzmann, D., Marshall, W.H., Rosenthal, A.R., and Kriss, J.P.: Computed tomography in Graves' ophthalmopathy, Radiology **118**:615, 1976.

31. Font, R.L., Naumann, G., and Zimmerman, L.E.: Primary malignant melanoma of the skin metastatic to the eye and orbit: review of ten cases and reveiw of the literature, Am. J. Ophthalmol. **63**:738, 1967.

32. Font, R.L., Yanoff, M., and Zimmerman, L.E.: Benign lymphoepithelial lesion of the lacrimal gland and its relationship to Sjögren's syndrome, Am. J. Clin. Pathol. **48**:365, 1967.

33. Frezzotti, R., and Guerra, R.: Sarcoma following irradated retinoblastoma: report of a case, Arch. Ophthalmol. **70**:471, 1963.

34. Gallie, B.L. Gene carrier detection in retinoblastoma, Ophthalmology **87**:591, 1980.

35. Gass, J.D.M.: Observation of suspected choroidal and ciliary body melanomas for evidence of growth prior to enucleation, Ophthalmology **87**:523, 1980.

36. Girard, L.J., Freeman, B.S., and Makk, L.: Plexiform neuroma of the periorbital area, Trans. Am. Acad. Ophthalmol. Otolaryngol. **66**:242, 1962.

37. Goldberg, F., Berne, A.S., and Oski, F.A.: Differentiation of orbital cellulitis from preseptal cellulitis by computed tomography, Pediatrics **62**:1000, 1978.

38. Green, W.R., and Zimmerman, L.E.: Ectopic lacrimal gland tissue, Arch. Ophthalmol. **78**:318, 1967.

39. Grove, A.S.: Orbital trauma and computed tomography, Ophthalmology **87**:411, 1980.

40. Guibert-Trainer, F., Piton, J., Calabet, A., and Caille, J.M.: Orbital syndromes: CT analysis of 100 cases, Comput. Tomogr. **3**:241, 1979.

41. Gyldensted, C., Lester, J., and Fledelius, H.: Computed tomography of orbital lesions: a radiologic study of 144 cases, Neuroradiology **13**:141, 1977.

42. Hart, W.M.: Metastatic carcinoma to the eye and orbit, Int. Ophthalmol. Clin. **2**:465, 1962.

43. Haverling, M., and Johanson, H.: Computed sagittal tomography of the orbit, AJR **131**:346, 1978.

44. Haye, C.: Lymphoid tumours of the orbit. In Bleeker, G.M., Garston, J.B., Kronenberg, B., and Lyle, T.K., editors: Modern problems in ophthalmology, Basel, 1975, S. Karger AG.

45. Henderson, J.W., editor, Orbital tumors, Philadelphia, 1973, W.B. Saunders Co.

46. Hesselink, J.R., Weber, A.L., New, P.F., et al.: Evaluation of mucoceles of the paranasal sinuses with computed tomography, Radiology **133**:397, 1979.

47. Hilal, S.K.: Computed tomography of the orbit, Ophthalmology **86**:864, 1979.

48. Hilal, S.K., and Trokel, S.L.: Computerized tomography of the orbit using thin sections, Semin. Roentgenol. **12**:137, 1977.

49. Hobbs, H.E.: Capillary and cavernous hemangiomata of the orbit, Trans. Ophthalmol. Soc. UK **81**:229, 1961.

50. Hogan, M.J.: Clinical aspects, management, and prognosis of melanomas of the uvea and optic nerve. In Boniuk, M., editor: Ocular and adnexal tumors: New and controversial aspects, St. Louis, 1964, The C.V. Mosby Co.

51. Hoyt, W.F., and Baghdassarian, S.A.: Optic glioma of childhood: natural history and rationale for conservative management, Br. J. Ophthalmol. **53**:793, 1969.

52. Hunsaker, J.N., Anderson, R.E., Van Dyk, H.J.L., and Wing, S.D.: A comparison of computed tomographic techniques in the diagnosis of Graves' ophthalmopathy, Ophthalmic Surg. **10**:34, 1979.

53. Jones, I.S.: Lymphangiomas of the ocular adnexa: an analysis of 62 cases, Trans. Am. Ophthalmol. Soc. **57**:602, 1959.

54. Jones, I.S., Reese, A.B., and Kraut, J.: Orbital rhabdomyosarcoma: an analysis of 62 cases, Am. J. Ophthalmol. **61**:721, 1966.

55. Katlan, N.R., and Griffin, W.R.: Osteoma of the orbit, Arch. Ophthalmol. **65**:542, 1961.

56. Kennerdell, J.S., and Maroon, J.C.: CT scan appearance of dysthyroid orbital disease, Ann. Ophthalmol. **10**:153, 1978.

57. Kollaritis, C.R., Di Chiro, G., Christiansen, J., et al.: Detection of orbital and intraocular foreign bodies by computerized tomography, Ophthalmic Surg. **8**:45, 1977.

58. Koornneef, L.: Orbital septa: anatomy and function, Ophthalmology **86**:876, 1979.

59. Ladekarl, S.: Von Recklinghausen's glioma of the optic nerve and chiasm, Acta Ophthalmol. **42**:127, 1964.

60. Lampert, V.L., Zelch, J.V., and Cohen, D.N.: Computed tomography of the orbits, Radiology **113**:351, 1974.

61. Leeds, N., and Seaman, W.B.: Fibrous dysplasia of the skull and its differential diagnosis: a clinical and roentgenographic study of 46 cases, Radiology **78**:570, 1962.

62. Lloyd, G.A.S.: CT scanning in the diagnosis of orbital disease, Comput. Tomogr. **3**:227, 1979.

63. Lobes, L.A., Grand, M.G., Reece, J., and Penkrot, R.J.: Computerized axial tomography in the detection of intraocular foreign bodies, Ophthalmology **88**:26, 1981.

64. Lombardi, G.: Orbitography with water-soluble contrast media, Acta Radiologica **47**:417, 1967.

65. Ludman, H., and Bulman, C.: The differential diagnosis of the orbital manifestations of paranasal disease, J. Laryngol. Otol. **90**:519, 1976.

66. MacCollum, D.W., and Martin, L.W.: Hemangiomas in infancy and childhood: a report based on 6479 cases, Surg. Clin. North Am. **36**:1647, 1956.

67. Manelfe, C. Pasquini, U, and Bank, W.O.: Metrizamide demonstration of the subarachnoid space surrounding the optic nerves, J. Comput. Assist. Tomogr. **2**:545, 1978.

68. Minton, L.R., and Elliott, J.H.: Ocular manifestations of infantile cortical hyperostosis, Am. J. Ophthalmol. **64**:902, 1967.

69. Momose, K.J., Weber, A.L., Goodman, M., et al.: Radiological aspects of inverted papilloma, Radiology **134**:73, 1980.

70. Moore, R.T.: Fibrous dysplasia of the orbit, Survey Ophthalmol. **13**(6):321, 1969.

71. Morgan, G.: Lymphocytic tumours of the orbit. In Bleeker, G.M., Garston, J.B., Kronenberg, B., and Lyle, T.K., editors: Modern problems in ophthalmology, Basel, 1975, S. Karger AG.

72. Moss, H.M.: Expanding lesions of the orbit: a clinical study of 230 consecutive cases, Am. J. Ophthalmol. **54**:761, 1962.

73. Nichols, C.W., Mishkin, M., and Yanoff, M.: Presumed orbital sarcoidosis: report of a case followed by computerized axial tomography and conjunctival biopsy, Trans. Am. Ophthalmol. Soc. **76**:67, 1978.

74. Nikoskelainen, E., Enzmann, D.R., Sogg, R.L., and Rosenthal, A.R.: Computerized tomography of the orbits: a report of 196 patients, Acta Ophthalmol. **55**:885, 1977.

75. Paul, E.V., Parnell, B.L., and Fraker, M.: Prognosis of malignant melanomas of the choroid and ciliary body, Int. Ophthalmol. Clin. **2**:387, 1962.

76. Pearl, R.M., and Vistnes, L.M.: Orbital blowout fractures: an approach to management, Ann. Plast. Surg. **1**:267, 1978.

77. Reese, A.B., and Ellsworth, R.M.: The evaluation and current concept of retinoblastoma therapy, Trans. Am. Acad. Ophthalmol. Otolaryngol. **67**:164, 1963.

78. Rodman, H.I., and Font, R.L.: Orbital involvement in multiple myeloma: review of the literature and report of three cases, Arch. Ophthalmol. **87**:30, 1972.

79. Salvolini, U., Menichelli, F., and Pasquini, U.: Computer assisted tomography in 90 cases of exophthalmos, J. Comput. Assist. Tomogr. **1**:81, 1977.

80. Saran, N., and Winter, F.C.: Bilateral gliomas of the optic discs, Am. J. Ophthalmol. **64**:607, 1967.

81. Smith, J.L., and Wheliss, J.A.: Ocular manifestations of nasopharyngeal tumors, Trans. Am. Acad. Ophthalmol. Otolaryngol. **66**:659, 1962.
82. Tadmor, R., and New, P.F.J.: Computed tomography of the orbit with special emphasis on coronal sections. I. Normal anatomy, J. Comput. Assist. Tomogr. **2**:24, 1978.
83. Tadmor, R. and New, P.F.J.: Computed tomography of the orbit with special emphasis on coronal sections. II. Pathological anatomy, J. Comp. Assist. Tomogr. **2**:35, 1978.
84. Trokel, S.L., and Hilal, S.K.: Submillimeter resolution CT scanning of orbital diseases, Ophthalmology **87**:412, 1980.
85. Trokel, S.L., and Hilal, S.K.: Recognition and differential diagnosis of enlarged extraocular muscles in computed tomography, Am. J. Ophthalmol. **87**:503, 1979.
86. Tym, R.: Piloid gliomas of the anterior optic pathways, Br. J. Surg. **49**:322, 1961.
87. Unsold, R., Norman, D., and Berninger, W.: Multiplanar evaluation of the optic canal from axial transverse CT sections, J. Comput. Assist. Tomogr. **4**:418, 1980.
88. Vail, D.T., Jr.: Orbital complications in sinus disease: review, Am. J. Ophthalmol. **14**:202, 1931.
89. Vermess, M., Haynes, B.F., Fauci, A.S., and Wolff, S.M.: Computer assisted tomography of orbital lesions in Wegener's granulomatosis, J. Comput. Assist. Tomogr. **2**:45, 1978.
90. Vignaud, J., and Aubin, M.L.: Coronal (frontal) sections in computerized tomography of the orbit, J. Neuroradiol. **5**:161, 1978.
91. Wende, S., Aulich, A., Nover, A., et al.: Computed tomography of orbital lesions: a cooperative study of 210 cases, Neuroradiology **13**:123, 1977.
92. Wolter, J.R., Bryson, J.M., and Blackhurst, R.T.: Primary orbital melanoma, Eye Ear Nose Throat J. **45**:64, 1966.
93. Wright, J.E., Lloyd, G.A.S., and Ambrose, J.: Computerized axial tomography in the detection of orbital space-occupying lesions, Am. J. Ophthalmol. **80**:78, 1975.
94. Youssefi, B.: Orbital tumors in children: a clinical study of 62 cases, J. Pediatr. Ophthalmol. **6**:177, 1969.
95. Zimmerman, R.A. and Bilaniuk, L.T.: CT of orbital infection and its cerebral complications, AJR **134**:45, 1980.
96. Zizmor, J., Fasano, C.V., Smith, B., and Rabbett, W.: Roentgenographic diagnosis of unilateral exophthalmos, JAMA **197**:343, 1966.

SECTION TWO

Topographic arteriography applied to the analysis of orbital masses and carotid cavernous fistulae

Jacques Moret and Jacqueline Vignaud

□ Basic aspects of pathologic orbital arteriography

Interpretation of orbital arteriography, which should always include exploration of both the internal and external carotid systems, must take into account two different elements of vascular anatomy that are visualized during serial angiography:

1. The arteries, notably the entire ophthalmic system, including its branches and collaterals.
2. The venous elements. These are divided into two groups: the first corresponds to a collecting system of large caliber vessels represented by the superior and inferior ophthalmic veins and their interconnections. The second group corresponds to the choroidal venous drainage (venae vorticosae system).

Displacements of normal vascular structures by relatively avascular intraorbital tumorous processes make up one type of basic pathologic pattern; pathology of purely vascular elements as well as hypervascular character of certain orbital tumors form a second kind of vascular alteration.

A brief review of arterial anatomy is appropriate before detailed analysis of pathologic material.

■ Normal anatomy

The ophthalmic artery most commonly takes its origin from the internal carotid artery, arising from the medial anterior aspect of its infraclinoid portion. In a little less than 10% of cases it arises from within the cavernous portion. Over 80% of the time, however, it arises from the extracavernous carotid, distal to the point of exit of the carotid artery from the cavernous sinus, but proximal (i.e., inferior) to the anterior clinoid process. In this circumstance it is subdural; it accompanies the internal carotid artery as that vessel penetrates the dura in its superiorward course. In rare instances, the ophthalmic artery may originate as a branch of the middle meningeal artery.

When the artery has its usual subdural point of origin, it enters the orbit by way of the optic canal, accompanying the optic nerve. When the origin is from the

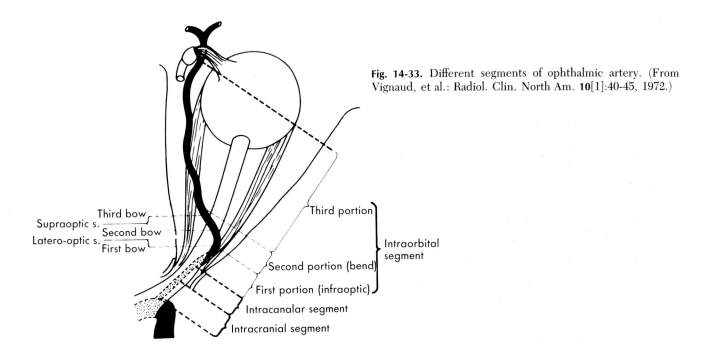

Fig. 14-33. Different segments of ophthalmic artery. (From Vignaud, et al.: Radiol. Clin. North Am. **10**[1]:40-45, 1972.)

Supraoptic s.
Latero-optic s.
Third bow
Second bow
First bow
Third portion
Second portion (bend)
First portion (infraoptic)
Intracanalar segment
Intracranial segment
Intraorbital segment

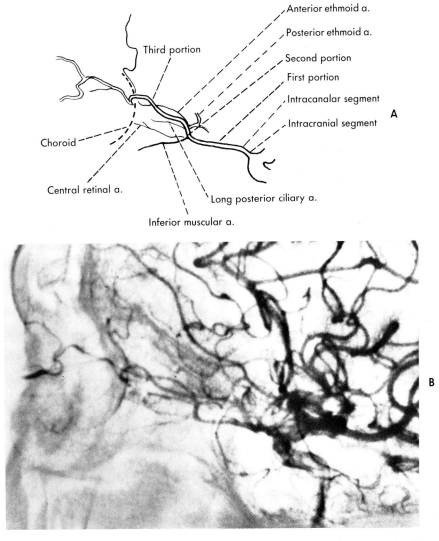

Third portion
Anterior ethmoid a.
Posterior ethmoid a.
Second portion
First portion
Intracanalar segment
Intracranial segment
Choroid
Central retinal a.
Inferior muscular a.
Long posterior ciliary a.
A

B

Fig. 14-34. Lateral view of normal ophthalmic artery. Internal carotid angiography (From Vignaud, et al.: Radiol. Clin. North Am. **10**[1]:40-45, 1972.)

cavernous portion of the carotid, it enters the orbit by way of the the superior orbital fissure.[13]

It is convenient to describe the ophthalmic artery as comprised of three segments: intracranial, intracanalicular, and intraorbital (Figs. 14-33 and 14-34).

Intracranial segment

The intracranial segment commences with the origin of the vessel and terminates as it enters the optic canal. The initial portion is both medial and inferior to the anterior clinoid process. The intracranial segment is divided into short and long limbs. The short limb has a superior course and the long limb, which is distal to it, has a more anterior-posterior course; the angle between the two limbs lies somewhere between 90° and 150°. The length of the short limb ranges from less than 1 mm to almost 3 mm; the length of the long limb varies from about 1.5 to 5 mm. The long limb is less than 3 mm in length more than two thirds of the time. According to the work of Hayreh and Dass,[4] in 85% of cases the whole of the intracranial course of the ophthalmic artery lies in the subdural space; in about 10% of cases it lies partly in the subdural space and partly within the substance of the dural sheath; and in 5% it is exclusively extradural.

As has been pointed out by Zimmerman and Vignaud[13] the site of origin of the ophthalmic artery in the lateral arteriogram is usually hidden because of the artery's origin from the medial aspect of the carotid. The origin may be seen, however, in coronal and oblique views. The intracranial segment runs obliquely upward and forward, nearly at right angles to the internal carotid artery. It is both medial and inferior to the anterior clinoid, lying beneath the midportion of the optic nerve and coursing relatively straight anteroposteriorly.

Intracanalicular segment

In most cases the ophthalmic artery accompanies the optic nerve within the optic canal. This segment of the vessel lies partly within the subdural space and partly within the substance of the dura and, occasionally, totally within the dural sheath. This latter fact may explain why the intracanalicular segment of the vessel may sometimes be slightly narrower than both the more proximal and distal segments.

Intraorbital segment

For descriptive purposes, Singh and Dass[11] have divided the intraorbital segment of the ophthalmic artery into three portions (Fig. 14-33).

The first portion extends from the point of entrance into the orbit to the point where the artery starts to bend around the nerve to become the second portion. This portion usually runs along the undersurface of the optic nerve.

The second portion crosses *over* the optic nerve, running in a medial direction from the inferolateral to the superomedial aspect of the nerve.

The third portion extends from the point at which the second part bends at the superomedial aspect of the optic nerve to its termination. It lies medial to the optic nerve.

The ophthalmic artery therefore, as seen in axial views, bends to change direction twice: the first bend is at the junction of the first and second portions as the vessel goes from an inferolateral to a superomedial position; the second bend occurs at the termination of the second portion, when the vessel angles sharply forward. At that point it has reached the medial wall of the orbit and travels forward beneath the lower border of the superior oblique muscle; it then divides into two terminal branches, the frontal and angular.

The intraorbital segment of the ophthalmic artery enters the orbit by passing through the annulus of Zinn and runs through the posterior portion of the muscle cone on the inferior aspect of the optic nerve. The first part of the intraorbital segment therefore has a course that merely continues the forward and lateral direction of the intracranial segment.

Of the three portions of the intraorbital ophthalmic artery, the second is the most useful in determining optic nerve enlargement by angiographic means. Rothman et al.[10] refer to this portion of the intraorbital ophthalmic artery as the *circumneural loop* because more than 80% of the time[5] the ophthalmic artery crosses over the optic nerve, going from the inferolateral aspect to superomedial aspect of the nerve. Theoretically, at least half the circumference of the nerve is capable of being outlined by the vessel (Fig. 14-35).

A number of variations exist, however; between 15% and 20% of the time the ophthalmic artery crosses under the optic nerve to reach the medial side. In a few circumstances it already lies on the medial aspect of the nerve at the commencement of the intraorbital segment.

The terminology regarding the crossing of the optic nerve by the second portion of the intraorbital segment is both redundant and confusing. As has been stated, in 75% to 80% of cases the intraorbital segment of the artery, which in its first portion lies beneath the midlongitudinal axis of the optic nerve, swings laterally, loops up and around the lateral aspect of the nerve to cross over the top, and then passes forward in a medial direction. This has been called either the supraoptic variety, the latero-optic variety, the externo-optic variety,

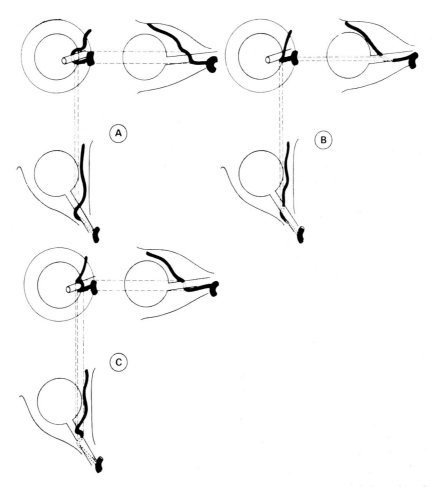

Fig. 14-35. Normal variations in configuration of ophthalmic artery. Frontal, lateral, and axial projections. **A,** Supraoptic variety. **B,** Infraoptic variety, type I. After infraoptic crossing, artery remains medial to optic nerve. **C,** Infraoptic variety, type II. After infraoptic crossing, artery passes around medial aspect of optic nerve, as in **B,** but also makes hook above nerve. Notice that only frontal projection allows recognition of variation in relation of artery to nerve. Semicircle formed around nerve is concave medially in infraoptic varieties. (From Vignaud, et al.: Radiol. Clin. North Am. **10**[1]:40-45, 1972.)

or finally, the inferolateral-superomedial variety.[12,13] These terms are synonymous.

In 17% of cases[12] the artery stays beneath the nerve while crossing from a line along the midlongitudinal axis of the nerve to a medial position above it. This type of crossing is known as the medio-optic, interno-optic, infraoptic, or inferomedial-superomedial variety. These again are synonymous terms.

There are two types of the infraoptic configurations (Fig. 14-35). In type I the artery leaves the undersurface of the optic nerve and passes forward and medially. In type II the artery leaves the lower aspect of the optic nerve, crosses its medial aspect obliquely, makes a curve above the optic nerve, and then passes forward and medially. Thus it comes to form a semicircle around the nerve, which is concave medially, in opposition to the more typical supraoptic crossing. The interested reader is referred to the works of Zimmerman and Vignaud[12] and Hayreh and Dass.[6]

The third division of the intraorbital segment runs medial to the optic nerve but is not always intimately related to it. It usually courses forward above the medial rectus and beneath the superior oblique muscles, reaching the medial wall of the orbit close to the foramen for the anterior ethmoid branches. It is usually anchored to the medial wall of the orbit by the anterior ethmoid artery, running forward close against the medial wall, passing below the trochlea, and then running upward and forward to lie nearly midway between the medial palpebral ligament and the orbital margin.

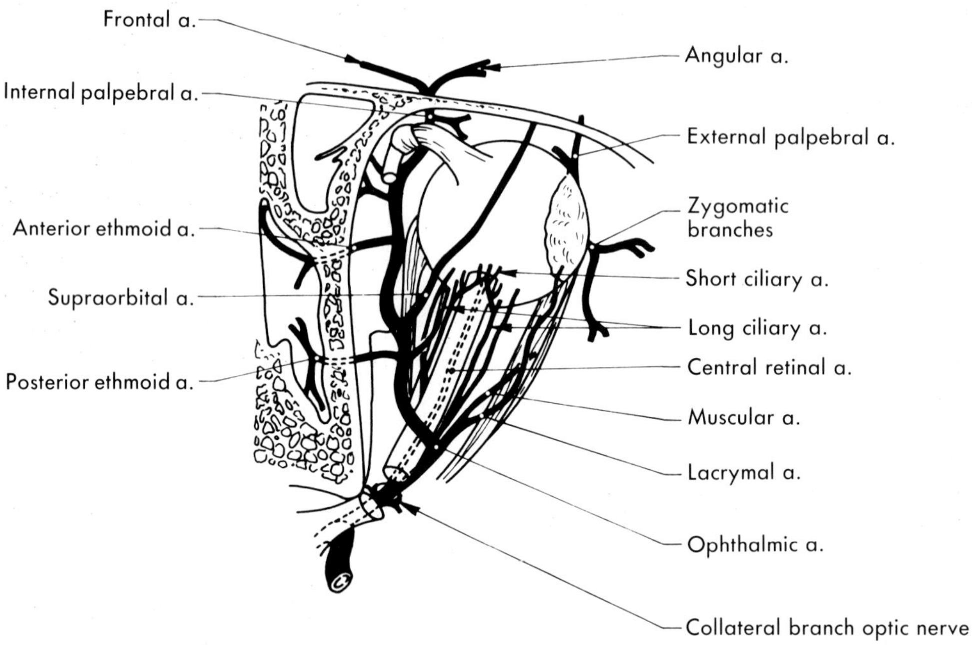

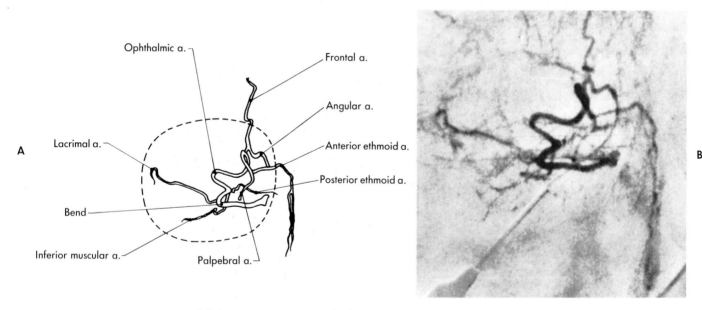

Frontal a.
Internal palpebral a.
Anterior ethmoid a.
Supraorbital a.
Posterior ethmoid a.

Angular a.
External palpebral a.
Zygomatic branches
Short ciliary a.
Long ciliary a.
Central retinal a.
Muscular a.
Lacrymal a.
Ophthalmic a.
Collateral branch optic nerve

Fig. 14-36. Ophthalmic artery and its branches. (From Vignaud, et al.: Radiol. Clin. North Am. **10**[1]:40-45, 1972.)

Ophthalmic a.
Lacrimal a.
Bend
Inferior muscular a.
Palpebral a.

Frontal a.
Angular a.
Anterior ethmoid a.
Posterior ethmoid a.

A

B

Fig. 14-37. Ophthalmic artery arteriography by catheterization of exposed angular artery, infraoptic variety; semicircle is concave medially. There is good visibility of ethmoid arteries. Notice opacification of mucosa of medial nasal wall by anterior ethmoid artery, and opacification of lacrimal artery, inferior muscular artery, and medial palpebral artery. No supraorbital artery is demonstrated. (From Vignaud, et al.: Radiol. Clin. North Am. **10**[1]:40-45, 1972.)

Branches of the ophthalmic artery
(Figs. 14-36 and 14-37)

Zimmerman and Vignaud[13] classify the branches of the ophthalmic artery into three groups.

Occular branches
  Central artery of retina
  Ciliary arteries
Orbital arteries
  Lacrimal
  Muscular
Extraorbital branches
  Anterior and posterior ethmoid arteries
  Supraorbital arteries
  Medial palpebral artery
  Supratrochlear artery
  Dorsal nasal artery
  Meningeal branches

Although any of these branches may serve as nutrient arteries for pathologic processes within the orbit and in the immediately surrounding area, they are not of significant localizing value.

■ **Analysis of basic pathologic angiograms with respect to displacement of the orbital vessels**

Angiography permits delineation of an orbital lesion's topography with respect to the adjacent anatomic elements, especially in relation to the orbital muscle cone.

With the advent of CT, the importance of detailed analysis of vascular displacements has considerably diminished because CT accurately localizes masses and determines their extension into adjacent tissues.

During a 1979 study of 310 orbital tumors, the use of arteriography in the diagnosis or localization of these lesions was indicated in less than 2% and involved only two types of pathologic conditions: (1) optic nerve pathologic conditions, in which case CT examination cannot always distinguish between an optic nerve tumor and one that has developed in close proximity to the optic nerve, and (2) much more rarely, lacrimal gland pathologic conditions, in which it is difficult to distinguish between intraglandular and extraglandular processes.

Topographic analysis of the effects of a mass on the ophthalmic arterial trunk

Except for several anatomic variants (Figs. 14-38 and 14-39), the ophthalmic artery enters the orbit via the optic canal accompanying the supra-adjacent optic nerve. No significant displacement of the intracranial or intracanalicular segments of the ophthalmic artery occurs.

The course of the second portion of the intraorbital ophthalmic artery has importance in tumor localization because displacements caused by optic nerve enlargement are the most easily discernible ones at that level,

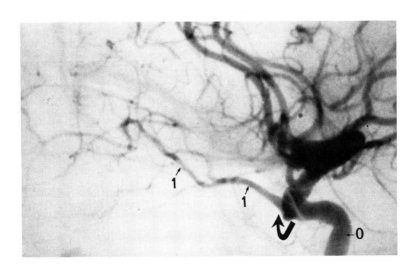

Fig. 14-38. Lateral internal carotid *(0)* angiogram. Ophthalmic artery *(1)* arises from intracavernous internal carotid at junction of portion C_3 and C_4 of carotid siphon *(curved arrow)*. In this variant, ophthalmic artery enters orbit through superior orbital fissure and not by optic canal.

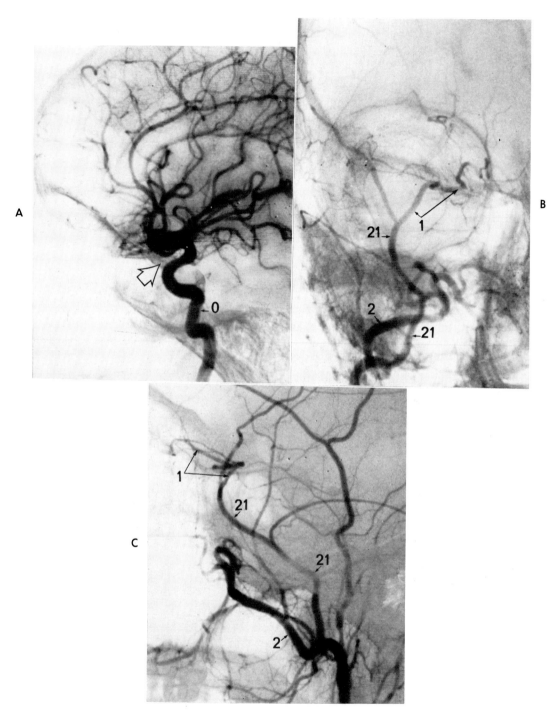

Fig. 14-39. A, Lateral internal carotid *(0)* angiogram. Ophthalmic artery is not seen *(open arrow).* **B** and **C,** AP **(B)** and lateral **(C)** external carotid angiogram in same patient as **A.** Ophthalmic artery *(1)* is well identified, arising from middle meningeal artery *(21)* and penetrating orbit by way of superior orbital fissure. *2,* Internal maxillary artery.

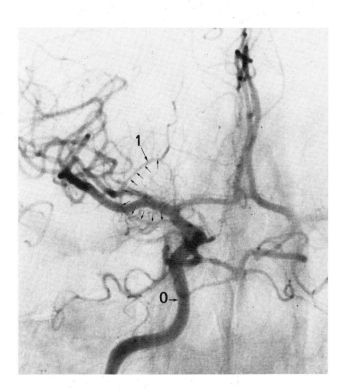

Fig. 14-40. AP internal carotid *(0)* angiogram. Ophthalmic artery *(1)* demonstrates uniform stretching *(small arrows)* around an optic nerve glioma.

provided that the configuration is of the inferolateral-superomedial type (the majority of cases). The increase in optic nerve volume (most often caused by glioma or meningioma) will appear as proportional enlargement of the arterial loop around the nerve (Fig. 14-40).

In the infraoptic type I variety, alterations of the second segment of the ophthalmic artery are not proportional to the size of the optic nerve and are therefore of no localizing value. Type II configurations may show openings of the circumneural loop, similar to the supraoptic variety.

Displacements of the third portion of the ophthalmic artery are essentially in the craniocaudal direction, thus providing information on the superior and inferior extent of a space-occupying process only (Fig. 14-41).

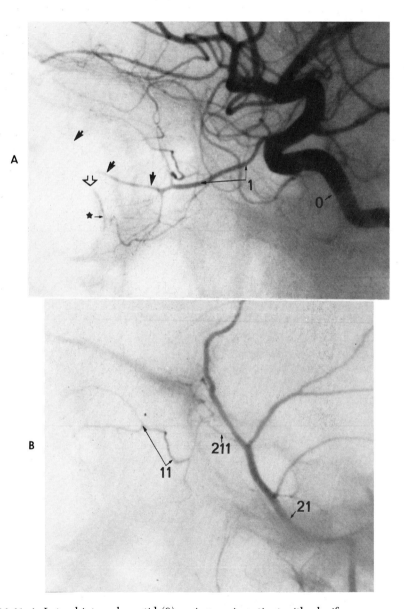

Fig. 14-41. A, Lateral internal carotid *(0)* angiogram in patient with plexiform neuroma. Third portion of ophthalmic artery *(1)* is clearly depressed in craniocaudal direction and protrudes at its superior concavity *(arrows).* This example illustrates extraconal, superior internal space-occupying process. Choroidal crescent *(star)* is displaced inferiorly *(open arrow).* **B,** Selective arteriography of middle meningeal artery *(21)* viewed laterally, in same patient as **A.** Lacrimal artery *(11)* is totally opacified by way of recurrent meningeal artery *(211)* Lacrimal artery is angiographically normal, indicating strictly superior and internal localization of intraorbital space-occupying process.

Analysis of mass effects at the level of the lacrimal artery

The lacrimal artery may arise either from the ophthalmic artery or from the middle meningeal artery. When the lacrimal artery originates from the ophthalmic artery (70% to 80% of cases), the relationships that it presents in its initial course along the optic nerve vary according to the manner of the crossing of the nerve by the ophthalmic artery. In the infraoptic variant the lacrimal artery usually originates from the second bend of the ophthalmic artery and proceeds laterally, crossing above the optic nerve. The "clamp" thus formed around the optic nerve by the second segment of the ophthalmic artery and the initial portion of the lacrimal artery trunk (Fig. 14-42) or of a meningoophthalmic artery permits the evaluation of the diameter of the nerve. This recreates "in reverse" anatomic conditions analogous to those shown by the ophthalmic artery when it crosses the optic nerve in the supraoptic manner.

After first proceeding in a transverse direction, the lacrimal artery takes an anterior course along the superior border of the lateral rectus muscle to reach the lacrimal gland, which it vascularizes in its entirety. At the heart of the glandular parenchyma the lacrimal artery gives rise to glandular and zygomatic branches that in turn anastomose with the anterior deep temporal artery (a collateral of the internal maxillary and transverse facial arteries).

Angiographically, most of the identifiable displacements of the lacrimal artery correspond to the effect of a craniocaudal mass, relating to a superoexternal orbital space-occupying process (Fig. 14-43).

All effects of a mass angiographically identified at the level of intraglandular collaterals of the lacrimal artery allow confirmation that a superoexternal anterior space-occupying process has developed within the glandular parenchyma (Fig. 14-44).

The topographic anatomy described above is also applicable to the lacrimal artery when it originates from the middle meningeal artery. In this case, it enters the

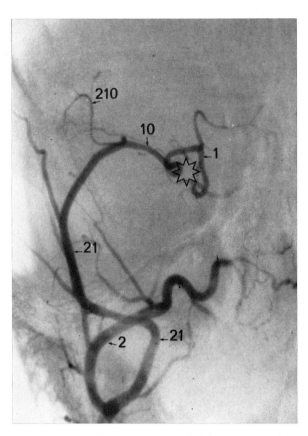

Fig. 14-42. AP internal maxillary *(2)* arteriogram. Ophthalmic artery *(1)*, opacified by way of prominent meningo-ophthalmic artery *(10)*, demonstrates infraoptic variation. In this anatomic condition, size of optic nerve *(star)* can be determined by deformations of "clamp" formed around nerve by these two arteries. *21,* Middle meningeal artery; *210,* meningolacrimal artery.

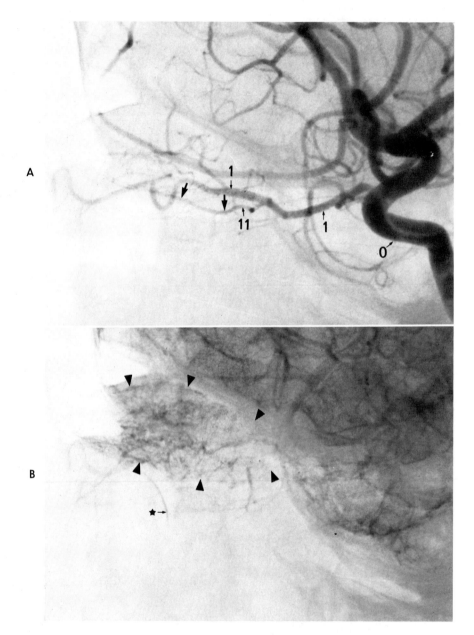

Fig. 14-43. A, Internal carotid *(0)* angiogram, lateral view, arterial phase. **B,** Venous phase, lateral view. Neovascularization *(black arrowheads)* caused by rhabdomyosarcoma is seen.

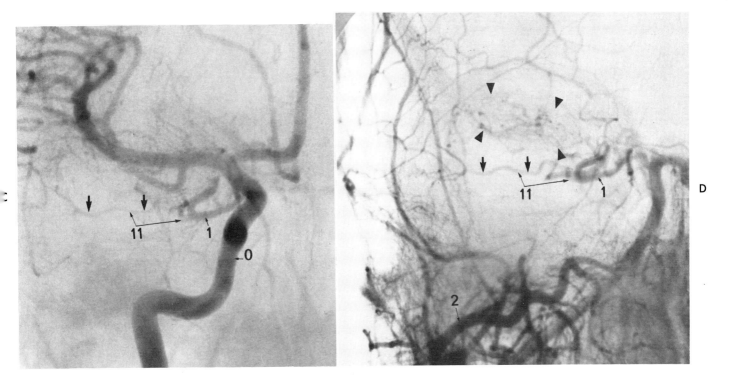

Fig. 14-43, cont'd. C, AP arterial phase. Downward displacement *(arrows)* of the lacrimal artery *(11)* is caused by intraorbital, extraconal space-occupying process, with superior and external extension. **D,** AP arteriography of internal maxillary artery *(2)* in same patient. Lacrimal artery *(11)* is nicely identified. It appears displaced inferiorly *(arrows)* in relation to superior external tumor, whose pathologic vascularization *(black arrowheads)* is evident. *1,* Ophthalmic artery; *star,* choroidal crescent.

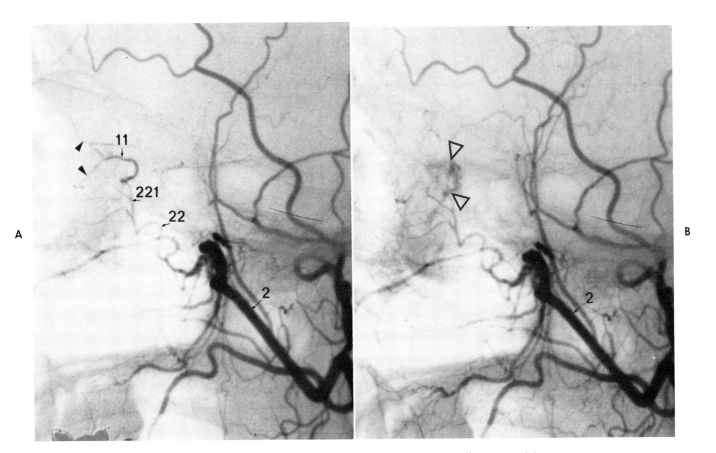

Fig. 14-44. A, Early, and **B,** late arterial phase studies of internal maxillary artery *(2)* in patient with mixed lacrimal gland tumor. The lacrimal artery *(11)* is opacified by way of lacrimal branch *(221)* of deep anterior temporal artery *(22).* Notice spreading apart and stretched appearance of lacrimal artery collaterals within glandular parenchyma. All these arteriographic signs together indicate mass within lacrimal gland.

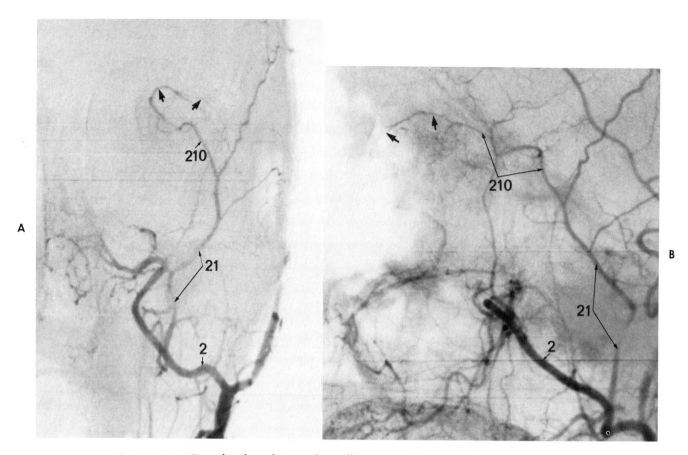

Fig. 14-45. A, AP, and **B,** lateral internal maxillary artery *(2)* angiogram in another patient with mixed lacrimal gland tumor. Lacrimal artery arises from the middle meningeal artery *(21)*; it penetrates orbit by way of canal of Hyrtl and represents meningolacrimal variety *(210)*. This meningolacrimal artery has focal protruberance of its glandular collaterals *(arrows)*, indicating mass lesion in lacrimal parenchyma. This arteriographic picture is similar to that observed when lacrimal artery arises from ophthalmic artery.

orbit by way of Hyrtl's canal (meningolacrimal artery) (Fig. 14-45). In the very rare cases in which the lacrimal artery arises from the deep anterior temporal artery, the topographic information supplied by the angiographic work-up concerns only the intraglandular localization of a space occupying process because the entire trajectory of the lacrimal artery trunk above the lateral rectus muscle is absent.

Topographic analysis of the effects of a mass at the supraorbital artery level

Most often arising independently from the ophthalmic arterial trunk at the level of its second bend (third segment), the supraorbital artery proceeds upward, passing between the oblique superior muscle (medially) and the lateral rectus and levator palpebrae superioris muscles (laterally). It then proceeds forward under the roof of the orbit to the level of the supraorbital fora-

men, where it penetrates the scalp and anastomoses with the external frontal collateral artery to the superficial temporal artery. Because of its very intimate anatomic relationships with the periosteum of the roof of the orbit, the supraorbital artery is an excellent indicator of mass lesions developing adjacent to the orbital roof. In such pathologic conditions it undergoes craniocaudal displacement along most of its course (Fig. 14-46).

Topographic analysis of the effects of mass lesions on the muscular arteries

Only the inferior muscular artery is visible 100% of the time, and it alone is therefore reliable as an indicator of significant angiographic displacements of the muscular arteries. There are three vascular territories of the orbital musculature: superior and internal, superior and external, and inferior.

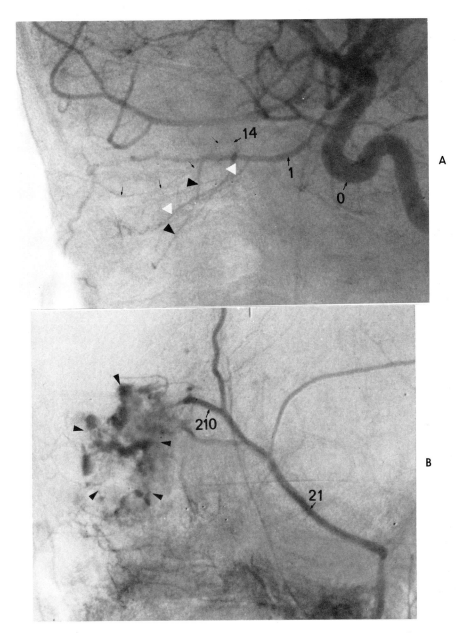

Fig. 14-46. A, Lateral internal carotid *(0)* angiogram. Craniocaudal displacement with superior concavity *(arrows)* at level of supraorbital artery *(14)* is seen. This pattern is associated with stretching and bowing of other ophthalmic artery branches, particularly at level of inferior and internal muscular artery *(solid arrowheads)*, and of posterior ciliary arteries *(white arrowheads)*. *1,* Ophthalmic artery. **B,** Selective middle meningeal artery *(21)* angiogram, lateral view, in same patient. Hypervascular tumoral process at orbital roof is supplied by middle meningeal artery, especially its meningolacrimal branch *(210)*. It was a bony angioma of orbital roof in 2-year-old child.

The inferior muscular artery is the principal feeding pedicle of the inferior territory, which always includes the inferior rectus, inferior oblique, and often a portion of the lateral rectus muscles. In 70% to 90% of cases the inferior muscular artery arises from a single trunk, and in the remaining cases from a trunk in common with the posterointernal ciliary artery (when the ophthalmic artery is in the supraoptic variation) or with the posteroexternal ciliary artery (when the ophthalmic artery is of the infraoptic variety). In nearly 95% of cases in which the ophthalmic artery crosses the nerve in supraoptic fashion, the inferior muscular artery is situated medial to the optic nerve during its early course (descending from inside to outside, and from back to front).

After this first segment it typically divides into three branches, one posterior and the other two anterior. It encloses the right inferior muscle along its external and internal borders, thus appearing like a "goose foot" on lateral views and like a "pitchfork" planted on the inferior rectus muscle as seen on the AP projection. There-fore the inferior muscular trunk accurately reflects an intraconal space-occupying process.

At the level of its first segment, the inferior muscular artery can indicate the existence of an intraconal process developing alongside the optic nerve. If the displacement is associated with an enlargement of the crossing loop of the ophthalmic artery with the optic nerve, this is an additional argument in favor of an increase in the volume of this nerve (Fig. 14-47).

Uniform stretching and displacement of all its branches indicates a space-occupying process developed within the inferior rectus muscle itself (Fig. 14-48); all displacements in the vertical plane with a superior concavity indicate most often a supraoptic, intra-conal space-occupying process (Fig. 14-49).

Vertical displacements (other than the diffuse mass effect described above) cause an inferior concavity corresponding to an extraconal space-occupying process that has developed at the orbital floor and pushed the inferior rectus muscle upwards (Fig. 14-50).

There is no other muscular pedicle that is consis-

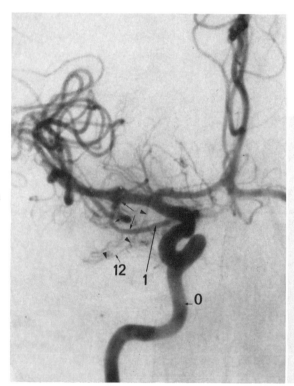
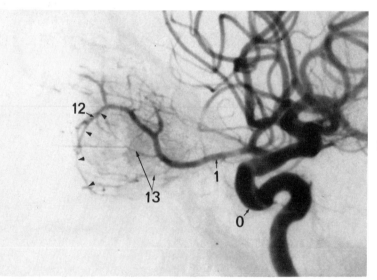

Fig. 14-47. A, AP, and **B,** internal carotid artery (0) angiogram in patient with optic nerve sheath meningioma. Ophthalmic artery loop (1) is enlarged around optic nerve (arrows) in example of external latero-optic crossing. Inferior muscular artery (12) is bowed in opposite direction (arrowheads), visible on AP study but most striking on lateral view. Mass effect is also noticeable at level of posterior ciliary arteries (13). These arteriographic signs together indicate definite increase in volume of optic nerve. Notice characteristic radial neovascularization contained in concavity of inferior muscular artery, seen particularly well on lateral view (**B**).

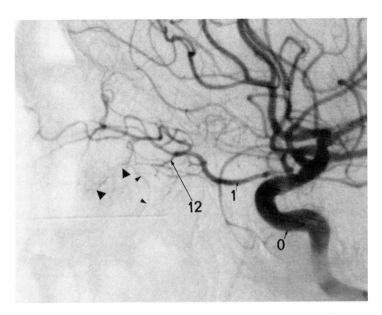

Fig. 14-48. Internal carotid artery *(0)* angiogram, lateral view. Uniform bowing of anterior *(large arrowheads)* and posterior *(small arrowheads)* branches of inferior muscular artery *(12)* is seen. This arteriographic pattern is characteristic of mass in inferior rectus muscle. Mass was a tumor. *1,* Ophthalmic artery.

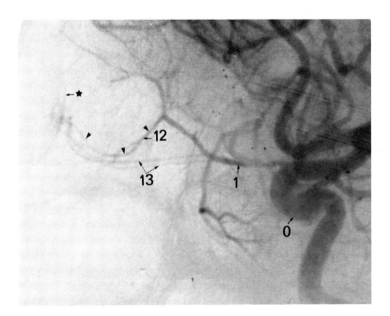

Fig. 14-49. Internal carotid artery *(0)* angiogram, lateral view. Inferior muscular artery *(12)* displays craniocaudal displacement with superior concavity at level of posterior ciliary arteries *(13).* Patient had superior intraconal echinococcal cyst. 1, Ophthalmic artery.

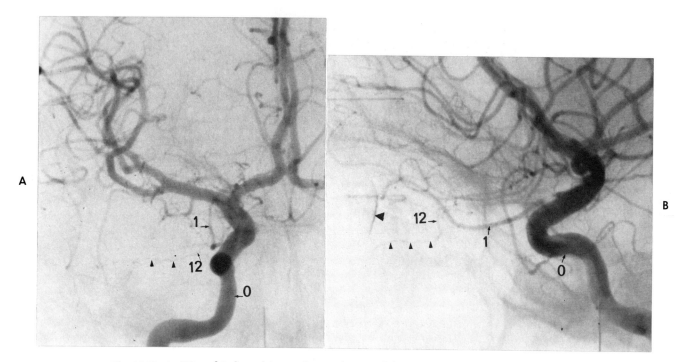

Fig. 14-50. A, AP, and **B,** lateral internal carotid artery *(0)* angiogram in patient with maxillary sinus epithelioma that extended into inferior orbital wall. Anterior branches of inferior muscular artery *(12)* demonstrate stretching and curve with inferior concavity *(small arrowheads).* Mass effect of mass is not uniform at level of the inferior muscular artery branches, which indicates inferior, intraorbital, extraconal mass. Notice focal flattening *(large arrowhead)* of choroidal crescent. *1,* Ophthalmic artery.

tently identified angiographically. However, in certain cases it is possible to recognize an external muscular artery, particularly when the lacrimal artery originates from the middle meningeal artery (meningolacrimal variant); in this case the information furnished by the effects of a mass on the external muscular artery is comparable to those described at the level of the lacrimal artery.

Topographic analysis of the effects of a mass on the posterior ciliary arteries

The posterointernal and posteroexternal ciliary arteries are routinely identified. They correspond to the vestiges of the distal embryonic ventral and dorsal ophthalmic arteries. They can originate from either a single or a common trunk or a collateral of the ophthalmic artery (most often the central retinal artery, more rarely the muscular lacrimal artery). The ciliary arteries follow the direction of the optic nerve up to the level of the papilla and then give off numerous short ciliary arteries that penetrate the sclera around the optic nerve.

The posterointernal and posteroexternal ciliary arteries are easily identified on lateral angiograms; they al-

ways have a sinuous trajectory and are well demonstrated in the lateral projection. The external ciliary artery often forms a large loop behind the globe before penetrating the sclera. Because they accompany the optic nerve during much of its course, the ciliary arteries can reflect displacement or morphologic alterations of this nerve, at least in the vertical direction (Figs. 14-46, 14-47, and 14-49). Infiltrating processes such as pseudotumor or orbital cellulitis can cause uniform stretching of the ciliary arteries without focal displacement.

Most other collateral branches of the ophthalmic artery are identifiable too inconsistently to be helpful in localizing intraorbital masses. One exception is the anterior ethmoid artery. In almost 7% of cases this vessel is in direct continuity with the ophthalmic arterial trunk and consequently can demonstrate the same type of displacement as the third portion of the ophthalmic artery.

In addition to the collateral arteries arising from the ophthalmic artery itself, the anastomotic branches between the ophthalmic system and the external carotid system (particularly at the level of the internal maxillary artery) must also be considered. The meningolacrimal

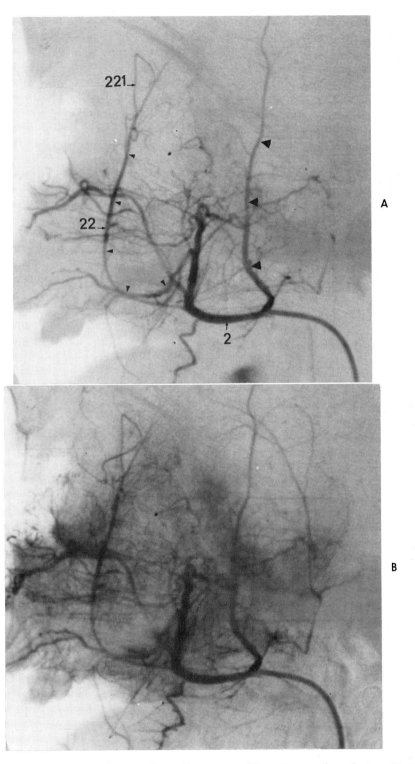

Fig. 14-51. A, Selective distal internal maxillary artery *(2)* angiogram, lateral view. Notice marked mass effect *(small arrowheads)*, with posterior concavity of anterior deep temporal artery *(22)* from its origin to level of its lacrimal branch *(221)*. Less prominent mass effect at level of the middle deep temporal artery is also seen *(large arrowheads)*. **B,** Late arterial phase, same patient as **A.** Large hypervascular tumor of external temporal fossa exends to external wall of orbit, producing displacements evident in **A.** Tumor was sarcoma in 2-year-old child.

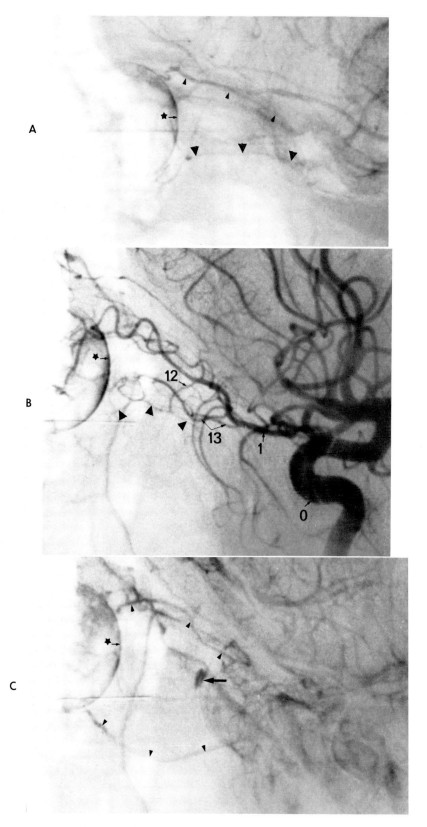

Fig. 14-52. A, Normal venous phase, internal carotid angiogram. Superior *(small arrowheads)* and inferior *(large arrowheads)* vorticose veins draining choroid (shown in form of choroidal crescent) *(star)* are perfectly identified. They delimit muscular cone. **B,** Arterial, and **C,** venous phase, internal carotid artery *(0)* angiogram in patient with cavernous angioma. In arterial phase, smooth protruberance *(large arrowheads)* of inferior muscular artery branches *(12)* is seen. In venous phase, symmetric bowing of superior and inferior vorticinous veins is present. These arterial and venous signs are characteristic of intraconal space-occupying process. Note abnormal puddle of contrast material *(black arrow). 1,* Ophthalmic artery; *13,* posterior ciliary arteries; *star,* choroidal crescent.

artery demonstrates mass effects that are identical to those described for the lacrimal artery. Alterations in the position of the vertical branch of the suborbital artery can also be identified when a mass develops at the level of the orbital floor (or at the level of the maxillary sinus when it extends to the orbit). Anteroposterior displacements or transverse displacements of the deep anterior temporal artery and of its lacrimal branch are seen when an orbital tumor extends into the infratemporal fossa (Fig. 14-51).

■ The venous system

To the arterial topography must be added the analysis of mass effects on the venous system. The superior and inferior ophthalmic veins are not particularly useful in identifying small focal tumor processes. The ophthalmic veins drain not only the orbit but also the nasal cavity territory and parts of the face. The nasal cavity is drained by way of ethmoid veins, and parts of the face medially are drained by way of the angular veins.

Venous drainage of the structures that have to do with the visual apparatus itself is by way of vorticose veins. The choroidal venous drainage is classically by way of a circle of four vorticose veins that perforate the sclera just behind the equator of the eye. They are designated as internal and external superior vessels and internal and external inferior vessels, respectively. These veins drain into lacrimal and superior ophthalmic veins; the central retinal vein drains into the inferior ophthalmic vein. The lacrimal vein and muscular veins also drain into the ophthalmic veins.[13]

In the venous phase of an internal carotid angiogram, the vorticose venous drainage is, in 70% to 80% of cases, visible in the form of two veins, one superior and the other inferior. They appear as a rectilinear trajectory, outlining the muscular cone to its apex (Fig. 14-52, *A*).

The normal concavity between the superior and inferior vorticose veins (Fig. 14-52, *B* and *C*) is easily recognizable and is of great assistance in affirming the intraconal localization of an intraorbital space-occupying process. The vorticose system can also exhibit the same mass effects as the muscular cone and appear displaced vertically from top to bottom or the reverse.

■ The choroidal crescent

The choroidal crescent is always visible angiographically. It is a layer composed of vascular elements—veins, capillaries, and arteries—that embrace the posterior two thirds of the globe.[2] The blood supply from the choroid comes from the posterior ciliary arteries and to a minor extent from the recurrent branches of the major circulosis arteriosis. On angiography the choroid is first seen in the late arterial phase, but it assumes its greatest prominence during the early venous phase. This reflects the composition of the choroid by a rich capillary network with multiple small veins.[13] It is possible to discern focal flattenings of the choroid crescent. Localized flattening at the center of the crescent is a good indication of an intraconal space-occupying process (Fig. 14-53). Any superior or inferior segmental flattening indicates the existence of a superior or infe-

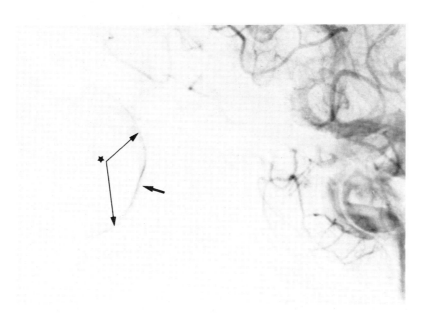

Fig. 14-53. Venous phase of internal carotid arteriogram. Choroidal crescent *(star)* is perfectly opacified. Focal flattening *(black arrow)* suggests mass at level of optic nerve. Glioma was found during surgery.

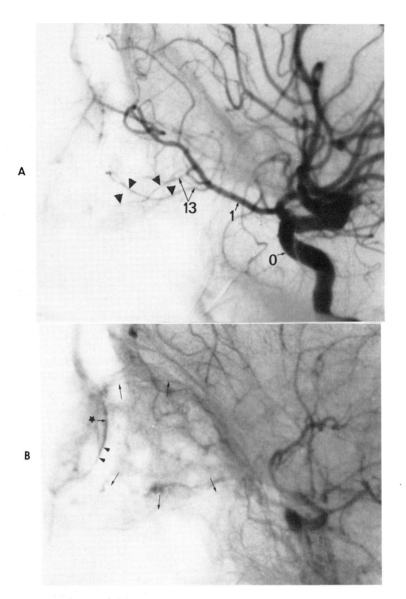

Fig. 14-54. Internal carotid *(0)* angiogram in **A,** arterial, and **B,** venous phases. Evidence of mass lesion with opposite concavity of superior and inferior vorticinous veins is seen in **B** (arrows). Also notice segmental flattening of choroidal crescent *(star)* in its inferior part *(black arrowheads).* This appearance is characteristic of superior intraconal space-occupying process seen in **A** *(arrowheads).* Cavernous angioma was present. *1,* Ophthalmic artery; *13,* posterior ciliary arteries.

rior process that in most cases will be extraconal and intraorbital (Figs. 14-54 to 14-58).

■ Summary

The topographic interpretation of mass effects on an angiographic workup must first attempt to identify the different signs at the levels of the various anatomic elements. Once this is accomplished, the individual signs should be considered together as a constellation of findings. Reliability of placing the lesion correctly within the orbit will be enhanced by use of these methods. Thus the following signs and processes can be correlated.

Uniform stretching of the inferior muscular artery branches, together with bowing of the superior and inferior vorticose veins, indicates an intraconal space-occupying process near the inferior rectus muscle (Fig. 14-52, *B* and *C*).

A mass with superior concavity of the posterior ciliary arteries associated with opposite displacement of

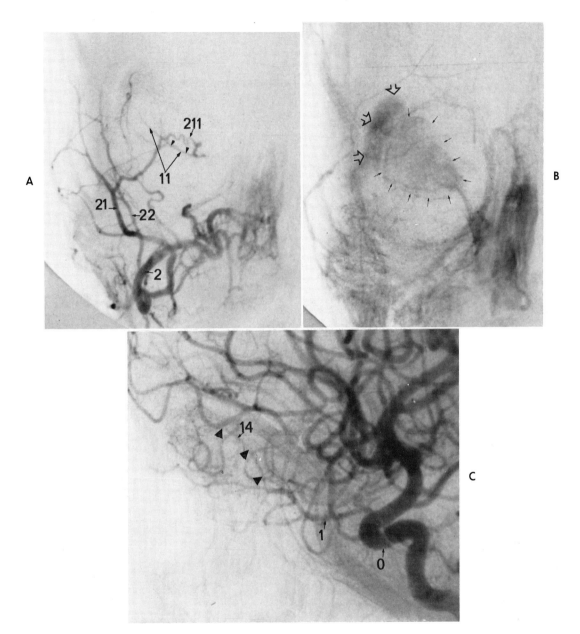

Fig. 14-55. Arteriography in AP view of internal maxillary artery *(2)* in **A**, early, and **B**, late arterial phases. Recurrent meningeal artery *(211)* opacifies lacrimal artery *(11)*, which has superior concavity *(small arrowheads)*. **C**, Contrast material injection of internal carotid artery *(0)*, lateral view. Supraorbital artery *(14)* shows corresponding inferior concavity *(large arrowheads)*. These arteriographic signs indicate space-occupying process developed at level of superior rectus or levator palpebrae superioris muscle. This diagnosis is confirmed by evidence of tumor stain *(dark arrows)* fully visible in **B**, clearly separate from physiologic opacification of lacrimal gland *(open arrows)*. Tumor was rhabdomyosarcoma. *1*, Ophthalmic artery; *21*, middle meningeal artery; *22*, deep anterior temporal artery.

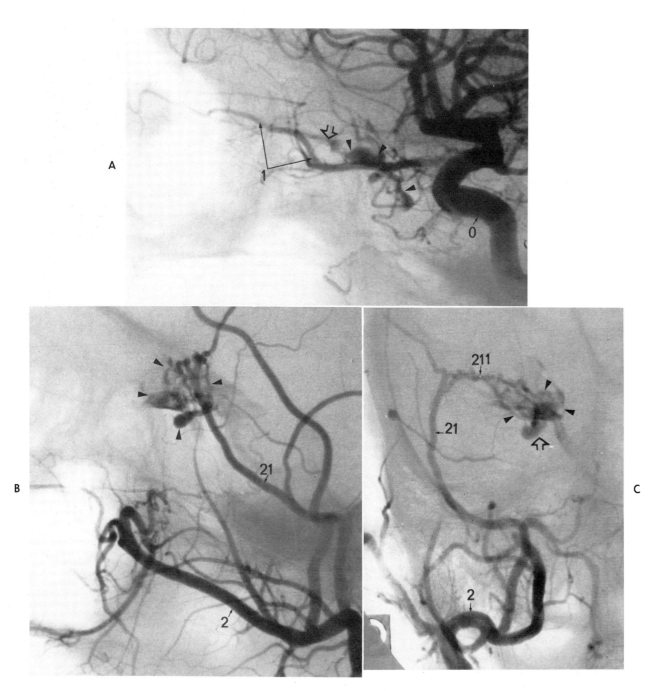

Fig. 14-56. A, Arteriography of internal carotid *(0)* viewed laterally. **B** and **C,** Arteriography of the internal maxillary artery *(2)* viewed laterally and in AP projection, respectively. An arteriovenous intraorbital fistula *(dark arrowheads)* has developed between recurrent meningeal artery *(211)* and superior ophthalmic vein *(open arrow). 1,* Ophthalmic artery; *21,* middle meningeal artery.

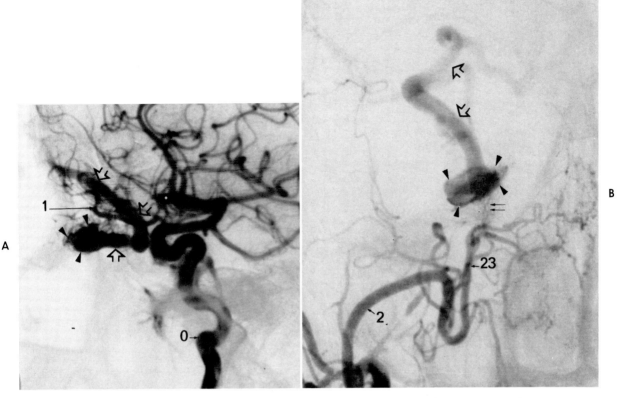

Fig. 14-57. A, Internal carotid *(0)* aniogram, lateral view. **B,** Internal maxillary artery *(2)* angiogram, AP view; both views in patient with intraorbital arteriovenous malformation developed within inferior rectus muscle *(dark arrowheads)*. This malformation drains at level of superior and inferior ophthalmic veins *(open arrow)*. It is supplied by ophthalmic artery *(1)* and by orbital branches passing through sphenomaxillary cleft *(small arrows)* that arose from sphenopalatine artery *(23)*.

the superior and inferior vorticose veins indicates an intraconal mass above the optic nerve (Fig. 14-54).

Inferior concavity of the supraorbital artery, associated with superior concavity of the initial portion of the lacrimal artery (intraconal portion), indicates a space-occupying process at the level of the superior rectus muscle or of the levator palpebrae superiosis muscle (Fig. 14-55).

A protrusion with a superior concavity of the third portion of the ophthalmic artery, associated with displacement of the choroidal crescent downward and forward and a normal course of the lacrimal artery, indicates an intraorbital, extraconal, superior, and internal space-occupying process (Fig. 14-41).

Numerous basic topographic patterns of intraorbital vessel displacement can thus be recognized even though there are many anatomic variations in the development of an orbital space-occupying process. In all fairness, however, it should be noted that all intraorbital

tumors are not necessarily accompanied by significant vascular displacement, for two fundamental reasons: (1) the tumor may be small and the displacements unidentifiable, and (2) the tumor may be located in an angiographically "silent" region (such as the inferoexternal quadrant of the orbit), in which case no vascular displacements will be identified. In these cases the hypervascular character of even a small tumor, however, can sometimes permit its localization.

□ Hypervascular orbital lesions

The diagnosis of a vascular orbital lesion belongs, by definition, to angiography. In our series of 310 patients with orbital lesions (excluding those of endocrine causes) 13% were of vascular origin.

The angiographic aspects of vascular orbital lesions are often characteristic, permitting a precise diagnosis. Typical lesions include ophthalmic artery aneurysms, arteriovenous intraorbital fistulae, arteriovenous malformations, cavernous angiomas, malignant neoplasms of vasoformative tumors, and other hypervascular tumors.

■ Ophthalmic artery aneurysms

Aneurysms of the ophthalmic artery usually arise at the site of origin of the artery and about 10% of these may eventually be responsible for a subarachnoid hemorrhage. In the rarest of circumstances the aneurysm may arise from within the intraorbital segment rather than from the intracranial segment. Under that condition the aneurysm may simulate an expanding neoplasm, being responsible for diminished visual acuity, papilledema, etc. An intraorbital hematoma ensues in the circumstance of rupture of the aneurysm. Zimmerman and Vignaud[13] point out that when an intraorbital ophthalmic aneurysm is discovered, an inflammatory process or a connective tissue disease should be ruled out.

■ Arteriovenous intraorbital fistulae

Arteriovenous fistulae develop most often between the superior ophthalmic vein and lacrimal artery or with the recurrent meningeal artery. A history of trauma is usually elicited. These fistulae are to be distinguished from the carotid cavernous variety (Fig. 14-56).

■ Arteriovenous malformations

Arteriovenous malformations are multipedicular, involving both the internal carotid system (through the ophthalmic artery and its collaterals) and the external carotid system (through orbital collaterals of the internal maxillary artery) (Fig. 14-57). These are usually of dural origin.

■ Cavernous angiomas

Cavernous angiomas are the most common angiomas of the orbit. Usually seen in infants and children, they represent a benign vascular malformation. They are most often intraconal and well encapsulated. They appear as pool-like vascular opacifications seen late on serial angiograms. The vascular blush frequently represents only a small portion of the total tumor volume. The venous drainage appears normal and the feeding arteries demonstrate no change in caliber (Fig. 14-58). For discussion of the radiologic features of other less common angiomas of the orbit the interested reader is referred to Dilenge.[3]

■ Hemangiopericytomas—malignant neoplasms or vasoformative tumors

Hemangiopericytomas appear as well-delineated hypervascular tumors. Early-draining veins are often present and the tumor frequently has enlarged arterial pedicles (Fig. 14-59). Hemangiopericytomas may arise wherever capillaries are found. About 5% of the total number of reported hemangiopericytomas arise from around the orbit and oronasopharyngeal region and paranasal sinuses.

■ Other hypervascular tumors

Of the true neoplasms that produce tumor stain, the most common are meningioma, rhabdomyosarcoma, paraganglioma, metastatic tumor, and neurinoma. In our series, hypervascular orbital tumors (with the exception of angiomas) represented 11% of cases. Only

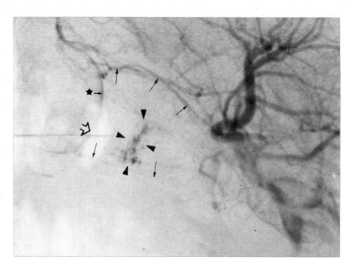

Fig. 14-58. Venous phase of internal carotid angiogram. Intraconal "vascular pools" (*black arrowheads*) between opposite concavities of superior and inferior vorticinous veins (*black arrows*) are seen. This is characteristic of intraconal cavernous angioma. Notice focal flattening (*open arrow*) of choroidal crescent (*star*).

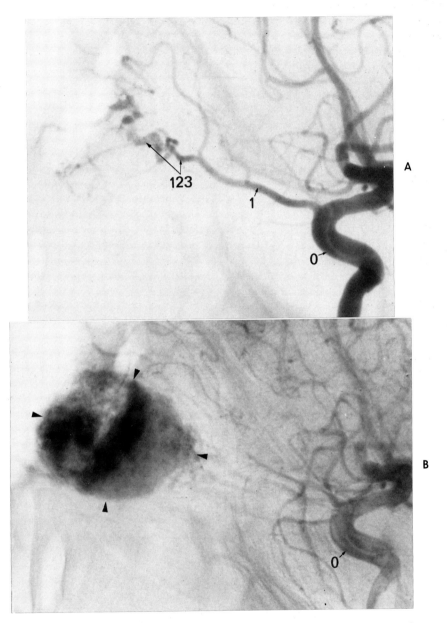

Fig. 14-59. Internal carotid *(0)* angiogram in lateral view in **A,** early and **B,** late arterial phases. Dilation of ophthalmic artery *(1)* and of its musculociliary collateral *(123)* is present. Well-demarcated hypervascular tumor *(black arrowheads)* with dense vascularization is seen. This is characteristic of hemangiopericytoma.

two types of tumors have characteristic arteriographic findings: meningiomas and osseous angiomas.

Meningiomas can arise from the optic nerve sheath (Fig. 14-60), or osseous wall of the orbit (usually the greater and lesser sphenoid alae) (Fig. 14-61, A to C). Hypervascularization of these tumors classically appears early in the angiographic series and has a typically radial appearance (Fig. 14-61, D). Homogeneous opacification and early draining veins are characteristic. The intensity of vascularization varies from one meningioma to another. In markedly hypervascular meningiomas, the arteriovenous shunting caused by the tumor can cause significant dilation of the feeding arterial pedicles (Fig. 14-61, A and B).

The second characteristic type of tumor corresponds to osseous angiomas, uncommon lesions that develop within the orbital walls (Fig. 14-62). The vascularization is seen as "pools" of contrast medium filling the osseous alveoli. Tumor circulation is slow and neither early venous return nor nourishing pedicular dilation is characteristic.

Other hypervascular orbital tumors do not have any particular pathognomonic angiographic characteristics, although differentiation between malignant and benign vascularization is sometimes possible. Vascular atypia (microthromboses, arteriovenous microshunts) on histologic examination associated with a poorly marginated lesion angiographically favors the diagnosis of malignant tumor. Typical examples are rhabdomyosarcoma arising from the orbital muscle cone (Figs. 14-55 to 14-63), some mixed tumors of the lacrimal gland (Fig. 14-44, B), some orbital metastases, primitive mesenchymal tumors (Fig. 14-64), and some epitheliomas that extend to the orbit (Fig. 14-65).

Conversely, homogeneous vascularization and well-defined borders without vascular atypia are suggestive of a benign tumor such as neurinoma (isolated or associated with a neurofibroma) or chemodectoma. Intraorbital neurinoma usually occurs at the bifurcations of the occulomotor nerve, and classically in the upper half of the orbit (Fig. 14-66). Chemodectoma (nonchromaffin paraganglioma) arises from the ophthalmic ganglion. This tumor type is rare. It has many of the angiographic characteristics of a glioma, i.e., massive homogeneous hypervascularization associated with significant arteriovenous shunting.

It should also be noted that diffuse hyperemia can occur with inflammatory pseudotumor. CT and orbital ultrasonography are usually the diagnostic procedures of choice. *Text continued on p. 650.*

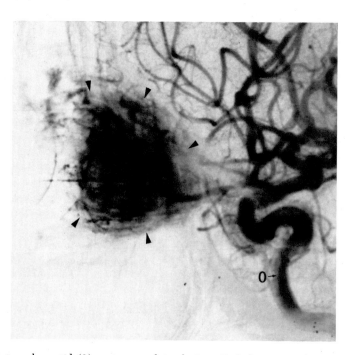

Fig. 14-60. Internal carotid *(0)* angiogram, lateral view. Pathologic vascularization *(black arrowheads)*, characterized by its radial nature, is seen in optic nerve sheath meningioma. Notice anterior displacement of choroidal crescent.

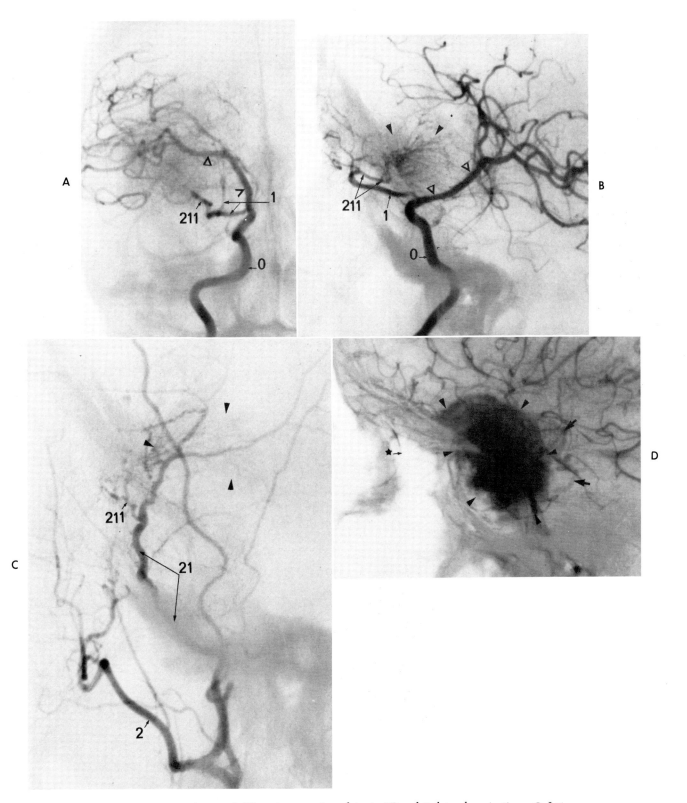

Fig. 14-61. Internal carotid *(0)* angiogram viewed in **A**, AP and **B**, lateral projections. **C**, Lateral arteriogram of external carotid in the same patient as **A** and **B**, Radial or "sunburst" vascularization characteristic of meningioma *(black arrowheads)* of anterior temporal fossa is seen. Large "mass effect" elevates middle cerebral artery axis *(open arrowheads)*. Extension of this meningioma into orbital apex at sphenoid cleft is affirmed by dilation of recurrent meningeal artery *(211)*, which is main feeding pedicle of tumor. Notice also dilation of middle meningeal artery *(21)* in **C**. *1*, Ophthalmic artery; *2*, internal maxillary artery. **D**, Internal carotid injection, lateral view, of another hypervascular meningioma of orbital apex *(black arrowheads)* in parenchymal phase. Notice early draining vein *(arrows)*. *Star*, Choroidal crescent.

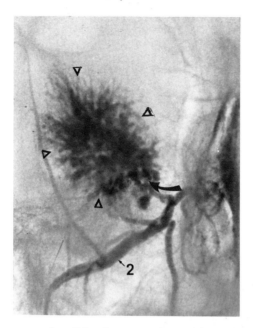

Fig. 14-62. Selective arteriography of distal portion of internal maxillary artery *(2)*, AP view. Pools of contrast media *(open arrowheads)* filling alveolar cavities of bony angioma of great wing of sphenoid are seen. *Curved arrow,* artery of foramen rotundum, sole feeding pedicle of angioma.

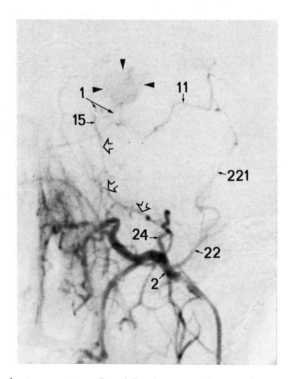

Fig. 14-63. Superselective arteriography of distal portion of internal maxillary artery *(2)*, AP view. Evidence of poorly marginated pathologic vascularization *(black arrowheads)* consisting of atypical microvessels in rhabdomyosarcoma of oblique muscle. Vascularization of this tumor is derived from distal portion of ophthalmic artery *(1)*, opacified in turn by way of anastomosis *(open arrowheads)* between infraorbital artery *(24)* and inferior palpebral artery *(15)*. *22,* Anterior deep temporal artery; *221,* lacrimal branch of anterior deep temporal artery.

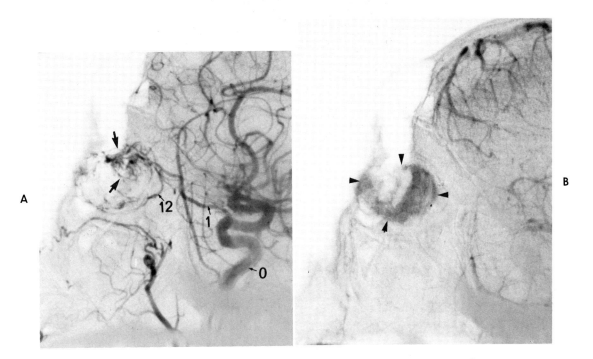

Fig. 14-64. Internal carotid *(0)* angiogram in lateral view in **A,** early arterial and **B,** venous phases. Pathologic vascularization from ophthalmic artery *(1)* and its inferior muscular collateral *(12)* is present *(arrows)*. In venous phase, parenchymal opacification of tumor is clearly evident *(arrowheads)*. Tumor was malignant orbital schwannoma.

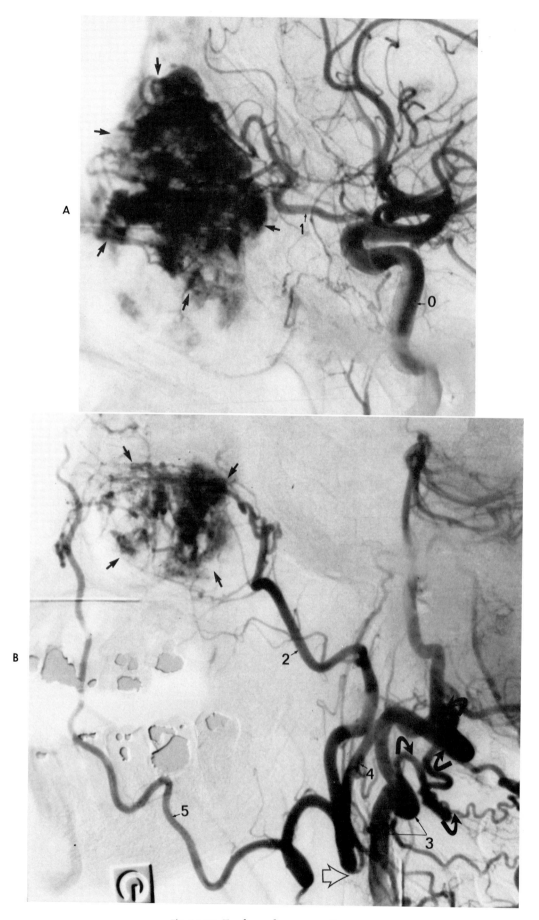

Fig. 14-65. For legend see opposite page.

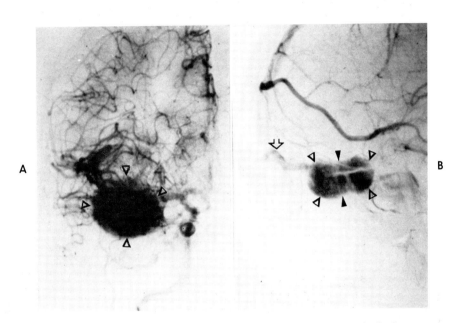

Fig. 14-66. A, AP and **B,** lateral views of internal carotid angiogram. Thick, homogeneous, pathologic opacification *(open arrowheads)* with "hourglass" configuration is seen. Narrow part of tumor *(solid arrowheads)* corresponds to its narrowing at level of sphenoid cleft. It was benign neurinoma, extending into temporal fossa and orbit. *Open arrow,* Superior ophthalmic vein.

Fig. 14-65. A, Internal carotid *(0)* angiogram, lateral view. Marked increase in caliber of ophthalmic artery *(1)* supplying large vascular tumor *(arrows)* is seen. Tumor was hypervascular adenocarcinoma involving maxillary sinus, ethmoid sinuses, and orbit. **B,** Vertebral artery *(3)* angiogram, lateral view. External carotid artery, which had been surgicaly ligated *(open arrow),* is totally revascularized by way of intervertebral collaterals *(curved arrows)* between vertebral *(3)* and occipital *(4)* arteries. *2,* Internal maxillary artery; *5,* facial artery; *black arrows,* tumoral extension at level of maxillary sinus.

□ Miscellaneous pathologic patterns

Lesions considered in this section represent variation in caliber or defects in opacification of the ophthalmic artery.

■ Variations in caliber

Excluding atheromatous narrowing localized at the ophthalmic artery origin, no diminution in arterial caliber can be definitely interpreted as pathologic. In certain rare cases, a hypoplastic ophthalmic artery occurs as an anatomic variant (Fig. 14-67). Dilations in arterial caliber occur with hypervascular tumors (Fig. 14-59, *A*), arteriovenous fistulae (Fig. 14-56, *A*), or arteriovenous malformations (Fig. 14-57, *A*). In addition, increased collateral flow with internal carotid artery occlusions may occur. In this case the ophthalmic artery revascularizes the supraclinoid internal carotid artery by way of its anastomosis with the orbital collaterals of the internal maxillary artery.

■ Defects in opacification

Partial or total absence of ophthalmic artery opacification is pathologic if the arteriographic evaluation is complete (both the internal and external carotid arteries are studied). It is usually occluded by migratory emboli. Absence of opacification is usually segmental because the numerous physiologic anastomoses often permit revascularization of a portion of the ophthalmic arterial trunk.

□ Spurious images
■ Patterns mimicking hypervascular lesions

The normal nasal mucosal blush partially overlaps the choroidal crescent in the lateral projection. The blush may be striking, especially following contrast material injection of the internal maxillary artery (because of its sphenopalatine branch). Occasionally, injection of contrast material into the internal carotid artery produces

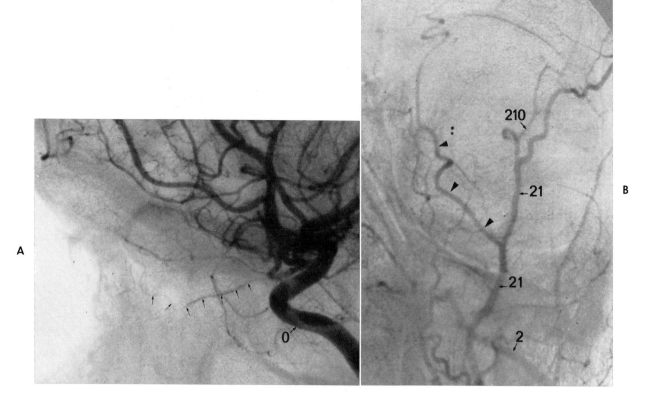

Fig. 14-67. A, Arteriography of internal carotid artery *(0)*, viewed laterally. Ophthalmic artery *(small arrows)* arises normally from portion C₂ of internal carotid artery, but appears thinned. This is anatomic variant. Ophthalmic artery in this patient, visible on contrast medium injection of internal carotid artery, only vascularizes neurosensory structures. Another ophthalmic branch arises from external carotid and supplies muscular and glandular structures. **B,** Arteriography of internal maxillary artery *(2)* in AP view, in same patient as **A.** Ophthalmic branches supplying muscular and glandular structures *(arrowheads)* arise from middle meningeal artery *(21)* and enters orbit by way of sphenoid cleft. *210,* Meningolacrimal artery.

a prominent blush because the internal nasal artery (a collateral of the anterior ethmoid) vascularizes the mucosa (Fig. 14-68). This appearance should not be confused with a hypervascular tumor.

An intense but physiologic parenchymogram of the lacrimal gland occasionally can be identified on internal maxillary studies if the lacrimal artery is of the meningolacrimal variety (Fig. 14-69). This opacification can be easily differentiated from a true hypervascular lesion by its homogeneous character, its typical superolateral location, and the anatomic variety of the feeding artery.

■ Absence of ophthalmic artery opacification

Complete absence of ophthalmic artery visualization during internal carotid injection can be caused by an ophthalmic artery arising from the middle meningeal artery (Fig. 14-39) or by an ophthalmic artery preferentially opacified by the external carotid (most commonly by means of a recurrent meningeal or meningo-ophthalmic artery (Fig. 14-69). When only partial visualization of the ophthalmic arterial trunk can be identified on internal carotid studies, examination of the homolateral internal maxillary trunk usually demonstrates a recurrent meningeal or meningo-ophthalmic artery supplying the distal ophthalmic artery.

■ Patterns mimicking an increase in ophthalmic artery caliber

Enlargement of the first and second portions of the ophthalmic artery are commonly identified. If no local

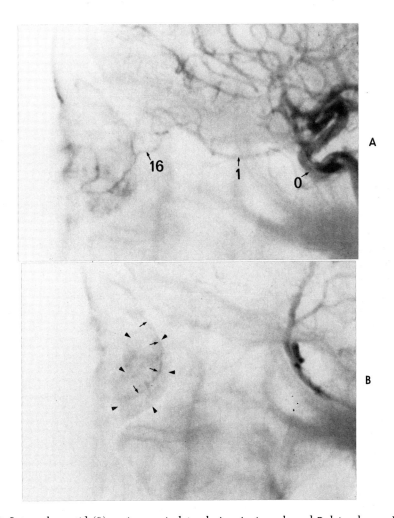

Fig. 14-68. Internal carotid *(0)* angiogram in lateral view in **A**, early and **B**, late phases. Large internal nasal artery *(16)* is an indirect collateral of ophthalmic artery *(1)*. In late phase, well-defined opacification *(dark arrowheads)* is superimposed over choroidal crescent *(arrows)*. This represents normal opacification of nasal fossa mucosa, supplied in this case in preferential manner by internal nasal artery.

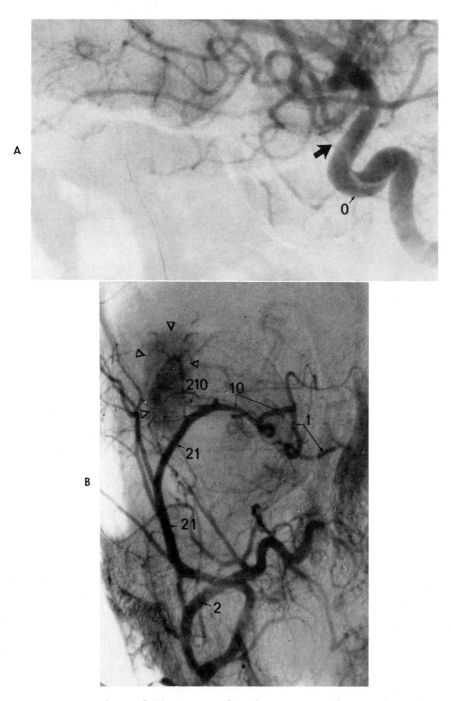

Fig. 14-69. A, Internal carotid *(0)* angiogram, lateral view. Notice absence of opacification of ophthalmic artery *(dark arrow).* **B,** Same patient in AP view of contrast medium injection of internal maxillary artery *(2).* Ophthalmic artery *(1)* is completely opacified by way of voluminous meningo-ophthalmic artery *(10).* Ophthalmic artery does not arise from middle meningeal artery *(21)* but is entirely dependent on external carotid system *210,* Meningolacrimal artery; *open arrowheads,* opacification of lacrimal gland.

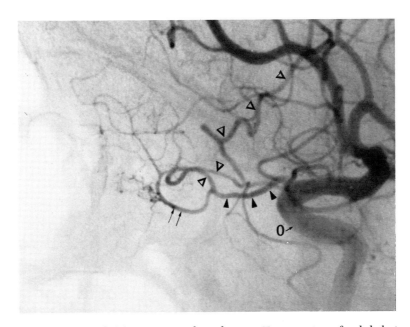

Fig. 14-70. Internal carotid *(0)* angiogram, lateral view. First portion of ophthalmic artery *(black arrowheads)* appears to have larger caliber than rest of ophthalmic artery *(double arrows).* This appearance is caused by taking over of meningeal territory of convexity by ophthalmic artery, as indicated by opacification of middle meningeal artery *(open arrowheads),* which appears as collateral of ophthalmic artery.

or regional pathologic process is present to account for this increase in flow, augmentation in the vascular bed is its cause. An example is when the middle meningeal artery arises from the ophthalmic artery and the meningeal territory of the convexity is annexed by the ophthalmic system (Fig. 14-70).

□ Carotid cavernous fistulae

Carotid cavernous fistulae are arteriovenous communications between an artery in the cavernous sinus and the cavernous venous plexus. The arterial anatomy of the cavernous sinus is an anatomic crossroad at the skull base, with numerous anastomoses between the internal carotid, external carotid, and vertebral arteries. The cavernous sinus itself is also a midline anastomotic crossroad between numerous draining cerebral veins and dural venous sinuses at the skull base. These two complex anatomic sustrates demand precise angiographic exploration of the three potential sources of arterial supply and also explain why the venous drainage can be homolateral, bilateral, or strictly contralateral.

■ Radioanatomic forms of carotid cavernous fistulae
Isolated internal carotid fistulae

Most frequently posttraumatic, internal carotid fistulae are related to a tear in the arterial wall at the level of the siphon in its C5, C4, or C3 portions. The C5 portion is the one most frequently involved, particularly with associated fractures at the skull base (Fig. 14-71). Rupture of an aneurysm in the cavernous sinus, which may be either traumatic or spontaneous, is another possible cause of this type of fistula (Fig. 14-72).

Isolated external carotid fistulae

External carotid fistulae are related to a rupture of the cavernous branches of the internal maxillary artery when these are not anastomosed with the cavernous branches of the carotid siphon (20% of anatomic cases). The accessory meningeal artery (Fig. 14-73) is the quasiexclusive pedicle of this type of fistula, the middle meningeal artery being the other possible source. In most cases, these fistulae are spontaneous, i.e., there is no significant history of trauma.

Mixed fistulae

Mixed fistulae correspond to lesions of the intracavernous collaterals of the internal carotid artery that anastomose with branches of the external carotid system. The supply to these fistulae will always be mixed, i.e., by way of both the external and internal carotid systems.

Fistulae caused by a rupture of the collaterals of the posterior group and those caused by a rupture of the

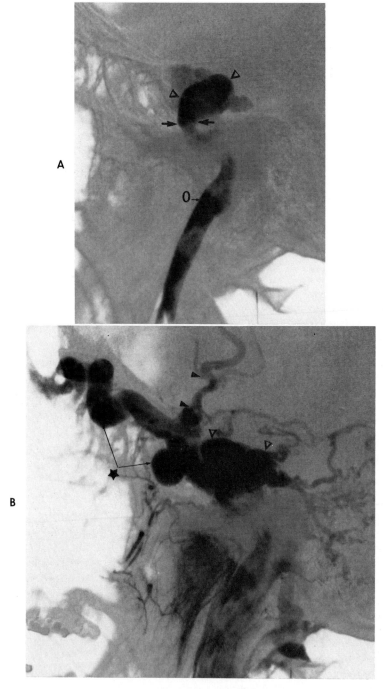

Fig. 14-71. Internal carotid *(0)* angiogram in lateral view in **A,** early and **B,** late arterial phases. Notice immediate opacification of the cavernous sinus *(open arrowheads)*, indicating a tear in carotid wall *(arrows)*. Superior ophthalmic vein *(star)* is dilated, and there is reflux into superficial middle cerebral veins *(solid arrowheads)*. Hemispheric vascularization distal to fistula is not visible, indicating a complete steal.

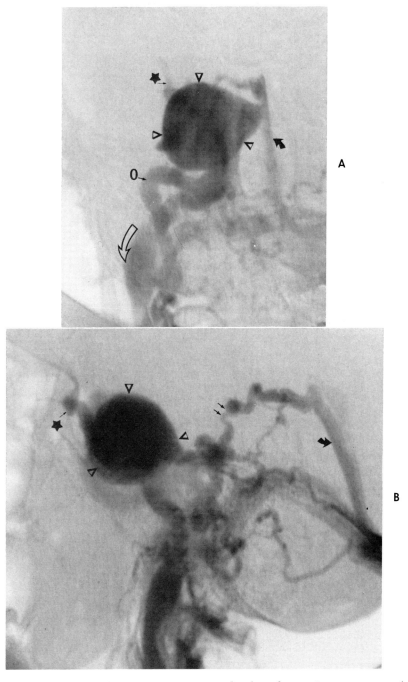

Fig. 14-72. Internal carotid *(0)* angiogram in **A,** AP and **B,** lateral view. Large aneurysm *(open arrowheads)* has ruptured in cavernous sinus. This is indicated by rapid opacification of superior ophthalmic vein *(star),* of lateral mesencephalic veins *(arrows),* of right sinus *(black curved arrow),* and of internal jugular vein *(open curved arrow).* Absence of hemispheric vascularization distal to fistula indicates high-flow shunt.

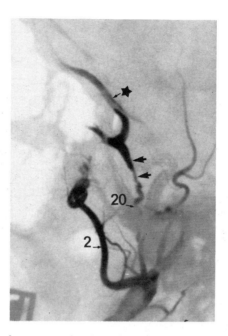

Fig. 14-73. External carotid arteriography, lateral view. Pure external carotid fistula *(arrows)* between meningeal artery *(20)* and cavernous sinus is present. Notice preferential drainage into superior ophthalmic vein *(star)*. *2,* Internal maxillary artery.

branches of the lateral group must be distinguished from one another.

Fistulae caused by rupture of the collaterals of the posterior group. The posterior collaterals originate from the C5 portion of the carotid siphon, either independently or from a common trunk. They correspond to the medial arteries of the clivus and the inferior and lateral hypophyseal arteries of the clivus. The first two have in common the fact that they anastomose with their contralateral homologues. A fistula deriving from these vessels can be supplied by both internal carotid arteries (Fig. 14-74). The external carotid supply to this group is usually derived from the ascending pharyngeal artery, whose jugular and hypoglossal branches always anastomose with the clivus arteries, particularly the lateral clival artery (Fig. 14-75, *A* and *B*). The prominent anastomotic network along the clivus between the arterial systems explains the frequently bilateral participations of the two ascending pharyngeal systems in supplying a fistula of the posterior group.

Fistulae caused by rupture of the arteries of the lateral group. The radioanatomic appearance of fistulae arising in the lateral group is a function of the site of the arterial rupture. Lesions of the inferolateral trunk near its origin on the C4 portion of the carotid siphon can be distinguished. In this type (Fig. 14-76) the supply is from multiple sources, by way of the internal carotid artery through the proximal end of the inferolateral trunk, and by way of the external carotid system by all the cavernous branches of the internal maxillary artery (artery of the foramen rotundum and accessory and middle meningeal arteries).

Lesions of the anterior collaterals of the inferolateral trunk can also be identified. In this type, the external carotid supply comes from the artery of the foramen rotundum (Fig. 14-77). The internal carotid supply comes from the proximal stump of the anterior branch of the inferolateral trunk. As this branch can anastomose with the ophthalmic artery through the recurrent deep ophthalmic artery, an ophthalmic supply is therefore also possible.

Lesions of the posterior collaterals of the inferolateral trunk can be distinguished. In this type, the external carotid supply comes from the cavernous branch of the middle meningeal artery or from the cavernous branch of the accessory meningeal artery. The internal carotid supply always arises from the proximal stump of the posterior group of the inferolateral trunk.

In 5% of cases the collaterals of the posterior group and the inferolateral trunk arise from a common source, the meningohypophyseal trunk. In this anatomic variety, a mixed fistula is supplied by all the cavernous branches of the internal maxillary artery and by the ascending pharyngeal artery (Fig. 14-78). It can also be

Text continued on p. 663.

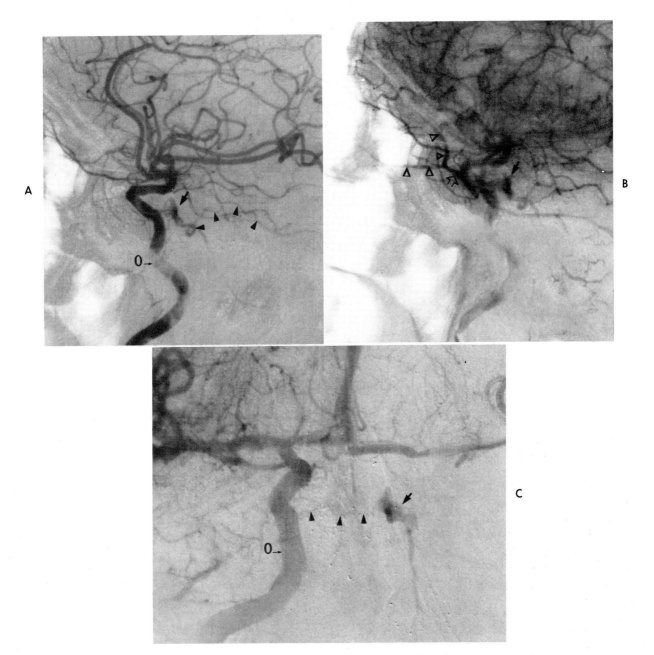

Fig. 14-74. Internal carotid *(0)* angiogram in lateral view in **A,** early and **B,** late arterial phases. Carotid cavernous fistula *(black arrow)* has developed from posterior collaterals of intracavernous carotid. Superior cerebellar artery *(dark arrowheads)* arises from this trunk. **B,** On late phase there is focal opacification of cavernous sinus *(open arrow)* as well as of superior and inferior ophthalmic veins *(open arrowheads)*. **C,** Contralateral internal carotid (0) angiogram, AP view, in the same patient as **A** and **B.** Notice that anastomoses between median arteries of clivus *(black arrowheads)* permit opacification of fistula *(arrow)*.

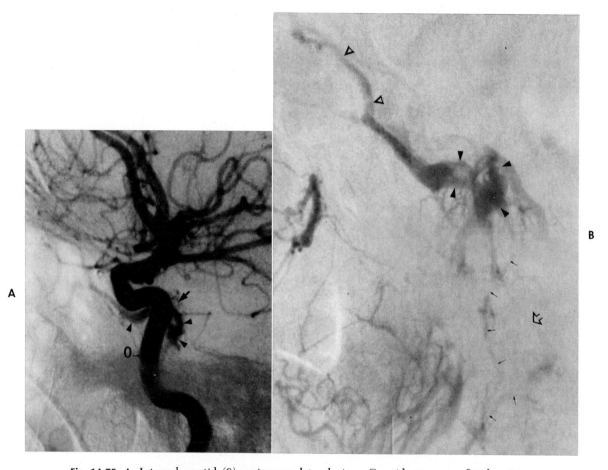

Fig. 14-75. A, Internal carotid *(0)* angiogram, lateral view. Carotid cavernous fistula arising from posterior branches of intracavernous carotid artery *(arrow)* is present. Notice early opacification of cavernous sinus *(black arrowheads).* **B,** Lateral view, selective contrast media injection of ascending pharyngeal artery in same patient as **A.** Notice early opacification of cavernous sinus *(black arrowheads)* and of superior ophthalmic vein *(open arrowheads)* by way of anastomoses between lateral artery of clivus and jugular branch of ascending pharyngeal artery *(small arrows).* Fistula was mixed carotid cavernous variety arising from posterior collaterals of intracavernous carotid artery. *Open arrow,* Inferior petrosal sinus. (Courtesy Mayo Clinic.)

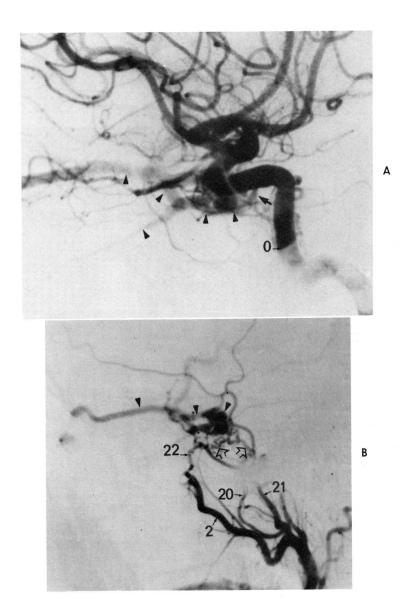

Fig. 14-76. A, Internal carotid *(0)* angiogram, lateral view. Early opacification of cavernous sinus and of superior and inferior ophthalmic veins *(solid arrowheads)* is associated with rupture of inferolateral trunk of intracavernous carotid *(arrow)* at its origin. **B,** External carotid angiogram, lateral view, in same patient as **A.** Note early opacification of cavernous sinus and superior ophthalmic vein *(solid arrowheads)* by way of cavernous branches *(open arrows)* of internal maxillary artery *(2). 20,* Accessory meningeal artery; *21,* middle meningeal artery; *22,* artery of foramen rotundum.

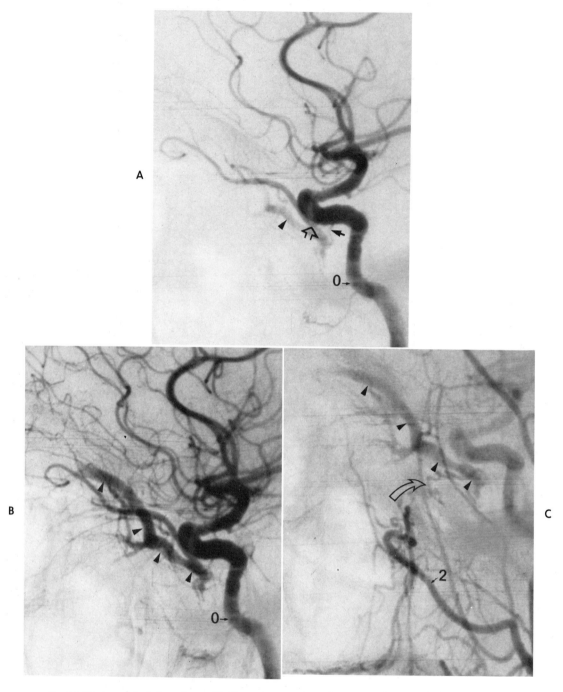

Fig. 14-77. A and **B,** Internal carotid (0) angiogram, lateral view, early, **A,** and late, **B,** arterial phases. Early opacification of cavernous sinus and superior ophthalmic vein *(solid arrowheads)* with rupture of anterior branches of inferolateral trunk *(dark arrow)* are seen. Notice abnormal origin of ophthalmic artery at level of junction of parts C_3 and C_4 of intracavernous corotid artery *(open arrow)*. **C,** External carotid angiogram, lateral view, in same patient as **A** and **B.** Cavernous sinus and superior ophthalmic vein *(black arrowheads)* are equally visible, supplied by artery of foramen rotundum *(curved open arrow)*, which is distal branch of internal maxillary artery *(2)*.

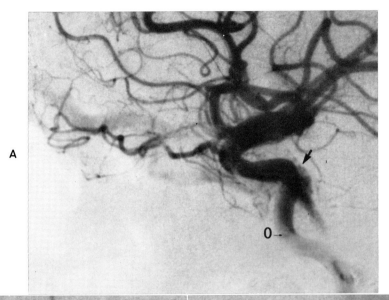

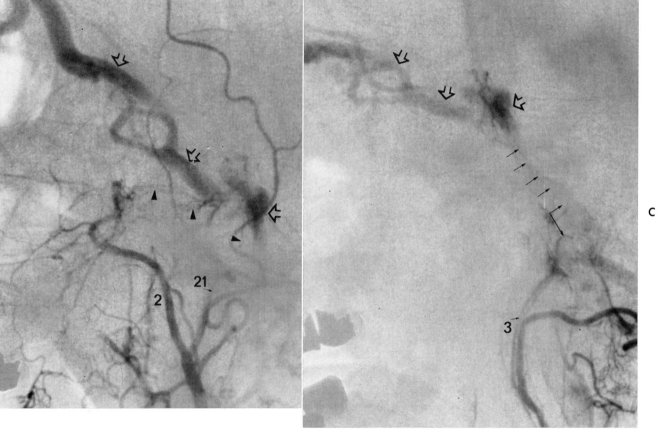

Fig. 14-78. A, Internal carotid *(0)* angiogram, lateral view, showing carotid cavernous fistula arising from the collaterals of posterior group of intracavernous carotid artery *(arrow)*. **B,** Contrast media injection of internal maxillary artery *(2)* in same patient as **A**. Notice early opacification of cavernous sinus and superior ophthalmic vein *(open arrows)* by way of all cavernous branches of internal maxillary artery *(black arrowheads)*. *21,* Middle meningeal artery. **C,** Selective contrast media injection, lateral view, of common occipitopharyngeal trunk in same patient as **A** and **B**. Identical opacification of cavernous sinus and superior ophthalmic vein *(open arrows)* as seen in **B** is present. This opacification is by way of anastomoses *(small arrows)* between median branch of lateral artery of clivus and jugular branch of ascending pharyngeal artery *(3)*. Therefore this is mixed carotid cavernous fistula arising from trunk common to posterior and lateral collaterals of intracavernous carotid artery, also known as meningohypophyseal trunk.

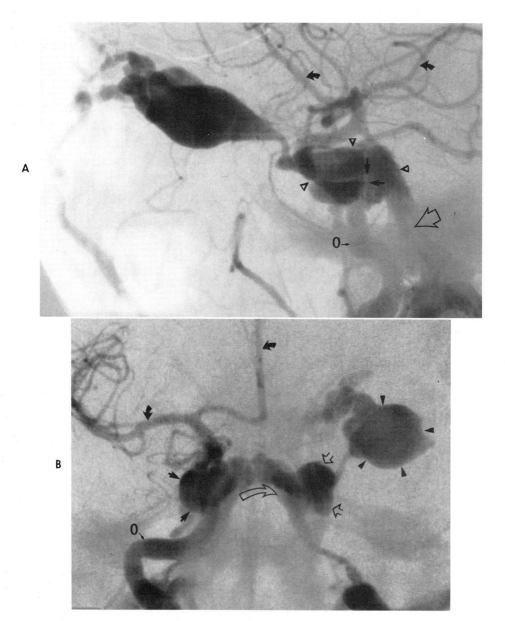

Fig. 14-79. A, Internal carotid *0* angiogram, lateral view. Carotid cavernous fistula is seen arising from tear in arterial wall of portion C5 of carotid siphon *(black arrows)*. Early opacification of cavernous sinus *(open arrowheads)* and of inferior (petrosal)sinus *(open arrow)* is seen. Notice that vascularization distal to fistula is present *(curved arrows)*. **B,** Internal carotid *(0)* angiogram, AP view in same patient as **A.** Immediate opacification of right cavernous sinus *(black arrows)* is present. Opacification of contralateral cavernous sinus *(open arrows)* by way of posterior venous confluence *(curved open arrow)*, and then contralateral superior ophthalmic vein is present. Second and third segments of contralateral superior ophthalmic vein are markedly dilated *(black arrowheads)*. Also notice normal cerebral vascularization distal to fistula *(curved arrows)*. This was pure internal carotid fistula, posttraumatic, with paradoxal ophthalmic venous drainage, leading to exophthalmos contralateral to carotid cavernous fistula.

supplied by both internal carotid arteries (by way of the median arteries of the clivus); the homolateral internal maxillary artery (by way of the artery of the foramen rotundum, accessory meningeal, and middle meningeal arteries); the two ascending pharyngeal arteries; and even the basilar trunk, if a persistent primitive trigeminal artery is present.

The great majority of these mixed fistulae are spontaneous. They appear in older subjects and are likely related to arterial aging and other predisposing factors such as arterial hypertension. Trauma may also be a contributing factor.

■ Venous drainage of carotid cavernous fistulae

Pure internal carotid fistulae, pure external carotid fistulae, and mixed fistulae must be distinguished from one another.

Pure internal carotid fistulae use nearly all the affer-

ent and efferent tributaries (mostly superior ophthalmic vein and inferior petrosal sinus) of the homolateral cavernous sinus (Figs. 14-71 and 14-72). They can also drain into contralateral veins. It is even possible to observe paradoxical venous drainage (i.e., right fistula to left venous drainage) leading to contralateral symptoms (Fig. 14-79).

The pure external carotid fistulae and the mixed fistulae preferentially drain into the superior ophthalmic system. For the pure external carotid fistulae the drainage will always be into the homolateral superior ophthalmic vein (Fig. 14-73). For mixed fistulae the drainage, while often involving the homolateral ophthalmic system, can also be bilateral (Fig. 14-80) or even contralateral.

The pathophysiology of the venous drainage of carotid cavernous fistulae is not well known. One possible explanation, particularly of paradoxical ophthalmic

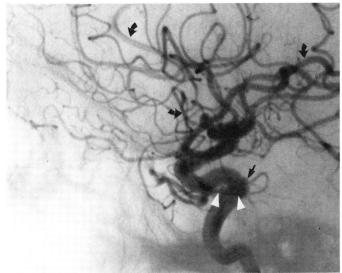

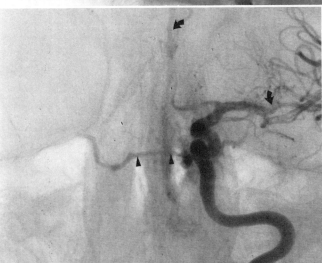

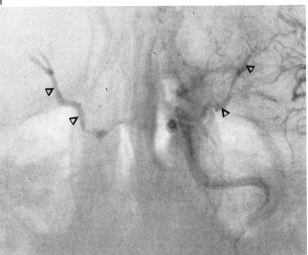

Fig. 14-80. Internal carotid angiogram. **A,** Lateral phase. **B,** Early AP phase. **C,** Late AP phase. Carotid cavernous fistula has developed from collaterals of posterior group of internal carotid artery *(black arrow)*. Venous drainage takes place initially by way of homolateral cavernous sinus in its posterior portion *(white arrowheads)* to enter opposite end of fistula through inferior coronary sinus *(black arrowheads)*. Two ophthalmic veins are also opacified *(open arrowheads)*. This was a spontaneous mixed carotid-cavernous fistula arising from collaterals of posterior group of intracavernous carotid, and presenting both bilateral and anterior venous drainage.

drainage, would be the presence of partial venous thrombosis of the ipsilateral cavernous plexus, necessitating contralateral drainage.

■ Hemodynamic aspects of carotid cavernous fistulae—high-flow, low-flow fistulae

Schematically, one must distinguish between the fistulae with high and low flow.

The high-flow fistulae create a complete hemodynamic steal of the arterial blood below the fistula. Angiographically, injection of the internal carotid artery shows rapid, early opacification of the cavernous sinus as well as its afferent and efferent channels, with total absence of distal (i.e., cephalic) vascularization (Figs. 14-71 and 14-72).

In these high-flow fistulae the hemodynamic steal also involves the vertebral and the contralateral carotid systems, as shown by opacification of the fistula during vertebral or contralateral carotid internal contrast material injection, even without compression during the angiography (Fig. 14-81). The external carotid is also frequently involved. It is thus possible to observe striking dilation of the cavernous branches of the ascending pharyngeal and internal maxillary arteries (Fig. 14-82), even though those same collaterals are not directly in-

volved in the fistula. The same is true of the ophthalmic steal, in which the Doppler effect produces complete reversal of the arterial flow (Fig. 14-83).

The low-flow fistulae direct little blood from the downstream arterial system. Internal carotid arteriography thus shows not only opacification of the fistula but also quasinormal cephalic flow (Fig. 14-84, *A*). In this type of fistula the opacification of the fistula by vertebral or contralateral carotid internal injection can be obtained only by compression of the common carotid artery on the side of the fistula (Fig. 14-84, *B* and *C*) (assuming the circle of Willis is complete).

The spontaneous evolution of carotid cavernous fistulae is a separate issue, although again one must contrast high-flow and low-flow fistulae.

The high-flow fistulae are mostly traumatic fistulae; i.e., they are usually strictly internal carotid fistulae and show no spontaneous tendency for regression.

On the contrary low-flow fistulae, which are most often spontaneous mixed fistulae, can regress spontaneously because of a decrease in the arterial pressure. These spontaneous regressions can be explained by thrombosis, which occurs inside the cavernous sinus during a local diminution in perfusion (Fig. 14-85).

Text continued on p. 669.

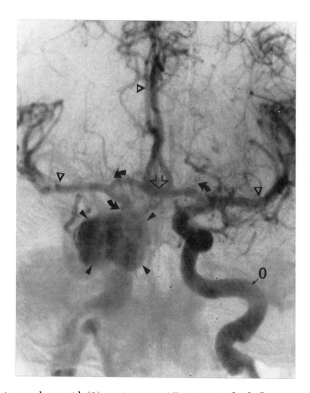

Fig. 14-81. Left internal carotid *(0)* angiogram, AP view, in high-flow contralateral carotid cavernous fistula *(black arrowheads)*. Notice that without compression on side of fistula there is shunt from left to right *(curved arrows)* by way of anterior communicating artery *(open arrow)*. Distal cerebral hemispheric vascularization is normal bilaterally *(open arrowheads)*.

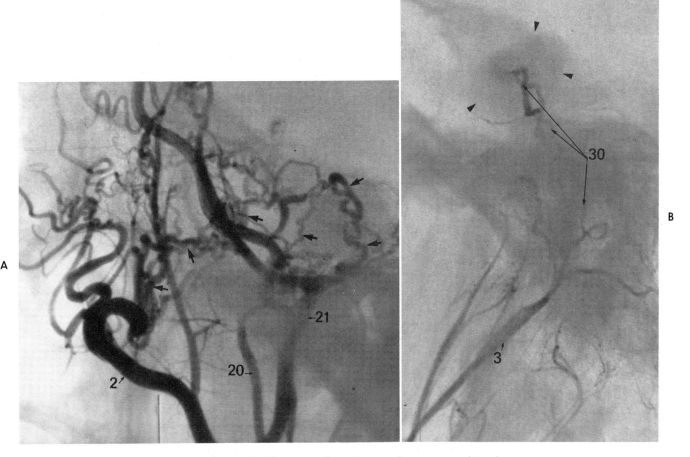

Fig. 14-82. A, External carotid and **B,** ascending pharyngeal angiograms, lateral view, in same patient as Fig. 14-71. Notice striking dilation of intracavernous collaterals *(arrows)* of internal maxillary artery *(2)* and of ascending pharyngeal artery *(3)*, in conjunction with marked increase in flow secondary to shunt caused by carotid cavernous fistula *(black arrowheads)*. In this case, false carotid external supply is present; fistula described in Fig. 14-71 remains pure internal carotid fistula. *20,* Accessory meningeal artery; *21,* middle meningeal artery; *30,* anastomosis between jugular branch of ascending pharyngeal artery and median branch of lateral artery of clivus.

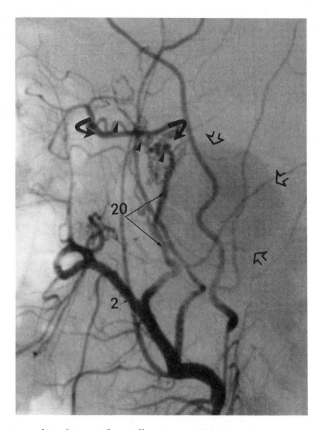

Fig. 14-83. Arteriography of internal maxillary artery *(2)* in same patient as Fig. 4-72, who developed high-flow carotid cavernous fistula caused by traumatic rupture of carotid siphon aneurysm. Notice that aneurysmal and fistulous sac *(open arrow)* is opacified by way of ophthalmic artery *(curved arrows)*, which itself is vascularized by anastomosis *(black arrowheads)* between recurrent tentorial artery and cavernous branch of accessory meningeal artery *(20)*. Hemodynamically, this appearance corresponds to ophthalmic steal and not to direct participation of ophthalmic artery in vascularization of fistula.

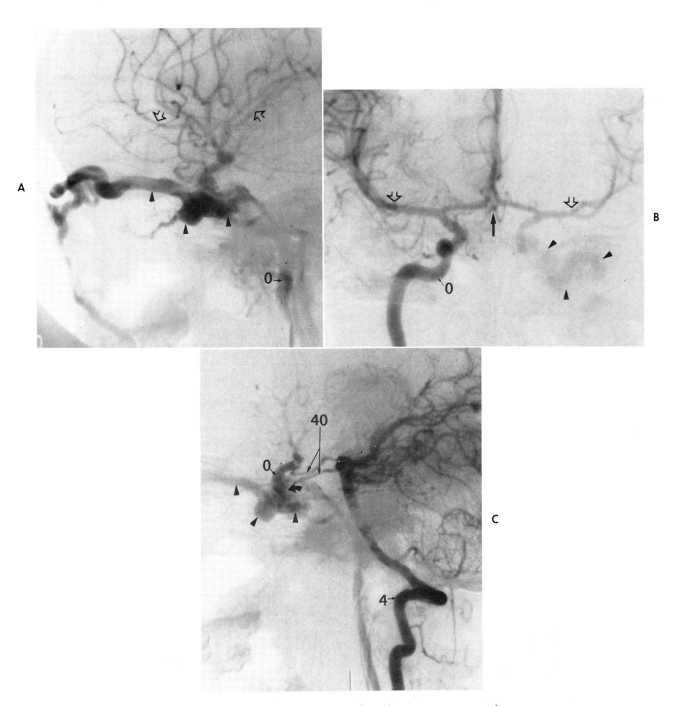

Fig. 14-84. A, Left internal carotid *(0)* angiogram, lateral view, in patient with traumatic carotid cavernous fistula developed at junction of portions C$_3$ and C$_4$ of carotid siphon. Notice early opacification of cavernous sinus and superior ophthalmic vein *(black arrowheads)*. Distal cerebral blood flow appears perfectly normal *(open arrows)*. **B,** Contralateral internal carotid *(0)* angiogram, AP view, in the same patient as **A.** Because of low-flow fistula, compression of homolateral common carotid is necessary to obtain faint opacification of fistular sac *(black arrowheads)* by way of anterior communicating artery and circle of Willis *(black arrow)*. Notice excellent bilateral hemispheric vascularization *(open arrows)*. **C,** Vertebral artery *(4)* angiogram, lateral view, with compression of ipsilateral common carotid artery in same patient as **A** and **B.** Notice excellent opacification of cavernous sinus and of superior ophthalmic vein *(black arrowheads)* by way of posterior communicating arteries *(40)* opacifying internal carotid *(0)* in retrograde fashion. This method also allows precise localization of fistular orifice *(curved arrow)* at level of part C$_3$ of carotid siphon.

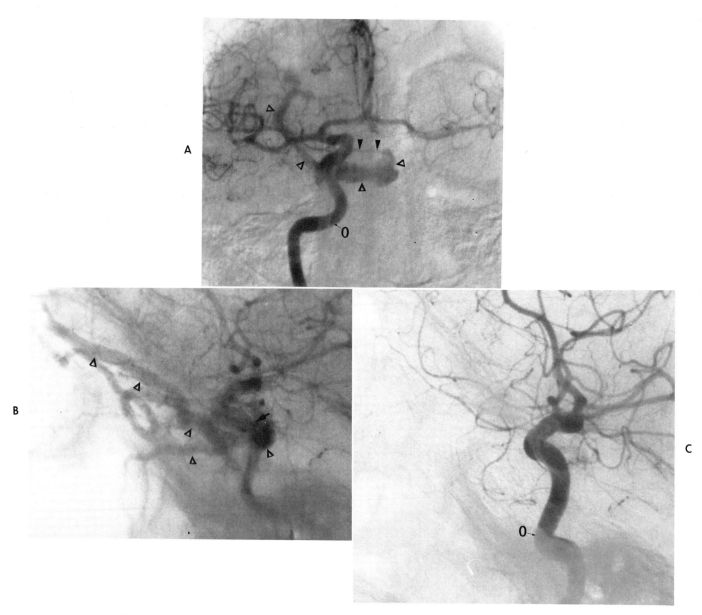

Fig. 14-85. Internal carotid *(0)* angiogram in **A,** AP and **B,** lateral views. Carotid cavernous fistula arising from meningohypophyseal trunk *(arrow)* is drained successively by posterior coronary sinus *(black arrowheads),* contralateral cavernous sinus, posterior venous confluence, and finally cavernous sinus and homolateral superior ophthalmic vein *(open arrowheads).* **C,** Immediately following angiogram, patient's symptoms spontaneously regressed. Internal carotid *(0)* angiogram made two months after first examination shows complete resolution of fistula.

■ Arteriographic evaluation in carotid cavernous fistulae

Arteriography is necessary for a precise causal and topographic diagnosis as well as therapy. This arteriographic evaluation will ideally comprise (inasmuch as the anatomic conditions and the age of the patient permit) the following procedures.

1. Injection of the ipsilateral internal carotid artery in AP and lateral views. It should also include selective lateral injections of the internal maxillary and ascending pharyngeal arteries, or, if not possible, injection of the main external carotid trunk. Finally, a lateral injection of the right or left vertebral artery with compression of the primary carotid artery homolateral to the fistula should be performed. This last injection facilitates blood flow diversion through the posterior connections towards the fistula, and gives the best view of the tear at the level of the carotid wall. It reduces superimposition of contrast material in the cavernous sinus and internal carotid artery (Fig. 14-84, C).

2. Injection of the contralateral internal carotid artery in the AP view, with compression of the homolateral common carotid. If a fistula involves the posterior group of the intracavernous collaterals of the internal carotid artery, examination of the external carotid artery and, if possible, selective injections of the internal maxillary artery and of the ascending pharyngeal artery are required.

Advances in superselective arterial catheterization and magnification-subtraction angiography are such that phlebographic studies done in the past (either by anterior opacification, using a vein of the forehead, or by posterior opacification by way of the inferior petrosal sinus) have limited use. They can be helpful in aged subjects, for whom there is a contraindication to arteriographic evaluation. They can occasionally be useful in evaluating thrombosis of the central retinal vein.

Precise topographic analysis and a complete hemodynamic study of the circle of Willis will permit evaluation and optimization of subsequent therapy.

□ **References**

1. Derreumaux, C.: Branches sensorielles et musculaires de l'artère ophthalmique. Etude embryologique et radio anatomique. Thesis for Doctorate in Medicine. Paris, 1976, Université Saint Louis Loribosiere.
2. DiChiro, G.: Angiographic topography of the choroid, Am. J. Ophthalmol. **54:**232-237,1962.
3. Dilenge, D.: Arteriography in angiomas of the orbit, Radiology **113:**355-361, 1974.
4. Hayreh, S.S., and Dass, R.: The Ophthalmic artery. I. Origin and intracranial and intracanalicular course, Br. J. Ophthalmol. **46:**65-98, 1962.
5. Hayreh S.S., and Dass, R.: The Ophthalmic Artery. II. Intraorbital course, Br. J. Ophthalmol. **46:**165-185, 1962.
6. Hayreh, S.S., and Dass, R.: The Ophthalmic artery. III. Branches, Br. J. Ophthalmol. **46:**212-247, 1962.
7. Lasjaunias, P., Vignaud, J., and Hasso, T.H.: Maxillary artery blood supply to the Orbit: normal and pathologic aspect, Neuroradiology **9:**87-97, 1975.
8. Moret, J., Lasjaunias, P., Theron, J., and Merland, J.J.: L'artère méningée moyenne: on apport à la vascularisation de l'orbite, J. Neuroradiol. **4:**225-248, 1977.
9. Padget, D.H.: Development of the cranial arteries in the human embryo, Contrib. Embryol. Carneg. Instit. **32:**205-262, 1948.
10. Rothman, S.L.G., Kier, D.L., Allen, W.E., and Pratt, A.G.E.: Arteriographic topography of orbital lesions, AJR **122:**607-620, 1974.
11. Singh, S., and Dass, R.: The central artery of the retina. I. Orgin and course, Br. J. Ophthalmol. **44:**193-211, 1960.
12. Vignaud, J., Clay, C., and Aubin, M.L.: Orbital arteriography, Radiol. Clin. North Am. **10**(1):39-61, 1972.
13. Zimmerman, R.A., and Vignaud, J.: Ophthalmic arteriography. In Arger, P.H., editor: Orbit Roentgenology, New York, 1977, John Wiley & Sons, Inc.

SECTION THREE

Dacryocystography

Charles J. Schatz

The radiographic evaluation of the lacrimal drainage system was first described by Ewing[5] and is of great value in the evaluation of patients with tearing (epiphora). Epiphora is commonly encountered by general ophthalmologists, and surgery is often indicated to relieve the symptom. Dacryocystography is capable of determining patency of the canaliculi, lacrimal sac, and nasolacrimal duct. When disease is present, the site and degree of obstruction and the presence of fistulae, diverticula, and concretions are evaluated with a dacryocystogram.

This chapter will detail the use of dacryocystography,

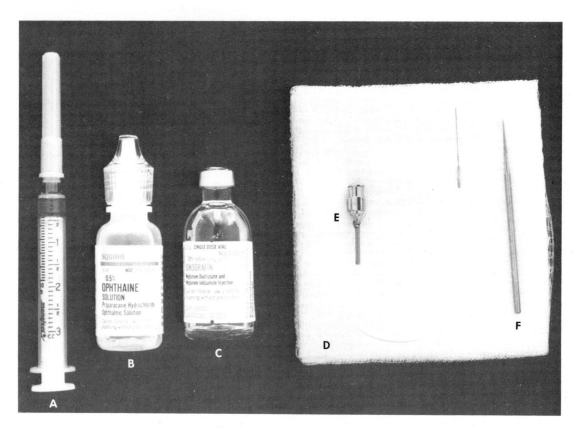

Fig. 14-86. Equipment used in dacryocystography: *a*, 3 ml syringe with 20 gauge needle; *b*, topical ophthalmic anesthetic; *c*, aqueous contrast material; *d*, gauze pads; *e*, blunt-tipped 27 gauge needle with approximately 25 cm of polyethylene tubing; *f*, lacrimal dilator.

including equipment, contrast materials, radiographic methods, and normal and pathologic conditions of the nasolacrimal apparatus.

□ Equipment

The equipment I used is shown in Fig. 14-86. The dacryocystogram needle can be made by grinding off the sharp point of a 27 gauge lymphangiogram needle on a grinding stone. The tip of the modified needle should be rounded and polished so that no metallic burrs remain. An alternative to this needle is a tapered catheter as described by Iba and Hanafee[7] made from no. 18 Teflon tubing.

□ Contrast materials

Ewing[5] used bismuth subnitrate in liquid petrolatum as the contrast material. Since then, many different opaque media have been described. Ethiodized oil (Ethiodol) was used by Campbell, Carter, and Doub.[2] Iodized oil (Lipiodol) was used by Hourn.[6] Iophendylate (Pantopaque) was used by Milder and Demorest.[12] Neohydriol was used by Agarwal.[1]

Oily materials, however, have disadvantages in the nasolacrimal system. Firstly, if they are extravasated, they can remain in the soft tissues for many years. Sargent and Ebersole[13] reported such a case that revealed a considerable amount of residual contrast material more than 3 years after oily contrast material was extravasated into the periorbital tissues. Secondly, oily opaque material is not completely miscible with tears and can fail to fill the entire nasolacrimal system, causing limitations diagnostically. Thirdly, it is more viscous than tears and often requires heating to reduce the viscosity before injecting, especially with iodized oil as described by Law.[8] When not heated, oily material requires a greater injection pressure than aqueous contrast material. "Physiologic" aqueous solution in the form of methylglucamine diatrizoate 40% (methylglucamine iodipamide 20%, Sinografin) has been used by Sargent and Ebersole[13] for dacryocystography. This material is nonirritating, water soluble, miscible with tears, and similar in viscosity and pH to tears. Sinografin is an excellent contrast material for dacryocystography. It can be used with all of the techniques used in this procedure.

□ Radiographic techniques

Since the original description of Ewing[5] many radiographic techniques for dacryocystography have been described. The commonly used techniques will be mentioned.

Macrodacryocystography, first described by Campbell,[3] uses a magnification technique after van der Plaat's description[15] of radiographic magnification technique.

Kinetic dacryocystography, used by Epstein[4] and Trokel and Potter,[14] uses a cinematography format for evaluating the anatomy and function of the nasolacrimal apparatus.

Distention dacryocystograph, described by Iba and Hanafee,[7] involves plain radiographs that are obtained during injection of the contrast material.

Intubation macrodacryocystography, described by Lloyd, Jones, and Welham,[9] combines distention dacryocystography and macrodacryocystography.

Subtraction dacryocystography, described by Lloyd and Welham,[10] combines intubation macrodacryocystography with a standard photographic subtraction technique.

Tomographic dacryocystography, which uses complex-motion tomography, is the technique used by the author. This technique gives excellent detail of the nasolacrimal apparatus, and both the frontal and lateral planes are obtained. The technique demonstrates filling defects, obstruction, fistulae, and diverticula with improved detail over all other techniques because of the thin scan sections that complex-motion tomography can produce. Most of the illustrations in this section were obtained from examinations using this technique.

□ Injection techniques

The injection procedure for dacryocystography requires local ophthalmic anesthesia. This is done after placing the patient on the examination table in the supine position. Following scout films, a few drops of the anesthetic agent are instilled into the conjunctival sac. Approximately 2 ml of the radiopaque material is drawn into the syringe and the lacrimal cannula and tubing are connected. The syringe, tubing, and cannula should be freed of all air bubbles. The lower lid is then slightly everted and the lower punctum is dilated with the lacrimal dilator. The region of the lacrimal sac is palpated; any fluid present in the sac should be expressed through the punctum or into the nose. The lacrimal cannula is then placed into the inferior punctum, where it should remain for the remainder of the procedure. The tubing is taped to the patient's face. The injection is then made and films are taken immediately. If distention dacryocystography or intubation dacryocystography is used, the films are obtained during the injection.

□ Indications for dacryocystography

Dacryocystography is indicated in patients with epiphora when a mechanical obstruction, lacrimal apparatus fistula or diverticulum, lacrimal concretion, lacrimal sac operative failure, or recurrent inflammatory disease of uncertain cause is suspected after the clinical examination. When there is a definite chronic obstruction on the clinical examination, the only treatment is surgery. The dacryocystogram is used to determine the site of obstruction and the presence of fistulae or diverticula so that the appropriate surgical procedure can be performed. This procedure is usually a dacryocystorhinostomy.

□ The normal dacryocystogram

The lacrimal system consists of the inferior canaliculus, superior canaliculus, common canaliculus, lacrimal sac, and nasolacrimal duct (Fig. 14-87). Tears from the conjunctival sac enter the inferior or superior canaliculi through their respective puncta in the eyelids immediately lateral to the medial canthus. After a short vertical segment there is a horizontal segment of each canaliculus. The superior and inferior canaliculi merge medially to form the common canaliculus (sinus of Maier). The common canaliculus is from 1 to 3 mm in length and enters the lateral aspect of the nasolacrimal sac near the junction of the upper and middle thirds. Radiographic measurements of the nasolacrimal apparatus were reported by Malik et al.[11] (Table 14-3). Any distention of the sac greater than 4 mm on the frontal radiograph is considered pathologic. The lacrimal sac ends in a slight taper caused by a mucosal fold (valve of Krause) slightly above the rim of the orbit. At this level the nasolacrimal duct begins. There is a central mucosal construction called the valve of Taillefer and a distal constriction called the valve of Hasner. The duct ends at the inferior meatus of the nose, beneath the inferior turbinate.

Table 14-3. Normal lacrimal passage dimensions*

Area	Dimension	Mean (in mm)	Range (in mm)
Lacrimal sac	Vertical diameter	11.10	6-14
	Lateral diameter	2.43	1-4
	Anteroposterior diameter	4.00	1-6
Nasolacrimal duct	Vertical diameter	20.97	13-26
	Lateral diameter	2.30	1-4
	Anteroposterior diameter	2.84	1-4

*From Malik, S.R.K., Gupta, A.K., Chaterjee, S., et al.: Br. J. Ophthalmol. **53:**174, 1964.

Fig. 14-87. Anatomy of normal lacrimal system. (After Campbell, W.: The radiology of the lacrimal system, Br. J. Radiol. **37:**1, 1964.)

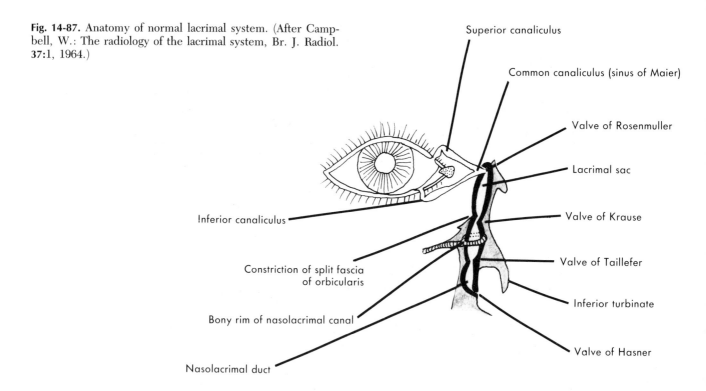

Superior canaliculus

Common canaliculus (sinus of Maier)

Valve of Rosenmuller

Lacrimal sac

Valve of Krause

Valve of Taillefer

Inferior turbinate

Valve of Hasner

Inferior canaliculus

Constriction of split fascia of orbicularis

Bony rim of nasolacrimal canal

Nasolacrimal duct

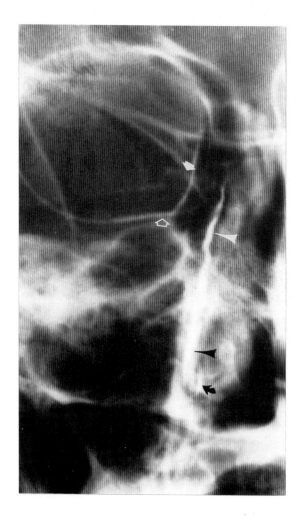

Fig. 14-88. Normal plain film dacryocystogram on right side. Superior canaliculus *(white arrow)*, inferior canaliculus with cannula in place *(open arrow)*, lacrimal sac *(white arrowheads)*, nasolacrimal duct *(black arrowhead)*, contrast material in nose *(curved arrow)*.

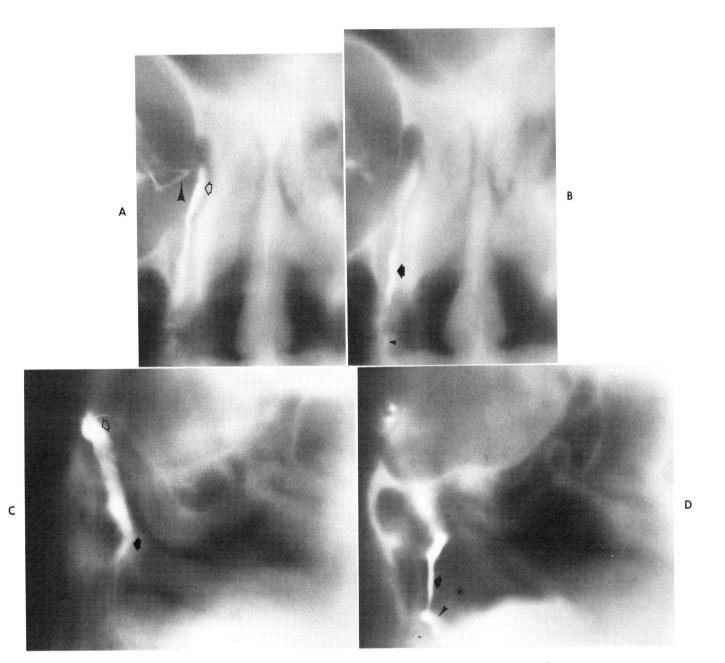

Fig. 14-89. Normal right tomographic dacryocystogram. **A,** AP view, anterior section; showing canaliculi *(arrowhead)* and lacrimal sac *(open arrow)*. **B,** AP view, posterior section, showing nasolacrimal duct *(arrow)* and contrast material in nose *(arrowhead)*. **C** and **D,** Lateral views, showing lacrimal sac *(open arrows)*, nasolacrimal duct *(closed arrow)*, and contrast material in nose *(arrowhead)*.

In the normal dacryocystogram the canaliculi, lacrimal sac, and nasolacrimal duct are not dilated, and contrast material is identified in the nose (Figs. 14-88 and 14-89). The lacrimal sac and nasolacrimal duct have a linear configuration. Frequently the patient will taste the contrast material within a few seconds of the injection because the contrast material drains from the nose into the pharynx and onto the base of the tongue in an unobstructed system.

□ Pathology of the nasolacrimal system

Tears are secreted by the lacrimal gland situated laterally and superiorly to the globe. Under normal circumstances the tears either evaporate from the surface of the globe or drain into the lacrimal passages, where they pass into the inferior meatus of the nose. Epiphora has two causes, as described by Campbell.[3] The first is excessive lacrimation, which results in inadequate evaporation and drainage for the greater volume of tears. Dacryocystography in this entity is normal. The second cause is obstructive epiphora, which results from complete or incomplete obstruction of the lacrimal system. A normal flow of tears cannot be adequately handled by the diseased drainage system. Dacryocystography of these lesions is abnormal.

■ **Obstruction**

Complete or incomplete obstruction can occur. In my series, approximately 90% of obstructions are complete and 10% are incomplete. The most common site of obstruction is at the junction of the lacrimal sac and nasolacrimal duct (Figs. 14-90 and 14-91). The second

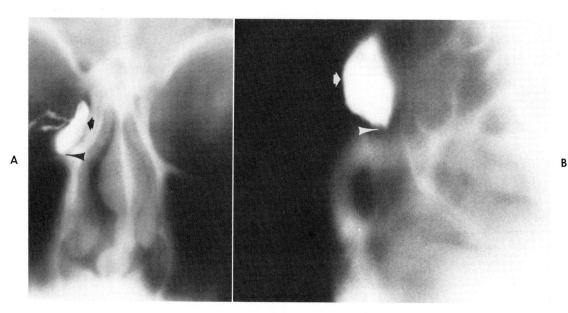

Fig. 14-90. Right tomographic dacryocystogram, showing typical configuration of lacrimal drainage system in patient with history of chronic dacryocystitis and radiographic findings of obstruction at junction of lacrimal sac and nasolacrimal duct. **A,** Frontal tomogram. **B,** Lateral tomogram. *Arrowhead,* Obstruction; *arrow,* dilated lacrimal sac.

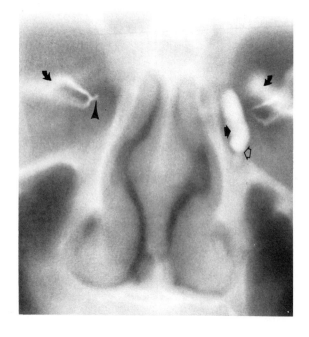

Fig. 14-91. Bilateral tomographic dacryocystogram revealing obstruction of common canaliculus *(arrowhead)* on right and obstruction at junction of lacrimal sac and nasolacrimal duct on left *(open arrow).* Dilated lacrimal sac is seen on left *(arrow).* Contrast material is seen in conjunctival sacs *(curved arrows)* from reflux through superior canaliculi.

most common site is at the common canaliculus (Fig. 14-91). These conclusions agree with Campbell[3] and Malik et al.[11] Less frequently the obstruction occurs within the lacrimal sac (Fig. 14-92).

Radiographically, the lacrimal sac above the obstruction will usually be dilated and will have an ovoid or rounded configuration (Figs. 14-90 to 14-92) rather than the normal linear configuration. Because the dilated sac is palpable below the medial canthus, the lesion has been called a "mucocele of the lacrimal sac" by Campbell.[3] Rarely, the sac will be constricted above the obstruction (Fig. 14-93).

When there is obstruction, there is usually reflux of the contrast material into the conjunctival sac through the uncannulated punctum (Figs. 14-91 to 14-93). This will be seen during the injection of a small volume of contrast material if the conjunctival sac is observed.

Again, the obstruction may be incomplete (Fig. 14-94). The dacryocystogram usually demonstrates a dilated lacrimal sac above the incomplete obstruction. Also, contrast material must be visualized in the nose to confirm the incomplete obstruction.

Various factors cause obstruction and include congenital stenosis, inflammatory processes, trauma, including

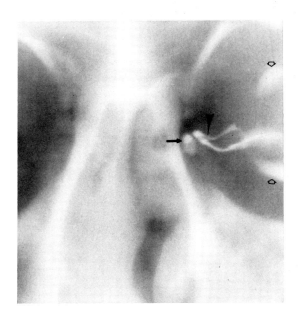

Fig. 14-92. Left tomographic dacryocystogram revealing obstruction in lacrimal sac *(arrow)*. *Arrowhead,* Canaliculi; *Open arrows,* contrast material in conjunctival sac.

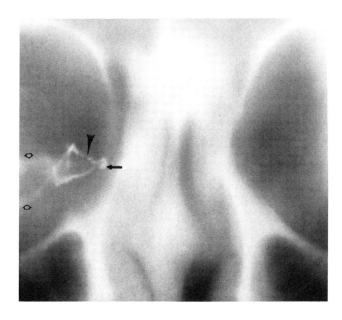

Fig. 14-93. Right tomographic dacryocystogram revealing high obstruction of lacrimal sac *(arrow)*. Notice that lacrimal sac is not dilated above obstruction. *Arrowhead,* Canaliculi; *open arrows,* contrast material in conjunctival sac.

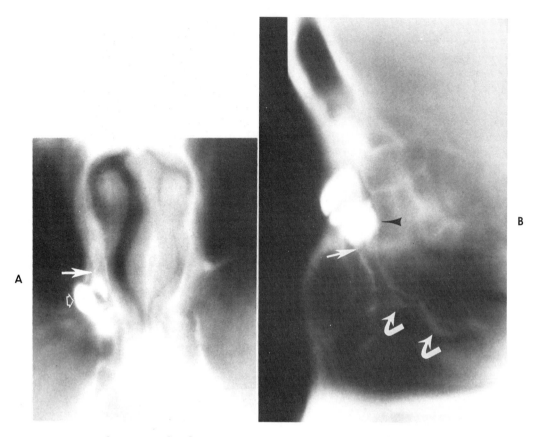

Fig. 14-94. Right tomographic dacryocystogram. **A,** AP view. **B,** Lateral view. Partial obstruction *(arrow)* is seen at junction of lacrimal sac and nasolacrimal duct. Notice dilated lacrimal sac *(arrowhead)* proximal to obstruction. Also notice diverticulum *(open arrow)* on AP view. Contrast material in nose (curved arrows) is seen on lateral view.

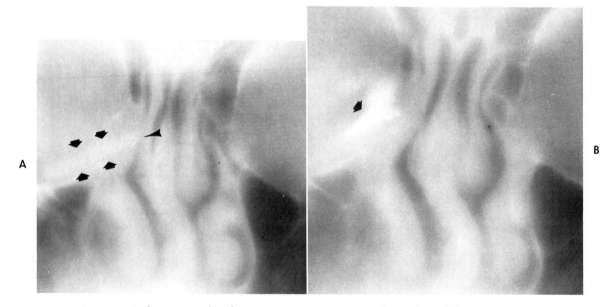

Fig. 14-95. Right tomographic dacryocystogram in patient with epiphora following operative repair of inferior "blow-out" fracture. **A,** Scout film showing silastic implant *(arrows)* with its medial end over nasoacrimal area *(arrowhead).* **B,** Contrast in obstructed and distorted lacrimal sac *(arrow)* at medial end of silastic implant.

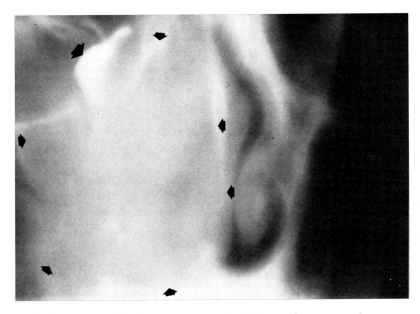

Fig. 14-96. Right tomographic dacryocystogram in 68-hear-old woman with squamous cell carcinoma of right maxillary sinus and nasal airway. Patient had epiphora caused by tumor's invasion into lacrimal bone and lacrimal sac. Tumor *Small arrows,* Tumor; *large arrow,* Dilated lacrimal sac.

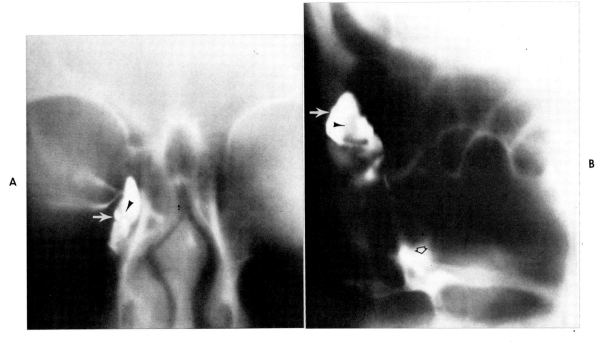

Fig. 14-97. Right tomographic dacryocystogram in patient with 10-year history of epiphora. **A,** AP view. **B,** Lateral view. Filling defect *(arrowhead)* in dilated lacrimal sac *(arrow)* represents concretion of *Actinomyces israelii* found at surgery. Obstruction was seen to be incomplete because contrast material is seen in inferior meatus on lateral view *(open arrow).*

foreign bodies (Fig. 14-95), and tumors (Fig. 14-96). Occasionaly with an inflammatory obstruction, a filling defect is seen in the canaliculi or obstructed nasolacrimal sac. This filling defect frequently represents a mycotic concretion of *Actinomyces israelii* (Fig. 14-97). A frequent artifact simulating a concretion is an air bubble injected into the nasolacrimal system during the dacryocystogram (Fig. 14-98). A cross-table lateral view will demonstrate the air bubble floating in the lacrimal sac (Fig. 14-98, *B*). In contradistinction, a concretion should not float in the contrast material.

■ Fistulae and diverticula

Fistulae and diverticula of the canaliculi or lacrimal sac are usually the result of longstanding obstruction (Fig. 14-94). An obstruction following trauma and facial fractures may result in a lacrimal sac–cutaneous fistula (Fig. 14-99).

Fistulae and diverticula are seen only in obstructed or partially obstructed nasolacrimal systems and will remain until adequate drainage is restored. In addition, it is not possible to diagnose a diverticulum preoperatively without a dacryocystogram.

■ Surgical devices

Occasionally, surgery for epiphora is unsuccessful or the obstruction is too high in the nasolacrimal apparatus to allow for a dacryocystorhinostomy. In many of these cases a drainage tube is placed between the medial canthus and the nasal cavity, allowing relief of the epiphora. These tubes are radiopaque and should be recognized as iatrogenic foreign bodies (Fig. 14-100).

□ Acknowledgement

I wish to thank Mrs. Barbara Chapman for her secretarial assistance in typing this manuscript and Mr. Steven Y. Shapiro for his photographic assistance.

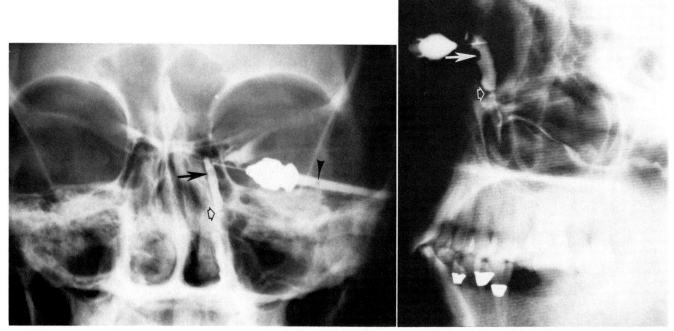

Fig. 14-98. Plain left dacryocystogram: **A,** Frontal view. **B,** Cross-table lateral view. Filling defects are air bubbles in dilated acrimal sac *(arrow)* and in plastic tubing *(arrowhead).* Notice appearance of air bubble on cross-table lateral view. Partial obstruction is present *(open arrow).*

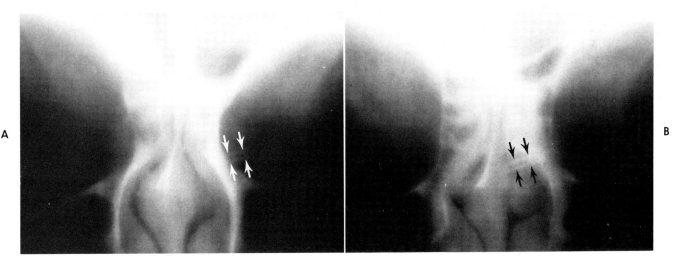

Fig. 14-99. Right dacryocystogram of 19-year-old patient with epiphora and dacryocystocutaneous fistula draining below inferior orbital rim. **A,** Frontal plain film view. **B,** Frontal tomographic view *Arrow,* dilated lacrimal sac; *arrowheads,* fistula; *curved arrow,* metallic marker on skin surface at cutaneous end of fistula.

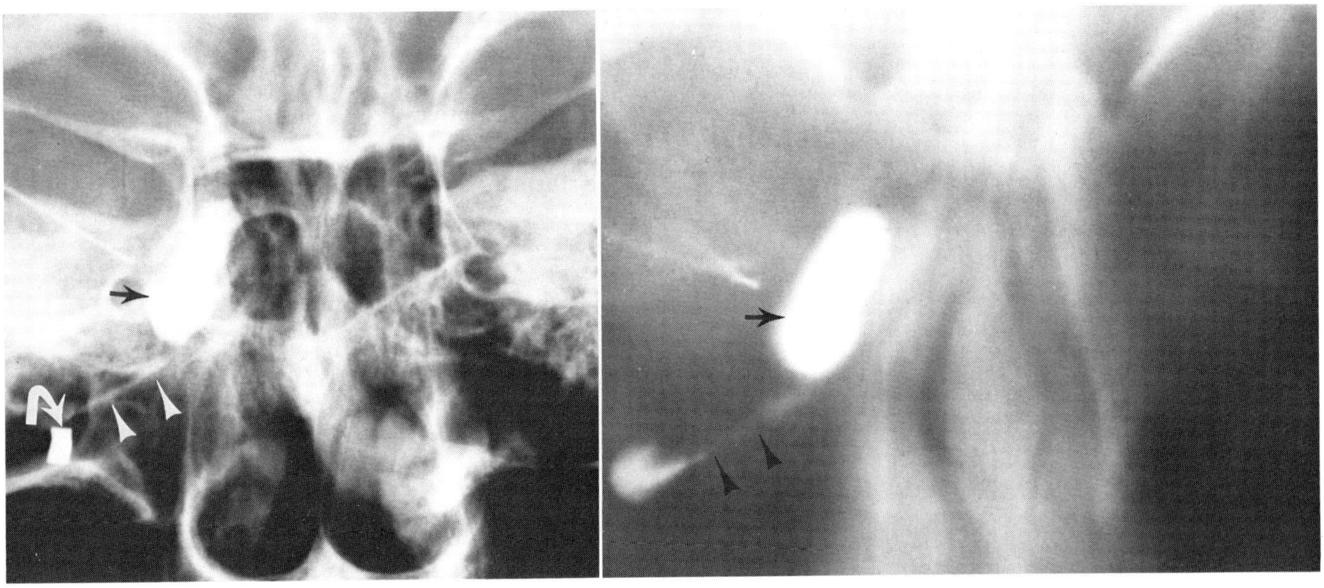

Fig. 14-100. AP tomograms demonstrating lacrimal drainage tube *(arrows)* between medial canthus and nose on left side. Patient had history of epiphora with unsuccessful dacryocystorhinostomy, requiring placement of drainage tube.

□ References

1. Agarwal, M.L.: Dacryocystography in chronic dacryocystitis, Am. J. Ophthalmol. **52**:245, 1961

2. Campbell, D.M., Carter, J.M., and Doub, H.P.: Roentgen ray studies of the nasolacrimal passageways, Arch. Ophthalmol. **51**:462, 1922.

3. Campbell, W.: The radiology of the lacrimal system, Br. J. Radiol. **31**:1, 1964.

4. Epstein, E.: Cine dacryocystography, Trans. Ophthalmol. Soc. UK **81**:284, 1961.

5. Ewing, A.E.: Roentgen ray demonstration of the lacrimal abscess cavity, Am. J. Ophthalmol. **26**:1, 1909.

6. Hourn, G.E.: X-ray visualization of the naso-lacrimal duct, Ann. Otol. Rhinol. Laryngol. **46**:962, 1937.

7. Iba, G.B., and Hanafee, W.N.: Distention dacryocystography, Radiology **90**:1020, 1968.

8. Law, F.W.: Dacryocystography, Trans. Ophthalmol. Soc. UK **87**:395, 1967.

9. Lloyd, G.A.S., Jones, B.R., and Welham, R.A.N.: Intubation macrodacryocystography, Br. J. Ophthalmol. **56**:600, 1972.

10. Lloyd, G.A.S., and Welham, R.A.N.: Subtraction macrodacryocystography, Br. J. Radiol. **47**:379, 1974.

11. Malik, S.R.K., Gupta, A.K., Chaterjee, S., et al.: Dacryocystography of normal and pathological lacrimal passages, Br. J. Ophthalmol. **53**:174, 1969.

12. Milder, B., and Demorest, B.H.: Dacryocystography. I. The normal lacrimal apparatus, Arch. Ophthalmol. **51**:180, 1954.

13. Sargent, E.N., and Ebersole, C.: Dacryocystography: the use of Sinografin for visualization of the nasolacrimal passages, AJR **102**:831, 1968.

14. Trokel, S.L., and Potter, G.D.: Kinetic dacryocystography, Am. J. Ophthalmol. **70**:1010, 1970.

15. van der Plaats, G.F.: X-ray enlargement technique, J. Belg. Radiol. **33**:89, 1950.

15 □ Head and neck lesions in children

C. KEITH HAYDEN, Jr., and LEONARD E. SWISCHUCK

A wide variety of head and neck lesions, both congenital and acquired, may be encountered in infants and children. Some of these lesions are similar to those encountered in adults but many others are unique to the pediatric patient. Although the value of conventional tomography, contrast laryngography, xeroradiography, and computerized tomography in the evaluation of upper airway disease in adults has been stressed, the vast majority of childhood conditions can be diagnosed with simple plain film radiography.* The reason for this is that air within the structures of the upper respiratory tract provides a natural contrast medium for the accurate delineation and evaluation of the adjacent soft tissues of the neck.[4] Most of these assessments are made on the lateral neck film obtained during inspiration, with the patient's neck partially extended. A lesion will rarely go undetected if these criteria are met. However, additional views (i.e., lateral films in expiration or frontal views in inspiration or expiration) or additional studies (i.e., esophagrams or fluoroscopic examination in the frontal and lateral projections) can be employed as the need arises. Improved visualization of the airway on both frontal and lateral views can be accomplished by combining increased filtration of the x-ray beam, a higher kilovoltage technique, and magnification.[227,401] However, these added parameters to the standard roentgenographic examination are not required in most cases.

□ Normal anatomy
■ Upper airway

On the properly obtained roentgenographic examination of the upper airway, all of the normal structures are readily identified (Fig. 15-1). It might be noted, however, that the prevertebral soft tissues and the airway in general are extremely pliable in infants; thus with expiration and flexion of the neck a wide variety of distortions and bizarre configurations can result (Figs. 15-2 and 15-3). In addition, the retropharyngeal soft tissues appear proportionately thicker in the newborn and young infant than in the older infant. The reason for this is that the vertebral bodies are not yet fully ossified and part of their mass is included in the prevertebral soft tissue space. It is therefore difficult to outline precise prevertebral soft tissue measurements for this age group. Nevertheless, a good rule of thumb for the young infant is that in the lateral view during inspiration, with the infant's neck fully extended, the soft tissue space from C1 to C4 (level of the larynx) can normally be up to one and one half times the width of the neighboring vertebral bodies.[423] As the infant matures the space is proportionately decreased so that in the older child these same soft tissues do not measure over 3 mm in thickness. In children of all ages the prevertebral soft tissue space normally doubles in thickness at the level of the larynx. This represents the point at which the esophagus separates from the airway (cricopharyngeus muscle). Nasopharyngeal adenoidal tissue is sparse in the newborn, but as the infant grows older this tissue becomes more abundant. Usually it first appears at about the age of 3 months[68] (Table 15-1).

■ Paranasal sinuses

Contrary to popular belief, sinuses are present in the young infant and can become infected. Of course, not all of the paranasal sinus cavities are developed at birth; the ethmoid and maxillary sinuses are primarily examined in the infant.* Because of their size, they often are

*References 67, 110, 247, 423.

*References 27, 292, 357, 372, 436.

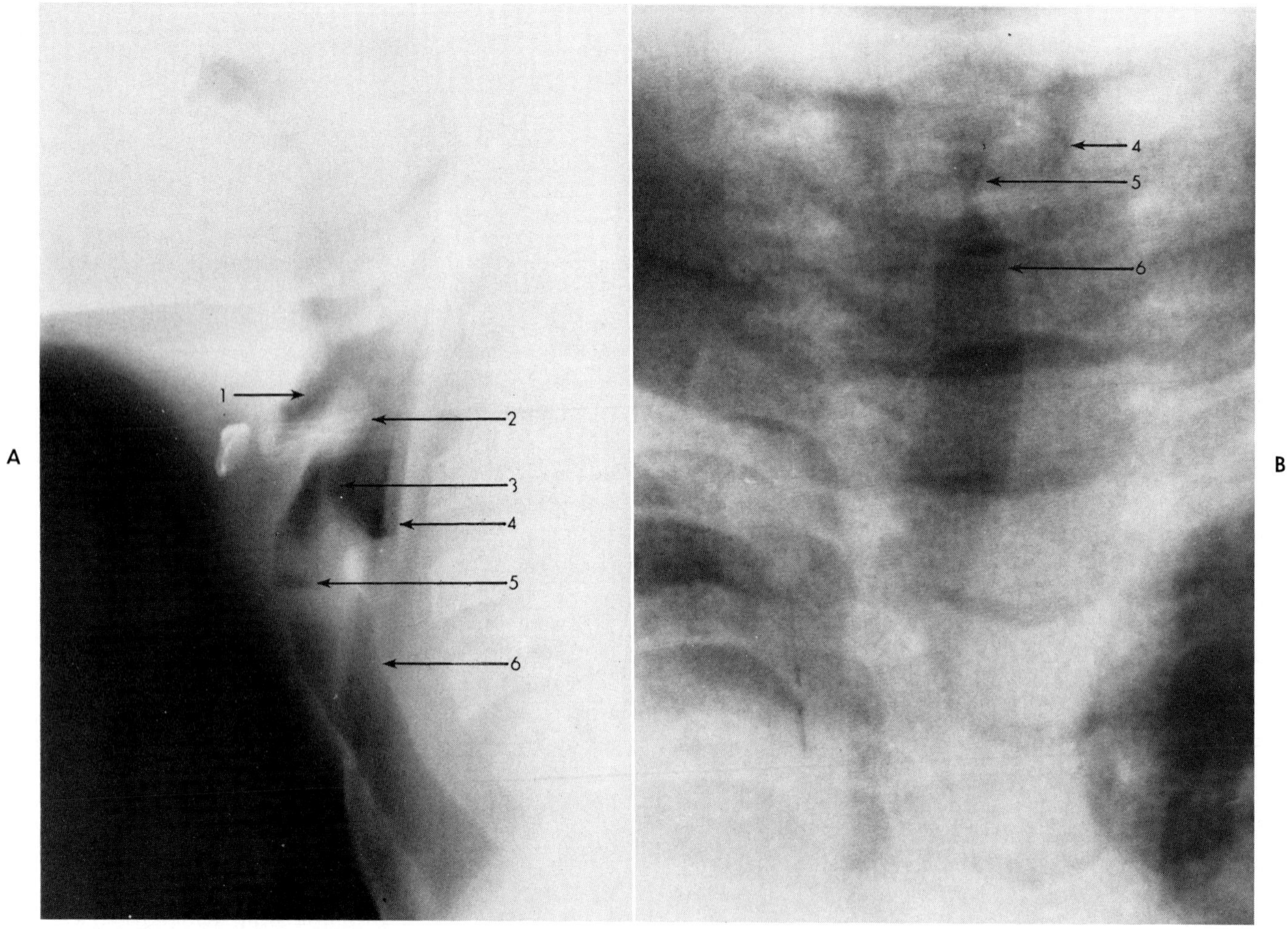

Fig. 15-1. Normal anatomy. **A,** Lateral view demonstrating, *1*, valleculae; *2*, epiglottis; *3*, aryepiglottic folds; *4*, pyriform sinuses, *5*, laryngeal ventricle; and, *6*, subglottis and upper trachea. False and true cords are above and below ventricle, respectively. **B,** Frontal view demonstrating, *4*, pyriform sinuses; *5*, true vocal cords; and, *6*, subglottis.

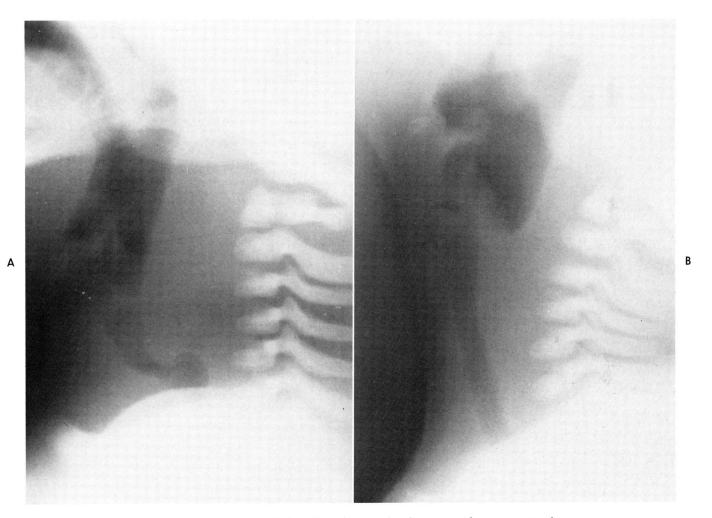

Fig. 15-2. A, Lateral view reveals buckling of airway, producing pseudomass in retropharyngeal region. **B,** Properly positioned study during full inspiration demonstrates normal airway and retropharyngeal soft tissues.

Fig. 15-3. A, Lateral poor inspiratory film reveals lack of distension of upper airway. Retropharyngeal mass is suggested *(arrows)* that is continuous with lower margin of adenoids and which represents normal lymphoid tissue. **B,** During deep inspiration pseudomass disappears.

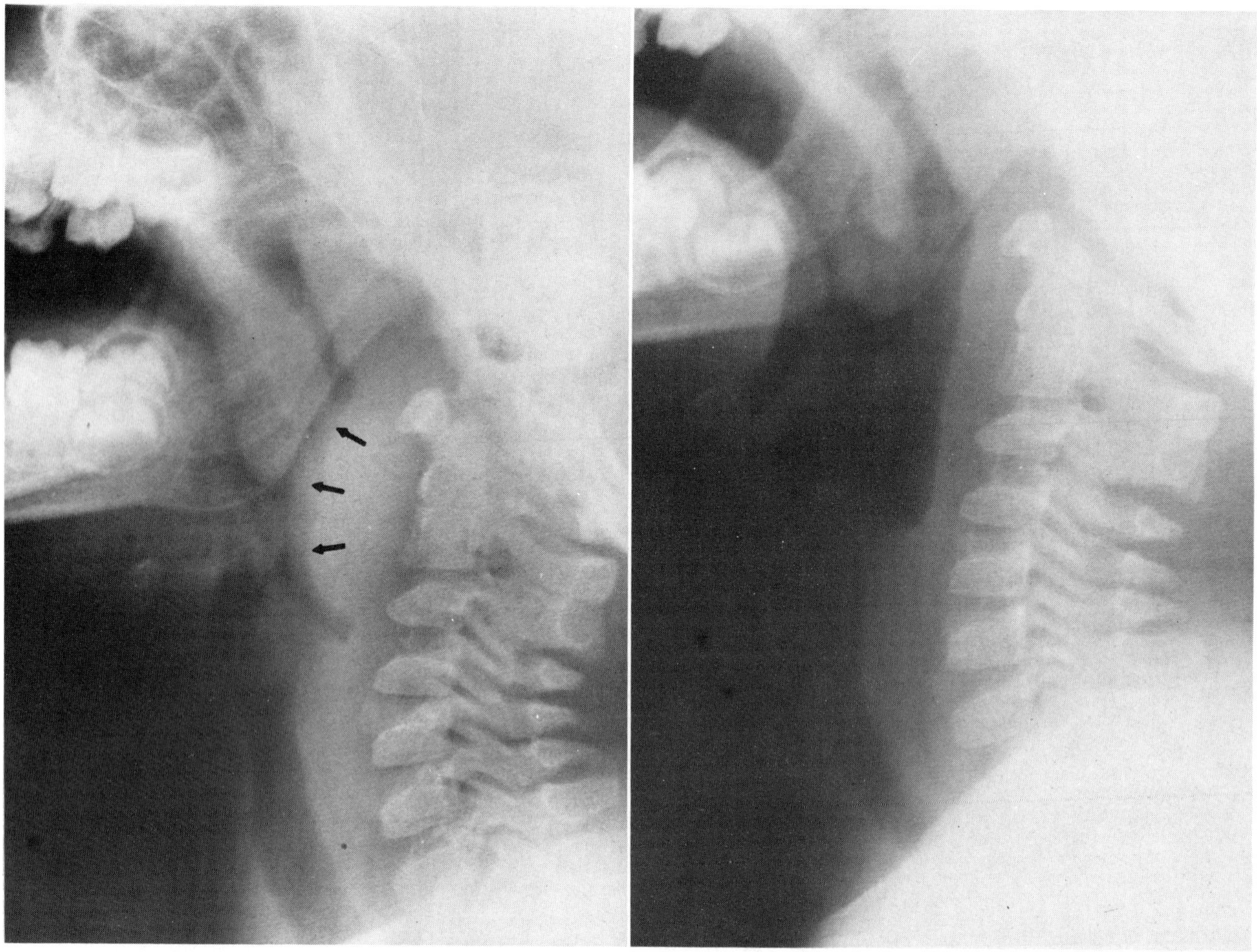

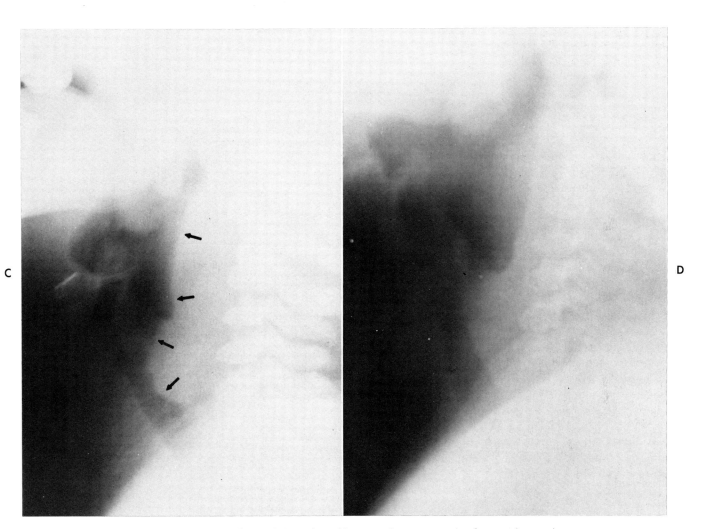

Fig. 15-3, cont'd. C, Another infant with similar pseudomass in retropharynx *(arrows).* **D,** During full inspiration pseudomass disappears. Notice, however, faint soft tissue density projecting into posterior hypopharynx. This represents lymphoid tissue projecting into distended hypopharynx.

Table 15-1. Normal nasopharyngeal lymphoid tissue*

| | | Thickness of soft tissue | | |
Age	No. of infants	0.0 cm	0.5 cm or less	Over 0.5 cm
1 day to 1 month	36	36	0	0
1 to 3 months	76	36	39	1
3 to 6 months	47	7	25	15
6 to 12 months	56	0	16	40
12 to 24 months	42	0	3	39

*From Capitanio, M.A., and Kirkpatrick, J.A.: Radiology, **96**(3):389-391, 1970.

not clearly visualized radiographically. With proper positioning, however, it is surprising how often they are demonstrable. In terms of positioning the lateral views pose no problem, but the Waters view can be quite critical. Typically, the Waters view in the adult is made by placing the oribitomeatal line at an angle of 37° with the plane of the film. In the older child this angle must be decreased to about 28°; otherwise the projection will be too steep for proper evaluation of the maxillary antrae. In the young infant the angle must be even less and the view is actually almost a PA view, with the forehead being only slightly off the cassette (1 to 2 cm). Using this technique, the maxillary and ethmoid sinuses are well visualized (Fig. 15-7, *B*). Other views are probably of no real value in children, at least for the evaluation of inflammatory disease.

The maxillary sinuses develop as evaginations from the fetal nasal chamber and are first recognizable anatomically at 85 days of embryonic life.[218,372] At birth the maxillary sinus is an elongated cavity measuring approximately 8 to 10 mm in length, 3 to 4 mm in width, and 3 to 5 mm in height.[27] Because of their small size, one can appreciate readily that proper positioning is most critical to antral visualization and assessment.

The ethmoid sinuses begin their development at about 6 months of fetal age, originating from recesses in the lateral walls of the middle, superior, and supreme meati of the fetal nasal chamber.[357,372,436] These sinuses, like the maxillary sinuses, are radiographically visualized at birth. The anterior ethmoid group of sinus cavities average 5 mm in height, 2 mm in width, and 2 mm in depth, while the posterior group average 5 mm, 4 mm, and 2 mm, respectively.[372] By contrast, the frontal and sphenoid sinuses develop after birth, with the sphenoid sinuses often being visualized by 2 years of age, but more generally being demonstrable (90%) by the age of 4 years.[145] The frontal sinuses are not demonstrable radiographically until approximately 4 to 8 years of age.

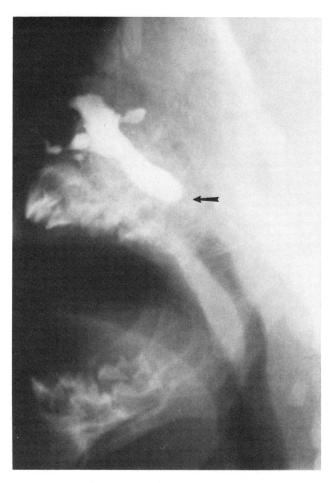

Fig. 15-4. Choanal atresia. Lateral view reveals obstruction of oily contrast material at level of posterior nares *(arrow).*

□ The nose, face, and sinuses
■ Choanal atresia

Choanal atresia represents a congenital obstruction of the nasal passage that can be either membranous or bony,[457] high or low, unilateral or bilateral. The atresia, or stenosis, can be complete or partial. With bilateral atresia immediate postnatal respiratory distress occurs because the normal newborn infant does not know how to breath through the mouth. After 2 to 6 weeks of life, mouth-breathing is learned[23,119,462]; but in the meantime, insertion of an oral airway can avoid a tracheostomy.[136,279,393] Unilateral choanal atresia, on the other hand, generally poses much less of a clinical problem[23,393] and usually goes unnoticed until either the unaffected nostril is blocked by mucous or mucosal swelling or the patient becomes aware that he cannot blow his nose on one side. When involvement is unilateral it is generally rightsided.[136]

Plain film examination of the nasal passages shows no

abnormal finding, whereas contrast studies quickly and easily demonstrate the abnormality. The instillation of a small amount of oily iodinated contrast material into the nose quickly demonstrates the level of obstruction. In a normal nasal passage the contrast material quickly passes into the nasopharynx, but in choanal atresia it remains in the obstructed nasal passage (Fig. 15-4).

■ Nasal masses

Nasal masses in infants and children generally appear with symptoms of nasal obstruction, rhinorrhea, or epistaxis. Masses encountered include developmental lesions (i.e., encephaloceles, dermoid clefts, or cysts), inflammatory lesions, and benign or malignant neoplasms. Both encephaloceles and dermoid clefts or cysts most commonly are located in the midline. Encephaloceles, it might be recalled, are more common in the occipital region; when they occur in the frontal area they are classified as nasofrontal, nasoethmoid, nasoorbital, transethmoid, or sphenomaxillary. They usually appear at birth; however, a second peak of incidence occurs at about age 5, and previously undiagnosed encephaloceles have even been discovered in patients as old as 60 years.[38,470]

Radiographically, CT scanning is most productive in the assessment of frontal encephaloceles.[63] In investigating this lesion it is particularly important to determine whether it is nasofrontal or nasoethmoid in type because this facilitates proper neurosurgical correction.[184] The nasofrontal encephaloceles occur above the nasal bones while the nasoethmoid encephaloceles occur under the nasal bones. Thus in the latter the nasal bones are elevated, while in the former they are depressed. In addition, the cribriform plate is depressed in nasofrontal encephaloceles, and a large V-shaped defect is present in the frontal bone. This causes a slanting lateral displacement or bowing of the superior aspect of the medial orbital wall but no true hypertelorism. With nasoethmoid encephaloceles a circular defect is present between the orbits and under the nasal bones, and definite hypertelorism is present.

The other developmental mass occurring in the region of the nose is the midline cleft, a lesion almost always associated with a sinus tract (i.e., congenital dermal sinus) or dermoid cyst. Indeed, both may be present, and the classical clinical sign of a dermoid cyst is the presence of a small dimple overlying the lesion. Histologically, the cysts are walled with squamous epithelium containing pilosebaceous material,[52] and both the tracts and the cysts have varying relationships to the nasofrontal bones and the nasal septum. Intracranial connections are not as common as when the lesion occurs in the occiput.[309,339]

Tumors of the nose are not particularly common in children; however, occasionally either a benign inflammatory or more commonly an allergic polyp will be encountered.[275] Polyps also occur with cystic fibrosis; various authors have shown an incidence ranging from 10% to 25%.[216,300,377] Such polyps have been shown to be present in children as young as 2 years of age but usually are seen between the ages of 4 and 12 years. They tend to be less common in adolescents.[408] No correlation between the severity of cystic fibrosis and the incidence of polyps has been demonstrated.[217] Surgery is the treatment of choice for the nasal polyps of cystic fibrosis,[408] but local steroid application can be useful in the treatment of allergic polyposis.[299] The diagnosis of nasal polyps is clinical, and the main radiographic findings center around associated sinus disease.

Chronic hypertrophic polypoid rhinosinusitis is a condition undoubtedly related to allergic nasal polyps but representing severe disease. This condition affects the entire upper respiratory epithelium and is characterized by vasomotor instability, polypoid mucosal hypertrophy, and superimposed infection.[460] The polyps may be unilateral or bilateral and most frequently occur in the nose and ethmoid sinuses. Other sinuses can also be involved. The resulting expansion of the ethmoid sinuses and nasal cavities can be so marked that hypertelorism and widening of the nasal bridge result.

A final type of nasal polyp is the antrochoanal polyp. This polyp usually is a solitary benign growth that arises in the maxillary antrum of a nonatopic patient and then passes through the ostium of the sinus, back through the nose, and finally into the posterior nasopharynx (Fig. 15-5). Approximately 71% of patients with antrochoanal polyps are between the ages of 10 and 29 years,* and histologically the polyps are similar to benign inflammatory polyps.

Radiographically the paranasal sinuses in these patients have a very high incidence of associated abnormality. Ipsilateral sinus opacification was present in 57.4% of patients, and bilateral or multiple sinus involvement was seen in 42%.[187] A nasopharyngeal soft tissue mass was demonstrated in only 11.4% of patients. In another study,[182] associated ipsilateral sinus disease was present in 69.2% of patients, and bilateral or multiple sinus disease was found in 23% of patients. In only one patient, however, was a choanal mass demonstrable.

Generally, this benign soft tissue polyp does not erode or destroy contiguous soft tissue or bony structures, but various authors[75,189,433] have described a few cases showing evidence of expansion of the involved maxillary antrum and erosion of the lateral antral wall. As far as treatment of these patients is concerned, it has

---

*References 182, 187, 400, 424.

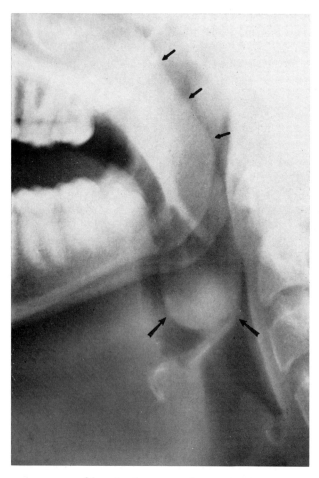

Fig. 15-5. Antrochoanal polyp. Lateral view reveals soft tissue mass *(lower arrows)* hanging down into hypopharynx. Notice that it extends from maxillary sinus into posterior nasal cavity *(upper arrows)*.

been shown that the best results are obtained with either intranasal antrostomy or a Caldwell-Luc operation.[433] When simple snare or avulsive polypectomy is performed, there is a recurrence rate of approximately 20%.[182,187]

True neoplasms of the nasal fossa in childhood are very uncommon. A variety of benign lesions can be encountered, including teratomas, fibrous histiocytomas,[389] chondromas, and neurofibromas. Nasal glioma is a relatively rare congenital neural malformation of the nasofrontal region[2,190,262] that consists of a mass of extracranial glial tissue enclosed in a fibrous capsule. The tumor may be connected to the brain by a pedicle of glial tissue, which is estimated to occur in 15% to 25% of cases.[262,402] However, the tumor does not connect with the cerebrospinal fluid space and thus is different from a frontal encephalocele.[34] Thirty percent of these tumors are intranasal, 60% extranasal, and 10% com-

bined.[245] Often these lesions appear with a progressively enlarging mass over the bridge of the nose. Hypertelorism and localized bone erosion can occur. CT scanning or tomography of the cribriform plate and cristi galli can determine whether or not these lesions communicate intracranially.

Malignant neoplasms can also be encountered; the most common one is the rhabdomyosarcoma.[105,112] Other malignant lesions very infrequently encountered are the olfactory neuroblastoma,[132,310] malignant teratoma,[101] and lymphoma. Radiographically, these tumors have about the same appearance, except for the possible presence of calcification in teratomas.

■ Sinusitis

Contrary to popular belief, sinusitis is a common problem in infancy and early childhood. Although it has been stated that the roentgenographic examination of the paranasal sinuses for inflammatory disease is rather futile in children[395] some valuable information can be obtained with proper filming. In addition, we do not believe that normal sinuses can be opacified simply by tears entering them in a crying infant. When one accepts the fact that the ethmoid and maxillary sinuses generally are present at birth and certainly are present in young infants,[357,372,436] then one should not be surprised to see sinus infection in this age group. Of course, this is not to say that the roentgenographic diagnosis of such infection is easy but only that it is possible.

Further complicating the problem is the fact that symptoms of sinusitis in infants and children often are less severe than they would be in the older child and adult.[240,281,366] Adults with sinusitis usually have pain over the involved area, headaches, and fever; however, in infants and children, more insidious signs such as chronic rhinorrhea, persistent cough (usually at nighttime because of a postnasal drip), and recurrent bouts of otitis media are more common.[240] In addition, there is clinical confusion between the symptoms of congestive rhinitis and actual sinusitis. For example, in the early stages of a viral upper respiratory tract infection, the patient feels congested. The nasal mucosa and the mucosa of the sinuses are congested, but not to the point at which obliteration of the sinus cavities occurs. For this reason the sinuses usually are clear radiographically at this stage of the infection, and the main problem is rhinitis. Later on, however, after the acute infection has subsided, residual sinus disease remains, often with superimposed bacterial infection. Indeed, the major predisposing factor to suppurative sinus infection is ostium occlusion, and the most common cause of such occlusion is viral upper respiratory infection or allergy.[214,216,343] Less frequently, mechanical abnormali-

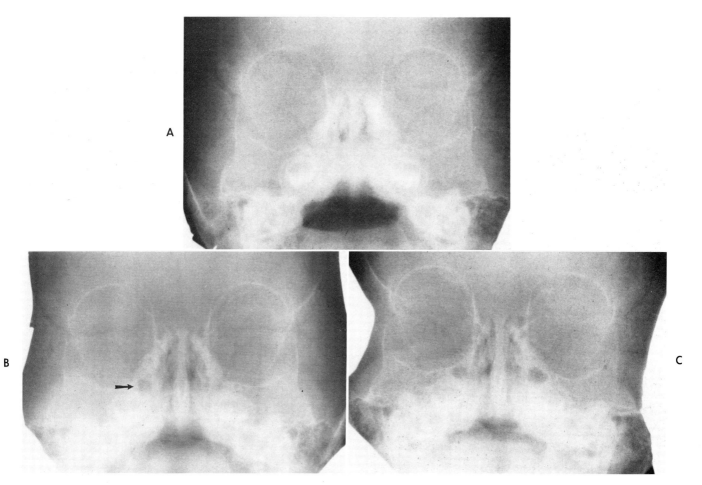

Fig. 15-6. Sinusitis in infant. **A,** Waters view reveals maxillary sinuses totally obliterated, as are anterior ethmoid sinus cavities. Erroneous interpretation of absence of maxillary and ethmoid sinus cavities can be made. **B,** With treatment, there was aeration of right maxillary sinus *(arrow)* and both ethmoid sinus cavities. Left maxillary sinus cavity still is obliterated. **C,** With completion of treatment both maxillary sinus cavities and both ethmoid air cell groups are aerated. This is normal appearance.

ties such as septal dislocation as a result of birth trauma,[216] unilateral choanal atresia,[142] and cleft palate[214] may be causative factors associated with sinusitis. Patients with cystic fibrosis commonly also have sinus disease,[243] and radiographic evidence of sinusitis in these children has been documented in 90% to 100% of cases.[152,305,377]

Since the introduction of antimicrobial agents, most of the acute infections involving the paranasal sinuses are treated successfully, and complications are few. However, complications still can occur.[75,150,186] In some cases infection spreads by way of anastomosing veins or by direct extension to nearby structures such as the orbit and central nervous system, and it has been suggested recently that anaerobic infections may be important contributing factors to these complications.[49] In

children, maxillary and ethmoid sinus disease frequently leads to proptosis because of associated orbital cellulitis and edema. In most of these patients true osteomyelitis of the bones of the orbit is not present, but the soft tissues are markedly inflamed. CT scanning can be extremely useful in defining the problem in these patients.

Radiographically, the findings of sinusitis vary according to the patient's age. In the very young infant, inflammatory changes are more of a challenge to assess because the sinuses are smaller and proper positioning of the patient is more difficult to attain. Nevertheless, with a properly obtained Waters view (not too steep) both the maxillary and ethmoid sinuses can be seen with clarity; when they are not radiolucent (Figs. 15-6 and 15-7) they are diseased. In younger infants the

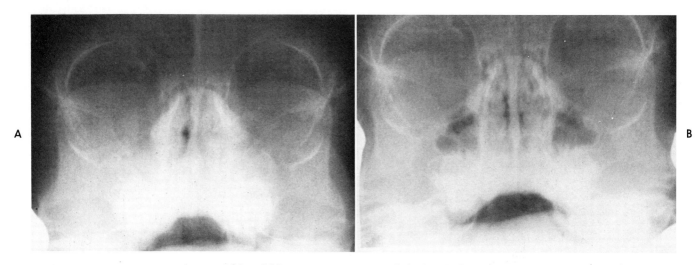

Fig. 15-7. Sinusitis in older child. **A,** Waters view reveals both maxillary sinus cavities totally obliterated. Erroneous interpretation of their being absent could be made. Notice that ethmoid air cells are aerated. **B,** After treatment all sinus cavities are normally radiolucent.

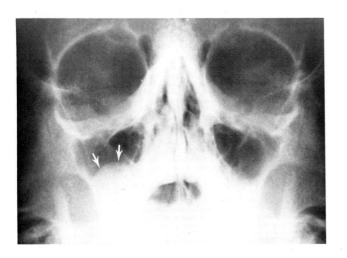

Fig. 15-8. Waters view reveals characteristic appearance and location of retention cyst in right maxillary sinus *(arrows).*

sinus cavities usually become airless, but as the child becomes older degrees of mucoperiosteal thickening can be distinguished. In the acute phases of infection, air-fluid levels and total sinus opacification can be seen. Variable bony wall demineralization occurs, and in some patients there are residual mucous retention cysts. Most often these latter lesions occur in the maxillary sinuses and appear as smooth, mucous-filled epithelial cysts arising from the floor or wall of the sinus cavity (Fig. 15-8). Most of them eventually disappear.

■ Paranasal sinus masses

Tumors of the paranasal sinuses are uncommon. Most often the lesion is some type of sarcoma (i.e., rhabdo-

myosarcoma, lymphosarcoma) although occasionally one encounters an odontogenic tumor. Roentgenographic changes in these patients depend on the demonstration of bone destruction, calcification, and associated soft tissue change. Polyps of the sinuses also are not particularly common but can be seen in patients with allergic conditions, in those with chronic infections, and in patients with cystic fibrosis. Secondary involvement of the sinuses can occur with tumors arising in the nasopharynx, such as angiofibromas and chordomas. In addition, sinus involvement can occur on a secondary basis with leukemia, lymphoma, reticuloendotheliosis, and metastatic neuroblastoma.

Mucoceles of the paranasal sinuses are uncommon in

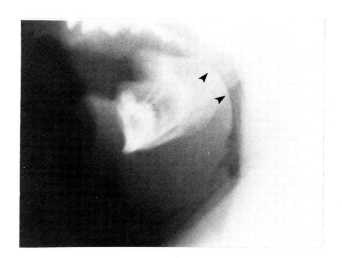

Fig. 15-9. Mandibular hypoplasia. Lateral view reveals very small mandible in infant with Treacher-Collins syndrome. Notice how retropositioned mandible and tongue cause compression of airway *(arrows)*.

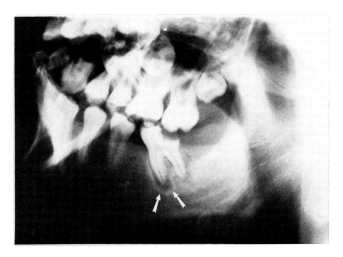

Fig. 15-10. Lateral view reveals characteristic appearance of root abscess or so-called radicular cyst *(arrows)*. Also notice caries in molar.

children. They represent complete filling of the sinus cavity with mucoid secretion as a result of obstruction of the sinus ostium. Most occur in the frontal or ethmoid sinuses, and the roentgenographic findings consist of complete opacification of the sinus with expansion of the sinus cavity. In the far advanced lesions erosion of the sinus wall can occur.[295,399]

□ Mandible

■ Hypoplasia (micrognathia)

Hypoplasia of the mandible can involve the entire mandible or just one side. When unilateral underdevelopment is present the condition is referred to as hemifacial microsomia. In such cases, associated temporomandibular joint hypoplasia, facial hypoplasia, and congenital hearing defects can occur.[73,88,413]

Generalized hypoplasia of the mandible results from abnormal development of the first and second branchial arches[160,161] and can be seen with a variety of syndromes, including Pierre Robin syndrome, Goldenhar's syndrome, Weyers mandibulofacial dysostosis,[453] and Treacher Collins syndrome.[280,359,413] It can also be seen with a number of chromosomal abnormalities, including trisomy 17-18, trisomy 13-15, and cri-du-chat syndrome. Because of the underdevelopment of the mandible in these cases, there is mandibular underbiting and recessing of the mandible into the oropharynx (Fig. 15-9). All of these factors, in addition to the tongue being displaced posteriorly, lead to severe airway compromise with marked respiratory distress[365] and on occasion to cor pulmonale with pulmonary edema.[80] Pharyngeal hypoplasia has been described[396] in addition to mandibular hypoplasia in Treacher Collins syndrome.

As the infant grows older the mandible usually becomes larger, more normal in position, and less prone to produce airway obstruction. Nevertheless, in early life mandibular hypoplasia and its associated posterior displacement of the tongue can produce profound respiratory distress, particularly if the infant is kept in the recumbent position. Therefore these infants should be kept in a prone position, and it has been suggested that prolonged nasotracheal intubation be used.[412]

Numerous variations of mandibular hypoplasia exist, including isolated hypoplasia of the mandibular rami and smallness of the mandible with a pointed symphysis menti (a deformity usually seen with aglossia).

■ Infection or inflammation

Osteomyelitis of the mandible can be seen in association with infected teeth or as part of a widespread hematogenous osteomyelitis. When part of a widespread infection, the organisms most frequently involved are the same as those seen with osteomyelitis involving the long bones (*Staphylococcus aureus, Haemophilus influenzae,* and *Streptococcus*).

Actinomycosis uncommonly involves the mandible, and when it does it usually arises from an adjacent gum infection. Radiographically, the findings of osteomyelitis usually consist of irregular bony destruction, localized osteopenia, and occasionally periosteal new bone reaction. In chronic infections, such as those usually seen with actinomycosis, bone sclerosis is often present. The radiographic appearance of osteomyelitis may be difficult to differentiate from that of other destructive lesions of the mandible.

Apical periodontal (radicular) cysts result from tooth

infection. Invariably there are caries in the crown of the involved tooth, and an area of bony destruction around the tooth root is seen radiographically. This results in a periapical granuloma that then can undergo cystic transformation and produce a typical apical periodontal cyst (Fig. 15-10).

As pointed out earlier, periostitis involving the jaw may be seen secondary to osteomyelitis; however, the most common cause of periostitis in the pediatric age group is Caffey's disease (infantile cortical hyperostosis). In the early stages the periosteal reaction may be layered, and in the latter stages one may see massive deposition of periosteal new bone. Almost all patients with Caffey's disease develop periosteal reaction along the mandible sooner or later; this is usually considered a hallmark of the condition.

A lesser known cause of periostitis is that seen with inflammation of the adjacent soft tissues (cellulitis).[421] In these cases there is no osteomyelitis; the findings represent a reactive periostitis that disappears with appropriate antibiotic therapy.

■ Trauma

Fractures involving the mandible result from direct blows and often involve two sites, as in the adult. This is probably because of the ringlike configuration of the mandible. Single fractures also commonly occur and usually are not too difficult to detect radiographically. In the adult, these fractures may occur through the body or the condylar process, but in the young infant condylar fractures very frequently are of the greenstick variety. They are best demonstrated on the Towne or Caldwell views of the head. Dislocation of the mandible is not particularly common in the pediatric age group although it can occur.

■ Tumors and tumorlike lesions

Primary tumors of the mandible are uncommon in children.* In contrast to the adult, in whom odontogenic lesions predominate, fibro-osseous lesions and giant cell granulomas make up the majority (about 64%)[96] of the primary mandibular tumors in childhood. Fibro-osseous lesions of the mandible include fibrous dysplasia,[91,154,204] ossifying fibromas,[3,376] and cementifying fibromas. Of these, fibrous dysplasia is the most common and usually is discovered in children or adolescents as a painless, slowly developing facial asymmetry.[440] Radiographically the lesion is cystic in appearance and somewhat bubbly and multiloculated; it causes expansion and cortical thinning of the mandible. Teeth in the involved area generally do not show resorption or displacement. When the lesion occurs bilat-

*References 29, 96, 225, 256.

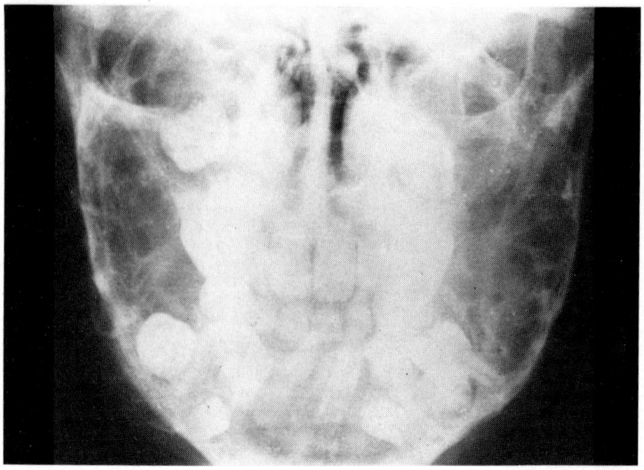

Fig. 15-11. PA view reveals the typical multiloculated appearance and associated malpositioning of teeth in patient with bilateral fibrous dysplasia (cherubism).

erally it often has a familial pattern, and the term *cherubism* is used (Fig. 15-11).

Ossifying and cementifying fibromas appear as unilocular defects with distinct margins and variable amounts of calcification within the tumor. Histologically, the calcified material formed by the tumor can be typical bone or can resemble cementum.[440] There continues to be debate concerning the origin of these tumors, although many authors think the tumors arise from the primitive mesenchyma surrounding the tooth.[178]

The other more common primary tumor encountered in the mandible is the giant cell granuloma or reparative granuloma, a lesion that usually occurs in childhood. Painless swelling is the most frequent initial symptom encountered with this lesion.[96] There is some confusion as to whether this lesion represents a true neoplasm[441] or represents reactive changes in response to trauma.[29,217] Most authors now seem to favor the latter concept. Radiographically the changes are distinctive but not diagnostically specific. Generally there is evidence of a large, well-circumscribed osteolytic defect, most commonly involving the posterior body and ramus of the mandible (Fig. 15-12).

Other nonodontogenetic tumors are rarely encountered. They include fibrosarcomas, osteogenetic sarcomas, and a variety of benign tumors such as fibromas, fibromyxoid fibromas, osteomas, and osteoblastomas.[62,235,242]

Most of the odontogenetic tumors of the mandible are either ameloblastomas* or a variety of cementomas or odontomas. Ameloblastomas usually produce multi-

*References 71, 107, 208, 466.

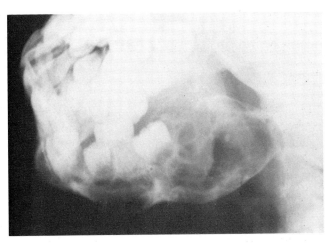

Fig. 15-12. Oblique view of mandible reveals multiloculated lesion expanding mandibular ramus and body. There is associated malpositioning of teeth. Findings are not pathognomonic but are characteristic of large reparative granuloma.

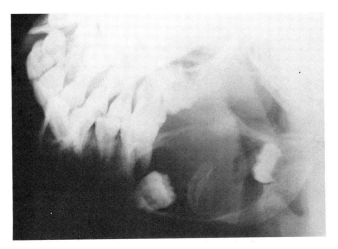

Fig. 15-13. Oblique view of mandible reveals typically unilocular, well-demarcated appearance of dentigerous cyst. Also notice displaced teeth.

locular expanding cystic radiolucent lesions, and cementomas or odontomas produce lesions with varying degrees of increased radiodensity.

Finally, there are a variety of other tumorlike primary lesions that can be seen to involve the jaw. These include various solitary odontogenic and aneurysmal bone cysts of the jaw.* Odontogenic cysts are basically either primordial or dentigerous (follicular) cysts. Primordial cysts are rare. They arise in the developing tooth bud before the crown is formed and thus represent an unformed tooth. They are detected when such a cyst is present and there is an absence of an adult

tooth in an adjacent location. Dentigerous cysts, on the other hand, arise in the tooth after the crown is formed but before the tooth erupts. The usually displaced unerupted tooth always lies in the wall of the cyst. Radiographically the cyst's margins are well defined, and the impacted or unerupted tooth is clearly visible (Fig. 15-13). Occasionally the roots of the involved tooth have been eroded. As a rule it is believed that when the normal tooth bud cyst (which surrounds all of the unerupted teeth in the child) becomes larger than 2 cm in diameter the involved tooth will become part of a dentigerous cyst and therefore never erupt. A small but definite number of dentigerous cysts will develop into ameloblastomas. Radiographically this malignant degeneration may be impossible to detect, and the roentgenographic picture is that of a routine dentigerous cyst. Finally, it should be noted that dentigerous cysts can be common manifestations of the basal cell nevus syndrome.

■ Systemic disease with mandibular involvement

Mandibular involvement may be seen with a variety of systemic disease processes. Bone marrow tumors in children not infrequently will involve the mandible; these include leukemia, lymphoma,* and metastatic malignancy (the most common being neuroblastoma, although a number of other sarcomas also can involve the mandible on a secondary basis). All these lesions produce mottled destruction of the mandible and destruction or disruption of the adjacent teeth. With leukemia and lymphoma there is a lesser tendency to produce periosteal new bone formation, while with metastatic neuroblastoma, spiculated new bone formation and periosteal layering are more common.

Lytic destructive lesions are a more common feature of histiocytosis,[117] and the mandible is an often involved site.[285,381,399] Most commonly this is seen with Letterer-Siwe's disease in infants or Hand-Schuller-Christian disease in young children. In the early stages the bone destruction may be difficult to differentiate from that produced by other lesions. In the more advanced cases, however, the mandible literally disappears and the teeth seem to float in the destroyed mandibular tissue; Thus the term *floating teeth* sign.

Generally speaking, mandibular abnormalities associated with metabolic diseases are seen with hyperparathyroidism (either primary or secondary) and rickets. In hyperparathyroidism the early findings usually consist of demineralization of the mandible and disappearance of the lamina dura. In more advanced cases, however, the mandible can become very mottled and absorption of the tips of the teeth roots can occur. In rickets the

*References 28, 31, 99, 385.

*References 58, 79, 81, 133.

mandible also shows demineralization and loss of the lamina dura, and in advanced cases the mandible appears to be washed out. The enamel of the teeth, however, remains very dense and the teeth appear to float in the demineralized mandible.

A number of bone dysplasias may show relatively characteristic findings. In ectodermal dysplasia the mandible may be underdeveloped, but the characteristic finding is absence or dysplasia of the teeth.[67,174] In osteogenesis imperfecta the teeth frequently are underdeveloped, with both the deciduous and permanent teeth being smaller than normal and demonstrating poorly formed roots. In osteopetrosis the mandible usually is not involved in the early stages. However, the mandible later becomes thickened and sclerotic. In these cases the teeth often become loose and are lost prematurely.

Not infrequently the temporomandibular joint is involved in juvenile rheumatoid arthritis. There may be ankylosis of the temporomandibular joint, which causes marked limitation of jaw motion. Eventually, condylar resorption and destruction can lead to underdevelopment of the mandibular ramus.[22,116,360]

□ Tongue
■ Macroglossia

Most abnormalities of the tongue leading to its enlargement can be diagnosed without radiographic assistance, but a large tongue can be seen with primary tumors such as rhabdomyosarcoma,[257] hemangioma, or lymphangioma. Non-neoplastic tumor enlargement of the tongue can be seen with ectopic thyroid tissue,[350] enteric duplication cysts,* cretinism, and Beckwith-Wiedemann syndrome.

■ Microglossia

A small tongue is seen less commonly and often is associated with a small mandible (see discussion of mi-

---

*References 51, 122, 151, 159, 258.

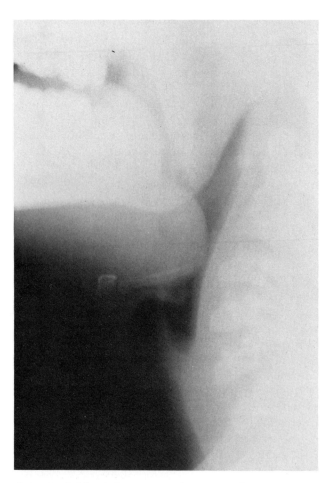

Fig. 15-14. Sublingual cyst. Lateral view reveals smoothly surfaced mass projecting into anterior portion of hypopharynx.

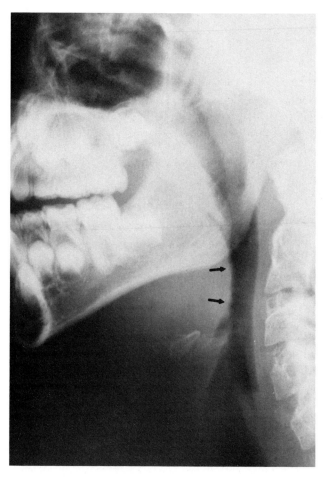

Fig. 15-15. Pseudovallecular mass—normal lymphoid tissue. Lateral view shows that normal, nodular lymphoid tissue can encroach on and fill valleculae *(arrows)*.

crognathia). Absence of the tongue can be part of the aglossia-adactylia syndrome.[221]

■ Tumors and tumorlike lesions involving the base of the tongue

A variety of mass lesions may be found to involve the base of the tongue. These include congenital lingual cysts,[261] thyroglossal cysts, dermoid cysts, and lingual thyroid masses. All of these lesions can appear clinically with airway obstruction. Radiographically, these lesions can be easily identified on the lateral view of the upper airway (Fig. 15-14) but cannot be differentiated from one another. In addition, one must be very careful in making a diagnosis of pathologic lesions involving the base of the tongue because normal lingual tonsils can bulge the base of the tongue, mimicking a tumor that can partially fill the vallecula (Fig. 15-15). This is particularly true of films obtained in expiration.

□ **Nasopharynx and hypopharynx**

■ Masses, tumors, and tumorlike lesions

When examining the nasopharynx and hypopharynx one should be aware of a number of normal structures that can simulate masses. For example, the posterior ends of the inferior turbinates not infrequently are nicely demonstrated on a good lateral inspiratory film (Fig. 15-16), and one must be aware of their presence so as not to mistake them for a tumor process. If the film was not obtained in a true lateral projection, the ear lobe projecting over the pharynx can also simulate a mass.

Other normal structures found in the pharynx include the nasopharyngeal adenoids, the palatine tonsils, and the soft palate and uvula. A tremendous variation in the size and bulk of normal nasopharyngeal adenoids and palatine tonsils exists, which can frequently cause them to appear enlarged (Fig. 15-17). This enlarged appearance does not necessarily mean, however, that they

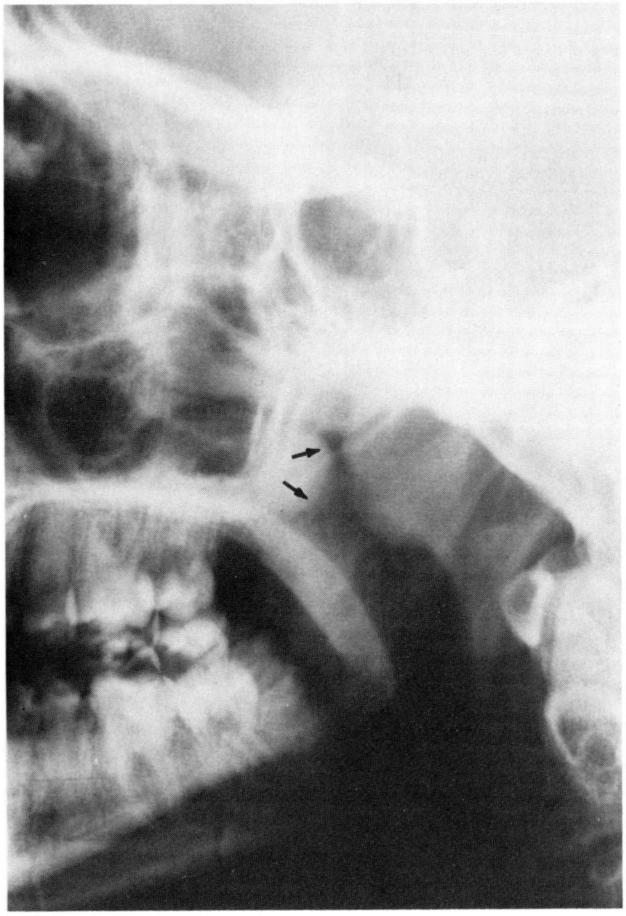

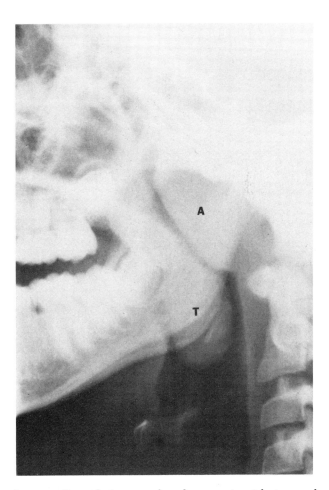

Fig. 15-16. Lateral view reveals masslike appearance of posterior portion of inferior turbinates (arrows). Also note normal adenoids and soft palate.

Fig. 15-17. Lateral view reveals rather prominent but normal tonsils (T) and adenoids (A).

are a clinically significant problem to the patient; most often they are not. Measurements have been developed to evaluate adenoid size,[146] but it must be appreciated that radiographically one is evaluating a three dimensional structure in only two dimensions. Because of this, the clinical evaluation and more recently evaluation with pressure transducers in the hypopharynx are more accurate in determining whether or not apparent adenoidal enlargement is responsible for symptoms. Nevertheless, it has been shown that large palatine tonsils and nasopharyngeal adenoids can in some cases lead to chronic airway obstruction and cor pulmonale.* Such chronic, severe obstruction of the airway results in hypoxia, hypercapnia, and acidosis, which in turn result in constriction of the peripheral arterioles and pulmonary hypertension. The entire symptom complex is usually alleviated after removal of the obstructing lymphoid tissue, although a complete return to a normal condition may take some time.

In the newborn infant[67] adenoidal tissue is very

*References 74, 118, 255, 265, 278, 284.

sparse, but by 3 months of age a half centimeter or so of thickness is usually present (see Table 15-1). Thereafter, the amount of soft tissue continues to increase; however, there is considerable variability in the size of this mass from patient to patient. If adenoidal tissue is not visualized after 6 months of age, one should consider an underlying immunologic deficiency such as hypogammaglobulinemia or agammaglobulinemia or the ataxia telangiectasia syndrome.[321] It should also be noted that in some patients the adenoidal tissue may extend into the retropharyngeal space. Such extensions may be nodular or smooth and may at first suggest a retropharyngeal mass or abscess.

Tumors involving the tonsils in children primarily consist of malignant neoplasms of lymphoid origin, such as lymphosarcoma and Hodgkin's disease.[215] Other tumors of the tonsils are rare, but teratomas in the neonate have been described.[386]

A variety of other nasopharyngeal tumors, cysts, and masses can also be encountered in the pediatric age group and most are readily detectable on the lateral neck film. For the most part one mass appears much

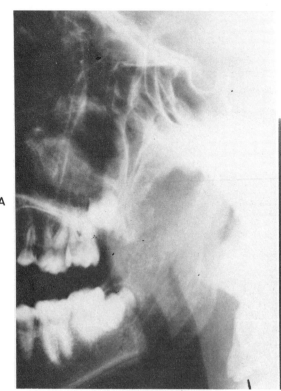
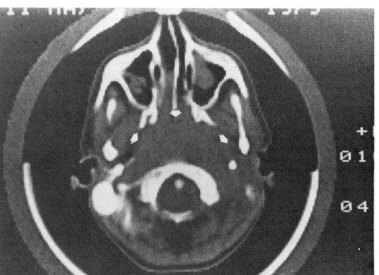

Fig. 15-18. Lymphoepithelioma in nasopharynx. **A,** Lateral view reveals total obliteration of normal nasopharyngeal airway. Although anterior margin of mass is not clearly defined, complete obliteration of nasopharyngeal anatomy should alert one to its presence. **B,** CT scan demonstrates same mass obliterating normal air passages *(arrows)*. Also notice probable retention cysts in both maxillary sinuses.

like the other, except that teratomas and neuroblastomas may contain calcifications. Tumors encountered in the newborn and young infant include teratomas,[25,141,236] dermoids,[39,210,259] neurofibromas,[331] neuroblastomas, hemangiomas,[250] and benign polyps.[102]

Many of these lesions, of course, also can be seen in the older child; however, more commonly the problem is a juvenile nasopharyngeal angiofibroma,* a lymphoepithelioma[215,329] (Fig. 15-18), or a soft tissue sarcoma such as a rhabdomyosarcoma.[105,215] Of these, the most common is the nasopharyngeal angiofibroma.

Characteristically, angiofibromas develop in adolescent boys and appear with airway obstruction, sinusitis, epistaxis, or occasionally evidence of intracranial spread. This benign tumor is extremely locally invasive and frequently extends into the pterygomaxillary fossa, paranasal sinuses, or base of the skull. Multidirectional

---

*References 203, 215, 362, 384.

tomography and CT of the skull base are usually required to define the exact limits of the tumor's extension. On lateral plain films of the nasopharynx a variable-sized nasopharyngeal mass is seen. When the mass is small it is difficult to differentiate from normal adenoidal tissue. Larger tumors usually obliterate the entire nasopharynx, and most patients demonstrate a characteristic anterior bulging of the posterior wall of the maxillary sinus (Fig. 15-19, A). This is called the antral sign. Angiographic studies must be performed to identify the precise source of blood supply to the tumor. Generally, the primary supply is from the internal maxillary branch of the external carotid artery but can also be derived from the internal carotid system, depending on the size of the tumor and in what direction extension has occurred. In addition, in those far advanced cases that reach the cervical region there may be additional blood supply from the muscular branches of the vertebral arteries.[362] The angiographic appearance generally

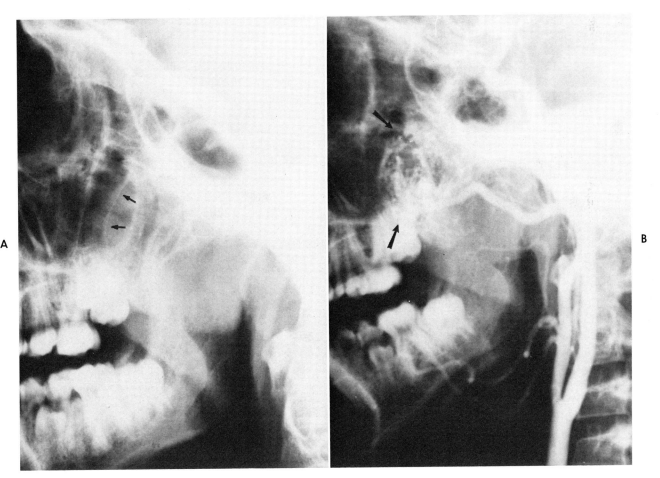

Fig. 15-19. Juvenile angiofibroma. **A,** Lateral view demonstrates large nasopharyngeal mass completely obliterating nasopharynx. There is no air gap in front of mass. There is anterior bulging (so-called antral sign) of posterior wall of maxillary sinus *(arrows)*. **B,** Lateral common carotid angiogram demonstrates rather vascular nature of these tumors *(arrows)*.

is quite characteristic, with evidence of dilated nodular tumor vessels with a hypertrophied internal maxillary artery* (Fig. 15-19, *B*). Only rarely are similar findings seen in lymphoepitheliomas or fibromas in this area.[384]

Surgical resection of the angiofibroma is considered the therapy of choice in those lesions without intracranial involvement. If there is associated intracranial extension, surgical resection of as much as possible of the extracranial component and irradiation of the intracranial portion is the treatment of choice. Because the tumor is such a vascular lesion, careful and complete surgical removal is very challenging. In the last several years preoperative embolization at the level of the external carotid artery system has been used to temporarily decrease the vascular supply of the tumor.[332,358]

Swelling of the uvula is an uncommon cause of respiratory distress or airway obstruction in children, but it can be seen with angioneurotic edema. Milder degrees of uvular swelling are seen with pharyngitis but are generally not severe enough to cause airway symptoms.

■ Velopharyngeal incompetence

The radiographic evaluation of the function of the soft palate in normal speech has proved to be of great value in the management of the patient with a cleft palate and poor speech. It also has been of considerable value in analyzing cases of abnormal speech caused by poliomyelitis, cerebral palsy, postadenoidectomy complications, etc. The roentgenographic examination is able to yield vital information that aids in decisions on whether the patient should have an operative procedure, a dental prosthesis, or further intensive speech therapy.

The action of the soft palate is easily studied in the lateral projection;[229,311] however, more extensive evaluation of the entire pharyngeal sphincter can be accomplished with studies in the frontal and basal projections.† Although cineradiography can be employed, this method results in greater radiation to the child; thus examination under fluoroscopic control with videotape and audio tape recording is the method of choice. Examination in the lateral projection can be performed without contrast material injection, although frontal and basal evaluations require coating the pharynx with barium through a nasal tube placed over the hard palate. It should also be pointed out that ultrasonography has been demonstrated to be of value in assessing lateral pharyngeal wall motion during speech.[185,234]

On examination of the pharynx on the lateral view one is able to determine the thickness and length of the soft palate, its relationship to the posterior nasopharyngeal wall, and the thickness of the adenoidal pad. In addition, by studying the action of the soft palate with certain test sounds, the range of motion of the velum can be determined and the position of the tongue studied with each sound.

During normal phonation the soft palate extends posteriorly and upward, assuming a high right-angle configuration and fitting snugly against the posterior pharyngeal wall (Fig. 15-20, *A*). If velopharyngeal incompetence is present, the soft palate lacks the high right-angle configuration and fails to reach the posterior pharyngeal wall (Fig. 15-20, *B*). Obviously many variations between these two extremes exist, and in children with prominent adenoidal tissue, even when the soft palate is somewhat short, apposition against the posterior pharyngeal wall still is possible. In other children a compensatory localized anterior bulge of the posterior pharyngeal wall can be seen. This is an adaptive mechanism and is called Passavant's ridge[229] (Fig. 15-20, *B*). In those patients with borderline velopharyngeal incompetence the use of a barium pharyngogram in the lateral projection is recommended for the most accurate assessment.[394] This type of examination is also useful in evaluating palatal fistulae and detecting a fistula in a pharyngeal flap.

■ Pharyngeal incoordination

This condition is a relatively common problem in the neonate but is for the most part transient.[94,139,353] A more permanent form, however, can be seen in conjunction with cerebral damage, with other neurologic or neuromuscular disturbances,[435] and with familial dysautonomia or the Riley-Day syndrome.*

Clinically, these patients demonstrate difficulty in eating, regurgitation of food into the nose, and repeated aspirations. Esophageal obstruction can be profound,[26] and in some cases it may be necessary to dilate the spastic cricopharyngeal muscle[35] or to perform a sphincterotomy or gastrotomy.[289] The majority of the affected infants, however, do not have this much difficulty, and usually as the newborn infant matures the degree of incoordination diminishes and slowly disappears. In these cases there is failure of cricopharyngeal and upper esophageal sphincter relaxation and hypertrophy of the cricopharyngeus muscle. On barium swallow examination there is evidence of massive reflux into the nasal passages; not infrequently barium also will spill over into the trachea.

■ Pharyngeal diverticula

Congenital pharyngeal diverticula are rare and may arise laterally or in the midline posteriorly (Fig. 15-21).† Most pharyngeal diverticula are believed to result

---

*References 203, 215, 304, 362, 429, 459.
†References 7, 163, 176, 229, 238, 325, 392, 467.

*References 75, 238, 272, 306, 356.
†References 48, 78, 267, 428.

Fig. 15-20. Velopharyngeal incompetence. **A,** Lateral view reveals normal soft palate *(P)* during phonation, showing high right-angle configuration and snug apposition against posterior pharyngeal wall *(arrows)*. There is no air gap between soft palate and posterior pharyngeal wall. **B,** Abnormal soft palate during phonation (sounding the letter "E"). Although soft palate has moved posteriorly and superiorly, it has failed to meet posterior pharyngeal wall and assume normal, sharp, high right-angle configuration. Air gap *(arrows)* persists. Also notice localized bulging of posterior pharyngeal wall (Passavant's ridge) *(R)*, an accommodative measure to further narrow air gap.

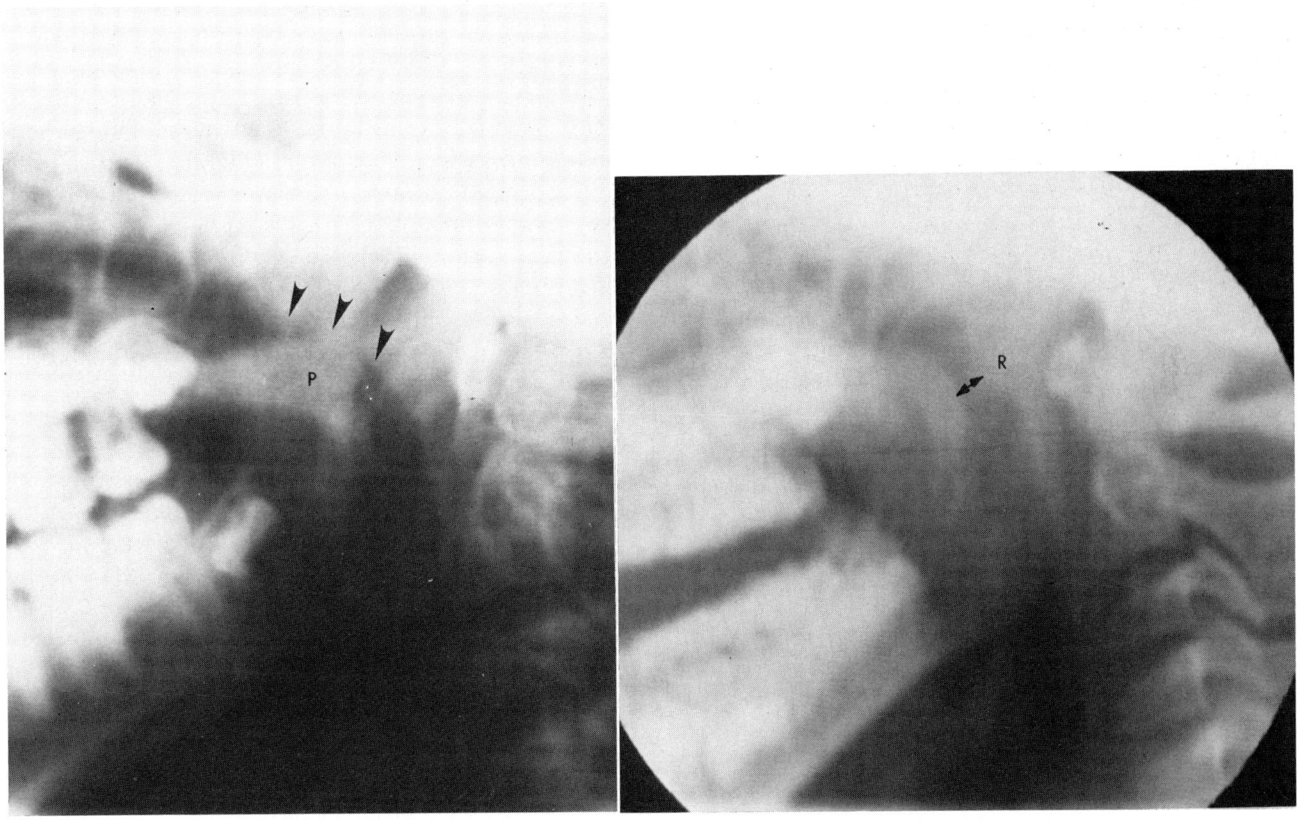

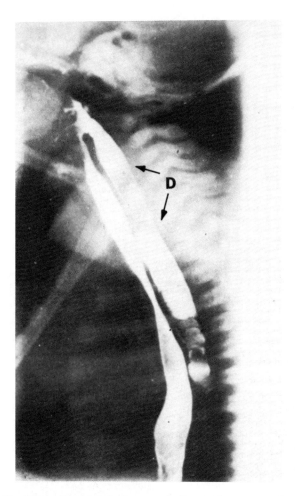

Fig. 15-21. Congenital pharyngeal diverticulum. Lateral view reveals large diverticulum *(D)* arising from above cricopharyngeus muscle. (From MacKellar, A., and Kennedy, J.C.: J. Pediatr. Surg. 7[9]:408-411, 1972.)

from iatrogenic perforation of the pharynx. These perforations occur above the cricopharyngeus muscle during intubation of neonates and young infants.* In such cases a submucosal passage is created that passes posteriorly or laterally to the esophagus and can reach as far distally as the diaphragm. In time it may dilate to form a diverticulum, or more correctly a pseudodiverticulum, which may be difficult to distinguish from the congenital type.

It is interesting to note that in older children such pharyngeal perforation often results in mediastinitis;[307] in the neonate, however, the perforation usually remains remarkably silent. In other infants the initial clinical findings may be those of dysphagia, regurgitation, respiratory distress, or even a clinical picture simulating esophageal atresia.[48,188,267]

---

*References 95, 113, 156, 173, 263, 319, 432, 450.

■ Foreign bodies

Infants and young children are like human vacuum cleaners, attempting to put in their mouth and often swallowing practically any small object they can find. Small, smooth articles generally pass through the pharynx and esophagus without difficulty, but many of the larger, more irregular or elongated objects become lodged in the hypopharynx (Fig. 15-22), pyriform recesses of the pharynx, or cervical portion of the esophagus. A foreign body in the hypopharynx may remain surprisingly asymptomatic after the initial coughing episode. It rarely results in an acute respiratory catastrophe unless there is total occlusion of the hypopharynx. By contrast, a laryngeal foreign body usually causes an acute respiratory catastrophe.[410,452] If such foreign bodies are radiopaque, they are readily identified[62,298] but if they are radiolucent (i.e., aluminum, wood, plastic), they may be almost impossible to detect without the use of contrast material.

If the foreign body causes a perforation, a retropharyngeal abscess may result. Rarely, a false aneurysm of the external carotid artery can develop following impaction of a foreign body in the adjacent pharynx.[312]

■ Sleep apnea

The hypersomnia or sleep apnea syndrome in adults has been and still is under intense investigation.[41,264,317,354] The most important underlying cause is incomplete airway obstruction caused by laxity of the supporting hypopharyngeal muscles during sleep. Sleep apnea in children bears some similarities to the syndrome in adults but has been less well studied. In the past it was generally attributed to hypertrophy of the tonsils and adenoids,[171,244,293] but recent investigation is more supportive of the lax muscle theory.[128]

Generally speaking, air flow monitoring techniques used on adults are difficult to perform on children and thus lateral view cine fluoroscopy has been advocated as a substitute.[128,405] In the normal patient there is minimal movement of the soft tissues of the hypopharynx during sleep,[5] but with the flaccid hypopharynx,[128] hypopharyngeal collapse has been observed on inspiration. More specifically, there was posterior movement of the tongue and forward bulging of the prevertebral soft tissues. The approximation of these two structures partially occluded the hypopharynx and larynx, and similar fluoroscopic findings have been documented in two adult patients with the hypersomnia sleep apnea syndrome.[443] The reason for this abnormal posterior movement of the tongue is not known. Newborn infants with partial nasal obstruction have been shown to have a similar fluoroscopic picture.[431] The hypothesis therefore is that an increase in negative pressure occurs in the posterior pharyngeal airway when the nose is partially blocked during nasal breathing.

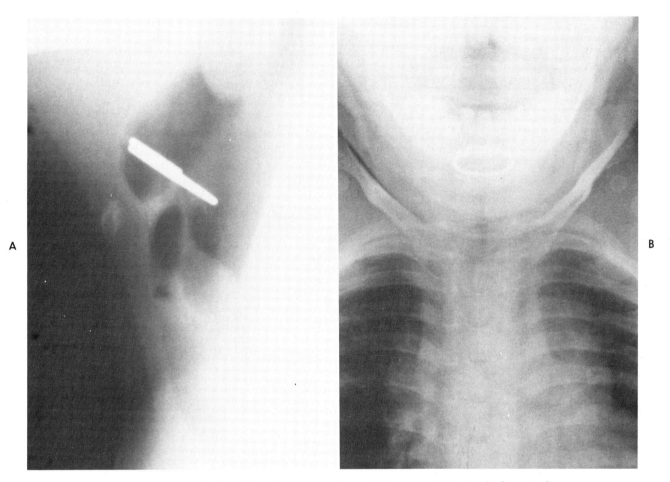

Fig. 15-22. Foreign body in hypopharynx. **A,** Lateral view reveals foreign body encircling epiglottis. Patient was drooling but had no real symptoms of airway obstructions. **B,** Frontal view demonstrates ring and confirms its position over epiglottis.

It is also interesting that a number of authors have suggested a link between the sudden infant death syndrome (SIDS) and sleep apnea in infants. The sudden infant death syndrome is a semidistinct clinical pathologic entity for which numerous hypotheses have been proposed. It would appear that there are a number of pathologic conditions that can produce the syndrome, including cardiac arrhythmias, gastric aspiration with laryngeal spasm, and chronic hypoxemia related to sleep apnea. One investigation[301] found an increased mass of muscle in the small pulmonary arteries in one half of the SIDS victims studied, and similar alterations in the pulmonary circulation of victims of SIDS have been confirmed by other observers.[276,455] These changes also have been described in other situations in which alveolar hypoxia occurs, such as the Pickwickian syndrome and in individuals living at high altitudes.[134,155] Thus it has been hypothesized that at least some of the patients with SIDS have alveolar hypoxia caused by hypoventilation such as that seen in patients with chronic sleep apnea; in one study, there was noted an increased incidence of prolonged sleep apnea and its associated intermittent alveolar hypoventilation among victims of crib death.[144] Similar findings of such apnea were also found in five hospitalized infants who were either "near misses" or siblings of victims of SIDS.[411]

□ **Retropharyngeal space (abnormal thickening)**

In assessing the retropharyngeal space, the radiologist's primary task is to determine whether or not it is of normal thickness. However, it must again be stressed that it is important to obtain the lateral neck film with the neck extended and the patient in deep inspiration. If these criteria are not met, the films either will be uninterpretable or will result in erroneous conclusions. The reason for this is that in the infant and young child the airway and prevertebral soft tissues are extremely pliable and therefore can become distorted and bizarre in configuration during expiration or flexion of the neck.[5,47,423] If, however, there still remains doubt as to whether or not a mass is present, a barium swallow examination can be made.

■ Infection

Patients with retropharyngeal cellulitis, adenitis, or frank abscess formation usually have a history of an upper respiratory tract infection followed by high fever, neck pain, stiffness (wry neck), and dysphagia.[67,110,423] Although stridor can also occur it usually is not the predominant clinical feature. When a retropharyngeal abscess is present it usually is the result of suppurative adenitis (upper respiratory infection); however, occasionally it can be the result of a pharyngeal or upper esophageal perforation caused by a foreign body.

Radiographically, the findings consist of thickening of the retropharyngeal soft tissues, with a forward bulging and displacement of the airway (Fig. 15-23). Gas may be present if an actual abscess is present.[471] Not infrequently there is straightening or reversal of the normal cervical lordosis. This is secondary to intense muscle spasm and can produce a pseudodislocated appearance of the upper cervical vertebrae. In less severe cases the findings are less striking, and a barium swallow examination may be required to determine whether or not any soft tissue swelling is present.

■ Trauma

Prevertebral soft tissue thickening as a result of edema or a hematoma can be a very important ancillary finding in cervical spine injuries. However, these changes are present only in those cases in which anterior spinal ligament or vertebral body injuries are present; thus in a good many significant cervical spine injuries the prevertebral soft tissues appear normal. In the lower cervical spine region, anterior displacement of the prevertebral fat stripe[454] can provide a clue to the presence of otherwise unnoticed edema; however, this fat stripe is not always readily visible in the infant or younger child.

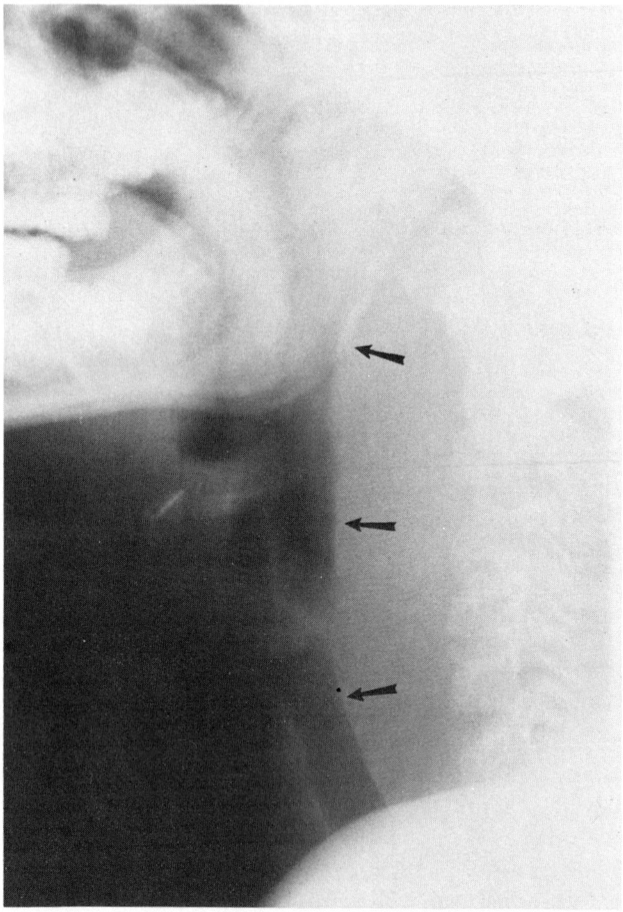

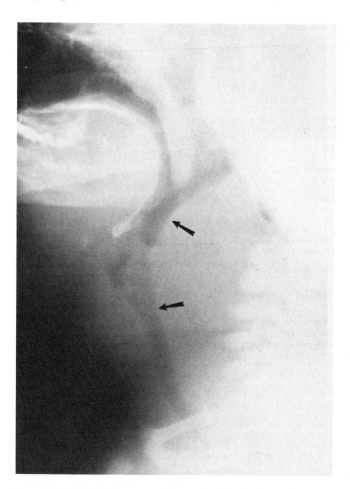

Fig. 15-23. Retropharyngeal abscess. Lateral view reveals typical curving anterior displacement of airway *(arrows)*, thickening of retropharyngeal soft tissues, and straightening of cervical spine.

Fig. 15-24. Lateral view reveals marked thickening of retropharyngeal soft tissues and anterior displacement of airway *(arrows)*. Findings are nonspecific, but were caused by myxedema in this hypothyroid newborn.

■ Tumor and tumorlike lesions

The most common tumor to occur in the retropharyngeal region in the infant and young child is the cystic hygroma.[13,14,239] In the vast majority of cases it does not arise primarily from the retropharyngeal space, but rather represents an extension of a more lateral lesion. Other tumors or tumorlike lesions occurring in the retropharynx include ectopic goiterous thyroid tissue,[67,70,183] teratomas, hemangiomas, neurofibromas,[409] primary or secondary neuroblastomas,[361,364] and enlarged lymph nodes from a variety of problems such as histiocytosis X, tuberculosis of the neck (scrofula), and lymphoma or leukemia.

When a retropharyngeal goiter is present in an infant, the infant usually is the offspring of a mother with hyperthyroidism or a mother who ingested iodine during pregnancy. Although the plain film radiographic findings are nonspecific, the goiter can be identified with radioisotope studies. In addition, it should be noted that myxedematous thickening of the retropharynx also can occur in hypothyroid infants (Fig. 15-24). The thickening in these cases is not a result of a goiter.[170]

Retropharyngeal soft tissue thickening can also occur as a result of enlargement of the internal jugular veins in infants with vein of Galen aneurysms[422] and we have recently seen a case of retropharyngeal edema in a patient with idiopathic thrombosis of the superior vena cava and innominate veins.

□ **The larynx**
■ Epiglottitis

Acute epiglottitis represents a true medical emergency, with sudden death being not at all uncommon. In most cases the infectious agent is *Haemophilus influenzae* type B, although various other strains of *Haemophilus influenzae*, as well as *Haemophilus parainfluenzae*, may be the cause.* The peak incidence of epiglottitis occurs in children between the ages of 3 and 6 years, although reports of epiglottitis in adults (also caused by *Haemophilus influenzae*) have also appeared.[44,472]

Clinically, patients with epiglottitis have a sore throat and a fever. These symptoms are followed by a rapid progression to severe supraglottic obstruction, stridor, and dysphagia. On direct examination, the pharynx is edematous and the epiglottis appears as a swollen cherry-red structure. It must be remembered that forceful attempts to see the epiglottis can result in catastrophic complete airway obstruction. Because of this possibility, the radiographic evaluation of the epiglottis, using the lateral view of the upper airway, is considered

to be the examination of choice in patients suspected of having epiglottitis.[67,110,423]

Because epiglottitis is a bacterial infection, antibiotics are indicated in its treatment. However, because of the emergence of strains of *Haemophilus influenzae* resistant to ampicillin, chloramphenicol is advocated as the drug of choice by some authors.[193] Of even greater importance in the treatment of epiglottitis is the establishment of an airway.[21,82] Although it was once advocated that tracheostomy be performed[274,348] many authors currently advocate the establishment of a secure airway by nasotracheal intubation.* The argument for this method is that it is quicker, less traumatic, and of lower morbidity. In addition, the nasotracheal tube can be removed sooner.[387] The primary advantage of the tracheostomy tube is that it has less of a chance of being accidentally dislodged or coughed out and requires less specialized nursing care.

Radiographically, the findings of epiglottitis consist of swelling or thickening of the epiglottis and aryepiglottic folds (Fig. 15-25, A). This leads to considerable supraglottic edema, which may reach such a magnitude that it completely obliterates the pyriform sinuses and the valleculae.† In many cases, mild to moderate hypopharyngeal overdistension occurs, but rarely to the degree seen with croup. In most authors' experience, the glottis, subglottis, and upper trachea are normal. However, 5 of 20 children with proven acute bacterial epiglottitis were demonstrated to have subglottic narrowing caused by subglottic edema,[383] which resulted in roentgenographic findings similar to those seen in croup. This, however, represents a rather rare situation because most patients with epiglottitis have a normal glottic and subglottic region.

The demonstration of the aforementioned findings in most cases virtually assures the diagnosis of epiglottitis. However, there are a few other conditions that can mimic these findings, and they include disorders such as angioneurotic edema,[93,180,446] reaction to a foreign body,[67,446] neurofibromatosis,[85] hemorrhage,[446] hot air or smoke inhalation, and burns caused by lye ingestion. There also have been several cases described of a chronic form of epiglottitis in which the clinical findings are not dissimilar from acute epiglottitis but in which no organism was isolated.[375,446] In addition, we have seen one case of epiglottitis caused by *Candida* infection in an immunologically compromised infant (Fig. 15-25, B).

Finally, it is most important not to misinterpret the normal so-called omega epiglottis for epiglottitis. Radiographically, the omega epiglottis may appear to be a

---

*References 44, 109, 110, 224, 247, 273, 337, 451.

---

*References 19, 46, 288, 349, 387, 448.
†References 67, 110, 168, 247, 347, 423.

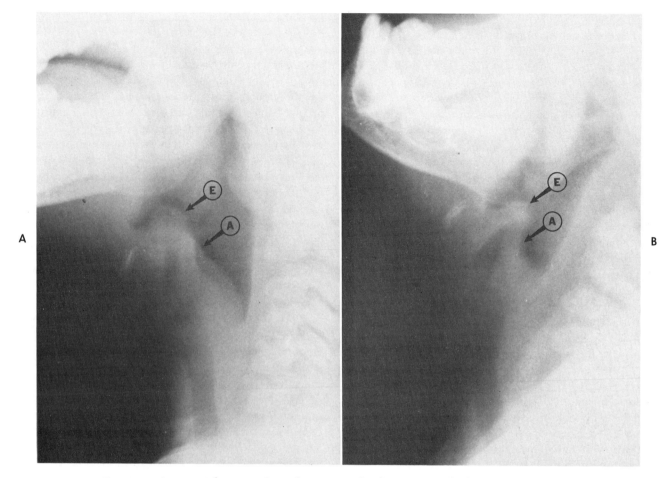

Fig. 15-25. Acute epiglottis. **A,** Lateral view reveals characteristic thickening of epiglottis (*E*) and aryepiglottic folds (*A*). **B,** Another infant with epiglottitis but with less swelling of epiglottis (*E*) and aryepiglottic folds (*A*).

little thickened in these patients on the lateral view (Fig. 15-26), but the impression is erroneous. It is caused by a floppy epiglottis with prominent downward curving lateral flaps that result in an inverted U or omega-shaped epiglottis. There is, however, no real thickening of the aryepiglottic folds or epiglottis in these patients, and this roentgenographic finding should rule out a diagnosis of acute infectious epiglottis. If one is not able to make this distinction on a lateral film of the neck it usually is because the inspiratory effort is not deep enough, and thus the study should be repeated with a deeper inspiration by the patient.

■ Croup (laryngotracheobronchitis)

The most common cause of acute upper airway obstruction in infants and young children is laryngotracheobronchitis or croup, and the peak age of incidence is between 6 months and 3 years. It almost always is viral in origin, with various strains of parainfluenza

being the most common agents involved. Other viruses implicated include strains of adenoviruses, respiratory syncytial viruses, and influenza viruses.[93,109,245] Bacterial croup is rather uncommon but does occur.[179,245] Generally, it is more severe and refractory than viral croup, and because the purulent exudates in these infections can produce subglottic and tracheal membranes, it has been called "membranous" croup.[179] In general these patients demonstrate radiographic findings similar to viral croup, although their course tends to be more severe and less responsive to supportive therapy. In 20 of 28 patients, pathogenic bacteria (hemolytic *Staphylococcus aureus*) were isolated,[179] although the author of the study points out that it is not clear whether membranous croup is caused primarily by bacterial infection or is a severe form of ordinary croup with superimposed bacterial infection. We have seen a few similar cases and can attest to its more refractory nature.

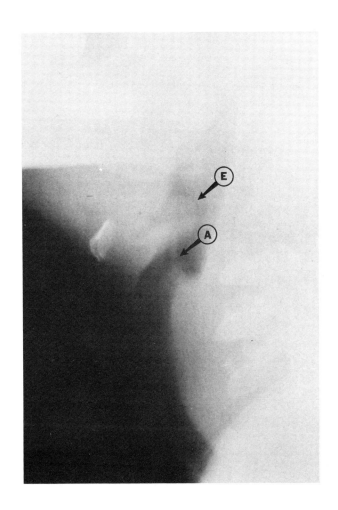

Fig. 15-26. Omega epiglottis—pseudoepiglottitis. Notice rather plump-appearing epiglottis *(E)*. This is erroneous impression caused by prominent side flaps on epiglottis. Notice that aryepiglottic folds *(A)* are thin in this patient; they are usually thickened with epiglottitis (see Fig. 15-25).

As the name would imply, laryngotracheobronchitis may involve the entire airway, although the subglottis is usually most critically involved. Clinically, most of these children demonstrate signs and symptoms of a full-blown viral respiratory tract infection, often preceding the actual onset of stridor. The stridor is primarily inspiratory in nature and can be very severe. Croup having onset without an associated viral respiratory tract infection often is termed spasmodic or allergic croup. It has also been called night croup because these infants can have very sudden onset of symptoms in the evening, yet there will be an absence of fever and a complete, or almost complete, remission of symptoms during the day. Furthermore, older children may have an acute onset of croup in the absence of a viral respiratory tract infection, and these instances are believed to represent an allergic phenomenon. Epinephrine has been shown to be effective in the treatment of these patients, as well as the early use of diphenhydramine hydrochloride.[93] The radiographic findings are indistinguishable from those of typical viral croup.

Radiographically, the findings of croup are characteristic and easily differentiated from those of epiglottitis.* The reason for this is that croup involves the glottic and subglottic structures, while epiglottitis involves the supraglottic area. Consequently, in croup the vocal cords usually appear thickened and fuzzy and on inspiration there is marked hypopharyngeal overdistension and concomitant subglottic tracheal narrowing (Figs. 15-27 and 15-28). These findings are demonstrated best on lateral views on the neck but also can be seen on frontal views. Hypopharyngeal overdistension simply reflects the presence of glottic obstruction, but subglottic narrowing is paradoxical and represents tracheal collapse as a result of negative intraluminal pressures that develop in this area during inspiration.[283,423] The finding is not particularly specific because it can occur with any paraglottic obstruction, but it is a hallmark of croup. On expiration, however, the narrowing will be seen not to be fixed, a point attesting to its paradoxical nature. Only in the more severe cases of croup and in those caused by bacterial infection does edema cause the nar-

*References 67, 98, 110, 123.

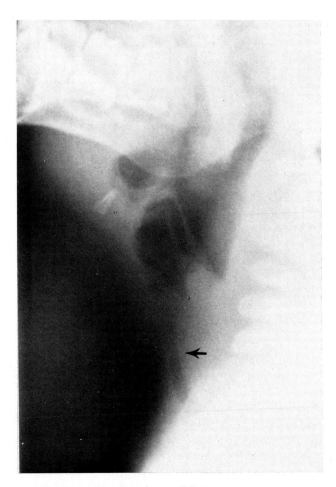

Fig. 15-27. Croup. Lateral view reveals characteristic findings consisting of marked hypopharyngeal overdistension, thin epiglottis, and aryepiglottic folds coupled with indistinctness of vocal cords, prominence of laryngeal ventricle, and paradoxical subglottic narrowing *(arrow)*.

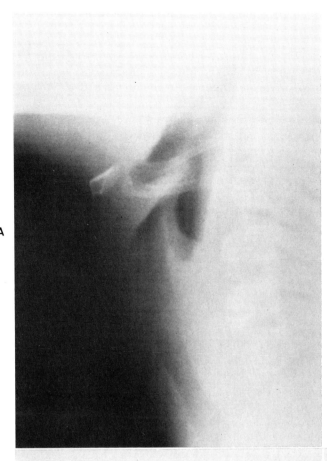

A

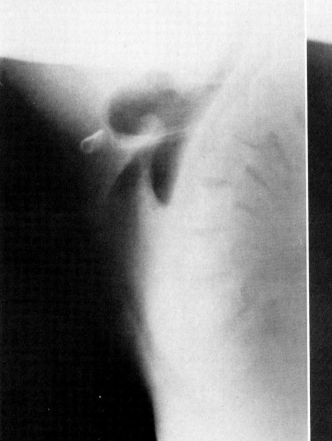

B

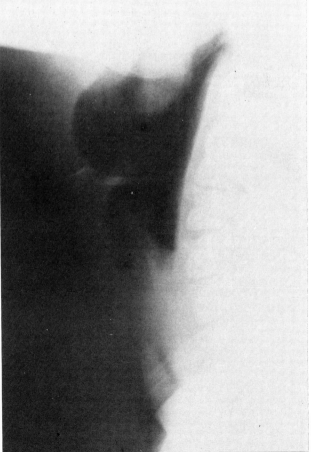

C

Fig. 15-28. Croup—changes with degree of inspiration. **A,** Lateral view taken in early inspiration shows no overaeration of hypopharynx and no subglottic narrowing. However, vocal cord area is fuzzy and indistinct. **B,** With more inspiration hypopharynx is beginning to overdistend; there is now subglottic narrowing of trachea. **C,** With deep inspiration hypopharynx is grossly overdistended and subglottis is markedly narrowed. Also notice continued indistinctness and fuzziness of vocal cords, and very prominent laryngeal ventricle.

rowing to be more fixed. In addition to these findings of croup, very often the laryngeal ventricles are overly prominent, and in bacterial croup membranes can be seen in the trachea.

A recent case report has also decribed a 13-month-old child with coccidioidomycosis involving the subglottic larynx.[149] On a lateral plain film of the neck there was evidence of symmetric narrowing of the subglottic airway, apparently representing primary involvement of the region. There have been other reports of granulomatous involvement of the larynx in adults as well as in children[330,445,461] but these occurred in association with pulmonary coccidioidomycosis and were thought to result from innoculation by organism-laden sputum. In a few patients with tracheitis the mucosa and exudate can be so thick that it can be seen on plain films.

On frontal views the vocal cords and subglottis appear thickened and funnellike in configuration (Fig. 15-29). Normally, the vocal cords abduct during inspiration

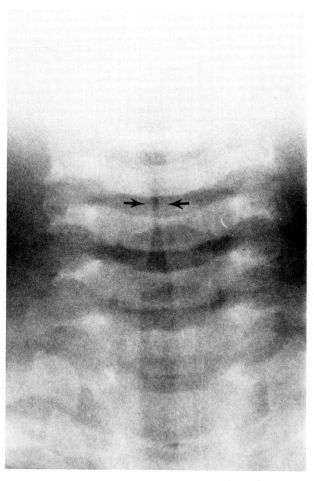

Fig. 15-29. Croup—frontal view. Frontal view reveals typical slitlike or funnel-shaped glottic region *(arrow)*. This configuration is seen on both inspiration and expiration. Compare this with normal appearance of vocal cords in Fig. 15-1, *B*.

or quiet breathing and reveal a wide-open airway. With crying or forced expiration (i.e., a modified Valsalva maneuver), the angle between the undersurface of the true vocal cords and the subglottic larynx (subglottic arch) becomes acute or squared-off (see Fig. 15-1, *B*). Because the vocal cords are edematous and in spasm in croup, there is little change between inspiration and expiration, and the funnel-shaped configuration is almost always present. Indeed, it is often best visualized on the ordinary frontal chest film.

Not all children with croup display the classical findings just described because to a great extent the findings depend on the degree of inspiration present. If the inspiratory effort is not deep, less hypopharyngeal overdistension occurs and less subglottic tracheal collapse is seen. In these patients the only roentgenographic finding may be thickening or fuzziness of the vocal cords, and the funnel-shaped glottis-subglottis as seen on frontal views becomes an even more important diagnostic finding.

Finally, it should be pointed out that if croup tends to be recurrent or if it occurs under the age of 6 months, one should consider some underlying lesions such as congenital subglottic stenosis, a laryngeal web, or a subglottic hemangioma. Laryngeal webs usually are diagnosed only with endoscopy, but subglottic stenosis and subglottic hemangioma can be radiographically differentiated from croup. All of these lesions are dealt with in greater depth later in this chapter.

■ Tumors and tumorlike lesions of the larynx

Tumors of the larynx are uncommon in children and the vast majority are benign. Sporadic reports of malignant lesions of the larynx include lymphosarcoma,[86] fibrosarcoma,[137,338,355] rhabdomyosarcoma,* and epidermoid carcinoma.[223,318] Benign tumors of the larynx consist of chondroma,[16,207] granular cell myoblastoma,[40] rhabdomyosarcoma,† plasma cell granuloma,[12] chemodectoma,[430,439] neurofibroma, and fibroma. Fibroma can occur either in an isolated form or as part of a congenital generalized fibromatosis.[233,295]

Neurofibromas and schwannomas also can occur in an isolated form or can be associated with von Recklinghausen's disease.‡ However, by far the most common laryngeal tumor in children is the so-called juvenile papilloma.[199,271,313] Although these lesions occur chiefly on the true and false cords, the anterior commissure, and in the subglottis, they also may be found throughout the entire respiratory tract; they have been recorded from the nose to the bronchi.[232, 245, 404] It is rare, however, for these lesions to occur in the trachea

---

*References 15, 16, 157, 374.
†References 20, 287, 314, 465.
‡References 85, 104, 153, 344, 345, 406, 437.

and bronchi without also being present in the larynx. The majority of patients with juvenile papillomatosis are between the ages of 18 months and 7 years[166] and characteristically they demonstrate an insidious onset of hoarseness. Dysphonia or aphonia also may be present in infants.

The cause of this condition is thought to be a virus,[43,209,434] although there has yet to be successful culturing of the virus in vivo. On the other hand, it has been demonstrated with electron microscopy that intranuclear viral particles of a size and morphology similar to the genital wart virus were present in patients with juvenile papillomatosis.[43] Overall then, although not definitely proven, a viral cause is presently the best consideration.

In terms of treatment of juvenile papillomatosis, it is interesting to note that there is a tendency for the papillomas to recede spontaneously by adolescence.[125] However, in most patients airway compromise becomes so severe that some form of treatment must be initiated. A wide variety of therapeutic approaches have

been developed, including direct surgical resection, autogenous vaccine administration,[201,415] intralaryngeal application of ultrasonography[121] intralaryngeal, submucosal injection of estradiol,[425] and destruction of the papillomas by carbon dioxide laser beam.[333,416,417] Unfortunately, none of these measures are completely successful, and recurrences of papillomas are common. A new approach that seems to have considerable promise, although not yet unequivocally endorsed, is the use of transfer factor in the immunologic treatment of the papillomas.[340]

An important point about juvenile papillomas is that seeding of the papillomas throughout the airway can occur as a result of surgical trauma to the mucosal membrane.[126] Indeed, chronic pulmonary disease may develop from these distally seeded lesions and result in death from pulmonary failure.[120, 363] Another important point to be remembered is that radiation therapy should be discouraged because of the resultant increased incidence of thyroid carcinoma. Furthermore, malignant degeneration of juvenile papillomas has been

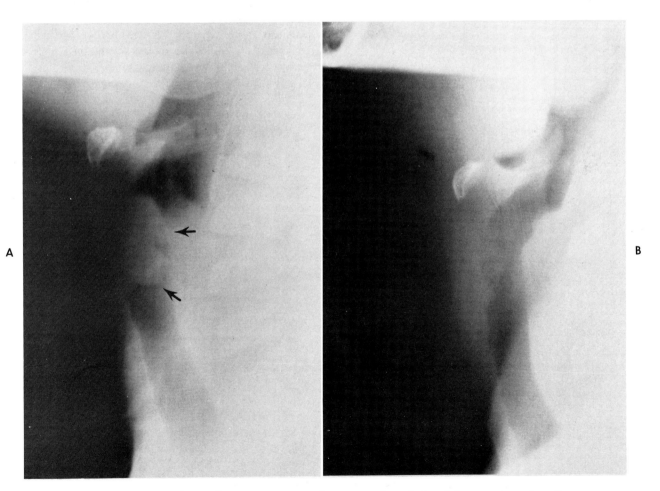

Fig. 15-30. Juvenile papillomatosis. **A,** Lateral view reveals typical nodular mass in region of glottis *(arrows).* **B,** Another patient with smaller mass but more discrete nodules.

demonstrated only in those patients previously treated with radiation therapy.[125,270]

Radiographically, the tumor appears as a nodular or lumpy mass best demonstrated on lateral neck films (Fig. 15-30). Its appearance is highly suggestive, but not pathognomonic, because any of the previously mentioned benign tumors can produce a similar picture, as can a variety of infiltrating diseases. These infiltrating diseases include conditions such as lipoid proteinosis,[449] amyloidosis,[471] and mucopolysaccharidosis. We have seen one patient with the last problem in whom infiltration of the larynx and the trachea led to considerable tracheal stenosis. Vocal nodules (singer's nodes) are not to be confused with juvenile papillomas. These nodules develop on the true vocal cords as a result of chronic vocal abuse and are the most common cause of hoarseness in childhood. They tend to regress spontaneously and are not visible radiographically.

■ **Foreign bodies in the larynx**

The aspiration of foreign bodies is not an uncommon problem in children. Although smooth or small objects usually pass through the larynx into the trachea and lower bronchi, larger, more irregular objects may lodge in the larynx. Many of these are ejected back into the pharynx during a paroxysm of coughing, but occasionally a foreign body may become persistently impacted in the larynx. Usually this occurs at the level of the vocal cords,[297,336,351] and in most instances the foreign body is slender and flat. An eggshell fragment is one such foreign body[303] frequently aspirated by children, but chicken bones, etc., also can be encountered. It should be noted that chicken and turkey bones usually are visible radiographically, while most fish bones are not.

In contrast to hypopharyngeal foreign bodies, laryngeal foreign bodies commonly cause severe respiratory distress, stridor, and even apnea. Frequently the problem is so acute that there is no time for plain films to be obtained.[410,452] In other instances, prolonged impaction of foreign bodies in the glottis can lead to edema, ulceration, and eventually stenosis.[200] If the foreign body is radiopaque, it usually is readily identified radiographically (Fig. 15-31). On the other hand, if it is nonopaque (e.g., fish bones, wood, plastic, aluminum, vegetable fiber), endoscopy usually is required for diagnosis and localization. However, one may use high-kilovoltage magnification techniques and CT for visualization of some of these nonopaque foreign bodies.[228,401]

■ **Congenital laryngeal web, stenosis, and atresia**

Overall, congenital laryngeal web, stenosis, and atresia are uncommon causes of upper respiratory tract obstruction in infancy. Laryngeal atresia[438] is of course a catastrophe, and diagnosis usually is made by endoscopy or not until after death. The same can be said for severe laryngeal stenosis. Both atresia and stenosis usually are isolated anomalies. They have been reported to occur, however, with esophageal atresia and tracheoesophageal fistula.[249,369] In a series of 158 cases of subglottic stenosis accumulated between the years of 1964 and 1974, 115 cases were congenital and 43 were acquired.[202] However, over the last 6 to 8 years, with the commonplace intubation of neonates in intensive care nurseries, acquired subglottic stenosis has become the more common variety.[59,324,418] Congenital laryngeal stenosis may be glottic, supraglottic, or subglottic, and may be membraneous (a laryngeal web) or cartilaginous.[9,196,197] Of these, glottic webs are the most common,[197] with the web consisting of a membrane across the anterior portion of the true cords. The degree to which the glottis is covered varies from mere anterior commissure webbing to almost complete occlusion of the airway. In the majority of cases, however, only the anterior two thirds of the glottis is involved.[197]

The symptoms of congenital subglottic stenosis are not always present at birth or in the neonatal period;

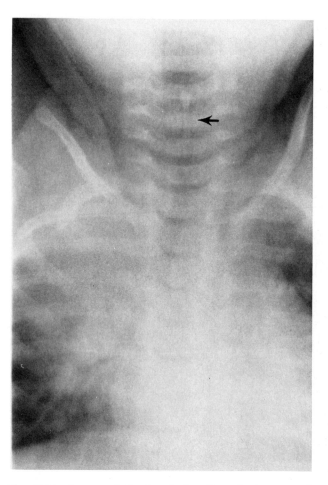

Fig. 15-31. Laryngeal foreign body. Frontal view reveals chicken bone stuck at level of vocal cords *(arrow)*.

however, invariably they become evident during the first few weeks or months of life. Stridor is the most common initial symptom, and although it generally is both inspiratory and expiratory, the inspiratory component predominates. These findings frequently are associated with dyspnea and a barking or brassy cough. Because of this, many patients with congenital subglottic stenosis may have what appears to be prolonged or multiple episodes of ordinary croup.[202] The problem can be even more complicated because ordinary croup aggravates the symptoms of congenital subglottic stenosis. Radiographically, laryngeal webs cannot be seen without the use of contrast material, and this is seldom employed. The characteristic findings of stenosis consist of a circumferentially smooth narrowing of approximately 1 to 1.5 cm of the subglottic portion of the larynx.* Actually, the findings are similar to those seen in

*References 67, 89, 110, 169, 245, 247, 423.

croup; however, a differentiating point is that in the cases of stenosis the narrowing persists on both inspiration and expiration (Fig. 15-32).

■ Acquired laryngeal stenosis

Acquired laryngeal stenosis may be a result of external or internal injury of the larynx. In the older child and adolescent the cause most often is external trauma.[135,302,315] As in the adult, the insult usually results from more severe injuries that cause crushing fractures of the thyroid, cricoid, or tracheal cartilages, avulsion of the larynx or trachea, tears of the thyrohyoid membrane, or dislocation of the arytenoid cartilages.[200] In many of these patients the diagnosis and proper treatment are delayed, and varying degrees of stenosis can occur as a result of scar tissue formation. Actual atresia can result if injury occurs to the developing larynx.

The most common cause of internal injury of the up-

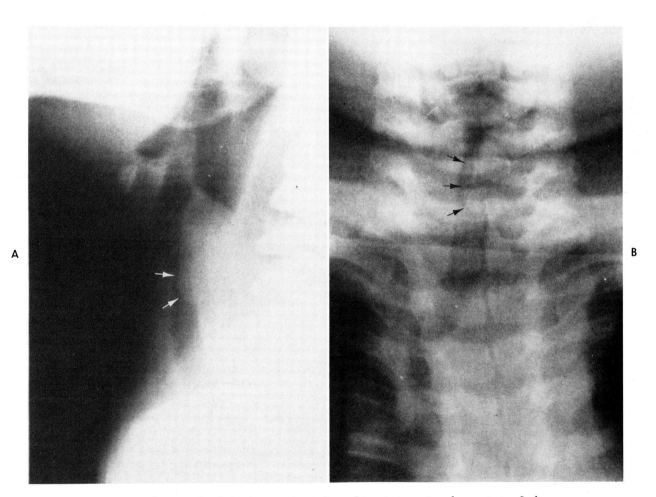

A

B

Fig. 15-32. Congenital subglottic stenosis. **A,** Lateral inspiratory view demonstrates findings similar to croup, with hypopharyngeal overdistension and subglottic narrowing *(arrows)*. **B,** On expiration, notice that area of subglottic stenosis remains narrow *(arrow)*. With croup this area usually dilates on expiration.

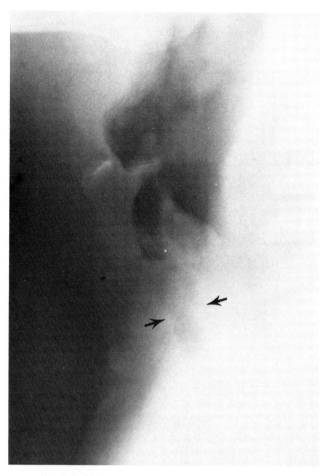

Fig. 15-33. Acquired subglottic stenosis. Lateral view reveals nodular subglottic stenosis *(arrows)* that resulted from previous intubation.

per airway is iatrogenic trauma related to intubation (Fig. 15-33) and tracheostomy.[108,162] This is particularly true in neonates who are in the intensive care nursery. Subglottic stenosis with exuberant granuloma formation is the most common form of postintubation stenosis, but glottic stenosis, as well as unilateral or bilateral vocal cord paralysis, can also occur. Laryngeal injury as a result of an aspirated or impacted upper airway foreign body can also cause stenosis if not recognized early.[200] A variety of toxic agents such as intense heat, steam, smoke, chemical corrosives (lye), acids, and poisons[200] can also cause internal injuries of the larynx and trachea with ultimate scarring and stenosis.[162] Laryngeal stenosis has also been reported with epidermolysis bullosa.[83]

■ Laryngeal cysts and laryngoceles

Congenital cysts of the larynx are rare, and virtually all of these patients exhibit inspiratory stridor at birth,

or shortly thereafter.[197,382] The cause of these cysts is unknown, although most authors regard them as simple retention cysts.[10,130,245] They are filled with mucoid secretions, contain no air, and are submucosal.[100,419] The majority involve the aryepiglottic folds, although they may also involve the epiglottis, ventricles, and pyriform sinuses.[130,419]

Radiographically, a cyst appears as a localized, homogeneously dense, smoothly marginated, rounded expansion of that portion of the larynx that is involved (i.e., the aryepiglottic fold, epiglottis, etc.). Although not diagnostic, the lateral plain film of the neck is extremely valuable in the identification of these masses.[110,197,382] The importance of early diagnosis and treatment of these lesions cannot be overemphasized. Almost 50% of them are diagnosed at autopsy in infants who died of asphyxia.[419] The treatment of choice is aspiration of the cyst and then removal of the cyst wall to prevent reaccumulation of secretions.[382]

Laryngoceles in infants and young children are extremely uncommon.[9,197,442] In the adult, laryngoceles have been reported in people whose vocations are associated with chronically increased intralaryngeal air pressure, e.g., glass blowers and musicians who play wind instruments.[427] The pathogenesis in infants is less clear, but the laryngoceles probably are congenital in origin. Two types of laryngoceles are classicially described, the internal and external laryngoceles.[197] The internal laryngocele represents about 60% of all laryngoceles and arises from the laryngeal ventricle. It enlarges in the supraglottic larynx to bulge the aryepiglottic fold medially and may extend posteriorly up to the arytenoid cartilage. The external laryngocele extends more cephalad and bulges externally through the thyrohyoid membrane to appear clinically as a mass in the neck.

■ Laryngotracheoesophageal cleft (persistent esophagotrachea)

This anomaly represents a spectrum ranging from a simple posterior laryngeal cleft to persistence of a common tube for the trachea and esophagus.* Clinically, these infants generally have an abnormal cry, are mute, and have a tendency to aspirate food into the larynx. In the more extensive, persistent esophagotrachea there is a complete lack of separation of the trachea from the esophagus, and symptoms resembling those of esophageal atresia or tracheoesophageal fistula occur. In addition, mutism, because of the excessive posterior laryngeal abnormality, is the rule. On plain lateral chest and neck films it is difficult to separate the tracheal air column from that of the esophagus. Definitive diagnosis

———
*References 37, 60, 127, 140, 147, 164, 269, 308, 327, 388, 468.

requires injection of contrast material into the combined laryngotracheoesophageal tube.

■ Laryngomalacia

Laryngomalacia is the most commonly encountered abnormality of the larynx in the young infant. In most cases the condition is caused by laxity of the aryepiglottic folds and the epiglottis;[110,195] however, in the more severe cases the entire larynx is involved. During inspiration the larynx, because of its laxity tends to collapse on itself. Symptoms most often appear shortly after the neonatal period and consist primarily of inspiratory stridor and a variable degree of intercostal and substernal retractions. Usually the stridor improves with activity and crying[282] and tends to worsen when at rest. The cry is generally normal, which distinguishes these infants from those with laryngeal tumors and vocal cord paralysis. Many infants with laryngomalacia can also have feeding difficulties. These consist of vomiting after feeding and taking an excessively long time to feed.[110,282] Overall, the prognosis is good, and with time stridor lessens. By the age of 1 year it usually has completely disappeared, although in some cases stridor has persisted for up to 5 years.[391]

The diagnosis of laryngomalacia is usually made on the basis of clinical and laryngoscopic findings. Fluoroscopic examination of these patients in the lateral position can also yield diagnostic information. In the resting, recumbent position, one can see hypopharyngeal overdistension, partial collapse and flattening of the base of the aryepiglottic folds, downward and backward bending of the epiglottis, and paradoxical narrowing of the subglottis.[110]

■ Vocal cord paralysis

Vocal cord paralysis, or paresis, in the infant or young child is not an uncommon cause of obstruction of the upper airway.[458] In the neonate it can be related to brain injury, intracranial hemorrhage, or perinatal anoxia resulting in brain damage.[131] It also has been associated with neurologic abnormalities such as the Arnold-Chiari malformation,[198,407] cerebral agenesis, and posterior fossa meningoceles.[36,131] In one study[458] 16 of 21 previously healthy patients, ranging in age from 1 day to 14 years, developed sudden respiratory distress as a result of vocal cord paralysis. The cause of the paralysis in the majority of these patients could not be discerned, but 11 of the children demonstrated improvement of vocal cord function within 1 month. The remaining 5 patients never did improve. Vocal cord paralysis is usually unilateral. It can also occur as a result of stretching of the recurrent laryngeal nerve during birth injury or stretching of the nerve by mediastinal vascular rings or masses. Bilateral vocal cord paralysis

has also been described in congenital cutis laxa and cystic fibrosis.[371]

Vocal cord paralysis is easily demonstrated with routine films and fluoroscopic examination of the larynx.[458] On the lateral view there will be indistinctness of the cords and less definition of the ventricle, and on deep inspiration there can be paradoxical collapse of the subglottis. The most definitive examinations, however, are frontal quiet breathing and phonation films and fluoroscopic examination of the cords in the frontal view. The paralyzed vocal cord(s) extends toward the midline with little variation during resting and phonation. When both cords are involved a narrow slitlike air passage is seen between them; however, if only one cord is paralyzed it will fail to reach the midline on phonation and fail to relax completely during quiet breathing.

A final disorder indirectly involving the vocal cords and producing upper airway obstruction is cricoarytenoid arthritis associated with juvenile rheumatoid arthritis. Although it has been estimated to be present in 26% of adults with rheumatoid arthritis[261] it has been reported only twice in the pediatric literature.[212,373] The cricoarytenoid joints are true diarthroidal articulations and demonstrate pathologic changes identical to those found in other such joints.* When the cricoarytenoid joint is involved it becomes rigidly fixed and thus immobilizes the vocal cord. Most adults with this manifestation of rheumatoid arthritis have inspiratory stridor that may be manifest only when they are inactive, relaxed, or asleep.[334] Very frequently, however, they have exacerbations of these symptoms with intercurrent respiratory infections. In one pediatric case described by Jacobs,[212] the child had a high spiking temperature, generalized rash, polyarthritis, inspiratory stridor, and progressively labored respirations. Radiographically, there was evidence of nonspecific hyperexpansion of the hypopharyngeal area (suggesting a glottic obstruction), and the final diagnosis was established by direct laryngoscopy.

□ Subglottic larynx and trachea
■ Tumors and tumorlike lesions

A wide variety of tumors and tumorlike lesions may be encountered in the upper trachea and subglottic larynx. The subglottic hemangioma is by far the most common lesion.† Other less common lesions include inflammatory histiocytomas,[83,397] mucoceles,[90] ectopic endotracheal thyroid tissue,[181,346] lipomas,[469] and fibromas.[10] All of these lesions appear as endotracheal masses and may be radiographically indistinguishable. Subglottic hemangiomas occur directly below the glottis

---

*References 33, 167, 328, 423.
†References 11, 66, 77, 110, 206, 247, 253, 420, 456.

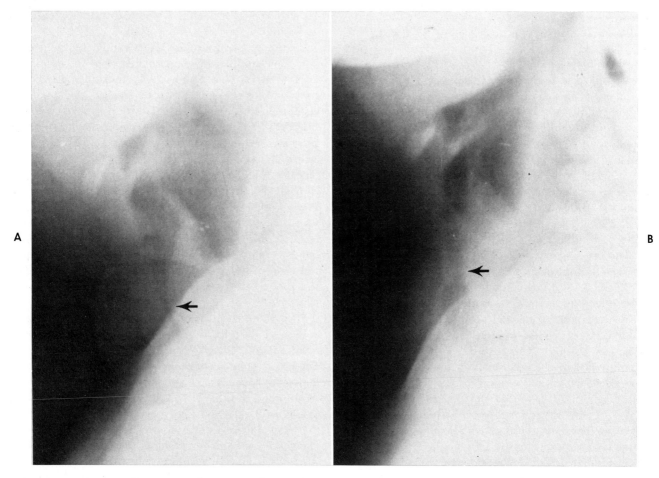

Fig. 15-34. A, Lateral view reveals typical appearance and location of mass produced by subglottic hemangioma *(arrows)*. **B,** Lateral view in another patient, demonstrating eccentric subglottic mass *(arrow)*.

and most often are posterior or lateral in position. Roentgenographically, they usually appear as rounded masses that encroach on the airway or glottis (Fig. 15-34), and although the finding is not pathognomonic, it is highly suggestive of a hemangioma.

The treatment of choice for subglottic hemangiomas remains controversial. Mist and oxygen may temporarily alleviate acute respiratory distress, but a tracheostomy should be performed if there is severe compromise of the airway.[253] Subsequent therapy depends on the risk at hand for any given patient. The reason for this is that these hemangiomas eventually involute in an analogous manner to the classic strawberry nevus hemangioma of the skin.[248] Before involution occurs, however, there may be a rapid growth spurt during infancy, which causes these patients to have more severe problems.

Because subglottic hemangiomas tend to involute spontaneously, it is difficult to thoroughly evaluate var-

ious treatment regimens. In the past, external radiation was used most frequently,[129,426] but the well-known relationship between thyroid malignancy and anterior neck radiation[45,352, 367] speaks against this form of therapy. To minimize radiation risk a technique was described[42] involving the intralaryngeal application of beta radiation. The placement of radioactive gold grains directly into the lesion has also been described.[23] In recent years, however, the use of systemic corticosteroids has been demonstrated to be successful by a number of authors.[87,138,320] This form of treatment evolved from the observation that there was marked regression of large visceral and skin hemangiomas when steroids were used in the treatment of thrombocytopenia.[230] A trial of steroid therapy for a 3-week period is advocated[253]; however, it is pointed out that steroid therapy will not replace the need for a tracheostomy if there is a significant airway obstruction.

Finally, surgical excision may be used although it is

usually advocated only after the failure of steroid therapy.[253] Surgical removal by means of thyrotomy in those patients with a symptomatic lesion that remains unchanged or has enlarged during a 1-year period of observation has also been advocated.[64]

■ Tracheal webs

Although webs are identified fairly frequently in the larynx, congenital tracheal webs not associated with any deformities of the cartilage or the wall of the trachea are extremely uncommon.[194,290] Inspiratory and expiratory stridor are the hallmarks of the clinical diagnosis of this entity. Rarely, a thin, faint transverse shadow of the web may be seen radiographically,[290] but most often the diagnosis is only made endoscopically.

☐ **Miscellaneous lesions of the neck**

■ Ectopic thyroid

Ectopic or aberrant thyroid tissue may occur at numerous locations in the neck or chest and in so doing lead to displacement or obstruction of the airway. Usually the ectopic thyroid tissue is situated in or near the midline, either in the lower retropharyngeal area or in the substernal region.[110] Radiographically, the soft tissue mass can easily be demonstrated with plain films of the lateral neck, but the findings are nonspecific. Nevertheless, the demonstration of a soft tissue mass in these locations should certainly bring up the possibility of ectopic thyroid tissue being present. Definitive diagnosis usually is made by radioisotope thyroid scanning.[110]

■ Thyroglossal duct cysts and sinuses

During the fourth week of fetal development the thyroid anlage[6,177,326] appears as a thickening of the entoderm in the floor of the pharynx. Shortly thereafter, this structure grows into a bilobate diverticulum that descends in the midline through the region, where the tongue muscles and hyoid bone later develop. Once it reaches the level of the thyroid cartilage it may deviate to one side or the other. Statistically it most often deviates to the left side.[172,266,335] As the diverticulum descends it remains attached to the pharynx by a hollow tubular stalk called the thyroglossal duct. Normally this duct becomes a solid core that disintegrates by the sixth week. The point or origin in the base of the tongue remains as the foramen cecum, and its termination remains as the pyramidal lobe of the thyroid gland.

Remnants and rests of the thyroglossal duct may persist from embryonic life, eventually proliferate, and give rise to thryoglossal cysts or sinus tracts.[286] Thyroglossal tract remnants have been found in more than 50% of cadavers examined[18] and radionuclide studies[103] have shown functioning thyroid tissue along the thyroglossal tract in one third of asymptomatic control patients; thus most of these remnants appear to be asymptomatic. Overall, clinically apparent thyroglossal duct cysts and fistulae are quite uncommon.

Accumulated secretions can produce a cyst at any level, although most occur just above or below the body of the hyoid bone.[10] These cysts may vary in size from 1 to 5 cms[251,368] and in most cases do not spontaneously communicate with the skin. Occasionally, however, they may do so after becoming infected,[341] but most external communications are the result of incision or incomplete excision of the cyst. Under these circumstances it is the residual secreting thyroglossal mucosa that produces a draining sinus tract. Carcinoma has been reported to develop in these ducts or cysts in a number of cases.[30]

Radiographically, thyroglossal duct cysts are best visualized on lateral views of the neck and appear as sharply circumscribed round to oval soft tissue masses. Demonstration of a fistulous tract can be accomplished by an injection of contrast material. A modified lacrimal duct cannula is gently inserted into the drainage site on the skin.[341] This is followed by the injection of several milliliters of water-soluble contrast material that nicely outlines the tract. The injection is not painful and thus no anesthesia is required.

■ Branchial cleft cysts, sinuses, and fistulae

Most authors[54,122] believe that branchial cleft cysts, sinuses, and fistulae arise from branchial cleft remnants and that all are lined with stratified squamous epithelium. Branchial cleft cysts constitute approximately 20% of all neck masses in children[97] and arise from the second branchial cleft. Other second branchial cleft anomalies include cutaneous sinuses that drain externally along the anterior border of the sternocleidomastoid muscle near the angle of the mandible, fistulae between the pharynx and the neck, and pharyngeal diverticula arising from the tonsillar fossa, pyriform sinuses, or valleculae.[97] Most cysts are located in the upper third of the neck, and fistula formation is present in only 10% to 15% of cases.[322]

Defects of the first branchial cleft are of two types[97]: type I consists of duplication of the membranous external auditory canal (cystic mass anterior and inferior to the ear lobe), and type II consists of an anomalous external auditory canal with deformity of the ear cartilage (a large cystic mass over the parotid gland and upper neck).[464] Malformations of the third branchial cleft are extremely uncommon and can consist of cysts, sinuses, or fistulae. They occur in the lower one third of the neck and are located near the midline.[97]

Radiographically, the findings of a branchial cleft cyst are nonspecific, being those of a soft tissue mass. The course and extent of a sinus tract can easily be demonstrated by the injection of water-soluble contrast material. Generally speaking, branchial cleft cysts and sinuses are easily treated with surgical resection, but if there is delay in treatment, infection frequently complicates the clinical picture.[54]

■ Cystic hygromas

Cystic hygromas represent congenital malformations of the cervical lymph sacs, and the most common sites of involvement are the posterior triangle of the neck and the supraclavicular fossa. The exact cause of these tumors is unknown, although there are two theories of origin. One suggests that the lymphatic endothelium sends out buds that later cannulize and form cysts, while the other theory suggests that the hygroma is the product of sequestration of the primitive jugular sac.[106] The histologically benign appearance of these tumors erroneously hides their invasive capabilities, and in most cases extensive infiltration into adjacent structures occurs. Symptoms depend on the structures involved, and the patient can have severe respiratory distress, dysphagia, or compression of the great vessels. In addition, large cystic hygromas arising from the neck can extend into the mediastinum or dissect posteriorly into the retropharyngeal space. Indeed, in the retropharyngeal space cystic hygromas are the most common tumor in children.[13,14,239]

In approximately 30% to 50% of patients, cystic hygromas appear as soft tissue masses at birth or shortly thereafter. In the remainder of patients the tumors appear clinically in the early years of life.[14,148] Spontaneous disappearance has been reported[50] but is not the general rule. Usually the tumor grows in proportion to the infant's growth; however, a rapid increase in size generally is the result of infection or hemorrhage.[97]

The treatment of choice for cystic hygromas is surgical excision,[13,14] although there is no agreement on the age at which the operation should be undertaken.[50,165,444] Other therapeutic approaches that have proven unsatisfactory include radiation therapy and the use of sclerosing agents. Aspiration of the cysts affords temporary improvement but also provides an entrance for infection.[13] Radiographically, the plain film findings depend on the size of the mass, its location, and its extent. More recently, CT has been advocated as the method of choice for demonstrating the exact extent of these low-attenuation tumors.[291]

■ Malignant tumors of the head and neck

Of 178 children with tumors of the head and neck, lesions of the lymphoid tissue accounted for almost 50% of the malignant ones.[215] Of these, Hodgkin's disease appeared as a neck mass approximately twice as com-

monly as did lymphosarcoma, even though lymphosarcoma, in general, was almost twice as common as Hodgkin's disease in children. On the other hand, extranodal sites in the head and neck occured more frequently with lymphosarcoma than with Hodgkin's disease in children.

Rhabdomyosarcoma is the second most common pediatric malignancy occurring in the head and neck,[215,268] and the most common sites of involvement are the nasopharynx, middle ear, and mastoid bone.[215] Fibrosarcomas and neurofibrosarcomas have an increased predilection in children for the head and neck (25% of all fibrosarcomas occur in this region) and occur in approximately 6% all patients.[215] Most occur in the mandible, cheek, and neck. Thyroid malignancies account for 5% of the tumors[25] and generally occur twice as commonly in girls as in boys. The occurrence of a thyroid malignancy following radiation therapy of the neck (even in the very low dose range of 200 rads) has been documented 10 to 20 years after the time of therapy. Other types of childhood malignancies involving the head and neck are neuroblastomas (primary and secondary) squamous cell carcinomas, melanomas, Ewing's sarcomas, malignant histiocytomas, osteogenetic and chondrogenetic sarcomas, malignant hemangiopericytomas, malignant hemangioendotheliomas, parotid malignancies, malignant Schwann cell tumors, and malignant teratomas.

■ Salivary glands

With the exception of viral parotitis, diseases of the salivary glands are rare in children. In the vast majority of cases of parotid gland infection the cause is the mumps virus;[254] however, the cytomegalic virus, the parainfluenza virus,[56] and the Coxsackie virus[205] also have been incriminated. Suppurative parotitis (most often a result of *Staphylococcus aureus* infection) may occur as a primary disease or more commonly as a complication of viral parotitis. Usually it is unilateral and accompanied by fever, swelling, and tenderness.[92] Neonatal suppurative parotitis, although rare, also has been documented;[252] and *Staphylococcus aureus* again is the causative organism.[252]

Recurrent idiopathic swelling of the parotid glands (autoimmune recurrent parotitis) may occur in otherwise healthy children. In most patients involvement is unilateral, although bilateral involvement, either simultaneously or alternatively, also has been noted.[226] Of 35 patients in one series[226] the vast majority of patients had their first episode before the age of 5; the initial episode usually subsided after 1 to 3 days. After a remission ranging from weeks to months the symptoms and swelling tend to recur.[370]

A complete remission or a significant improvement

occurs in about 60% of patients by 5 to 10 years of age.[370] Radiographically, plain film findings demonstrate nonspecific soft tissue masses. Sialography demonstrates various degrees of sialectasis, but no evidence of parotid duct stenosis[226] (see Chapter 4).

Although rare in childhood, Sjögren's syndrome has been described by a number of authors* and as in the adult the syndrome is considered a chronic autoimmune disorder. It is characterized by the triad of dry eyes, dry mouth, and connective tissue disease (most commonly juvenile rheumatoid arthritis). Bilateral enlargement of the salivary glands may occur in a variety of disorders including cystic fibrosis,[53] malnutrition and transiently during acute asthmatic attacks. Salivary gland tumors in the general population constitute less than 3% of all neoplasms[115] and malignancies of the salivary glands in children are even more rare.[231] However, mixed tumors, adenocystic carcinomas, and mucoepidermoid tumors can occur in adolescents. Only 1.28% to 5% of all salivary gland tumors occur in children.†

---

*References 8, 111, 241, 296, 316, 390.
†References 32, 61, 72, 192.

■ High esophageal foreign bodies

Esophageal foreign bodies are not uncommon in the young child, and the most frequent site of impaction is the cervical segment of the esophagus just below the cricopharyngeus muscle. One series[191] documented 90% of esophageal foreign bodies located in this area. It has been postulated[211] that large objects tend to lodge in the upper esophagus because of the poor peristalsis that exists immediately below the cricopharyngeus muscle.

The usual clinical symptoms of an esophageal foreign body consist of excessive drooling, poor feeding, and dysphagia. With high esophageal foreign bodies, however, patients frequently have symptoms suggesting respiratory disease (i.e., stridor, wheezing, chronic pneumonia).* Esophageal symptoms if present can be completely overshadowed by the respiratory difficulties. Failure to recognize this evidence of a high esophageal foreign body can lead to a late diagnosis and complications such as esophageal ulceration or perforation, chronic aspiration pneumonia, and failure to thrive.

---

*References 55, 57, 67, 114, 123, 142, 158, 191, 195, 211, 404.

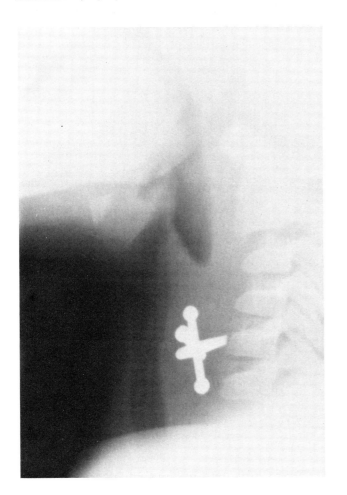

Fig. 15-35. Foreign body in upper esophagus. Lateral view reveals jack lodged in upper esophagus.

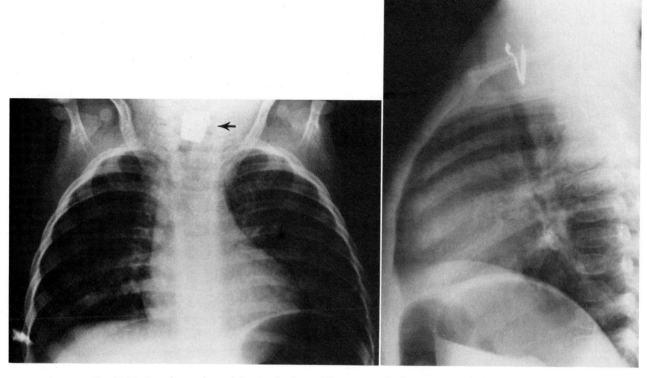

Fig. 15-36. Occult esophageal foreign body. **A,** This patient had symptoms of recurrent pneumonia. Metallic foreign body *(arrow)* was noted as incidental finding on chest film. **B,** Lateral view demonstrates location of foreign body (high esophagus) and the associated inflammatory edema that caused anterior displacement and compression of tracheal airway.

Radiographically, the diagnosis of radiopaque esophageal foreign bodies can be easily made with plain films of the chest and neck (Figs. 15-35 and 15-36). If the foreign body is not radiopaque (e.g., objects of plastic, aluminum, or wood), secondary soft tissue changes or focal overdistension of the upper airway may lead one to suspect its presence. In many cases only a barium swallow examination will reveal the foreign body. As previously mentioned, lateral films should be obtained in inspiration with the neck hyperextended. The arms also should be pulled downward. High-kilovoltage technique films with filtration and magnification can improve the radiographic imaging of some of the more elusive foreign bodies[228] as can CT scanning.

□ **References**

1. Abbott, T.R.: Complications of prolonged nasotracheal intubation in children, Br. J. Anaesth. **40**:347-353, 1968.
2. Alexander, T.A.: Nasal glioma, J. Pediatr. Surg. **13**:522-524, 1978.
3. Amies, A., and Fleming, W.E.: Central ossifying fibroma of the jaws, Oral Sug. **15**:1409-1414, 1962.
4. Ardran, G.M., and Kemp, F.H.: The mechanism of changes in form of the cervical airway in infancy, Med. Radiogr. Photogr. **44**:26-38, 1968.
5. Ardran, G.M., and Kemp, F.H.: The nasal and cervical airway in sleep in the neonatal period, AJR **108**:537-542, 1970.
6. Arey, L.B.: Developmental anatomy, Philadelphia, 1974, W.B. Saunders Co.
7. Astley, R.: The movements of the lateral walls of the nasopharynx: a cineradiographic study, J. Laryngol. Otol. **72**:325-328, 1958.
8. Athreya, B.H., et al.: Sjögren's syndrome in children, Pediatrics **59**:931-938, 1977.
9. Atkins, J.P.: Laryngeal problems of infancy and childhood, Pediatr. Clin. North Am. **9**:1125-1135, 1962.
10. Bachman, A.L.: Benign non-neoplastic conditions of the larynx and pharynx, Radiol. Clin. North Am. **16**:273-290, 1978.
11. Baden, M., et al.: Upper airway obstruction in a newborn secondary to hemangiopericytoma, Can. Med. Assoc. J. **107**:1202-1204, 1972.
12. Bahadori M., and Liebow, A.A.: Plasma cell granuloma of the lung, Cancer **31**:191-208, 1973.
13. Barnhart, R.A., and Brown, A.K., Jr.: Cystic hygroma of the neck, Arch. Otolaryngol. **86**:100-104, 1967.
14. Barrand, K.G., and Freeman, N.V.: Massive infiltrating cystic hygroma of the neck in infancy, Arch. Dis. Child **48**:523-531, 1973.
15. Batsakis, J.G.: Tumors of the head and neck: clinical and pathological considerations, Baltimore, 1974, The Williams & Wilkins Co.
16. Batsakis, J.G., and Fox, J.E.: Rhabdomyosarcoma of the larynx: report of a case, Arch. Otolaryngol. **91**:136-140, 1970.

17. Batsakis, J.G., and Fox, J.E.: Supporting tissue neoplasms of the larynx, Surg. Gynecol. Obstet. **131**:989-997, 1970.
18. Batson, O.V.: The adult thyroglossal duct, Anat. Rec. **94**:449-450, 1946.
19. Battaglia, J.D., and Lockhart, C.H.: Management of acute epiglottitis by nasotracheal intubation, Am. J. Dis. Child **126**:334-336, 1975.
20. Battifora, H.A., Eisenstein, R., and Smith, J.A.: Rhabdomyoma of larynx, Cancer **23**:183-190, 1969.
21. Baxter, J.D., and Pashley, N.R.T.: Acute epiglottitis: 25 years' experience in management. The Montreal Children's Hospital, J. Otolaryngol. **6**:473-476, 1977.
22. Becker, M.H., Coccaro, P.J., and Converse, J.M.: Antegonial notching of the mandible: an often overlooked mandibular deformity in congenital and acquired disorders, Radiology **121**:149-151, 1976.
23. Benjamin, B.: Choanal atresia, Adv. Otorhinolaryngol. **23**:65-72, 1978.
24. Benjamin, B.: Treatment of infantile subglottic hemangioma with radioactive gold grain, Ann. Otol. Rhinol. Laryngol. **87**:18-21, 1978.
25. Berger, A., Altman, M., and Winter, S.T.: Neonatal asphyxia caused by teratoma of pharynx, Am. J. Dis. Child **109**:584-585, 1965.
26. Bergman, A.B., and Lewicki, A.M.: Complete esophageal obstruction from cricopharyngeal achalasia, Radiology **123**:289-290, 1977.
27. Bernstein, L.: Pediatric sinus problems, Otolaryngol. Clin. North Am. **4**:127-142, 1971.
28. Berry, M., Krishan, A., and Bhargava, S.: An aneurysmal bone cyst of the mandible: a case report, Australas. Radiol. **17**:196-198, 1973.
29. Bhaskar, S.N.: Oral tumors of infancy and childhood: a survey of 293 cases, J. Pediatr. **63**:195-210, 1963.
30. Bhagavan, B.S., Rao, D.R.G., and Weinberg, T.: Carcinoma of thyroglossal duct cyst, Surgery **67**:281-292, 1970.
31. Bhaskar, S.N., Bernier, J.L., and Godby, F.: Aneurysmal bone cyst and other giant cell lesions of the jaws: report of 104 cases, J. Oral Surg. **17**:30-41, 1959.
32. Bianchi, A., and Cudmore, R.E.: Salivary gland tumors in children, J. Pediatr. Surg. **13**:519-521.
33. Bienenstock, H., Ehrlich, G.E., and Freyberg, R.H.: Rheumatoid arthritis of the cricoarytenoid joint: a clinico-pathologic study, Arthritis Rheum. **6**:48-63, 1963.
34. Black, B.K., and Smith, D.E.: Nasal glioma: two cases with recurrence, Arch. Neural. Psychiatr. **64**:614-630, 1950.
35. Blank, R.H., and Silbieger, M.: Cricopharyngeal achalasia as a cause of respiratory distress in infancy, J. Pediatr. **81**:95-98, 1972.
36. Bleustone, C.D., E'elerme, A.N., and Samuelson, G.H.: Airway obstruction due to vocal cord paralysis in infants with hydrocephalus and meningomyelocele, Ann. Otol. Rhinol. Laryngol. **81**:778-783, 1972.
37. Blumberg, J.B., et al.: Laryngotracheoesophageal cleft: the embryologic implications—review of the literature, Surgery **57**:556-559, 1965.
38. Blumenfeld, R., and Skolnik, E.M.: Intranasal encephaloceles, Arch. Otolaryngol. **82**:527-531, 1965.
39. Boies, L.R., Jr., and Harris, D.: Nasopharyngeal dermoid of the newborn, Laryngoscope **75**:763-767, 1965.
40. Booth, J.B., and Osborn, D.A.: Granular cell myoblastoma of the larynx, Acta Otolaryngol. **70**:279-293, 1970.
41. Borowiecki, B., et al.: Fibro-optic study of pharyngeal airway during sleep in patients with hypersomnia obstructive sleep apnea syndrome, Laryngoscope **88**:1310-1313, 1978.
42. Bourne, R.G., and Taylor, R.G.: Treatment of juvenile laryngeal angioma with a beta-ray therapy applicator, Radiology **103**:423-426, 1972.
43. Boyle, W.F., Riggs, J.L., and Oshino, L.S.: Electron microscopic identification of papovavirus in laryngeal papilloma, Laryngoscope **83**:1102-1108, 1973.
44. Branfors, H.P., and Jeppsson, P.H.: Acute epiglottitis: a clinical, bacteriological and serological study, Scand. J. Infect. Dis. **7**:103-111, 1975.
45. Braverman, L.: Consequences of thyroid radiation in children, N. Engl. J. Med. **292**:204-206, 1975.
46. Breivik, H., and Klaastad, O.: Acute epiglottitis in children: review of 27 patients, Br. J. Anaesth. **50**:505-510, 1978.
47. Brenner, G.H.: Variations in the depth of the cervical prevertebral tissues in normal infants studied by cinefluorography, AJR **91**:573-577, 1964.
48. Brintnall, E.S., and Kridenbaugh, W.W.: Congenital diverticulum of the posterior hypopharynx stimulating atresia of the esophagus, Ann. Surg. **131**:564-574, 1950.
49. Brook, I., et al.: Complications of sinusitis in children, Pediatrics **66**:568-572, 1980.
50. Broomhead, I.W.: Cystic hygroma of the neck, Br. J. Plast. Surg. **17**:225-244, 1964.
51. Brown, S., and Keer-Wilson, R.: Intra-oral duplication cyst, J. Pediatr. Surg. **13**:95-96, 1978.
52. Brownstein, M.H., Shapiro, L., and Stevin, R.: Fistula of the dorsum of the nose, Arch. Dermatol. **109**:227-229, 1974.
53. Bruns, W.T., and Tang, T.T.: Submandibular sialolithiasis in a cystic fibrosis patient, Am. J. Dis. Child **126**:685-686, 1973.
54. Buckingham, J.M., and Lynn, H.B.: Branchial cleft cysts and sinuses in children, Mayo Clinic Proc. **49**:172-175, 1975.
55. Buckler, J.M.A., and Stool, S.E.: Failure to thrive: exogenous cause, Am. J. Dis. Child **114**:652-653, 1967.
56. Buckley, J.M., Poche, P., and McIntosh, K.: Parotitis and parainfluenza 3 virus, Am. J. Dis. Child **124**:789, 1972.
57. Bunker, P.G.: Foreign body complications, Laryngoscope **71**:903-917, 1961.
58. Burkitt, D., and O'Connor, G.T.: Malignant lymphoma in African children, Cancer **14**:258-269, 1961.
59. Burmann, O.H., Jr.: Subglottic stenosis: a new epidemic in children, Contemp. Surg. **13**:9-13, 1978.
60. Burroughs, N., and Leape, L.L.: Laryngotracheoesophageal cleft: report of a case successfully treated and review of the literature, Pediatrics **53**:516-522, 1974.
61. Byars, L.T., Ackerman, L.V., and Peacock, E.: Tumors of salivary gland origin in children: a clinical pathologic appraisal of 24 cases, Ann. Surg. **146**:40-51, 1957.
62. Byers, P.D.: Solitary benign osteoblastic lesions of bone: osteoid osteoma and benign osteoblastoma, Cancer **22**:43-57, 1968.
63. Burd, S.E., Harwood-Nash, D.C., Fitz, C.R., and Rogovitz, D.M.: Computed tomography in the evaluation of encephaloceles in infants and children, J. Comput. Assist. Tomogr. **2**:81-87, 1978.
64. Calcaterra, T.C.: An evaluation of the treatment of subglottic hemangioma, Laryngoscope **78**:1956-1964, 1968.
65. Campbell, D.R., Brown, S.J., and Manchester, J.S.: An evaluation of the radio-opaque of various ingested foreign bodies in the pharynx and esophagus, J. Can. Assoc. Radiol. **19**:183-186, 1968.
66. Campbell, J.S., et al.: Congenital subglottic hemangiomas of the larynx and trachea in infants, Pediatrics **22**:727-737, 1958.
67. Capitanio, M.A., and Kirkpatrick, J.A., Jr.: Upper respiratory tract obstruction in infants and children, Radiol. Clin. North Am. **6**:265-277, 1968.

68. Capitanio, M.A., and Kirkpatrick, J.A., Jr.: Nasopharyngeal lymphoid tissue: roentgen observations in 257 children two years of age or less, Radiology 96:389-391, 1970.
69. Capitanio, M.A., et al.: Congenital anhidrotic ectodermal dysplasia, AJR 103:168-172, 1968.
70. Carswell, F., Kerr, M.M., and Hutchinson, J.H.: Congenital goiter and hypothyroidism produced by maternal ingestion of iodides, Lancet 1:1241-1243, 1970.
71. Castner, D.V., Jr., McCully, A.C., and Hiatt, W.R.: Intracystic ameloblastoma in the young: report of a case, Oral Surg. 23:127-137, 1967.
72. Castro, E.B., et al.: Tumors of the major salivary gland in children, Cancer 29:312-317, 1972.
73. Cavom, J.W., Jr., Pratt, L.L., and Alonso, W.A.: First brachial cleft syndromes and associated congenital hearing loss, Laryngoscope 86:739-745, 1976.
74. Cayler, G.G., et al.: Heart failure due to enlarged tonsils and adenoids, Am. J. Dis. Child 118:708-717, 1969.
75. Chandler, J.R., Langenbrunner, D.J., and Stevens, E.R.: The pathogenesis of orbital complications in acute sinusitis, Laryngoscope 80:1414-1428, 1970.
76. Chhangani, D.L., Agarwai, K.K., and Popli, S.P.: Expansion of antrum and erosion of lateral nasal wall: antrochoanal polyps, J. Laryngol. Otol. 81:1049-1051, 1967.
77. Christiaens, L., et al.: Hemangiomas of the larynx and of the trachea in infants: six cases, Arch. Fr. Pediatr. 22:513-531, 1965.
78. Clay, B.: Congenital lateral pharyngeal diverticulum, Br. J. Radiol. 45:863-865, 1972.
79. Cockshott, W.P.: Radiological aspects of Burkitt's tumor, Br. J. Radiol. 38:172-180, 1965.
80. Cogswell, J.J., and Easton, D.M.: Cor pulmonale in the Pierre-Robin syndrome, Arch. Dis. Child 49:905-908, 1974.
81. Cohen, M.H., et al.: Burkitt's tumor in United States, Cancer 23:1259-1272, 1969.
82. Cohen, S.R., and Chai J.: Epiglottitis: twenty-year study with tracheostomy, Ann. Otol. Rhinol. Laryngol. 87:461-467, 1978.
83. Cohen, S.R., Landing, B.H., and Isaacs, H.: Epidermolysis bullosa associated with laryngeal stenosis, Ann. Otol. Rhinol. Laryngol. Suppl. 87(5 pt. 2 suppl. 52):25-28, 1978.
84. Cohen, S.R., Landing, B.H., and Isaacs, H.: Fibrous histiocytoma of the trachea, Ann. Otol. Rhinol. Laryngol. Suppl. 87(5 pt. 2 suppl. 52):2-4, 1978.
85. Cohen, S.R., Landing, B.H., and Isaacs, H.: Neurofibroma of the larynx in a child, Ann. Otol. Rhinol. Laryngol. Suppl. 87(5 pt. 2 suppl. 52):29-31, 1978.
86. Cohen, S.R., and Wang, C.: Steroid treatment of hemangiomas of the head and neck in children, Ann. Otol. Rhinol. Laryngol. 81:584-590, 1972.
87. Cohen, S.R., et al.: Primary lymphosarcoma of the larynx in a child, Ann. Otol. Rhinol. Laryngol. 87:20-24, 1978.
88. Converse, J.M., et al.: On hemifacial microsomia: the 1st and 2nd branchial arch syndrome, Plast. Reconstruct. Surg. 51:268-279, 1973.
89. Cundy, R.L., and Bergstrom, L.B.: Congenital subglottic stenosis, J. Pediatr. 82:282-284, 1973.
90. Dagan, R., et al.: Subglottic mucocele in an infant, Pediatr. Radiol. 8:119-121, 1979.
91. Dahlgren, S.E., et al.: Fibrous dysplasia of jaw bones: a clinical, roentgenographic and histopatholic study, Acta Otolaryngol. 68:257-270, 1969.
92. David, R.B., and O'Connell, E.J.: Suppurative parotitis in children, Am. J. Dis. Child 119:332-335, 1970.
93. Davidson, F.W.: Acute laryngeal obstruction in children: a fifty year review, Ann. Otol. Rhinol. Laryngol. 87:606-613, 1978.
94. Decarlo, J., Tramer, A., and Startzman, H.H.: Congenital iodized oil aspiration in the newborn, Am. J. Dis. Child 84:442-445, 1952.
95. DeEspinosa, H., and de Paredes, C.G.: Traumatic perforation of the pharynx in a newborn baby, J. Pediatr. Surg. 9:247-248, 1974.
96. Dehner, L.P.: Tumors of the mandible and maxilla in children. I. Clinicopathologic study of the 46 histologically benign lesions, Cancer 31:364-384, 1973.
97. Dehner, L.P.: Jaws and somatic structures of neck. In Kissane, J.M., editor: Pathology of infancy and childhood, ed. 2, St. Louis, 1975, The C.V. Mosby Co.
98. DeLevie, M., Nogrady, M.B., and Spence, L.: Acute laryngotracheobronchitis (croup) with correlation of clinical severity with radiologic and virologic findings, Ann. Radiol. 15:193-200, 1972.
99. DeMartino, A., Sorbellini, F., and Parrini, C.: Hemangiomatous aneurysmal cyst of the jaw, Osp. Ital. Pediatr. 12:586-596, 1977.
100. DeSanto, L.W., Devine, K.D., and Weiland, L.H.: Cysts of the laryngoclassification, Laryngoscope 80:145-176, 1970.
101. Dicke, T.E., and Gate, G.A.: Malignant teratoma of the paranasal sinuses, Arch. Otolaryngol. 91:391-394, 1970.
102. Dieter, R.A., Jr., Hollinger, P.H., and Maurizi, D.G.: Angiofibromatous polyp of the pharynx, Am. J. Dis. Child 119:91-93, 1970.
103. Dische, S., and Berg, P.K.: An investigation of the thyroglossal tract using the radioisotope scan, Radiol. Clin. North Am. 14:293-303, 1963.
104. Dixon, J.W.: Solitary neurilemmomata presenting in the larynx, pharynx and neck, J. Laryngol. Otol. 73:819-829, 1959.
105. Donaldson, S.S., Castro, J.R., and Jesse, R.H.: Rhabdomyosarcoma of the head and neck in children, Cancer 31:26-35, 1973.
106. Dowd, C.N.: Hygoma cysticum colli, Ann. Surg. 58:112-132, 1913.
107. Dresser, W.J., and Segal, E.: Ameloblastoma associated with a dentigerous cyst in a 6 year old child, Oral Surg. 24:388-391, 1967.
108. Duc, T.V., et al.: Laryngotracheal lesions induced by endotracheal intubation in children: anatomic study of 53 cases, Nouv. Presse Med. 3:365-371, 1974.
109. Dunbar, J.S.: Epiglottitis and croup, J. Can. Assoc. Radiol. 12:86-95, 1961.
110. Dunbar, J.S.: Upper respiratory tract obstruction in infants and children, AJR 109:225-246, 1970.
111. Duncan, H., Epker, B.N., and Sheldon, G.M.: Sjögren's syndrome in childhood: report of a case, Henry Ford Hosp. Med. J. 17:35, 1969.
112. Dupin, C.L., and LeJoune, F.E., Jr.: Nasal masses in infants and children, South Med. J. 71(2):124-128, 1978.
113. Edison, B., and Hollinger, P.H.: Traumatic pharyngeal pseudodiverticulum in the newborn infant, J. Pediatr. 82:483-485, 1973.
114. Emerson, E.B.: Foreign bodies in airways and esophagus, Am. J. Surg. 105:522-523, 1963.
115. Eneroth, C.M.: Histological and clinical aspects of parotid tumors, Acta Otolaryngol Suppl. 191:1-19, 1964.
116. Engle, M.B., Richmond, J.B., and Brodie, A.G.A.: Mandibular growth disturbance in rheumatoid arthritis of childhood, Am. J. Dis. Child 78:728-743, 1949.
117. Ennis, J.T., et al.: The radiology of the bone changes in histiocytosis X, Clin. Radiol. 24:212-220, 1973.
118. Epstein, E.S., Sternberg, J., and Shapiro, E.: Acute respiratory distress in an infant produced by hypertrophied tonsils, AJR 91:571-572, 1964.
119. Evans, J.N.G., and MacLachlan, R.F.: Choanal atresia, J. Laryngol. Otol. 85:903-929, 1971.

120. Fagan, C.J., and Swischuk, L.E.: Juvenile laryngeal papillomatosis with spread to the lung, Am. J. Dis. Child 123:139-140, 1972.

121. Fairman, H.D.: Papillomatosis of the larynx, Proc. Roy. Soc. Med. 65:619-624, 1972.

122. Favara, B.E., Francios, R.A., and Akers, D.R.: Enteric duplications, Am. J. Dis. Child 122:501-506, 1971.

123. Fearon, B.: Acute laryngotracheobronchitis in infancy and childhood, Pediatr. Clin. North Am. 9:1095-1112, 1962.

124. Fearon, B.: Acute airway obstruction. In Ferguson, C.F., and Kendig, E.L., editors: Otolaryngology II, ed. 2, Philadelphia, 1972, W.B. Saunders Co.

125. Fearon, B., and MacRae, D.: Laryngeal papillomatosis in children, J. Otolaryngol. 5:493-496, 1976.

126. Fearon, B., et al.: Airway problems in children following prolonged endotracheal intubation, Ann. Otol. Rhinol. Laryngol. 75:975-986, 1966.

127. Felman, A.H., and Talbert, J.H.: Laryngotracheoesophageal cleft: description of a combined laryngoscopic and roentgenographic diagnostic technique and report of two patients, Radiology 103:641-644, 1972.

128. Felman, A.H., et al.: Upper airway obstruction during sleep in children, AJR 133:213-216, 1979.

129. Ferguson, C.F., and Flake, C.G.: Subglottic hemangioma as a cause of respiratory obstruction in infants, Ann. Otol. 70:1095-1112, 1961.

130. Ferguson, C.F., and Kendig, E.L., editors, Pediatric otolaryngology, Philadelphia, 1971, W.B. Saunders Co.

131. Ferguson, C.F., and Kendig, E.L.: Disorders of the respiratory tract in children. In Pediatric otolaryngology, vol. 2, Philadelphia, 1972, W.B. Saunders Co.

132. Ferlito, A., and Micheau, C.: Infantile olfactory neuroblastoma: A clinicopathological study with review of the literature, ORL 41(1):40-50, 1979.

133. Ferris, R.A., Hakkal, H.G., and Cigtay, O.S.: Radiological manifestations of North American Burkitt's lymphoma, AJR 123:614-620, 1975.

134. Fishman, A.P.: Hypoxia on the pulmonary circulation: how and where it acts, Circ. Res. 38:221-231, 1976.

135. Fitz-Hugh, G.S., Wallenborn, W.M., and McGovern, F.H.: Injuries of the larynx and cervical trachea, Ann. Otol. Rhinol. Laryngol. 71:419-442, 1962.

136. Flake, C.G., and Ferguson, C.F.: Congenital choanal atresia in infants and children, Ann. Otol. Rhinol. Laryngol. 73:458-473, 1964.

137. Flanagan, P., Cross, R., and Libcke, J.H.: Fibrosarcoma of the larynx, J. Laryngol. Otol. 79:1049-1056, 1965.

138. Fost, N.C., and Esterly, N.B.: Successful treatment of juvenile hemangiomas with prednisone, J. Pediatr. 72:351-357, 1968.

139. Frank, M.M., and Gatewood, O.M.B.: Transient pharyngeal incoordination in the newborn, Am. J. Dis. Child 111:178-181, 1966.

140. Frates, R.E.: Roentgen sign in laryngotracheoesophageal cleft, Radiology 88:484-486, 1967.

141. Frech, R.S., and McAlister, W.H.: Teratoma of nasopharynx producing depression of the posterior hard palate, J. Can. Assoc. Radiol. 20:204-205, 1969.

142. Friedberg, J.: Maxillary sinus disease and the pediatric patient, Otolaryngol. Clin. North Am. 9:163-173, 1976.

143. Friedberg, S.A., and Bluestone, C.D.: Foreign body accidents involving air and food passages in children, Otolaryngol. Clin. North Am. 3:395-403, 1970.

144. Froggatt, P., Lyneas, M.A., and MacKenzie, G.: Epidermiology of sudden unexpected death in infants ("cot death"), Br. J. Prev. Soc. Med. 25:119-134, 1971.

145. Fujioka, M., and Young, L.W.: The sphenoidal sinuses: radiographic patterns of normal development and abnormal findings in infants and children, Radiology 129:133-136, 1978.

146. Fujioka, M., Young, L.W., and Girdayn, B.R.: Radiographic evaluation of adenoidal size in children: adenoidal nasopharyngeal ratio, AJR 133:401-404, 1979.

147. Fuzesi, K., and Young, D.G.: Congenital laryngotracheoseophageal cleft, J. Pediatr. Surg. 11:933-937, 1976.

148. Galofre, M., et al.: Results of surgical treatment of cystic hygroma, Surg. Gynecol. Obstet. 115:319-326, 1962.

149. Gardner, S., et al.: Subglottic coccidioidomycosis presenting with persistent stridor, Pediatrics 66:623-625, 1980.

150. Gellady, A.M., Shulman, S.T., and Ayoub, E.M.: Periorbital and orbital cellulitis in children, Pediatrics 62:272-277, 1978.

151. Gellis, S.S., and Feingold, M.: Picture of the month—enteric cyst of tongue, Am. J. Dis. Child 134:985-986, 1980.

152. Gharib, R., Allen, R., and Jons, H.A.: Paranasal sinuses in cystic fibrosis, Am. J. Dis. Child 108:499-502, 1964.

153. Gibbs, N.M., Taylor, M., and Young A.: Von Recklinghausen's disease in the larynx and trachea of an infant, J. Laryngol. Otol. 71:626-630, 1957.

154. Gibson, M.J., and Middlemiss, J.H.: Fibrous dysplasia of bone, Br. J. Radiol. 44:1-13, 1971.

155. Gillam, P.M.S., and Mymin, D.: Hypoventilation and heart disease, Lancet 2:853-855, 1961.

156. Girdany, B.R., Sieber, W.K., and Osman, M.Z.: Traumatic pseudodiverticulum of the pharynx in newborn infants, N. Engl. J. Med. 280:237-240, 1969.

157. Glick, H.N.: Unusual neoplasm in larynx of child (rhabdomyomyxosarcoma), Ann. Otol. Rhinol. Laryngol. 53:699, 1944.

158. Glass, W.M., and Goodman, M.: Unsuspected foreign bodies in young child's esophagus presenting with respiratory symptoms, Laryngoscope 76:605-615, 1966.

159. Gorlin, R.J., and Gorlin, J.B.: Developmental anomalies of the jaws, Semin. Roentgenol. 6(4):426-440, 1971.

160. Gorlin, R.J., Kalnins, V., and Izant, R.J.: Occurence of heterotopic gastric mucosa in the tongue, J. Pediatr. 64:604-606, 1964.

161. Grabb, W.C.: The first and second branchial arch syndrome, Plast. Reconstr. Surg. 36:485-508, 1965.

162. Greene, R., and Stark, P.: Trauma of the larynx and trachea, Radiol. Clin. North Am. 16:309-320, 1978.

163. Griffith, B.H., et al.: Motion of the lateral pharyngeal walls during velopharyngeal closure, Plast. Reconstr. Surg. 41:338-342, 1968.

164. Griscom, N.T.: Persistent esophagotrachea, AJR 97:211-215, 1966.

165. Gross, R.E.: The Surgery of infancy and childhood, principles and techniques, Philadelphia, 1953, W.B. Saunders Co.

166. Gross, W.E., and Crocker, T.R.: Current management of juvenile laryngeal papillomata, Laryngoscope 80:532-543, 1970.

167. Grossman, A., Martin, J.R., and Root, H.S.: Rheumatoid arthritis of the cricoarytenoid joint, Laryngoscope 71:530-544, 1961.

168. Grunebaum, M.: Respiratory stridor—a challenge for the paediatric radiologist, Clin. Radiol. 24:485-490, 1973.

169. Grunebaum, M.: The roentgenologic investigation of congenital subglottic stenosis, AJR 125:877-880, 1975.

170. Grunebaum, M., and Moskowitz, G.: The retropharyngeal soft tissues in young infants with hypothyroidism, AJR 108:544-545, 1970.

171. Guilleminault, C., Eldridge, F.L., and Simmons, F.B., et al.: Sleep apnea in eight children, Pediatrics 58(1):23-30, 1976.

172. Guimaraes, S.B., Uceda, J.E., and Lynn, H.B.: Thyroglossal duct remnants in infants and children, Mayo Clin. Proc. 47:117-120, 1972.

173. Gwinn, J.L., and Lee, F.A.: Radiological case of the month: pseudodiverticulum of the pharynx, Am. J. Dis. Child 121:329-333, 1971.

174. Gwinn, J.L., and Lee, F.A.: Radiological case of the month: congenital anhidrotic ectodermal dysplasia, Am. J. Dis. Child 128:215-216, 1974.

175. Gyepes, M.T., and Linde, L.M.: Familial dysautonomia: the mechanism of aspiration, Radiology 91:471-475, 1968.

176. Gyepes, M.T., and Desilets, D.T.: The submentovertical projection: a new approach to the study of laryngeal and pharyngeal function in infants, Radiology 92:758-762, 1969.

177. Hamilton, W.J., and Mossman, H.W.: Hamilton, Boyd and Mossman's human embryology, Baltimore, 1972, The Williams & Wilkins Co.

178. Hamner, J.E., III, Scofield, H.H., and Cornyn, J.: Benign fibro-osseous jaw lesions of periodontal membrane origin: an analysis of 249 cases, Cancer 22:861-878, 1968.

179. Han, B.K., Dunbar, J.S., and Striker, T.W.: Membranous laryngotracheobronchochitis (membranous croup), AJR 133:53-58, 1979.

180. Hansel, F.J.: Clinical allergy, St. Louis, 1953, The C.V. Mosby Co.

181. Hardwick, D.F., Cormode, E.J., and Riddell, D.G.: Respiratory distress and neck mass in a neonate intratracheal thyroid, J. Pediatr. 89:591-605, 1976.

182. Hardy, G.: Choanal polyps, Ann. Otol. Rhinol. Laryngol. 66:306-326, 1957.

183. Hassan, A.I., Aref, G.H., and Kassem, A.S.: Congenital iodide-induced goiter with hypothyroidism, Arch. Dis. Child 43:702-704 1968.

184. Haverson, G., Bailey, I.C., and Kiryabwire, J.W.M.: The radiological diagnosis of anterior encephaloceles, Clin. Radiol. 25:317-322, 1974.

185. Hawkins, C.F., and Swisher, W.E.: Evaluation of a real-time ultrasound scanner in assessing lateral pharyngeal wall motion during speech, Cleft Palate J. 15:161-166, 1978.

186. Haynes, R.E., and Crambleth, H.G.: Acute ethmoiditis—its relationship to orbital cellulitis, Am. J. Dis. Child 114:261-267, 1967.

187. Heck, W.E., Hallberg, O.E., and Williams, H.L.: Antrochoanal polyps, Arch. Otolaryngol. 52:538-548, 1950.

188. Heller, R.M., Kirchner, S.G., and O'Neill, J.A.: Perforation of the pharynx in the newborn: a new look-alike for esophageal atresia, AJR 128:335-337, 1977.

189. Hiranandani, L.H., and Malgiri, R.D.: Expansion of antrum by antrochoanal polyps, J. Laryngol. Otol. 80:175-177, 1966.

190. Hirsh, L.F., Stool, S.E., Langfitt, T.W., and Schut, L.: Nasal glioma, J. Neurosurg. 46:85-91, 1977.

191. Hoeksma, P.E., and Huizinga, E.: On foreign bodies and perforations of esophagus, Ann. Otol. Rhinol. Laryngol. 80:36-41, 1971.

192. Hoffman, K., and Block, M.A.: Tumors of major salivary glands in children, Mich. Med. 67:1461-1464, 1968.

193. Holdaway, M.D.: Croup and epiglottitis: diagnosis and action, Drugs 13(6):452-457, 1977.

194. Holinger, P.H., Johnston, K.C., and Basinger, C.E.: Benign stenosis of the trachea, Ann. Otol. Rhinol. Laryngol. 59:837-859, 1950.

195. Holinger, P.H., and Johnston, K.C.: Infant with respiratory stridor, Pediatr. Clin. North Am. 2:403-411, 1955.

196. Holinger, P.H., Johnston, K.C., and Schild, J.A.: congenital anomalies of the tracheobronchial tree and of the esophagus: diagnosis and treatment, Pediatr. Clin. North Am. 9:1113-1124, 1962.

197. Holinger, P.H., and Brown, W.T.: Congenital webs, cysts, lar-yngoceles, and other anomalies of the larynx, Ann. Otol. Rhinol. Laryngol. 76:744-752, 1967.

198. Holinger, P.C., et al.: Respiratory obstruction and apnea in infants with bilateral abductor vocal cord paralysis, meningo-mye-locele, hydrocephalus, and Arnold-Chiari malformation, J. Pediatr. 92:368-373, 1978.

199. Holinger, P.H., and Schild, J.A.: Laryngeal papilloma: review of etiology and therapy, Laryngoscope 78:1462-1474, 1968.

200. Holinger, P.H., and Schild, J.A.: Pharyngeal, laryngeal, and tracheal injuries in the pediatric age group, Ann. Otol. Rhinol. Caryngol. 81:538-545, 1972.

201. Holinger, P.H., Shipkowitz, N.L., and Holper, J.C.: Studies of the etiology of laryngeal papilloma to an autogenous vaccine, Acta Otolaryngol. 65:63-69, 1968.

202. Holinger, P.H., et al.: Subglottic stenosis in infants and children, Ann. Otolaryngol. 85:591-599, 1976.

203. Holman, C.B., and Miller, W.E.: Juvenile nasopharyngeal fibroma: roentgenologic characteristics, AJR 94:292-298, 1965.

204. Houston, W.O., Jr.: Fibrous dysplasia of maxilla and mandible: clinicopathologic study and comparison of focal bone lesions with lesions affecting general skeleton, J. Oral Surg. 23:17-39, 1965.

205. Howlett, J.G., Somlo, F., and Kalz, F.: A new syndrome of parotitis with herpangina caused by the Coxsackie virus, Can. Med. Assoc. J. 77:5-7, 1957.

206. Hudson, H.L., and McAlister, W.H.: Obstructing tracheal hemangioma in infancy, AJR 93:428-431, 1965.

207. Hyams, V.J., and Rabuzzi, D.P.: Cartilaginous tumors of the larynx, Laryngoscope 80:755-767, 1970.

208. Hylton, R.P. Jr., McKena, T.W., and Albright, J.E.: Simple ameloblastoma: report of case, J. Oral Surg. 30:59-62, 1972.

209. Incze, J.S., Lui, P.S., and Strong, M.S.: The morphology of human papillomas of the upper respiratory tract, Cancer 39:1634-1646, 1977.

210. Ingram, D.R., and Poznanski, A.K.: Nasopharyngeal dermoid: a case demonstrated by contrast radiography, Radiology 92:297-298, 1969.

211. Jackson, C., and Jackson, C.L.: Bronchoesophagology, Philadelphia, 1950, W.B. Saunders Co.

212. Jacobs, J.C., and Hui, R.M.: Cricoarytenoid arthritis and airway obstruction in juvenile rheumatoid arthritis, Pediatrics 59:292-294, 1977.

213. Jaffe, B., and DeBlanc, B.: Sinusitis in children with cleft lip and palate, Arch. Otolaryngol. 93:479-482, 1971.

214. Jaffe, B.F.: Chronic sinusitis in children, Clin. Pediatr. 13(11):944-948, 1974.

215. Jaffe, B.F., and Jaffe, N.: Diagnosis and treatment of head and neck tumors in children, Pediatrics 51:731-740, 1973.

216. Jaffe, B.F., Stome, M., Khaw, K.T., and Schwachmann, H.: Nasal polypectomy and sinus surgery for cystic fibrosis, Otolaryngol. Clin. North Am. 10(1):81-86, 1977.

217. Jaffe, H.L.: Giant cell reparative granuloma, traumatic bone cyst, and fibrous (fibro-osseous) dysplasis of the jaw bones, Oral Surg. 6:159-175, 1953.

218. Jazbi, B.: Subluxatin of the nasal septum in newborn: etiology and treatment, Otolaryngol. Clin. North Am. 10:125-138, 1977.

219. Jazbi, B.: Nasopharyngoscopy and sinoscopy in children, Adv. Otorhinolaryngol. 23:73-86, 1978.

220. Jazbi, B.: Sinusitis in infants and children. In Pediatric otorhinolaryngology, New York, 1980, Appleton-Century-Crofts.

221. Johnson, G.F., and Robinow, M.: Aglossia-adactylia, Radiology 128:127-132, 1978.

222. Johnsen, S.: What is prolonged intubation? Acta Otolaryngol. 75:377-378, 1973.

223. Jones, D.G., and Gabriel, C.E.: The incidence of carcinoma of

the larynx in persons under twenty years of age, Laryngoscope **79**:251-255, 1969.

224. Jones, H.M.: Acute epiglottitis and supraglottitis, J. Laryngol. **72**:932-939, 1958.

225. Jones, J.H.: Non-odontogenic oral tumors in children, Br. Dent. J. **119**:439-447, 1965.

226. Jones, P.G., and Heller, H.G.: Recurrent parotitis and saliectasis, Aust. Paediatr. J. **4**:290-292, 1968.

227. Joseph, P.M., et al.: Upper airway obstruction in infants and small children: improved radiographic diagnosis by combining filtration, high kilovoltage, and magnification, Radiology **121**:143-148, 1976.

228. Joseph, P.M., et al.: Upper airway obstruction in infants and small children: improved radiographic diagnosis by combining filtration, high kilovoltage, and magnification, Year Book Diag. Radiol. (abst.), Chicago, 1978, Year Book Medical Publishers, Inc.

229. Kamdar, K.N., and Ozo, R.K.: Palatography ("A study of velopharyngeal closure"), Australas. Radiol. **17**:26-31, 1973.

230. Katz, H.P., and Askin, J.: Multiple hemangiomata with thrombopenia: an unusual case with comments on steroid therapy, Am. J. Dis. Child **115**:351-357, 1968.

231. Kaufman, G., and Klopstock, R.: Papillomatosis of the respiratory tract, Am. Rev. Respir. Dis. **88**:839-846, 1963.

232. Kauffman, S.L., and Stout, A.P.: Tumors of major salivary glands in children, Cancer **16**:1317-1331, 1963.

233. Kauffman, S.L., and Stout, A.P.: Congenital mesenchymal tumors, Cancer **18**:460-476, 1965.

234. Kelsey, C.A., Crummy, A.G., and Schulman, E.Y.: Comparison of ultrasonic and cineradiographic measurements of lateral pharyngeal wall motion, Invest. Radiol. **4**:241-245, 1969.

235. Kent, J.N., Castro, H.F., and Girotti, W.R.: Benign osteoblastoma of the maxilla: case report and review of the literature, Oral Surg. **27**:209-219, 1969.

236. Kesson, C.W.: Asphyxia neonatorum due to a nasopharyngeal teratoma, Arch. Dis. Child **29**:254-255, 1954.

237. Kirkpatrick, J.A., and Olmsted, R.W.: Cinefluorographic study of pharyngeal function related to speech, Radiology **73**:557-559, 1959.

238. Kirkpatrick, R.H., and Riley, C.M.: Roentgenographic findings in familial dysautonomia, Radiology **68**:654-700, 1957.

239. Kittredge, R.D., and Finby, M.: The many facets of lymphangioma, AJR **95**:56-66, 1965.

240. Kogutt, M.S., and Swischuk, L.E.: Diagnosis of sinusitis in infants and children, Pediatrics **52**:121-124, 1973.

241. Koivukangas, T., et al.: Sjögren's syndrome and achalasia of the cardia in two siblings, Pediatrics **51**:943-945, 1973.

242. Kramer, H.S.: Benign osteoblastoma of the mandible: report of a case, Oral Surg. **24**:842-851, 1967.

243. Kramer, R.: Otolaryngologic complications of cystic fibrosis, Otolaryngol. Clin. North Am. **10**:203-208, 1977.

244. Kravath, R.E., Pollak, C.P., and Borowiecki, B.: Hypoventilation during sleep in children who have lymphoid airway obstruction treated by nasopharyngeal tube and T and A, Pediatrics **59**:865-871, 1977.

245. Kudo, A., and Lewis, J.S.: Nasal gliomas, Arch. Otolaryngol. **94**:351-355, 1971.

246. Kushner, D.C., and Harris, G.B.C.: Obstructing lesions of the larynx and trachea in infants and children, Radiol. Clin. North Am. **16**:181-194, 1978.

247. Lallemand, D., Sauvegrain, J., and Mareschal, J.L.: Laryngotracheal lesions in infants and children: detection and follow-up studies using direct radiographic magnification, Ann. Radiol. **16**:293-304, 1973.

248. Lampe, I., and Latourette, H.B.: Management of hemangiomas in infants, Pediatr. Clin. North Am. **6**:511-528, 1959.

249. Landing, B.H.: Anomalies of the respiratory tract, Pediatr. Clin. North Am. **4**:73-102, 1957.

250. Lavigna, D.M., Jr., and Birck, H.G.: Hemangioma of pharynx in a newborn, Arch. Otolaryngol. **92**:282-283, 1970.

251. Lawson, V.G., and Fallis, B.A.: Surgical treatment of thyroglossal duct cysts, Can. Med. Assoc. J. **100**:855-858, 1969.

252. Leake, D., and Leake, R.: Neonatal suppurative parotitis, Pediatrics **46**:203-207, 1970.

253. Leikensohn, J.R., Benton, C., and Cotton, R.: Subglottic hemangioma, J. Otolaryngol. **5**:487-492, 1976.

254. Levitt, L.P., et al.: Mumps in a general population: seroepidemiologic study, Am. J. Dis. Child **120**:134-138, 1970.

255. Levy, A.M., et al.: Hypertrophied adenoids causing pulmonary hypertension and severe congestive heart failure, N. Engl. J. Med. **277**:506-511, 1967.

256. Lewin, M.L.: Non-malignant maxillofacial tumors in children, Plast. Reconstr. Surg. **38**:186-196, 1966.

257. Liebert, P.S., and Stool, S.E.: Rhabdomyosarcoma of the tongue in an infant: results of combined radiation and chemotherapy, Ann. Surg. **178**:621-624, 1973.

258. Lister, J., and Zachary, R.B.: Cystic duplication in the tongue, J. Pediatr. Surg. **3**:491-493, 1968.

259. Loeb, W.J., and Smith, E.E.: Airway obstruction in a newborn by pedunculated pharyngeal dermoid, Pediatrics **40**:20-23, 1967.

260. Lofgren, R.H.: Respiratory distress from congenital cysts, Am. J. Dis. Child **106**:610-612, 1963.

261. Lofgren, R.H., and Montgomery, W.W.: Incidence of laryngeal involvement in rheumatoid arthritis, N. Engl. J. Med. **267**:193-195, 1962.

262. Lowe, R.S., et al.: Nasal glioma, Plast. Reconstr. Surg. **47**:1-5, 1971.

263. Lucaya, J., Herrera, M., and Salcedo, S.: Traumatic pharyngeal pseudodiverticulum in neonates and infants: two case reports and review of the literature, Pediatr. Radiol. **8**:65-69, 1979.

264. Lugaresi, F., et al.: Snoring, Electroencephalogr. Clin. Neurophysiol. **39**:59-64, 1975.

265. Luke, M.J., et al.: Chronic nasopharyngeal obstruction as a cause of cardiomegaly, cor pulmonale, and pulmonary edema, Pediatrics **37**:762-768, 1966.

266. MacDonald, D.M.: Thyroglossal cysts and fistulae, Int. J. Oral. Surg. **3**:342-346, 1974.

267. MacKellar, A., and Kennedy, J.C.: Congenital diverticulum of the pharynx simulating esophageal atresia, J. Pediatr. Surg. **7**:408-411, 1972.

268. Mahour, G.H., et al.: Rhabdomyosarcoma in infants and children: a clinicopathologic study of 75 cases, J. Pediatr. Surg. **2**:402-409, 1967.

269. Mahour, G.H., Cohen, S.R., and Woolley, M.M.: Laryngotracheoesophageal cleft associated with esophageal atresia and multiple tracheoesophageal fistulas in a twin, J. Thorac. Cardiovasc. Surg. **65**:223-226, 1973.

270. Majoros, M., Devine, K.D., and Parkhill, E.M.: Malignant transformation of benign laryngeal papillomas in children after radiation therapy, Surg. Clin. North Am. **43**(4):1049-1061, 1963.

271. Majoros, M., Parkhill, E.M., and Devine, K.D.: Papilloma of the larynx in children: a clinico-pathologic study, Am. J. Surg. **108**:470-475, 1964.

272. Margulies, S.L., et al.: Familial dysautonomia: a cineradiographic study of the swallowing mechanism, Radiology **90**:107-112, 1968.

273. Margolis, C.Z., Colletti, R.B., and Grundy, G.: *Hemophilus influenzae* type B: the etiologic agent in epiglottitis, J. Pediatr. **87**:322-323, 1975.

274. Margolis, C.Z., Ingram, D.O., and Meyer, J.H.: Routine tracheotomy in *Hemophilus influenzae*, type B, epiglottitis, J. Pediatr. **81:**1150-1153, 1972.

275. Marsden, D.: Nasal polyposis in children, South Med. J. **71**(8):911-913, 1978.

276. Mason, J.M., et al.: Pulmonary vessels in SIDS, N. Engl. J. Med. **292:**479, 1975.

277. Mattila, M.A.K., Suutarinen, T., and Sulaman, M.: Prolonged endotracheal intubation of tracheostomy in infants and children, J. Pediatr. Surg. **4:**674-681, 1969.

278. McCartney, F.J., Panday, J., and Scott, O.: Cor pulmonale as a result of chronic nasopharyngeal obstruction due to hypertrophied tonsils and adenoids, Arch. Dis. Child **44:**585-592, 1969.

279. McGovern, F.H.: Bilateral choanal atresia in the newborn—a new method of medical management, Laryngoscope **71:**480-483, 1961.

280. McKenzie, J., and Craig, L.: Mandibulofacial dysostosis (Treacher-Collins syndrome), Arch. Dis. Child **30:**391-395, 1955.

281. McLain, D.C.: Sinusitis in children: lessons from 25 patients, Clin. Pediatr. **9:**342-345, 1970.

282. McSwiney, P.F., Cavanagh, N.P.C., and Languth, P.: Outcome in congenital stridor (laryngomalacia), Arch. Dis. Child **52:**215-218, 1977.

283. Meine, F.J., et al.: Pharyngeal distention associated with upper airway obstruction: experimental observations in dogs, Radiology **111:**395-398, 1974.

284. Menashe, V.D., Farrehi, C., and Miller M.: Hypoventilation and cor pulmonale due to chronic upper airway obstruction. J. Pediatr. **67:**198-203, 1965.

285. Meranus, H., et al.: Histiocytosis X: problems in diagnosis, Oral Surg. **26:**759-768, 1968.

286. Meyer, H.W.: Congenital cysts and fistulae of the neck, Ann. Surg. **95:**1-26; 26-248, 1932.

287. Mikulowski, P.: Extracardiac rhabdomyoma, Acta Pathol. Microbiol. Scand. **80:**222-224, 1972.

288. Milko, D.A., Marshak, G., and Striker, T.W.: Nasotracheal intubation in the treatment of acute epiglottitis, Pediatrics **53:**674-677, 1974.

289. Mills, C.P.: Dysphagia in pharyngeal paralysis treated by cricopharyngeal sphincterotomy, Lancet **1:**455-457, 1973.

290. Miller, B.J., and Morrison, M.D.: Congenital tracheal web—a case report, J. Otolaryngol. **7:**218-222, 1978.

291. Miller, E.M., and Norman, D.: The role of the computed tomography in the evaluation of neck masses, Radiology **133:**145-149, 1979.

292. Miller, J.H.: Roentgen anatomy of the developing paranasal sinuses, Scientific exhibit, Sixty-sixth Scientific Assembly and Annual Meeting of The Radiological Society of North America, Dallas, Texas, Nov. 16-21, 1980.

293. Moffat, D.A.: Postural apnea due to large tonsils and adenoids, J. Pediatr. **89:**510, 1976.

294. Moller, N.E., and Thomsen, J.: Mucocele of the paranasal sinuses in cystic fibrosis, J. Laryngol. Otol. **92**(11):1025-1027, 1978.

295. Morettin, L.B., Mueller, E., and Schreiber, M.: Generalized hamartomatosis (congenital generalized fibromatosis), AJR **114:**722-734, 1972.

296. Morgan, W.S.: The probable systemic nature of Mikuliez's disease and its relation to Sjögren's syndrome, N. Engl. J. Med. **251:**5-10, 1954.

297. Morioka, W.T., et al.: Unexpected radiographic findings related to foreign bodies, Ann. Otol. Rhinol. Laryngol. **84:**627-630, 1975.

298. Muroff, L.R., and Seaman, W.B.: Normal anatomy of the larynx and pharynx and the differential diagnosis of foreign bodies, Semin. Roentgenol. **9:**267-272, 1974.

299. Mygind, N.: Nasal allergy, London, 1978, Blackwell Scientific Publications, Ltd.

300. Mygind, N., Thomsen, J., and Winge-Flensborg, E.: Nasal immunoglobulins in cystic fibrosis, ISIAN Proceedings (Tokyo) **120,** 1977.

301. Naeye, R.L.: Pulmonary artery abnormalities in the sudden infant death syndrome, N. Engl. J. Med. **289:**1167-1170, 1973.

302. Nahum, A.M.: Immediate care of acute blunt trauma, J. Trauma **9:**112-125, 1969.

303. Naveh, Y., Friedman, A., and Altmann, M.: Eggshell aspiration in infants, Am. J. Dis. Child **129:**498-499, 1975.

304. Neel, H.B., III, et al.: Juvenile angiofibroma: review of 120 cases, Am. J. Surg. **126:**547-556, 1973.

305. Neeley, J., et al.: The otolaryngologic aspects of cystic fibrosis, Trans. Am. Acad. Ophthalmol. Otolaryngol. **76:**313-324, 1976.

306. Neuhauser, E.B.D., and Harris, G.B.C.: Familial dysautonomia of Riley-Day: roentgenographic features, Tenth International Congress of Radiology (abstr.), 1962.

307. North, J., and Emanuel, B.: Mediastinitis in a child caused by perforation of pharynx, Am. J. Dis. Child **129:**962-963, 1975.

308. Novoselac, M., Dangel, P., Fisch, U.: Laryngotracheoesophageal cleft, J. Pediatr. Surg. **8:**963-964, 1973.

309. Nydell, C.C., and Marson, J.K.: Dermoid cysts of the nose, a review of 39 cases, Ann. Surg. **150:**1007-1016, 1959.

310. Ogura, J.H., and Schnenck, N.L.: Unusual nasal tumors, problems in diagnosis and treatment, Otolaryngol. Clin. North Am. **6:**813-837, 1973.

311. O'Hara, A.E.: Roentgen evaluation of patients with cleft palate, Radiol. Clin. North Am. **1:**1-11, 1963.

312. Okafor, B.C.: Aneurysm of the external carotid artery following a foreign body in the pharynx, J. Laryngol. Otol. **92:**429-434, 1978.

313. Oleske, J.M., and Kushnick, T.: Juvenile papilloma of the larynx, Am. J. Dis. Child **121:**417-419, 1971.

314. Olofsson, J.: Extracardiac rhabdomyoma, Acta Otolaryngol. **74:**139-144, 1972.

315. Olson, N.R., and Miles, W.K.: Treatment of acute blunt laryngeal injuries, Ann. Otol. Rhinol. Laryngol. **80:**704-709, 1971.

316. O'Neill, E.M.: Sjögren's syndrome with onset at ten years of age, Proc. R. Soc. Med. **58:**689-690, 1965.

317. Orem, J., Norris, P., and Lydic, R.: Laryngeal abductor activity during sleep, Chest **73:**300-301, 1978.

318. Orton, H.B.: Carcinoma of the larynx: clinical report of case age 13½ years, Laryngoscope **57:**299-303, 1947.

319. Osman, M.Z., and Girdany, B.R.: Traumatic pseudodiverticulum of the pharynx in infants and children, Ann. Radiol. **16:**143-147, 1973.

320. Overcash, K.E., and Putney, P.J.: Subglottic hemangioma of the larynx treated with steroid therapy, Laryngoscope **83:**679-682, 1973.

321. Ozonoff, M.B.: Ataxia-telangiectasis: chronic pneumonia, sinusitis, and adenoidal hypoplasia, AJR **120:**297-299, 1974.

322. Paley, W.G., and Keddie, N.C.: The etiology and management of branchial cysts, Br. J. Surg. **57:**822-824, 1970.

323. Paparo, G.P., and Symchych, P.S.: Postintubation subglottic stenosis and cor pulmonale, J. Pediatr. **90:**97-98, 1977.

324. Parkin, J.L., Stevens, M.H., and Jung, A.L.: Acquired and congenital subglottic stenosis in the infant, Ann. Otolaryngol. **85:**573-581, 1976.

325. Patriquin, H.B.: The roentgen evaluation of childhood speech disorders: basic principles and techniques, with special reference to movements of the lateral pharyngeal walls, Ann. Radiol. **16:**273-279, 1973.

326. Patten, B.M.: Human embryology, New York, 1968, McGraw-Hill Book Co.

327. Petersson, G.: Inhibited separation of the larynx and upper part of trachea from the esophagus in a newborn: report of a case successfully operated upon, Acta Chir. Scand. **110:**250-254, 1955.

328. Phelps, J.A.: Laryngeal obstruction due to cricoarytenoid arthritis, Anesthesiology **27:**518-522, 1966.

329. Pick, T., Maurer, H.M., and McWilliams, N.B.: Lymphoepithelioma in childhood, J. Pediatr. **84:**96-100, 1974.

330. Platt, M.A.: Laryngeal coccidioidomycosis, JAMA **237:**1234-1235, 1977.

331. Pleasure, J., and Geller, S.A.: Neurofibromatosis in infancy presenting with congenital stridor, Am. J. Dis. Child **113:**390-393, 1967.

332. Pletcher, J.D., et al.: Preoperative embolization of juvenile angiofibromas of the nasopharynx, Ann. Otol. **84:**740-746, 1975.

333. Polayani, T.G., Bredemeier, H.C., and Davis, T.W.: A CO_2 laser for surgical research, Med. Biol. Eng. **8:**541-548, 1970.

334. Polisar, I.A., et al.: Bilateral midline fixation of cricoarytenoid joints as a serious medical emergency, JAMA **172:**901-906, 1960.

335. Pollock, W.F., and Stevenson, E.O.: Cysts and sinuses of the thyroglossal duct, Am. J. Surg. **112:**225-232, 1966.

336. Ponniah, R.D., and Singh, G.: Foreign bodies in the larynx in infancy, Practitioner **217:**789-791, 1976.

337. Poole, C.A., and Altman, D.H.: Acute epiglottitis in children, Radiology **80:**798-805, 1963.

338. Prasad, J.N.: Fibrosarcoma of the larynx, J. Laryngol. Otol. **86:**267-274, 1972.

339. Pratt, L.W.: Midline cysts of the nasal dorsum: embryologic origin and treatment, Laryngoscope **75:**968-980, 1965.

340. Quick, C.A., et al.: Treatment of papillomatosis of the larynx with transfer factor, Ann. Otol. Rhinol. Laryngol. **84:**607-613, 1975.

341. Rabinov, K., and Joffe, N.: A blunt-tip side-injecting cannula for sialography, Radiology **92:**1438, 1969.

342. Rabinov, K., van Orman, P., and Gray, E.: Radiologic findings in persistent thyroglossal tract fistulas, Radiology **130:**135-139, 1979.

343. Rachelefsky, G.S., et al.: Sinus disease in children with respiratory allergy, J. Allergy Clin. Immunol. **65:**310-314, 1978.

344. Raffensperger, J., and Cohen, R.: Plexiform neurofibromas in childhood, J. Pediatr. Surg. **7:**144-151, 1972.

345. Ralis, Z., and Emery, J.L.: Congenital plexiform neurofibroma of the vagus with cardiac, pulmonary, and visceral involvement, J. Pathol. **17:**55-57, 1972.

346. Randolph, J., Grunt, J.A., and Vawter, G.F.: The medical and surgical aspects of intratracheal goiter, N. Engl. J. Med. **268:**457-461, 1963.

347. Rapkin, R.H.: Diagnosis of epiglottitis: simplicity and reliability of radiographs of neck in differential diagnosis of croup syndrome, J. Pediatr. **80:**96-98, 1972.

348. Rapkin, R.H.: Tracheostomy in epiglottitis, Pediatrics **52:**426-429, 1973.

349. Rapkin, R.H.: Nasotracheal intubation in epiglottitis, Pediatrics **56:**110-112, 1975.

350. Reaume, C.E., and Sofie, V.L.: Lingual thyroid: review of the literature and report of a case, Oral Surg. **45:**841-845, 1978.

351. Reed, M.H.: Radiology of airway foreign bodies in children, J. Can. Assoc. Radiol. **28:**111-118, 1977.

352. Refetoff, S., et al.: Continuing occurrence of thyroid carcinoma after irradiation to the neck in infancy and childhood, N. Engl. J. Med. **242:**171-175, 1975.

353. Reichert, T.J., et al.: Congenital cricopharyngeal achalasia, Ann. Otol. Rhinol. Laryngol. **86:**603-610, 1977.

354. Remmers, J.E., et al.: Pathogenesis of upper airway occlusion during sleep, J. Appl. Physiol. **44:**931-938, 1978.

355. Rigby, R.A., and Holinger, P.H.: Fibrosarcoma of the larynx in an infant, Arch. Otolaryngol. **37:**425-429, 1943.

356. Riley, C.M., et al.: Central autonomic dysfunction with defective lacrimation: report of five cases, Pediatrics **3:**468-478, 1949.

357. Ritter, F.N.: The paranasal sinuses: anatomy and surgical technique, ed. 2, St. Louis, 1978, The C.V. Mosby Co.

358. Roberson, G.H., et al.: Therapeutic embolization of juvenile angiofibroma, AJR **133:**657-663, 1979.

359. Rogers, B.O.: Berry-Treacher-Collins syndrome: a review of 200 cases (mandibulofacial dysostosis: Franceschetti-Swahlen-Klein syndromes), Br. J. Plast. Surg. **17:**109-137, 1964.

360. Ronning, O., and Valiaho, M.L.: Involvement of facial skeleton in juvenile rheumatoid arthritis, Ann. Radiol. **18:**347-353, 1975.

361. Rosedale, R.S.: Neuroblastoma of nodose ganglion of infant vagus nerve, Arch. Otolaryngol. **80:**454-459, 1964.

362. Rosen, L., Hanafee, W., and Nahum, A.: Nasopharyngeal angiofibroma: an angiographic evaluation, Radiology **86:**103-107, 1966.

363. Rosenbaum, H.D., Alavi, S.M., and Bryant, L.R.: Pulmonary parenchymal spread of juvenile laryngeal papillomatosis, Radiology **90:**654-660, 1968.

364. Rosenfield, L., Graves, H., Lawrence, R.: Primary neurogenic tumors of the lateral neck, Ann. Surg. **167:**847-855, 1968.

365. Rouledge, R.T.: The Pierre-Robin syndrome: a surgical emergency in the neonatal period, Br. J. Plast. Surg. **13:**204-218, 1960.

366. Rulon, J.T.: Sinusitis in children, Postgrad. Med. **48:**107-112, 1970.

367. Saenger, G.L., and Silverman, F.M.: Neoplasia following therapeutic irradiation for benign conditions in childhood, Radiology **74:**889-904, 1960.

368. Sammarco, G.J., and McKenna, J.: Thyroglossal duct cyst in the elderly, Pediatrics **25:**98-101, 1970.

369. Sayre, J.W., and Hall, E.G.: Anomalies of the larynx associated with tracheoesophageal fistula, Pediatrics **13:**150-154, 1954.

370. Sazama, L.: Pathogenesis and treatment of recurrent juvenile parotitis, Rev. Stomatol. Chir. Maxillofac. **69:**309-314, 1968.

371. Scanlin, T.F., Shapiro, R.S., and Rosenlund, M.L.: Vocal cord paralysis in cystic fibrosis, J. Pediatr. **86:**984-985, 1975.

372. Schaeffer, J.P.: The embryology, development and anatomy of the nose, paranasal sinus, nasolacrimal passageways and olfactory organ in man, Philadelphia, 1920, Blakiston.

373. Schlesinger, B.E., et al.: Observations on the clinical course and treatment of one hundred cases of Still's disease, Arch. Dis. Child **36:**65-76, 1961.

374. Schoder, H.J., Kressin, J., and Ziehe, K.R.: Maligne tumoren des kindes im HNO, Gebiet. Z. Laryngol. Rhinol. Otol. **47:**135-140, 1968.

375. Schrottenbaum, U.M.: Rare chronic inflammation of the epiglottis, Z. Allg. Path. Anat. **104:**255-257, 1963.

376. Schauman, A., Smith, F., and Ackerman, L.V.: Benign fibroosseous lesions of the mandible and maxilla: a review of 35 cases, Cancer **26:**303-312, 1970.

377. Schwachman, H., Kulezyki, L.L., and Mueller, H.L.: Nasal polyps in patient with cystic fibrosis, Am. J. Dis. Child **102:**768-769, 1961.

378. Schwachman, H., et al.: Nasal patients with cystic fibrosis, Pediatrics **30:**389-401, 1962.

379. Scott, J.O., and Kramer, S.S.: Pediatric tracheostomy. I. Radiographic features of difficult decannulations, AJR **130:**887-891, 1978.

380. Scott, J.R., and Kramer, S.S.: Pediatric tracheostomy. II. Radiographic features of difficult decannulations, AJR **130:**893-898, 1978.

381. Sedano, H.O., et al.: Histiocytosis X: clinical, radiologic and histologic findings with special attention to oral manifestations, Oral Surg. **27**:760-771, 1969.

382. Shackelford, G.C., and McAlister, W.H.: Congenital laryngeal cyst, AJR **114**:289-292, 1972.

383. Shackelford, G.D., Siegel, M.J., and McAlister, W.H.: Subglottic edema in acute epiglottitis in children, AJR **131**:603-605, 1978.

384. Shaffer, K., et al.: Pitfalls in the radiographic diagnosis of angiofibroma, Radiology **127**:425-428, 1978.

385. Shafer, W.G.: Cysts, neoplasms, and allied conditions of odontogenic origin, Semin. Roentgenol. **6**:403-413, 1971.

386. Shah, B.L., Vasan, U., Raye, J.R.: Teratoma of the tonsil in a premature infant, Am. J. Dis. Child **133**:79-80, 1979.

387. Shann, F.A., et al.: Prolonged nasotracheal intubation of tracheostomy in acute laryngotracheobronchitis and epiglottitis, Aust. Paediatr. J. **11**:212-217, 1975.

388. Shapiro, M.J., and Falla, A.: Congenital posterior cleft larynx, Ann. Otol. **75**:961-967, 1966.

389. Shearer, W.T., et al.: Benign nasal tumor appearing as neonatal respiratory distress: first reported case of nasopharyngeal fibrous histiocytoma, Am. J. Dis. Child **126**:238-241, 1973.

390. Shearn, M.A.: Sjögren's syndrome. In Smith, L.H., Jr., editor: Major problems in internal medicine series, vol. 2, Philadelphia, 1971, W.B. Saunders Co.

391. Shulman, J.B., et al.: Familial laryngomalacia: a case report, Laryngoscope **86**:84-91, 1976.

392. Skolnick, M.L.: Video velopharyngography in patients with nasal speech, with emphasis on lateral phyaryngeal motion in velopharyngeal closure, Radiology **93**:747-755, 1969.

393. Skolnik, E.M., Kotler, R., and Hanna, W.A.: Clinical atresia, Otolaryngol. Clin. North Am. **6**(3):783-789, 1973.

394. Skolnik, M.L., Glaser, E.R., and McWilliams, B.J.: The use and limitations of the barium pharyngogram in the detection of velopharyngeal insufficiency, Radiology **135**:301-304, 1980.

395. Shopfner, C.E., and Rossi, J.O.: Roentgen evaluation of the paranasal sinuses in children, AJR **118**:176-186, 1973.

396. Shprintzen, R.J., et al.: Pharyngeal hypoplasia in Treacher-Collins syndrome, Arch. Otolaryngol. **105**:127-131, 1979.

397. Siegel, M.J., and McAlister, W.H.: Tracheal histiocytoma, and inflammatory pseudotumor, J. Can. Assoc. Radiol. **29**:273-274, 1978.

398. Siegel, M.J., Shackelford, G.D., and McAlister, W.H.: Paranasal sinus mucoceles in children, Radiology **133**:623-626, 1979.

399. Sigala, J.L., et al.: Dental involvement in histiocytosis, Oral Surg. **33**:42-48, 1972.

400. Sirola, R.: Choanal polyps, Acta Otolaryngol. **61**:42-48, 1965.

401. Slovis, T.L.: Non-invasive evaluation of the pediatric airway: a recent advance, Pediatrics **59**:872-880, 1977.

402. Smith, K.R., Jr., et al.: Nasal gliomas: a report of five cases with electron microscopy for one, J. Neurosurg. **20**:968-982, 1963.

403. Smith, L., and Gooding, C.A.: Pulmonary involvement in laryngeal papillomatosis, Pediatr. Radiol. **2**:161-166, 1974.

404. Smith, P.C., Swischuk, L.E., and Fagan, C.J.: An elusive and often unsuspected cause of stridor or pneumonia (the esophageal foreign body), AJR **122**:80-89, 1974.

405. Smith, T.H., et al.: Sleep apnea syndrome: diagnosis of upper airway obstruction by fluoroscopy, J. Pediatr. **93**:891-892, 1978.

406. Smith, T.T.: Solitary neurofibroma of the larynx, Arch. Otolaryngol. **39**:144-151, 1944.

407. Snow, J.B., Jr., and Rogers, K.A.: Bilateral adductive paralysis of vocal cords secondary to Arnold-Chiari malformaton and its management, Laryngoscope **75**:316-321, 1965.

408. Sorensen, H.: Rhinologic aspects of cystic fibrosis. In Jazbi B., editor: Pediatric otorhinolaryngology, a review of the ear, nose and throat problems in children, New York, 1980, Appleton-Century-Crofts.

409. Steichen, F.M., et al.: Congenital retropharyngeal neurofibroma causing laryngeal obstruction in a newborn, J. Pediatr. Surg. **6**:480-483, 1971.

410. Steichen, F.M., Fellini, A., and Einhorn, A.H.: Acute foreign body laryngotracheal obstruction: a cause of sudden and unexplained death in children, Pediatrics **48**:281-285, 1971.

411. Steinschneider, A.: Prolonged apoxea and the sudden infant death syndrome: clinical and laboratory observations, Pediatrics **50**:646-654, 1972.

412. Stern, L.M., et al.: Management of Pierre-Robin syndrome in infancy by prolonged nasoesophageal intubation, Am. J. Dis. Child **124**:78-80, 1972.

413. Stovin, J.J., Lyon, J.A., Jr., and Clemmens, R.L.: Mandibulofacial dysostosis, Radiology **74**:225-231, 1960.

414. Striker, T.W., Stool, S., and Downes, J.J.: Prolonged nasotracheal intubation in infants and children, Arch. Otolaryngol. **85**:106-109, 1967.

415. Strome, M.: Analysis of an autogenous vaccine in treatment of juvenile papillomatosis of the larynx, Laryngoscope **79**:272-279, 1969.

416. Strong, M.S., et al.: Laser surgery in the aerodigestive tract, Am. J. Surg. **126**:529-533, 1973.

417. Strong, M.S., et al.: Recurrent respiratory papillomatosis: management with carbon dioxide laser, Ann. Otol. Rhinol. Laryngol. **85**:508-516, 1976.

418. Strong, R.M., and Rassy, V.: Endotracheal intubation: complications in neonates, Arch. Otolaryngol. **103**:329-335, 1977.

419. Suehs, O.W., and Powell, D.P., Jr.: Congenital cysts of the larynx in infants, Laryngoscope **77**:654-663, 1967.

420. Sutton, T.J., and Nogrady, M.B.: Radiologic diagnosis of subglottic hemangioma in infants, Pediatr. Radiol. **1**:211-215, 1973.

421. Suydan, M.J., and Mikity, V.G.: Cellulitis with underlying inflammatory periostitis of the mandible, AJR **56**:133-135, 1969.

422. Swischuk, L.E.: Large vein of Galen aneurysms in the neonate (a constellation of diagnostic chest and neck radiologic findings), Pediatr. Radiol. **6**:4-9, 1977.

423. Swischuk, L.E., Smith, P.C., and Fagan, C.J.: Abnormalities of the pharynx and larynx in childhood, Semin Roentgenol. **9**:283-300, 1974.

424. Syme, W.S.: Choanal polyps, J. Laryngol. Otol. **31**515-518, 1916.

425. Szpunar, J.: Laryngeal papillomatosis, Acta Otolaryngol. **63**:74-86, 1967.

426. Tefft, M.: Radiotherapeutic management of subglottic hemangioma in children, Radiology **86**:207-214, 1966.

427. Thawley, S.E., and Bone, R.C.: Laryngopyocele, Laryngoscope **83**:362-368, 1973.

428. Theander, G.: Congenital posterior midline pharyngoesophageal diverticula, Pediatr. Radiol. **1**:153-155, 1973.

429. Thomas, M.L., and Mowat, P.D.: Angiography in juvenile nasopharyngeal haemangiofibroma, Clin. Radiol. **21**:403-406, 1970.

430. Tobin, H.A., and Harris, H.H.: Non-chromaffin paraganglioma of the larynx, Arch. Otolaryngol. **96**:154-157, 1972.

431. Tonkin, S.L., et al.: The pharyngeal effect of partial nasal obstruction, Pediatrics **63**:261-271, 1979.

432. Touloukian, R.J., et al.: Traumatic perforation of the pharynx in the newborn, Pediatrics **59**:1019-1022, 1977.

433. Towbin, R., Dunbar, J.S., and Bove, K.: Antrochoanal polyps, AJR **132**:27-31, 1979.

434. Ullman, E.V.: On the etiology of laryngeal papilloma, AcTA otolaryngol. **5**:317-334, 1923.

435. Utian, H.L., and Thomas, R.G.: Cricopharyngeal incoordination in infancy, Pediatrics **43**:402-406, 1969.

436. Van Alyea, O.E.: Nasal sinuses, anatomical and clinical Considerations, Baltimore, 1942, The Williams & Wilkins Co.
437. Van Loon, E.L., and Diamond, S.: Neurofibroma of the larynx, Ann. Otol. Rhinol. Laryngol. **51:**122-126, 1942.
438. Vargas, F., and Patron, M.: A case of atresis of the larynx, Ann. Chir. Infant. **12:**355-358, 1971.
439. Vetters, J.M., and Toner, P.G.: Chemodectoma of larynx, J. Pathol. **101:**259-265, 1970.
440. Waldron, C.A.: Non-odontogenic neoplasms, cysts, and allied conditions of the jaws, Semin. Roentgenol. **6:**414-425, 1971.
441. Waldron, C.A., and Shafer, W.G.: The central giant-cell reparative granuloma of the jaws: an analysis of 38 cases, Am. J. Clin. Pathol. **45:**437-447, 1966.
442. Walpita, P.R.: Laryngocele in an infant, J. Pediatr. Surg. **10:**843-844, 1975.
443. Walsh, R.E., et al.: Upper airway obstruction in obese patients with sleep disturbance and somnolence, Ann. Internal. Med. **76:**185-192, 1972.
444. Ward, P.H., Harris, P.F., and Downey, W.: Surgical approach to cystic hygroma of the neck, Arch. Otolaryngol. **91:**508-514, 1970.
445. Ward, P.H., et al.: Coccidiomycosis of the larynx in infants and adults, Ann. Otol Rhinol. Laryngol. **86:**655-660, 1977.
446. Watt, F.B., Jr., and Slovis, T.L.: The enlarged epiglottis, Pediatr. Radiol. **5:**133-136, 1977.
447. Weber, A.L., and Grillo, H.C.: Tracheal stenosis: an analysis of 151 cases, Radiol. Clin. North Am. **16:**291-308, 1978.
448. Weber, M.L., et al.: Acute epiglottitis in children: treatment with nasotracheal intubation: report of 14 consecutive cases, Pediatrics **57:**152-155, 1976.
449. Weidner, W.A., Wenzi, J.E., and Swischuk, L.E.: Roentgenographic findings in lipoid proteinosis: a case report, AJR **110:**457-461, 1970.
450. Wells, S.D., et al.: Traumatic prevertebral pharyngoesophageal pseudodiverticulum in the newborn infant, J. Pediatr. Surg. **9:**217-222, 1974.
451. Wenner, H.A.: Airway obstruction: acute infections and hypersensitivity reactions. In Jazbi, B.: Pediatric otorhinolaryngology, a review of ear, nose and throat problems in children, New York, 1980, Appleton-Century-Crofts.
452. Weston, J.T.: Airway foreign body fatalities in children, Ann. Otol. Rhinol. Laryngol. **74:**1144-1148, 1965.
453. Weyers, H.: Mandibular facial dysostosis, a new syndrome of multiple degeneration, Acta Paediatr. **40:**143-164, 1951.
454. Whalen, J.P., and Woodruff, C.L.: The cervical prevertebral fat stripe, AJR **109:**445-451, 1970.
455. Williams, A., Vawter, G., and Reid, L.: Increased muscularity of the pulmonary circulation in victims of sudden infant death syndrome, Pediatrics **63:**18-23, 1979.
456. Williams, H.E., et al.: Hemangiomas of the larynx in infants: diagnosis, respiratory mechanics, and management, Aust. Paediatr. J. **5:**149-154, 1968.
457. Williams, H.J.: Posterior choanal atresia, AJR **112:**1-11, 1971.
458. Williams, J.L., Capitanio, M.A., and Turtz, M.G.: Vocal cord paralysis; radiologic observations in 21 infants and young children, AJR **128:**649-651, 1977.
459. Wilson, G.H., and Hanafee, W.N.: Angiographic findings in 16 patients with juvenile nasopharyngeal angiofibroma, Radiology **92:**279-284, 1969.
460. Wilson, M.: Chronic hypertrophic polypoid rhinosinusitis, Radiology **120:**609-613, 1976.
461. Winter, B., Villaveces, J., and Spector, M.: Coccidioidomycosis accompanied by acute tracheal obstruction in a child, JAMA **195:**1001-1004, 1966.
462. Winther, L.K.: Congenital choanal atresia, Arch. Dis. Child. **53:**338-340, 1978.
463. Wolman, L., Darke, C.S., and Young, A.: Larynx in rheumatoid arthritis, J. Laryngol. Otol. **79:**403-434, 1965.
464. Work, W.P.: Newer concepts of first branchial cleft defects, Laryngoscope **82:**1581-1593, 1972.
465. Wyatt, R.B., Schochet, S.S., Jr., and McCormick, W.F.: Rhabdomyoma: light and electron microscopic study of a case with intranuclear inclusions, Arch. Otolaryngol. **92:**32-39, 1970.
466. Young, D.R., and Robinson, M.: Ameloblastoma in children: report of a case, Oral Surg. **15:**1155-1162, 1962.
467. Yules, R.B., and Chase, R.A.: Quantitive cine-evaluation of palate and pharyngeal wall mobility in normal palates, in cleft palates, and in velopharyngeal incompetency, Plast. Reconstr. Surg. **41:**124-128, 1968.
468. Zachary, R.B., and Emery, J.L.: Failure of the separation of larynx and trachea from the esophagus: persistent esophagotrachea, Surgery **49:**525-529, 1961.
469. Zakrzewski, A.: Subglottic lipoma of the larynx, J. Laryngol. Otol. **79:**1039-1048, 1965.
470. Ziter, F.M.H., Jr., and Bramwit, D.N.: Nasal encephaloceles and gliomas, Br. J. Radiol. **43:**136-138, 1970.
471. Zizmor, J., and Noyek, A.M.: Some miscellaneous disorders of the larynx and pharynx, Semin. Roentgenol. **9:**311-322, 1974.
472. Zwahlen, A., and Regamey, C.: Acute epiglottitis in the adult, Schweiz. Med. Wochenschr. **108**(13):477-482, 1978.

16 □ The temporal bone

□ Embryology and developmental anatomy

R. Thomas Bergeron

Each of the organs of special sense has a fascinating phylogeny. None surpasses the ear, however, in demonstrating the resourcefulness and richness of invention of a biologic system in making adaptive modifications so as to deal successfully with a changing environment.

The ear began as an organ of balance. In the fish of 350 million years ago it existed as a fluid-filled pocket, sunken beneath the surface of the skin on either side of the head. The pocket communicated directly with the ocean water in which the ancient fish swam, providing a mechanism whereby the fish could sense its orientation in the sea. It is physically possible for such a structure to be sensitive to low-frequency vibrations transmitted through the water, and indeed such was likely the case. Hearing nonetheless was only incidental, if not accidental, to a structure primarily developed to provide balance.

By the time evolution had produced creatures that existed on land the vestibular system had become much more highly developd. But in so doing, it lost its continuity with the external environment, becoming deeply encased and sealed off within the base of the skull. To become successful land dwellers, however, perception of sound had become important to survival. The economy of nature prevailed. Connection between the external environment and the inner ear was reestablished and the middle and externl ear were evolved. Concurrently, the hearing portion of the inner ear structure became much more highly specialized (Fig. 16-1).

The following is the story of the development of the ear as we know it. It bears great relevance to the understanding of congenital anomalies, malformations, anatomic variations, and the "normal" state.

Streeter[138] provides the definitive account of the embryologic development of the inner ear. Numerous others have also studied the development of the ear in this and previous centuries but the most complete single source of information relating to development of all portions of the temporal bone remains in Bast and Anson[9], *The Temporal Bone and Ear*. Shambaugh[125] presents the essence of their work in abbreviated form in *Surgery of the Ear*. Iurato[69] presents an even more concise precis in *Submicroscopic Structure of the Inner Ear*.

■ Inner ear

Inner ear development may be considered in three stages: (1) endolymphatic (otic or membranous) labyrinth, (2) perilymphatic (periotic) labyrinth, and (3) bony labyrinth.

Inner ear formation commences about the third week of fetal life. A platelike thickening of ectoderm on either side of the head forms near the hind brain; this is called the *optic placode*. This invaginates in a few days and forms the *optic pit*. By the fourth week of embryonic life the pit has deepened and narrowed and its lips have fused to form the *otocyst* (otic vessicle). The otocyst is fluid filled and ectodermal lined and constitutes the primitive endolymphatic (otic), or membranous, labyrinth.

By 4½ weeks the otocyst has elongated and starts to divide into two sections, the utricular-saccular portion and the smaller endolymphatic duct portion. The *utricle* and *semicircular canals* differentiate from the posterolateral aspect of the otocyst, while the *saccule* and *cochlear duct* and the communication betwen the two, the *ductus reuniens*, arise anteromedially.

In early development the posterior, superior, and lateral semicircular canals are three compressed semispherical, disclike pouches at about right angles one to another. As the discs enlarge the epithelial walls of their centers fuse and then disappear. The remaining peripheral portions give rise to the definitive semicircular ducts. The region into which the semicircular ducts open becomes the utricle.

The saccule originates from the anteromedial portion of the otocyst. At the sixth developmental week the future cochlea makes its first appearance in the form of the cochlear duct, which developes as an evagination of the saccule. By 8 weeks the duct is elongated and beginning to coil; by 11 weeks it has formed 2½ turns.

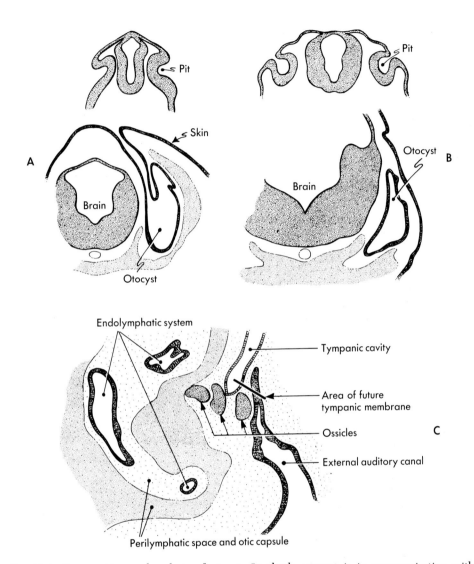

Fig. 16-1. Comparative embryology of ear. **A,** In shark, otocyst is in communication with circumambiant water. **B,** Human endolymph contained within membranous labyrinth is surrounded by another fluid, perilymph. Aqueous system of human progenitors is restored in this way and equilibratory function of inner ear is maintained. **C,** Auditory function, which is subserved by wave transmitting system, is brought about in humans by conversion of branchial arch apparatus of shark. (Modified from Anson, B., Harper, D., and Winch, T.: The vestibular and cochlear aqueducts: developmental and adult anatomy of their contents and parietes, Third Symposium on the Role of the Vestibular Organs in Space Exploration, NASA SP **152:**125, 1967.)

Later, the communication between the cochlear duct and the saccule becomes narrowed to form the ductus reuniens. Similarly, parts of the utricle and saccule become constricted to form the *utricular duct* and the shorter *saccular duct*, which eventually join together to form the common *endolymphatic duct.*

The endolymphatic or membranous labyrinth enlarges within its cartilaginous encasement until midterm, by which time it has reached its complicated adult form. The surrounding cartilaginous otic capsule then ossifies. No further growth of these structures occurs for the lifetime of the individual, with the exception of the endolymphatic duct and sac. Interestingly, these structures are the earliest appendages of the otic vessicle to appear; but unlike the rest of the membranous labyrinth, which reaches adult shape and size by midterm, the endolymphatic duct and sac continue to change throughout infancy and childhood until after puberty. At full adulthood the endolymphatic sac is three times larger than at birth. Its function will be discussed later.

As the mature anatomic configuration of the labyrinth develops (by approximately 6 to 7 months of fetal age the membranous labyrinth is completely developed) its sensory end-organs emerge, appearing in the utricle and saccule between 7 and 8 weeks, within the semicircular ducts by 8 weeks, and within the cochlea at 12 weeks. Differentiation in the cochlear duct goes on at the slowest rate, not being completed until after midterm. It is noteworthy that the cochlea not only is the last of the labyrinth to differentiate but also is less stable and more subject to developmental malformations and acquired disease than are the phylogenetically older vestibular end-organs.

▪ Perilymphatic (periotic) labyrinth

Concomitant with the differentiation of the otocyst, the mesenchyme surrounding it undergoes changes.[136,137] By 7 weeks of fetal age it has become precartilage. At 8 weeks the precartilage changes to an outer zone of true cartilage that forms the *otic capsule*, while the inner zone begins to loosen and vacuolize and forms the *perilymphatic space*. Fluid-filled cavities appear around the vestibule and cochlear duct and finally surrond the semicircular ducts. These spaces all eventually fuse and become confluent, forming a continuous perilymphatic labyrinth containing a delicate matrix composed of arachnoid-like connective tissue. The perilymph circulates within the interstices of the filaments as they traverse the distance between the membranous labyrinth and the endosteum of the otic capsule. This filamentous matrix is present to some degree in all portions of the perilymphatic space, except around the cochlear duct in the spaces known as the *scala tympani* and *scala ves-*

tibuli. The absence of filaments within the scalae permits undampened pulsatile movement of the perilymph between the oval and round windows. The kinetic energy of the sound waves is absorbed by the membranes of the cochlear duct and the "secondary tympanic membrane" of the round window.

The perilymphatic space has three prolongations into the surrounding osseous otic capsule; the *cochlear aqueduct* (perilymphatic duct), the small *fissula ante fenestram*, and the *fossula post fenestram*. These latter two structures are of only remote radiologic interest; however, either or both of them may be involved as a focus of diseased bone in otosclerosis.

The cochlear aqueduct extends from the scala tympani near the round window to the subarachnoid space near the emergence of the glossopharyngeal nerve on the inferior surface of the petrous pyramid. It will be described in further detail in the section on anatomy.

▪ Bony labyrinth

Ossification of the otic capsule commences only when the cartilage has attained maximum growth and maturity. Once the membranous labyrinth has become encased by enchondral bone all growth of the inner ear structures ceases and there is no possibility for future expansion of this rigid structure. The enchondral bone formed in the cartilage of the otic capsule is never removed and replaced by haversion bone; i.e., there is no remodeling. Along with the ossicles, the otic capsule is unique within the human body. They remain as a primitive, relatively avascular type of bone that is exceptionally hard and poor in osteogenic response.[125]

Ossification occurs between the sixteenth and twenty-third weeks of fetal life, with 14 separate centers identifiable. No suture lines are visible because ossification begins only after all growth has ceased. The bony otic capsule is complete except for an area over the lateral semicircular canal, a narrow rim of cartilage that remains around the oval window, and the fissula ante fenestram.

The otic capsule is made up of concentric layers of dense enchondral bone with a thin uniform layer of endosteal bone being laid down against the endoendosteal membrane that lines the labyrinth. Outside the enchondral layer, periosteal bone is laid down in parallel lamellae.

The endosteal layer and the thick middle enchondral layer of the capsule remain relatively inert and unchanged through life. In response to infection or trauma the endosteal membrane lining the labyrinth may proliferate, obliterating the lumen of the labyrinth (see section on infections of the temporal bone: obliterative labyrinthitis).

The enchondral layer participates very poorly in osteogenic repair, so fractures of the labyrinth may remain completely unhealed except by fibrous union. However, there are also advantages to this poor bone repair. The poor osteogenic response made possible the construction of a labyrinthine fenestra that remained permanently open in early operations for stapedial otosclerosis. One of the conditions that prompted the development of stapes prosthesis implantation surgery following stapes mobilization procedures in early otosclerosis surgery was the failure of fractured stapedial crura or footplates to heal.

The periosteal bone of the labyrinthine capsule, i.e., the bone that lies peripheral to the dense middle endochondral bone, continues to be added to by apposition during infancy and up until early adult life. In due course this periosteal bone is removed and replaced by haversion bone. Eventually pneumatic cells invade most of the periosteal layer of the capsule along with much of the remainder of the temporal bone. As with other periosteal bone, that of the otic capsule reacts readily to infection or trauma with osteogenesis. Rarely, there may be a profound response such as that occurring with a meningioma.

As has been noted, ossification about the entire otic capsule is relatively uniform and complete with the exception of three areas: the area around the oval window, the area of the fissula ante fenestram, and an area over the lateralmost bulge of the lateral semicircular canal. Ossification in this latter region is unique because in early stages it is the same as in the remainder of the otic capsule, with the production of three layers of bone; however, at approximately midterm the portion covering the lateralmost sweep of the lateral semicircular canal undergoes dissolution. By the thirteenth week the periosteal layer and varying amounts of the middle enchondral layer have been removed. Eventually there is reconstitution with varying thickness of the periosteal bone. In some circumstances this reconstitution is (normally) very thin and for that reason it can appear radiographically as a site of bony dehiscence; this can be misinterpreted as a sign of labyrinthine fistula when occurring in the presence of cholesteatoma. One should therefore be circumspect and not overinterpret this finding on radiographs.

■ Outer and middle ear

Although it is apparent that the sound-perceiving neurosensory apparatus of the inner ear comes from the ectodermal otocyst, the sound-conducting mechanism arises from totally different and widely separated anlages. The sound-conducting mechanisms of the outer and middle ear are derived from the branchial or gill apparatus of the embryo.

At 4 weeks of fetal age three branchial arches sepa-rated by two branchial grooves have developed on either side of the embryo head. The second branchial groove and the third arch make only an evanescent appearance in the embryo, disappearing except in those rare circumstances in which a branchial cleft or branchial cleft cyst persists in the neck behind and below the external auditory meatus, sometimes extending inward as far as the palatine tonsils.

The first branchial groove deepens to become the primitive external auditory meatus, while the corresponding evagination from the pharynx, the first pharyngeal pouch, grows outward and upward toward it. For a brief moment in embryologic time the epithelium of the first branchial groove touches the endoderm of the first pharyngeal pouch, but soon mesoderm grows between and separates these two layers. This is the region of the future tympanic membrane.

Over the next 5 fetal months the first branchial groove contributes to the development of the mature configuration of the *external acoustic meatus*, the outer, cuticular layer of the *tympanic membrane*, and the *tympanic ring*.

The auricle develops from around the first branchial groove from six knoblike outgrowths or hillocks arising from the first and second branchial arches, appearing at the sixth week of embryonic life and fusing by the third month.

The first pharyngeal pouch becomes the *eustachian tube* and *middle ear cavity*; the cartilages of the first and second branchial arches form the ossicles. The first branchial arch forms most of the *malleus* and *incus;* the second branchial arch forms the *stapes*, the *lenticular process* and *incus*, and the *handle* of *malleus*. With further development the ossicles separate from their parent cartilages and fuse. These separate processes develop independent growth.

The ossicles, similar to the otic capsule and labyrinth, grow only through the first half of uterine life and then ossify. Each of these bones ossifies from a single center; the incus appears at 16 weeks, the malleus at 16½ weeks, and the stapes at 18 weeks. The ossicles are formed of enchondral bone that persists for the rest of the individual's life, as does the enchondral layer of the labyrinthine capsule. The malleus and incus remain solid and relatively constant in size and shape. The stapes, however, undergoes a process of erosion and thinning soon after it ossifies. The adult stapes is less bulky and considerably more delicate and fragile than it is in mid-fetal life. With this diminution in bulk and weight there develop exceptional variations in size, shape, and strength of the adult crura and footplate. A normal adult footplate varies from thick and uniform to thin and irregular. It even may be dehiscent in its central portion. One therefore should abstain from characterizing an irregular, thick, thin, or dehiscent footplate as abnormal.

As the ossicles differentiate and ossify, the surrounding mesenchymal connective tissue becomes less dense and less cellular; by 18 to 21 weeks the tissue filling the space of what is to become the middle ear is very loose, somewhat vacuolated, and mucoid in character. By 22 weeks this vacuolated, mucoid connective tissue gives way to the upward expanding tympanic epithelium of the pharyngeal pouch. The latter encroaches on and wraps around the ossicles and their tendons and ligaments, investing them with epithelial tissue derived from endoderm. Communication between the pharynx and middle ear is thus established. At maturity only the eustachian tube remains as an anatomic reminder of the upward migration of the first pharyngeal pouch in the formation of the tympanic cavity and communicating spaces.

By the thirtieth week "pneumatization" of the tympanum proper is almost complete. Pneumatization of the antrum soon follows and progresses rapidly from the thirty-fourth to the thirty-fifth week, but in the epitympanum it lags and is not completed until the last month of fetal life.

The reader should understand that pneumatization at this stage of development has nothing to do with the actual presence of air in the ear; used in this context it relates rather to the process of focal dissolution and displacement of mesenchymal connective tissue with eventual formation of the space that comes to be lined by an advancing layer of entodermal (respiratory) epithelium arising from the first pharyngeal pouch. This space will become the aerated cavities of the eustachian tube, the middle ear, antrum, etc., at term. Pneumatization thus comes to refer to the creation of an epithelial-lined space to be aerated later.

■ Pneumatic cells of the temporal bone

The air cells of the temporal bone develop as outpouchings of the antrum, epitympanum, tympanic cavity, and eustachian tube. Despite tentative epithelial evaginations appearing from the antrum as early as 34 weeks, no significant pneumatic cellular expansion into the remainder of the temporal bone occurs until after birth, with the stimulation caused by the presence of air within the middle ear. The pneumatizing process then goes into a period of high activity, proceeding over several years. The petrous apex may demonstrate continued pneumatization into early adult life.

Pneumatization occurs as a result of epithelial-lined projections arising from the lining of the middle ear and its extensions. These evaginations probe the spaces between spicules of new bone that are forming and the spaces created by the degeneration of bone marrow into a loose connective tissue stroma. The air cells will invade bone only after the marrow has been converted into a loose mesenchymal tissue. It is averred by Wittmaack[154] that the presence of middle ear infections in infancy causes the embryonic subepithelial connective tissue to fibrose; this prevents its condensation and thinning and impedes the progress of the advancing fingers of evaginating pneumatic cells. This would explain pneumatization arrest following otitis media in infants and children.

■ The neonatal temporal bone

At birth the anatomic portions of the hearing and vestibular system are virtually fully developed with the exception of the formation of the osseous portion of the external acoustic canal. Even the internal acoustic canal (which is not part of the bony labyrinth but is by common clinical practice considered to be part of the inner ear because of its juxtaposition and functional relationship to the labyrinth) is of nearly adult vertical dimension and will grow probably no more than 1 mm in height during the remainder of the individual's life. (The length of the internal acoustic canal, however, will increase substantially during childhood.)

Shambaugh[126] emphasizes that the remainder of the neonatal temporal bone, however, is small and differs from the adult both in shape and position, occupying the inferolateral surface of the skull rather than the lateral aspect as in mature individuals. He notes that as viewed from the side the infant temporal bone consists of a large squamous portion, a diminutive tympanic portion, and no mastoid. Whereas in the adult the mastoid lies posterior to the tympanic ring, in the child the petrous portion lies behind the tympanic ring and below the squamous portion.

■ Formation of the mastoid process

The mastoid process is a postnatal structure and begins to develop during the second year of life as a result of downward extension of cells arising from the squamous portion and partially by extensions of cells from the petrous portions. These two parts of the mastoid process come together at the petrosquamous suture line. Within the mastoid process air cells grow down from the antrum vertically in the petrous portion to the mastoid tip and laterally and radially into the squamous portion. A dividing bridge of bone separating these two cell tracks is known as *Koerner's septum*. This is visible radiographically as a pointed bony spicule directed obliquely downward, originating from the antral roof.

With further maturation of the mastoid, the thin, incomplete infantile ring that constitutes the tympanic portion of the bone grows laterally and inferiorly to form the osseous extension of the (heretofore) cartilaginous auditory canal. Two suture lines are formed: the *tympanosquamous suture* arising in the anterosuperior meatal wall and the posteriorly positioned *tympanomastoid suture.*

□ Normal anatomy

R. Thomas Bergeron

The traditional presentation of anatomy of the ear in a radiologic text has been confined to that of bony anatomy alone, frequently as demonstrated solely on radiographs. CT, with its capability of demonstrating soft tissue as well as bone, provides reason enough to broaden the description to include soft tissue structures. Much more important, however, is the fact that bony changes reflect the eventual (and often late) result of antecedent soft tissue disease. To provide more meaningful consultative interpretation of temporal bone radiographs and CT at least some familiarity with soft tissue anatomy in conjunction with bony landmarks is essential. Additionally, the mechanics of the ear bear so heavily on understanding the functions of the ear that it is virtually impossible to proceed in that enterprise without a good anatomic foundation.

The anatomy of the temporal bone is complex and in many circumstances confusing. Part of the complexity has to do in dealing wih 350 million years of evolutionary modification of this organ and part has to do with unfortunate anatomic terminology, ambiguity, imprecision, and redundancy that has become fixed in scientific nomenclature. The following section is a compendium gathered from many anatomic sources.*

■ Temporal bone

The temporal bones are situated at the sides and base of the skull. Each consists of five parts: squamous, mastoid, petrous, tympanic, and styloid process.

Squamous portion

The squamous portion forms the anterolateral and upper part of the bone; it is shell-like and thin. The external surface is smooth and convex, giving attachment to the temporalis muscle; it forms part of the wall of the temporal fossa. A gently arching *zygomatic process* arises from the lower portion of the squama and is directed anteriorly. Its lateral surface is convex and lies directly beneath the skin and subcutaneous tissue. The medial surface is concave and serves as the origin of the masseter muscle. The anterior end of the zygomatic process articulates with the zygomatic bone. The posterior portion of the zygomatic process is divided into an anterior and posterior root. The posterior root lies above the external audiory canal and becomes continu-

ous with the temporal line posterior to the external auditory canal.

The anterior root becomes the articular tubercle of the condylar (mandibular) fossa. The condylar fossa is bound posteriorly to the anterior surface of the tympanic bone.

The mandibular fossa is cleaved in the sagittal plane by the tympanosquamous suture laterally and by that suture's inward extension, the petrotympanic (glaserian) fissure, medially. The portion of the condylar fossa anterior to the fissure is the articular portion of the joint; that portion posterior to the glaserian fissure is the nonarticular portion.

The internal surface of the squama is concave and irregular. Meningeal vessels groove the inner surface. The superior border articulates with the parietal bone and the anteroinferior border articulates with the greater wing of the sphenoid.

Mastoid portion

The mastoid portion has a rough outer surface and serves as origin to a portion of the occipital and the posterior auricular muscles. In the adult the mastoid portion is continued inferiorly into a conical projection, the mastoid process. This process gives attachment to the sternocleidomastoid, splenius capitis, and longissimus capitis muscles. On the medial side of the process is a deep groove, the mastoid notch or digastric groove, for the attachment of the digastric muscle. Medial to this is a shallow furrow, the occipital groove, which lodges the occipital artery.

The inner or intracranial surface of the mastoid presents a deeper groove, the sigmoid sulcus, which lodges part of the transverse sinus.

The superior border is broad and serrated and articulates with the parietal bone. The posterior border, similarly serrated, articulates with the inferior border of the occipital bone. Anteriorly and above, the mastoid portion is fused with the descending process of the temporal squama; below, it enters into the formation of the external acoustic meatus and the tympanic cavity.

The mastoid process is hollowed to form a number of spaces, the mastoid cells, which exhibit great variety in size and number. In the upper and front part of the process these cells are large and irregular, toward the middle part they diminish in size, and those in the apex of the process are frequently small. In addition to these cells there occurs a large irregular cavity, the tympanic antrum, that is situated at the upper and anterior part of the mastoid portion of the bone. The antrum communicates with the remainder of the mastoid cells and with the epitympanum (attic), which is situated anteroinferiorly and medially by way of the *additus ad antrum.*

---

*References 4, 9, 49, 59, 60, 118, 119, 125, 152.

Petrous portion

The petrous pyramid is wedged in at the base of the skull between the sphenoid bone anteriorly and the occipital bone posteriorly. It is directed medially, forward, and slightly upward. It contains the inner ear.

The petrous portion resembles a toppled three-sided pyramid lying on the flat surface of one of its sides. Its base is laterally positioned and is fused with the internal surfaces of the squamous and mastoid portions. The apex points medially and forward and is inserted into the angular interval between the posterior border of the greater wing of the sphenoid bone and the basilar part of the occipital bone. The anterior (middle fossa) face of the petrous pyramid has a more horizontal orientation and is "longer" than the posterior surface, which is relatively vertical and "shorter."

The anterior face (surface) forms the posterior limit of the middle cranial fossa and is continuous laterally with the inner surface of the squamous portion; it is united at these edges by the petrosquamous suture. Its surfaces are somewhat irregular and marked by depressions for convolutions of the brain and by a shallow depression medially for the reception of the semilunar ganglion (Meckel's cave) of the fifth cranial nerve. The arcuate eminence, which marks the site of the underlying superior semicircular canal, is near its midportion. In front of and slightly lateral to this eminence is a depression that marks the position of the tympanic cavity. The layer of bone that separates the tympanic and cranial cavities is usually very thin and is known as the *tegmen tympani*. A nearby groove leads laterally and posteriorly to an oblique opening, the hiatus of the facial canal, which transmits the greater superficial petrosal nerve and the petrosal branch of the middle meningeal artery.

The posterior face (surface) of the petrous pyramid forms the anterior bony limit of the posterior fossa and is continuous with the inner surface of the mastoid portion of the temporal bone at the petromastoid suture. To reiterate, this face has a more vertical orientation than the anterior surface. Near the center of this surface is the opening to the internal auditory (acoustic) canal (meatus), which transmits the seventh and eighth cranial nerves, the nervus intermedius, and the internal auditory artery. The opening of the internal auditory canal is known as the *porus acusticus.*

The lateral end of the internal auditory canal is closed by a vertical plate of bone, the *lamina spiralis*, which separates the fundus of the canal from the vestibule. The fundus is divided by a transverse crest of bone, the *crista falciformis*, into unequal upper and lower compartments. The crista, which arises anteriorly, usually extends medially no more than 2 to 3 mm. The upper compartment occupies about 40% and the lower about

60% of the vertical dimension of the canal. In the upper compartment the facial nerve (VII) lies anteriorly and the superior vestibular division of cranial nerve VIII lies posteriorly. The branches of the latter go to the utricle and superior and lateral semicircular canals. In the compartment beneath the crista falciformis there are three sets of foramina. Anteriorly, a set is arranged spirally about the central canal of the cochlea (the *modiolus*) to accommodate the cochlear division of the eighth cranial nerve. Posteriorly, branches of the inferior division of the vestibular nerve take their exit, one set of foramina leading to the saccule and the remainder leading to the posterior semicircular canal.

Posteroinferior to the internal acoustic meatus is a small slit that leads to the vestibular aqueduct. This transmits the endolymphatic duct along with the accompanying artery and vein.

The inferior face (surface) of the petrous pyramid is a rough and irregular surface and forms part of the exterior of the base of the skull. It furnishes partial attachment for the *levator veli palatini* and the cartilaginous portion of the eustachian tube. It is pierced anteriorly by the aperture of the carotid canal. The cochlear aqueduct opens on the inferior surface, lying almost vertically beneath the porus acousticus. Behind the opening of the cochlear aqueduct lies the jugular fossa.

There are two minute canals that perforate the inferior surface of the petrous portion within or near the jugular fossa.

The *inferior tympanic canaliculus*, which accommodates the tympanic branch of the glossopharyngeal nerve (Jacobson's nerve). This lies between the carotid canal and the jugular fossa.

The *mastoid canaliculus*, which serves as entrance for the auricular branch of the vagus nerve (Arnold's nerve). This is located within the lateral part of the jugular fossa.

The styloid process originates from the inferior face of the pyramid. The *stylomastoid foramen* is situated between the downward projections of the mastoid process and the styloid process. This foramen constitutes the terminus of the bony facial canal.

The superior angle (border) of the petrous portion of the temporal bone is grooved for the superior petrosal sinus and gives attachment to the tentorium cerebelli. This superior angle commonly is referred to as the "petrous ridge"; it represents the line of the intersection between the anterior and posterior surfaces of the pyramid. The anteromedial extremity of the ridge is notched for the reception of the roots of the trigeminal nerve.

The posterior angle of the pyramid is defined by the junction of the lower aspect of the posterior surface with the posterior limits of the inferior surface. From the perspective of the inner surface of the skull within the posterior fossa, the posterior angle is marked by a sulcus of the petrous portion that along with a corresponding sulcus on the occipital bone forms the channel for the inferior petrosal sinus. An excavation on the inferior and medial aspect of the posterior surface of the pyramid, in continuity with this sulcus, is known as the *jugular fossa*. The corresponding depression, in continuity with the sulcus arising from the occipital bone, is known as the *jugular notch*. These semilunar cavities face one another and together form the *jugular foramen*. The dilated portion of the internal jugular vein that occupies the foramen is the *jugular bulb*.

The anterior angle of the pyramid marks the junction between the pyramid and the bones of the floor of the middle cranial fossa. The anterior border is divided into two parts: the medial part, which articulates with the greater wing of the sphenoid, and the lateral portion, which adjoins the squamous part at the petrosquamous suture.

At the angle of the junction of the petrous and squamous portions, two (semi) canals are placed one above the other and separated by a thin plate of bone. This septum is known as the *septum canalis musculotubarii* (cochleariform process). The upper canal contains the tensor tympani muscle, and the lower canal is the bony portion of the eustachian tube.

Tympanic portion

The tympanic portion of the temporal bone is a curved plate lying below the squamous part and in front of the mastoid process. Its *posterior* surface is somewhat C-shaped and forms the *anterior* wall, the floor, and the posteroinferior aspect of the bony external auditory canal. At the medial end of the canal there is a narrow furrow, the *tympanic sulcus,* for the attachment of the tympanic membrane. The lateral border of the tympanic portion of the temporal bone is roughened, forming a large part of the margin of the opening of the external auditory canal; this is continuous with the cartilaginous part of the canal. The lateral part of the upper border is fused with the back of the postglenoid tubercle. Its medial extension forms the posterior boundary of the petrotympanic fissure.

There is considerable ambiguity in anatomic descriptions regarding the terms *petrotympanic fissure, tympanosquamous fissure,* and *glaserian fissure.* Many anatomic depictions point unassailably to a junction between the *squamous* and tympanic portions, labeling the area "petrotympanic fissure." This is more easily understood if one recognizes that the tympanosquamous fissure "squamotympanic" is merely the lateral extension of the petrotympanic fissure. The glaserian fissure is the medial fissure, the petrotympanic. This

serves as a passageway for the anterior tympanic branch of the internal maxillary artery. In the medialmost extreme portion of the petrotympanic fissure is the small canal for the chorda tympani, the *iter chordae anterius (anterior tympanic aperture).*

The lower border of the tympanic bone encloses the root of the styloid process. Posteriorly, the tympanic portion blends with the squamous and mastoid portions, forming the anterior boundary of the tympanomastoid fissure.

Styloid process

The styloid process of the temporal bone averages about 2.5 cm in length and projects downward and forward from the undersurface immediately anterior to the stylomastoid foramen. It gives origin to muscles and ligaments of the hyoid and tongue regions.

■ External auditory canal

The walls of the external auditory canal (meatus) are formed laterally of fibrocartilage and medially of bone, while both parts are lined by skin reflected inward. The osseous portion of the meatus, which comprises slightly more than half of the canal, is a tunnel through the temporal bone. The bony canal is about 16 mm long and directed inward, forward, and downward. On a sagittal scan section the canal is oval or elliptical in shape, with its long axis directed downward and slightly backward. The anterior wall, floor, and lower part of the posterior wall are formed by the tympanic component of the temporal bone; the remainder of the posterior wall and the roof arise from the squamousal portion.[118]

The tympanic membrane makes a compound angle with the external acoustic meatus. The inferior border of the tympanic membrane lies closer to the midsagittal plane than does the superior border. Additionally, the anterior border lies closer to the midsagittal plane than does the posterior border. This means that the tympanic membrane is sloping both downward and inward. The posterosuperior wall of the external auditory meatus measures about 25 mm in the adult while the anteroinferior wall is over 30 mm.

Vessels and nerves

The arteries of the external auditory meatus are derived from the external carotid artery through branches from the posterior auricular, superficial temporal, and internal maxillary arteries. The veins and lymphatics connect with those of the auricle. The veins ultimately empty into the internal and external jugular veins and occasionally into the sigmoid sinus by way of mastoid emissary veins.

The lymphatics of the external acoustic canal and auricle empty into all adjacent regional nodes including the parotid, superficial cervical, and retroauricular groups.

Because the development of the external ear is embryologically complex, the cutaneous enervation is similarly complex and subject to considerable variation. Enervation is derived from the auriculotemporal branch of the mandibular division of the trigeminal nerve and from cutaneous branches of the cervical plexus, primarily the greater auricular nerve from C2 and C3. There are also contributions from sensory fibers originating in the eighth, ninth, and tenth cranial nerves.

■ The middle ear

The middle ear or tympanic cavity is an irregular, laterally compressed space within the temporal bone. It is filled with air that is conveyed to it from the nasopharynx through the eustachian tube. It is traversed by the ossicular chain, which connects the lateral and medial walls. The ossicles both transmit and amplify the vibrations incident on the tympanic membrane across the cavity to the inner ear.

The tympanic cavity consists of three parts: the *tympanic cavity proper* opposite the tympanic membrane, the *attic* or epitympanic recess above the level of the membrane, and the *hypotympanum*, a variable inferior and medial extension occurring below the level of the tympanic membrane.

Shaped more like a cleft than a box, the vertical dimension (including the attic) and the anteroposterior dimension of the cavity are each about 15 mm. The transverse dimensions measure about 6 mm superiorly and 4 mm inferiorly. Opposite the center of the tympanic membrane it may measure only about 2 mm. The lateral extent of the cavity is defined by the tympanic membrane or *membranous wall* and the medial or *labyrinthine wall* by the otic capsule. The roof is known as the *tegmental wall* and the floor, which is separated from the jugular fossa by a thin plate of bone, is known as the *jugular wall*. Anteriorly the space is delimited by the *carotid wall* and posteriorly by the *mastoid wall*.

Roof or tegmental wall

The tegmen tympani is a plate of bone that arises from the petrous portion of the temporal bone. Its forward prolongation becomes the roof of the canal for the tensor tympani muscle and its backward continuation forms the roof of the mastoid antrum. The tegmen tympani separates the middle ear cavity from the middle cranial fossa. The lateral margin of the tegmen interdigitates with the squamous portion of the temporal bone at the petrosquamous suture. In children this may be unossified and may allow a direct passage of infection from the middle ear to the epidural space of the middle

cranial fossa. In adults, veins from the middle ear perforate this suture to end in the petrosquamous sinus (present in about 50% of cases) and the superior petrosal sinus. They may transmit infection directly into the cranial venous sinuses.[59]

Floor or jugular wall

The floor or jugular wall of the middle ear cavity lies either at or slightly below the level of the floor of the external auditory meatus and is usually a very thin plate of bone that separates the cavity from the internal jugular vein. If the jugular bulb is particularly small, then the floor may be correspondingly thick—even as much as a centimeter—and it may contain air cells intervening between the middle ear cavity and the internal jugular vein. The inferior extent of the tympanic cavity below the level of the inferior attachment of the tympanic membrane, along with its medial extension, is known as the *hypotympanum.*

If the jugular bulb is very large it may bulge upward into the floor of the tympanic cavity, giving it a convex margin. This bulging reduces the potential size of the hypotympanum. Occasionally the bone may be dehiscent (see section on high jugular bulb), with the jugular bulb present within the hypotympanum. The importance of recognition of this anatomic variation is obvious in the differential diagnosis of glomus tumor, jugular diverticulum, aberrant position of the carotid canal, etc.

A small aperture for the passage of the tympanic branch of the glossopharyngeal nerve (Jacobson's nerve) is present within the jugular wall near the labyrinthine wall.

Mastoid or posterior wall

The mastoid or posterior wall is wide above and below and presents the *additus ad antrum* (entrance to the tympanic antrum), the *pyramidal eminence*, and the *incudal fossa*. The additus ad antrum is a large, irregular aperture that leads posteriorly from the epitympanic recess to the mastoid antrum. The pyramidal eminence is situated immediately behind the oval window and in front of the vertical (mastoid) portion of the facial canal; it is hollow and contains the origin and belly of the stapedius muscle. Its summit projects forward toward the oval window and it is pierced by a small aperture that transmits the tendon of the muscle. The cavity of the pyramidal eminence is prolonged downward and backward in front of the facial canal and communicates with it by a minute aperture that transmits a twig from the facial nerve to the stapedius muscle.

There are two important recesses in the posterior wall, the *sinus tympani* and the *facial recess* (see Fig. 16-77). They may be the sites of occult extension of disease within the middle ear. They are demonstrated with ease by means of horizontal plane cuts in CT.

The tympanic sinus is a space that is bounded by the labyrinthine wall medially and by the pyramidal eminence laterally.

The facial recess is bounded by the pyramidal eminence, styloid complex, and facial canal medially and by the bony tympanic annulus laterally. The facial recess is an important surgical landmark when the middle ear cavity is entered from the posterior aspect by means of a mastoid approach.

The incudal fossa is a small depression in the lower and posterior portion of the epitympanic recess; this is the site of attachment of the posterior ligament of the short process of the incus.

Just lateral and usually slightly inferior to the aperture transmitting the tendon of the stapedius muscle is the aperture for the chorda tympani nerve as it separates from the mastoid portion of the facial nerve.

Carotid or anterior wall

The carotid or anterior wall is wider above than below and corresponds with the carotid canal, from which it is separated by a thin plate of bone that is perforated by the tympanic branch of the internal carotid artery and also by the caroticotympanic nerve. At the upper part of the anterior wall are the orifice of the semicanal for the tensor tympani muscle and the tympanic orifice of the eustachian tube, separated from each other by the septum canalis musculotubarii. These semicanals run from the tympanic cavity forward and downward to the angle between the squamous and petrous portion of the temporal bone. These semicanals lie one above the other rather than side by side.

The semicanal for the tensor tympani is the superior and smaller of the two; it is cylindrical and lies beneath the tegmen tympani. It extends on to the labyrinthine wall of the tympanic cavity and ends immediately above the oval window. In current usage the septum canalis musculotubarii is more commonly known as the *processus cochleariformis*. This bony structure forms the lateral wall and floor of the semicanal for the tensor tympani.

The eustachian tube. The eustachian tube is the lower of the two channels and the one through which the tympanic cavity communicates with the nasopharynx. Its length is about 3.5 cm and its direction is downward, forward, and medialward. It forms an angle of about 45° with the sagittal plane and one of about 30° to 40° with the horizontal plane. Part of the eustachian tube is composed of bone and part is composed of fibrous tissue and cartilage.

The osseous portion is a little over a centimeter in length. It begins in the carotid wall below the process cochleariformis and, tapering slowly, ends at the angle of junction of the squamous and petrous portions of the temporal bone. Its distalmost end has a serrated margin for the attachment of the cartilaginous portion.

The cartilaginous portion is around 2.5 cm in length. The cartilage lies in a groove between the petrous part of the temporal bone and the greater wing of the sphenoid. This groove ends opposite the middle of the medial pterygoid plate.

The tube is not of uniform diameter; its narrowest portion (the isthmus) lies at the junction of the bony and cartilaginous portion. It is at its widest diameter at the pharyngeal orifice. The cartilaginous and bony portions of the tube are not in the same vertical plane, the cartilaginous portion being slightly more steeply inclined than the bony portion.

Lateral or membranous wall

The tympanic cavity extends above the level of the tympanic membrane as the epitympanic recess. The lateral boundary of the tympanic cavity proper therefore is the tympanic membrane together with the small rim of the temporal bone to which it is attached. The osseous tympanic ring is complete superiorly at the notch of Rivinus. Close to this notch are three small apertures: the petrotympanic (glaserian) fissure and the anterior and posterior tympanic apertures (iter chordae anterius and posterius).

The petrotympanic fissure transmits the tympanic branch of the internal maxillary artery and houses the anterior process of the malleus and its anterior ligament.

The chorda tympani nerve gains entrance and finds egress from the tympanic cavity by way of the posterior and anterior tympanic apertures, respectively. The chorda tympani traverses the tympanic cavity but gives off no branches to it.

The tympanic membrane is directed obliquely downward and inward, forming an angle of about 50° with the floor of the external acoustic canal and about 15° with the midsagittal plane. The manubrium of the malleus is attached to the medial surface of the tympanic membrane at its center and pulls the membrane inward; the lateral surface of the membrane therefore appears concave and the central depression of this concavity is called the *umbo*.

Medial or labyrinthine wall

The medial wall of the tympanic cavity is that part of the petrous portion of the temporal bone that surrounds the internal ear and separates the cavities of the middle and internal ears.[59] Several bulges and depressions are apparent, reflecting the various contours of the inner ear structures.

Posteriorly and superiorly, in what would be considered the medial wall in the region of the additus, is the prominence produced by the anterior limb of the lateral semicircular canal. Below this and extending more anteriorly is the prominence of the facial canal produced by the bone overlying the intratympanic portion of the facial nerve. Anterior to the prominence of the facial canal is the curving terminus of the septum canalis musculotubarii; this also serves as a landmark for the position of the geniculum of the facial nerve, which lies immediately anterior to the knee of the facial nerve.

Immediately below the mesotympanic facial canal is the oval window niche, which contains the oval window at its medial terminus. Below the oval window lies the promontory, a convexity that bulges into the tympanic cavity and represents a portion of the basal turn of the cochlea. Below and behind the back part of the promontory is the round window niche, which leads to the round window. The round window has an orientation very close to the coronal plane. Posterior to the promontory is a smooth bony projection, the *subiculum promontorii*, which forms the inferior border of the deep depression known as the *tympanic sinus*. Inferior to the subiculum lies the round window niche.

The superior border of the sinus tympani is bounded by another smooth, bony bridge, the ponticulus. The oval window niche lies superior to the ponticulus.

To recapitulate: there are two bony bridges, the upper or ponticulus and the lower or subiculum. Between the two lies the sinus tympani. Above the ponticulus lies the oval window niche. Below the subiculum lies the round window niche.

Epitympanic recess

That portion of the tympanic cavity that extends above the level of the tympanic membrane is known as the epitympanic recess, or attic. This is a chamber having a height about one third that of the entire tympanic cavity; the attic projects lateral to the plane of the tympanic membrane. This small portion of the tympanic cavity therefore has as its lateral wall a part of the squamous portion of the temporal bone; the inferior, medially directed pointed terminus of the lateral attic wall is known as the *scutum*.

The attic contains the head of the malleus and the body and short process of the incus. Superiorly the epitympanic recess is bounded by the tegmen tympani; medially by the prominence of the lateral semicircular canal and the prominence of the facial nerve; laterally by the scutum; and inferiorly the incudal fossa and the bony surface just behind it. The boundary line between the tympanic cavity proper and the epitympanic recess is marked by the prominence of the facial canal medially, the inferior limit of the incudal fossa inferiorly, and

the scutum laterally. The additus ad antrum originates from the posterosuperior aspect of the epitympanic recess.

Contents of tympanic cavity

Auditory ossicles. Three small bones span the width of the tympanic cavity. The *malleus* consists of a head, a neck (manubrium), and two processes. The head lies within the epitympanum. The *manubrium* is attached to the tympanic membrane. The *lateral process* abuts against the tympanic membrane immediately below the pars flaccida. The *anterior process* is a slender spicule of bone that passes forward and downward into the petrotympanic fissure.

The *incus* is shaped somewhat like a premolar tooth, with two widely diverging roots that differ in length. The *body* is somewhat cuboid but compressed transversely. On its anterior surface is a deeply concavoconvex facet that articulates with the head of the malleus. The body of the incus and the head of the malleus are bound to one another by a thin capsular ligament, forming a diarthroidial joint known as the *incudomalleolar articulation*.

The two crura of the incus diverge from one another narrowly at right angles. The *short crus* or short process projects almost horizontally backward and is attached to the incudal fossa in the lower and posterior portion of the epitympanic recess.

The *long crus* (long process) descends nearly vertically behind and parallel to the manubrium of the malleus and bends medially to end in a rounded projection, the *lenticular process*, which is tipped with cartilage and articulates with the head of the stapes. This is also a diarthroidal joint and is called the *incudostapedial articulation*.

From its articulation with the incus, the stapes passes almost horizontally across the tympanic cavity to meet the wall of the labyrinth at the oval window.

The *stapes* resembles a stirrup and consists of a head, a neck, two crura, and a base. The *head* has a depression that is covered by cartilage and articulates with the lenticular process of the incus. The *neck* is the constricted part of the bone succeeding the head, and its posterior aspect gives insertion to the tendon of the stapedius muscle.

The *anterior* and *posterior crura* diverge from the neck and are connected at their ends to the flattened oval plate known as the *base*, which forms the footplate of the stapes and is fixed to the margin of the oval window by the annular ligament. The anterior crus is shorter and less curved than the posterior. The edge of the stapedial base is covered with cartilage, as is the rim of the oval window; the junction thereof constitutes the *tympanostapedial syndesmosis*.

Ligaments. The ossicles are connected with the walls of the tympanic cavity by ligaments: three for the malleus, and one each for the incus and stapes.

The *anterior ligament* goes from the neck of the malleus just above the anterior process to the carotid wall near the petrotympanic fissure. The *superior ligament* descends from the roof of the epitympanic recess to the head of the malleus. The *lateral ligament* goes from the posterior part of a notch of Rivinus to the head of the malleus.

The *posterior ligament* of the incus is a short, thick band connecting the neck and end of the short crus to the posterior wall of the incudal fossa.

The *annular ligament* of the base of the stapes has been described previously. It represents the fibrous ring that encircles the base of the stapes and attaches to the margin of the oval window.

Muscles. The muscles of the tympanic cavity have already been alluded to; one each arises from the anterior and posterior walls.

The *tensor tympani*, the larger muscle, is contained in the bony canal above the osseous portion of the eustachian tube, from which it is separated by the processus cochleariformis. It passes backward through the canal and ends in a slender tendon that enters the tympanic cavity; it makes a sharp bend around the terminus of the process cochleariformis and is inserted into the manubrium of the malleus near its root. It is supplied by a branch of the mandibular nerve that passes through the otic ganglion.

The *stapedius* muscle rises from the walls of the conical cavity hollowed out of the interior of the pyramidal eminence; its tendon emerges from the orifice at the apex of the pyramidal eminence and as it moves forward it is inserted into the posterior surface of the neck of the stapes. It is supplied by a branch of the facial nerve.

By their actions both the tensor tympani and stapedius muscles reduce the efficiency of the sound-conducting mechanism. The tensor tympani accomplishes this by tightening the drum of the tympanic membrane and thereby diminishing the amplitude of excursion of the malleus. The stapedius muscle exerts its action by pulling the head of the stapes backward, which causes the base of the bone to rotate on a vertical axis drawn through its own center. The posterior part of the base is pressed inward toward the vestibule and the forward portion is withdrawn from it. This reduces the amount of area effectively transmitting the vibration at the footplate and diminishes the mechanical advantage of the lever mechanism. Both of these muscles therefore serve to protect the inner ear from excessive amplitude oscillations of the footplate of the stapes when there is a very loud noise. This protective reflex is invoked with low-frequency vibration only and is most effective at frequencies under 5000 Hz.

Nerves and vessels. The nerves of the middle ear cavity are represented by the tympanic plexus, which lies on the cochlear promontory under the mucosa, within grooves or canals in the bone. This plexus is formed chiefly by the tympanic branch (nerve of Jacobson) of the ninth cranial nerve but is reinforced by one or more caroticotympanic nerves derived from the internal carotid sympathetic plexus. The facial nerve also makes a minor contribution to the tympanic plexus. These fibers are mostly parasympathetic secretomotor fibers. The tympanic branch of cranial nerve IX supplies sensory enervation to the mucosa of the middle ear.

Glomus tympanicum tumors take their origin in cell groups associated with the tympanic branch of the ninth cranial nerve.

The chorda tympani arising from cranial nerve VII traverses the middle ear cavity but is not a source of enervation to the cavity.

The tympanic cavity derives its arterial supply from a number of vessels, most of which are branches of the external carotid artery. These include the *anterior tympanic* artery arising from the internal maxillary artery; the *inferior tympanic* artery arising from the ascending pharyngeal artery; the *stylomastoid* artery arising from either the posterior auricular or the occipital artery, which gives off a *posterior tympanic* artery; a superior *tympanic* and *petrosal* artery arising from the middle meningeal artery; and *caroticotympanic* branches arising from the internal carotid artery.

The veins roughly parallel the arteries and empty into the superior petrosal sinus and pterygoid plexus. The lymphatics begin as a network in the mucous membrane and end chiefly in the retropharyngal carotid lymph nodes.

■ Route of the facial nerve (cranial nerve VII)

The facial or seventh cranial nerve emerges from the brainstem as two roots, *motor* and *sensory*. The motor root is the larger. It leaves the medulla oblongata at the inferior border of the pons, medial to the acoustic nerve. The smaller sensory root or *nervus intermedius* (of Wrisberg) contains efferent and visceral efferent fibers. It emerges from the medulla between the motor root of the facial nerve and the acoustic nerve.

Motor root

As the motor root leaves the medulla it pierces the pia mater and receives its sheath. The bundle then continues forward and laterally in the posterior fossa to the internal auditory meatus, where it enters in conjunction with the nervus intermedius and acoustic nerve. As it spans the distance between the medulla and the porus acousticus the motor root aligns itself in a groove on the superior surface of the cochlear division of the acoustic nerve. This intracranial segment is 23 to 24 mm in length.

The internal auditory canal segment is 7 to 8 mm in length and lies in a superior relationship to the cochlear nerve, passing above the crista falciformis. While within the canal, the motor root is separated from the acoustic bundle by the nervus intermedius, but the three nerve bundles are all surrounded by one sheath or arachnoid and dura and by continuations of the subarachnoid and subdural spaces. While still within the canal, the motor root and the nervus intermedius unite to form the combined nerve trunk.

The labyrinthine segment of the nerve measures 3 to 4 mm in length and passes forward and laterally within its own bony channel, the *fallopian canal*. When it reaches a point just lateral and superior to the cochlea it angles sharply forward, nearly at a right angle to the long axis of the petrous pyramid, to reach the geniculate ganglion. At the ganglion the direction of the nerve reverses itself, executing a hairpin turn so that it runs posteriorly. This is the so-called first knee or *first genu* of the facial nerve. At this point the facial nerve is lying just above the base of the cochlea, i.e., above and medial to the promontory.

The first genu of the facial nerve, in the limb distal to the geniculate ganglion, delineates the anteriormost extent of the tympanic segment of the nerve. This tympanic segment is around 12 mm in length and passes posteriorly and laterally, perpendicular to the long axis of the petrous bone on the medial wall of the tympanic cavity. It lies above the oval window and below the bulge of the lateral semicircular canal. At the level of the sinus tympani the nerve changes its direction at the *second genu*. At this point the nerve assumes a vertical position, dropping downward in the posterior wall of the tympanic cavity and the anterior wall of the mastoid to exit at the base of the skull from the stylomastoid foramen. This mastoid segment is about 15 to 20 mm in length.[119]

There are three primary branches of the facial nerve: the greater superficial petrosal nerve, the nerve to the stapedius muscle, and the chorda tympani.

The greater superficial petrosal nerve arises from the geniculate ganglion and exits the petrous bone and facial canal just anterior to the geniculate ganglion by way of the facial hiatus along the anterior aspect of the petrous pyramid. The greater superficial petrosal nerve is a mixed nerve containing both parasympathetic fibers (from the nervus intermedius) and sympathetic fibers.

The nerve to the stapedius muscle is a small twig given off from the facial nerve as it descends in the posterior wall of the tympanic cavity behind the pyramidal eminence.

The chorda tympani takes its origin about 5 mm above the stylomastoid foramen and is composed mainly of sensory fibers, although it also contains a few motor fibers and is therefore a mixed nerve. As it leaves the trunk of the facial canal it pursues a slightly recurrent course upward and forward in the canaliculis chorda tympani (*iter chordae posterius*), a minute canal in the posterior wall in the tympanic cavity. It enters the tympanic cavity close to the border of the tympanic membrane. It then crosses the cavity running on the medial surface of the tympanic membrane at the junction of its upper and middle thirds. It is covered by mucous membrane lining of the tympanic cavity and passes to the medial side of the manubrium of the malleus above the tendon of the tensor tympani. It therefore passes *between* the malleus and the incus. It leaves the tympanic cavity by way of a canal in the petrotympanic fissure to pass to the base of the skull through a small foramen, the *iter chordae anterius* (anterior tympanic aperture). It eventually joins the lingual nerve in the parapharyngeal space to supply taste sensation to the anterior two thirds of the tongue.

Bony dehiscences

It is customary to consider the facial canal to be a closed bony tube except where branches make their exit. Such is not invariably the case. Baxter[10] reported dehiscence in more than half of over 500 temporal bones studied microscopically. Dehiscences in the canal were most common in the tympanic portion near the oval window region and were occasionally present in the mastoid segment and near the region of the geniculate ganglion. The average dimension of these dehiscences was less than 1 mm. The radiologic demonstration of a substantial loss of bone in any region of the facial canal therefore should be considered abnormal.

Anomalous course in petrous bone

Although the course of the facial nerve through the temporal bone is one of the most constant of anatomic relationships, anomalous courses do occur. Such a circumstance may be extremely treacherous for a surgeon, and everyone involved in the interpretation of temporal bone images must be alert to the possibility of such an anomaly.

An anomalous course of the mastoid portion is to be expected in the presence of atresia of the external acoustic canal (discussed later), but numerous such courses have been reported in the absence of any other significant developmental abnormality.

Most of the anomalous courses reported are involved in that part of the nerve peripheral to the geniculate ganglion. The interested reader is referred to the work of Basek,[8] Dunkin et al.,[33] Shambaugh,[125] Wright et al.,[156] and Schucknect.[119]

The main trunk of the facial nerve in its tympanic portion may take an anomalous course along the medial wall of the tympanic cavity, the most common having a position anterior and inferior to the oval window rather than above it. More importantly, the nerve may divide into two or more branches at any position along its course and these two branches may either parallel one another or diverge.

An anomalous course of the facial nerve within the tympanic cavity is a diagnosis unlikely to be made other than by direct inspection by the operating surgeon. On the other hand, an unusual course or absence of an identifiable canal in the mastoid portion of the facial nerve canal is an observation that should be made by the interpreter of either complex motion tomograms or CT scans. Otherwise, the surgeon may inadvertently injure the abnormally positioned nerve during a mastoidectomy.

■ The inner ear (Fig. 16-2)
Bony labyrinth

The bony labyrinth consists of the *vestibule, semicircular canals,* and *cochlea.*

Vestibule. The central portion of the cavity of the bony labyrinth is the vestibule. The vestibule is a relatively large ovoid perilymphatic space measuring approximately 4 mm in diameter, leading anteriorly into the cochlea and posteriorly into the semicircular canals. There are cribrose areas, minute openings for the entrance of the nerve branches from the vestibular nerve on the medial wall and floor of the vestibule, where it abuts on the lateral end of the internal acoustic canal. The vestibule has two other openings: the oval window for the footplate of the stapes, and the vestibular aqueduct.

Semicircular canals. The three semicircular canals are continuous with the vestibule. Each of the canals makes about two thirds of a circle and measures about 1 mm in cross-section diameter. Each is enlarged at one end to form the *bony ampulla.* The nonampulated ends of the superior and posterior semicircular canals join to form the bony *common crus.*

A portion of the superior (anterior) semicircular canal usually forms a ridge (arcuate eminence) on the anterior surface of the petrous bone (the posterior delimitation of the middle cranial fossa). The lateral (horizontal) semicircular canal projects as a ridge on the medial wall of the additus.

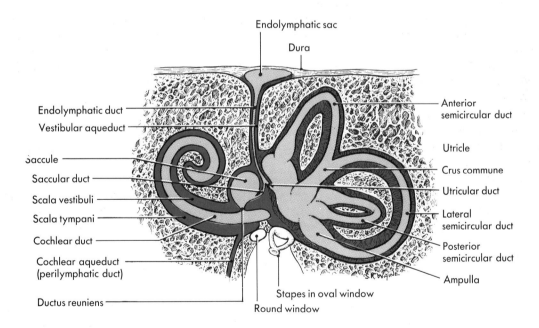

Fig. 16-2. Inner ear, schematic drawing. Membranous labyrinth is enclosed within bony labyrinth and separated from it by perilymphatic space. Cochlear and vestibular portions of membranous labyrinth are surrounded by perilymph. Vestibule and semicircular canals tend to be suspended from walls of bony labyrinth by myriad tiny arachnoid-like filaments. No such filaments exist around cochlear duct. Membranous labyrinth encloses endolymphatic space and is filled with endolymph. Endolymphatic sac and duct are in continuity with endolymphatic space. Cochlear aqueduct communicates with subarachnoid space and is in continuity with perilymphatic space. Oval window abuts against vestibule; round window is located at commencement of basilar turn of cochlea. Perilymphatic space is in color.

The perilymphatic space of the semicircular canals opens and communicates freely with the vestibule at both their ends.

The superior (anterior) and posterior semicircular canals are both arranged in a vertical orientation at approximately right angles to one another. The anterior canal is directed anterolateraly at an angle about 45° to the midsagittal plane, and the posterior canal is directed posterolaterally at a corresponding angle. It should be noted therefore that the angles of the vertical canals are oriented within both temporal bones so that the superior (anterior) semicircular canal of one side has the same sagittal orientation as the posterior canal of the opposite side, and vice versa.

The lateral semicircular canal does not occupy a horizontal plane and for this reason the older terminology ("horizontal") has been discarded. The anterior limb of the lateral semicircular canal lies in the plane higher than the posterior limb, making an angle of about 30° with the horizon. In the erect position therefore the neck would have to be flexed about 30° for the lateral semicircular canal to be "horizontal."

Cochlea. The perilymphatic cavity of the vestibule is also continuous with the cochlea anteriorly. The cochlea is a conical structure, its base lying on the internal auditory canal and its apex or *cupola* directed anteriorly, laterally, and slightly downward. The base measures around 9 mm and its axis height is about 5 mm. The base is perforated by numerous apertures for the passage of the cochlear nerve.

The cochlea consists of a conical central axis, the modiolus; a bony canal wound spirally around the central axis for a little more than 2½ turns; and a delicate *osseous spiral lamina*, which projects from the modiolus into the canal and partially divides it. In the living state the division of the canal is completd by the *basilar membrane*, which stretches from the free border of the osseous spiral lamina to the outer wall of the bony cochlea. The two passages into which the cochlear canal is thus divided communicate with each other at the apex of the modiolus by a small opening, the *helicotrema*.

The modiolus is the conical central pillar of the cochlea. Its base is broad and appears at the lateral end of the internal acoustic canal, where it corresponds with the cochlear outflow of the eighth cranial nerve. It is perforated by numerous orifices for the transmission of the branches of the nerve.

The bony *cochlear canal* takes between 2½ and 2¾ turns around the modiolus. The first turn bulges toward the tympanic cavity and this elevation on the medial wall of the tympanic cavity is known as the *promontory*. The bony cochlear canal is about 30 mm long and diminishes gradually in diameter from the base to the

summit, where it ends in the cupola, which forms the apex of the cochlea. The cross-sectional diameter of the beginning of the canal is about 3 mm. The openings in or near the first portion of the cochlear canal include the round window, which is covered by the secondary tympanic membrane; the oval window (actually an opening of the vestibule), which is covered by the footplate of the stapes; and the aperture of the *cochlear canaliculus*, which leads to a small canal that communicates with the subarachnoid space by an opening on the inferior surface of the petrous portion of the temporal bone. The cochlear canaliculus, also known as the *cochlear aqueduct* or *perilymphatic duct*, allows at least theoretical equilibration between the perilymphatic space and the subarachnoid space.

Membranous labyrinth (Fig. 16-3)

The interconnecting spaces of the membranous labyrinth constitutes the endolymphatic cavity. The labyrinth consists of the cochlear duct, the vestibular sense organs, the endolymphatic duct and sac, the round window membrane, and the vascular system.

Cochlear duct. The *cochlear duct* is a spiral tube lying within the cochlea and attached to its outer wall. The cochlear duct is a blind pouch; it cleaves the perilymphatic space within the bony labyrinth and divides it into two portions, the scala vestibuli and the scala tympani. The cochlear duct is triangular, its roof being formed by Reisner's membrane, its outer wall by the endosteum lining the bony canal, and its floor by the

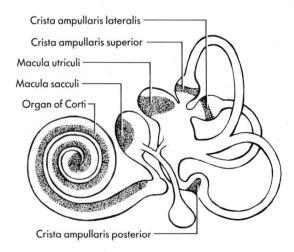

Fig. 16-3. Specialized sensory areas of membranous labyrinth. Sensory cells mediating hearing are located in organ of Corti within cochlear duct. Sensory organs of vestibular labyrinth are located in maculae of utricle and saccule and within ampullae of semicircular canals. Macula of utricle mediates most of sensations having to do with linear acceleration of head; ampullary cristae are sensitive to changes in angular acceleration of head.

basilar membrane and the outer part of the osseous spiral lamina. It contains the organ of Corti, which is the site of placement of the supporting and sensory (hair) cells that mediate hearing.

The vestibular sense organs. The sensory organs of the vestibular labyrinth are located in the maculae of both the utricle and saccule and within the ampullae of the semicircular canals. The epithelium consists of supporting and hair cells (sensory cells) covered by a gelatinous layer into which the cilia project.

Vestibular physiology is complex. The maculae are referred to as organs of static balance because the otoliths, under the influence of gravity (they have a specific gravity of 2.71), exert traction on the cilia of the hair cells in varying positions of the head. The macula of the utricle mediates most of the sensations that have to do with linear acceleration of the head. The ampullary crests located within the semicircular canals are called organs of kinetic balance because they are stimulated by the movement of or pressure changes in the endolymph caused by the angular acceleration of the head; this produces deviation of the cupulae.

The utricle resides within the elliptical recess of the vestibule. The sensory cells of the utricle lie within the *macula*. The semicircular ducts all open into the utricle. From the anteromedial part of the utricle the *ductus utriculosaccularis* takes its origin and opens into the endolymphatic duct.

The saccule lies in the spherical recess near the opening of the scala vestibuli of the cochlea. The macula of the saccule is located along its anterior wall.

The saccule communicates with the sinus of the endolymphatic duct by way of the saccular duct and with the cochlear duct by way of the ductus reuniens. From the lower part of the saccule the ductus reuniens communicates with the basal end of the cochlear duct.

The semicircular ducts are about one quarter of the diameter of the semicirular canals. Each has an ampulla at one end, which lies within the ampulla of the corresponding bony canal. The semicircular ducts open by five orifices into the utricle, the common crus being a single opening for the junction of the medial end of the superior and the upper end of the posterior semicircular ducts. A crestlike septum, the *ampullary crest*, crosses the base of each ampulla and is made up of sensory epithelium distributed on a mound of connective tissue and covered by a gelatinous cupola.

Endolymphatic duct and sac. The *endolymphatic duct* begins within the vestibule as a dilated portion, the *endolymphatic sinus*. It arises at the confluence of the utricular and saccular ducts. As it leaves the vestibule it narrows into an isthmus and passes through the vestibular aqueduct. As the endolymphatic duct reaches the dural opening of the vestibular aqueduct it widens

again into the flat *endolymphatic sac*. The remainder of the sac lies between the periosteum of the petrous bone and the dura mater.

Round window membrane. The round window membrane (secondary tympanic membrane) measures about 3 mm in its horizontal axis and about 1.5 mm in its transverse axis. The round window membrane is of particular importance in acoustic energy transfer within the inner ear, where it performs as a yielding area of the bony labyrinth to permit movement of the perilymph in association with excursions of the stapedial footplate. Movements of these two diaphragms should be typically 180° out of phase with one another.

Vascular system. The arterial blood supply to the membranous labyrinth originates within the cranial cavity and effectively is distinct from the vessels that supply the otic capsule in the tympanic cavity, although there are a few terminal branches that penetrate the endosteal layer. In a study of 100 human specimens Mazzoni[85] reported finding a consistent arterial loop in the region of the internal auditory canal. This loop is either the main trunk or a branch of the anterior inferior cerebellar artery in 80% of cases, of the accessory anterior cerebellar artery in 17%, or a branch of the posterior inferior cerebellar artery in 3%. The loop was found inside the internal auditory canal in 40%, at the porus in 37%, and within the cerebellopontine angle cistern in 33% of cases.

The anterior inferior cerebellar artery arterial loop gives rise to the *internal auditory artery* (labyrinthine artery) and also frequently to the *subarcuate artery*. It then takes a recurrent course to the cerebellum. The internal auditory artery distributes to the dura and nerves in the internal auditory canal to adjacent bone of the canal and to the medial aspect of the inner ear before dividing into the *common cochlear artery*.[84] The further ramifications of these arteries to the membranous labyrinth are discussed by Hawkins[56] and further elaborated on by Schuknecht.[119]

The main venous channels of the cochlea are the *posterior* and *anterior spiral veins*. These join together near the base of the cochlea to form the *common modiolar vein*. The common modiolar vein is joined by the vestibulocochlear vein to become the *vein of the cochlear aqueduct*. This main channel enters a bony canal near (but not within) the cochlear aqueduct to empty into the inferior petrosal sinus.

The semicircular canals are drained by vessels that pass toward the utricular end to form the *vein of the vestibular aqueduct*, which accompanies the endolymphatic duct and drains into the lateral venous sinus.

Bast and Anson[9] describe an *internal auditory vein* that traverses the internal auditory canal and drains into the inferior petrosal sinus, but this is an inconstant vessel.

Perilymphatic spaces and fluid systems

The perilymphatic space (see Fig. 16-3) of each semicircular canal is continuous at both ends with the perilymphatic space of the vestibule, and this space is in turn continuous widely with that of the scala vestibuli. The scala vestibuli is continuous with the scala tympani at the helicotrema. All the perilymphatic spaces therefore open widely into each other.

The total volume of fluid contained within the developmentally mature periotic space is estimated to be approximtely 0.2 ml—about 3 drops. Without those three drops of fluid, however, the transmission of sound waves from the oval window to Reissner's membrane in the cochlea could not be mediated.

There are several actual or potential dehiscences in the compact bone of the petrous portion of the temporal bone that could theoretically permit communcation between the perilymphatic space and the middle and internal ears.[59] These include (1) the oval window, normally sealed off from the middle ear cavity by the foot plate of the stapes and its annular ligament, (2) the round window, normally sealed off from the middle ear by the secondary tympanic membrane, (3) the *fissula ante fenestram* and the *fossula post fenestram,* two small extensions of the perilymphatic space extending from the vestibule toward the tympanic cavity that are usually obliterated by connective tissue, and (4) the vestibular aqueduct, a channel that extends through the otic capsule from the vestibule to the posterior cranial fossa and transmits the endolymphatic duct and accompanying vein. The duct, vein, and connective tissue surrounding them so fill the aqueduct that there is no perilymphatic *space* and therefore no actual communication between the perilymphatic space of the vestibule and the epidural space. (5) The fifth actual or potential dehiscence is the cochlear aqueduct (perilymphatic duct, cochlear canaliculus), a normally minute canal that opens on the inferior surface of the petrous part of the temporal bone and permits communication between the subarachnoid space and the scala tympani. Occasionally the cochlear aqueduct is very patulous, and this provides at least a theoretical possibility of free communication of the perilymphatic space with the subarachnoid space. Whether this is physiologically important in the transport of potentially noxious substances to the inner ear from the violated subarachnoid space is yet unproved.

■ How the ear amplifies sound

Once the inner ear becomes sequestered within the base of the skull it becomes necessary in the evolutionary sense to reestablish continuity with the external environment so as to provide a suitable apparatus for the reception of sound. Evolution elegantly fashioned a method based on the simplest of hydraulic principles, solving the problem of acoustical impedance mismatch between sound waves traveling in the air and those same waves traveling in the fluid of the inner ear—the ossicular lever mechanism vibrating in an air chamber and attached to the large area diaphragm (tympanic membrane) on one side and the small area diaphragm (stapes footplate) on the fluid side.

Sound waves are amplified by three different mechanisms by the time the vibrations in the air of the external acoustic canal are changed to fluid pulsations of the perilymph within the membranous labyrinth.

The first mechanism is the "organ pipe" resonance of the external canal. The resonant frequency of the column of air enclosed within the external acoustic canal accounts for approximately doubling of the pressure at the tympanic membrane compared to that at the entrance to the canal for frequencies between 2000 and 5400 Hz.

Secondly, the area of the tympanic membrane varies between 15 and 30 times the area of the oval window. This concentration of force at the stapes footplate amplifies the incoming vibrations of sound approximtely 15 to 30 times.

Finally, the lever mechanism of the ossicular chain reduces the amplitude of the excursion of the bone at the footplate of the stapes in comparison to the long handle of the malleus and thereby increases the force by a factor of 2 to 3.

The sound waves therefore may be amplified by a factor of up to 180 by the time that they encounter the perilymph.[134]

□ Temporal bone imaging

R. Thomas Bergeron

The radiology of the temporal bone need not be difficult. The radiographic anatomy, while compact, is neither disorderly nor unduly complex. Diseases affecting the area are not unique and therefore lend themselves to traditional cataloging. Moreover, complex motion tomography renders most of the anatomic structures as separable, distinct, and readily identifiable shadows, and their small size is not an unsuperable impediment to their recognition when seen in isolation from other structures. CT is supplanting virtually all other imaging modalities, providing bony detail equivalent to or greater than complex motion tomography and giving the indisputable added advantage of demonstrating soft tissue anatomy.

■ Patient history

Before commencing a radiographic examination of the temporal bone it is our practice to obtain a history from the patient. Ideally, this information should be submitted by the referring physician with the x-ray request, but this is so often not the case that we have chosen to use the form shown above. This short, detailed history is solicited from the patient either by the x-ray technologist or the radiologist and usually offers adequate clinical information on which to make a judgment regarding the correct anatomic parts necessary to be particularly addressed in the examination. "Routine" views may thus serve as both a start and finish of the examination in some diseases, but perhaps only as a start in others. For example, plain film study of the mastoids would be sufficient in a suspected acute mastoiditis but likely inadequate in the search for an elusive fracture following trauma. Outpatients are asked to complete the above form by themselves before the examination.

It is important that the technologist review this material with the patient before beginnng the examination. This helps the technologist become schooled in neurotologic diagnosis and provides guidance so that the roentgenographic examination is properly tailored for that particular patient. This information is also available to the radiologist at the time of interpretation of the films; it will help him to make a correct judgment as to whether the radiographic endpoint has been reached in that specific patient.

■ Radiographic devices and techniques

Although good plain film temporal bone studies may be obtained using almost any radiographic equipment,

the various commercially available head units seem to give better films more consistently than ceiling-mounted tubes. The smaller, less complicated devices (such as the Compere Head Unit) offer the greatest ease of examination because of easy maneuverability. In addition, beam restriction is optimal because the cones and diaphragms are specifically designed for temporal bone radiography in these units. In contradistinction to the more modest head units, some of the larger, more "versatile," more complicated (automated? remote?), and more expensive devices seem to control the technologist rather than vice versa. They frequently render inferior films, although the complex machinery is admittedly very impressive.

Fractional focal spots should be used if available. A fine line grid with an 8:1 ratio is adequate. Higher grid ratios are of dubious value for imaging this part of the body when using standard monoplane radiographic technique with high-speed screens. Film-screen technology has advanced to the point that par speed screen use is no longer appropriate.

It goes almost without saying that techniques and views must be adjusted, depending on the anatomic area of interest in any particular projection and patient. For example, exposure values for the Stenvers view used to visualize the labyrinth will differ from the Stenvers view used to visualize the air cells in the mastoid tip. As another example, a base view is not obtained in our routine mastoid views for a case of suspected acute mastoiditis, yet it is unfailingly obtained in our same examination entitled "mastoid views" in a suspected glomus jugulare tumor.

To reiterate, roentgenographic examination must take heed of the patient history or else face the likelihood of missing the mark. The "purist" clinician (or radiologist) who believes that radiographs must be interpreted on the basis of shadows alone, without "prejudice" or benefit of knowledge of the clinical problem makes the dangerous (and often incorrect) assumption that all necessary and appropriate views are available for inspection. This attitude reveals a failure to understand that an important contribution that radiologists have to offer is the direction of the examination in order to provide diagnostic films so that even the most difficult case becomes self-evident. It is the radiologist's responsibility and duty to be aware of the patient history in order to achieve this end. In many circumstances it is an absolute necessity.

■ Plain film examination—standard views

The reader is referred to *Merrill's Atlas of Radiologic Positions and Radiologic Procedures*[6] for patient position and tube angulation in order to obtain routine mastoid series. We find the following projections useful.

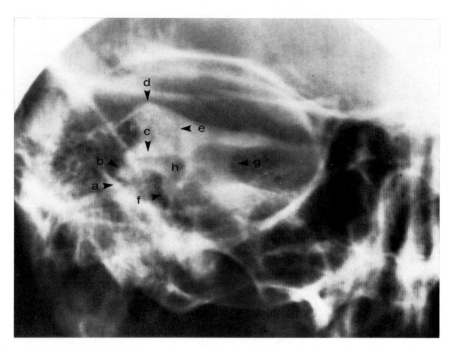

Fig. 16-4. Transorbital AP view. *a*, Scutum; *b*, combination shadow of malleus and incus; *c*, lateral semicircular canal; *d*, arcuate eminence; *e*, superior semicircular canal; *f*, basal turn of cochlea; *g*, posterior lip of internal acoustic canal; *h*, vestibule.

Frontal projections—nonrotated (Fig. 16-4)

Transorbital AP view. The internal acoustic canals are projected through the middle portion of the orbit. Radiographic technique must take into account the fact that the bony labyrinth constitutes the densest bone in the body. A film that is correctly exposed for a standard Caldwell projection of the skull will be underexposed for adequate penetration of the labyrinthine structures.

This is the single most valuable plain film view for delineating the internal acoustic canal, cochlea, vestibule, and semicircular canals. Additionally, the middle ear structures are well seen, including the attic, malleus and incus, scutum, and medial one third to two thirds of the external acoustic canal. The floor of the external acoustic canal is frequently obscured by mastoid air cells. The medial one half to two thirds of the petrous ridge is also seen, as well as the antrum if not obscured by overlying mastoid air cells.

In assessing the length of the internal acoustic canals on plain film radiography, the transorbital AP view is the only view that should be used for measurement. Although the Stenvers view may show the posterior lip of the internal acoustic canal more clearly, rotation of the head causes foreshortening of the canal and thereby renders an inaccurate measurement. Because of rectilinear distortion, the Towne view only infrequently provides adequate spatial resolution for identification of the structures to be measured.

Towne projection *(Fig. 16-5).* The Towne view gives an

excellent projection of the petrous ridge and antrum. It is frequently the best view for showing transverse (vertical) fractures of the petrous portion and the possible extension of these fractures to the foramen magnum. It may also be the most sensitive view for delineating antral cholesteatoma.

In order to improve resolution by diminishing scatter (which is considerable in the Towne view), it is advisable to use a slit diaphragm so that the projected image on the film is no more than about 6 cm high.

Lateral views

The anatomy best delineated in the various lateral views (Fig. 16-6) includes the mastoid air cells and their septa within the temporal squama and the anterior and posterior surfaces of the petrous pyramid.

The three most common projections used for this purpose are the Henschen, the Schuller, and the Laws views (Table 16-1). All of these views embody caudal angulation of the tube with or without rotation of the head in an effort to project one temporal bone separate from the opposite one.

Table 16-1. Three common lateral projections

Projection	Caudal angulation	Rotation
Henschen	15°	0°
Schüller	30°	0°
Laws	15°	15°

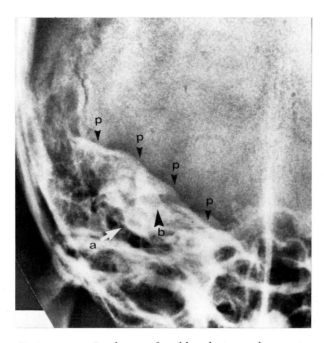

Fig. 16-5. Towne Projection. *a*, Basal turn of cochlea; *b*, internal acoustic canal; *p*, petrous ridge.

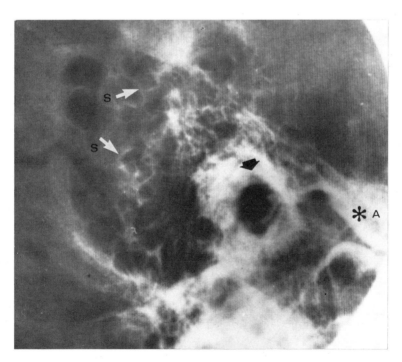

Fig. 16-6. Lateral projection, Henschen view. **A*, Anterior; *short black arrow*, external acoustic canal; *S*, bony septa between adjacent cells.

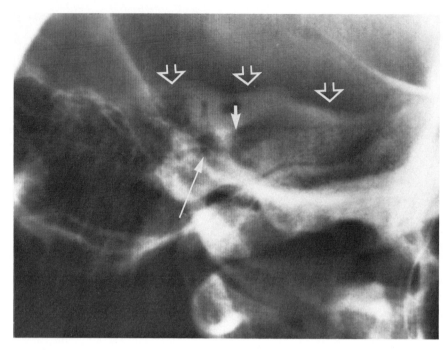

Fig. 16-7. Stenvers view. *Long arrow,* Vestibule; *short arrow,* posterior lip of internal acoustic canal; *open arrows,* petrous ridge.

These views are some of the most sensitive for delineating diminished aeration in the presence of acute mastoiditis, as well as defining the integrity of the tegmen, the sinodual plate, etc.

Because a near-axial view of the external acoustic canal is provided in these projections, the detection of atresia of the external acoustic canal and other lesions affecting the external acoustic canal may be provided.

Parallel view of petrous ridge—Stenvers projection

Although the Stenvers view (Fig. 16-7) gives a profile view of the mastoid tip, it is important to remember that it gives an undistorted, unforeshortened view of the entire petrous ridge because the entire petrous ridge is parallel to the plane of the film. Thus it is an excellent view for the examination of the integrity of the entire length of the petrous ridge and also provides good definition of the posterior lip of the internal acoustic canal and both superior and inferior tips of the petrous bone medial to the porus acusticus. As has been mentioned previously, the Stenver's view gives a foreshortened and therefore inaccurate length to the internal acoustic canal.

Axial views of petrous ridge—Owen and Mayer projections

The Owen and Mayer views (Fig. 16-8) provide projections at a 90° angle to the Stenvers projection and thus represent attempts at axial views of the petrous ridge. These views appear to be particularly difficult for most technologists to position properly and also difficult for the radiologist to interpret because of rectilinear distortion. In judging the correctness of positioning and tube angulation in these views, the following facts may be useful to bear in mind.

The purpose of these views includes visualization of the malleus and incus within the attic; the attic should appear as an upward extension of the ovoid lucency of the external acoustic canal. If the ossicles are projected too far inferiorly, there is excessive caudal angulation of the tube. Similarly, if they remain hidden within the roof of the attic, there is inadequate caudal angulation. Inappropriate rotation of the head will cause the ossicles to be projected either anterior or posterior to the attic space.

These views are particularly useful in assessing attic cholesteatoma and the integrity of the malleus and incus. In our experience the Owen view, which we define as 30° rotation and 30° caudal angulation, is usually insufficient in both planes of movement in order to define the anatomic structures above. The Mayer view, which calls for 45° rotation and 45° caudal angulation of the tube, is usually too much. As a result, the correct angle is usually obtained by an intermediate Owen-Mayer view.[117]

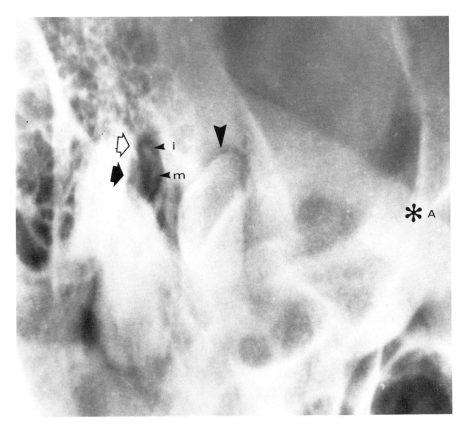

Fig. 16-8. Owen-Mayer projection. *A, Anterior; *long black arrow,* temporomandibular joint; *open black arrow,* attic; *closed black arrow,* external acoustic canal; *i,* incus; *m,* malleus.

Frontal axial view of tympanic cavity and attic—Guillen projection

Because the sagittal plane of the tympanic cavity is angled 12° to 15° toward the midline anteriorly, a frontal projection obtained with the head rotated 12° to 15° toward the side of interest will provide a true frontal axial view of this space[51] (Fig. 16-9). This view is the most sensitive one for demonstrating displacement of the malleus and incus, either toward or away from the lateral attic wall by attic cholesteatoma formation. This is uncommonly used in plain film examination of the temporal bone in the United States, but is gaining increased acceptance in frontal tomography for middle ear disease.

Submentovertex (base) view

Although the submentovertex projection (Fig. 16-10) is not part of our routine mastoid series, it is always included for those patients who are candidates for erosive lesions around the base of the skull, including glomus jugulare tumors, cranial nerve neuromas, and basal meningiomas. The internal acoustic canals are also frequently well delineated in this projection and their en-

largement and possible erosion by an acoustic neuroma may be well seen. As with the Towne view, a slit diaphragm should be used to provide a maximum width of the projected image not to exceed approximately 8 centimeters.

Special projections—Chausee III, IV

These special views enjoy lessening popularity with the increased availability of complex motion tomography and CT. The interested reader is referred to *Merrill's Atlas of Radiographic Positions.*[6]

■ Tomography (Fig. 16-11)

Before CT, complex motion tomography provided the best form of temporal bone imaging. All other techniques represented compromises, some providing a better "make do" than others, but nonetheless still inferior. Linear tomography can be useful in delineating larger lesions, such as antral cholesteatomas and larger acoustic neuromas, and glomus jugulare tumors, but it is inadequate for examinations requiring good definition of small bony structures without streak artifacts.

Text continued on p. 754.

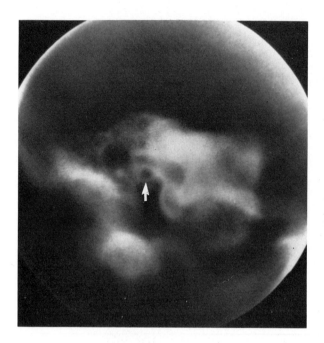

Fig. 16-9. Guillen projection. Because tympanic cavity is inclined 15° toward midsagittal plane, patient's head must be turned about 15° toward side of interest in order to obtain true axial view of middle ear cavity and its contents. This is best view to evaluate cleft of air interposed between lateral attic wall and malleus and incus and optimum projection for defining intratympanic facial nerve canal (*arrow*).

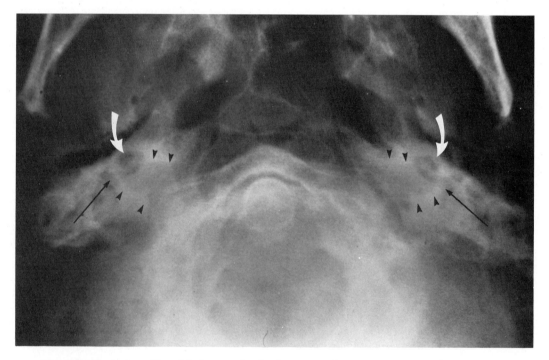

Fig. 16-10. Base view. *Short black arrowheads,* Anterior and posterior margins of the internal acoustic canals; *curved white arrows,* cochleae; *long black arrows,* vestibules.

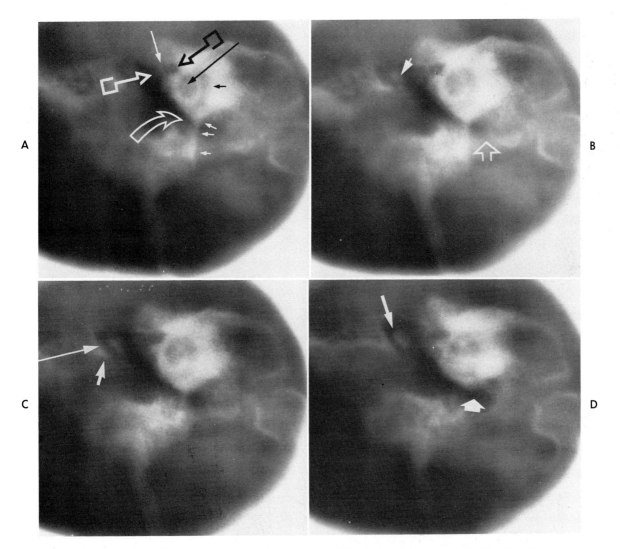

Fig. 16-11. Complex motion tomography of temporal bone: important anatomical landmarks in frontal and lateral projections. Frontal projections are obtained from anterior to posterior and sagittal projections are obtained from lateral to medial. **A** to **G**, Frontal; **H** to **M**, lateral. **A,** *Small white arrows,* Cortical margin of lateral aspect of carotid canal; *curved white arrow,* hypotympanum; *hooked white arrow,* intratympanic portion of facial canal; *long white arrow,* bony septum separating labyrinthine portion from intratympanic portion of facial nerve canal. This section is immediately posterior to region of geniculate ganglion. *Hooked black arrow,* Labyrinthine segment of facial canal; *long black arrow,* apical turn of cochlea; *short black arrow,* middle turn of cochlea. **B,** *Short white arrow,* Head of malleus; *open white arrow,* carotid canal. **C,** *Long white arrow,* Lateral wall of attic; *short arrow,* scutum. **D,** *Long arrow,* Body of incus within attic; *short white arrow,* hypotympanum.

Continued.

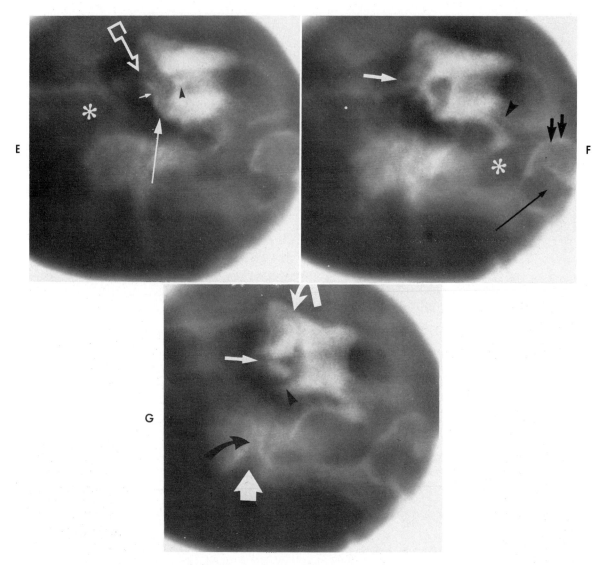

Fig. 16-11, cont'd. E, *Short black arrow,* Crista falciformis within internal acoustic canal; *long white arrow,* round window in basal turn of cochlea. This portion of cochlea is known to surgeon as "promontory." *Short white arrow,* Oval window; *hooked white arrow,* anterior limb of lateral semicircular canal; *asterisk,* external acoustic canal. **F,** *White arrow,* Lateral-most sweep of lateral semicircular canal; *short black arrow,* aperture of cochlear aqueduct; *double arrows,* jugular tubercle; *long black arrow,* hypoglossal canal; *asterisk,* jugular foramen. **G,** *Curved white arrow,* Superior semicircular canal and arcuate eminence; *short white arrow,* posterior limb of lateral semicircular canal; *black arrow,* posterior semicircular canal; *broad white arrow:* stylomastoid foramen; *curved black arrow,* inferior limit of mastoid portion of facial canal.

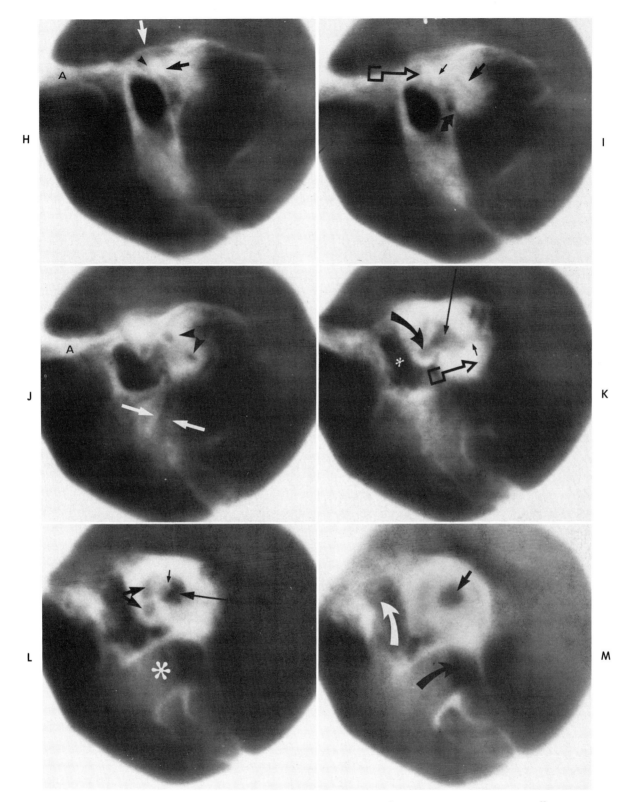

Fig. 16-11, cont'd. H to **M,** Lateral projections. *A,* Anterior; *white arrow,* tegmen antri; *small black arrow,* lateralmost aspect of head of malleus; *larger black arrow,* incus. **I,** *Hooked arrow,* Malleus; *small black arrow,* incus; *larger black arrow,* lateral sweep of lateral semi-circular canal; *curved black arrow,* second genu of facial nerve. **J,** *Black arrows,* Anterior and posterior limbs of lateral semicircular canal; *white arrows,* distal mastoid portion of facial canal just above stylomastoid foramen; *A,* anterior. **K,** *Short black arrow,* Crus commune; *hooked black arrow,* vestibular aqueduct; *long black arrow,* vestibule; *curved black arrow,* basal turn of cochlea (axial view); *asterisk,* hypotympanum. **L,** *Long black arrow,* Internal acoustic canal; *short black arrow,* crista falciformis; *double arrows,* basal and middle turns of cochlea; *asterisk;* jugular foramen. **M,** *Curved white arrow,* Carotid canal; *curved black arrow,* jugular foramen; *straight black arrow,* internal acoustic canal.

Rigorous beam restriction is essential. The best definition is obtained in frontal tomography by filming one temporal bone at a time. If necessary to obtain both temporal bones simultaneously, a midline lead diaphragm should be placed at the tube end and a lead mask on the cassette holder. The patient's eyes should be protected with either lead ellipses or leaded glass eyeglasses. The interposition of this metal on the face will diminish the definition of the anatomic structures in the plane of the temporal bone only to a slight degree; it will afford excellent protection to the eyes, diminishing the exposure to them by more than 90% if a lead sheet of only 0.3 mm is used (Dobrin, R., et al., 1973).

It is our practice to obtain AP tomographic sections in the temporal bone at 1 mm intervals, with the carotid canal as the anterior landmark and the jugular fossa marking the posterior limits. This calls for approximately 12 exposures. Lateral tomograms are obtained on a case-by-case basis. We usually obtain these at 2 mm intervals. The lateral boundary is dependent on the anatomy under study; the medial boundary is usually the posterior lip of the internal acoustic canal. For a detailed discussion of the tomographic anatomy of the normal temporal bone the interested reader is referred to the publication by Valvassori and Buckingham.[147]

□ CT of the temporal bone

Ir. F.W. Zonneveld, P.F.G.M. van Waes, H. Damsma, P. Rabischong, and J. Vignaud

Since the introduction of high-resolution computed tomography (with which details significantly smaller than 1 mm can be resolved), CT has been applied more and more to examinations of the petrous bone.[32,78,123] Basically, such applications have been restricted to the transverse and the coronal planes.[27,141] Other planes of interest, as they are known in classical otoradiology,[24] have not been explored by means of direct CT scanning.

The following section* considers direct CT scanning images in seven different otoradiological planes[157]: transverse, coronal, sagittal, semi-axial, semi-longitudinal, axio-petrosal and longitudinal. Although limited to seven planes, it is obvious that other planes can also be scanned directly, for example, the inclined sagittal plane.[92] Direct scanning is to be preferred since this technique avoids the degradation of image quality which results from multiplanar reformatting.[67,144]†

The visualization matrix (Table 16-2) and nomenclature guide (see box) refer to Figs. 16-12 to 16-70. This matrix shows which anatomical detail can be visualized best in which plane. Longitudinal visualization means that the longitudinal extent of the anatomical structure is visible (the course of the facial nerve or the spiral of the cochlea).

Transverse visualization means that the anatomical structure is seen in cross-section (plane perpendicular to facial nerve or plane through the modiolus of the cochlea).

*Reprinted from Zonneveld, F.W., van Waes, P.F.G.M., Damsma, H., Rabischong, P., and Vignaud, J.: Direct multiplanar CT of the petrous bone, with permission of Philips Medical Systems. Some of these illustrations were originally published in Zonneveld, F.W. and Albrecht, C.: Medicamundi **26**:81-92, 1981 and in Zonneveld, F.W.: Neuroradiology **25**(1):1-10, 1983.

†Technique: Scans were performed with a Philips TOMOSCAN 310 at the Utrecht University Hospital. This scanner was equipped with an experimental table swivel mechanism and with three special headrests.

The principle of geometrical enlargement was used in order to obtain a spatial resolution of 0.6 mm. The temporal bone was enlarged to an 8 cm square field of view by means of a zoom reconstruction.

Other factors contributing to the sharpness of the image were the use of 1200 projection directions in a 9.6 second scan time and a Ramp convolution filter. To avoid degradation of the sharpness by partial volume averaging a slice thickness of 1.5 mm was used.

For display and photography a window level of 300 H and a window width of 3200 H were selected. The scans were made at 120 kV and 360 mAs, resulting in a peak skin dose of about 5R (50 mGy).

Table 16-2. Visualization matrix

L / T	Longitudinal visualization / Transverse visualization	Transverse	Coronal	Sagittal	Semi-axial	Semi-longitudinal	Axio-petrosal	Longitudinal
6	Tegmen tympani		T	T	T	T	T	T
7	Pyramidal eminence	T		T				
8	Tympanic membrane	T	T		T	T	T	
9	Promontory		T		T		T	
10	Oval window	T	T		T	T	T	
11	Round window	T		T		T		T
12	Facial canal (first part)	L			L		L	T
15	Facial canal (second part)	L		T				
16	Facial canal (third part)	T	L	L	L	L	L	L
17	External auditory meatus	L	L	T		L		
20	Manubrium of malleus	L			L		L	T
21	Incudo-malleolar articulation	T						T
24	Long process of incus	T			L		L	T
25	Incudo-stapedial articulation	T					T	
26	Stapes	L		T				
27	Tendon of tensor tympani muscle	L	L	T	L			

L / T	Longitudinal visualization / Transverse visualization	Transverse	Coronal	Sagittal	Semi-axial	Semi-longitudinal	Axio-petrosal	Longitudinal
28	Processus cochleariformis		T		T		T	
29	Tensor tympani muscle	L					T	L
30	Stapedius muscle	T		L	L	T	T	T
31	Vestibule	T	T	T	T	T	T	T
32	Cochlea (first turn)	T				L	T	L
33	Cochlea (second turn)	T				L	T	L
34	Lateral semicircular canal	L	T	T	T	T	T	T
35	Superior semicircular canal	T			L		L	
36	Posterior semicircular canal	T				L		L
37	Aqueduct of vestibule	T		T	T		T	
38	Aqueduct of cochlea	L	L	T	L		L	
39	Internal auditory meatus	L	L	T				
41	Canal of internal carotid artery	L		T		L	T	L
43	Eustachian tube	L						L
44	Petro-mastoid canal	L	L	T			T	L

NOMENCLATURE

1. Antrum
2. Tegmen antri
3. Tympanic cavity
4. Attic (epitympanic recess)
5. Lateral wall of the attic
6. Tegmen tympani
7. Pyramidal eminence
8. Tympanic membrane
9. Promontory
10. Oval window
11. Round window
12. Facial canal (first part)
13. Geniculate ganglion
14. Canal of superficial petrosal nerve
15. Facial canal (second part)
16. Facial canal (third part)
17. External auditory meatus
18. Head of malleus
19. Neck of malleus
20. Manubrium of malleus
21. Incudo-malleolar articulation
22. Body of incus
23. Short process of incus
24. Long process of incus
25. Incudo-stapedial articulation
26. Stapes
27. Tendon of tensor tympani muscle
28. Processus cochleariformis
29. Tensor tympani muscle
30. Stapedius muscle
31. Vestibule

32. Cochlea (first turn)
33. Cochlea (second turn)
34. Lateral semicircular canal
35. Superior semicircular canal
36. Posterior semicircular canal
37. Aqueduct of vestibule
38. Aqueduct of cochlea
39. Internal auditory meatus
40. Falciform crest
41. Canal of internal carotid artery
42. Jugular bulb
43. Eustachian tube
44. Petro-mastoid canal
45. Aditus ad antrum
46. Tympanic sinus
47. Common crus
48. Ampulla of lateral s.c. canal
49. Ampulla of superior s.c. canal
50. Ampulla of posterior s.c. canal
51. Second genu of facial canal
52. Chorda tympani nerve
53. Canal of chorda tympani nerve
54. Petrotympanic suture*
55. Petro-occipital suture
56. Glaserian fissure*
57. Morgagni canal
58. Koërner spur
59. Styloid process
60. Marrow of styloid process
61. Sigmoid sulcus
62. Mastoid process

*Author's note: The petrotympanic and Glaserian fissures are identical anatomic structures.

■ Transverse plane

In distinction from polytomography, CT allows the transverse or the horizontal plane (Figs. 16-12 to 16-21) to be obtained with the patient in a comfortable supine position. The gantry is tilted slightly to adjust the scan plane parallel to the nasion-biauricular plane.

Patient comfort, the possibility of comparing both ears, and the fact that the majority of the anatomical details are imaged make the transverse plane the ideal plane for the baseline study of the petrous bone.

This plane is of special interest for the visualization of both the incudomalleolar and the incudostapedial articulations, both the first and the second part of the facial canal, the internal auditory meatus, the lateral semicircular canal and the round window. In general the examination area extends to between the first turn of the cochlea and the superior semicircular canal. A disadvantage of the transverse plane is the radiation dose received by the eye lenses.

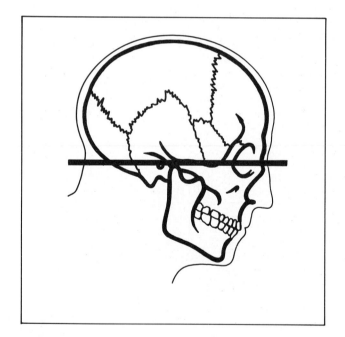

Fig. 16-12. Section position of transverse plane. Scans are parallel to plane through nasion and superior margin of external orifice of external auditory meatus.

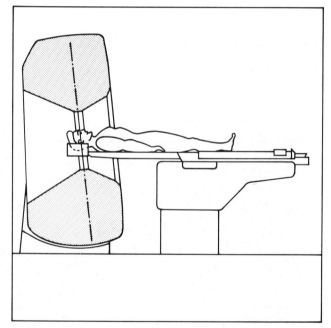

Fig. 16-13. For examination of transverse plane, patient is in supine position with gantry slightly tilted backward. Variants with more tilt are possible (to avoid radiation dose to eye).

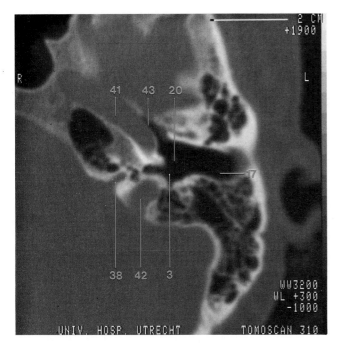

Fig. 16-14. Transverse scan at level of orifice of cochlear aqueduct.

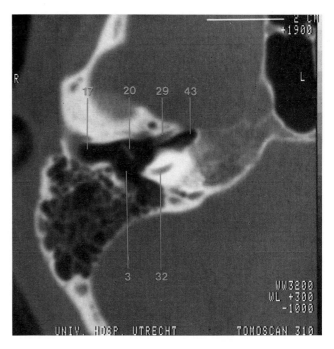

Fig. 16-15. Transverse scan at level of manubrium of malleus and first turn of cochlea.

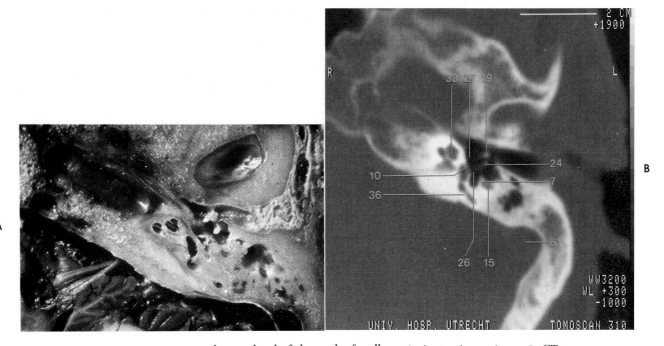

Fig. 16-16. Transverse plane at level of the neck of malleus. **A,** Anatomic specimen. **B,** CT scan.

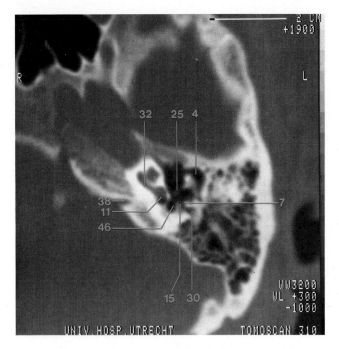

Fig. 16-17. Transverse scan at level of round window.

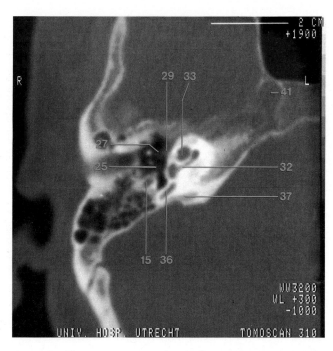

Fig. 16-18. Transverse scan at level of tensor tympani muscle and ligament.

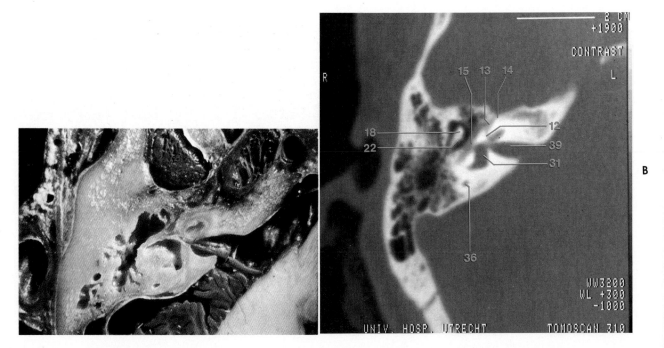

Fig. 16-19. Transverse plane at level of internal auditory meatus and vestibule. **A,** Anatomic specimen. **B,** CT scan.

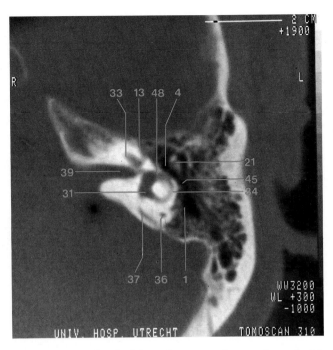

Fig. 16-20. Transverse scan at level of lateral semicircular canal, geniculate ganglion, and incudomalleolar articulation.

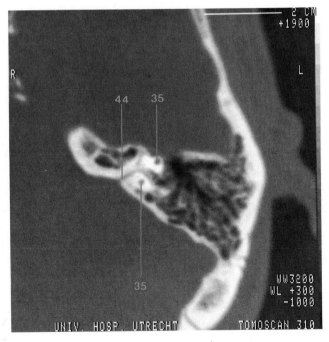

Fig. 16-21. Transverse scan at level of petromastoid canal (also called subarcuate tract).

■ Coronal plane

The coronal plane (Figs. 16-22 to 16-28) is relatively easy to obtain with the patient in the prone position and the head tilted upwards, i.e., extended.

Good general views of the three parts of the ear are possible, especially when visualization of the tegmen tympani is required. This, and the possibility of com-

paring both ears, make this plane also suitable as a basic tomographic plane.

The coronal plane is of special interest for imaging the internal auditory meatus and the vestibule.

The examination area extends to between the anterior margin of the attic and the posterior semicircular canal.

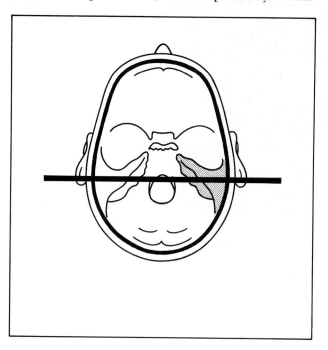

Fig. 16-22. Section position of coronal plane as indicated for right ear. However, both ears can be scanned simultaneously.

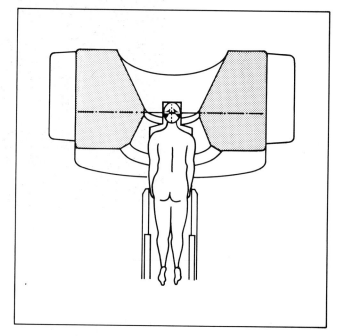

Fig. 16-23. For examination of coronal plane patient is in supine position with head tilted upward.

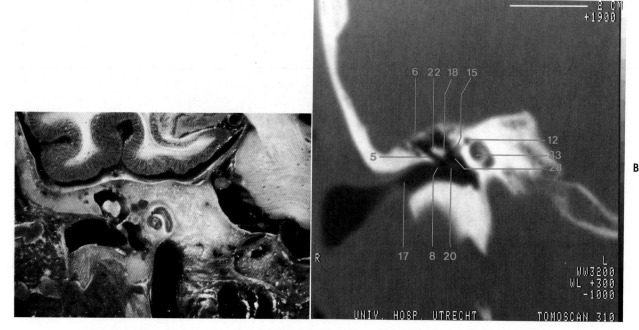

Fig. 16-24. Coronal plane at level of ossicles and second turn of cochlea. **A,** Anatomic specimen. **B,** CT scan.

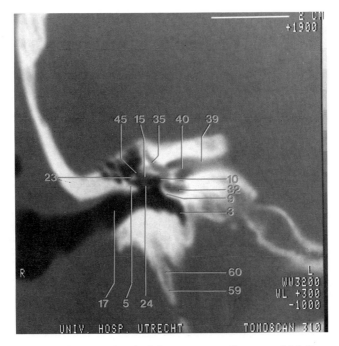

Fig. 16-25. Coronal scan at level of short process of incus and falciform crest.

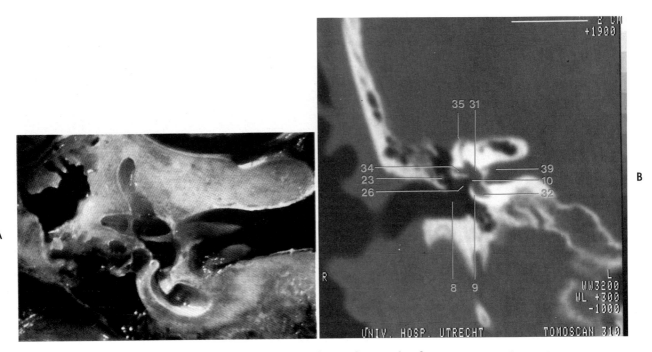

Fig. 16-26. Coronal plane at level of oval window and internal auditory meatus. **A,** Anatomic specimen. **B,** CT scan.

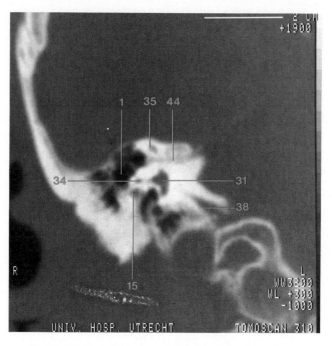

Fig. 16-27. Coronal scan at level of cochlear aqueduct.

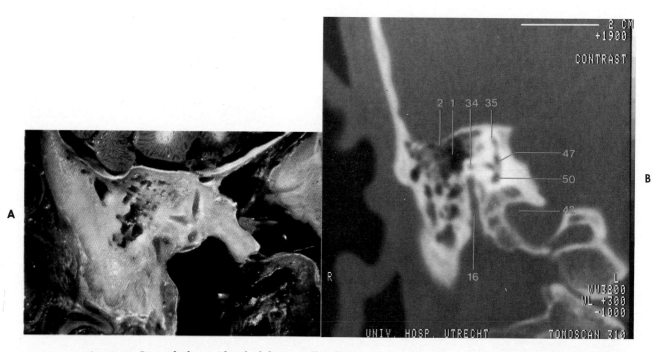

Fig. 16-28. Coronal plane at level of the ampulla of posterior semicircular canal. **A,** Anatomic specimen. **B,** CT scan.

■ Sagittal plane

In CT the sagittal plane (Figs. 16-29 to 16-36) is more difficult to obtain than it is in polytomography. Positioning of the patient in this plane is possible only with a few types of scanner because of the importance of the shape of the patient aperture cone.

The patient is in a semi-prone/semi-decubitus position on a separate support behind the gantry.

His head is turned upward and sideways and his cheek, on the side to be examined, rests against a head support which is attached to the table in order to perform the slice incrementation. This technique was developed by Blumm.[15] The sagittal plane is of special interest for the visualization of the vestibular aqueduct, the third part of the facial canal including the elbow, both the internal and the external auditory meati in cross-section, and the mastoid.

The examination area extends to between the internal and the external auditory meati.

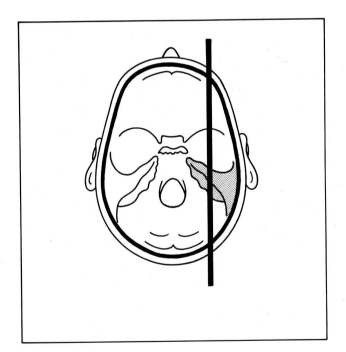

Fig. 16-29. Section position of sagittal plane as indicated for right ear.

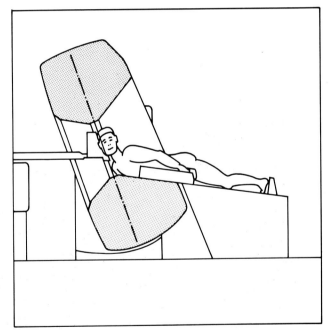

Fig. 16-30. For examination of sagittal plane, patient is in semi-prone-semidecubitus position on special support behind gantry, with head tilted upward and turned with cheek of side to be examined leaning aginst a special headrest. Shoulder is retracted from scan plane.

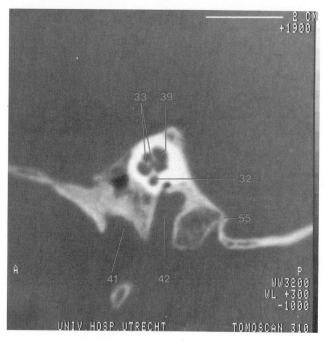

Fig. 16-31. Sagittal scan at level of modiolus of cochlea.

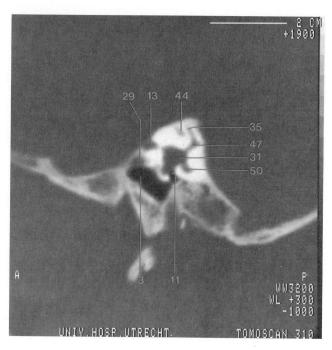

Fig. 16-32. Sagittal scan at level of the crus commune, geniculate ganglion, and round window.

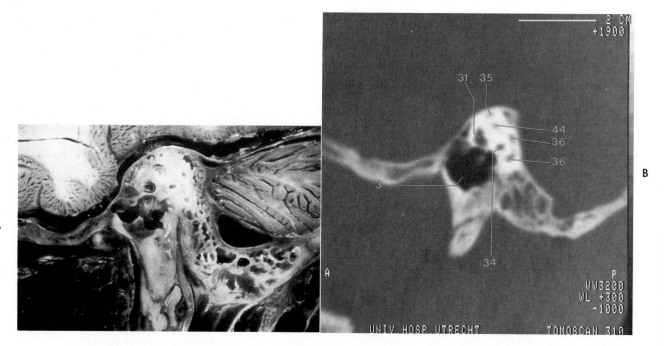

Fig. 16-33. Sagittal plane at level of ampulla of lateral semicircular canal. **A,** Anatomic specimen; **B,** CT scan.

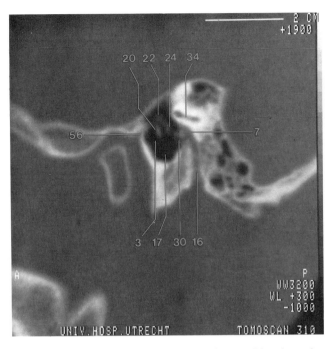

Fig. 16-34. Sagittal scan at level of third part of facial canal.

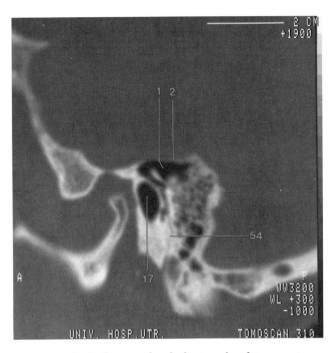

Fig. 16-35. Sagittal scan at level of external auditory meatus.

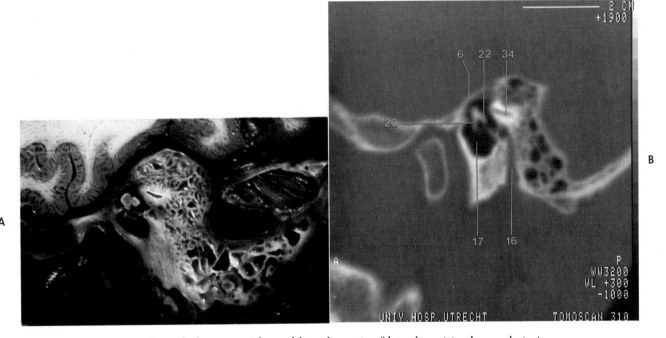

Fig. 16-36. Sagittal plane at ossicles and lateral margin of lateral semicircular canal. A, Anatomic specimen. B, CT scan.

■ Semi-axial plane

The semi-axial plane[51] (Figs. 16-37 to 16-45) is derived from the coronal plane by rotating the latter through an angle of approximately 20° about a vertical axis, in such a direction that the plane will subtend an angle of approximately 55° with the axis of the petrous pyramid. The patient is prone and his head is tilted upward. The 20° angle of the plane is obtained by making use of either a special swivelled headrest or a combination of table swivel with a standard coronal headrest. The gantry is tilted until the scan plane is perpendicular to the nasion-biauricular plane.

The semi-axial plane is of special interest for the visualization of the lateral and medial tympanic walls with the oval window, promontory and the second part of the facial canal in cross-section.

The examination area extends to between the geniculate ganglion and the posterior semicircular canal.

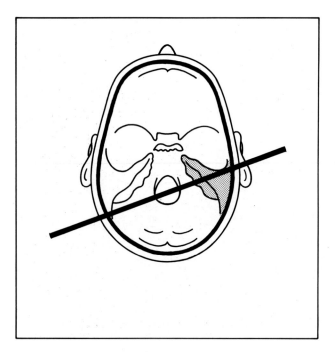

Fig. 16-37. Section position of semiaxial plane as indicated for right ear.

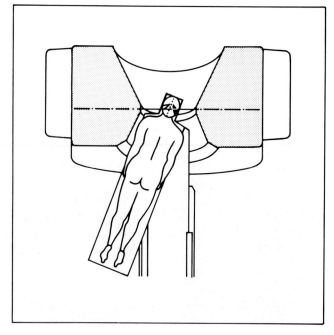

Fig. 16-38. For examination of semiaxial plane, patient is in prone position with head tilted upward while table is swiveled about 20° in direction opposite to side of patient that is to be examined.

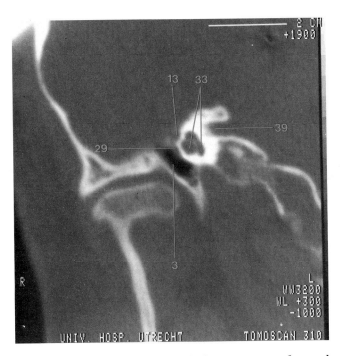

Fig. 16-39. Semiaxial scan at level of anterior part of second turn of cochlea.

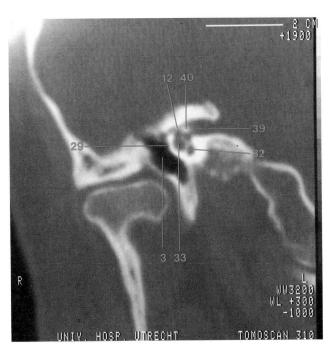

Fig. 16-40. Semiaxial scan at level of first part of facial canal.

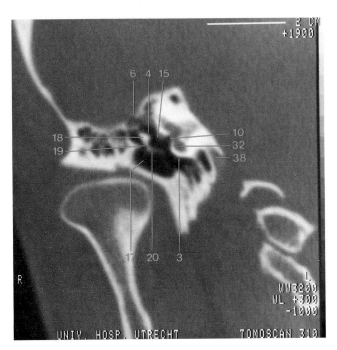

Fig. 16-41. Semiaxial scan at level of malleus.

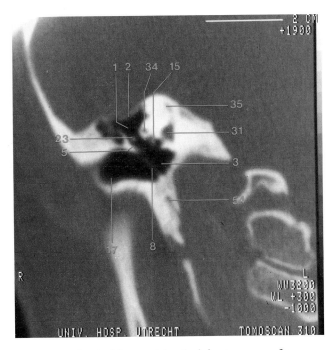

Fig. 16-42. Semiaxial scan at level of short process of incus.

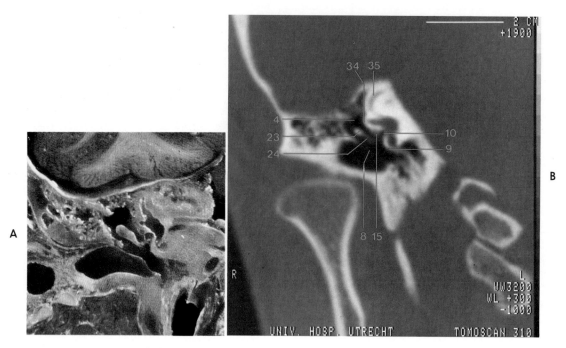

Fig. 16-43. Semiaxial plane at level of incus and oval window. **A,** Anatomic specimen. **B,** CT scan.

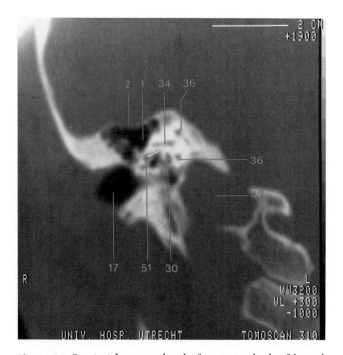

Fig. 16-44. Semiaxial scan at level of posterior limb of lateral semicircular canal.

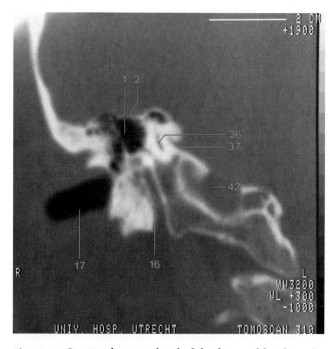

Fig. 16-45. Semiaxial scan at level of third part of facial canal.

■ Semi-longitudinal plane

The semi-longitudinal plane [157] (Figs. 16-46 to 16-54) is derived from the coronal plane by rotating the latter through an angle of approximately 20 ° about a vertical axis, in such a direction that the plane will subtend an angle of approximately 15° with the axis of the petrous pyramid. The patient is prone and his head is tilted upward. The 20° angle of the plane is obtained by making use of either a special swivelled headrest or a combination of table swivel with a standard coronal headrest.

The gantry is tilted until the scan is perpendicular to the nasion-biauricular plane. In radiography the projection perpendicular to the semi-longitudinal plane was introduced by Wullstein (Steep Stenvers) and Chausse (Chausse III), but was never used in polytomography.

However, the semi-longitudinal plane is of special interest for the visualization of the first and second turns of the cochlea, the external auditory meatus, the canal of the internal carotid artery and the posterior semicircular canal.

This plane is also helpful in imaging the surgical pathways, both endaural as well as retro-auricular, to the middle ear. The examination area extends to between the head of the malleus and the posterior semicircular canal.

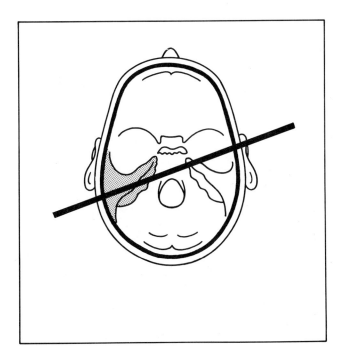

Fig. 16-46. Section position of semilongitudinal plane as indicated for left ear.

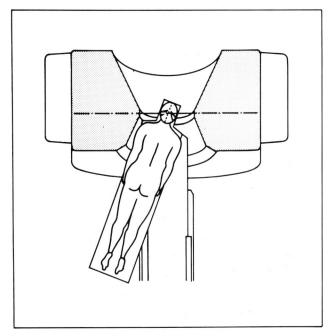

Fig. 16-47. For examination of semilongitudinal plane, patient is in prone position with head tilted upward while table is swiveled about 20° in direction toward side of patient that is to be examined.

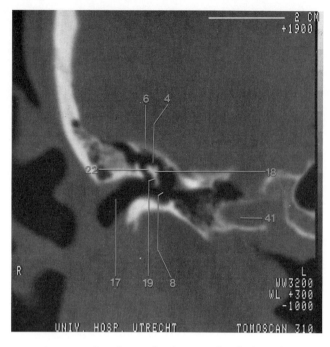

Fig. 16-48. Semilongitudinal scan at level of ossicles.

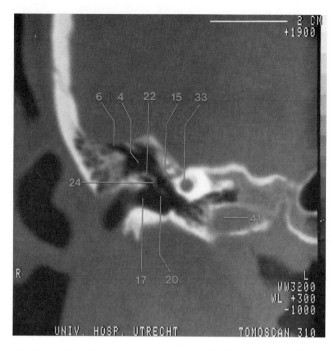

Fig. 16-49. Semilongitudinal scan at level of cupula of cochlea.

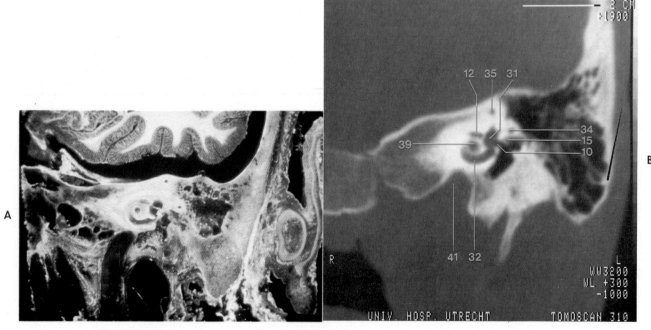

Fig. 16-50. Semilongitudinal plane at level of first turn of cochlea and oval window. **A,** Anatomic specimen. **B,** CT scan.

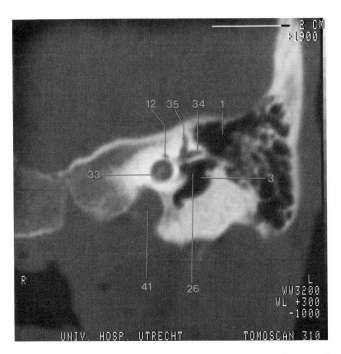

Fig. 16-51. Semilongitudinal scan at level of second turn of cochlea.

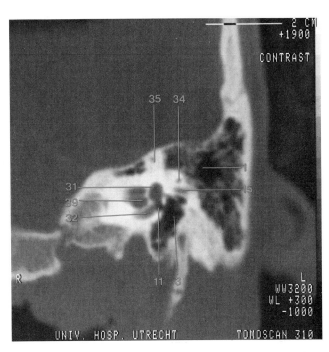

Fig. 16-52. Semilongitudinal scan at level of round window niche.

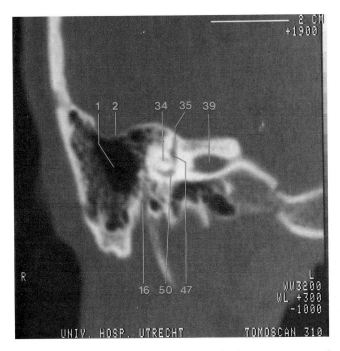

Fig. 16-53. Semilongitudinal scan at level of crus commune of posterior and superior semicircular canals.

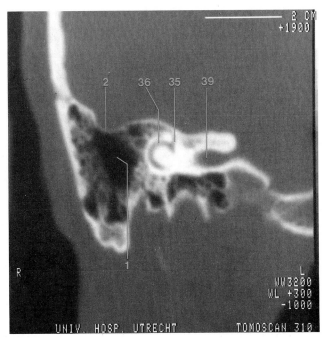

Fig. 16-54. Semilongitudinal scan at level of posterior semicircular canal.

■ Axio-petrosal plane

The axio-petrosal plane[107] (Figs. 16-55 to 16-62) is derived from the coronal plane by rotating the latter through an angle of 40° about a vertical axis in such a direction that the plane is more or less perpendicular to the axis of the petrous pyramid. The "official" angle is 55° but we are of the opinion that the ossicles can be visualized better at an angle of 40°. The patient is prone and his head is tilted upward.

The 40° angle of the plane is obtained by combining a 20° swivelled headrest with a 20° table swivel.

The gantry is tilted until the scan plane is perpendicular to the nasion-biauricular plane.

The axio-petrosal plane is of special interest for the visualization of the cochlea in cross-section, the longitudinal shape of the malleus and incus, including the incudo-stapedial articulation, and the oval window. The superior semicircular canal, the vestibular aqueduct and the first part of the facial canal are also well imaged. The examination area extends to between the cochlea and the posterior semicircular canal.

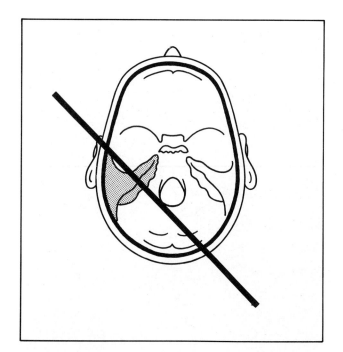

Fig. 16-55. Section position of axiopetrosal plane as indicated for left ear.

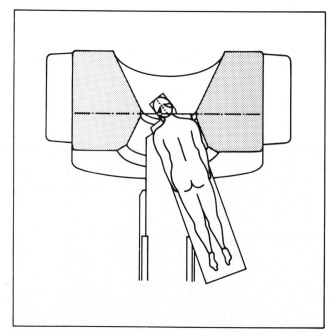

Fig. 16-56. For examination of axiopetrosal plane, patient is in prone position with head tilted upward and turned toward side to be examined (about 20°) while table is swiveled about 20° in direction opposite side of patient that is to be examined.

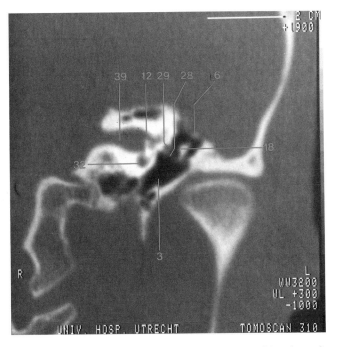

Fig. 16-57. Axiopetrosal scan at level of first part of facial canal.

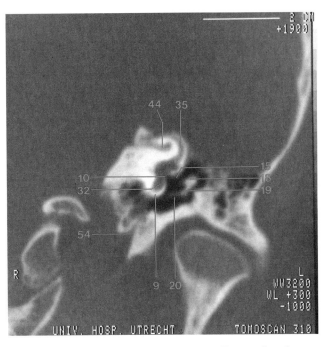

Fig. 16-58. Axiopetrosal scan at level of malleus and oval window.

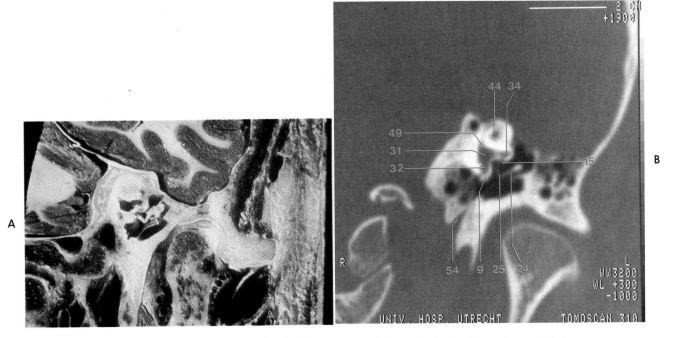

Fig. 16-59. Axiopetrosal plane at level of long process of incus. **A,** Anatomic specimen. **B,** CT scan.

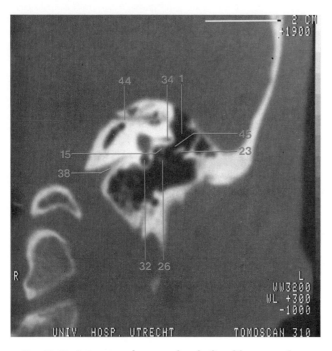

Fig. 16-60. Axiopetrosal scan at level of cochlear aqueduct.

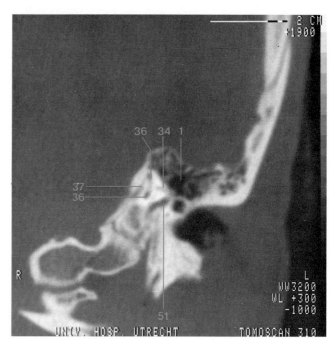

Fig. 16-61. Axiopetrosal scan at level of second genu of facial canal.

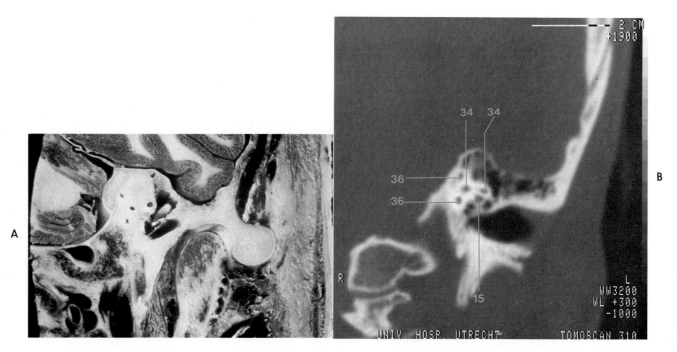

Fig. 16-62. Axiopetrosal plane at level of midcross-section of posterior and lateral semicircular canals. **A,** Anatomic specimen. **B,** CT scan.

■ Longitudinal plane

The longitudinal plane[133] (Figs. 16-63 to 16-70) is derived from the coronal plane by rotating the latter through an angle of 40° about a vertical axis, in such a direction that the plane is more or less parallel to the axis of the petrous pyramid. The patient is prone and his head is tilted upward. The 40° angle of the plane is obtained by combining a 20° swivelled headrest with a 20° table swivel. The gantry is tilted until the scan is perpendicular to the nasion-biauricular plane.

The longitudinal plane is of special interest for the visualization of the spiral of the cochlea, the posterior semicircular canal, the canal of the internal carotid artery, the mastoid and the bony part of the Eustachian tube. The examination area extends to between the ossicles and the posterior semicircular canal.

A disadvantage of this plane is that the image quality may be impaired by molar teeth filling artifacts.

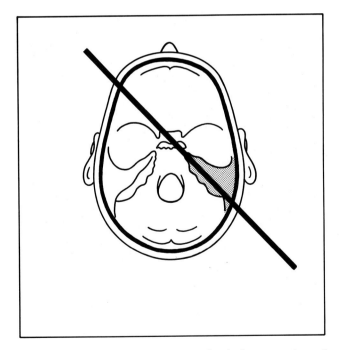

Fig. 16-63. Section position of longitudinal plane as indicated for right ear.

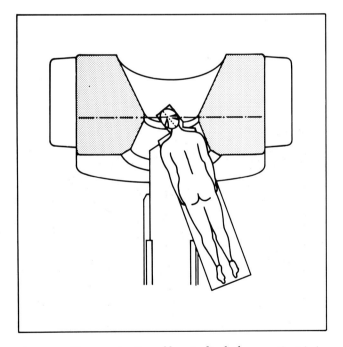

Fig. 16-64. For examination of longitudinal plane, patient is in prone position with head tilted upward and turned toward side opposite one to be examined (about 20°) while table is swiveled about 20° in direction toward side of patient to be examined.

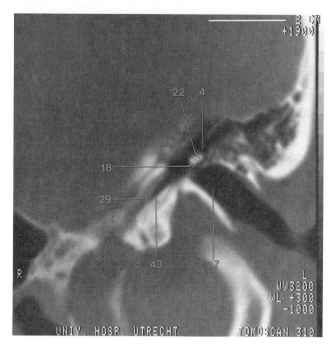

Fig. 16-65. Longitudinal scan at level of eustachian tube and tensor tympani muscle.

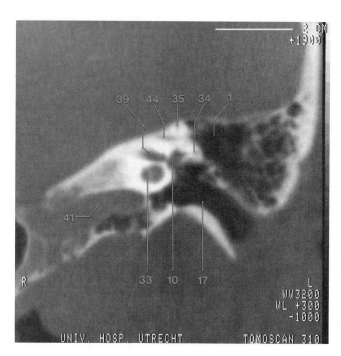

Fig. 16-66. Longitudinal scan at level of siphon of internal carotid artery and oval window.

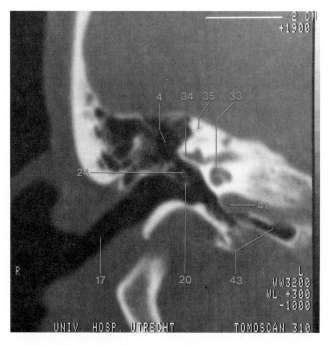

Fig. 16-67. Longitudinal scan at the level of the second turn of the cochlea.

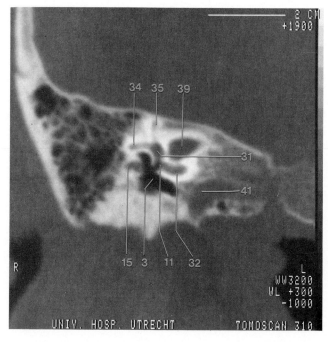

Fig. 16-68. Longitudinal scan at level of round window niche.

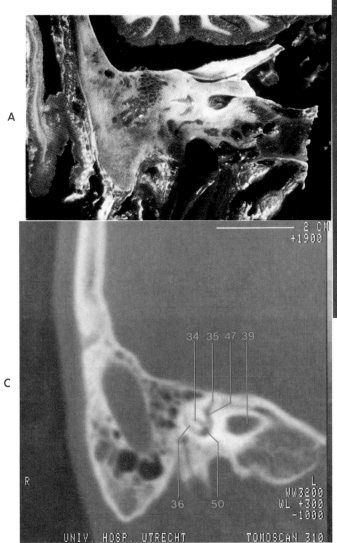

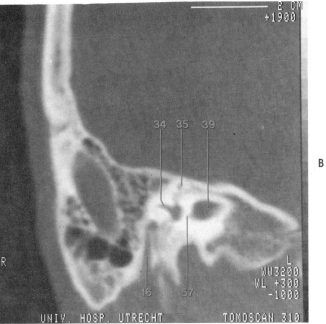

Fig. 16-69. Longitudinal plane at level of posterior limb of lateral semicircular canal. A, Anatomic specimen; B, CT scan through third part of facial canal; C, CT scan through crus commune.

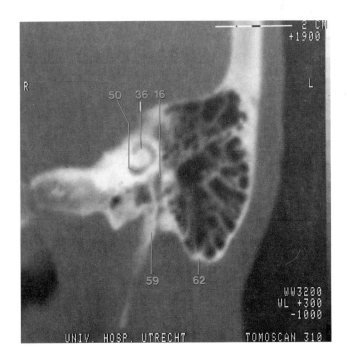

Fig. 16-70. Longitudinal scan at level of posterior semicircular canal.

■ Conclusion

The transverse plane appears to be the most suitable for the baseline study. Usually one other plane, perpendicular to the transverse plane, is selected on the pathology and the anatomical details to be imaged (see visualization matrix). This is especially the case when tissue interfaces of interest are parallel to the transverse plane, or when the particular anatomical detail can be imaged only with the help of a perpendicular plane; for example the following supplemental planes should be obtained: (1) an axio-petrosal to visualize the ossicles, (2) a coronal-plane to visualize the internal auditory meatus, (3) a sagittal plane to visualize the vestibular aqueduct and third part of the facial canal, and (4) a longitudinal plane to visualize the Eustachian tube.

Direct scanning technique in other planes is by far superior to multiplanar reformatting since to achieve similar results with MPR it would be necessary to accumulate 30 1 mm scans at 0.5 mm intervals within 1 minute (to avoid the effects of patient motion). Even then, the image would be only a 15 mm wide strip instead of an image covering the complete temporal bone.

□ Acknowledgment

We wish to express our appreciation for the assistance of technicians Anneke Hamersma and Wilma M. Pauw in carrying out the patient examinations.

□ **Anatomic variations and developmental anomalies**

R. Thomas Bergeron and Richard S. Pinto

The outer and middle ear structures have an embryologic development distinct from the labyrinth. They develop from the first and second branchial arch-groove complex, while the labyrinth arises from the ectodermal plate. Anatomic variations, anomalies, and congenital malformations reflect that fact; one part of the ear structure (the labyrinth, for example) may be normal while another portion is grossly malformed. Because outer and middle ear development are more closely linked, significant malformations of the external acoustic canal usually are accompanied by middle ear deformity and vice versa. Admittedly, inner ear malformations are seen more frequently among patients who have anomalies of the other two compartments as compared to the normal population, but this is substantially less than a one to one correlation. The toxic embryopathy subsequent to maternal ingestion of thalidomide is a well-recognized exception; in this circumstance all three compartments of the ear are regularly (but not invariably) involved.[142]

Additionally, the internal acoustic canal (which is not part of the ear at all) may be normal in the presence of a grossly deformed inner ear. Cases of dysplasia or aplasia of the internal acoustic canal have been reported in the presence of a normal labyrinth[112] (Fig. 16-82), but extreme hypoplasia or aplasia of the internal acoustic canal is more commonly associated with significant bony malformation of the inner ear.[106] The development of the internal acoustic canal is distinct from that of the labyrinth and the underlying, unifying mechanism explaining the coexistence of these congenital deformities is not apparent.

Uncommonly, all portions of the ear structures and the internal acoustic canal are developmentally malformed, but this is decidedly rare and always accompanied by severe functional impairment.

From the point of view of radiology of the temporal bone, benign anatomic variations comprise the range of dimensions, contours, and spatial orientation of the bony structures within that region encountered in a normal population that demonstrates neither functional impairment nor anatomic substrate carrying the potential for imperiling the well-being of the individual. These two tests provide the crucial distinction between a "variation" and an anomaly or malformation.

The subject of discussion in this section will include (1) bony developmental abnormalities of the outer, middle, and inner ear, (2) arterial and venous vascular abnormalities, and (3) developmental cerebrospinal fluid fistulae.

■ Causes of congenital deafness

Any discussion on congenital malformations of the ear should be prefaced by a study of the causes of congenital deafness. Ormerod[96] reviews this most succinctly, classifying the pathology as follows:

1. Failure to develop (occurring during the first 3 weeks of pregnancy)
   Of the bony cochlea
   Of the membranous cochlea
   Of the organ of Corti and the tectorial membrane
   Of the conducting mechanism
      the middle ear and ossicles
      the external auditory meatus

These types of abnormalities are the result of inherited factors or might be a result of toxic influences caused by certain forms of maternal illness during the first 3 weeks of pregnancy.

2. Interruption in development (occurring during the first 3 months of pregnancy)
   Of the organ of Corti and the tectorial membrane
   Of the ossicles of the middle ear
   Of the external canal

These types of abnormalities are the result of inherited factors, toxic influences caused by maternal illness, or endocrine insufficiency.

3. Degeneration of parts of the auditory apparatus

that have already developed to some degree or have reached maturity

Of the canal of the cochlea or scala media

Of the sensory end organ including the tectorial membrane

Of the nerve elements, including the spiral ganglion and the basal nuclei

It goes without saying that the contribution of radiology in defining pathologic processes in congenitally deaf individuals is primarily confined to demonstrating only those pathologic processes that are manifested by bony abnormalities.

■ External acoustic canal

Variations

The bony external acoustic canal shows considerable variation in both size and configuration. It comprises the medial two thirds of the complete external acoustic canal, the lateral one third being cartilaginous. The total length of the canal is approximately 2.5 cm as measured from the bottom of the concha. The length of the bony canal thus usually falls within the range of 1.5 to 1.7 cm. The bony portion is usually narrower than the cartilaginous part and it is directed medially, anteriorly, and slightly inferiorly, forming in its course a slight curve, the convexity of which is posterosuperior in position. Its medial end is smaller than the lateral end and it is obliquely placed, with the anterior wall projecting medially about 4 mm beyond the posterior wall.[152]

Eckerdal and Ahlquist[34] reported on sagittal sections of the bony external acoustic canal in 53 autopsy specimens. They found that the canal frequently had continuous changes of caliber as well as shape when analyzed in succeeding sagittal layers. They divided the canals into three groups: conical, hourglass-shaped, and ovoid. The mean value for the surface area of a sagittal section

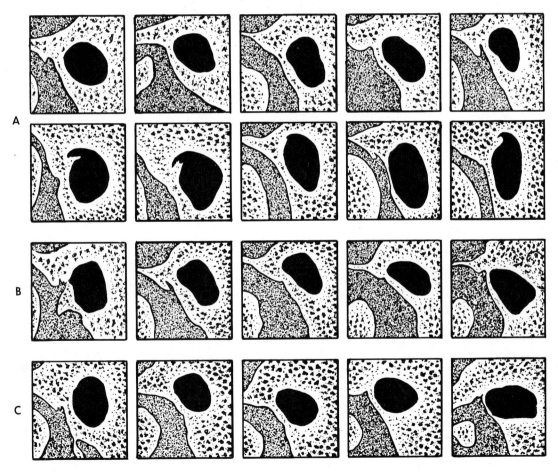

Fig. 16-71. Variations in external acoustic canal. **A,** Various configurations in bony external acoustic canal as seen in different specimens. **B,** Progressive thinning of anterior wall of external canal as one progresses from lateral to medial (left to right). Bony wall separating external acoustic canal from temporomandibular joint at medial end of canal is usually less than 1 mm. **C,** Change in orientation of long axis of ovoid canal as one progresses from lateral to medial. This spiraling configuration is not uncommon. (Based on Eckeral and Ahlquist.[34])

at the medial aspect of the bony canal is only 75% of a similar section at the lateral aspect of the canal.

There is a wide spectrum of shapes of the external acoustic canal, varying from circular to oval to heart-shaped or triangular. The long axis of an oval canal may change its orientation, spiraling from medial to lateral.

The bone that forms the anterior wall of the canal and separates it from the temporomandibular joint averages about 1.5 mm in thickness but is always less than that at its extreme medial end. The range varies from about 0.2 mm in thickness to almost 4 mm (Fig. 16-71).

Viraponge et al.[150,151] studied 38 temporal bones in the axial projection as demonstrated with CT. Thirty-seven percent (14 of 38) showed a generally uniform AP diameter throughout the length of the bony canal. Sixty-three percent (24 of 38) showed variations in both size and contour. Narrowing either from the posterior wall or narrowing of both the anterior and posterior walls just lateral to the tympanic membrane was demonstrated in 14 of 24 patients who showed variations.

Malformations—atresia of external acoustic canal

Atresia of the external acoustic canal may be of varying degree. There is microtia or a deformed pinna. At otoscopy there may be merely a shallow dimple in the place of the external acoustic canal or a small, blind pouch. The radiologic points to be addressed include the following.

Presence of a bony "atresia" plate and presence of a soft tissue "plug"

Status of the middle ear cleft
Status of the ossicles
Evidence of an acquired cholesteatoma
Position of the facial canal in its mesotympanic and mastoid portions
Position and size of the oval and round windows
Status of the labyrinth and internal acoustic canal

Atresia plate and soft tissue plug. The fundamental defect in atresia of the external acoustic canal arises from hypoplasia of the tympanic portion of the temporal bone or from hyperplasia of Reichert's cartilage (base of the styloid process) or of the squamous portion of the temporal bone. In the latter two circumstances the lateral wall of the tympanic cavity is occluded by an osseous block or "atretic" plate.[110] Thickness of the plate should be assessed (Figs. 16-72 to 16-75).

Developmental failure of recannulation of the soft tissue plug between the middle ear space and the concha results in a solid soft tissue mass interposed between those two structures. Thickness of the plug should be assessed.

Middle ear cleft. The middle ear cavity (Figs. 16-72 and 16-74) may be normal in isolated, unilateral atresia of the external acoustic canal. At the opposite extreme, the middle ear cavity may be completely absent (Fig. 16-73). Usually, however, there is narrowing of the middle ear cleft (Fig. 16-75). This is generally caused by encroachment laterally from the atretic bony plate. Occasionally the vertical dimension of the middle ear space is also diminished either by upward migration of

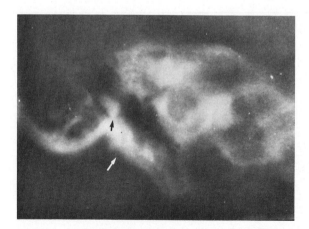

Fig. 16-72. Atresia of external acoustic canal. Notice thick atretic plate. Ossicles are malformed and fused to plate. Middle ear cleft is narrowed.

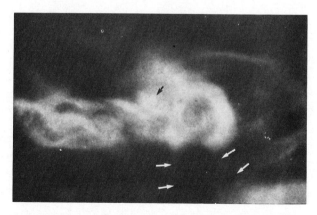

Fig. 16-73. Atresia of external acoustic canal. Notice dense bony ledge that leads from side of skull to labyrinth. No identifiable middle ear cleft is seen. Deformed ossicular mass is fused to atretic plate *(black arrow).* White arrows indicate carotid canal.

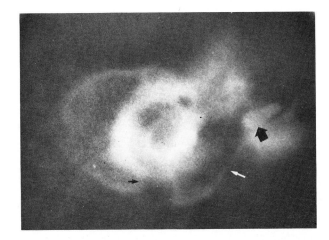

Fig. 16-74. Atresia of external acoustic canal. There is very thin atretic plate *(white arrows)*. Ossicular mass is deformed and fused to lateral attic wall *(black arrow)*. Hypoplastic carotid canal *(short black arrow)* can also be seen.

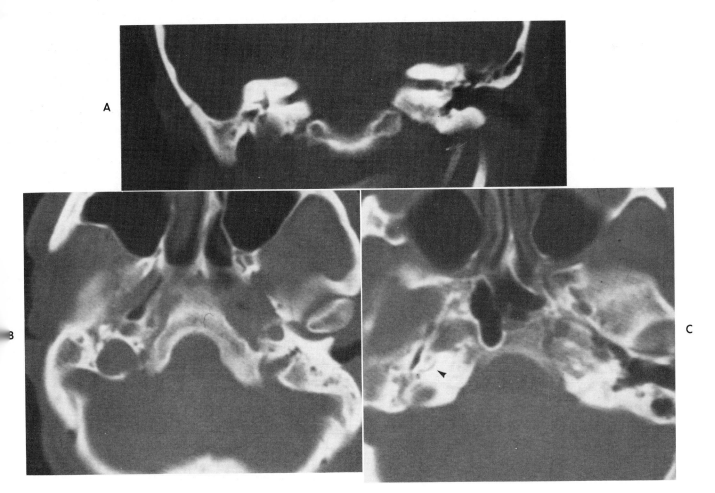

Fig. 16-75. Atresia of external acoustic canal. **A,** There is complete atresia of right external acoustic canal. No middle ear cleft is identifiable. No ossicular mass can be identified, although sections at other levels suggested their possible presence. **B,** There is high, large jugular bulb. **C,** Inner ear structures are normal *(arrow)*. (Case courtesy Peter Som, M.D., New York.)

the jugular bulb intruding on the hypotympanum or by descent of the tegmen superiorly. Occasionally both circumstances occur.[103] In mandibulofacial dysostosis the attic and antrum are also typically absent or slit-like.[103]

The middle ear space occasionally contains bony septa and the lateralmost portion subsequently may be the site of an acquired cholesteatoma. Pulec and Freedman[110] report such a case. The epithelial cells arise from the tympanic membrane. Phelps et al.[103] report several other cases of "acquired" cholesteatoma associated with a congenital developmental defect.

Ossicles. All three ossicles (Figs. 16-72 to 16-75) may be deformed. Because normal maturation of the stapes involves dissolution of bone and an eventual paring away to its ultimate diminutive adult state, maturation arrest may result in a huge, bulky stapes. Alternately it may be small, deformed, or totally absent.

Malleus and incus deformities are easier to recognize because they are usually larger than the stapes. They may be fused to one another or to either wall of the attic. When there is a large atretic plate, the long handle of the malleus is frequently bent laterally and fused with the atretic plate.

Facial canal. In anomalies of the atresia group the facial nerve (Fig. 16-76) may be expected to have an abnormal course within a deformed middle ear cavity. In those cases in which there is severe hypoplasia of the tympanic portion of the temporal bone, the mastoid portion migrates forward toward the temporomandibular joint, usually carrying the facial nerve with it.[62,103] The mastoid portion of the facial nerve often has a short vertical course with an abrupt turn anteriorly, crossing the inferior aspect of the middle ear and exiting in the area of the temporomandibular joint itself. In one of Jahrsdoerfer's[62] atresia patients the nerve had no vertical (mastoid) segment whatsoever and was represented by a horizontal knuckle of soft tissue that crossed the lower third of the middle ear. In a second patient the facial nerve itself compartmentalized the middle ear into superior and inferior sections.

The nerve frequently has an aberrant intratympanic segment as well. The bony canal may be in an abnormal position, it may be partially dehiscent, or the nerve may travel outside the bony canal altogether. The stapes and the facial nerve are both of second branchial arch origin; malformations of one are commonly associated with malformations of the other.[63]

In summary, the intratympanic course of the facial nerve is frequently aberrant and may be associated with a deformed stapes; the mastoid portion is usually foreshortened and anteriorly placed, with the nerve exiting somewhere near the temporomandibular joint. The radiologist should make every attempt to assess the position of the mastoid portion of the facial nerve in the event that a corrective plastic surgery procedure is to be performed.

Position and size of oval and round windows. The oval and round windows may have an abnormal position, may be smaller than usual, or may be totally absent.[105] This is of considerable surgical significance, particularly with regard to the oval window, because operative maneuvers are possible to correct conductive deafness caused by an absent oval window. The round window is difficult to define radiologically and for that reason its radiologic absence should not be considered an anatomic certainty. Normal diameters of the oval window have a range of 2.5 to 4 mm by 1.5 to 2 mm. Normal diameter for the round window ranges from 1.9 to 2.5 mm.[3]

Labyrinth and internal acoustic canal. The status of the inner ear is of quintessential importance to the surgeon contemplating a procedure to correct the conductive mechanism in a patient with atresia of the external acoustic canal. In patients who have a radiologically demonstrable inner ear abnormality a coexisting sensorineural hearing deficit is almost a certainty. In patients with radiographic evidence of inner ear malformation or hypoplastic internal auditory canals, corrective surgery for the conductive impairment may be open to question.[79]

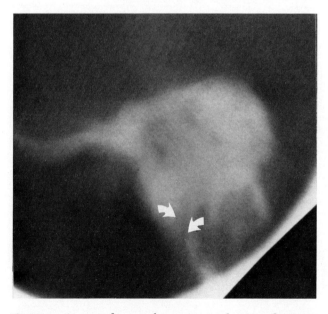

Fig. 16-76. Atresia of external acoustic canal. Mastoid portion of temporal bone has migrated anteriorly and its anterior surface forms posterior margin of temporomandibular joint. Mastoid portion of facial canal is also anterior and nerve exits from anteriorly placed stylomastoid foramen *(curved arrows).*

■ Middle ear

Including the epitympanic recess, the vertical and anteroposterior diameters of the middle ear cleft are each about 15 mm. The transverse diameter measures about 6 mm above and about 4 mm below; opposite the center of the tympanic cavity it is only about 2 mm.

The hypotympanum is the pneumatized inferior extension of the middle ear cleft below the level of the tympanic ring. This is variable both in depth and in medial extension. The bone of the floor of the tympanic cavity, which separates it from the jugular bulb below, is thick when the hypotympanum is underdeveloped and small and thin when it is deep. Air cells of the mastoid group variably pneumatize this bony separation if the floor of the cleft is some distance removed from the jugular bulb.

An important variation exists in the depth and angle of the *sinus tympani*, the bony pocket that lies between the bony labyrinth medially and pyramidal eminence laterally.[116] The tympanic sinus is of surgical significance in that it may contain diseased tissue (most commonly an acquired cholesteatoma) that is not visible by the usual surgical approach. The difficulty in approach depends on how deeply and in what direction the sinus tympani extends (Fig. 16-77).

To approach the sinus tympani through the mastoid the surgeon must enter between the facial nerve and the posterior or lateral semicircular canals or both. The distance between the sinus tympani and facial nerve is therefore important, as is the distance between the facial nerve and the posterior semicircular canal. The

normal measurements for the sinus tympani are a depth of 3 mm (range 0.6 to 6.0 mm) and a width of 2 mm (range 1 to 3 mm). The deepest and widest portion of the sinus tympani is usually located at the level of the round window membrane.

The distance between the sinus tympani and facial nerve is about 1 mm (range 0.1 to 1.6 mm). The distance between the facial nerve and the posterior semicircular canal is about 3 mm (range 2.0 to 3.5 mm, mean 2.9 mm) at a distance between 2 mm and 3 mm below the inferior border of the footplate of the stapes.

Although such minute differences may seem to be of interest only to the microsurgeon, they emphasize the need for precision diagnostics in this field of imaging. One may hope to see the sinus tympani on at least two contiguous sections on axial CT of the middle ear.

Isolated middle ear anomalies as a cause of congenital conductive hearing loss are rare. In a study of polytomography of 63 ears demonstrating congenital conductive hearing loss,[61] only four had isolated middle ear anomalies. In contradistinction, 9 of the 63 had isolated external canal atresia, 34 had combined external canal and middle ear anomalies, 2 had anomalous external and inner ear structures, and 5 had deformities of all three compartments. For the interested reader this subject is considered in greater detail in the work of Bergstrom.[13]

The various abnormalities that may be encountered in malformations of the middle ear associated with atresia of the external canal have been discussed in the previous section. Occasionally one may encounter ossicular

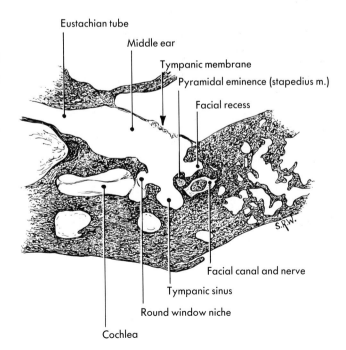

Fig. 16-77. Relationships of sinus tympani, facial recess, and facial canal within posterior wall of middle ear. Axial section through temporal bone at level of round window niche. These relationships are of paramount importance to operating surgeon because they affect surgeon's ability to gain access to diseased tissue. Tympanic sinus may be site of occult disease. Primary facial nerve pathologic processes may also obliterate these spaces. This minute anatomy is exquisitely defined on axial computed tomography.

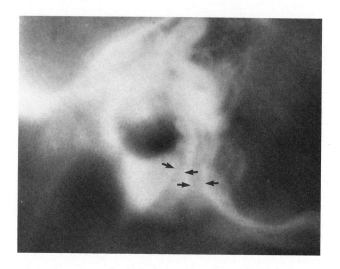

Fig. 16-78. Congenital malformation of middle ear and facial nerve. Malleus was deformed. Intratympanic and mastoid portions of facial nerve were duplicated. There are two facial canals.

abnormality as an isolated finding in association with facial nerve anomaly (Fig. 16-78).

■ The inner ear

Variations

There is essentially no range of normal in size or shape of the osseous labyrinth.[65,143] The cochlea is conical, measuring about 5 mm from base to apex, and its breadth across the base is about 9 mm. It normally has 2½ to 2¾ coils, appearing as three "stories." Polvogt and Crowe[104] published the photomicrographs of temporal bones of one patient with only two coils within the cochlea and another patient with three coils, both ostensibly in subjects with normal hearing. It is difficult to evaluate these findings because they are at such great variance with the experience of others, but nonetheless one must recognize that probably some small variation does exist in the number of cochlear turns, though not in the size of the cochlea itself.

The vestibule is ovoid but flattened transversely. It measures about 5 mm from before backward, the same from above downward, and about 3 mm across. No normal variants exist.

Each of the semicircular canals is about 0.8 mm in diameter, each with a dilation at one end called the ampulla. The superior semicircular canal is oriented transversely to the long axis of the petrous portion of the temporal bone and measures about 15 to 20 mm in length. The posterior semicircular canal is also vertically placed and is directed backward, nearly parallel with the posterior surface of the petrous portion. It is the longest canal, measuring from 18 to 22 mm. The lateral semicircular canal is the shortest of the three, its arch being directed horizontally backward and laterally. It is inclined 30° with the horizontal, the anterior limb of which lies in the superior plane. As with the vesti-

bule there are no normal variants, although the anatomically abnormal may be without clinical symptoms.

Malformations

Abnormalities of the inner ear (Figs. 16-79 to 16-82) may be both bony and membranous or membranous alone; they may be of varying severity and may involve the vestibule and semicircular canals alone, the cochlea alone, or a combination of both with differing degrees of abnormality.* For these reasons it is useless to attempt to classify developmental abnormalities on the basis of eponyms; each individual case tends to be "one of a kind." It is preferable to describe the anatomic abnormality as such. Two exceptions exist because these particular eponyms denote the severity of the labyrinthine defect in one term: the Michel defect and the Mondini defect.

The Michel defect. The Michel defect is the most severe bony dysplasia and is characterized by a total lack of development of the inner ear structures.[101] The defect may involve the labyrinth alone (cochlear and vestibular portions) or the labyrinth and the remainder of the petrous portion as well. The other two compartments of the ear are usually normal.

The Mondini defect. The Mondini defect is described traditionally as a cochlea having only 1½ turns, with the middle and apical turns being incorporated into a single sac. There is a variable amount of hearing loss. Although the 1½ turn cochlea is the essence of the eponymic connotation, Mondini's dysplasia covers a wide spectrum of morphologic and functional abnormalities, including a flattened cochlea, shortened cochlear duct, immature auditory and vestibular sense organs and

---

*References 13, 36, 65, 66, 96, 99, 120, 128, 145.

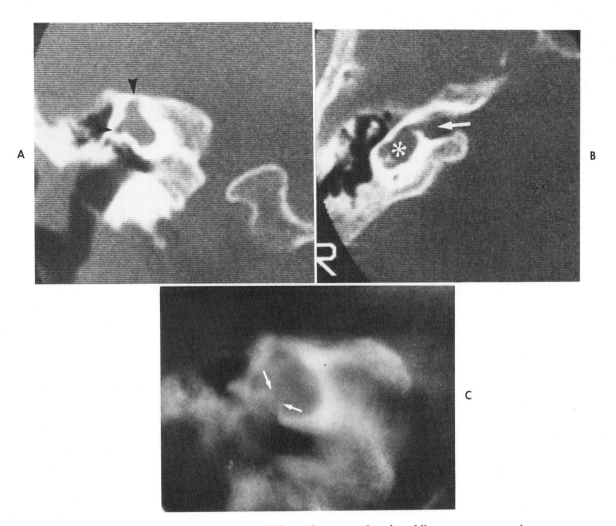

Fig. 16-79. Congenital abnormality of labyrinth. External and middle ear were normal. **A,** Coronal CT. Cochlea and vestibule are contained within single membranous sac. Tiny stumps represent superior and lateral semicircular canals *(arrows)*. **B,** Axial view. Asterisk indicates common vestibulocochlear chamber. Arrow lies within internal acoustic canal. **C,** Frontal view made on complex motion tomogram. Notice patulous oval window of vestibulocochlear chamber *(arrows)*.

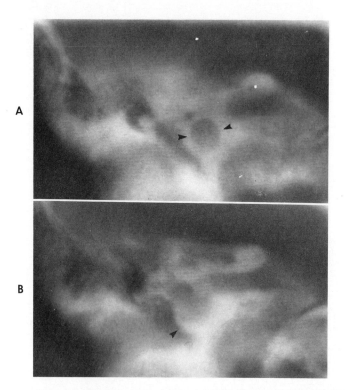

Fig. 16-80. Mondini defect. **A,** Separation between apical and middle turns of cochlea is missing. **B,** More posterior cuts show presence of basilar turn. (Courtesy Peter Som, M.D., New York.)

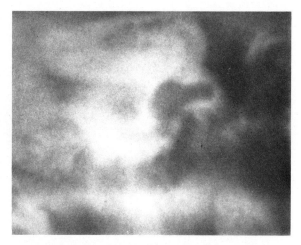

Fig. 16-81. Minor developmental abnormality of inner ear. Lateral semicircular canal is truncated and broad and tends to be incorporated into larger space of vestibule. Other two semicircular canals were normal as was cochlea. Minor variations in size of lateral semicircular canal are most common anomaly of vestibular system. Patients are frequently asymptomatic.

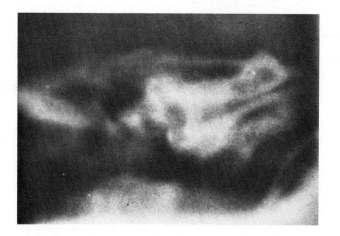

Fig. 16-82. Hypoplasia of internal acoustic canal. Vertical dimension of canal measured less than 2 mm. Patient was born deaf. Labyrinth and middle and external ears were normal. (Courtesy G. Wortzman, M.D., Toronto.)

nerves, enlarged vestibule, deformed semicircular canals, and bulbous endolymphatic sac.[120] Incomplete expressions of the disorder can occur with little or no loss of auditory or vestibular function, while severe forms show complete deafness and lack of vestibular response. It may occur either in isolation or in association with anomalies in other organs, such as Klippel-Feil syndrome, Pendred's syndrome, and trisomy syndrome. It may be bilateral or unilateral. A recent radiologic paper on the subject is that of Som et al.[128]

■ Congenital fistulae between subarachnoid space and middle ear cavity

Developmental defects of the ear may lead to abnormal communications with the subarachnoid space, resulting in the presence of cerebrospinal fluid within the middle ear cavity. With an intact tympanic membrane this may be responsible for cerebrospinal fluid rhinorrhea and may simulate serous otitis media.[155] If the tympanic membrane is perforated, the patient will experience spontaneous cerebrospinal fluid otorrhea. The clinical diagnosis is not always readily apparent. Meningitis may ensue.[69,93,139]

The anatomic substrate varies. Although there may be isolated defects, such as in the tegmen of the antrum or of the tegmen tympani and in the roof of the external auditory canal,[69,155] it is more commonly seen in patients who have developmental abnormalities in the region of the oval window and the medial wall of the vestibule[23] (Fig. 16-79, C). It is postulated that the cerebrospinal fluid traverses the cochlear aqueduct from the subarachnoid space and leaks into the middle ear at the fistula site, which is located in one of the following areas: in the stapedial footplate, around the edges of the stapedial footplate, under the bony facial canal, or in a dehiscence in the medial wall of the tympanic cavity.

Cerebrospinal fluid may leak into the middle ear as a result of developmental deficiencies in both the lateral and medial walls of the labyrinth.[23,127] The cerebrospinal fluid gains access to the labyrinth from the internal acoustic canal by way of a deficiency in the medial wall of the labyrinth and leaks into the middle ear cleft by way of deficiency in the lateral wall of the labyrinth.

Congenital deafness, with demonstrable evidence of middle or inner ear developmental abnormality, should always raise the possibility of a coexisting abnormal fistulous communication between the middle ear and the labyrinth or the middle ear and the subarachnoid space. Otitis media coupled with recurrent serous mastoiditis and isolated or repeated episodes of meningitis should raise the question of a possible congenital fistula between the middle ear cavity and the subarachnoid space.

■ Vascular anomalies

There are a number of vascular anomalies that impinge on temporal bone imaging. These have to do with the persistence of fetal arterial vessels and anastomoses. The importance of some anomalies lies mostly in their recognition on angiography but in others there is a direct clinical implication.

The otic artery is a persistent carotid basilar connection and may be seen as a large vessel emerging from the internal acoustic canal.[113] A persistent stapedial artery has been reported as causing pulsating tinnitus.[46] A persistent embryologic vascular loop of the middle meningeal artery that arose from a persistent stapedial artery, internal carotid artery, and ophthalmic artery has been reported in causing an audible bruit over the external acoustic canal in a 10-year-old boy.[83]

Nontraumatic, nonatheromatous aneurysms of the intracranial arteries probably take their origins at the points of obliteration of embryologic arterial vessels. Therein lies the importance in understanding the embryology of the vessels subserving the temporal bone.[72,73]

Anderson et al.[2] reported on 10 congenital aneurysms of the carotid artery in the carotid canal within the petrous portion of the temporal bone, and Moffat and O'Connor[87] recorded a case of bilateral intrapetrous internal carotid aneurysms. If the aneurysms in the intrapetrous portion of the temporal bone enlarge sufficiently they may erode the bone and appear as a mass within the middle ear. Such a case was reported by Connley and Hildeyard in 1969.[28]

A case of complete absence of both internal carotid arteries has been reported, with no carotid canals present within either temporal bone.[40] The blood supply to the brain was through enlarged basilar and vertebral arteries.

Aberrant position of carotid artery within temporal bone

Although the intrapetrous portion of the carotid artery may be the site of a congenital aneurysm that enlarges and eventually erodes the carotid canal and decompresses into the middle ear space, a more common cause for presentation of the carotid artery within the middle ear (Figs. 16-83 and 16-84) is its aberrant position, without aneurysm, as a result of a bony developmental deficiency in the carotid canal.

In such a circumstance the carotid artery lies superior, lateral, and posterior to its normal position as it enters the base of the skull and resides within the middle ear space. This may be responsible for a pulsating tinnitus and conductive hearing loss. It may mimic a glomus jugulare, glomus tympanicum, or other "vascular" tumor at otoscopic examination. Lapayowker[71] re-

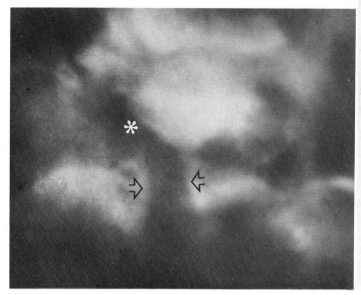

A

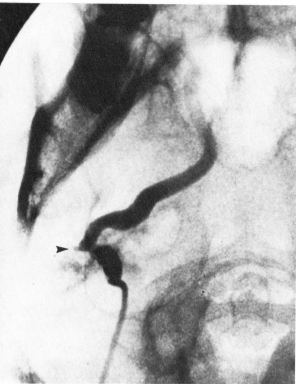

Fig. 16-83. Aberrant position, internal carotid artery. **A,** Coronal view, complex motion tomogram. Bony septum separating carotid canal (*arrows*) from hypotympanum (*asterisk*) is deficient. This finding alone suggests that internal carotid artery lies in an aberrant position within tympanic cavity. **B,** Selective internal carotid arteriogram with subtraction, base view. Intrapetrous portion of carotid artery lies more lateral than normal; portion is within tympanic cavity. Arrow points to small traumatic aneurysm within tympanic cavity. It was demonstrated several days after attempted biopsy of vascular-appearing intratympanic "mass."

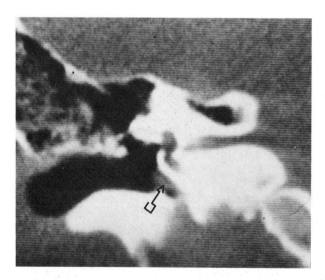

Fig. 16-84. Aberrant internal carotid artery. Bony septum separating carotid canal from hypotympanum is deficient. Soft tissue mass within hypotympanum (*arrow*) is internal carotid artery. Carotid canal is somewhat smaller than usual; artery was hypoplastic.

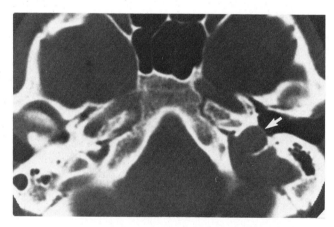

Fig. 16-85. High jugular bulb. Jugular bulb on left occupies superior and lateral position, separated from hypotympanum by paper-thin bony septum (*arrow*). Occasionally bone is totally dehiscent in these circumstances, and jugular bulb then comes to lie within tympanic cavity. In either circumstance, transmission of venous pulsations to tympanic cavity may result in pulsating tinnitus.

ported three cases of aberrant positioning of the internal carotid artery and made the observation that if one constructed a perpendicular line from the lateral aspect of the vestibule the lateralmost portion of the carotid artery on angiography should not lie lateral to this so-called *vestibular line*. Over the years this has proved to be a valid observation, although it is somewhat cumbersome and depends on angiography to make a diagnosis. The limiting lateral wall of the carotid canal that separates it from the hypotympanum is easily demonstrated on every coronal tomogram of the temporal bone in the normal patient. Its absence should be considered prima facie evidence of an aberrant internal carotid artery. The identification of the possible presence of an aberrant carotid artery in a patient with pulsating tinnitus is of paramount importance because this may prevent needless surgical exploration of the tympanic cavity with its attendant risks if the "mass" is biopsied.

Aneurysms of the carotid artery when it lies within an aberrant position are possible even in the absense of trauma, surgical or otherwise. Quisling and Rhoton[111] provide a contemporary radiologic-anatomic analysis of the intrapetrous carotid artery branches.

Abnormalities of jugular bulb and jugular foramen

The jugular bulb is usually separated from the hypotympanum by a plate of bone of varying thickness. There are two separate abnormal positions of the bulb that should be distinguished: (1) high jugular bulb and (2) jugular diverticulum.

High jugular bulb. The bulb (Fig. 16-85) occupies a superior lateral position, diminishing the separation between the hypotympanum and the venous structure. The bone may be totally deficient and the bulb may appear as a mass within the floor of the middle ear cleft. The patient may complain of pulsating tinnitus; at otoscopy the bulb may be confused with a vascular, tumorous mass.

Transaxial CT defines the thickness of the bony plate separating the jugular bulb from the hypotympanum to excellent advantage. Inspection of CT scans of many patients without ear complaints demonstrates that thinning of the bony plate that separates the middle ear cavity from the jugular bulb is commonplace.

Jugular bulb diverticulum. The jugular bulb diverticulum (Figs. 16-86 to 16-88) is distinct from the high jugular bulb in that there is not only superior but also medial extension of the bulb. A jugular diverticulum does not intrude on the middle ear space but rather extends upward to the petrous portion of the temporal bone, occasionally eroding into the internal acoustic canal. It may displace the vestibular aqueduct superiorly.

Patients with a pure (medial) jugular diverticulum may have hearing loss, but it is sensorineural and not conductive. They may have tinnitus, but this is episodic and not pulsatile. The tinnitus is likely related to the

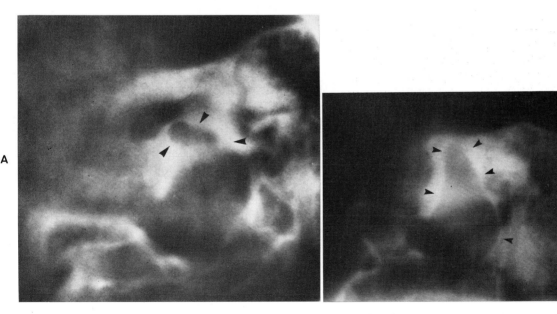

Fig. 16-86. Jugular diverticulum. **A,** Notice superior medial extension of diverticulum from enlarged jugular bulb. There is elevation and compression of floor of internal acoustic canal. **B,** Different case. Diverticulum extended superiorly, posterior to internal acoustic canal.

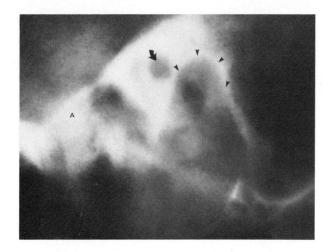

Fig. 16-87. Jugular diverticulum. Complex motion tomogram, lateral view. Jugular bulb has extended both medially and superiorly, lying posterior to internal acoustic canal. This position may elevate, compress, or obstruct endolymphatic duct. *Black arrows,* Huge jugular diverticulum; *curved arrow,* internal acoustic canal; *A,* anterior.

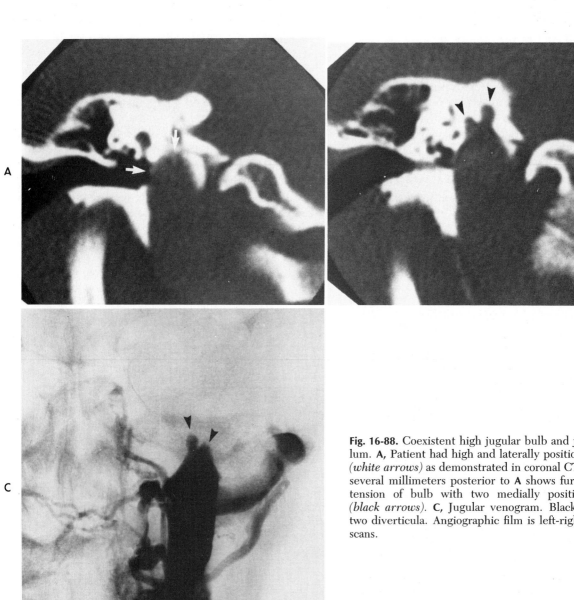

Fig. 16-88. Coexistent high jugular bulb and jugular diverticulum. **A,** Patient had high and laterally positioned jugular bulb *(white arrows)* as demonstrated in coronal CT scan. **B,** Section several millimeters posterior to A shows further superior extension of bulb with two medially positioned diverticula *(black arrows).* **C,** Jugular venogram. Black arrows point to two diverticula. Angiographic film is left-right reversal of CT scans.

alteration in hydrodynamic pressure within the vestibular system as a result of displacement of the vestibular aqueduct. Intrusion of the bulb into the internal acoustic canal causes direct pressure on the eighth cranial nerve itself and might be responsible for hearing loss or tinnitus.

It should be noted that the superiormost extension of a medial jugular diverticulum usually lies in a plane higher than the level of a high jugular bulb.

Jahrsdoerfer et al.[64] cite a case of classic Ménière's disease subsequent to obliteration of the endolymphatic duct by a medially positioned jugular diverticulum. Stern and Goldenberg distinguish between these two entities by referring to them as lateral and medial diverticula of the bulb. An additional example of a jugular diverticulum is cited by Noyek et al.[95]

An exhaustive discussion of the anatomy of the jugular bulb is presented in the work of Graham.[50] Reports on the lateral extension of the high-placed jugular bulb into the middle ear cavity may be found in the work of West and Bandy,[153] Robin,[114] Farrell and Hantz,[38] Lloyd et al.,[79a] Moretti,[88] Overton and Ritter,[98] and Gejerot.[45]

Pulsating tinnitus and its relation to developmental vascular displacements

Pulsating tinnitus is a complaint that alerts the clinician to the possibility of a vascular tumor within the middle ear. Glomus tympanicum and glomus jugulare tumors are the archetypal examples. However, a congenital aneurysm of the intrapetrous carotid artery may also appear as a pulsatile mass within the middle ear. An aberrant carotid artery secondary to a misplaced carotid canal (with a bony deficiency in its lateral aspect) may also appear as a middle ear "mass" with pulsating tinnitus. Further, a high-placed jugular bulb in association with a bony wall of the hypotympanum that is either exceedingly thin or dehiscent may cause pulsating tinnitus. With dehiscent bone the jugular bulb may come to lie partially within the middle ear and be seen as a mass at otoscopy. It is the radiologist's task to rule out all of these possibilities when encountering this clinical history.

□ Inflammatory disease
R. Thomas Bergeron
■ External auditory canal

Uncomplicated viral or bacterial otitis externa is probably the most frequent entity encountered by the otologist; the radiologist does not see these patients professionally. Patients with inflammatory conditions of the external ear are usually referred for radiologic work-up only when the disease is chronic and intractable or when the diagnosis or extent is in doubt. Otitis externa

may be part and parcel of chronic otitis media of either bacterial or mycobacterial origin and must always be considered in that light.

There are two conditions that appear to predispose toward a primary otitis externa progressing to a life-threatening conclusion: diabetes in the elderly and immunosupression.

Malignant otitis externa

The elderly diabetic may develop an external otitis caused by the gram-negative organism, *Pseudomonas aeruginosa*. This condition is referred to as "malignant" otitis externa (Figs. 16-89 and 16-90) because of the relentless, progressive, potentially lethal course leading to death in over one half of the patients with this disease. There is no neoplasia. The infection spreads to the soft tissues beneath the skin in the external acoustic canal and if not successfully treated may lead to mastoiditis, sepsis, osteomyelitis of the base of the skull, sigmoid sinus thrombosis, multiple cranial nerve palsies, meningitis, and death.[18,20] In Chandler's series of 72 patients who had a median age of 71 years there were only four who did not have diabetes. Two of the four had chronic lymphatic leukemia and another had granulocytopenia secondary to hypersplenism. The remaining patient was an 80-year-old nondiabetic man who appeared otherwise healthy.

Coser et al.[29] reported two cases of malignant external otitis in infant boys 5 and 6 months of age. Both were undernourished, anemic, and in generally poor health. Both children survived after vigorous treatment against gram-negative pathogens.

The spread of the osteomyelitis dictates the onset of the various clinical signs. Posterior spread into the mastoid may cause a facial palsy as a result of involvement of the mastoid (vertical) portion of the seventh cranial nerve. Medial spread through the tympanic membrane may cause an otitis media with destruction of the ossicles and a facial nerve palsy as a result of involvement of the intratympanic (mesotympanic) portion of the facial canal.

There may be a sigmoid sinus thrombosis and a jugular foramen syndrome as a result of posterior extension.

Anterior extension represents disease in the temporomandibular joint. There may be abscess formation in the subtemporal space. There may be paralysis of cranial nerves III, V, and VI.[18,19,35]

An excellent review of the subject was published by Mendez et al.,[86] providing radiographic clinical correlation. These authors divided the radiologic manifestation of the disease into early and late stages. The early stage is manifested by soft tissue mass within the external acoustic canal or clouding of the mastoid air cells

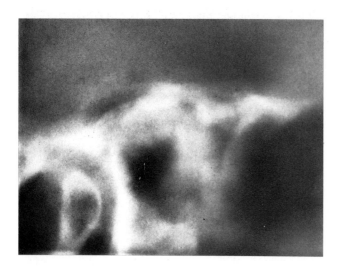

Fig. 16-89. Malignant otitis externa. Complex motion tomogram, lateral view. There is marked destruction of roof and posterior wall of external acoustic canal in association with thickening of soft tissue. Ostium of meatus is reduced in caliber. This condition is seen in elderly diabetics and almost invariably is caused by *Pseudomonas aeruginosa* infection.

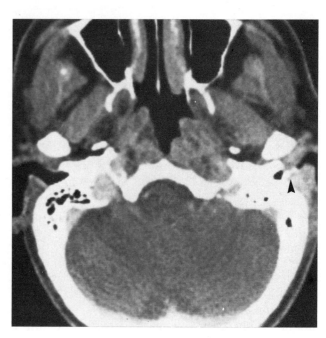

Fig. 16-90. Malignant otitis externa. There is soft tissue swelling of external acoustic canal and immediately adjacent area. Bony sequestrum is present *(arrow)*. Lesion enhanced with contrast medium. (Courtesy Peter Som, M.D., New York.)

with no bone destruction. In the late stage, bone destruction may extend into the middle ear cavity, temporomandibular joint, base of the skull. There is good correlation between the radiographic stages and the clinical findings. Their material was derived from a study of nine patients.

Osteomyelitis of the external acoustic canal and temporal bone secondary to immunosuppression

Immunosupressed patients are likely candidates for the progression of minor infections into life-threatening ones. These patients, while free of the microangiopathy of the diabetic, are nonetheless rendered peculiarly susceptible to intractable infections in the external acoustic canal, leading to osteomyelitis of the base of the skull (Figs. 16-91 and 16-92). The course may be particularly fulminant.

CT in the axial plane is the premier technique for demonstrating soft tissue mass and bone destruction, particularly when it is extensive.

Very early destruction of the walls of the external acoustic canal is difficult to demonstrate with certainty; complex motion tomography in the lateral projection is sometimes helpful. The interpreter must be mindful that (1) The anterior tympanic wall tends to be normally

thinner as one progresses from lateral to medial (Fig. 16-71), and (2) because the squamosal roof of the external acoustic canal normally extends farther lateral than does the tympanic floor, a straight sagittal tomogram of the side of the head will always show a "destroyed" floor in the lateralmost section with an intact roof. This is a normal finding.

■ The middle ear

The middle ear and communicating air spaces of the temporal bone are in continuity with the respiratory epithelium of the pharynx by way of the eustachian tube and are subject to bacterial and viral invasion through this communication. Mild infections may cause hyperemia of the mucosa, edema, and serous effusion. The radiologist normally does not see acute otitis media patients (Fig. 16-93).

Mastoiditis

Acute serous mastoiditis is characterized radiographically by clouding of the mastoid cells and thickening of the mucous membrane of the bony septa, without evidence of bone destruction (Figs. 16-94 and 16-95). This is seen well on the Towne view. In order to evaluate the bony septa, however, lateral views of the mastoid

Text continued on p. 797.

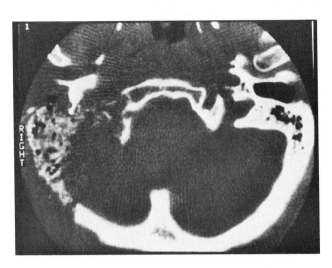

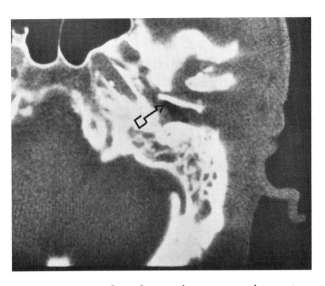

Fig. 16-91. Osteomyelitis of temporal bone in immunosuppressed patient. There was massive destruction of right temporal bone and adjacent base of skull. Patient was middle-aged, immunosuppressed alcoholic. There was no diabetes.

Fig. 16-92. Osteomyelitis of external acoustic canal in conjunction with acute mastoiditis. There is small bony sequestrum *(arrow)*. Patient was immunosuppressed. Notice massive soft tissue swelling.

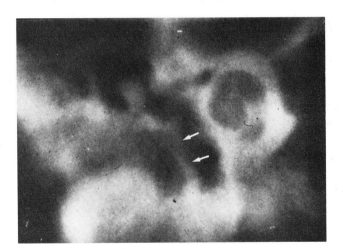

Fig. 16-93. Chronic otitis media with retracted, thickened tympanic membrane *(arrows)*. Acute otitis media would bulge tympanic membrane in opposite direction.

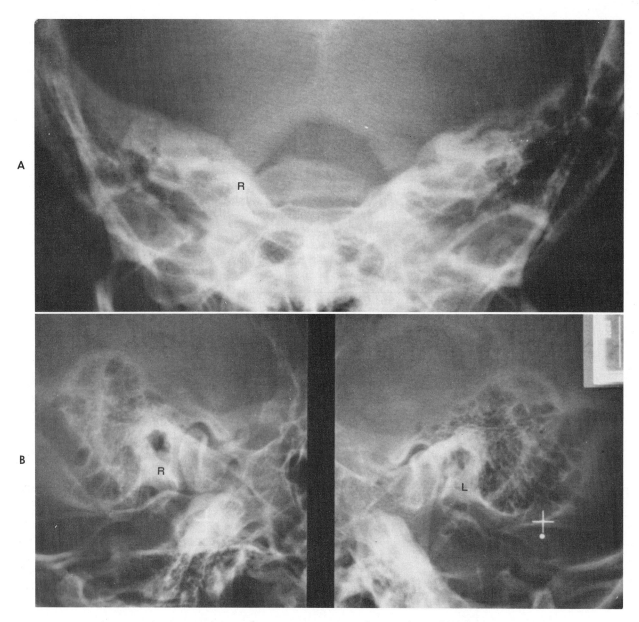

Fig. 16-94. Acute serous mastoiditis. **A,** Towne view. There is diminished lucency of mastoid air cells on right *(R)* without evidence of bone destruction. **B,** Modified Schuller view confirms presence of clouding within mastoid cells on right *(R)*. Bony septa are maintained and there is no evidence of sclerosis. These findings are consistent with diagnosis of acute serous mastoiditis. *L,* Left.

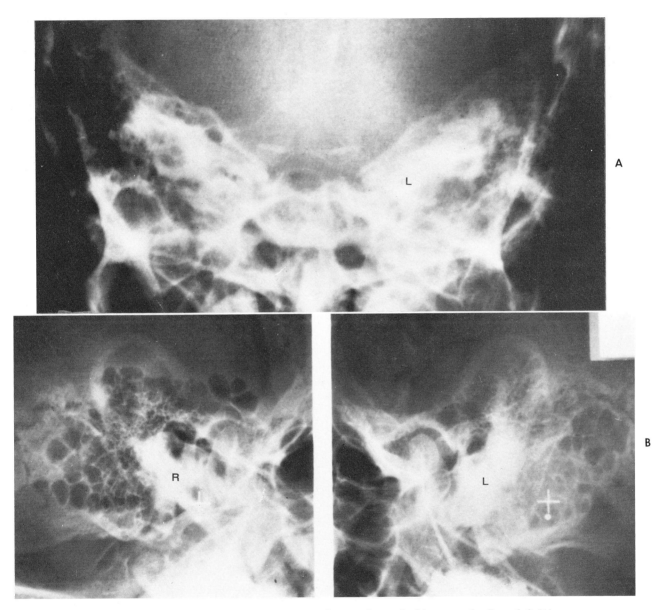

Fig. 16-95. Acute mastoiditis. **A,** Towne view. There is diminished lucency of cells on left *(L)*, without evidence of septal destruction. **B,** Law view. Effusion within mastoid air cells is well demonstrated, as is maintenance of bony septa. *R,* Right; *L,* left.

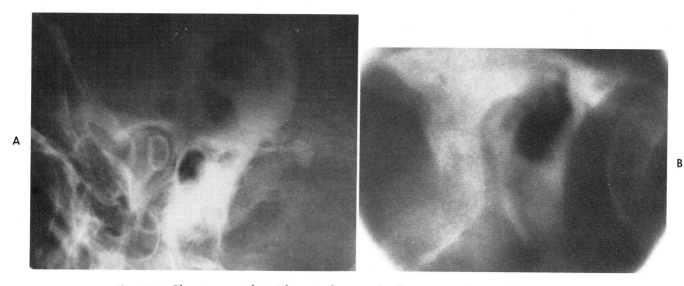

Fig. 16-96. Chronic mastoiditis. There is absence of cells. Bone is dense and sclerotic. **A,** Routine mastoid view. **B,** Lateral projection, complex motion tomogram. Mastoid portion of facial canal is well outlined because air cells that usually surround it are sclerotic.

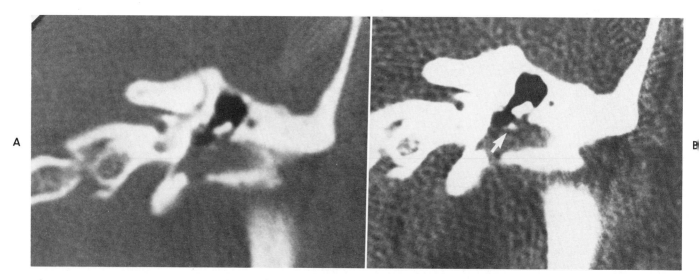

Fig. 16-97. Granulation tissue, external acoustic canal and middle ear. Patient had long-standing chronic otitis externa. Polypoid soft tissue mass eventually filled entire canal. **A,** Coronal CT scan shows soft tissue mass filling external acoustic canal, tympanic cavity, and hypotympanum. Attic is aerated. Incus appears normal. **B,** Manipulation of window level and window width permits identification of small, calcified fragment *(arrow)* that represents only remaining portion of malleus. Biopsy showed mass to be granulation tissue. True soft tissue tumors of middle ear or external acoustic canal could cause similar CT image. Acquired cholesteatoma would be expected to show coexistent soft tissue disease within attic.

are essential; the Schuller view probably shows this area to best advantage. CT will show this even better but rarely is indicated in the acute process unless some other coexisting disease is suspected. Complex motion tomographic studies are difficult to interpret insofar as the presence of fluid within the cells because of the blurring inherent in the technique. There may be false positive interpretations.

Acute coalescent mastoiditis is characterized radiographically by the presence of clouded cells with evidence of progressive lysis of bony septa. If the antrum is involved, "sagging" of the posterosuperior osseous external canal may ensue because of destruction of the bony superstructure of that portion of the canal.

In severe and persisting infections the mucous membrane may become ulcerated, polypoid, or granulomatous. Prolonged infection may be associated with resorption of the ossicles and mastoid bone by demineralization and osteoclastic activity.[121]

The infectious process may break through the cortex of the mastoid to form subperiosteal accumulations of purulent exudate and granulation tissue. The process may extend to the epidural space of the posterior and middle cranial fossae, break through the mastoid tip into the neck (Bezold's abscess), or evacuate through a fistula into the external acoustic canal.

Chronic mastoiditis follows repeated bouts of otitis media with accompanying mastoid infection. There is gradual reduction in the number of air cells, with thickening of the mucous membrane and reactive scleroris of the bony septa (Fig. 16-96). Mucosal edema may lead to the formation of polyps. Occasionally these polyps may become so large that they deliver through the external acoustic canal because the tympanic membrane is almost routinely destroyed as a consequence of the purulent otitis media. Persistent suppuration also may be accompanied by mucosal ulceration and the formation of granulation tissue. The granulation may also appear as a polypoid mass within the external canal (Fig. 16-97).

Chronic inflammation is commonly associated with rarefying osteitis of the ossicles, otic capsule, and mastoid bone. Resorption of the otic capsule may occur even in the absence of an acquired cholesteatoma.[68] Under that circumstance the suppurative process may lead to invasion and destruction of the inner ear, with fistulization usually by way of the lateral semicircular canal. This may lead to obliterative labyrinthitis (see below).

Acquired cholesteatoma

One of the common complications of chronic mastoiditis is the development of an acquired cholesteatoma. Schucknect[121] prefers the term *keratoma* and defines

this as the accumulation of exfoliated keratin in the middle ear or other pneumatized area of the temporal bone, arising from keratinizing squamous epithelium that has invaded these areas from the external auditory canal. It usually becomes infected.

Acquired cholesteatoma arises most commonly in the epitympanum as a consequence of epidermal invasion through a perforation of the superior portion of the tympanic membrane.

Although antral cholesteatomas are the object of much radiologic interest, attic cholesteatomas are more frequent and are often an important component of the conductive hearing loss that accompanies chronic otitis media.

An attic cholesteatoma may take origin from either the lateral (frequent) or the medial (less frequent) attic wall (Figs. 16-98 to 16-100). Lateral attic wall lesions commonly show destruction of the scutum. The malleus and incus may be displaced either laterally or medially, depending on where the bulk of the cholesteatoma exists. If there is significant displacement, there is reasonable expectation that the ossicles themselves will be involved in the cholesteatoma. In flagrant cases the ossicles may be completely destroyed. Medial extensions may erode the capsular bone surrounding the lateral semicircular canal and produce a fistula.

An attic cholesteatoma may extend posteriorly into the antrum, periantral cells, and central mastoid tract or inferiorly into the middle ear. Rarely, it is found behind an intact tympanic membrane. This occurs only when the perforation has been followed by spontaneous healing of the membrane. Adults with acquired cholesteatomas usually have minimal pneumatization as the result of multiple childhood infections and reactive osteitis; children with acquired cholesteatomas frequently have extensively pneumatized temporal bones with extensive invasion of the cell tracts by the epidermal ingrowth.

Rarefying osteitis with or without acquired cholesteatoma

The bone destruction that occurs peripheral to an acquired cholesteatoma (Fig. 16-101) is commonly explained on the basis of pressure necrosis arising from the expanding necrotic mass, but Schucknect[121] disputes this, stating that the presence of the epidermal tissue alone causes bone resorption. Nonetheless, the propensity for an acquired cholesteatoma to be accompanied by local bone destruction leads to destruction of the ossicles, fistulization or invasion of the bony labyrinth, erosion of the bony canal about the facial nerve, and extension into areas adjacent to the temporal bone. Acquired cholesteatomas are usually infected and when accompanied by bone erosion they can lead to exten-

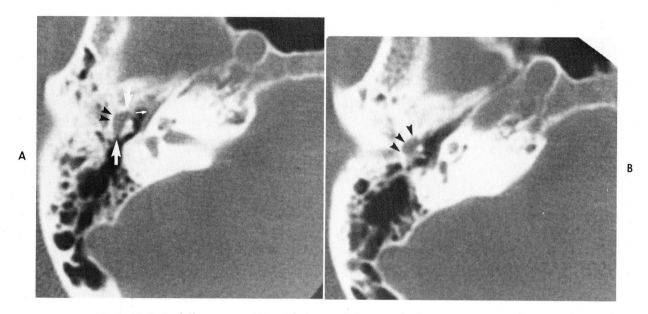

Fig. 16-98. Attic cholesteatoma. CT, axial view. **A,** Soft tissue shadow separates air within attic from surrounding bone *(arrows)*. Notice soft tissue shadow interposed between lateral attic wall and combination shadow of malleus and incus *(double arrows)*. This represents small attic cholesteatoma. **B,** Same patient at level several milimeters inferior to **A.** Notice inferior extension of cholesteatoma *(arrows)* that envelops long handle of malleus (seen in cross-section). There may be no bone destruction early in course of attic cholesteatomas.

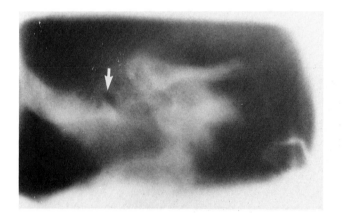

Fig. 16-99. Acquired cholesteatoma. Complex motion tomography, frontal view. Mass is seen within attic and middle ear. Ossicles cannot be identified. Otic capsular bone about lateral semicircular canal is markedly rarefied inferiorly and is absent superiorly. Thin cleft of air *(arrow)* remains between lateral margin of soft tissue mass and lateral wall of upper portion of attic. This acquired cholesteatoma, which had its maximum growth within medial aspect of attic, had displaced ossicles laterally and destroyed most of them. Fistula was present between middle ear space and lateral semicircular canal.

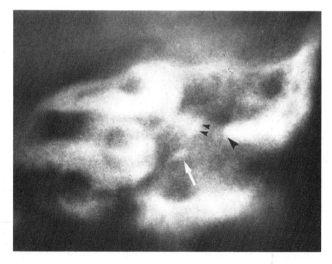

Fig. 16-100. Acquired cholesteatoma. There is amputation of scutum *(arrow)* and soft tissue mass that displaces ossicular remnants medially *(double arrows)*. Separated fragment of lower portion of malleus is present *(large arrow)*. Soft tissue fills external ear canal, middle ear, and antrum. Bone destruction is widespread.

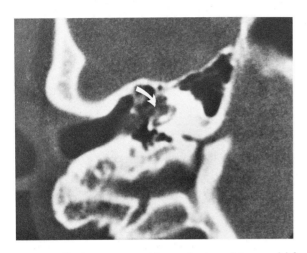

Fig. 16-101. Cholesteatoma with rarefaction of bone of labyrinth. Notice bony rarefaction along lateral aspect of labyrinth. Soft tissue mass fills most of middle ear cleft from anterior to posterior.

sion into the epidural space and its consequent sequelae.

The presence of an identifiable soft tissue mass with a focal area of bone destruction within the middle ear–mastoid complex should lead reasonably to the radiologic diagnosis of an acquired cholesteatoma if occurring in the presence of chronic mastoiditis (Figs. 16-102 to 16-106). Occasionally the histologist will prove the radiologist wrong, finding no evidence of keratinization—no cholesteatoma—within the soft tissue mass. The radiologist should not be dismayed; such a distinction is plainly beyond the capability of the imaging modalities in current use. The clinical and surgical implications remain the same, however, and such an "error" on the part of the radiologist does not render a disservice to the patient.

On plain film examination the Owen-Mayer view is the single most helpful projection to demonstrate attic wall destruction and ossicular destruction or displacement. CT has supplanted complex motion tomography for more thorough radiographic investigation.

The combination of soft tissue mass in association with focal bone destruction in a patient with chronic mastoiditis is good radiologic evidence of the presence of an acquired cholesteatoma. Although rarifying osteitis as part of otitis media may occur in the absence of a cholesteatoma, the odds are 3:1 that bone destruction

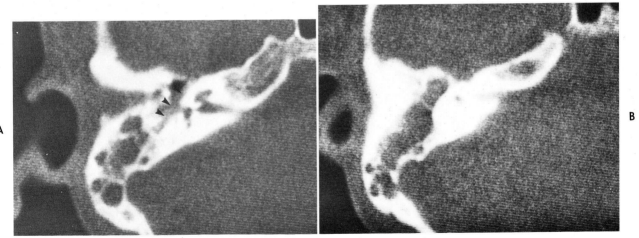

Fig. 16-102. Cholesteatoma involving intratympanic facial nerve. **A,** Notice that soft tissue mass completely fills middle ear cleft and is continuous with shadow of intratympanic facial nerve canal *(arrows)*. Patient had progressive facial nerve palsy. There was no evidence that mastoid portion of facial canal was involved. **B,** Cholesteatomatous mass fills attic-antral area; there is marked destruction of septa between adjacent air cells. Tegmen is preserved anteriorly, although thinned.

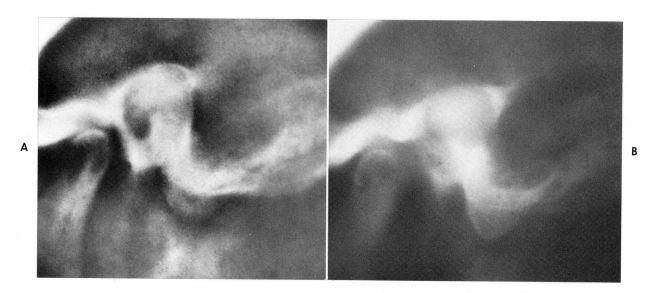

Fig. 16-103. Acquired cholesteatoma with marked bone destruction. Complex motion tomogram, lateral view. **A,** Soft-tissue mass fills upper portion of tympanic cavity, epitympanum, additus ad antrum, and attic. There has been marked destruction of separating bony septa, and large cavity now exists. Excavation of bone has resulted in paper-thin tegmen as well as reduction of bone separating mastoid cavity from posterior fossa. Sigmoid portion of lateral sinus rests against this wall of bone, known as "dural sinus plate." If its integrity is breached, then there is possibility of lateral venous sinus thrombosis. **B,** Section taken several millimeters lateral to **A** shows upward bulging and further thinning of tegmen with disruption of dural sinus plate.

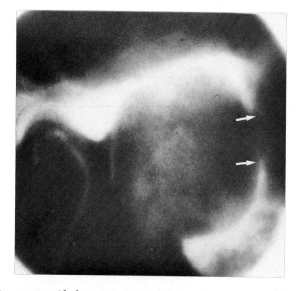

Fig. 16-104. Cholesteatoma. Complex motion tomogram, lateral view. Progression of this acquired cholesteatoma without treatment has resulted in massive excavation of mastoid portion of temporal bone. This constitutes the so-called automastoidectomy of cholesteatomatous disease. Notice breach in dural sinus plate *(arrows).*

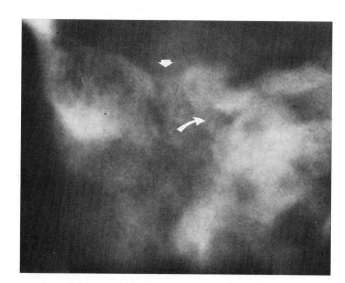

Fig. 16-105. Chronic mastoiditis with cholesteatoma formation. There is massive acquired cholesteatoma that has filled attic-antral area, destroyed lateral attic wall, and perforated tegmen *(straight arrow).* Ossicles have been destroyed along with bony labyrinth about lateral semicircular canal. Destruction has progressed to involve lateral wall of vestibule *(curved white arrow),* medial aspect of roof of external acoustic canal, and part of its floor.

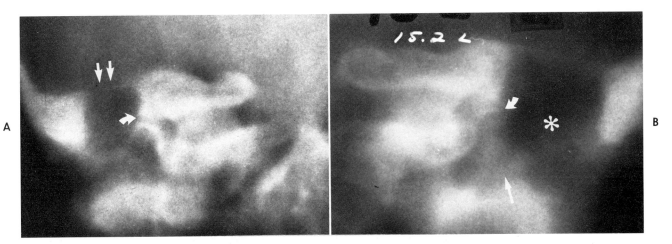

Fig. 16-106. Acquired cholesteatoma with labyrinthine fistula. **A,** Cholesteatoma within mastoid antrum has caused marked destruction with thinning of tegmen *(double arrows).* Destruction has continued medially and involved otic capsular bone surrounding lateral semicircular canal *(curved white arrow).* Fistula has developed between lateral semicircular canal and cholesteatoma cavity. Patient developed violent nystagmus and vertigo when pressure was applied to external ear canal. **B,** Similar case, with greater destruction of bone about lateral semicircular canal *(arrow),* and greater erosion of lateral attic wall and scutum. There is massive bony defect *(asterisk).* Notice soft tissue mass in middle ear *(long arrow).*

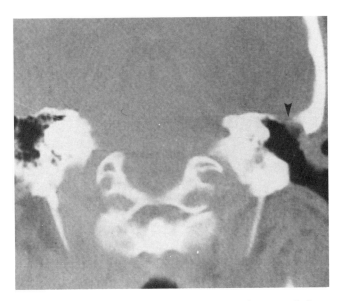

Fig. 16-107. Brain herniation through mastoidectomy defect. Soft tissue mass appearing beneath tegmen defect is brain. Patient had recurrent meningitis following mastoidectomy for chronic mastoiditis. (Courtesy Peter Som, M.D., New York.)

in the presence of chronic otitis media will be accompanied by cholesteatoma.[68] Occasionally a cholesteatoma may be present without any bone destruction whatsoever.

A rare complication of cholesteatoma with destruction of the tegmen is the herniation of brain tissue into the middle ear mastoid region (Fig. 16-107). Paparella et al.[100] reported 10 such cases that were insidious in onset. The soft tissue mass within the temporal bone was brain rather than cholesteatoma: no cholesteatoma coexisted. Six of his ten patients had no previous mastoid surgery and none had a history of trauma.

Unusual manifestations of cholesteatomas

There are several manifestations of acquired cholesteatoma that are unusual.

Mastoid cholesteatomas. Mastoid cholesteatomas fill all of the air systems within the entire pneumatized portion of the temporal bone, causing no bone destruction in the majority of cases. They occur more frequently in younger age groups and account for about 3% of all acquired cholesteatomas.

Cholesteatoma in the petrous apex. Chronic petrositis (Fig. 16-108) is a complication of chronic middle ear and mastoid suppuration with osteitis. Osteitis occurring about the bony portion of the eustachian tube in the peritubal cells may lead to inflammatory changes in the carotid canal and in rare instances can result in thrombosis and obliteration of the internal carotid ar-

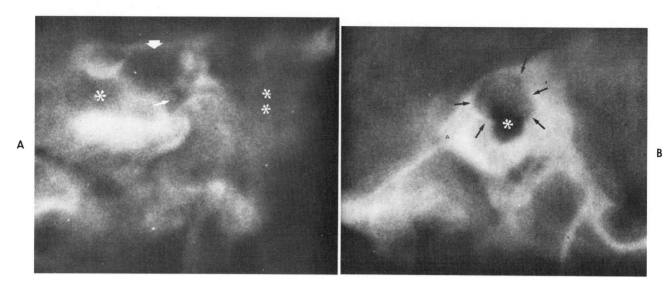

Fig. 16-108. Acquired cholesteatoma eroding internal acoustic canal. Large acquired cholesteatoma fills middle ear. Ossicles have been destroyed as well as lateral attic wall and part of tegmen. Cholesteatoma has spread medially into petrous apex cells, lying medial to semicircular canals. Patient had progressive facial nerve palsy and sensorineural as well as conductive hearing defect. Surgery showed cholesteatoma had extended well into internal acoustic canal and had invested itself about both seventh and eighth cranial nerves. **A,** Frontal tomogram. *Asterisk.* Internal auditory canal; *Broad white arrow,* apex cholesteatoma; *Small white arrow,* vestibule; *Double asterisks,* middle and external ear destruction. **B,** Lateral tomogram. A, Anterior; *Asterisk,* internal auditory canal; *Arrows,* cholesteatoma.

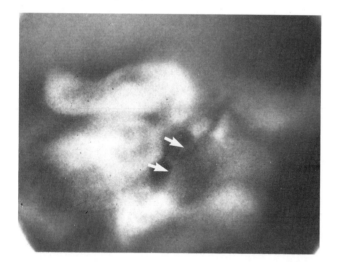

Fig. 16-109. Cholesteatoma, external acoustic canal. There is expansile, destructive lesion within medial aspect of external acoustic canal. Tympanic membrane is displaced medially *(arrows).* Acquired cholesteatomas in external acoustic canal are rare and occur as result of inclusions with accumulation of epithelial debris. They are seen more commonly in patients who have atresia of external acoustic canal. In that circumstance only most medial portion of external acoustic canal is developed; cholesteatoma takes its origin from epithelial cells of tympanic membrane.

tery. Abscess formation may occur in this region or in the petrous apex area.

Acquired cholesteatomas can also occur in the petrous tip as a result of chronic apical petrositis. There may be erosion into the labyrinth with attendant seventh and eighth nerve dysfunction.

Cholesteatoma of the external acoustic canal. An acquired cholesteatoma can have origin within the external acoustic canal lateral to the tympanic membrane (Fig. 16-109). There is no association with middle ear disease. This topic is discussed further in the section on benign tumors of the external acoustic canal.

Tuberculous otitis media and mastoiditis

Tuberculosis of the middle ear and mastoid in adults usually has an insidious onset and a chronic course. The onset of suppurative otitis media in a patient known to be suffering from pulmonary tuberculosis should lead one to suspect the possibility of tuberculous otitis media. The radiologic manifestations of this may be rupture of the tympanic membrane with exuberant granulation tissue in the middle ear and extension into the external acoustic canal. There may be an accompanying tuberculous otitis externa. Bone destruction may become an eventual sequel. Lincoln and Selle[75] as cited

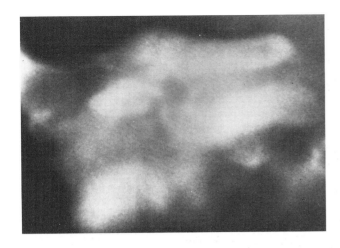

Fig. 16-110. Ossifying labyrinthitis. Patient had preceding acute suppurative otitis media and mastoiditis. Internal architecture of membranous and bony labyrinth of lateral semicircular canal is destroyed; there is marked sclerosis. Suppurative labyrinthitis is followed by complete, irreversible sensorineural deafness.

in Lucente et al.[81] point out that facial paralysis, as a result of involvement of either the intratympanic or mastoid portion of the facial canal, occurs in approximately 5% of cases of childhood tuberculous otitis media. This is somewhat higher than the incidence encountered in adults. There may be subperiosteal abscess and multiple periauricular sinuses. Sequestration of the external acoustic canal may become evident with concomitant neck abscesses by extension through the mastoid cortex.

Mastoid pneumatocele and mastoid cyst

Nomura et al.[94a] reported 1 case and reviewed 9 others of gas-filled epidural cysts that communicated with the mastoid air cells by way of a defect in the tegmen. It was presumed that the cyst had begun within the petrous portion and expanded into the epidural space through the bony defect. The authors postulated three causal factors: (1) chronic inflammation, (2) trauma, and (3) anomalous development of the petrous portion during the process of pneumatization. Madeira and Summers[82] published radiographic and CT depiction of a large epidural mastoid pneumatocele (mastoid cyst) that caused fluctuating, progressive amaurosis.

Mucocele

Osborn and Parkin[97] reported a case of mucocele of the petrous apex. The lesion was lytic with a sclerotic rim. It had eroded into the internal acoustic meatus and had developed a fistula with the cochlea. The patient had demonstrated a progressive sensorineural hearing loss and at the time of surgery had a complete absence of labyrinthine function. The lesion was radiographically indistinguishable from cholesteatoma. Its inflammatory basis was unclear.

Otogenic pneumocephalus

Mastoid pneumatoceles occur because of confinement of the air cavity within the epidural space by the overlying dura. In the event that there is a rent in the dura and a bony dehiscence of the tegmen, there may be free communication between the intracranial cavity and the mastoid–middle ear complex. These patients, in the absence of trauma, usually have a history of chronic otitis media and mastoiditis with cholesteatoma formation. In either event if there is free communication between intracranial space and the air cavities of the temporal bone, there may be air within the epidural, subdural, and subarachnoid spaces. The patient usually has recurring bouts of meningitis. A review of the literature and publication of plain film, complex motion tomographic, and CT manifestations of otogenic pneumocephalus was reported by Frankel et. al.[41]

■ The inner ear

Acute viral labyrinthitis has no radiologic correlate. The otic capsular bone may undergo rarefying osteitis insofar as it contributes to the medial wall of the middle ear cavity in the presence of otitis media. Fistulae into a semicircular canal as a result of cholesteatoma formation usually occur at the lateral semicircular canal.

Acute suppurative labyrinthitis may result in the development of a profound sclerosis, with complete radiologic obliteration of the internal architecture of the labyrinth.[58,76] This is known as obliterative labyrinthitis or labyrinthitis ossificans (Fig. 16-110).

Luetic osteitis

Syphilis may cause osteitis of the temporal bone as a predominant lesion, with secondary involvement of the membranous labyrinth in late congenital, latent, and

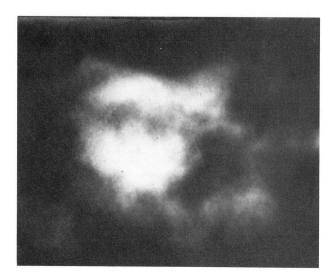

Fig. 16-111. Luetic osteitis. Left temporal bone, coronal section, complex motion tomography. Internal architecture of labyrinth has been destroyed. There is spotty rarefaction in matrix of sclerosis. Luetic osteitis shows more diffuse changes within labyrinth than are usually seen with otosclerosis.

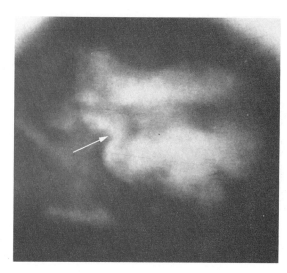

Fig. 16-112. Fenestral otosclerosis. Complex motion tomogram, frontal view. Oval window and oval window niche are obliterated by otosclerotic bone *(arrow)*. Except in advanced pathologic processes, radiologic diagnosis of footplate otosclerosis is difficult and subject to error.

tertiary syphilis.[119] The radiologic appearance is characterized by spotty rarefaction in an irregular matrix of sclerosis (Fig. 16-111). The disruption of the normal anatomic structure of the labyrinths appears much more profound than in labyrinthine otosclerosis as visualized radiologically. These patients have a so-called dead ear—total absence of hearing and labyrinthine function.

□ Disorders of growth, metabolism, and aging
■ Otosclerosis

Otosclerosis is a bony disease of the labyrinth and stapes that confines itself almost exclusively to caucasians and is an important aspect of hearing loss in that race. It occurs only in the human otic capsule.[77] The hearing loss usually has its onset in the second and third decade of life. It is seen slightly more frequently in women (about 60% to 70%) and appears to be activated by pregnancy.[119]

The disease is characterized by an early lytic (spongiotic) phase, followed by a reparative (sclerotic) phase. Eighty-five percent of otosclerotic foci are located in the oval window region. The round window niche, anterior wall of the internal auditory canal, and stapedial footplate are also common sites. When the oval window or round window is involved this may be referred to as fenestral otosclerosis. Lesions about the oval window that embrace the footplate may be referred to as footplate otosclerosis, even though the stapes itself is not

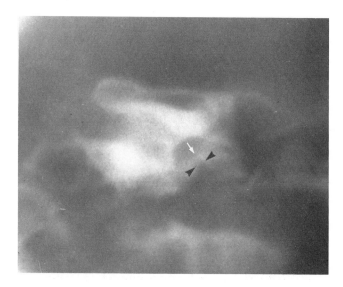

Fig. 16-113. Footplate otosclerosis. Oval window niche is easily visible *(black arrows)*. Oval window itself appears to be completely overgrown with otosclerotic bone *(white arrow)*.

involved. The incus is only rarely involved and this has not been defined radiologically.

The radiologic definition of oval window or footplate otosclerosis is possible only if the otosclerotic focus is substantial (Figs. 16-112 and 16-113). This pathologic process challenges the spatial resolution capability of contemporary roentgenographic equipment, including

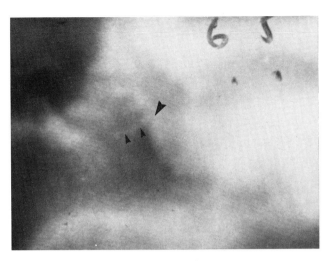

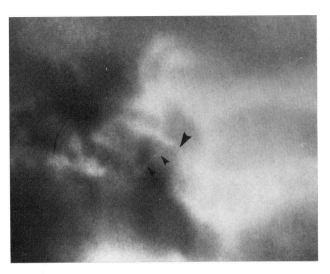

Fig. 16-114. Otosclerosis ("frozen" prosthesis). Patient had stapedectomy with insertion of prosthesis and transient improvement in hearing. Hearing loss recurred. Frontal tomogram shows bony overgrowth of otosclerotic process *(large arrow)* about stapes prosthesis *(small arrows)*.

Fig. 16-115. Malpositioned stapes prosthesis, fenestral otosclerosis. Following successful stapedectomy with placement of prosthesis, patient suffered acute conductive hearing loss after falling. Prosthesis *(small arrows)* has moved, with its tip lying superior to its desired position within region of oval window niche *(large arrow)*.

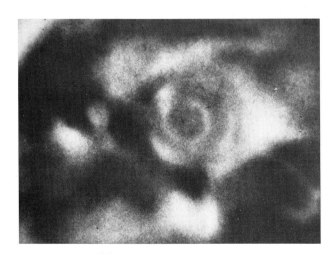

Fig. 16-116. Cochlear otosclerosis. Patient had marked footplate otosclerosis. Notice multiple areas of bone loss (otospongiosis) in turns of cochlea. Patient had profound sensorineural and conductive hearing loss.

the best complex motion tomography devices and the best CT machines.

Although the diagnosis of footplate otosclerosis usually falls more in the clinical rather than the radiologic domain, radiology may have a substantial contribution to make in the follow-up of patients with stapes prostheses who develop progressive hearing loss follow-

ing surgery. It is possible to demonstrate displacement of the prosthesis or bony overgrowth at the oval window, both of which findings are of use in the further clinical managment of the patient (Figs. 16-114 and 16-115).

■ Cochlear otosclerosis

There is very little debate that the cochlea may exhibit profound otosclerotic change in the presence of severe footplate otosclerosis. There is substantial controversy, however, about whether significant labyrinthine involvement may occur in the absence of significant fenestral (footplate) disease.[121,124,146]

The radiologic diagnosis of cochlear otosclerosis is difficult. Minor variations in x-ray exposure during complex motion tomography can make the labyrinth appear either spongiotic or sclerotic. Cochlear otosclerosis may be "created" almost at will. Additionally, minor irregularities on the surface of the basal turn of the cochlea as depicted radiologically are common in patients who have no hearing loss of any kind. In the absence of other compeling evidence of profound otosclerosis, especially fenestral otosclerosis, the radiologist should exercise great circumspection in making the diagnosis of labyrinthine otosclerosis.

In advanced pathologic processes the radiologic diagnosis of labyrinthine otosclerosis may be made with conviction (Fig. 16-116). The disruption in the normal bony architecture of the cochlea is much more confined in labyrinthine otosclerosis than may be seen with either luetic osteitis or Paget's disease, which tends to be

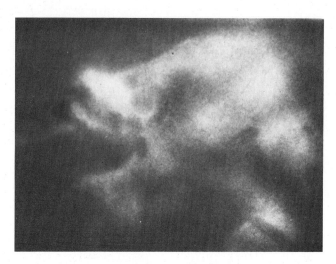

Fig. 16-117. Paget's disease. There is marked loss of mineral content in petrous tip, labyrinth, and adjacent floor of posterior cranial fossa. Loss of bone substance associated with Paget's disease is of far greater extent than with either luetic osteitis or labyrinthine otosclerosis.

much more widespread. We have not seen a convincing radiologic demonstration of labyrinthine otosclerosis affecting the otic capsular bone about the semicircular canals or vestibule.

In profound cochlear otosclerosis it may be possible to demonstrate abnormality of the otic capsule with CT, but this once again challenges the spatial resolution capability of the technology. A proposed radiologic diagnosis of this disease by CT should be viewed with informed scepticism except for those instances of widespread demineralization in the spongiotic phase.

■ **Paget's disease**

Paget's disease (Fig. 16-117) is a disorder of unknown cause that affects the older population, with a male/female ratio of 4:1.

Paget's disease may cause both sensorineural and conductive hearing loss. Because it involves the temporal bone, the lytic process is much more widespread and more profound than that seen in either otosclerosis or luetic osteitis. The petrous apices and the skull base are particularly involved. With progression of the disease the bony structure of the labyrinth may simply disappear from view. Eventually even the semicircular canals, vestibule, and internal acoustic canals may no longer be visible. Basilar invagination frequently is a concomitant.

Although the ossicles can be involved they are usually well preserved radiologically until the very late stages of the disease.[120]

■ **Fibrous dysplasia**

The fibro-osseous diseases (Figs. 16-118 and 16-119) can affect the bones of the skull and face, and the petrous bone is no exception.[25] Conductive hearing loss occurs as a result of occlusion of the external acoustic canal.

■ **Histiocytosis X**

Reticuloendothelioses may affect the temporal bone, being characterized by irregular lucent areas of bone destruction with scalloped margination. The diagnosis can only be suggested on the basis of radiologic characteristics, with histologic certainty arising only as a consequence of biopsy.

■ **Osteopetrosis**

Osteopetrosis is characterized by failure of resorption of calcified cartilage and primitive bone. It may be responsible for facial nerve palsy as a consequence of compression of the facial nerve anywhere within the facial canal. It is usually responsible for conductive deafness subsequent to diminished ossicular excursion by the osteopetrotic bone.[53]

□ **Trauma**

Trauma of the temporal bone has been the subject of numerous radiologic reports. Bergeron and Rumbaugh[11] and Davis and Rumbaugh[30] reviewed the salient clinical and radiologic features in roentgeno-

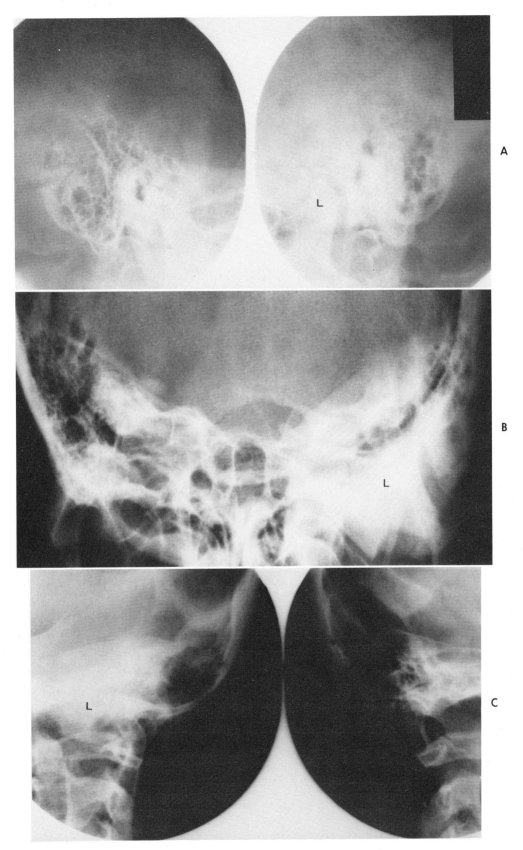

Fig. 16-118. Fibrous dysplasia masquerading as mastoiditis. Patient had narrowing of external acoustic canal that led to radiography. **A,** Law's projection showed diminished lucency to cells on left *(L)*, suggesting mastoiditis. **B,** Towne view shows thickening of squamosal and petrous portions characteristic of fibrous dysplasia. *L,* Left. **C,** Stenvers view shows petrous portion to best advantage. Mastoid portion of bone is normal. *L,* Left. (Courtesy Peter Som, M.D., New York.)

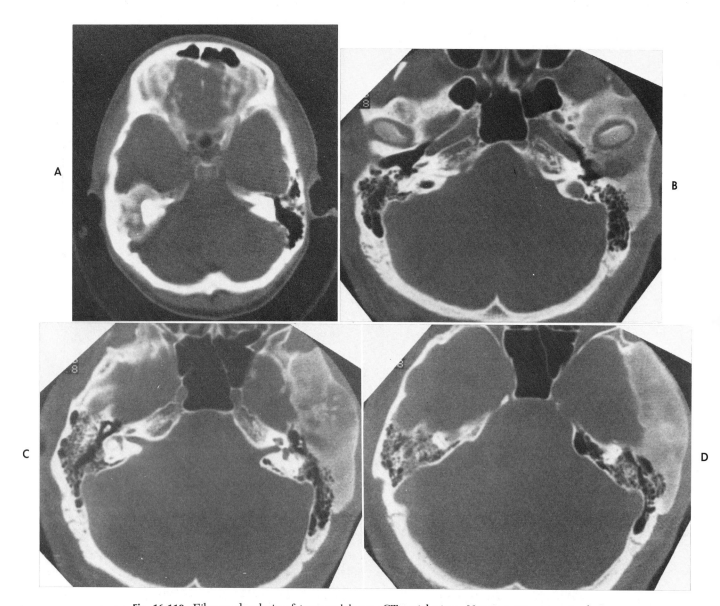

Fig. 16-119. Fibrous dysplasia of temporal bone. CT, axial view. Noncontrast scan reveals expansile process of petrous portion of temporal bone. Serial contiguous scans showed anterior and posterior cortices of petrous portion to be intact. Labyrinth gives appearance of "floating" within cystic lesion. It is not affected by process. Those who make distinctions on radiologic character of fibro-osseous dysplasias would call above cystic form "nonossifying fibroma," as opposed to more solid form (see Fig. 16-118), "fibrous dysplasia." **B** to **D,** Succeeding cephalad sections through skull of different patient with fibrous dysplasia involving squamous, tympanic, and mastoid portions of left temporal bone (and part of sphenoid). External auditory canal is occluded by fibro-osseous overgrowth. (**B** to **D** Courtesy Peter Som, M.D., New York.)

graphic diagnosis before the era of CT. There is no large series of cases reported employing CT alone in the radiologic diagnosis of temporal bone trauma, although it is evident that CT is now probably the technology of choice. The availability of the axial projection alone facilitates the detection of small endocranial fractures otherwise obscured. The course of fractures as they traverse the (temporal) bone may be followed with greater precision. Small ossicular dislocations may be identified. Focal collections of blood or cerebrospinal fluid within a single air cell or small group of mastoid cells may be shown. Most importantly, more fractures are identified because the temporal bone tends to shatter if it receives a severe blow and many of these fractures have not been identified with previous radiologic techniques.

Linear fractures of the squamous portion of the temporal bone are common sequelae to a sharp blow to the lateral aspect of the skull (Fig. 16-120). Occasionally the fracture will extend into the tympanic portion and involve the external acoustic canal. This should be distinguished from the tympanosquamous suture (glaserian fissure). The tympanosquamous suture itself is occa-

sionally involved in diastatic fractures, making identification more problematical (Figs. 16-121 and 16-122).

Fractures involving the petrous portion of the temporal bone are usually classified in a way that makes clear their orientation with respect to the long axis of the petrous portion of the temporal bone. Those that go along the axis are classified as longitudinal fractures; those at right angles to this are called transverse fractures. The latter are also referred to as vertical fractures.

Not all fractures of the petrous portion occur in the orthogonal planes. These are referred to as complex fractures. They are frequently multiple (Fig. 16-123).

The transverse (vertical) fractures are the type most often seen on plain films. They are demonstrated to best advantage in either the Caldwell or the Towne projection (Fig. 16-124). Although most transverse fractures are just lateral to or through the labyrinth, they may occur as far medially as the internal acoustic canal. Fractures that come to involve the more lateral portion of the petrous pyramid as it joins with either the squamosal or mastoid portions are usually longitudinal or complex.

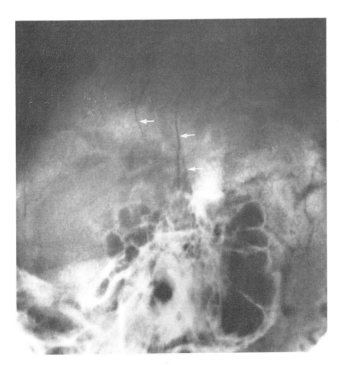

Fig. 16-120. Linear fractures of temporal squama. Blows to side of head may be associated with linear fractures of temporal squama. If fractures involve inner table of skull and course through air cells, there may then be communication between middle ear–mastoid region and subarachnoid space. Meningitis may follow.

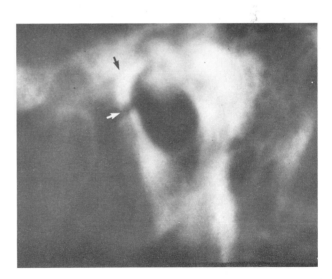

Fig. 16-121. Fracture of anterior wall of external acoustic canal and tympanic ring. Fracture (*white arrow*) has occurred several millimeters inferior to glaserian fissure (*black arrow*). Fragment has rotated slightly clockwise.

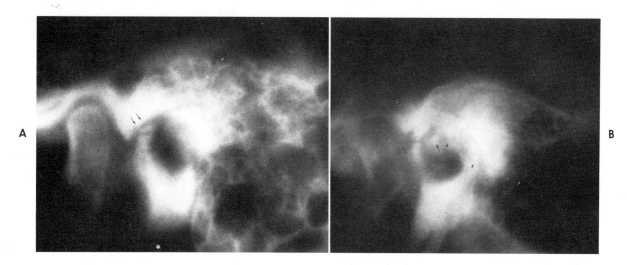

A B

Fig. 16-122. Complex fracture, temporal bone. Complex motion tomography, lateral view. **A,** Fracture commences anteriorly in region of glaserian fissure and continues posteriorly. There is separated fracture fragment involving upper portion of anterior wall of external acoustic canal. **B,** Section several milimeters medial to **A** shows fracture line entering mastoid portion of facial canal about 15 mm superior to stylomastoid foramen *(small posterior arrow)* and ossicular disruption *(small upper arrows).* Molar tooth configuration of normal maleoloincudal relationship has been lost.

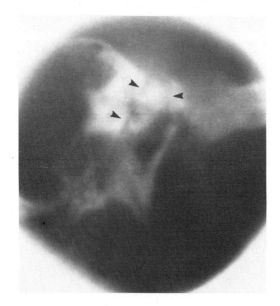

Fig. 16-123. Multiple fractures of temporal bone. Complex motion tomography, lateral view. Temporal bone has been comminuted by fractures *(arrows).* There is ossicular disruption and subluxation.

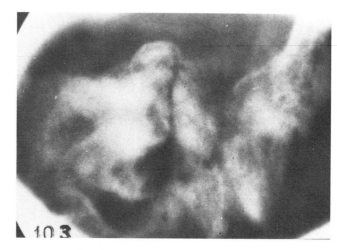

Fig. 16-124. Transverse fracture, left temporal bone. Complex motion tomography, frontal view. Fracture courses through labyrinth and at level slightly anterior to this entered vestibule. Patient had hearing loss and severe labyrinthine dysfunction.

Harwood-Nash[55] subdivides longitudinal fractures into anterior and posterior types. Anterior fractures tend to involve the parietotemporal regions of the skull and extend into the anterior aspect of the petrous bone through the tegmen tympani, terminating in the region of the labyrinth. The posterior type involves the posterior part of the parietal bone as well as the mastoid and posterosuperior portions of the petrous bone. The posterior type may also converge on the otic capsule.

As would be expected, anterior longitudinal fractures may enter the labyrinthine portion of the facial canal, and posterior longitudinal fractures may enter the facial canal in its mastoid portion. This may be helpful when attempting to identify the fracture site when a patient has head trauma and consequent facial nerve palsy.

Fractures through the middle ear–mastoid complex may cause submucosal hemorrhage and hemotympanum. The elevation of the mucous membrane as well as the presence of blood may be detected with CT.

Ossicular disruption may ensue. The incudostapedial joint is the most fragile of the articulations and is the one most frequently disrupted. Because of the small dimensions of the bones involved, however, it is the most difficult of the dislocations to identify radiologically.

The malleus is the most firmly anchored ossicle and it demonstrates the greatest stability.

Because of the medial inclination of the tympanic cavity, the Guillen projection is used to demonstrate possible ossicular subluxation or dislocation. With sufficient skull trauma the dislocation may be complete and the ossicles may lie free within the middle ear cavity or, if there is concomitant laceration of the tympanic membrane, they may lie even within the external acoustic canal (Fig. 16-125).

If CT is not available, lateral complex motion tomography is also useful in demonstrating possible malleoincudal dislocation. The "molar tooth configuration" described by Potter[107] in the lateral projection may be destroyed. Normally, the long handle of the malleus and the long process of the incus should subtend an angle with one another that resembles the diverging roots of a molar tooth. The head of the malleus and the body of the incus are normally held in close approximation by a relatively dense ligamentous investment. This combination shadow represents the crown of the "tooth" in the analogy used by Potter.

Fractures coursing through the semicircular canals or (rarely) the vestibule may be associated with acute lab-

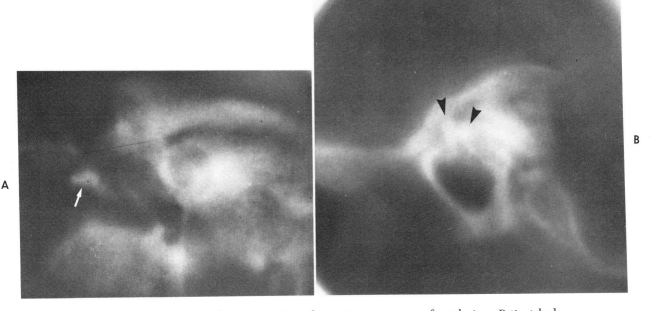

Fig. 16-125. Ossicular dislocation. **A,** Complex motion tomogram, frontal view. Patient had severe head trauma and suffered immediate, severe hearing loss on this side. Otoscopy showed a blood clot deep within external acoustic canal. Tomography shows malleus and incus to be dislocated from attic, lying within medial aspect of external acoustic canal. Inspection of "blood clot" at its removal from ear canal provided ossicles for later transplant. **B,** Different case, lateral tomogram. Note subluxation of body of incus with respect to head of malleus. (**A** Courtesy Charles Schatz, M.D., Los Angeles.)

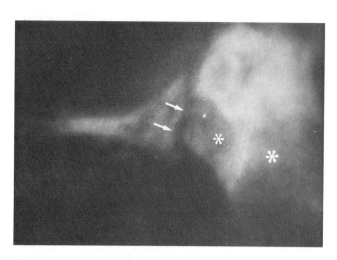

Fig. 16-126. Fracture through intrapetrous carotid canal. Patient had gunshot wound to head. There were multiple fractures, one of which went through intrapetrous carotid canal. Angiography showed traumatic occlusion of internal carotid artery secondary to fracture. *Large asterisk,* Jugular foramen; *small asterisk,* carotid canal; *arrows,* fracture.

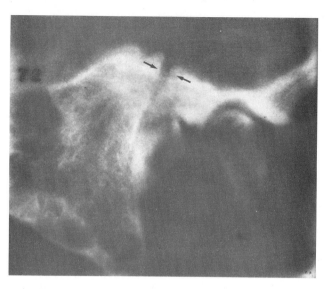

Fig. 16-127. Cleft Fracture, petrous bone. Lateral tomogram. Patient had head trauma several months previously and experienced cerebrospinal fluid otorrhea subsequently. Several tomographic examinations in frontal view alone failed to demonstrate fracture *(arrows)* because it lay largely parallel to plane of section. This film, which indicated diagnosis, was scout view on first tomographic examination in lateral projection.

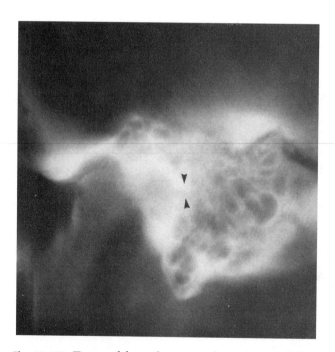

Fig. 16-128. Temporal bone fracture with cerebrospinal fluid leak. Lateral complex motion tomogram. There was complex fracture with multiple segments entering many different areas of temporal bone. Clouding of mastoid air cells was caused by cerebrospinal fluid. Notice fracture in posterior wall of external acoustic canal *(arrows)*. Patient had cerebrospinal fluid otorrhea and is candidate for meningitis.

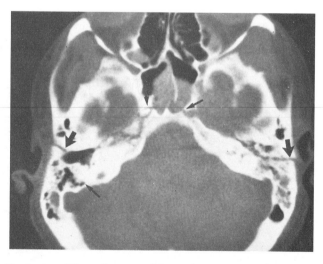

Fig. 16-129. Bilateral temporal bone fractures. CT axial view. Multiple fractures in each temporal bone are identified. Small endocranial fracture is also seen on right. Patients with cerebrospinal fluid within tympanomastoid complex may have cerebrospinal fluid rhinorrhea if tympanic membrane is intact or cerebrospinal fluid otorrhea if tympanic membrane is lacerated or perforated. They are candidates for meningitis. Notice unsuspected fractures in sphenoid sinus associated with fluid within sinus. This is also source for cerebrospinal fluid rhinorrhea and meningitis following head trauma. (Courtesy Peter Som, M.D., New York.)

yrinthine dysfunction. Fractures through the cochlea are associated with immediate, total, and irreversible deafness. Fractures through the internal acoustic canal may be associated with both seventh and eighth cranial nerve dysfunction. The eighth cranial nerve dysfunction is usually the more severe of the two.

Fractures that enter the facial canal either in its labyrinthine, intratympanic, or mastoid portions may be responsible for a delayed facial palsy with advancing edema.

Fractures that enter the carotid canal may cause traumatic occlusion of the internal carotid artery (Fig. 16-126).

Fractures that cause a communication between the middle ear mastoid complex and the cerebrospinal space may be responsible for the eventual development of cerebrospinal fluid otorrhea, cerebrospinal fluid rhinorrhea (if the tympanic membrane is intact), recurring meningitis, pneumocephalus, mastoid pneumatoceles, intracranial abscesses, and death (Figs. 16-127 to 16-129).

□ Tumors
R. Thomas Bergeron, Ajax E. George, and Richard S. Pinto

■ External auditory canal

Tumors which take their origin within the external acoustic canal are of the benign and malignant varieties. Two common benign *bony* lesions occuring within the external acoustic canal are exostoses and, far less frequently, osteomas.

Exostoses

Exostoses (Figs. 16-130 and 16-131, *A* and *B*) tend to be located in the medial end of the bony canal, near the tympanic membrane. They are usually multiple, bilateral, and variable in size. They represent ledges of periosteal bone that appear to be a response to periosteal irritation or stimulation and in a sense are a kind of osteophyte. They are seen most commonly in cold water swimmers.[1,48] Occasionally, a cholesteatoma (keratoma) may develop medial to an exostosis if it obstructs the external acoustic canal.

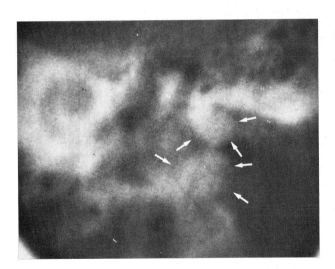

Fig. 16-130. Exostosis, external acoustic canal. Medial position of "kissing" exostosis within external acoustic canal is common. These patients may have conductive hearing loss. This lesion is most frequently encountered in cold water swimmers.

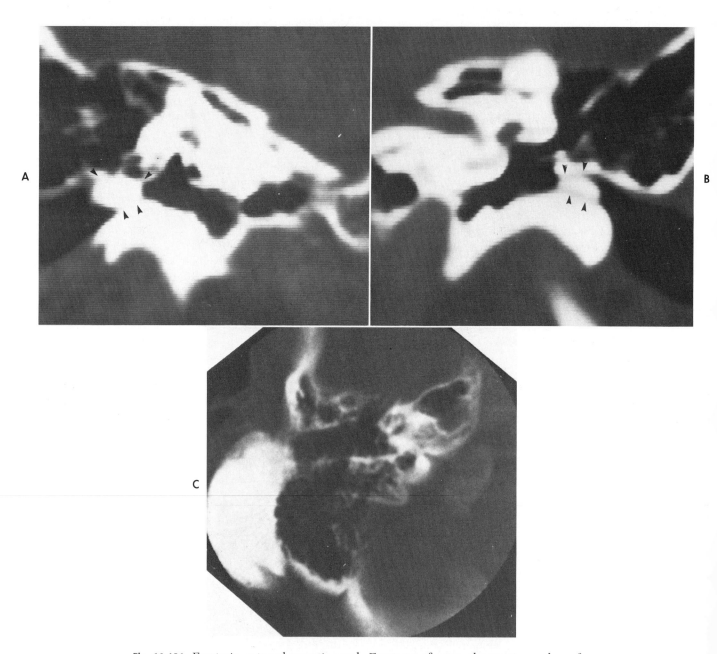

Fig. 16-131. Exostosis, external acoustic canal. Exostoses of external acoustic canal are frequently bilateral *(arrows)*. They are commonly seen in cold water swimmers and adjacent bone is always normal. **A,** Right side. **B,** Left side. **C,** Osteoma, extracanicular, involving mastoid portion. Depiction is with axial CT.

Osteomas

Osteomas (Fig. 16-131, *C*) of the external acoustic canal usually start at the junction between the cartilaginous and bony portions, i.e., at the junction of the lateral one third and medial two thirds of the external acoustic canal. Osteomas are composed of mature bone; they may grow into adjacent bone of the mastoid. Such growth is never demonstrated with exostoses.

Extracanalicular osteomas of the temporal bone have also been reported.[31] Their radiographic appearance is that of homogeneously dense bone with smooth contours. They occur in all portions of the temporal bone and because of their progressive increase in size have been responsible for eustachian tube obstruction and compression of the contents of the internal acoustic canal. The mastoid region is the most prevalent site (over 75%), with squama and the internal acoustic canal following in frequency. Osteomas are rare before puberty and there is a slight predilection in women. The tumors are usually asymptomatic.

Ceruminomas (benign ceruminous adenoma)

Tumors that arise from the modified cerumen-secreting sweat glands in the cartilaginous portion of the external auditory canal (lateral one third) of the external acoustic canal may be either benign or malignant. The benign ceruminomas show no evidence of bony invasion and appear purely as a soft tissue mass within the lateral aspect of the external acoustic canal. Some of these lesions tend to recur and in that sense have a malignant potential.

Keratomas (cholesteatomas)

Acquired keratomas (Figs. 16-109 and 16-132) within the tympanomastoid complex are a common consequence of chronic infection. Keratomas may exist in the medial portion of the external acoustic canal in the circumstance of incomplete recannulation of the canal, as a developmental defect, or as part of atresia of the external acoustic canal. Rarely, keratomas can begin within a normal external acoustic canal, lateral to the tympanic membrane. The cause is unknown but is probably related to epithelial metaplastic changes in the canal wall.[48] Excavations may occur in the inferior bony external canal reaching down to the jugular bulb, as well as anteriorly, posteriorly and superiorly, effectively skeletonizing the periannular regions of the external acoustic canal.

Benign skin tumors

Any of the benign skin neoplasms can occur in the skin overlying the cartilaginous portion of the external acoustic canal. These include lipomas, sebaceous cysts, and fibromas. Other than the presence of a soft tissue mass and possible low attenuation values associated with fatty content as demonstrated on CT, these lesions have no radiologic correlate. The underlying bone is normal.

Malignant neoplasms

Actinic keratoses and basal cell carcinomas are the most common malignant lesions of the pinna and auricle (Fig. 16-133). Squamous cell carcinomas are the

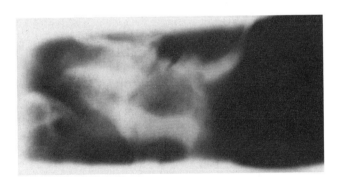

Fig. 16-132. Keratoma, acquired cholesteatoma, external acoustic canal. Frontal tomogram. Pale, nonpulsatile mass was demonstrated at otoscopy. Middle ear space was normal behind medially displaced, intact tympanic membrane. Process is both expansile and noninfiltrating.

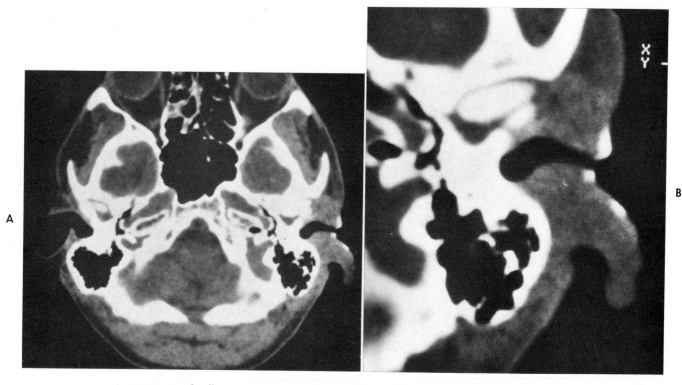

Fig. 16-133. Basal cell carcinoma, external ear. **A,** Notice diffuse soft tissue swelling of ear and adjacent soft tissue. Actinic keratoses and basal cell carcinomas are most common malignant lesions affecting pinna and auricle. **B,** Enlarged view of diseased ear.

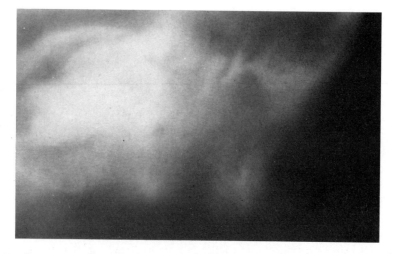

Fig. 16-134. Squamous cell carcinoma, external acoustic canal. Complex motion tomography, frontal view. There is soft-tissue mass filling external acoustic canal and middle ear. Floor of external acoustic canal and lateral aspect of floor of hypotympanum have been destroyed.

most common malignancy involving the skin of the external acoustic canal[21,22] (Fig. 16-134).

Next in incidence are the adenomatous tumors, which have varying degrees of malignant potential: the adenoma, pleomorphic adenoma, adenoid cystic carcinoma, and adenocarcinoma.

. . .

The radiologic distinction between benign and malignant tumors of the external acoustic canal is based purely on the evidence of bone destruction. This is an imperfect criterion because while the absence of destruction implies benignancy its presence does not necessarily guarantee cancer. Although bone destruction is a constant finding in malignant neoplasms of the external acoustic canal it may also be seen with malignant otitis externa, with osteomyelitis in the immunosuppressed patient, with granulomatous otitis (tuberculosis), with facial nerve neuroma, and as an extension of benign tumors within the middle ear that are destroying bone by pressure necrosis rather than invasion.

On the whole, patients with benign tumors in the external acoustic canal are asymptomatic with the exception of the finding of a soft tissue mass within the canal and having the possible complaint of (conductive) deafness. Patients with malignant tumors of the external acoustic canal usually have pain as a cardinal sign as well as a soft tissue mass and otorrhea.

The character of the bone destruction is important. In the inflammatory and malignant tumor lesions the destruction tends to be more infiltrative and there is more widespread rarefaction. In the destruction associated with pressure from the advancing edge of a benign tumor the bone adjacent to that which is destroyed appears normal.

■ The middle ear
Benign neoplasms

Primary benign tumors of the middle ear space are rare and are usually of the adenomatous variety. As with similar lesions in the external acoustic canal, benign tumors arising within the middle ear cleft have no characteristic radiologic feature other than soft tissue mass. These patients may be treated for otitis media and the radiologist may be unable to distinguish between a true neoplasm and an acquired cholesteatoma without bone destruction, polypoid proliferation of the tympanic mucosa, and other signs of acquired cholesteatoma.

The choristoma is a benign middle ear tumor that is an embryologic curiosity. It is composed of ectopic mature salivary gland tissue that lies within the middle ear space. It is the tympanic analog of the Stafne cyst of the mandible. The salivary tissue is functional and the pa-

tient is often treated for chronic otitis media. Although histologically benign, choristomas may come to fill the middle ear cleft and invest the ossicles. They may eventually incorporate the intratympanic facial nerve and complete resection of the tumor may be impossible without sacrifice of the nerve[132,140] (Fig. 16-135).

Malignant neoplasms

Primary malignant neoplasms of the middle ear include squamous cell carcinoma, the adenomatous glandular carcinomas (including adenoid cystic carcinoma, ceruminous adenocarcinoma), and mucoepidermoid carcinoma[37] (Fig. 16-136). Malignant lymphomas may involve the mucous membrane diffusely or may appear as a soft tissue mass. Reticulum cell sarcoma, appearing as a middle ear cleft mass, has been reported as the initial complaint of a patient who died 14 months later of disseminated malignant lymphoma.[44]

Embryonal rhabdomyosarcoma is an uncommon disease that is seen almost exclusively in young children, and the middle ear is one of the sites of predilection when it arises in the head and neck region.[42] In its early stages the clinical course may mimic that of intractable otitis media, with otorrhea or bleeding from the ear; the seventh cranial nerve is frequently involved early in the course of the disease. The propensity for local invasion and destruction of bone is characteristic of rhabdomyosarcoma, and the rapid regional spread is pathognomonic.[17] The tumor may spread in a retrograde fashion through the fallopian canal, traverse the internal acoustic canal, and escape into the posterior cranial fossa.[47,89]

Although bone destruction is the hallmark of a malignant tumor arising within the middle ear in children, massive bone destruction with multiple cranial nerve neuropathies, evidence of soft tissue mass within the pharynx, and possible skeletonization of the cochlea should indicate the immediate possibility of an embryonal rhabdomyosarcoma. Schwartz et al.[122] have published the CT depiction of this lesion in the temporal bone.

Glomus tympanicum

Glomus tympanicum tumors (Figs. 16-137 and 16-138) originate from the paraganglionic bodies about the tympanic plexus arising from Jacobson's nerve as it ramifies over the cochlear promontory.[120] Although glomus tumors are histologically malignant in only about 10% of cases they tend to be locally invasive and to enlarge inexorably. They tend to recur if incompletely excised.

Patients with a glomus tympanicum tumor may have pulsating tinnitus. At otoscopy there is a bluish mass. Either complex motion tomography or CT will show that the mass lies within the hypotympanum and cannot

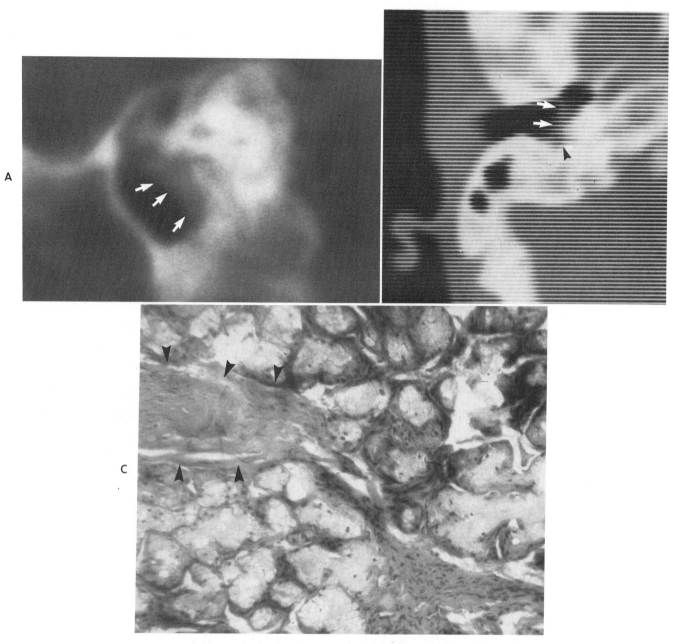

Fig. 16-135. Choristoma of tympanic cavity. Patient had long-standing history of otitis media. **A,** Complex motion tomogram, lateral view. Soft tissue mass *(arrows)* is identified within tympanic cavity and extends into epitympanum. There is possible posterior extension into adjacent bone. **B,** Axial CT projection shows soft tissue mass that spans sagittal dimension of middle ear cleft and hugs labyrinthine wall. Sinus tympani and facial recess are also filled with tumor. **C,** Photomicrograph of operative specimen. Mature salivary gland tissue had surrounded facial nerve *(arrows)* and was inseparable from it. Choristoma of middle ear is example of histologically benign lesion (ectopic mature salivary gland tissue) that has caused bone destruction. (Courtesy Y.B. Choo, M.D., Daniel Rabuzzi, M.D., and A. Liebeskind, M.D., New York.)

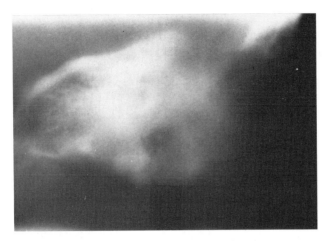

Fig. 16-136. Squamous cell carcinoma, external ear and middle ear. There is destruction of external acoustic canal, middle ear, tegmen, and otic capsule. Bone destruction is hallmark of malignant soft tissue tumors of both middle ear and outer ear.

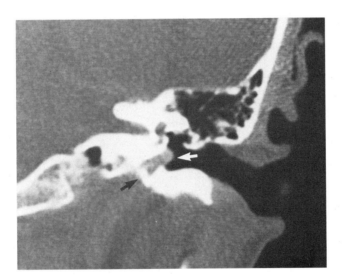

Fig. 16-137. Glomus tympanicum. Notice soft tissue mass filling hypotympanum and lower portion of tympanic cavity *(white arrow)*. Mass cannot be separated from labyrinthine wall. Notice that remainder of tympanic cavity and mastoid air cells appear normal. Of special importance is fact that bony margin that delineates lateral superior border of carotid canal is present *(black arrow)*. This finding rules out possibility of aberrant internal carotid artery. Most likely radiologic diagnosis is glomus tympanicum tumor. (Compare with Fig. 16-84.)

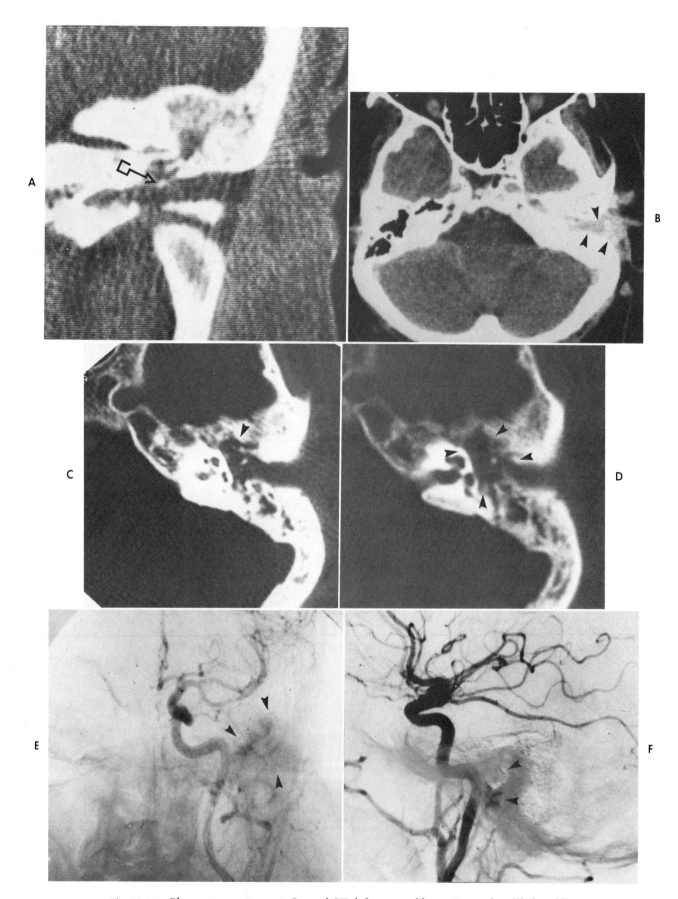

Fig. 16-138. Glomus tympanicum. **A,** Coronal CT, left temporal bone. Tumor has filled middle ear and excavated into external acoustic canal. There is some erosion and fragmentation of ossicles *(arrow)*. Soft tissue shadow within mastoid could be consequent to obstruction of drainage or tumor extension. **B,** Axial CT with contrast material. Notice enhancing mass filling left external acoustic canal *(arrows)*. **C** to **D,** Progressively cephalad CT views through middle ear. Notice destruction *(arrows)*. **E** and **F,** Frontal and lateral angiograms, respectively. Notice tumor blush *(arrows)*.

be separated from the medial wall of the middle ear cleft inferiorly. When the tumor is large it fills the middle ear cleft totally and may excavate into the adjacent external acoustic canal. By this stage there is usually bony erosion. The tumor is intensely vascular on contrast-enhanced CT.

In addition to glomus tympanicum, the differential diagnosis of a pulsating vascular tumor within the hypotympanum includes dehiscent jugular bulb, aberrant internal carotid artery, and glomus jugulare tumor that has eroded into the middle ear. Jugular venography and cerebral angiography may be required to distinguish among them.

■ The inner ear

There are no known primary tumors, either benign or malignant, arising from the membranous labyrinth.

■ Other tumorous lesions in the temporal bone and adjacent skull base

Glomus jugulare

The CT appearance of glomus jugulare tumors (Figs. 16-139 to 16-143) is discussed in Chapter 13.

The paraganglionic cells or so-called glomus bodies exist in the jugular bulb along Jacobson's nerve, especially at the site of the tympanic plexus, and along the vagus nerve, especially near the nodose ganglion. Vascular tumors of these structures are termed glomus jug-

ular tumors, glomus tympanicum tumors, and glomus vagale tumors, respectively.[26]

The most common symptoms of glomus tumors originating or extending into the middle ear are hearing loss and pulsating tinnitus. Other symptoms, in order of decreasing frequency, are nerve palsies, vertigo, and pain.

Common nerve involvements are the seventh cranial nerve from invasion of the mastoid portion of the facial canal, the eighth cranial nerve from erosion of the cochlea, the ninth, tenth, and eleventh cranial nerves (jugular foramen syndrome) from extension into the jugular foramen, and not infrequently the twelfth cranial nerve as a result of involvement of the hypoglossal canal. Twelfth cranial nerve palsy occasionally may be seen in isolation. Fifth and sixth cranial nerve palsies are unusual but may occur in cases of tumor invasion of the middle cranial fossa.

Glomus jugulare tumors tend to grow along the planes of least resistance by following preexisting pathways in the temporal bone, i.e., fissures, air-cell tracts, vascular channels, and foramina.[130] These pathways are followed preferentially because they provide adequate blood supply to support continued tumor growth.

Glomus tumors grow in a centripetal pattern, following multiple pathways and simultaneously extending to the protympanum, hypotympanum, or mesotympanum.

When reaching the protympanum a glomus jugulare

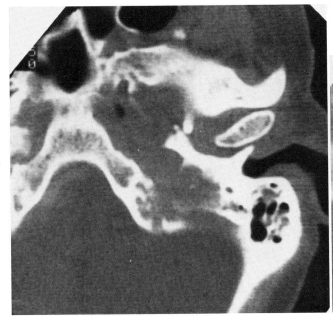

A

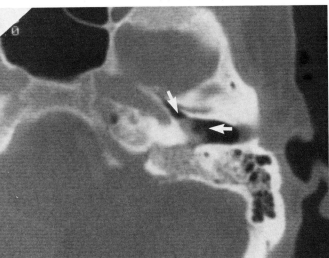

B

Fig. 16-139. Glomus jugulare tumor. **A,** Notice destructive lesion in region of jugular foramen. Foramen is enlarged, but irregularly so, with loss of cortical margination. **B,** Tumor has extended into middle ear cavity *(arrows)*. Patient complained of pulsating tinnitus.

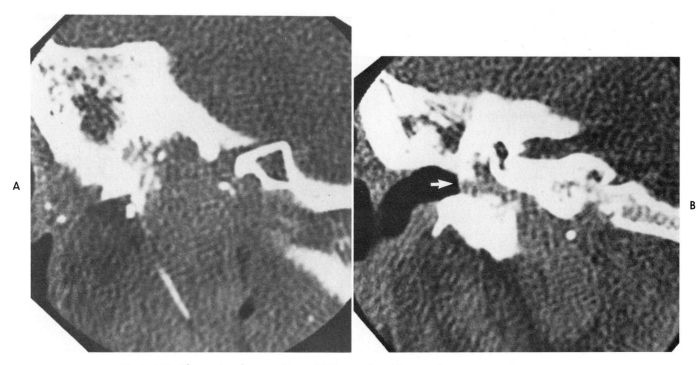

Fig. 16-140. Glomus jugulare. **A,** Coronal CT scan shows large soft tissue mass that has eroded superiorly into mastoid and laterally to erode upper one half of styloid process. **B,** Tumor has eroded bony partition between hypotympanum and jugular foramen and has come to fill entire tympanic cavity and bulge tympanic membrane laterally *(arrow)*. Patient complained of pulsating tinnitus and had paresis of ninth, tenth, and twelfth cranial nerves.

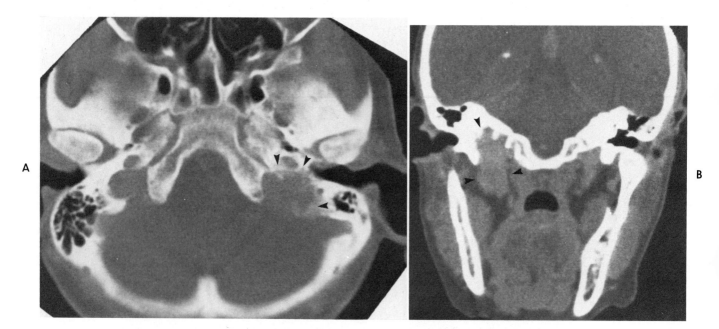

Fig. 16-141. Glomus jugulare tumor. **A,** There is enlargement of jugular foramen with loss of normal cortication and irregular margination *(arrows)*. **B,** Scan in coronal view shows inferior extent of lesion *(arrows)*. CT scan of lesions at base of skull should always include coronal views in order to define inferior and superior limits of lesion.

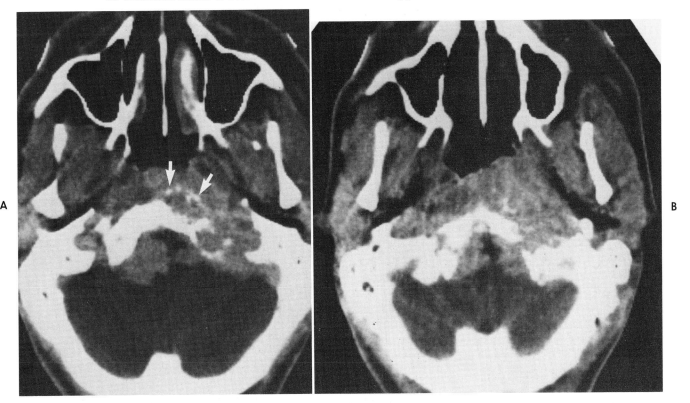

Fig. 16-142. Glomus jugulare. **A,** Axial CT scan at level of internal acoustic canals shows densely enhanced lesion within right cerebellopontine angle cistern. Lesion has broad attachment to posterior surface of petrous portion. There is no evidence of widening of internal acoustic canal. These findings are consistent with highly vascular cerebellopontine angle meningioma. **B,** Sections taken few milimeters inferior to **A** show true origin of lesion; there is marked enlargement of jugular foramen with erosion laterally, posteriorly, and anteriorly into tympanic cavity. Glomus jugulare tumor is now most likely radiologic diagnosis. Vascular metastatic lesions to base of skull could cause similar appearance.

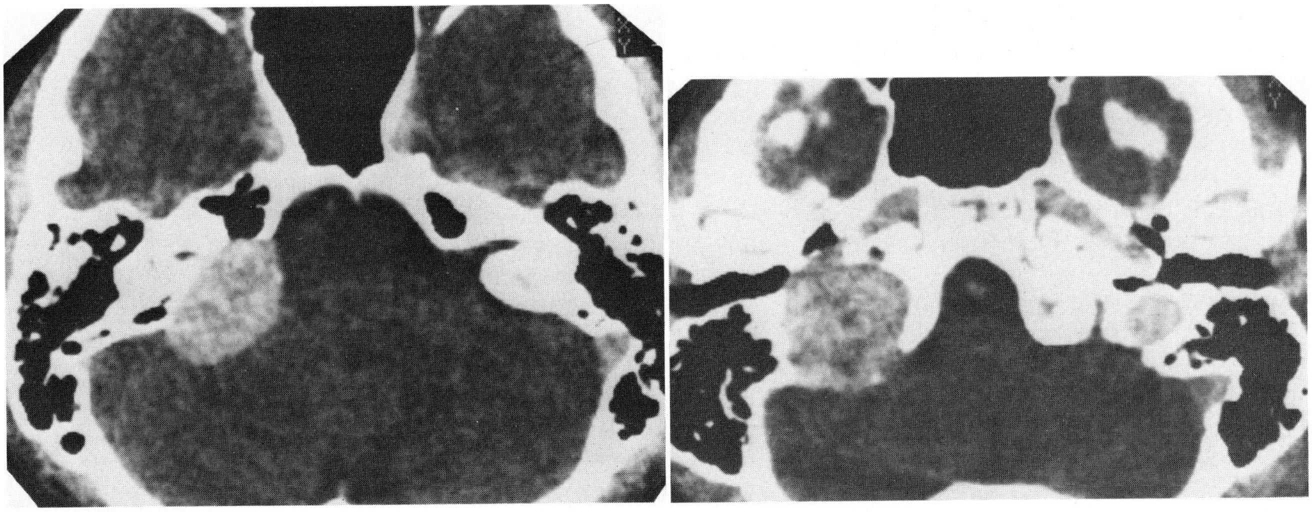

Fig. 16-143. Malignant glomus jugulare tumor. **A,** There is extensive destruction at base of skull with calcific debris *(arrows)*. Tumor mass may be identified on both sides of midline within posterior fossa. **B,** Section few milimeters from **A** shows enhanced nasopharyngeal mass. Patients with this manifestation of glomus jugulare tumor may have epistaxis. Patient also had multiple metastatic lesions to lung. About 10% of glomus jugulare tumors are malignant.

tumor may follow three different pathways. First, the tumor may grow into the lumen of the eustachian tube and present as a mass in the nasopharynx or in the lateral pharyngeal recess; the patient may have epistaxis. Second, there may be invasion of the petrous apex by way of peritubal air cells or an anterior cell tract. Finally, the tumor may follow the internal carotid artery to the middle cranial fossa. This latter circumstance is the most common form of spread from the protympanum.

When glomus tumors reach the hypotympanum they may spread into the temporal bone further, using an additional three pathways of egress. First, they may enter the lumens of the great veins and extend intraluminally. Second, they may extend extraluminally into the carotid sheath, growing inferiorly into the neck. Finally, they may grow under the base of the skull and enter the cranial nerve foramina. Generally they follow the cranial nerves into the foramina and produce cranial nerve palsies prior to massive central nervous system invasion.

When the tumor enters the mesotympanum it acts again as a central locus from which the tumor further invades the temporal bone. Additional extension is common, particularly into the facial recess and sinus tympani. Spread into the mastoid by way of perifacial air cells occurs. The sinus tympani also provides access for growth beneath the facial nerve.

Superior extension into the epitympanum involves the ossicular heads; progression posterosuperiorly by way of the additus ad antrum leads into the mastoid antrum and adjacent cells. Medial extension from the mesotympanum will cause cochlear destruction. Rarely, the tumor may erode anteriorly through the tegmen tympani and appear as a middle cranial fossa mass.

Radiology has a pivotal role in both diagnosis and management of patients with glomus jugulare tumors. Complex motion tomography may show soft tissue mass in the mesotympanum or hypotympanum in conjunction with erosion of the jugular foramen. The bony plate that separates the jugular foramen from the middle ear cavity may be destroyed. If the tumor is advanced there may be a soft tissue mass within the lateral pharyngeal space and evidence of further destruction about the base of the skull, petrous apex, etc.

Jugular venography may define intraluminal or extraluminal growth into the adjacent veins, indicate venous obstruction, indicate extension into or around the carotid sheath, and locate the inferior extent of the lesion.

Arteriography, particularly subselective arteriography, has now become standard in the assessment of glomus jugulare tumors because a comprehensive understanding of the vascular supply is requisite before embolization and indeed before surgical management even if embolization is not carried out. Besides demonstrating the size, borders, various nutrient vessels, and almost virtually certain histologic diagnosis, arteriography provides for demonstration of the presence or absence of multiple lesions. Most importantly, arteriography gives a precise, accurate map for the selective embolization of the tumor.[58] The subject is also covered in detail in Chapter 9.

Nonglomus tumors of the jugular foramen— Schwannomas

Erosive tumors other than those of the glomus jugulare may occur at the skull base in the region of the jugular foramen (Figs. 16-144 and 16-145). The differences in biology, extension, and position of the epicenter of the lesion may render the similarity between these nonglomus tumors and the true paraganglion cell tumors only superficial.

Schwannoma of the ninth, tenth, or eleventh cranial nerves may cause enlargement of the jugular foramen.[43] Neuromas enlarging any of the foramina at the base of the skull, including the jugular foramen, may cause a smooth-walled defect with preservation of the cortical margin. The leading edge may be scalloped. Large lesions cause more extensive and more erosive destruction.

Although schwannomas may appear "vascular" at angiography or on CT, the degree of vascularity usually does not approach that of glomus tumors. Difficulty in

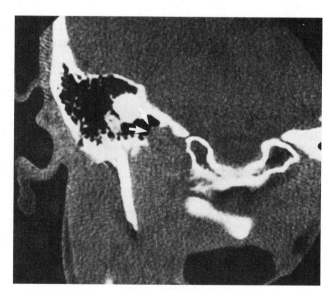

Fig. 16-144. Ninth cranial nerve neuroma. Coronal CT section. Soft tissue tumor extends into parapharyngeal space. There is erosion of bone delimiting inferior peritubal cells *(arrows)*.

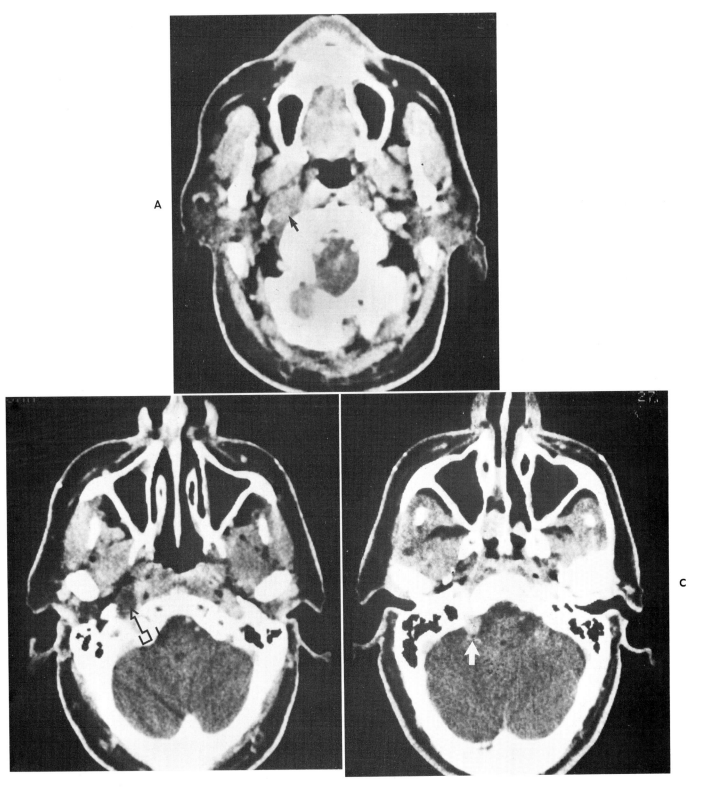

Fig. 16-145. Tenth cranial nerve neuroma. **A,** Soft tissue mass lateral to longus colli muscles is visible on right *(arrow)*. **B,** At slightly different level mass *(arrow)* has diminished attenuation values, suggesting either cystic necrosis or fatty degeneration. **C,** A small nubbin of tumor *(arrow)* intrudes into posterior fossa.

differential diagnosis could arise in the very small tumor that has just eroded into the mesotympanum from the region of the jugular foramen. In this circumstance the arteriographic differences between a glomus jugulare and a vascular neuroma could pose a diagnostic problem. Subselective arteriography, however, might help distinguish the two on the basis of vascular supply.

Congenital epidermoidomas (cholesteatomas)

Congenital epidermoidomas (cholesteatomas) (Figs. 16-146 and 16-147) arise from ectodermal rests and may show diminished attenuation at CT. There is no enhancement. The lesions are typically expansile, with scalloped borders and significant cortical bone disruption if the lesion is sufficiently large. These lesions are uncommon. As of 1975 only 36 cases had been reported in the petrous apex.[102]

Primary cholesteatomas arising in the skull base near the jugular foramen may mimic glomus jugulare tumors or metastases. The fact that cholesteatomas are avascu-

lar lesions may be helpful in the differential diagnosis. Primary cholesteatomas arising in the middle ear cleft are radiologically indistinguishable from acquired cholesteatomas.

Meningiomas

It is well accepted that meningiomas arising from adjacent arachnoid villi may invade the temporal bone as a secondary manifestation of the disease. Occasionally they may appear as ear neoplasms. The site of invasion into the temporal bone depends on the site of the primary tumor.[52,90] The invasion can be through the tegmen, the petrous apex, the internal acoustic canal, or the hypotympanum by way of the jugular foramen or other nearby structures. Having reached the middle ear cleft, the meningioma may appear as a soft tissue mass within the ear. Perforation of the tympanic membrane can result in presentation of the tumor in the external acoustic canal.

Primary meningiomas arising within the middle ear

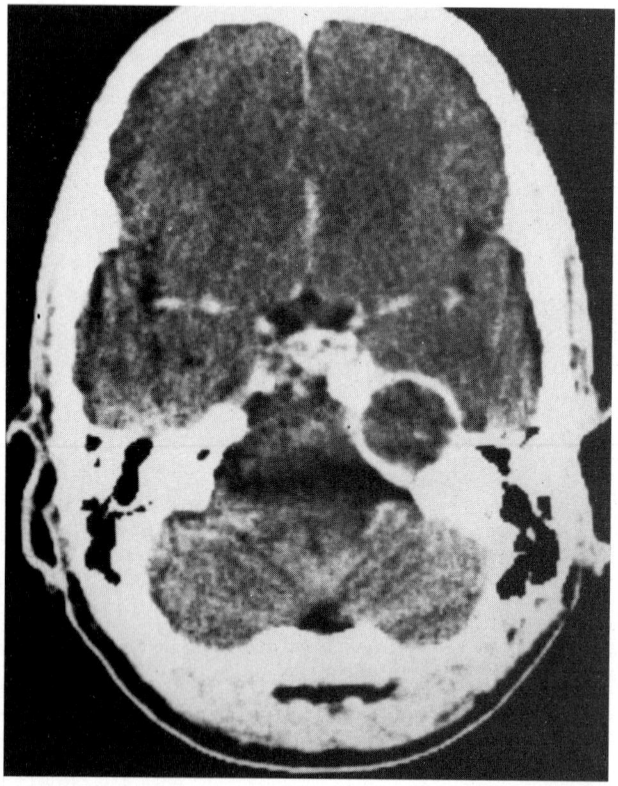

Fig. 16-146. Primary cholesteatoma (epidermoidoma) of petrous apex. There is expansile lesion within apex that has remodeled medial tip of petrous portion of temporal bone. Attenuation values of mass were slightly below that of brain; it was not enhanced. Remainder of temporal bone was free of inflammatory disease. This represents primary epidermoidoma of temporal bone. (Courtesy Peter Som, M.D., New York.)

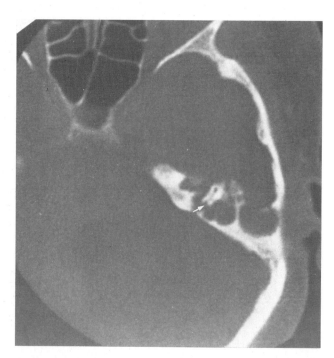

Fig. 16-147. Primary cholesteatoma. Lesion involves temporal bone extensively. There is expansion with scalloped margination at leading edges of tumor. Capsular bone has been destroyed about posterior limb of superior semicircular canal (*arrow*). Primary cholesteatomas are developmental inclusion tumors; cholesterin crystals may cause them to have fatlike density on CT scanning. More commonly their attenuation values resemble that of adjacent brain. In absence of infection there is little likelihood of enhancement on CT.

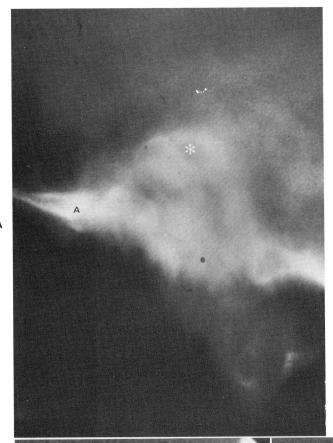

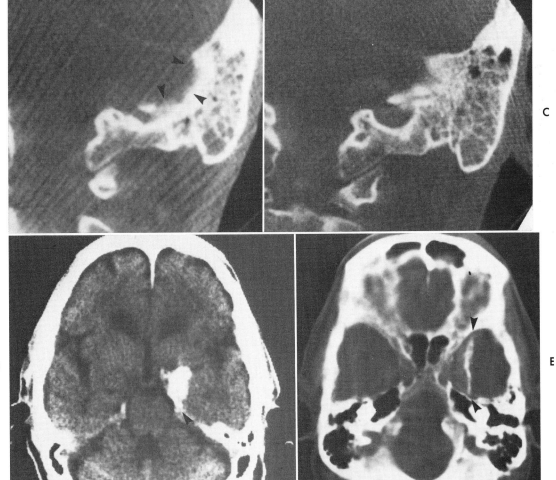

Fig. 16-148. Primary meningioma. **A,** Lateral tomogram, left temporal bone. Normal bony architecture has been destroyed. Lesion is infiltrative and lytic. Tumor was confined to temporal bone. *A,* Anterior; *asterisk,* internal acoustic canal. **B,** Axial tomogram, different case. Meningioma arose from petrous ridge, eroding it and invading mastoid cells. **C,** Section anterior to **B.** Mastoid cells are filled with tumor. **D,** Axial tomogram, different case. Calcified tumor has attachment to petrous apex. **E,** Scan section inferior to **D.** Meningioma extends along medial aspect of middle fossa, abutting on lesser wing of sphenoid.

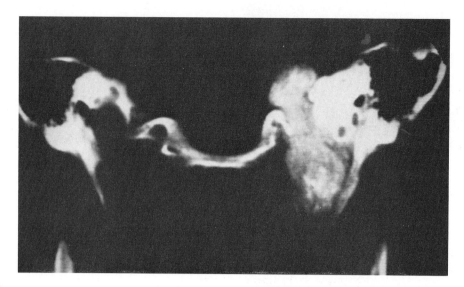

Fig. 16-149. Primary meningioma of temporal bone. CT, frontal view. Calcified transcranial lesion extends from posterior fossa through petro-occipital cleft into parapharyngeal space. This primary meningioma probably arose from arachnoid granulations located about jugular foramen.

cleft itself arise from ectopic arachnoid granulations (Figs. 16-148 and 16-149). Guzowski et al.[52] studied 200 temporal bones histopathologically and found the presence of arachnoid granulations in a surprising number of specimens. Their distribution is located primarily in four sites: along the greater superficial petrosal nerve, in the internal acoustic meatus, in the area around the geniculate ganglion, and in the jugular foramen.[90] Each of these sites therefore serves as a possible locus for the development of a primary temporal bone meningioma. Four such cases of primary meningioma of the temporal bone arising either within the middle ear cleft or mastoid are reported by Guzowski et al.[52]

Fibro-osseous lesions—fibrous dysplasia, ossifying fibroma

The fibro-osseous lesions (see Figs. 16-118 and 16-119) affect the temporal bone as an isolated finding only rarely. Barrionuevo[7] reviewed 27 cases from the world literature and added three more. Twenty-four of the thirty were of the monostotic form, five were polyostotic, and one was associated with the McCune-Albright syndrome (polyostotic fibrous dysplasia with skin hyperpigmentation and endocrine disturbances [precocious puberty or hyperthyroidism]).

The mastoid and petrous portions of the bone are more commonly affected than the squamous portion. There may be areas of sclerosis or, alternatively, bone resorption with expansion. The mastoid cortex may be enlarged and the rarefaction of the septa of the air cells may create the impression of a large cystic lesion. The inner ear, internal auditory canal, fallopian canal, and vestibular aqueduct usually are not involved.

Levine et al.[75] believe that both histologic and radiologic distinction may be made between fibrous dysplasia and ossifying fibroma. It is their belief that ossifying fibroma is characterized radiologically by an ovoid or circular expansile lesion with distinct boundaries and thinning of the cortical bone, giving an eggshell appearance. Their case report includes a CT scan showing an expansile lesion of the temporal squama. Other contemporary workers in the field categorize all lesions—both sclerotic and cystic—under the broader term *fibro-osseous dysplasias*.

The progress of fibrous dysplasia is slow, and enlargement of the temporal bone region and hearing loss are the usual clinical complaints. There is frequent obstruction of the external acoustic canal and this may be responsible for cholesteatoma formation.

Metastatic disease of the temporal bone

Metastasis to the base of the skull in the region of the jugular foramen can mimic a glomus jugulare tumor (Fig. 16-150).

Metastatic disease of the temporal bone is rare.[138] In the age group most vulnerable to metastatic spread, the temporal bone marrow has been largely replaced by rather avascular fat.[80] The pathogenesis of tumor spread is from petrous apex bone marrow, essentially the only functioning marrow site in an older individual's temporal bones; there is extension later into the mesotympanum and antrum.[1,14]

Meningeal carcinomatosis is characterized by a peculiar predilection for invasion of the internal acoustic canal, often bilaterally, with destruction of cranial nerves VII and VIII. There may be growth into the

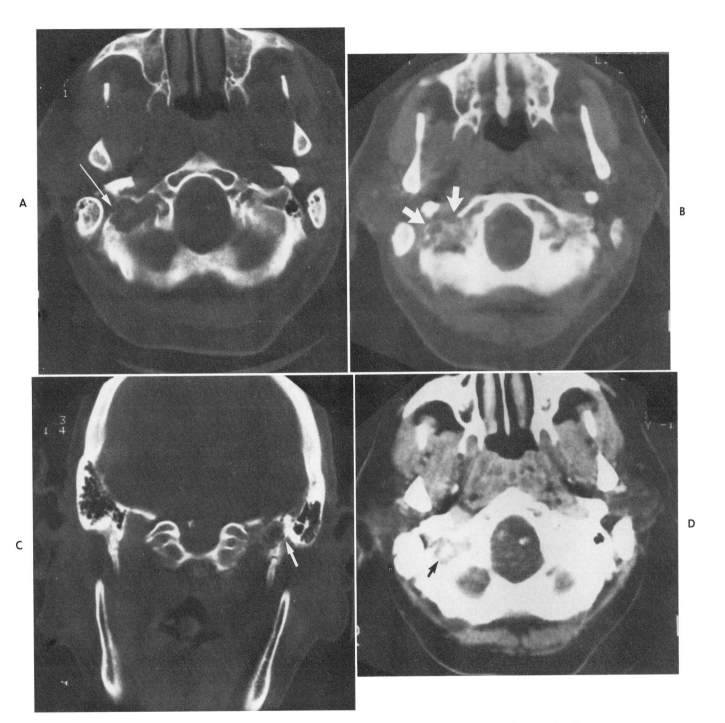

Fig. 16-150. Metastatic adenocarcinoma. Destructive lesion in skull base involves jugular foramen. Epicenter of lesion, however, is more laterally placed than usual glomus jugulare tumor and extension is chiefly lateral, involving stylomastoid foramen. **A,** Axial view. Arrow points to stylomastoid foramen. **B,** Section taken 5 mm from **A,** showing extensive destruction *(arrows).* **C,** Coronal view. Jugular tubercle and hypoglossal canal are intact. Destruction is both superior and lateral, involving base of styloid process and abutting against digastric groove *(arrow).* **D,** There is minimal enhancement of lesion. Some calcific debris lies within central portion *(arrow).* Patient's initial symptoms were that of facial nerve palsy; that finding alone speaks strongly against glomus jugulare tumor, despite superficial resemblance of two lesions on causal examination of CT scans.

cochlea, vestibule, and semicircular canals. The membranous labyrinth may be invaded as well as the cochlear and endolymphatic ducts.[54] Berlinger et al.[14] report metastatic malignant melanoma with bilateral eighth nerve involvement related to meningeal spread.

Leukemia may cause diffuse, random involvement of the temporal bone, with infiltration of the marrow spaces and the internal auditory and facial canals. Gapany-Gapanavicius et al.[44] reported an unusual case of histiocytic malignant lymphoma with a primary appearance in the middle ear cleft of a young woman. This is only the third case of primary lymphoma within the middle ear cleft reported. The patient died 14 months later of fulminant lymphoma.

Primary tumors that can metastasize to the temporal bone include breast, lung, thyroid, kidney, and prostate. Squamous cell lesions, adenocarcinomas, and sarcomas have been reported as metastasizing to the temporal bone (Fig. 16-151). Tumors of adjacent structures, the pinna, nasopharynx, sphenoid region, parotid, and central nervous system, can involve the temporal bone by direct extension.[138]

Facial neuromas

Facial nerve neuromas arise with equal frequency throughout the course of the nerve.[109] Once the nerve has left the brainstem and traversed the cisternal space it is enclosed within an osseous conduit throughout the remainder of its course in the temporal bone. Facial neuromas erode the bone and do so early in the natural history of the disease because of their intimate relationship within this protective bony tube. However, except for the portion that lies within the internal acoustic canal and the proximal labyrinthine segment, the bone

is not particularly thick surrounding the remainder of the nerve, at least not throughout its circumference. Through a large part of its course the nerve is in a thin-walled canal that lies adjacent to large "empty" spaces: the epidural space near its geniculate portion, the tympanic cavity in its mesotympanic portion, and the pneumatized mastoid in its vertical portion. Therefore while bone erosion may occur early, the tumor may grow to relatively large size, decompressing into adjacent "empty" spaces before clinical symptoms become sufficiently compeling to bring about investigation.

Facial neuromas are actually nerve sheath tumors, schwannomas, and usually arise from the sensory portion of the nerve. Symptoms produced depend on the site of origin and the size of the tumor. The most common symptom is facial paralysis. Paralysis is by no means always present, however, nor is it necessarily the earliest or most prominent symptom. Symptoms may be only disorders in tearing, salivation, or taste, or hearing loss.

Facial neuromas may cause (1) enlargement and erosion of the internal acoustic canal (internal acoustic canal segment) (Fig. 16-152), (2) destruction of the otic capsule near the geniculate ganglion with or without presentation of a soft tissue mass in the epidural space within the middle cranial fossa (labyrinthine segment), (3) the presence of a soft tissue mass with substantial erosion of ossicular structures and the otic capsule (intratympanic segment), (4) focal or diffuse enlargement of the facial canal (Fig. 16-153), and (5) destruction of the pneumatic cells within the mastoid with possible bony dehiscence into the posterior fossa and the region of the jugular foramen (mastoid segment). The tumor may break into the mesotympanum, eroding large por-

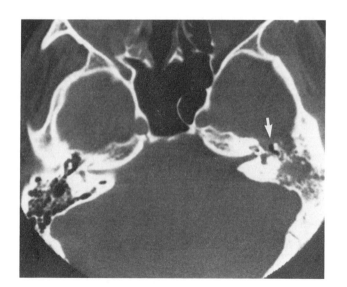

Fig. 16-151. Metastasis of tumor to temporal bone. Notice widespread destruction of temporal bone, with loss of tegmen (*arrow*) and destruction in region of antrum and in periantral area. Jugular foramen was normal. Primary lesion was esthesioneuroblastoma of nasal cavity that had been treated 18 months earlier.

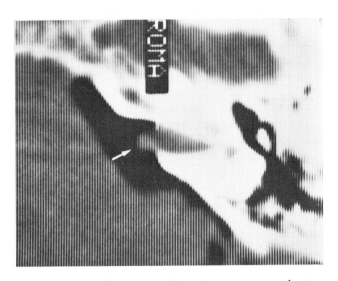

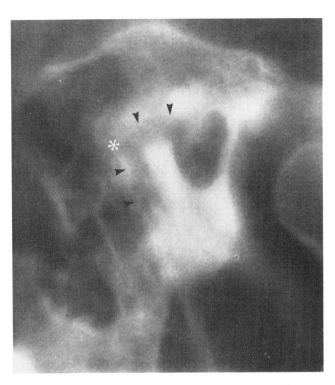

Fig. 16-152. Facial neuroma. Gas cisternogram, axial view. There is gas in cerebellopontine angle cistern, outlining soft tissue tumor within internal acoustic canal and protruding slightly into cistern *(arrow)*. Patient had sensorineural hearing loss. Surgery showed this to be facial neuroma involving segment within internal acoustic canal and immediately adjacent cisternal portion. Both clinical and radiologic findings suggested an acoustic neuroma.

Fig. 16-153. Facial neuroma in tympanic and mastoid portions. Complex motion tomogram, lateral view. Patient had extensive neuroma involving most of intratympanic portion, second genu, and mastoid segment of facial nerve. Asterisk is at level of second genu.

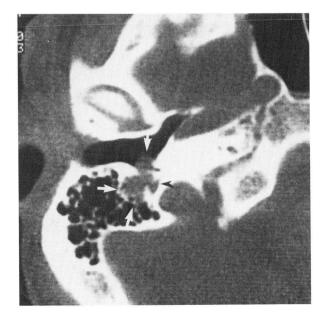

Fig. 16-154. Facial nerve neuroma. Patient is 24-year-old man who had been followed for Bell's palsy for 5 years. Symptoms were slow in onset and progressive. Tumor of mastoid portion of facial nerve eroded into posterior portion of middle ear cavity and filled both facial recess and sinus tympani. It is also expanded posteriorly into adjacent mastoid air cells.

tions of the posterior wall and roof and floor of the external acoustic canal (Fig. 16-154).

It should be noted that this tumor is a benign tumor that causes significant erosion in the middle and outer ear. Other than facial neuromas, most other neoplastic processes associated with bone destruction within the middle ear and external acoustic canal are malignant.

No radiologic pursuit of facial nerve neuroma is complete without examination of every portion of the nerve. The internal acoustic canal may be widened or flared as with an acoustic neuroma. On the other hand, the internal acoustic canal may be normal appearing and yet be the site of a small facial nerve neuroma. For this reason the diagnosis should not be ruled out radiologically without a gas cisternogram if clinical conviction is strong.

In the work-up of a patient for facial neuroma, the radiologist should be mindful of several facts.

1. The facial nerve lies in the superior compartment of the internal acoustic canal; the presence of a small facial nerve neuroma may be betrayed by erosion of the crista falciformis or inferior displacement thereof. The findings may be indistinguishable from those of a small acoustic neuroma.

2. An erosive lesion near the region of the geniculate ganglion should always raise the possibility of a facial neuroma. These patients need not necessarily have facial paralysis.

3. Soft tissue lesion within the middle ear associated with conductive hearing loss and ossicular destruction should also raise the possibility of a facial neuroma. Sensorineural loss associated with a middle ear mass may be caused by invasion of the cochlea.

4. Soft tissue lesions with bone destruction in the region of the mastoid portion of the facial canal, when the pneumatic cells remote from the area of abnormality show no evidence of chronic ear disease, should raise the possibility of a facial nerve neuroma.

5. Facial nerve neuromas may be relatively localized tumors or they may spread over substantial distances of the nerve. There can be generalized widening of the facial canal all the way from the geniculate ganglion through the stylomastoid foramen in extensive lesions. On the other hand, the lesion may be very localized. On occasion it may undergo fatty degeneration. Diminished attenuation values on CT scanning should alert the radiologist to the possibility of fatty degeneration of a facial nerve neuroma as well as raise the possibility of a nonneoplastic, cholesterin-bearing lesion. Reports confirming the use of radiologic studies in diagnosis of facial neuromas have been published by Shambaugh et al.[126] and by Pulec.[108]

Acoustic neuromas

The radiologic diagnosis of small acoustic neuromas has occupied the interest of clinicians and radiologists for decades. The task has become enormously simplified with the advent of CT. Large acoustic tumors have always been easy to diagnose because bony changes are frequently concomitant with most of the tumors.

Most (greater than 95%) acoustic neuromas take their origin at Scarpa's ganglion in the superior vestibular division of the acoustic nerve, located at the junction of the lateral and middle thirds of the upper compartment of the internal acoustic canal. The nerve is encased in thick, dense bone at this point and any circumferential growth is accompanied by remodeling and erosion of the contours of the canal (Figs. 16-155 to 16-157).

Tumor growth takes the path of least resistance and thus the neuroma grows medially toward the porus acusticus, finally escaping into the cerebellopontine angle cistern. Left undisturbed the tumor expands further. Depending on the vectors of tumor growth, the cistern may become filled with tumor and obliterated or may be widened. The cisternal space widens as a result of brainstem displacement toward the opposite side caused by the leading edge of the tumor. Eventually the tumor may indent the stem itself.

If there is anterior growth, the tumor slips through the incisural notch and grows in a dumbell configuration into the medial aspect of the middle cranial fossa.

Posterior growth may cause cerebellar edema and displacement, with or without rotation, effacement, or displacement of the fourth ventricle from the midline

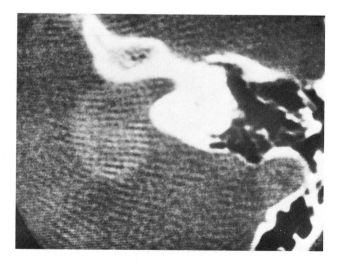

Fig. 16-155. Acoustic neuroma. Contrast-enhanced CT, axial view. Most acoustic neuromas take their origin from within lateral one third of internal acoustic canal. They grow medially, remodeling and widening canal and frequently amputating or foreshortening posterior lip. Tumor then disgorges into cerebellopontine angle cistern.

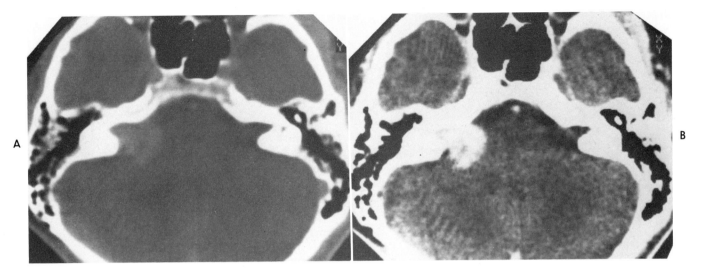

Fig. 16-156. Acoustic neuroma. **A,** CT scan, bone window. There is widening of internal acoustic canal on right with foreshortening of posterior lip. **B,** Manipulation of window level and window width demonstrates enhanced tumor that fills widened canal and spills into cerebellopontine angle cistern. These findings should suggest acoustic neuroma. Extremely rarely, facial neuroma beginning within internal acoustic canal can cause similar findings.

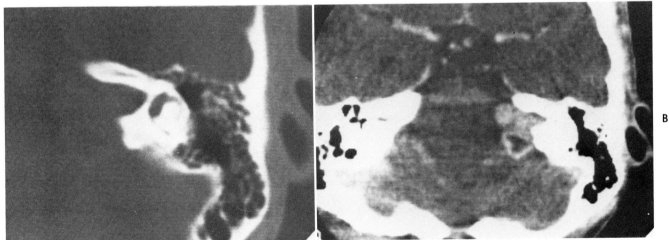

Fig. 16-157. Acoustic neuroma. **A,** Axial CT scan shows flaring of internal acoustic canal with amputation of posterior lip. **B,** Postcontrast study shows that part of tumor is solid and portion of it is cystic.

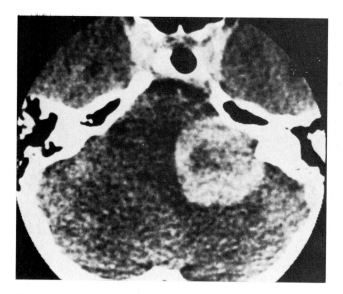

Fig. 16-158. Acoustic neuroma with central necrosis. Lesion extends almost to midline. There is cerebellar edema.

(Fig. 16-158). There is no significant anteroposterior displacement of the fourth ventricle.

Tumors reaching large size regularly displace and compress the aqueduct of Sylvius, causing obstructive hydrocephalus.

Radiologic diagnosis. The radiologic diagnosis of acoustic neuroma may be inferred on the basis of bone changes as evidenced either on plain films, complex motion tomographic studies, or CT with bone window review. Acoustic tumors may be diagnosed with greater certainty radiologically if the tumor mass itself and its attenuation characteristics are identified by CT.

Iophendylate (Pantopaque) cisternography, a mainstay in the diagnosis of small acoustic tumors since the 1960s,[16] has been largely superceded in contemporary imaging departments (Fig. 16-159). This is not because Iophendylate is a poor agent but rather because the technical failure rate of the examination is relatively high—there are false positive examinations and many equivocal results.[39,94,129] There is also the unlikely but remote specter of arachnoiditis attendant to the use of this agent in this clinical circumstance.[12] One of the chief objections to the use of intracranial Iophendylate since 1974 has been the artifacts that it generates with CT. Because CT is used in the follow-up and management of these patients postoperatively, its preoperative

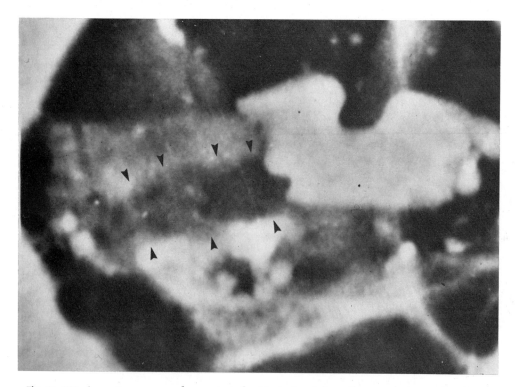

Fig. 16-159. Acoustic neuroma demonstrated with iophendylate (Pantopaque). Small-volume iophendylate study shows failure of contrast medium to enter internal acoustic canal *(arrows)*. Tumor measuring 9 mm was removed. Pantopaque remains, however.

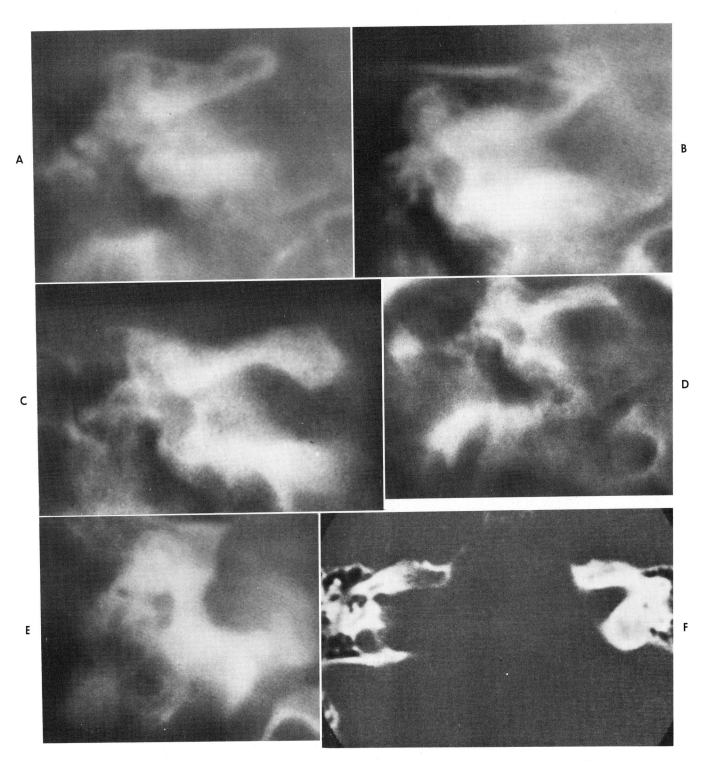

Fig. 16-160. Plain film manifestation of acoustic neuroma. **A,** Flaring of internal acoustic canal. **B,** Flaring of superior and inferior lips only of internal acoustic canal. Patient had tumor of extracannalicular origin. **C,** Ballooning of central portion of canal. **D,** Erosion of inferior portion of petrous tip. **E** and **F,** Agressive bone destruction.

use with the attendant, relatively permanent intracranial entrapment of the agent, should not be taken lightly.

Angiography is reserved only for the complicated case or when the underlying pathology is in doubt. Classical pneumoencephalography no longer has a place in contemporary acoustic neuroma radiologic workup.

Changes in the bone as demonstrated on plain films, complex motion tomography, and CT (Fig. 16-160).

INTRACANALICULAR LESIONS. The internal acoustic canal may be normal or may show one or more of the following:

1. Inferior displacement of the falciform crest
2. Erosion (disappearance) of the falciform crest
3. Enlargement of the internal acoustic canal

Regarding this enlargement, a 1 mm greater vertical dimension than the opposite side at a comparable measuring point may be present (may be a normal variant). In addition, there may be in excess of 2 mm greater vertical dimension than the opposite side at a comparable measuring point (likelihood of acoustic neuroma is great).[145]

Finally, a flared or trumpet-shaped internal acoustic canal may be present.

SMALL LESIONS. Lesions defined as intruding not more than 1.5 cm into the cisternal space may show any or all of the above findings but additionally will frequently show increased flaring of the canal and erosion of the posterior lip, with shortening of the internal acoustic canal.

INTERMEDIATE-SIZE AND LARGE TUMORS. There is a variable amount of bony change. Once the tumor enters the cisternal space one may not correlate tumor size with the degree of bone destruction. It is possible to have a massive tumor with only very moderate bony change. On the other hand, a large degree of bony change is almost always accompanied by a very large tumor.

Intermediate-size tumors may show the findings enumerated above, with exaggeration of degree, and early erosion of both the superior and inferior lips of the internal acoustic canal and posterior lip. There may be remodeling (excavation) of the posterior surface of the petrous pyramid. Large tumors may show extensive erosion of the petrous portion (variable) or minimal erosion of the petrous portion (variable).

Demonstration of soft tissue mass (Fig. 16-161). Contemporary radiologic work-up of acoustic neuromas dictates assessment of the internal acoustic canal and petrous portion of the temporal bone, preferably by CT. This is then followed by a CT scan performed both without and with intravenous iodinated compounds. The detection rate of acoustic neuromas with CT without contrast enhancement approaches 60%. With contrast enhancement virtually all of the intermediate-size and large tumors are identified. The majority of acoustic neuromas are enhanced; the enhancement may be homogeneous, nonhomogeneous, or rimlike. The latter circumstance is rare and occurs only with those tumors that have undergone significant cystic degeneration and necrosis.

METRIZAMIDE CISTERNOGRAPHY AND GAS CISTERNOGRAPHY (Figs. 16-162 to 1-169). An intracanalicular acoustic neuroma may demonstrate either no plain film

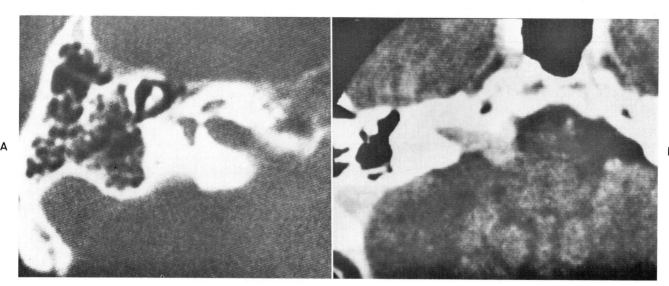

Fig. 16-161. Acoustic neuroma. **A,** "Bone window" CT showed no evidence of abnormal internal acoustic canal. **B,** Notice small enhanced tumor spilling from canal into cisternal space, as demonstrated following injection of intravenous iodinated contrast medium.

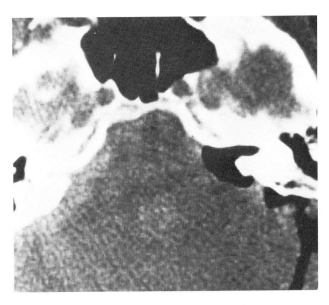

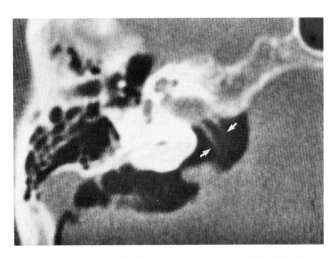

Fig. 16-162. Normal internal acoustic canal as demonstrated on gas CT cisternography. Internal acoustic canal and cerebellopontine angel cistern immediately adjacent to it are filled with gas. Even small canals usually fill with ease.

Fig. 16-163. Intracanalicular acoustic neuroma. Gas CT cisternogram. Tumor filled internal acoustic canal. Seventh *(anterior arrow)* and eighth *(posterior arrow)* cranial nerves are demonstrated as they cross cisternal space. Normally they are closer together but tumor had splayed them apart.

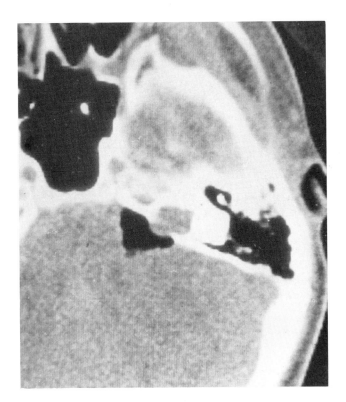

Fig. 16-164. Intracanalicular acoustic neuroma. CT cisternography. Leading edge of tumor barely intrudes into cisternal space.

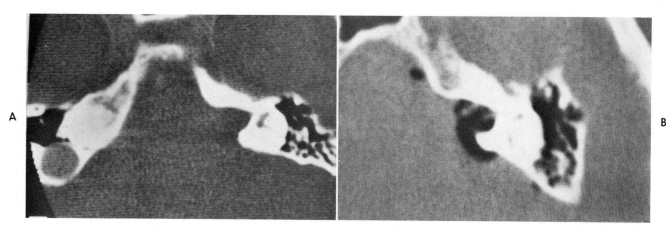

Fig. 16-165. Patulous internal acoustic canal. Gas CT cisternogram. **A,** Patient had sensori-neural hearing loss on left side and was thought to have acoustic neuroma. Complex motion tomography showed a widened canal. CT scan with bone review in axial projection confirmed presence of wide, flared canal. (Notice unrelated high jugular bulb on opposite side.) **B,** Gas CT cisternography shows that internal acoustic canal was merely patulous. Normal nerve structures are identified. There is no evidence of tumor. Gas CT cisternography is definitive in most circumstances when used to exclude presence of acoustic neuroma. Dependency on bone changes alone would have led to false positive diagnosis of acoustic neuroma in this patient.

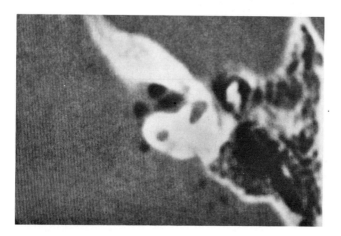

Fig. 16-166. Arachnoid adhesions. Gas CT cisternogram. Bubbles of gas are identified within widened internal acoustic canal. Multiple webs were demonstrated at various levels.

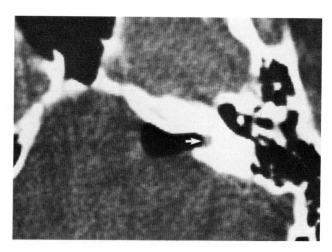

Fig. 16-167. Ganglioneuroma. Gas CT cisternogram. Tumor measuring 3 mm and arising from fundal portion of eighth nerve was identified at surgery *(arrow).*

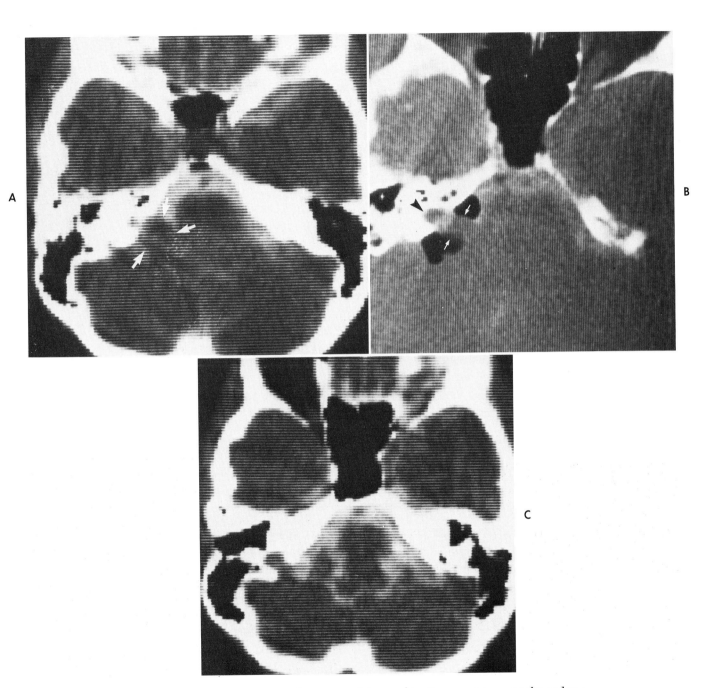

Fig. 16-168. Acoustic neuroma as demonstrated by combination gas cisternography and metrizamide. **A,** Cerebellopontine angle tumor demonstrated with metrizamide alone *(arrows)*. **B,** Cerebellopontine angle tumor demonstrated with gas alone *(arrows)*. **C,** Brainstem has been outlined by metrizamide. There is no evidence of deformity of stem by tumor.

Fig. 16-169. Acoustic neuroma, combination study. Gas and metrizamide cisternography. **A,** Small tumor within cerebellopontine angle cistern is outlined by gas *(arrows)*. **B,** Metriza-mide outlines brainstem and shows that there is no indenting of stem by tumor.

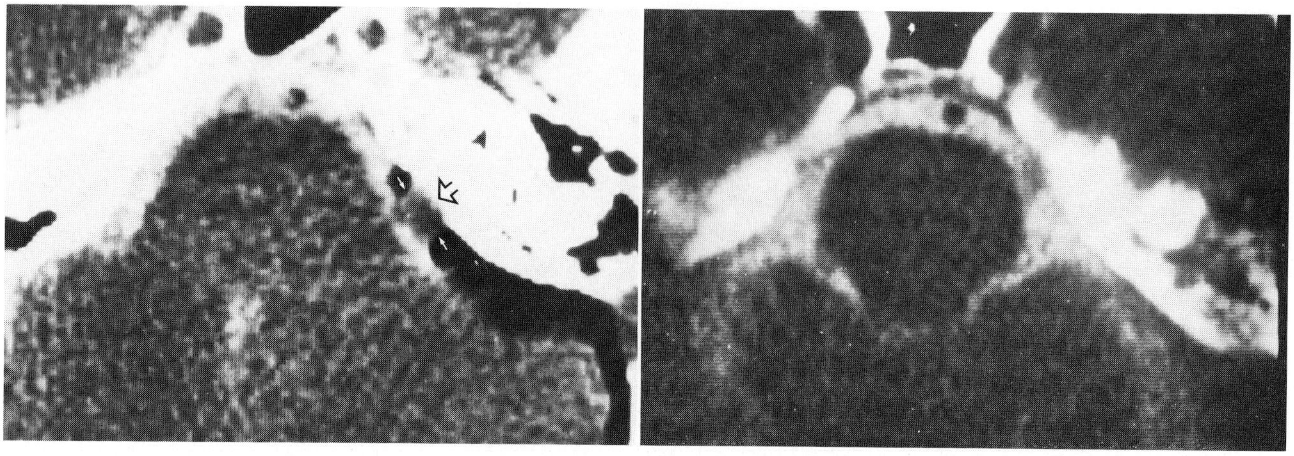

changes or only equivocal ones and may escape detection on routine CT with and without iodinated intravenous contrast medium. The small acoustic neuroma that protrudes less than 1 cm into the cisternal space may similarly prove elusive. These two circumstances prompted the development of alternative diagnostic studies that would alter the x-ray absorption in the subarachnoid space within both the cerebellopontine angle cistern and its extensions into the internal acoustic canal.

Metrizamide, an aqueous contrast agent miscible with cerebrospinal fluid, was introduced into clinical use in the United States in the late 1970.[115] This is a positive contrast agent. The use of a negative contrast agent, air or carbon dioxide, was introduced only slightly later.[70,130]

If the CT scan does not provide positive tumor identification in patients thought to have acoustic neuroma, the possibility that an intracanalicular or very small acoustic neuroma exists. We prefer negative contrast media and use carbon dioxide gas as the agent. Carbon dioxide is favored over air because the morbidity (headache) is reduced by the use of carbon dioxide.

Gas cisternography is a definitive examination for the presence of a tumor either within the cerebellopontine angle cistern or within the internal acoustic canal. Intracanalicullar tumors as small as 3 mm have been identified with this technique (Fig. 16-167).

Some workers prefer positive contrast agents rather than gas, recognizing that partial volume effects around the tumor edges are responsible for slight underestimation of tumor size when gas is used.

It is our practice to confine the use of an aqueous, positive contrast agent to the work-up of large tumor in order to define the relationship between the tumor and the brainstem. It is almost impossible to demonstrate this dependent anatomy when using a gaseous contrast agent. With the miscible water-soluble contrast agents, however, this is easily obtainable. In the equivocal case as well, when the diagnosis of an intra-axial versus an extra-axial tumor is in question, metrizamide may provide the best agent to demonstrate the relationship of the tumor to the brainstem.

Other tumors within the cerebellopontine angle

Three other tumors enter into the differential diagnosis of lesions within the cerebellopontine angle: (1) cerebellopontine angle meningioma, (2) epidermoidoma, and (3) fifth cranial nerve neuroma.

Cerebellopontine meningioma. Meningiomas (Figs. 16-170 to 16-172) tend to have a broader-based attachment to the posterior surface of the petrous bone as compared to acoustic neuromas. The principal distinction lies in the fact that the internal acoustic canal is not enlarged as compared to an acoustic neuroma. Meningiomas frequently calcify. Enhancement of the meningioma on the CT scan is usually more dense. Venous engorgement of the vessels on the free border of the tentorium tends to be more prominent with meningiomas than with acoustic neuromas.

Epidermoidomas. Epidermoidomas (congenital cholesteatomas) may arise within the cerebellopontine angle cistern and may reach enormous size. These lesions tend not to be enhanced and frequently have attenuation values below that of water because of their fat content. The internal acoustic canal is again normal.

Fifth cranial nerve neuromas. Fifth cranial nerve neuromas begin in the region of the semilunar ganglion on

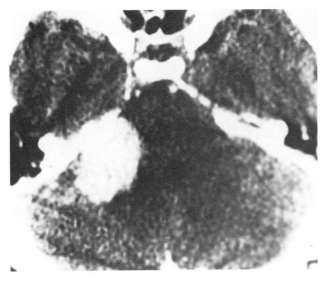

Fig. 16-170. Cerebellopontine angle meningioma. CT with contrast medium, axial projection. Intensely enhanced lesion was partially calcified on noncontrast study. Internal acoustic canal was normal.

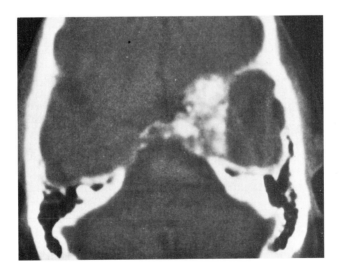

Fig. 16-171. Meningioma arising from petrous apex. Calcified lesion arose from apex and extended anteriorly along medial wall of middle cranial fossa.

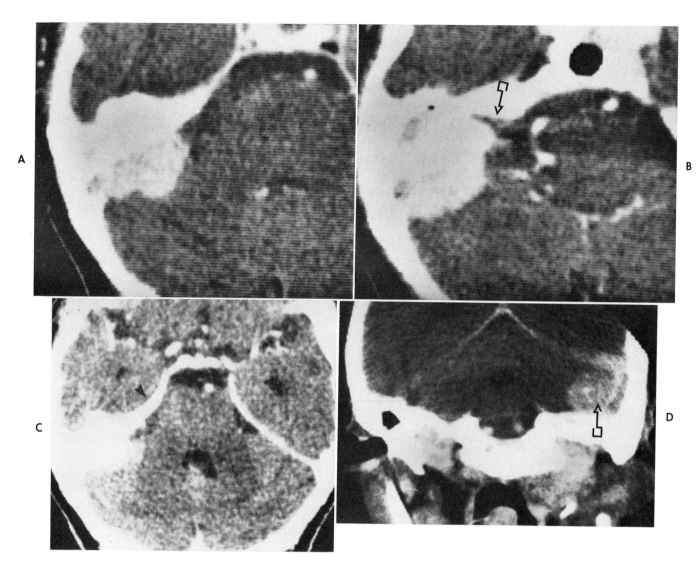

Fig. 16-172. Meningioma, cerebellopontine angle. **A,** CT, axial view after injection of contrast medium. Notice intense enhancement of lesion and its broad attachment to posterior surface of petrous portion. **B,** Epicenter of lesion is posterior to small internal acoustic canal *(arrow)*. **C,** Edge of tentorium on affected side *(arrow)* appears broader than on normal side. This is caused by engorgement of draining veins and is seen with meningiomas in this area, not acoustic neuromas. **D,** Coronal view. Notice position of lesion with respect to tentorium and cerebellopontine angle cistern.

the anteromedial surface of the petrous tip. On occasion these lesions will have a large posterior fossa component, sometimes far larger than the middle cranial fossa portion. Bone destruction involves the tip of the petrous apex and the anterior surface as well as the posterior surface. The internal acoustic canal is normal. The tumors tend to be enhanced on contrast CT scans.

It should be noted that the clinical finding of a fifth cranial nerve lesion is not always helpful in distinguishing fifth cranial nerve neuromas from acoustic neuro-

mas. Almost all acoustic neuromas, once they reach the intermediate size or larger, are accompanied by fifth cranial nerve findings as well as eighth cranial nerve disorders.

Tumors involving other cranial nerves at the base of the skull (neuromas of the ninth, tenth, eleventh, and twelfth cranial nerves) cause erosion of the inferior and posterior surfaces of the petrous portion. The soft tissue mass of the tumor is frequently enhanced on CT examination. A discussion of the diagnosis and differential diagnosis of these lesions is found in Chapter 13.

☐ **References**

1. Adams, W.: The etiology of swimmer's exostoses of the external auditory canals and of associated changes in hearing. J. Laryngol. Otol. **65**:133, 1951.

2. Anderson, R.D., Liebeskind, A., Schechter, M.M., and Zingesser, L.H.: Aneurysms of the internal carotid artery in the carotid canal of the petrous temporal bone, Radiology, **102**:639-642, 1972.

3. Anson, B.J., and Bast, T.H.: The surgical significance of stapedial and labyrinthine anatomy, Arch. Otolaryngol. **71**:188-206, 1960.

4. Anson, B.J., and Donaldson, J.A.: Surgical anatomy of the temporal bone, ed. 3, Philadelphia, 1981, W.B. Saunders Co.

5. Anson, B., Harper, D., and Winch, T.: The vestibular and cochlear aqueducts: developmental and adult anatomy of their contents and parietes. Third symposium on the role of the vestibular organs in space exploration, NASA SP **152**:125, 1967.

6. Ballinger, P.W., editor: Merrill's atlas of radiographic positions and radiographic procedures, ed. 5, St. Louis, 1982, The C.V. Mosby Co.

7. Barrionuevo, C.E., Marcallo, F.A., Coelho, A., et al.: Fibrous dysplasia and the temporal bone, Arch. Otolaryngol. **106**:298-301, 1980.

8. Basek, M.: Anomalies of the facial nerve in normal temporal bones, Ann. Otol. Rhinol. Laryngol. **71**:392, 1962.

9. Bast, T.H., and Anson, B.J.: The temporal bone and ear, Springfield, Ill., 1949, Charles C. Thomas, Publisher.

10. Baxter, A.: Dehiscence of the fallopain canal, J. Laryngol. Otol. **85**:587, 1971.

11. Bergeron, R.T., and Rumbaugh, C.L.: The temporal bone. In Newton, T.H., and Potts, D.G.: Radiology of the skull and brain, St. Louis, 1971, The C.V. Mosby Co.

12. Bergeron, R.T., Rumbaugh, C.L., Fang, H., and Cravioto, H.: Experimental pantopaque arachnoiditis in the monkey, Radiology 99:95-101, 1971.

13. Bergstrom, LaV.: Pathology of congenital deafness: present status and future priorities, Ann. Otol. Rhinol. Laryngol. **89**(suppl. 74):31-42, 1980.

14. Berliner, N.T., Koutroupas, S., Adams, G., and Maisel, R.: Patterns of involvement of the temporal bone in metastatic and systemic malignancy, Laryngoscope **90**:619-627, 1980.

15. Blümm, R.: Direct sagittal (positional) computed tomography of the head, Neuroradiology **22**:199-201, 1982.

16. Britton, B.H., Hitselberger, W.E., and Hurley, B.J.: Iophendylate examination of posterior fossa in the diagnosis of cerebellopontine angle tumors, Arch. Otolaryngol. **88**:60-71, 1968.

17. Buffin, J.T., and Buck-Barrett, R.: Sarcoma of the ear in children: two case histories, J. Laryngol. Otol. **87**:95-98, 1973.

18. Chandler, J.H.: Malignant external otitis, Laryngoscope **78**:1257-1294, 1968.

19. Chandler, J.H.: Pathogenesis and treatment of facial paralysis due to malignant external otitis, Ann. Otol. Rhinol. Laryngol. **81**:648, 1972.

20. Chandler, J.H.: Malignant external otitis: further considerations, Ann. Otol. Rhinol. Laryngol. **86**:417-428, 1977.

21. Chen, K.T., and Dehner, L.P.: Primary tumors of the external and middle ear: introduction and pathologic study of squamous cell carcinoma, Arch. Otolaryngol. **104**:247-252, 1978.

22. Chen, K.T., and Dehner, L.P.: Primary tumors of the external and middle ear. II. A clinicopathological study of 14 paragangliomas and three meningiomas, Arch. Otolaryngol. **104**:253-259, 1978.

23. Clark, J.L., DeSanto, L.W., and Facer, G.W.: Congenital deafness and spontaneous CSF otorrhea, Arch. Otolaryngol. **104**:163-166, 1978.

24. Claus, E., Le Mahieu, S.F., and Ernould, D.: The most used otoradiological projections, J. Belge Radiol. **63**:183-203, 1980.

25. Cohen, A., and Rosenwasser, H.: Fibrous dysplasia of the temporal bone, Arch. Otolaryngol. **89**:447-459, 1969.

26. Cole, J.M.: Glomus jugulare tumors, Laryngoscope **87**:1244-1258, 1977.

27. Collins, J.M., Forbes, G.S., Harner, S.G., et al.: Preferred scanning planes of the petrous bone in high resolution CT, Presented at The Sixty-seventh Annual Meeting of the Radiological Society of North America, Chicago, Nov. 15-20, 1981.

28. Conley, J., and Hildeyard, V.: Aneurysm of the internal carotid artery presenting in the middle ear, Arch. Otolaryngol. **90**:35-38, 1969.

29. Coser, P.L., Stamm, A.E.C., Lobo, R.C., and Pinto, J.A.: Malignant external otitis in infants, Laryngoscope **90**:312-316, 1980.

30. Davis, D.O., and Rumbaugh, C.L.: The temporal bone. Newton, T.H., and Potts, D.G., editors: Radiology of the skull and brain, St. Louis, 1971, The C.V. Mosby Co.

31. Denia, A., Perez, F., Canalis, R.R., and Graham, M.D.: Extracanalicular osteomas of the temporal bone, Arch. Otolaryngol. **105**:706-709, 1979.

32. De Smedt, E., Potvliege, R., Pimontel-Appel, B., et al.: High resolution CT-scan of the temporal bone: a preliminary report, J. Belge Radiol. **63**:205-212, 1980.

33. Dunkin, D., Shea, J., Sleecks, J., et al.: Bifurcation of the facial nerve, Arch. Otolaryngol. **86**:619, 1967.

34. Eckerdal, O., and Ahlquist, J.: External bony auditory canal and the tympanic bone, Acta. Radiol. fasc. 3 **21**:425-431, 1980.

35. Eldous, E.W., and Schinn, J.B.: Far advanced malignant external otitis: report of a survival, Laryngoscope **83**:1810-1815, 1973.

36. Everberg, G.: Investigations into unilateral total deafness and absence of vestibular function with a particular view to the x-ray appearances in the inner ear: polytomography of inner ear abnormalities, Acta. Otolaryngol. **52**:47-62, 1960.

37. Fairman, H.D.: Tumors of the middle ear cleft and temporal bone. In Ballantyne, J., and Groves, J. editors: Diseases of the ear, nose and throat, vol. 2, ed. 3, Philadelphia, 1971, J. B. Lippincott Co.

38. Farrell, F.W., and Hantz, O.: Protruding jugular bulb presenting as a middle ear mass: case report and brief review, AJR **128**:685-687, 1977.

39. Fisch, V.P., Neozoleki, J., and Wellaver, J.: Diagnostic value of meatocisternography, Arch. Otolaryngol. **101**:339-343, 1975.

40. Fischer, A.G.: A case of complete absence of both internal carotid arteries, J. Anat. Physiol. **48**:37-46, 1914.

41. Frankel, M., Fahey, D., and Alker, G.: Otogenic pneumocephalus secondary to chronic otitis media, Arch. Otolaryngol. **106**:437-439, July 1980.

42. Friedman, I., Harrison, D., Tucker, W., and Bird, E.: Electron microscopy of a rhabdomyosarcoma of the ear, J. Clin. Pathol. **18**:63, 1965.

43. Gacek, R.R.: Schwannoma of the jugular foramen, Ann. Otol. Rhinol. Laryngol. **85**:215-224, 1976.

44. Gapany-Gapanavicius, B., Chisin, R., and Weshler, Z.: Primary presentation of malignant lymphoma in middle ear cleft. Ann. Otol. Rhinol. Laryngol. **89**:180-183, 1980.

45. Gejrot, T.: Retrograde jugularography in the diagnosis of abnormality of the superior bulb of the internal jugular vein, Acta. Otolaryngol **57**:177-180, 1964.

46. Glassock, M.E., III, Dickins, J.R.E., Jackson, C.G., and Wiet, R.J.: Vascular anomalies of the middle ear, Laryngoscope **90**:77-88, 1980.

47. Goepfert, H., Cangir, A., Lindberg, R., and Ayala, A.: Rhabdomyosarcoma of the temporal bone: is surgical resection necessary? Arch. Otolaryngol. **105**:310-313, 1979.

48. Goodhill, V.: Ear diseases, deafness and dizziness, New York, 1979, Harper & Row, Publishers, Inc.

49. Goss and Mayo, editors: Gray's Anatomy, Philadelphia, 1959, Lea & Febiger.

50. Graham, M.D.: The jugular bulb: its anatomic and clinical considerations in contemporary otology, Laryngoscope 87:105-125, 1977.

51. Guillen, G.: Quelques apports aux techniques radio-otologiques modernes: l'incidence transorbitaire: la tomographie, Rev. Laryngol. 76:395-446, 1955.

52. Guzowski, J., Paparella, M.M., Rao, K.N., and Hoshino, T.: Meningiomas of the temporal bone, Laryngoscope 86:1141-1146, 1976.

53. Hamersmah, H.: Osteopetrosis (marble bone disease) of the temporal bone, Laryngoscope 80:1518, 1970.

54. Harbert, F., Liu, J.C., and Berry, R.G.: Metastatic malignant melanoma to both VIIIth nerves, J. Laryngol. Otol. 83:889-891, 1966.

55. Harwood-Nash, D.C.: Fractures of the petrous and tympanic parts of the temporal bone in children: a tomographic study of 35 cases, AJR 110:598-607, 1970.

56. Hawkins, J.: Vascular patterns of the membranous labyrinth, Third symposium on the role of the vestibular organs in space exploration, NASA SP 152:241, 1967.

57. Hesselink, J.R., Davis, K.R., and Taveras, J.M.: Selective arteriography of glomus tymanicum and jugulare tumors: techniques, normal and pathologic arterial anatomy, AJNR 2:289-297, 1981.

58. Hoffman, R.H., Brookler, K.H., and Bergeron, R.T.: Radiologic diagnosis of labyrinthitis ossificans, Ann. Otol. Rhinol. Laryngol. 88(2):253-257, 1979.

59. Hollinshead, W.H.: Anatomy for surgeons, vol. 1, The head and neck, ed. 2, New York, 1968, Harper & Row, Publishers, Inc.

60. Iurato, S.: Submicroscopic structure of the inner ear, New York, 1967, Pergamon Press, Inc.

61. Jafek, B.W., Nager, G.T., Strife, J., and Gayler, R.W.: Congenital aural atresia: an analysis of 311 cases, Trans. Am. Acad. Ophthalmol. Otolaryngol. 80:588-595, 1975.

62. Jahrsdoerfer, R.: Congenital malformations of the ear: analysis of 94 operations, Ann. Otol. Rhinol. Laryngol. 89:348-352, 1980.

63. Jahrsdoerfer, R.A.: The facial nerve in congenital middle ear malformations, Laryngoscope 91:1217-1225, 1981.

64. Jahrsdoerfer, R.A., Cail, W.S., and Cantrell, R.W.: Endolymphatic duct obstruction from a jugular bulb diverticulum, Ann. Otol. Rhinol. Laryngol. 90:619-623, 1981.

65. Jensen, J.: Malformations of the inner ear in deaf children, Acta. Radiol. 286:27-35, 1969.

66. Jensen, J., and Rovsing, H.: Tomography in congenital malformations of the middle ear, Radiology 90:268-275, 1968.

67. Johnson, G.A., and Korobkin, M.: Imaging techniques for multiplanar computed tomography, Radiology 144:829-834, 1982.

68. Kaneko, Y., Yuasa, R., Ise, I., et al.: Bone destruction due to the rupture of a cholesteatoma sac: a pathogenesis of bone destruction in aural cholesteatoma, Laryngoscope 90:1865-1871, 1980.

69. Kaseff, L.G., Nieberding, P.H., Shorago, G.W., and Huertas, G.: Fistula between the middle ear and subarachnoid space as a cause of recurrent meningitis: detection by means of thin-section, complex-motion tomography, Radiology 135:105-108, 1980.

70. Kricheff, I.I., Pinto, R.S., Bergeron, R.T., and Cohen, N.: Air-CT cisternography and canalography for small acoustic neuromas, AJNR 1:57-63, 1980.

71. Lapayowker, M.S., Liebman, E.P., Ronis, M.L., et al.: Presentation of the internal carotid artery as a tumor of the middle ear. Radiology 98:293-297, 1971.

72. Lasjaunias, P.: Craniofacial and upper cervical arteries, Baltimore, 1981, The Williams & Wilkins Co.

73. Lasjaunias, P., and Moret, J.: Normal and nonpathological variations in the angiographic aspects of the arteries of the middle ear, Neuroradiology 15(4):213-219, 1978.

74. Levine, P.A., Wiggins, R., Archibald, R.W.R., and Britt, R.: Ossifying fibroma of the head and neck: involvement of the temporal bone: an unusual and challenging site, Laryngoscope 91:720-725, 1981.

75. Lincoln, E., and Selle, M.: Tuberculosis in children, New York, 1963, McGraw-Hill Book Co.

76. Linthicum, F.H., Jr., Alonso, A., and Denia, A.: Traumatic neuroma: a complication of transcanal labyrinthectomy, Arch. Otolaryngol. 105:654-655, 1979.

77. Linthicum, F.H., Jr., and Schwartzman, J.A.: An atlas of micropathology of the temporal bone, Philadelphia, 1974, W.B. Saunders Co.

78. Littleton, J.T., Shaffer, K.A., Callahan, W.P., and Durizch, M.L.: Temporal bone: comparison of pluridirectional tomography and high resolution computed tomography, AJR 137:835-845, 1981.

79. Livingston, G.: Congenital ear abnormalities due to Thalidomide, Proc. R. Soc. Med. 58:493-497, 1965.

79a. Lloyd, T.V., van Aman, M., and Johnson, J.C.: Aberrant jugular bulb presenting as a middle ear mass, Radiology 131:139-141, 1979.

80. Lodge, W.O., Jones, H.M., and Smith, M.E.: Malignant tumors of the temporal bone, Arch. Otolaryngol. 61:535-541, 1955.

81. Lucente, F.E., Tobias, G.W., Parisier, S.C., and Som, P.M.: Tuberculous otitis media, Laryngoscope 88:1107-1114, 1978.

82. Madeira, J.T., and Summers, G.W.: Epidural mastoid pneumatocele, Radiology 122:727-728, 1977.

83. Marano, G.D., Horton, J.A., and Gabriele, O.F.: Persistent embryologic vascular loop of the internal carotid, middle meningeal, and ophthalmic arteries, Radiology 141:409-410, 1981.

84. Mazzoni, A.: Internal auditory artery supply to the petrous bone, Ann. Otol. Rhinol. Laryngol. 81:13, 1972.

85. Mazzoni, A.: Vein of the vestibular aqueduct, Ann. Otol. Rhinol. Laryngol. 88:759-767, 1979.

86. Mendez, G., Jr., Quencer, R.M., Post, J.D., and Stokes, N.A.: Malignant external otitis: a radiographic-clinical correlation, AJR 132:957-961, 1979.

87. Moffat, D.A., and O'Connor, A.F.F.: Bilateral internal carotid aneurysms in the petrous temporal bones, Arch. Otolaryngol. 106:172-175, 1980.

88. Moretti, J.A.: Highly placed jugular bulb and conductive deafness secondary to sinusojugular hypoplasia, Arch. Otolaryngol. 102:430-431, 1976.

89. Myers, E.N., Stool, S., and Weltschew, A.: Rhabdomyosarcoma of the middle ear, Ann. Otol. Rhinol. Laryngol. 77:949, 1968.

90. Nager, G.T.: Meningiomas involving the temporal bone, Springfield, Ill. 1964, Charles C Thomas, Publisher.

91. Naunton, R., and Valvassori, G.: Inner ear anomalies: their association with atresia, Laryngoscope 78:1041-1049, 1968.

92. Navez, J.P., and Cornelis, G.: Etude tomographique de la chaine ossiculaire de profil en inclinaison sélectionnée, J. Belge Radiol. 55:189-190, 1972.

93. Nenzelius, C.: On spontaneous cerebrospinal otorrhea due to congenital malformations, Acta Otolaryngol. 39:314-328, 1951.

94. Novy, S., and Jensen, K.M.: Filling defects and nonfilling of the

internal auditory canal in posterior fossa myelography, AJR **124**:265-270, 1975.

94a. Nomura, Y., Takemoton, K., and Komatsuzaki, A.: The mastoid cyst. Report of a case, Laryngoscope **81**:438-446, 1971.

95. Noyek, A.M., Holgate, R.C., Wortzman, G., et al.: Sophisticated radiology in otolaryngology, J. Otolaryngol. **6**:73-94, 1977.

96. Ormerad, F.C.: The pathology of congenital deafness, J. Laryngol. Otol. **74**:919-950, 1960.

97. Osborn, A.G., and Parkin, J.L.: Mucocele of the petrous temporal bone, AJR **132**:680-681, 1979.

98. Overton, S.B., and Ritter, F.N.: A high placed jugular bulb in the middle ear: clinical and temporal bone study, Laryngoscope **83**:1986-1991, 1973.

99. Paparella, M.M.: Mondini's deafness—a review of histopathology, Ann. Otol. Rhinol. Laryngol. **89**(2 pt. 3 suppl. 67):1-10, 1980.

100. Paparella, M.M., Meyerhof, W.L., and Oliviera, C.A.: Mastoiditis and brain hernia (mastoiditis cerebri), Laryngoscope **88**:1097-1106, 1978.

101. Paparella, M.M., and Shumrick, D.A.: Otolaryngology. Vol. 2, Philadelphia, 1973, W.B. Saunders Co.

102. Peron, D.L., and Schucknecht, H.: Congenital cholesteatoma with other anomalies, Arch. Otolaryngol. **101**:499-505, 1975.

103. Phelps, P.D., Lloyd, G.A.S., and Sheldon, P.W.E.: Congenital deformities of the middle and external ear, Br. J. Radiol. **50**:714-727, 1977.

104. Polvogt, L.M., and Crowe, S.J.: Anomalies of the cochlea in patients with normal hearing, Ann. Otol. Rhinol. Laryngol. **46**:579-581, 1937.

105. Pöschl, M.: La coupe tomographique à travers le rocher, Fortschr. Rüontgenstr. **68**:174, 1943.

106. Potter, G.D.: Inner ear abnormalities in association with congenital atresia of the external auditory canal, including a case of Michel deformity, Ann. Otol. Rhinol. Laryngol. **78**:598-604, 1969.

107. Potter, G.D.: Trauma to the ear, Otolaryngol. Clin. North Am. **6**:401-412, 1973.

108. Pulec, J.L.: Facial nerve tumors, Ann. Otol. Rhinol. Laryngol. **78**:962-982, 1969.

109. Pulec, J.L.: Symposium on ear surgery. II. Facial nerve neuroma, Laryngoscope **82**(2):1160-1176, 1972.

110. Pulec, J.L., and Freedman, H.M.: Management of congenital ear abnormalities, Laryngoscope **88**:420-434, 1978.

111. Quisling, R.G., and Rhoton, A.L., Jr.: Intrapetrous carotid artery branches: radioanatomic analysis, Radiology **131**:133-136, 1979.

112. Reisner, K.: Tomography in inner and middle ear malformations, Radiology **92**:11-20, 1969.

113. Reynolds, A.F., Jr., Stovring, J., and Turner, P.T.: Persistent otic artery, Surg. Neurol. **13**:115-117, 1980.

114. Robin, P.E.: A case of upwardly situated jugular bulb in the left middle ear, J. Laryngol. Otol. **86**:1241-1246, 1972.

115. Rosenbaum, A.E., Drayer, B.P., DuBois, P.J., and Black, O.: Visualization of small extracanalicular neurilemmomas by metrizamide cisternographic enhancement, Arch. Otolaryngol. **104**:239-243, 1978.

116. Saito, R., Igarashi, M., Alford, B., and Guilford, F.: Anatomical measurement of the sinus tympani, Arch. Otolaryngol. **94**:418, 1971.

117. Scanlan, R.: Personal communication, Los Angeles, Cal., 1973.

118. Schaeffer, and Parsons, J., editors: Morris' human anatomy, Philadelphia, 1942, Blakiston.

119. Schuknecht, H.F.: Pathology of the ear, Harvard University Press. Cambridge, Mass., 1974, Harvard University Press.

120. Schucknecht, H.F.: Mondini dysplasia—a clinical and pathological study, Ann. Otol. Rhinol. Laryngol. **89**(1 pt. 2 suppl. 65):3-23, 1980.

121. Schucknecht, H. and Kirchner, J.: Cochlear Otosclerosis: fact or fantasy, Laryngoscope **84**:766, 1974.

122. Schwartz, R.H., Movassaghi, N., and Marion, E.D.: Rhabdomyosarcoma of the middle ear: a wolf in sheep's clothing, Pediatrics **65**:1131-1133, 1980.

123. Shaffer, K.A., Haughton, V.M., and Wilson, C.R.: High resolution computed tomography of the temporal bone, Radiology **134**:409-414, 1980.

124. Shambaugh, G., Jr.: Clinical diagnosis of cochlear (labyrinthine) otosclerosis, Laryngoscope **75**:1588, 1965.

125. Shambaugh, G., Jr.; Facial nerve decompreson and repair, surgery of the ear, ed. 2, Philadelphia, 1967, W.B. Saunders Co.

126. Shambaugh, G.E., Jr.: Facial neurilemmomas: a study of four diverse cases, Arch. Otolaryngol. **90**:742-755, 1969.

127. Skolnik, E.M., and Ferrer, J.L.: Cerebrospinal otorrhea, Arch. Otolaryngol. **70**:795-799, 1959.

128. Som, P.M., Khilnani, M.T., Beranbaum, S.L., and Wolf, B.S.: Mondini defect: a variant, AJR **129**:1120-1122, 1977.

129. Sones, P.J., Cioffi, C.M., and Hoffman, J.C., Jr.: A practical approach to the diagnosis of cerebellopontine angle tumors, AJR **122**:554-559, 1974.

130. Sortland, O.: Computed tomography combined with gas cisternography for the diagnosis of expanding lesions in the cerebellopontine angle, Neuroradiology **18**:19-22, 1979.

131. Spector, G.J., Sobol, S., Thawley, S.E., et al.: Glomus jugulare tumors of the temporal bone: patterns of invasion in the temporal bone, Laryngoscope **89**:1628-1639, 1979.

132. Steffen, T.N., and House, W.: Salivary gland choristoma of the middle ear, Arch. Otolaryngol. **76**:74, 1962.

133. Stenvers, H.W.: Röntgenologie des Felsenbeines und des bitemporalen Schädelbildes, Berlin, 1928, Springer Verlag.

134. Stevens, S.S., and Warshowsky, F.: Sound and hearing, New York, 1965, Time-Life Books, Inc.

135. Streeter, G.L.: The factors involved in the excavation of the cavities in the cartilaginous capsule of the ear in the human embryo, Am. J. Anat. **22**(1):1917.

136. Streeter, G.L.: The development of the scala tympani, scala vestibuli and periaticular system in the human embryo, Am. J. Anat. **21**(299):1917.

137. Streeter, G.L.: The histogenesis and growth of the otic capsule and its contained periotic tissue spaces in the human embryo, Contrib. Embryol. **20**:5-54, 1918.

138. Stucker, F.J., and Holmes, W.F.: Metastatic disease of the temporal bone, Laryngoscope **86**:1136-1140, 1976.

139. Sykora, G.F., Kaufman, B., and Katz, R.L.: Congenital defects of the inner ear in association with meningitis, Radiology **135**:379-382, 1980.

140. Taylor, G., and Martin, H.: Salivary gland in the middle ear, Arch. Otolaryngol. **73**:651, 1961.

141. Taylor, S.: The petrous temporal bone (including the cerebellopontine angle), Radiol. Clin. North Am. **20**:67-86, 1982.

142. Terrahe, K.: Malformations of the inner and middle ear due to thalidomide embryopathy: results of tomography of the ear, Fortschr. Roentgenstr. **102**:14, 1965.

143. Turkewitsch, B.G.: Alters-und Geschlechtseigenschaften des anatomischen Baues des menichlichen knochernen Labyrinthes, Anat. Anz. **70**:225, 1930.

144. Turski, P.A., Norman, D., de Groot, J., and Capra, R.: High-resolution CT of the petrous bone: direct vs. reformatted images, AJNR **3**:391-394, 1982.

145. Valvassori, G.E.: The abnormal internal auditory canal: the diagnosis of acoustic neuroma, Radiology **92**:449-459, 1969.

146. Valvassori, G.E.: Otosclerosis, Otolaryngol. Clin. North Am. **6**:379-389, 1973.

147. Valvassori, G.E., and Buckingham, R.A.: Middle ear masses mimicking glomus tumors: radiographic and otoscopic recognition, Ann. Otol. Rhinol. Laryngol. **83**:606-612, 1974.

148. Valvassori, G., Naunton, R., and Lindsay, J.: Inner ear anomalies: Clinical and histopathological considerations, Ann. Otol. Rhinol. Laryngol. **78**:929-938, 1969.

149. Virapongse, C., Rothman, S.L.G., Kier, E.L., and Sarwar, M.: Computed tomographic anatomy of the temporal bone, AJNR **3**:379-389, 1982.

150. Virapongse, C., Sarwar, M., Sasaki, C., and Kier, E.L.: high resolution computed tomography of the osseous external auditory canal. I. Anatomy, JCAT 1983.

151. Virapongse, C., Sarwar, M., Sasaki, C., and Kier, E.L.: High resolution computed tomography of the osseous external auditory canal. II. Pathology, JCAT 1983.

152. Warwick and Williams, editors: Gray's anatomy, ed. 35, Philadelphia, 1973, W.B. Saunders Co.

153. West, J.M., Bandy, B.C., and Jatek, B.W.: Aberrant jugular bulb in the middle ear cavity, Arch. Otolaryngol. **100**:370-372, 1974.

154. Wittmaack, K.: Uber die normale und die pathologische Pneumatisation des Schlafenbeines, Jena, 1918, Fischer.

155. Wolfowitz, B.: Spontaneous CSF otorrhea simulating serous otitis, Arch. Otolaryngol. **105**:496-499, 1979.

156. Wright, J., Jr., Taylor, C., and McKay, D.: Variations in the course of the facial nerve as illustrated by tomography, Laryngoscope **77**:717, 1967.

157. Zonneveld, F.W., and Damsma, H.: Direct multiplanar CT of the petrous bone. Presented at The Sixty-eighth Annual Meeting of the Radiological Society of North America Chicago, Nov. 28-Dec. 3, 1982.

158. Zonneveld, F.W., van Waes, P.F.G.M., and Burggraaf, J.: CT of the semi-longitudinal plane in the petrous bone. Presented at The Sixty-seventh Annual Meeting of the Radiological Society of North America, 1981.

Index